Pulmonary Disease of the Fetus Newborn and Child

Pulmonary Disease of the Fetus Newborn and Child

EDITORS

EMILE M. SCARPELLI, M.D., Ph.D.,

Professor of Pediatrics, Associate Professor of Physiology,
Director, Pediatric Pulmonary Center,
Albert Einstein College of Medicine, New York

PETER A. M. AULD, M.D.,

Professor of Pediatrics and Obstetrics,
Cornell University Medical College, New York,
Director of Perinatology Center,
New York Hospital—Cornell Medical Center, New York

HAROLD S. GOLDMAN, M.D.,

Professor of Radiology,
Director, Division of Pediatric Radiology,
Albert Einstein College of Medicine, New York

LEA & FEBIGER · 1978 · PHILADELPHIA

Library of Congress Cataloging in Publication Data

Main entry under title:

Pulmonary disease of the fetus, newborn, and child.

Bibliography: p.
Includes index.
1. Pediatric respiratory diseases. 2. Lungs—Diseases. 3. Infants (Newborn)—Diseases. 4. Fetus—Diseases. I. Scarpelli, Emile M. II. Auld, Peter A. M. III. Goldman, Harold S. [DNLM: 1. Lung diseases—In infancy and childhood. 2. Fetal diseases. 3. Infant, Newborn, Diseases. WS280 P982]
RJ431.P84 618.9′22′4 78-8762
ISBN 0-8121-0606-7

Published in Great Britain by Henry Kimpton Publishers, London

Printed in the United States of America

Print Number 3 2 1

TO ALL OUR CHILDREN

Preface

This text is the promised "companion volume" to *Pulmonary Physiology of the Fetus, Newborn, and Child,* which appeared in 1975. More than a companion, it is the natural continuation of ideas and principles presented in that text. Indeed contemporary physiology provides the base that generates performance in clinical medicine. We present in this volume the constituents of performance—pathophysiology, diagnostics, and therapeutics—in the field of pulmonology of the fetus, newborn, and child.

When planning this enterprise, we were asked to consider the kind of "specialist" who might be concerned with the apparently diffuse array of interests that were suggested by the title of the book. Would it be the fetologist, obstetrician, or perinatologist; or would it be the anesthesiologist or pediatrician? Our answer was, "Hopefully one and all." In other words, all these specialties might be considered properly in the domain of one specialist, a kind of developmental pulmonologist whose concern is the pulmonary system and its aberrations before, during, and after birth and continuing to adulthood. We do not believe the array diffuse; we think it is natural—as natural for the developing lung to have a specialist as it is for the "adult" lung to have a single "chest physician." We know no rational course for pre-adult pulmonary medicine outside the hands of one "specialist" who will take it from fetal life through adolescence. If this idea comes through clearly in this book, the credit goes to the authors.

Again we must confess the book is incomplete, but the bibliographies will take the interested reader beyond its present limits. We are also aware of the seemingly uneven distribution of space among individual topics; but emphasis was placed on areas of active research and development, and on contemporary advances. We are grateful to our colleagues who have provided the material to realize these aims, and to our secretaries and the staff of our highly professional publishers, who have taken it from there to here.

EMILE M. SCARPELLI
PETER A. M. AULD
HAROLD S. GOLDMAN

New York, New York

Contributors

PETER A. M. AULD, M.D.
Professor of Pediatrics and Obstetrics,
Cornell University Medical College, New York,
Director of Perinatology Center,
New York Hospital-Cornell Medical Center, New York

BELLA C. CLUTARIO, M.D.
Assistant Professor of Pediatrics,
Clinical Director, Pediatric Pulmonary Division,
Albert Einstein College of Medicine, New York

CAROLYN R. DENNING, M.D.
Professor of Pediatrics,
New York University School of Medicine, New York,
Director, Cystic Fibrosis Center,
St. Vincent's Hospital and Medical Center, New York

CARL F. DOERSHUK, M.D.
Professor of Pediatrics,
Case Western Reserve University School of Medicine, Cleveland,
Director, Cystic Fibrosis and Pulmonary Disease Center,
Rainbow Babies' and Children's Hospital, Cleveland

JOHN J. DOWNES, M.D.
Professor of Anesthesia and Pediatrics,
University of Pennsylvania School of Medicine, Philadelphia,
Director of Anesthesiology,
Children's Hospital of Philadelphia, Philadelphia

ELLIOT F. ELLIS, M.D.
Professor and Chairman of Pediatrics,
State University of New York at Buffalo School of Medicine, Buffalo,
Pediatrician-In-Chief,
Children's Hospital of Buffalo, Buffalo

WILLIAM W. FRAYER, M.D.
Assistant Professor of Pediatrics,
Cornell University Medical College, New York,
Assistant Attending Pediatrician,
New York Hospital-Cornell Medical Center, New York

ALLEN I. GOLDBERG, M.D.
Assistant Professor of Anesthesiology,
University of Pennsylvania School of Medicine, Philadelphia,
Director, Pediatrics Intensive Care-Intermediate,
Children's Hospital of Philadelphia, Philadelphia

HAROLD S. GOLDMAN, M.D.
Professor of Radiology,
Director, Division of Pediatric Radiology,
Albert Einstein College of Medicine, New York

W. HARDY HENDREN, M.D.
Professor of Surgery,
Harvard Medical School, Boston,
Chief of Pediatric Surgery and Visiting Surgeon,
Massachusetts General Hospital, Boston

JULIEN I. E. HOFFMAN, M.D.
Professor of Pediatrics and Senior Member of Cardiovascular Research Institute,
University of California, San Francisco,
Attending Pediatrician,
H. C. Moffett Hospital, San Francisco

BERNARD H. HOLZMAN, M.D.
Assistant Professor of Pediatrics,
University of Miami School of Medicine, Miami,
Director, Pediatric Intensive Care Unit,
Jackson Memorial Hospital, Miami

SAMUEL H. KIM, M.D.
Assistant Professor of Surgery,
Harvard Medical Center, Boston,
Associate Visiting Surgeon,
Massachusetts General Hospital, Boston

ALFRED N. KRAUSS, M.D.
Associate Professor of Pediatrics,
Cornell University Medical College, New York,
Associate Director of Perinatology Center,
New York Hospital-Cornell Medical Center, New York

MARTIN I. LORIN, M.D.
Associate Professor of Pediatrics,
Baylor College of Medicine, Houston

MARVIN D. LOUGH, R.R.T.
Technical Director of Pediatric Respiratory Therapy and Pulmonary Functions,
Rainbow Babies' and Children's Hospital, Cleveland

LEROY W. MATTHEWS, M.D.
Gertrude Lee Chandler Tucker Professor of Pediatrics,
Case Western Reserve University School of Medicine, Cleveland,
Director of Laboratories,
Rainbow Babies' and Children's Hospital, Cleveland

H. IAN A. NISBET, M.D.
Professor of Anesthesia,
University of Dalhousie, Halifax,
Associate Anesthetist,
Victoria General Hospital, Halifax

STANLEY E. READ, M.D., Ph.D.
Assistant Professor of Pediatrics,
Cornell University Medical College, New York,
Assistant Professor,
Rockefeller University, New York,
Assistant Attending Pediatrician,
New York Hospital-Cornell Medical Center, New York

EMILE M. SCARPELLI, M.D., Ph.D.
Professor of Pediatrics, Associate Professor of Physiology,
Director, Pediatric Pulmonary Center,
Albert Einstein College of Medicine, New York

W. SHAIN SCHLEY, M.D.
Clinical Assistant Professor in Otolaryngology,
Cornell Medical College, New York,
Assistant Attending Otolaryngologist,
New York Hospital-Cornell Medical Center, New York

DAVID J. STEWARD, M.D.
Professor of Anesthesia,
University of Toronto, Toronto,
Chief of Anesthesia,
The Hospital for Sick Children, Toronto

PAUL SYMCHYCH, M.D.
Assistant Professor of Pathology,
Cornell University Medical College,
Pediatric Pathologist,
New York Hospital-Cornell Medical Center, New York

Contents

Examination of the Lung (Physiologic and Anatomic Basis)

EMILE M. SCARPELLI

1

Pulmonary activity may now be examined at most stages of human development. Examination of the fetus is a clinical practicality in which techniques are in an early stage of development but hold great promise for the future. Examination of the newborn infant often presents special problems to the responsible physician, whose initial analysis in the delivery room needs to be thorough but rapid, especially when there is neonatal distress or when prior examination of the fetus has forecast a neonate at risk. The more detailed examination of the infant in the relatively serene atmosphere of the nursery begins to approach the standard examination that one would plan for a more cooperative individual. Through infancy and childhood the techniques of pulmonary examination come to include all methods that require the assistance of the patient, in addition to those in which he need be only passive.

The Fetus and the Newborn

Special features of the examination of the fetus and newborn infant with regard to the respiratory system are mentioned in this section. General principles of pulmonary physical diagnosis, which may be applicable to both the newborn and child, are covered in the remaining sections of this chapter.

THE FETUS

Important clinical information may be obtained by examining amniotic fluid and by monitoring several parameters of fetal cardiovascular-pulmonary function.

Amniotic Fluid. Because morphologic and biochemical maturation of the lung are the determinants of pulmonary stability at birth and thus of susceptibility of the newborn to respiratory distress, the recently described *amniotic fluid tests for pulmonary maturation* are now widely used clinical laboratory procedures. The tests are based on observations that (1) the fetal lung synthesizes and secretes into fetal pulmonary fluid the surface active phospholipids that establish alveolar stability at birth; (2) development of these processes determines functional maturation of the lung; and (3) examination of the phospholipid content and/or surface activity of amniotic fluid can provide a reliable estimate of fetal lung development. The most popular tests are:

(1) The *L/S ratio,* in which amniotic fluid lipids are separated by thin layer chromatography and the relative amounts of lecithin (L) and sphingomyelin (S) are compared (Fig. 1-1).

(2) The *shake test,* in which serial dilutions of amniotic fluid in ethanol are prepared, the mixtures are shaken in test tubes to produce foam, and foam stability (persistence) is evaluated (Fig. 1-2).

An L/S ratio of 2.0 or more indicates pulmonary maturation and negligible risk of respiratory distress syndrome, whereas a ratio of 1.0 or less indicates high risk. Similarly a stable foam from amniotic fluid: ethanol, 1:2, signals low risk of respiratory distress syndrome, whereas an unstable foam from a 1:1 dilution indicates high risk. It should be noted that in complicated pregnancies the relationship of the L/S ratio to gestational age may be altered. Thus, certain conditions

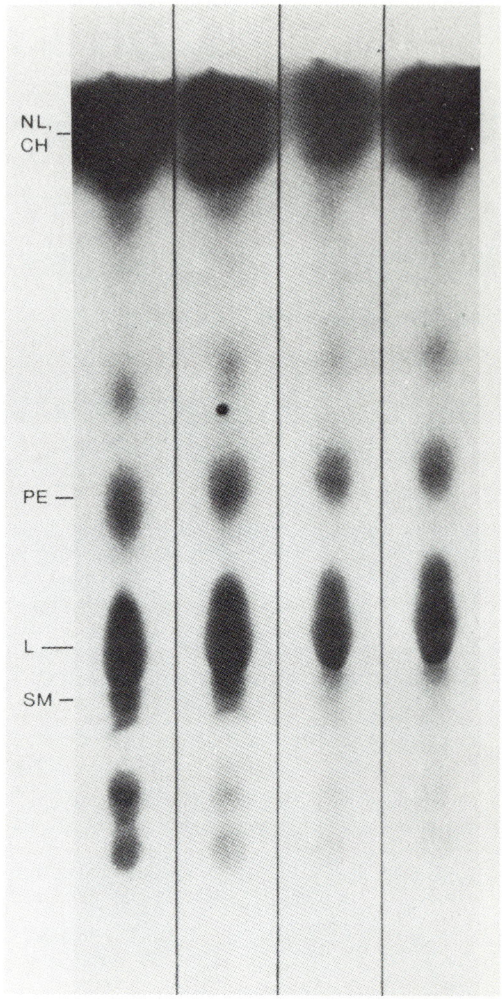

FIG. 1-1. Lecithin/sphingomyelin amniotic fluid test for fetal lung maturity. Duplicate thin layer chromatograms of lipid extracts of amniotic fluid of pregnant women. Iodine stain. NL = neutral lipids; CH = cholesterol; PE = phosphatidyl ethanolamine; L = lecithin; SM = sphingomyelin. Just below the large lecithin spot in the two chromatograms on the left is a relatively dense sphingomyelin spot, whereas the sphingomyelin spot is extremely light in the two chromatograms on the right. According to the amniotic fluid test, the lungs of the fetus in the amniotic fluid compartment of the right are more mature than those of the left. (From Scarpelli, E. M.: Physiology and pathology of pulmonary surfactants. *Triangle, The Sandoz Journal of Medical Science, 10:47,* 1971.)

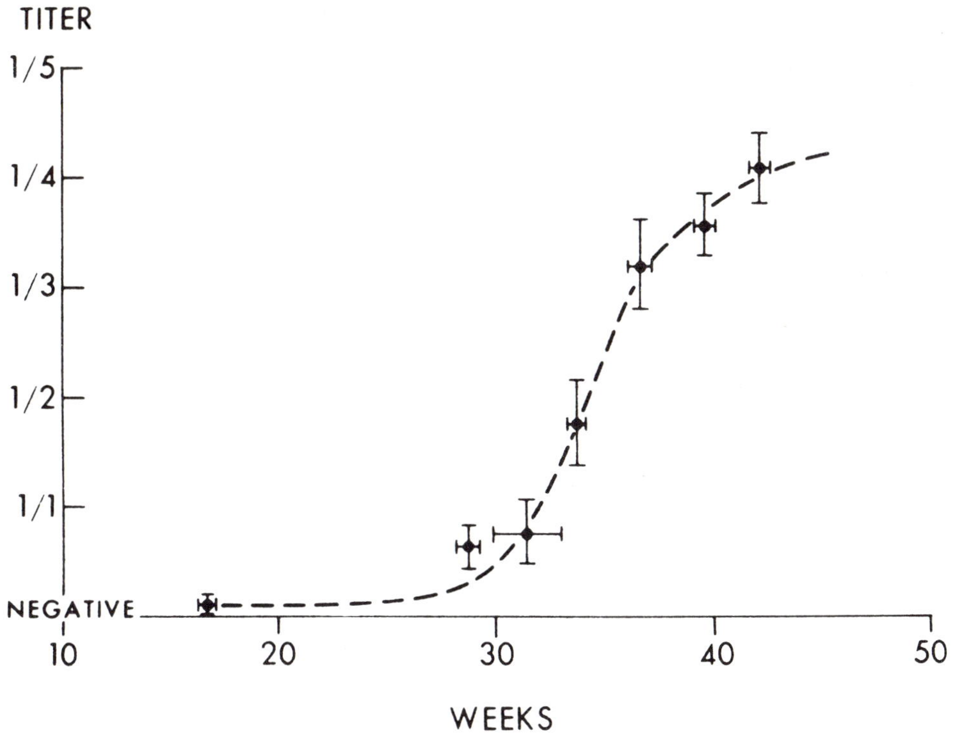

FIG. 1-2. The "shake test" of production of stable foam when amniotic fluid is diluted serially with 95% ethanol and the mixture is shaken vigorously for 15 sec. Fifteen minutes later the air-liquid interface is examined for small, stable bubbles. A complete ring of bubbles is a positive response. The diagram relates to gestational age, the titer (amniotic fluid/ethanol) at which a positive response was obtained. A negative test at 1/1 dilution is associated with high risk to respiratory distress syndrome, whereas a positive test at 1/2 dilution signals low risk. (From Clements, J. A. et al.: Assessment of the risk of the respiratory distress syndrome by a rapid test for surfactant in amniotic fluid. *N. Engl. J. Med. 286*:1077, 1972. Reprinted by permission from the publisher.)

(e.g., maternal hypertension, toxemia, renal disease, and severe isoimmunization) seem to accelerate maturation and increase the L/S ratio, whereas others (e.g., mild to moderate diabetes mellitus) may retard maturation and result in a low ratio.

Prenatal detection of genetic disorders by examination of cells from amniotic fluid has proved most successful for a number of hereditary diseases. To date prenatal detection of genetic disorders with a primary pulmonary component is not possible, but contemporary investigation in this area is promising (Table 1-1). For example, it has been shown that protease inhibitors such as α_1 and α_2 antitrypsin may be recovered from amniotic fluid and that a distinctive metachromasia is present in amniotic fluid cells in cystic fibrosis. Certain hereditary disorders in which pulmonary disease is a prominent complicating feature, such as Hunter's and Hurler's syndromes, are now diagnosable by analysis of the relevant enzyme activities of cultivated amniotic fluid cells.

The presence of *meconium* in amniotic fluid should always alert the physician to the possibility of serious pulmonary disease (meconium aspiration) at birth, since infants who have aspirated meconium are usually depressed at birth, and once meconium has

TABLE 1-1. Some Hereditary Diseases in Which Pulmonary Involvement May Be Present

Autosomal Dominant
Familial interstitial fibrosis
Familial spontaneous pneumothorax
Marfan's syndrome
Pulmonary arteriovenous fistula
Tuberous sclerosis
Autosomal Recessive
Agammaglobulinemia
α_1 antitrypsin deficiency (familial emphysema)
Ataxia-telangiectasia syndrome
Chronic granulomatous disease
Cystic fibrosis
Familial dysautonomia
Familial pulmonary alveolar microlithiasis
Hurler's syndrome
Kartagener's syndrome
Primary pulmonary hypertension
Sex-Linked Recessive
Agammaglobulinemia
Chronic granulomatous disease
Hunter's syndrome

reached the periphery of the lung, a life-threatening pneumonitis may result. It should also be noted that meconium-stained amniotic fluid is not always associated with neonatal distress. Nonetheless, all such infants must be considered to be at risk.

Cardiovascular-Pulmonary Status. Fetal distress, which often presages respiratory difficulties at birth, may be assayed by a number of clinical procedures. The most common method is to monitor *fetal heart rate* by phonocardiography, ultrasonography, or electrocardiography. Normally fetal heart rate is between 120 and 160 beats per minute; it slows in relationship to uterine contraction (Fig. 1-3). Cardiac deceleration that occurs early during contraction and lasts less than 90 seconds (early deceleration, type I dip) is normal; late deceleration (type II dip) that starts 30 to 40 seconds after the onset of contraction and persists for up to 60 seconds after the end of contraction may be associated with fetal acidemia and neonatal distress; variable decelerations may be due to umbilical cord occlusion and may be associated with fetal acidemia. Relatively recently it has been suggested that electronic averaging from the fetal electrocardiogram of beat-to-beat fetal heart rate variability provides a reliable index of fetal stability. Normally fetal heart rate variability ranges from 15 to 25 beats/min. If variability diminishes or is lost (i.e., beat-to-beat fetal heart rate is fixed), one must be suspicious of associated fetal immaturity, the effects of maternal drug administration, the presence of congenital malformation, or fetal asphyxia.

Direct sampling of *fetal capillary blood*, which has received wide acceptance as a clinical diagnostic method, has shown a good correlation between fetal acid-base status, the acid-base status of blood from the umbilical vessels, and the Apgar score of the infant at birth. Although a number of complicating factors militate against strict correlations between fetal capillary blood acid-base status and the neonatal condition, it is generally accepted that a fetal pH greater than 7.25 is usually benign, that pH from 7.20 to 7.25 should alert one to the possibility of neonatal depression and distress, and that pH less than 7.20 should be taken as a categoric sign of fetal distress and thus neonatal risk.

The fact that the mammalian fetus normally makes *breathing movements in utero* has been confirmed in a number of laboratories (Fig. 1-4), and it has been suggested that monitoring fetal breathing in human pregnancies by ultrasonography can (1) provide a valuable direct measure of fetal activity, (2) be a useful guide to fetal health during labor, and (3) have predictive value in the care of fetuses of hypertensive women and in the identification of those near-term fetuses who may experience distress during labor. Thus Boddy, Dawes, and Robinson, while stressing that their reported observations are preliminary findings that need to be confirmed at other centers, also indicate that a most serious prognostic sign is the appear-

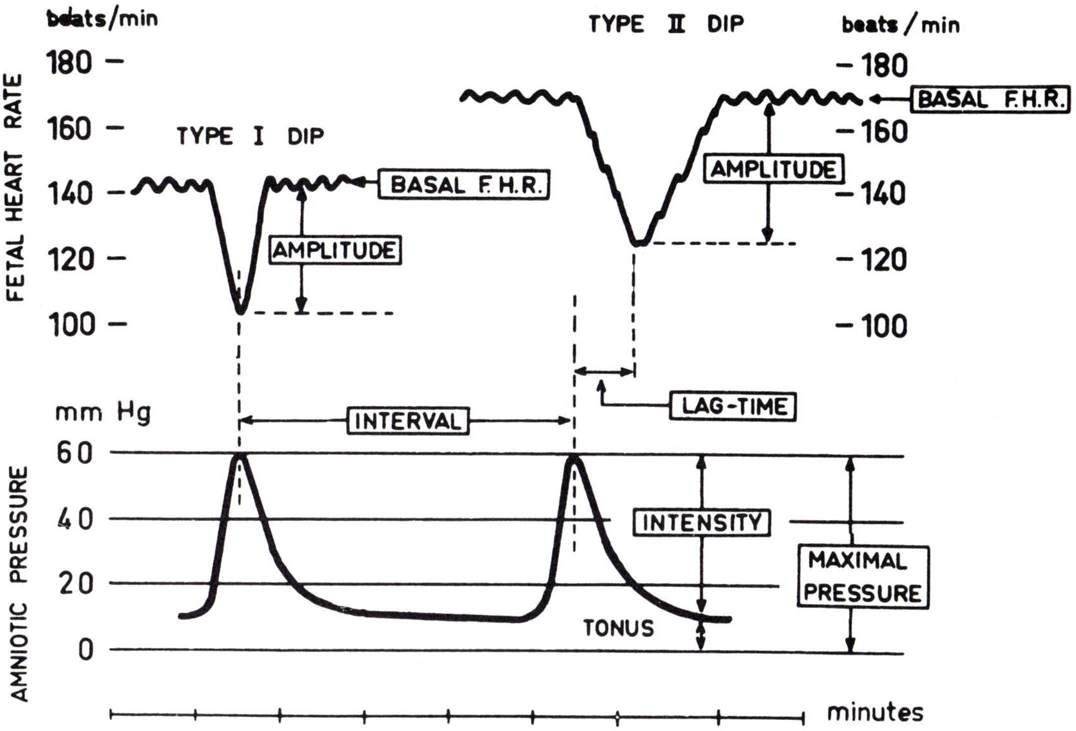

FIG. 1-3. Early (type I dip) and late (type II dip) decelerations of fetal heart rate associated with uterine contraction. (From Caldeyro-Barcia, R. et al.: Control of fetal heart rate during labor. In *The Heart and Circulation in the Newborn and Infant.* D. E. Cassels (Ed.). Grune & Stratton, New York, 1966.)

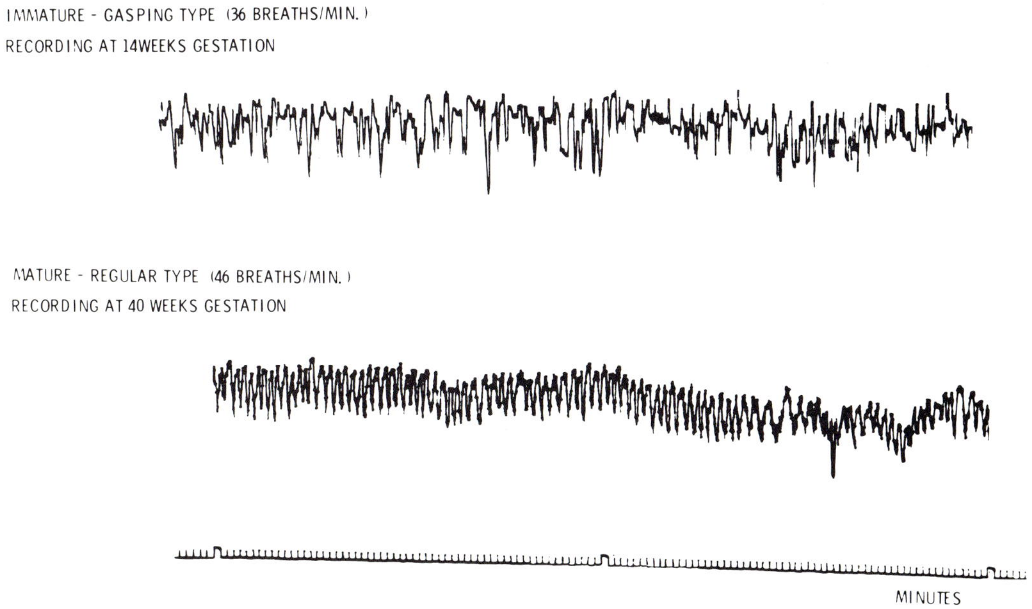

FIG. 1-4. Examples of immature (above) and mature (below) human fetal breathing movements in utero. (From Boddy, K., G. S. Dawes and J. Robinson: Intrauterine fetal breathing movements.[13])

ance of fetal gasping in association with diminution of normal breathing movements. They also report an association between late decelerations of fetal heart rate and fetal acidemia on the one hand, and the appearance of an increasing number of fetal gasping movements on the other hand. Conversely, it was noted that the continuation or reappearance of normal fetal breathing movements during labor provides direct evidence that the fetus is in good condition. Boddy and his colleagues warned that ultrasonography to monitor fetal breathing is not developed sufficiently for routine clinical examinations, that experience and practice are required, and that further development of relevant instrumentation is needed to facilitate clinical application. However, ultrasonographic recording of fetal breathing should become a valuable clinical research tool.

We have found that fetal breathing movements in utero may be seriously affected by barbiturate anesthetics administered into the maternal circulation (Fig. 1-5). Both short- and long-acting barbiturates cross the human and sheep placenta, and studies from sheep suggest that relatively low fetal levels can depress the respiratory center in utero (and thus presumably also at birth). Thus, absence of fetal breathing should lead to the suspicion of respiratory center depression.

THE NEWBORN IN THE DELIVERY ROOM

The immediate examination of the newborn infant in the delivery room is what Auld and Abramson have termed a screening procedure. The examination should be at once thorough, rapid, and educated insofar as careful prior monitoring of the fetus may have alerted the examiner to expected neonatal morbidity. In addition, careful prior attention to the maternal history during pregnancy and to the details of labor and delivery often provide essential clues to the origin of neonatal distress.

The Cry. Since most infants cry lustily after birth (and it is pertinent to recall that a cry can move a volume of air equivalent to the vital capacity of the infant), the absence of crying or weak crying, especially in association with muscle flaccidity, should alert the examiner to central nervous system depression—anesthetic, hemorrhagic, hypoxemic—and the need for oxygen therapy and resuscitation.

Posterior Pharynx. Aspiration of the poste-

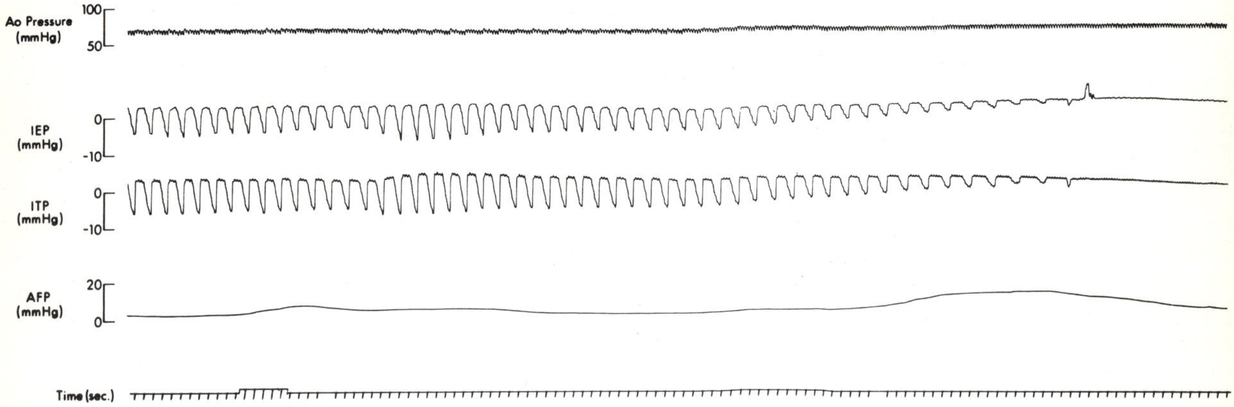

FIG. 1-5. Depression of spontaneous breathing movements of sheep fetus in utero by administration of sodium thiopental, 1.0 mg/kg intravenously, to the ewe: Ao = aortic; IEP = intraesophageal pressure; ITP = intratracheal pressure; AFP = amniotic fluid pressure of fetus. Mark on the time scale signals the injection period. (From Condorelli, S. and E. M. Scarpelli: Fetal breathing: induction in utero and effects of vagotomy and barbiturates. *J. Pediatr.* *88*:94, 1976.)

rior pharynx through both nares is a simple procedure that (1) confirms the patency of this obligatory airway of the neonate and rules out the rare congenital anomaly, choanal atresia, (2) clears the pharynx of material (e.g., amniotic fluid or gastrointestinal secretions and debris) that could be aspirated, and (3) provides material for inspection with regard to the possible nature of prior aspiration into the respiratory tract. For example, fetal distress is associated with gasping breathing movements in utero at which time fluid may be aspirated into the lung. Immediate examination of pharyngeal fluid could provide a clue regarding the aspirated material (blood, meconium, gastric contents, pus). In addition, recent studies indicate that phospholipid analysis of the posterior pharyngeal aspirate obtained immediately after birth can provide information about susceptibility to respiratory distress syndrome; such data are as reliable as the amniotic fluid tests described previously.

General Status. The infant's heart rate, respiratory effort, muscle tone, response to somatic stimulation, and color should be evaluated and scored according to the Apgar method (Table 1-2). This procedure ensures rapid and thorough examination of the vital parameters and, in addition, does have some prognostic significance. Thus infants who score less than 3 at 1 minute of age have higher mortality than those who score over 7. In addition, the Apgar score is a fair reflection of the degree of acidemia that accompanies asphyxia at birth.

Ventilation. Gross examination of the thorax provides the first indication of the relative ease with which air can enter the lung at the time that fetal pulmonary fluid is rapidly being absorbed. Marked intercostal, subcostal, and substernal retractions combined with diminished or absent breath sounds immediately alert the examiner to a major obstruction of the extrathoracic or intrathoracic airways that may require immediate surgical intervention (Table 1-3). If the obstruction is not complete, inspiratory stridor (usually with extrathoracic airway problems) or ex-

TABLE 1-2. Apgar Method for Evaluation of Infant in the First Minutes of Life

Sign	0	1	2
Heart rate	Absent	<100/min	>100/min
Respiratory effort	Absent	Weak cry; hypoventilation	Strong cry
Muscle tone	Limp	Some flexion of extremities	Well flexed
Response to stimulation of feet	None	Some motion	Cry
Color	Blue/pale	Pink body; blue extremities	Pink

TABLE 1-3. Some Conditions That May Require Early or Immediate Surgical Intervention*

Extrathoracic Segments of the Airway
Choanal atresia
Micrognathia
Macroglossia
Neck masses (e.g., tumors, congenital goiter, and hemangiomas)
Oropharyngeal masses (e.g., lingual cysts)
Lingual thyroid
Glottic and laryngeal masses, stenosis, and other malformations
Intrathoracic Structures
Great vessel malformations
Mediastinal masses
Esophageal atresia and fistula
Lung cysts
Lobar emphysema
Lung agenesis and hypoplasia
Pneumothorax
Pneumomediastinum
Chylothorax
Diaphragm: hernia and eventration; paralysis

*Derived from Coryllos, E.: Surgical emergencies in respiratory difficulties of newborn infants.[1]

piratory crackles or wheezes (usually with intrathoracic airway problems) may be heard with and sometimes without the stethoscope. Determination, by inspection, of the symmetry of diaphragmatic excursions often reflects the first sign of disease of a hemithorax, such as unilateral phrenic nerve paralysis and diaphragmatic hernia or eventration. Diminished or absent breath sounds in the hemithorax can fix the diagnosis.

Crackles and wheezes (p. 52) may be heard on occasion in the normal newborn infant immediately after air-breathing begins. These seemingly adventitious sounds, which are probably due to the flow of gas through airways from which fetal pulmonary fluid has not been absorbed completely, are not abnormal and disappear rapidly once sustained air-breathing is established. Persistence of these sounds should be a warning to the examiner of possible illness, e.g., pneumonia, aspiration either initially at birth or intermittently as in the case of fistulae, and bleeding.

Cardiac Findings. Examination of the heart should be directed toward determination of rate, rhythm, and sounds. The neonatal heart rate is generally between 100 and 160 beats/min. and variable. The beat-to-beat variability in the neonate generally is similar to that in the fetus (see p. 4). Cardiac rhythm is generally regular, although an occasional extrasystole may be heard, in which case an electrocardiogram should be recorded. Transient systolic murmurs, usually related to the ductus arteriosus, may be heard. They are ordinarily, but not invariably, physiologic.

The Skin. Examination of the skin is an essential component of pulmonary evaluation during the screening procedure. The skin of full-term infants is generally covered with vernix caseosa at birth, whereas vernix is usually absent in premature infants.

Some degree of generalized *cyanosis* is usually seen before the first breath, perhaps less in infants delivered by cesarean section than in those born by the vaginal route, but it normally clears rapidly once regular air-breathing is established. Acrocyanosis, i.e., cyanosis of the hands and feet, and perioral cyanosis may persist for a variable length of time. This condition is usually due to diminished vascular perfusion, perhaps as a result of the fall in skin temperature as the neonate enters his new environment, and should not be considered abnormal. Acrocyanosis must be distinguished from central cyanosis, which has more serious implications. Central or generalized cyanosis is apparent when *all* perfused surfaces are blue including, for example, those of the base of the tongue and oral pharynx where temperature change is not significant and perfusion should be normal. Persistent central cyanosis demands oxygen therapy, and the physician must consider that it may be of cardiopulmonary (shunts and/or inadequate ventilation) or central nervous system (depression leading to hypoventilation) origin. Rarely, the lower extremities may be cyanotic while the upper extremities appear normal (differential cyanosis) when there is a large right-to-left shunt through the ductus arteriosus. Occasionally the head, neck and shoulders may appear cyanotic, with the rest of the body normal. The latter "ecchymoses," which do not respond to oxygen therapy, have been attributed to excessive pressure over the thorax during delivery and thus have been termed traumatic cyanosis.

When there has been excessive blood loss and/or cardiovascular decompensation (e.g., anesthetic effect, fetal-maternal transfusion, ruptured umbilical vessels), the skin appears *pallid.* Determination of the hematocrit confirms whether blood loss has occurred and indicates the need for transfusion. A normal hematocrit associated with persistent skin pallor is sometimes seen in infants who require resuscitation and has been attributed to diminished cutaneous vascular perfusion, for example, in response to low cardiac output.

Icterus of the skin, fingernails, and toenails indicates staining by bile pigment, which is usually associated with meconium-stained amniotic fluid and thus should suggest the possibility of meconium aspiration.

THE NEWBORN IN THE NURSERY

Examination of the infant in the nursery can be more deliberate and detailed than the screening procedure of the delivery room. Many of the principles and procedures to be described in later sections may be applied to the infant in the nursery, so only the special features that pertain to examination of the respiratory system of the newborn are mentioned in this section.

Inspection. This check of the infant must take into account spontaneous activity and response to somatic stimulation (for signs of central nervous system depression); the quality and vigor of the infant's cry (for signs of depression and airway patency); the color of the skin and mucosa; and the symmetry and excursions of the thorax. Heart rate and rhythm and respiratory rate and rhythm must be recorded (Table 1-4).

Generally the *respiratory rhythm* of the newborn is variable, and the more immature the infant, the more irregular it is. Several breathing patterns have been characterized in the premature infant, including *periodic breathing*, in which periods of apnea alternate with periods of relatively rapid breathing (Fig. 1-6); *apneic breathing*, in which the periods of apnea are relatively longer; and *deep-sighing respirations*, in which deep in-

TABLE 1-4. Respiratory Rate, Pulse Rate, and Blood Pressure from the Newborn Period to 18 Years of Age

Age	Respiratory Rate*		Pulse Rate*		Blood Pressure†	
	Male	Female	Male	Female	Systolic	Diastolic
Newborn	—	—	—	—	80(16)	46(16)
6–12 mo	—	—	—	—	89(29)	60(10)§
0–1 yr	31(1.3)	30(0.8)	135(18)	126(21)	—	—
1–2 yr	26(0.5)	27(0.5)	105(16)	104(17)	96(30)‡	66(25)§
2–3 yr	25(0.4)	25(0.3)	93(12)	93(9)	99(25)‡	64(25)§
3–4 yr	24(0.2)	24(0.2)	87(9)	89(9)	100(25)‡	67(23)§
4–5 yr	23(0.2)	22(0.2)	84(8)	84(8)	99(20)‡	65(20)§
5–6 yr	22(0.2)	21(0.2)	79(7)	79(7)	94(14)	55(9)
6–7 yr	21(0.2)	21(0.3)	76(8)	77(8)	100(15)	56(8)
7–8 yr	20(0.2)	20(0.2)	75(8)	76(8)	102(15)	56(8)
8–9 yr	20(0.2)	20(0.2)	73(9)	73(7)	105(16)	57(9)
9–10 yr	19(0.2)	19(0.2)	70(7)	70(8)	107(16)	57(9)
10–11 yr	19(0.2)	19(0.2)	67(7)	69(8)	111(17)	58(10)
11–12 yr	19(0.2)	19(0.3)	67(7)	69(7)	113(18)	59(10)
12–13 yr	19(0.2)	19(0.3)	66(7)	69(8)	115(19)	59(10)
13–14 yr	19(0.2)	18(0.3)	65(8)	68(8)	118(19)	60(10)
14–15 yr	18(0.2)	18(0.4)	62(7)	66(8)	—	—
15–16 yr	17(0.3)	18(0.4)	61(8)	65(8)	—	—
16–17 yr	17(0.4)	17(0.5)	61(6)	66(8)	—	—
17–18 yr	16(0.5)	17(0.7)	60(8)	65(7)	—	—

*Data from Iliff, A. and V. A. Lee.: Pulse rate, respiratory rate, and body temperature of children between two months and 18 years of age. *Child Dev. 23:*238, 1952. Values are mean (± SD).

†Data from Nadas, A. S. and D. C. Fyler.[19] Authors adapted data in the literature and rounded figures to the nearest decimal place. Values are mean (±2 SD).

‡Systolic and diastolic pressures of these four groups are at the mean ages of 1, 2, 3, and 4 years respectively.

§Diastolic pressures were taken at the point of muffling of the sounds.

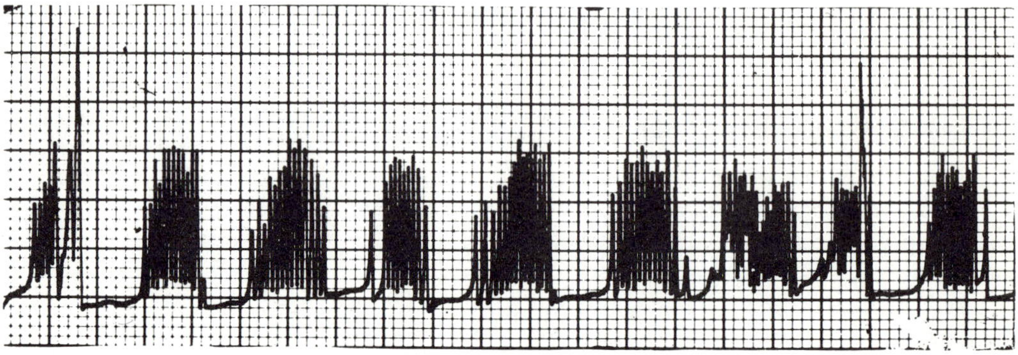

FIG. 1-6. A tracing of periodic breathing in the premature infant. (From Auld, P. A. M.: Pulmonary physiology of the newborn infant.[25])

spiratory efforts are interposed regularly in the basic regular or periodic breathing pattern. These irregular patterns of the premature infant have been attributed to hypoxemia and/or to the tendency of normal alveoli to collapse spontaneously. Evidence for this explanation comes from observations that irregular breathing may be converted to regular breathing by increasing the concentration of inspired oxygen or by increasing functional residual capacity with constant negative pressure around the thorax.

These irregular patterns may not be seen in the early neonatal premature infant, but may develop during the first day and may persist for several weeks. Infants with irregular (periodic) breathing may have periods of apnea up to 10 seconds alternating with periods of ventilation lasting 10 to 15 seconds; the average respiratory rate may be 30 to 40 breaths/min., while respiratory rate during the intervals of breathing may be 50 to 60 per minute. When the periods of apnea are excessive (e.g., longer than 10 to 20 seconds) and/or frequent (so that mean frequency per minute is compromised), one must suspect a pathologic process: The syndrome of excessive apneic episodes in the premature infant, *apnea of prematurity*, can be fatal, so the cause must be searched for carefully (e.g., aspiration, respiratory distress syndrome, pneumonia, hemorrhage). Often, however, the cause may not be apparent; nonetheless, the possibility of death remains high and the infant must be monitored and resuscitated diligently.

The relatively high compliance of the infant's chest wall (in contrast to lung compliance, which is about the same as that of the older child) results in a tendency of the *intercostal muscles* to draw inward and the costal margin to recede during inspiration. These movements of the chest wall may be exaggerated (retractions) in relation to the degree of prematurity, and they are most obvious when there is obstruction (airway) or high static resistance (alveolar) to inspiration. In fact, a method for relating the degree of retractions to the severity of pulmonary disease has been proposed (Fig. 1-7). Although this method is not strictly quantitative, it is most useful in that it focuses the examiner's attention on the extent and degree of retractions and on the use of the accessory muscles of respiration, including the alae nasa (nasal flaring).

Recently a noninvasive method for transillumination of the neonatal thorax with high-intensity light from a fiberoptic probe has been described by Kuhns and co-workers. Early results suggest that this aid may become valuable for the cribside detection of pneumothorax or pneumomediastinum in the newborn (see also Chapter 19).

Palpation, Percussion of the Thorax. These

techniques are as important in the examination of infants as they are in the examination of older individuals. In fact the infant presents certain advantages; because of his compliant chest wall and small mass of muscle and adipose tissue, a higher degree of examiner sensitivity may be achieved. Thus palpable crackles and wheezes (airway obstruction), crepitations (subcutaneous emphysema), and cardiac impulses may be appreciated. In addition, alterations of the percussion note may indicate extensive areas of effusion, consolidation, or collapse when the examination is done carefully. Because of the higher resonance of the infant's thorax, the percussion tap should be much lighter than that used for examination of older individuals.

Auscultation. Auscultatory sounds may be interpreted in the same way for infants as they are for older individuals. However, the rapid respiratory rate, the quick distribution of respired gas in the lung, and the natural anarchism of the infant can make characterization and timing of adventitious sounds a chore. Thus, whenever possible, judicious advantage should be taken of the long and deep inspiratory phase of the infant's cry.

Infants' breath sounds have been characterized as being "harsher" than those of adults. In fact, they are transmitted with less distortion because of the relatively short distance between their site of origin and the examiner's receiver.

Historic Perspective

Thorough history-taking is a skill that is perfected with time and practice. For the newborn infant, parental history, history of past and immediate pregnancies of his mother, and knowledge of her course of labor and delivery may provide important clues to the possibility of pulmonary disease. These same factors are important in reviewing the history of older infants and children, in addition to the attention that must be given to growth and development, feeding habits, immunizations, environment, performance and attendance at school, and previous visits to the physician.

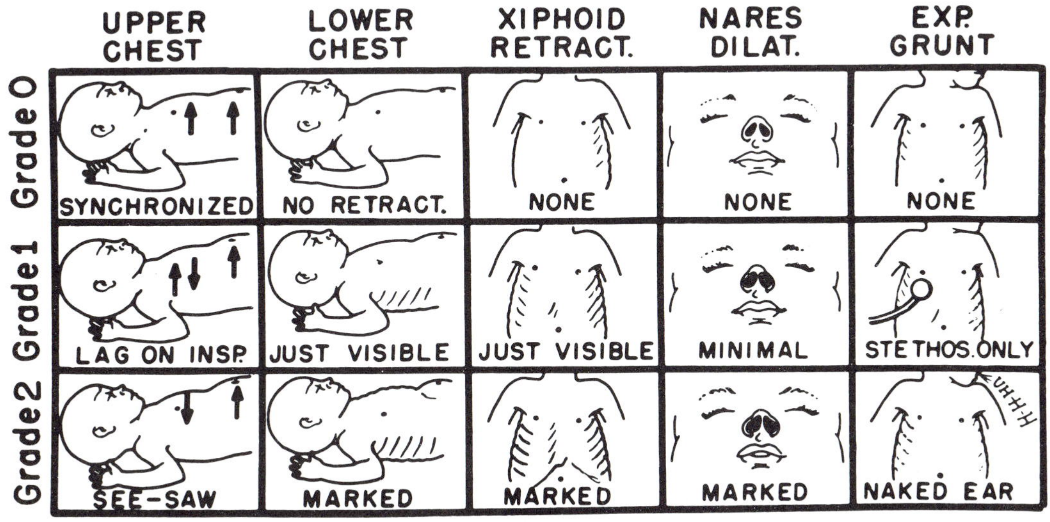

FIG. 1-7. A suggested system for grading retractions in infants. (Redrawn from Silverman, W. A. and D. H. Anderson: A controlled clinical trial of effects of water mist and obstructive respiratory signs, death rate and necropsy findings among premature infants. *Pediatrics 17*:1, 1956.)

When respiratory disease is acute and serious, careful inquiry about the onset of the illness is essential. For example, the sudden onset of difficult breathing suggests immediately either exposure of the respiratory tract to noxious materials, such as stomach contents, caustic chemicals, foreign particles, and untoward environmental contaminants, or sudden disruption of airway and/or alveolar integrity such as in pneumothorax, hemothorax, and injury to the lung parenchyma. The rapid development of respiratory distress with actual or imminent respiratory failure can be due to a variety of causes, the most common of which are asthma in children, pneumonia and upper airway obstruction in the infant and young child, and respiratory distress syndrome in the newborn (Table 1-5). The common association of cardiac failure and respiratory difficulties must be noted and considered whenever a patient is seen for "breathing problems." Chronic or recurrent respiratory illness should always bring to mind infection (e.g., tuberculosis, bronchiectasis), allergic or immunologic problems, congenital abnormalities, a foreign body, recurrent bleeding, and extrapulmonary disease including neoplasm.

Personal, Familial, and Environmental Background

Since pulmonary disease may be present without acute symptomatology or with evanescent and mild symptoms that are not considered serious—especially in the pediatric population in whom colds and slight fevers are common occurrences sometimes considered mundane by parents and physician—the lung problem may have been in a relatively stable state or only slightly progressive before the patient is seen by his doctor. Thus occasional colds and bouts of coughing may be the first sign of cystic fibrosis in a young child; tuberculosis, fungal diseases, and sarcoidosis may have been active previously but presently nonprogressive; asthma may have been considered as nothing more than an inordinate susceptibility to colds; and a pulmonary abscess from a prior pneumonia may have gone undetected until a careful history and physical examination are obtained. Careful review of the *personal history* of the patient is therefore essential and should include (1) genetic background; (2) perinatal history (labor, delivery, course in nursery); (3) prior

TABLE 1-5. Common Causes of Acute Respiratory Failure*

	Infants (1–24 mo)
Bronchopneumonia	Foreign body aspiration
Upper airway obstruction	Intrathoracic anomalies, e.g., diaphragmatic hernia, lobar emphysema
Congenital heart disease	Encephalitis
Status asthmaticus	Poisoning
Septicemia	Cystic fibrosis
	Children (2–12 yr)
Status asthmaticus	Trauma:
Congenital heart disease	thoracic
Bronchopneumonia	head
Encephalitis	shock
Peripheral polyneuritis	Drowning
Septicemia	Burns
Poisoning	Renal failure

*From Downes, J. J., T. Fulgencio and R. C. Raphaely: Acute respiratory failure in infants and children. *Pediatr. Clin. North Am.* *19*:423, 1972.

pulmonary and upper respiratory infections (including middle ear, sinuses, adenoids, tonsils); (4) prior and present use of medications; and (5) successful immunization.

The *environmental background* of the patient must be assessed carefully. Knowledge of past and present location of residences is important. For example, histoplasmosis is present in the Ohio River Valley, coccidioidomycosis in the southwestern United States, pulmonary eosinophilia in certain countries of Asia, and a seemingly high incidence of childhood sarcoidosis in Utah, Idaho, and North Carolina. The community environment of the patient should be determined with regard to its possible relation to pulmonary disease. Although pneumoconioses do not constitute a major problem in children, the list of known industrial toxins that may damage the lung is quite extensive and should be considered especially with regard to patients with chronic and diffuse pulmonary disease (Table 1-6). Since the patient's home or neighborhood can be a source of pulmo-

TABLE 1-6. Glossary of Pneumoconioses and Examples of Related Industrial Trades*

Conditions	Industrial Trades
Aluminum pneumoconiosis	Fireworks manufacturing
Asbestosis	Auto mechanics Carpentry Mill workers Miners
Baritosis	Barite miner Ceramics worker Paint manufacturing
Bagassosis	Paper manufacturing Sugar cane workers
Berylliosis	Ceramics worker Fluorescent lamp manufacturing Propellant manufacturing
Coal Miner's Pneumoconiosis	
Hard Metal Pneumoconiosis	Cutting tool worker
Kaolinosis	Brick manufacturing Ceramics worker Paper manufacturing
Shaver's Disease	Abrasives manufacturing
Siderosis	Flame cutter Foundry worker Welder
Silicosis	Bricklayer Ceramics worker Coal miner Sandblaster Stone cutter
Talcosis	Ceramics worker Cosmetics worker Miner Plastics worker Rubber worker

*Derived from Baum, G. L. (Ed.).[3]

nary disease, inquiry must be made regarding contact with mammals (tularemia from rabbits, brucellosis from domestic animals, hypersensitivity to animal dander), birds (psittacosis-ornithosis, pigeon breeder's lung disease), insects (hypersensitivity), rural irritants such as those from barns and hay (hypersensitivity—farmer's lung), and air conditioners and heating systems (irritant contaminants).

Tuberculosis clearly illustrates the need to investigate the *family background* as an essential part of the examination, since it is still the most frequently encountered contagious disease with a positive family history. Similarly, viral infections, whose clinical manifestations include a wide spectrum of respiratory involvement from upper respiratory tract infection through bronchitis and bronchiolitis to pneumonia, or other infections in subjects with whom the patient has had contact should be defined at the initial examination. A number of diseases show a familial predisposition that the examining physician must consider: (1) asthma, (2) cystic fibrosis, (3) sickle cell anemia, (4) interstitial pulmonary fibrosis, (5) pulmonary arteriovenous fistula and telangiectasis, and (6) agammaglobulinemia (see also Table 1-1). To this list should be added cardiac disease, renal disease, and pulmonary emphysema. Although the latter develops beyond the pediatric period, α_1 antitrypsin deficiency (which may be diagnosed in childhood) may be a predisposing feature in some patients.

The Symptoms

The major or key symptoms of pulmonary disease in adults are generally reported to be cough, sputum, hemoptysis, chest pain, dyspnea, and wheezing. One of the problems for the physician caring for an infant or young child is that although these patients may cough, sputum is not expectorated and a "sputum history" is difficult to ascertain. Similarly hemoptysis, unless there is profuse bleeding or bleeding in the upper airway, may be hidden, and chest pain often must be inferred from the anguish and posture of the patient whose verbal reports and signs may be misleading. Thus one is left with cough, dyspnea (i.e., difficult or labored breathing), and wheezing as the relatively easily realized symptoms that need to be evaluated carefully, and one must resign himself to the ambiguities of the others. To these key symptoms for the infant and young child, i.e., cough, dyspnea, and wheezing, should be added difficulty feeding, alterations in the state of activity, and phonation. By listing these parameters as "symptoms"—which may be defined as *subjective* evidence of disease—the assumption is that the patient would report them if he could.

COUGH

Cough is a reflex induced by stimulation of afferent end-organs in the epithelium of the pharynx, larynx, trachea, and bronchi—there are none apparently in the distal airways and alveoli; cough may be precipitated also by stimulation of the parietal pleura and of nerve endings in other viscera. In this reflex, a deep inspiratory effort is followed by contraction of the expiratory muscles against a closed glottis. Pleural and intrapulmonary pressures increase markedly, up to 300 mm Hg, before the glottis opens and air is propelled out of the lung. The simultaneous increase of arterial blood pressure and cerebrospinal fluid pressure (Fig. 1-8) indicates that forced coughing should not be encouraged unnecessarily during the examination of the patient.

Cough induced by irritation of the pharyngeal mucosa—as may occur in pharyngitis or with pharyngeal irritation from secretions or exudates from the sinuses—is usually dry and persistent, but may be paroxysmal and explosive. A laryngeal or tracheolaryngeal cough is harsh, sometimes brassy, and barking (the well-known croupy cough). When only the

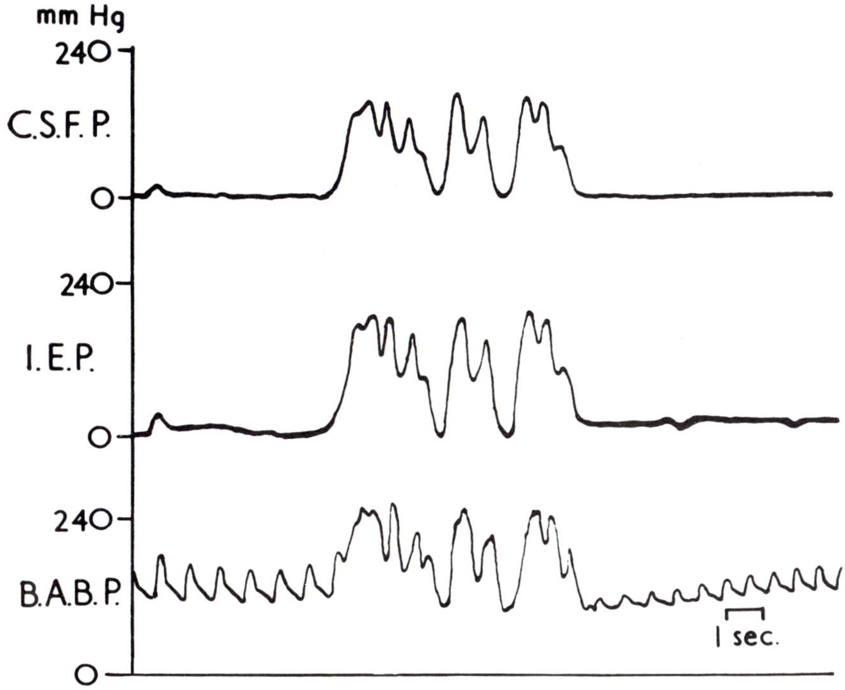

FIG. 1-8. Mechanical effects of coughing in man: CSFP = cerebrospinal fluid pressure; IEP = intraesophageal pressure; BABP = brachial arterial blood pressure. (From McIntosh, H. D., E. H. Estes and J. V. Warren: The mechanism of cough syncope. *Am. Heart J. 52:70,* 1956.)

trachea is involved, the cough may be harsh, dry, and painful at first, becoming loose and productive later. A similar cough may be present in association with bronchial disease, in which case, however, it may be preceded by a transient wheeze. Cough in association with diseases of the smaller airways (e.g., with asthma, cystic fibrosis, bronchiolitis) may include a more prominent high-pitched or wheezing component. Cough may come in prolonged paroxysms typical of pertussis, but is also seen with other conditions in which the mucosa is severely irritated such as in cystic fibrosis. It should be remembered that a paroxysm of coughing may sometimes (though rarely) produce cough syncope as a result of the concomitant changes in cerebrospinal fluid and blood pressure (see Fig. 1-8).

A chronic productive cough is always a sign of important bronchopulmonary disease such as tuberculosis, bronchiectasis (cystic fibrosis), fungal infection, atelectasis, foreign body, tracheal compression, congestive heart failure, and asthma or other allergy. Cough associated with deglutition should raise the possibility of aspiration that may be due to pharyngeal incoordination, tracheoesophageal fistula, achalasia, or hypopharyngeal disease. A nocturnal cough, including laryngeal cough, is often associated with allergy or viral infection, whereas productive cough on arising in the morning suggests a chronic condition such as bronchitis and bronchiectasis.

DYSPNEA

Dyspnea, which might be reported as "shortness of breath" by a reliable historian, indicates difficult or labored breathing. For the pediatric population, tachypnea is often the first indication of dyspnea, though the two terms are not synonymous. Similarly, although hypoxia and dyspnea often coexist, the association of the two is not invariable. In fact, hypoxia per se probably plays a small role in the production of "labored breathing," whereas it is a frequent contributory factor to tachypnea. In most clinical states dyspnea is due to multiple factors that vary according to the condition (Table 1-7).

In most conditions the complete basis for dyspnea is not established. Table 1-7 suggests that dyspnea may be associated with increased or decreased alveolar ventilation, an increase or decrease in any of the usual indices of chemical stimuli in arterial blood, and may occur even in the absence of known hematogenous or reflex stimuli. Chemoreceptor and central mechanisms of chemical stimulation are both indicated in Table 1-7 as potential causes of dyspnea where hypercapnia and acidosis exist. This is done because there is still uncertainty regarding the relative contribution of these mechanisms to respiratory stimulation by acid-base changes. When arterial hypocapnia exists in conjunction with a normally reactive CNS circulation (metabolic acidosis, fever, hyperventilation, stimulant drugs), it is presumed in Table 1-7 that central Pco_2 and $[H^+]$ have also been lowered. However, when CNS circulation is diminished (shock) or the buffer capacity of the blood is reduced (anemia), it is considered that central hypercapnia and acidosis may exist concurrently with the arterial hypocapnia and alkalosis indicated in Table 1-7.

TABLE 1-7. Conditions in Which Dyspnea Is a Prominent Symptom

					Basis for Dyspnea					
		Direction of Chemical Changes in Arterial Blood			Contribution of Reflex Factors (other than chemoreceptor)			Contribution of Chemical Factors		
								Chemo-receptor		Central
Condition*	Alveolar Ventilation at Rest	Pco_2	$[H^+]$	Po_2	*Hering-Breuer*	*Baro-receptors*	*Pain*	Po_2	Pco_2, (H^+)	Pco_2, $[H^+]$
Metabolic acidosis	↑	↓	↑	↑					+	+
Poliomyelitis	↓	↑	↑	↓				+	+	+
Myasthenia	↓	↑	↑	↓				+	+	+
Emphysema	↓	↑	↑	↓	+			+	+	+
Asthma	↓	↑	↑	↓	+			+	+	+
Pneumonia	±	±	±	↓	+		+	+	±	±
Atelectasis	±	±	±	↓	+			+	±	±
Cardiac decompensation	±	±	±	↓	+	+		+	?	?
Pulmonary embolism	±	±	±	±	+		+			
Anemia	↑	↓	↓	↑						?
Hemorrhage	↑	↓	↓	↑		+				?
Hyperventilation	↑	↓	↓	↑						
Fever	↑	↓	?	↑					?	?
Stimulant drugs	↑	↓	↓	↑						

Arrows indicate the direction of ventilatory and chemical changes usually observed in the conditions cited.

± indicates inconstant direction.

+ shows the probable contribution of a particular reflex or chemical factor.

? denotes factors suspected to be important but for which little or no evidence exists.

*From Lambertsen, C. J.: Abnormal types of respiration. In *Medical Physiology* Volume 2, (13th ed.), V. B. Mountcastle (Ed.). The C. V. Mosby Co., St. Louis, 1974.

Labored breathing may be acute, chronic, or intermittent. Acute dyspnea may be due to cardiac failure (and thus usually accompanied by widespread rales), pneumonia (and thus associated with other signs of pulmonary infection), pleural effusion (associated with pulmonary infection or secondary to systemic disease), pneumothorax (either spontaneous idiopathic, or during the course of other pulmonary disease or therapy), pulmonary thromboembolism (rare in pediatrics), massive atelectasis (e.g., following acute airway obstruction), and other acute obstructions of the airways in which airway resistance is increased (e.g., aspiration, asthma, bronchiolitis, laryngotracheitis, and epiglottitis).

Chronic and progressive dyspnea is usually the result of congestive heart failure in infants and children. It is exacerbated by the recumbent position, by sucking movements (which compromise minute ventilation) during feedings, and by a full stomach (which increases the "static" work of breathing after feeding). Chronic, progressive dyspnea is also one of the most distressing features of progressive airway disease in cystic fibrosis, and one may assume that it plays a role in the discomfort of patients with bronchopulmonary dysplasia. Patients with severe malcurvature of the spine (kyphosis, scoliosis) may find breathing labored when alveolar ventilation is compromised by the deformity.

Asthma is the most common cause of intermittent dyspnea in the pediatric population. Because it is so common, one may too easily attribute the labored breathing to bronchospasm exclusively and neglect investigation of those complications that may aggravate and accentuate the problem, e.g., pulmonary infection, pneumothorax, obstruction with atelectasis, and cardiac failure. Paroxysms of dyspnea that occur during the night (paroxysmal noctural dyspnea) may also be due to asthma, although cardiac failure should also be suspected. In a few other conditions intermittent dyspnea is a problem, such as episodes of active or recrudescent pulmonary infection in cystic fibrosis, so-called allergic bronchopulmonary aspergillosis with eosinophilia, and dyspnea of functional or psychoneurotic origin (usually producing a hyperventilation syndrome).

WHEEZING

The term wheezing as used in this section refers to the noises of breathing produced by diseased airways, as perceived by the patient or his associates. Thus it is a generic term for the audible sounds that are *symptomatic* of respiratory disease. "Wheezes" is also used to describe one class of adventitious sounds that are best characterized by stethoscopic examination of the lung: This *sign* of airway disease is discussed on page 53. Thus it is understood that the wheezes reported by the patient may be the crackles or wheezes (rales or rhonchi) heard by the examining physician through the stethoscope.

Assessments of the changes of airway caliber during breathing, including the direct measurement of airway dimensions during spontaneous breathing in dogs (Fig. 1-9), confirm the expectation, based on an understanding of airway transmural pressure gradients, that the intrathoracic airways dilate during inspiration and narrow during expiration and that the converse changes occur in the extrathoracic airway. Thus one would expect maximal resistance to airflow to occur in the extrathoracic trachea and larynx during inspiration, and in the intrathoracic airways during expiration. From this principle a general maxim, which has clinical relevance, may be proposed: Wheezes that are primarily expiratory suggest increased resistance to airflow through the intrathoracic airways (intrathoracic trachea, bronchi, and bronchioles), whereas adventitious sounds that are primarily inspiratory suggest increased airflow resistance in the extrathoracic airways (glottis, larynx, and extrathoracic portion of the trachea). Often wheezes are produced during both inspiration and expiration (especially

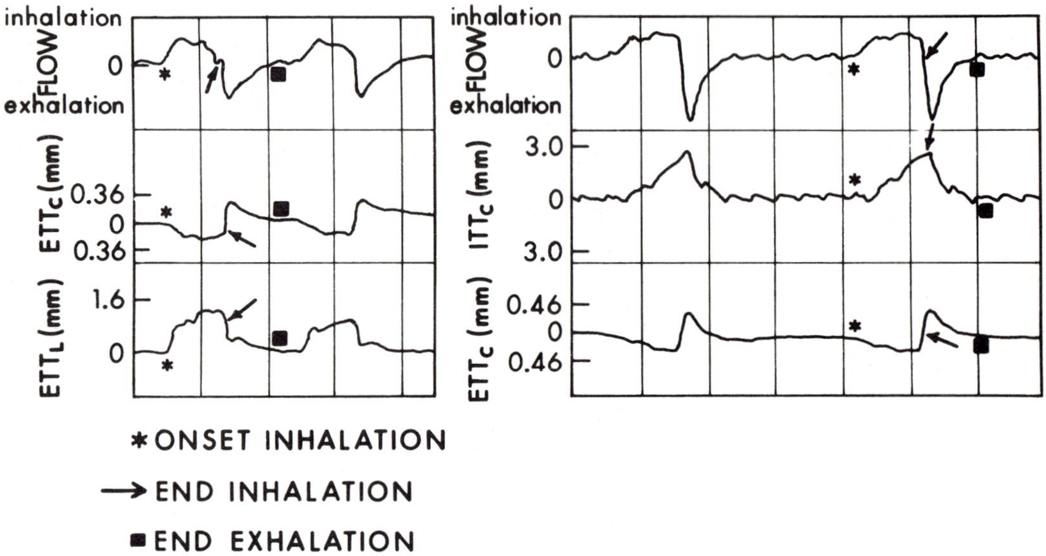

FIG. 1-9. Changes of airway caliber during spontaneous breathing, eupnea, in the dog. Upward deflections of "flow" = inspiration; downward deflections of "flow" = expiration: ITT_c = intrathoracic tracheal circumference; ETT_c = extrathoracic tracheal circumference; ETT_L = tracheal segment length, measured from mercury strain gauges fixed to the trachea. (Redrawn from Scarpelli, E. M., F. J. P. Real and A. M. Rudolph: Tracheal motion during eupnea. *J. Appl. Physiol. 20*:473, 1965.)

when there is serious narrowing of the airway); nonetheless the respiratory phase in which the sounds are loudest may provide a good clue to the location of the diseased airways. On the other hand, an airway that is only marginally patent or one that is closed entirely has little or no airflow and thus produces little or no sound—this mitigating factor must be kept in mind when applying the general maxim.

Wheezing, which is easily recognized by patient, parents, and physician, is characteristically high pitched and musical. Wheezes that are loudest on inspiration may be termed *inspiratory stridor* and, as mentioned, usually signify disease of the extrathoracic airway. Wheezes that are loudest on expiration, i.e., indicative of intrathoracic airway disease, are often associated with prolongation of the expiratory time. The tachypnea of respiratory disease may mask the latter symptom, but it can often be elicited during the physical examination. Unilateral wheezing sometimes may be recognized by the patient or his parents—it may even be accentuated when he lies on the ipsilateral side. This may provide the first clue to the location of a foreign body, for example. Wheezing that appears suddenly is suggestive of aspiration, but may also be associated with other causes of airway obstruction such as asthma (in which case the previous history of the patient is important), or laryngotracheitis, epiglottitis, and bronchiolitis (in which cases concurrent signs or immediate history of infection help in formulating a diagnosis). Chronic and/or progressive wheezing suggests extramural or intramural airway compression, e.g., from neoplasm, congenital abnormalities, or chronic infection.

DIFFICULTY FEEDING

Children with respiratory disease, like those with other illnesses, tend to reduce their food intake. In addition, feeding brings specific problems to the infant or child with respiratory disease. Since deglutition precludes concurrent breathing movements, sustained ingestion of foods—especially liquids—is difficult and may require frequent pauses to catch one's breath. This action may be especially obvious in the infant who cannot sustain sucking movements during feeding and thus becomes agitated and requires more time to complete his feedings. In addition, as the stomach begins to fill, the work of breathing increases, presumably because of the extra load that must be moved during each descent of the diaphragm. For a respiratory system that may already be at or near its limits of work production, the added load may prove difficult to handle and thereby aggravate tachypnea and dyspnea. For the infant or young child who is fed (incorrectly) in the recumbent position, the need to displace the load horizontally, i.e., without the aid of gravity, presents an added problem. For similar reasons, feeding may increase the stress on an overloaded cardiovascular system in patients with heart disease, so that it is important to consider this possibility as well when evaluating the effect of feeding. It is also necessary to remember these stresses of feeding when prescribing diet and feeding practices for the patient in hospital. Finally, intolerance to a full stomach may lead to vomiting and aspiration, which in turn may seriously aggravate respiratory distress in cardiopulmonary patients. For these reasons, maintenance of a decompressed stomach is an essential adjunct, too often forgotten, to the patient's overall treatment program.

ACTIVITY

Physical activity—whether feeding, sucking, crawling, or strenuous exercise—is curtailed in the presence of respiratory disease. Whereas the reliable historian is quick to mention changes in exercise tolerance, or the onset of exertional dyspnea, the infant or child cannot. Nevertheless, the observant parent can provide important relevant information to the physician. The first, even subtle, changes in eating or playing habits; an exaggerated, untoward response to ordinary colds; a changing enthusiasm for outdoor activities; and reports from school regarding patient participation in class activities may provide the earliest information regarding the onset of disease. Conditions that may influence physical activity should also be sought, such as environmental (smog, temperature) and emotional (including infant crying) factors, since they can provide insights into the nature and severity of the disease.

Alterations of spontaneous activity or emotional state may be symptoms of the hypoxemia that, to some extent, invariably accompanies respiratory disease. These symptoms depend on the degree of hypoxemia and the rapidity with which it has developed, i.e., the time available for compensatory adjustments to have taken place, including increased minute ventilation and cardiac output, and redistribution of blood volume. Chronic hypoxemia is usually expressed as a loss of physiologic reserve, in which the subject is easily fatigued and, as the condition becomes more profound, may become listless and inactive. When hypoxemia develops rapidly, emotions may become unstable, critical capacity may be lost, muscular incoordination and impairment of vision may occur, and a state of extreme restlessness or anxiety may ensue. These manifestations must alert the physician to frank or imminent respiratory failure and the need for corrective therapy. It should be noted that *hyperventilation* in response to respiratory disease, and perhaps exaggerated by emotional factors, can produce some of the symptoms described for hypoxemia as an effect of cerebral hypoxia induced by alkalemic cerebral vasoconstriction. Evaluation of arterial blood gas tensions and pH should place the two conditions in perspective.

PHONATION

Hoarseness is generally associated with viral laryngitis, which is usually short-lived. However, persistent hoarseness may be associated with chronic infection, neoplasm, granuloma, or compression of the recurrent laryngeal nerve from a mediastinal lesion. Snoring, nasal breathing, and nasal speech should lead to a suspicion of adenoidal hyperplasia, posterior choanal obstruction, or a nasal foreign body. These symptoms may also be present in Pierre Robin syndrome.

Expiratory grunting is a cardinal symptom (sign) of respiratory distress syndrome in the newborn infant. It may be due to the abnormally exaggerated tendency of the alveoli to collapse during expiration, although some physicians have suggested that it is related to severe hypoxemia in these babies. Grunting may also accompany pulmonary edema and pneumonia, perhaps for the same reasons that it is seen in neonatal respiratory distress, and it is a frequent concomitant of chest pain, perhaps for other reasons.

The muffled voice with drooling, which may or may not follow antecedent cough and hoarseness but has an acute onset and rather rapid progression, should always bring to mind the potentially fatal problem of acute epiglottitis.

SPUTUM AND HEMOPTYSIS

Sputum is an elusive commodity when dealing with infants and children; often it is only the word of the parent, regarding the sound of phlegm with coughing and the odor of the breath, upon which a judgment can be made regarding the duration or severity of productive coughing. When sputum production has been observed, it is important to estimate the amount produced daily (large, sometimes extraordinary amounts are produced by patients with cystic fibrosis), its color (mucoid sputum is clear or white; purulent sputum may be yellow or green), the presence of blood (frank or streaking), and the odor (foul-smelling sputum suggests infection from fusospirochetal and anaerobic organisms as is seen with lung abscesses).

Hemoptysis is spitting or coughing of blood from a lesion anywhere in the respiratory tract, from the pharynx to the lung parenchyma. It is an unusual symptom in pediatrics, often related to trauma, which must be taken most seriously because of the potential danger of hemorrhage and because—when its origin is bronchopulmonary—it signifies serious disease. The source of expectorated blood is usually the nasopharynx (epistaxis), mouth and oropharynx, and perhaps the larynx, whereas the source of coughed-up blood is the upper and lower airways (e.g., in bronchitis, bronchiectasis, erosion by aspirated material) and alveolar parenchyma (e.g., in lung abscess, tuberculosis, cardiac failure with edema, erosion from aspiration). Pulmonary hemosiderosis, in which there may be episodes of life-threatening massive parenchymal bleeding, should also be considered.

CHEST PAIN

It has been said that chest pain is one of the most difficult symptoms to evaluate in adults; it is even more complex the younger the patient and approaches virtual frustration when one deals with infants. The classification of chest pain as proposed by Baum is given with the understanding that careful observation of posture, attitude, and situations that seem to induce irritation or crying may provide the only means whereby the pediatrician can surmise chest pain.

The parietal pleura, unlike the visceral pleura, is well supplied with pain receptors that produce sharp, knifelike sensations when stimulated (*pleuropulmonary pain*). Whereas stimulation of the pleural surface (or peritoneal surface for that matter) of the outer margin of the diaphragm produces pain in the lower thoracic and upper abdominal regions (the T6 dermatome), stimulation of the pleural or peritoneal surface of the central diaphragm causes pain in the neck and shoulder, the regions supplied by the third and fourth spinal segments. (Although free nerve endings have been identified in alveolar septae, these are not pain receptors. Thus alveolar disease itself probably produces no pain.) Pleuropulmonary pain, which is intermittent and precipitated by breathing and other motion, is usually associated with bacterial pneumonia (when the pleural surface becomes involved) and sometimes with tuberculous pleural effusion. Viral and mycoplasma pneumonias rarely give pleuritic pain. In fact, viral pericarditis is the only documented viral infection that produces pleural effusion with any degree of frequency. Epidemic pleurodynia produces severe "pleuritic" pain due to pleural irritation from what is basically a muscular disease or due to basic pleural disease with overlying muscular involvement. Other diseases that may result in pleuropulmonary pain are spontaneous pneumothorax (acute pain) and pleural metastases (chronic); pulmonary infarction may also cause pleuritic pain.

Substernal burning and pain (e.g., from tracheitis) and similar pain in the parasternal regions (e.g., from bronchitis or aspiration of caustic material), which often is accentuated by deep breathing and cough, has been called *tracheobronchial pain.*

Deep thoracic pain that may be referred to corresponding somatic segments, sometimes associated with dysphagia or regurgitation, may be indicative of esophageal disease, and substernal pain that radiates to the neck and shoulder may be of cardiac or mediastinal origin (e.g., tumor, lymph nodes, mediastinal emphysema).

Localized pain in the chest cage may be muscular (e.g., from strain, trauma, inflammation), skeletal (e.g., from trauma, Tietze's syndrome, metastases) or neural (e.g., from intercostal neuritis as produced by herpes zoster. Its characteristic persistence and the associated tenderness along the course of the inflamed nerve permit differentiation from pleuropulmonary pain).

Physical Examination: Extrapulmonary

The extrapulmonary examination includes thorough evaluation of all systems, with particular attention to those discussed below.

MENTAL STATUS

The most important extrapulmonary evaluation concerns the mental functions of the patient, his level of awareness and his emotional status, since these factors are affected directly by the adequacy of alveolar ventilation and, conversely, they may alter respiratory activity. The prime example is the asthmatic child, who should breathe slowly and deeply for optimal ventilatory efficiency but tends to breathe rapidly and shallowly in response to respiratory reflexes and often also as a consequence of anxiety. Calm assurance and instruction may be the best therapy for some of these children.

The effects of hypoxemia on cerebral function were discussed earlier (p. 19). Whereas some degree of hypoxemia invariably accompanies pulmonary disease, one often finds arterial PCO_2 to be normal or even lower than normal. However, should *hypercapnia* develop, one must assume that respiratory failure has been established. Hypercapnia is always dangerous, since any disease capable of producing even mild hypercapnia has the potential for producing severe hypercapnia. The serious consequences of hypercapnia are increased intracranial pressure, lethargy, and coma. It is important to recognize that the clinical manifestations (1) may bear no exact relationship to the severity of hypercapnia, (2) are more likely to occur with marked increases of Pa_{CO_2} over brief periods of time, and (3) cannot be differentiated clearly from the effects of hypoxemia and thus require direct measurement of Pa_{CO_2} for confirmation.

THE SKIN

Inspection of the color and character of the skin is a sine qua non of the extrapulmonary physical examination. Generalized excessive redness—*erythema*—may be the first indication of overheating (iatrogenic or due to fever) or of polycythemia. *Pallor* may be due to anemia or to decreased peripheral vascular perfusion as an accompaniment of shock, exposure to cold, or local vascular occlusion. If there is concomitant hypoxemia, the skin color may be ashen.

Cyanosis, discussed earlier (p. 8), is usually due to hypoxemia in which case it is determined both by the degree to which hemoglobin is unsaturated and by the absolute hemoglobin concentration. Thus, for example, 80% saturation in a patient with 9.0 g of hemoglobin per 100 ml blood results in 1.8 g/100 ml of reduced hemoglobin, whereas the same saturation (and therefore, presumably, the same Pa_{O_2}) in a child with 16.0 g of hemoglobin per 100 ml results in 3.2 g/100 ml of reduced hemoglobin. In the first case cyanosis would probably be inapparent; in the second case it probably would be seen. All else being equal, however, the acyanotic child would be "sicker" than the cyanotic child in this example. Commonly, cyanosis is due to right-to-left shunt, ventilation-perfusion ($\dot{V}_A/\dot{Q}$) abnormality, or hypoventilation syndrome. The right-to-left shunt may be extrapulmonary (in which case breathing of 100% oxygen does not result in a marked increase of arterial Po_2), or it may be pulmonary (in which case 100% oxygen under positive pressure may produce a marked increase of arterial Po_2 if alveolar collapse is a prominent feature of the disease). When cyanosis is due to $\dot{V}_A/\dot{Q}$ abnormality or hypoventilation syndrome, arterial Po_2 increases markedly during 100% oxygen-breathing.

It should also be remembered that cyanosis may be apparent when there is methemoglobinemia or sulfhemoglobinemia (e.g., following ingestion of nitrites, nitrates, sulfonamides, phenacetin, or rarely due to an enzymatic defect producing congenital methemoglobinemia).

The presence of cutaneous *hemangiomas* should lead to a suspicion of possible, though rare, pulmonary arteriovenous malformations. *Petechiae* or larger hemorrhages in the skin may be associated with bleeding diathesis from a variety of causes and thus with pulmonary bleeding. Petechiae localized to the face may be the result of excessive coughing with or without associated bleeding diathesis.

Cutaneous *edema,* due to the accumulation of liquid in interstitial tissue, may be local (e.g., due to inflammation, trauma, lymphatic or venous obstruction), restricted to an area above the level of the diaphragm (e.g., with superior vena caval obstruction), or primarily below the level of the diaphragm (e.g., with congestive cardiac failure).

Subcutaneous emphysema is easily felt and often readily seen. The subcutaneous collection of air may be quite extensive (Fig. 1-10); it may originate from breaks in the peripheral pulmonary parenchyma with subsequent dissection of air along the airways to the medi-

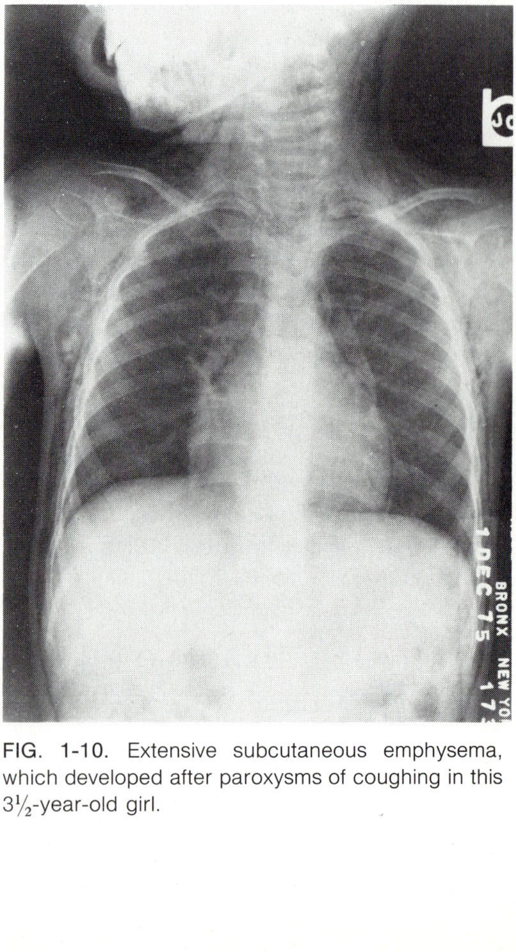

FIG. 1-10. Extensive subcutaneous emphysema, which developed after paroxysms of coughing in this 3½-year-old girl.

astinum and, ultimately, to subcutaneous tissue in the supraclavicular region. The subcutaneous air is not a problem in itself, but demands investigation into its cause (e.g., trauma, infection, or, as may be the case, unknown cause). One must also consider the possibility that air dissection has taken place along other viscera (e.g., periaortic, periesophageal) and ultimately into the thorax and/or peritoneum.

The classic review of Beerman and Kirschbaum includes a number of additional cutaneous manifestations of pulmonary disease.

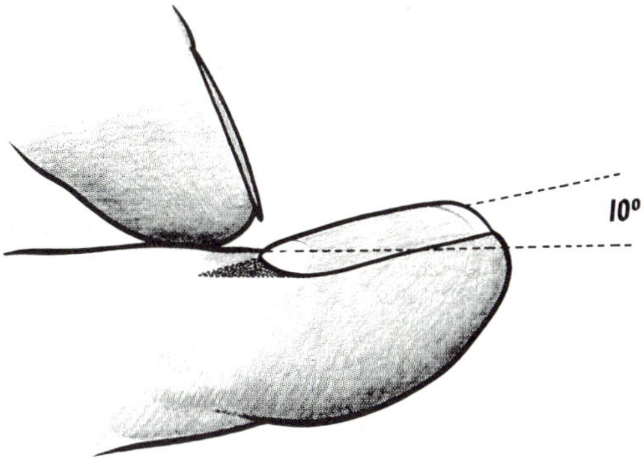

FIG. 1-11. Demonstration of the floating nail root in clubbing. (Redrawn after DeGowin, E. L. and R. L. DeGowin.[8])

OTHER SYSTEMS

The remainder of the extrapulmonary examination should pay particular attention to (1) middle ear and sinuses (for evidence of chronic and acute infection and for patency of the orifice of the eustachian tube); (2) oronasal pharynx (for evidence of enlarged tonsils and adenoids or other possible causes of upper airway obstruction); (3) the abdomen (noting liver size in relation to position of diaphragm; status of superficial veins; presence of ascites); (4) muscle tone; and (5) the extremities and digits (for evidence of clubbing and hypertrophic pulmonary osteoarthropathy).

Clubbing. This condition of the terminal phalanges probably results from an overgrowth of highly vascularized tissue, which is reversible if the cause is removed. Clubbing is usually painless and bilateral; rarely it may involve only one hand, e.g., in association with aortic aneurysm or arteriovenous fistula of the subclavian artery. In children with congenital heart disease and a different degree of hypoxemia between fingers and toes, an analogous discrepancy in the degree of clubbing may be observed.

The signs of clubbing are the floating nail (Fig. 1-11), the convex nail, and transverse broadening of the terminal phalanx (Fig. 1-12). The examiner can demonstrate the floating nail by pressing the mantle with the tip of his finger and finding the nail root to be resilient and springy. The normal response is for the nail plate to rest snugly against the bone without movement.

The first sign of increased curvature of the nail is obliteration of the unguophalangeal angle, which may be noted by inspection of the profile of the terminal digit. Normally the nail makes an angle of 20 degrees or more with the projected line of the digit. With clubbing this angle is diminished, and as clubbing progresses, the nail becomes convex (Fig. 1-12). Some authors have noted that the convex nail itself may be seen without clubbing, i.e., without the floating nail and obliteration of the unguophalangeal angle, in such conditions as rheumatoid arthritis, chronic paronychia, acromegaly, and so-called congenital clubbing. They have also noted that clubbing may occur without curving of the nail. Nonetheless, clubbing usually involves, sequentially, development of the floating nail, change in normal angle and change in normal curvature, followed by development of bulbous finger tips, sometimes called "drumstick fingers" (see Fig. 1-12).

The development of clubbing may be a rapid process; formation of the floating nail and change in the normal angle have been observed within 10 days after a tonsillectomy

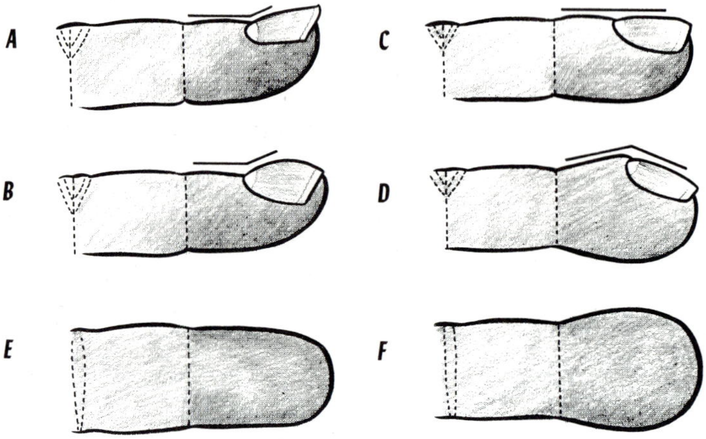

FIG. 1-12. Clubbing: *A*, normal flat nail; *B*, normal curved nail. (The angle in A and B is 20 degrees); *C*, early clubbing; *D*, severe clubbing. Viewed from the palmar surface, *E*, normal terminal phalanx narrower than middle phalanx; *F*, broad terminal phalanx with clubbing. (Redrawn after Hopkins, H. U.: *Leopold's Principles and Methods of Physical Diagnosis.* W. B. Saunders Co., Philadelphia, 1965.)

that induced a lung abscess. Nadas and Fyler noted that patients with congenital heart disease often have fiery red fingers and toes, which they recognize as the precursor of cyanosis and clubbing in subjects whose arterial oxygen saturation is permanently or paroxysmally low-normal. The cause of clubbing is not known; however, clubbing does occur in a number of cardiopulmonary and also noncardiopulmonary diseases (Table 1-8). Pulmonary disease is the most common cause.

Hypertrophic Pulmonary Osteoarthropathy (HPO). This disorder involves the formation of new bone along the phalanges and long bones in association with pulmonary disease. Although often associated with clubbing and perhaps etiologically related to it, HPO is not synonymous with clubbing. For example, the clubbing associated with congenital heart disease and biliary cirrhosis, as well as the clubbing of hepatogenic cyanosis, is rarely accompanied by HPO, and HPO may occur in some chronic pulmonary diseases without clubbing. Pathogenesis is not known, but it is generally felt that the earliest anatomic change in the limbs is an overgrowth of highly vascular connective tissue, followed by subperiosteal new bone formation. The stimulus for this reaction presumably comes directly from abnormal intrathoracic masses; a vagal reflex mechanism has been postulated, but the evidence is not conclusive. The most common cause of HPO is primary pulmonary tumor (rare in children). Suppurative lung

TABLE 1-8. Conditions That May Be Associated with Clubbing

Pulmonary Disease
Bronchiectasis
Lung abscess
Pulmonary tuberculosis (with cavitation)
Pulmonary neoplasm
Pulmonary emphysema ("adult type")
Cardiovascular Disease
Cyanotic congenital heart disease
Subacute bacterial endocarditis
Other Diseases
Hepatic cirrhosis
Chronic obstructive jaundice
Chronic ulcerative colitis
Regional enteritis
Chronic dysentery (amebic, bacillary)
Multiple polyposis
Thyrotoxicosis
Familial (benign)

disease, including that of cystic fibrosis, may be associated with HPO. In addition to the characteristic roentgenographic findings (Fig. 1-13), the extremities may be red and painful and the skin may be glistening. It should be noted that "familial osteoarthropathy" apparently bears no relationship to cardiopulmonary disease.

Physical Examination: Pulmonary Landmarks

The principles upon which examination of the cardiopulmonary system of the infant and child are based are essentially the same as those for examination of the adult, but have certain distinctive anatomic features.

LARYNX AND TRACHEA

The larynx is a series of articulated cartilages connected to the bony structures above, below, and behind it by muscles capable of lowering or raising it in the neck or tilting its axis in relation to that of the vertebral column (Fig. 1-14). Except during swallowing, the inferior constrictors of the pharynx hold the posterior border of the cricoid cartilage against the pharyngeal wall, thus preventing inspired air from entering the esophagus. The cartilages of the larynx (Fig. 1-15) include (1) the cricoid, the only complete cartilaginous ring in the respiratory tract; (2) the thyroid, which articulates with the posterior cricoid and from which arises the epiglottis anteriorly; and (3) the arytenoids, which articulate with the superior surface of the posterior portion of the cricoid (cricoarytenoid joints). Closure of the larynx during swallowing is its single vital function, the essence of which is strong adduction of the true vocal cords by movement of the arytenoids. Nonetheless, supplementary movements ensure complete closure of the airways, e.g., closure of the false cords, approximation of the aryepiglottic folds, and movement of the epiglottis backward and downward. The relevant anatomic landmarks in the fetus are shown in Figure 1-16.

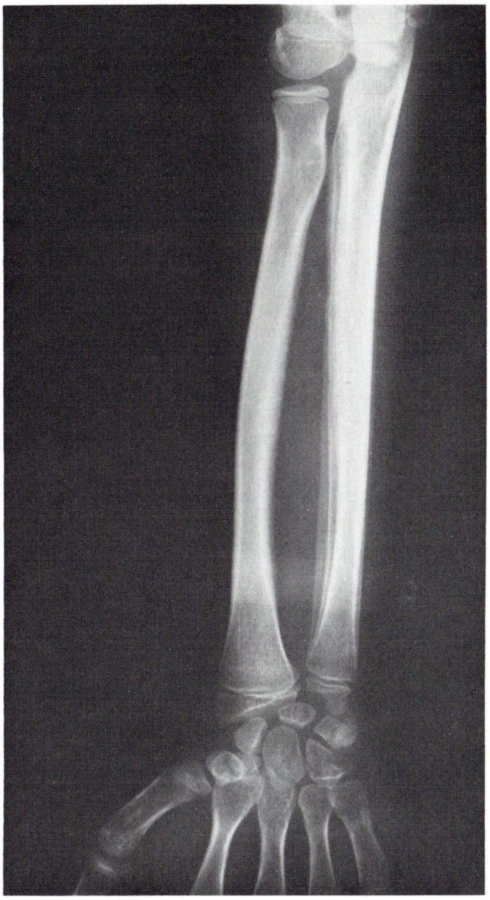

FIG. 1-13. Hypertrophic pulmonary osteoarthropathy. Periosteal new bone formation, in layers, is best seen in this radiograph along the shaft of the ulna. (Courtesy of Dr. Harold S. Goldman, Albert Einstein College of Medicine, New York.)

Since the newborn infant is an "obligatory" nasal breather, a major portion of the total resistance to airflow is accounted for by this airway. With growth of the head from infancy to adulthood, the structures of the face, including the nose and mouth, increase in size out of proportion to the contents of the cranial cavity (Fig. 1-17). Nonetheless the oronasal cavity, larynx, and trachea still constitute the sites of major resistance to

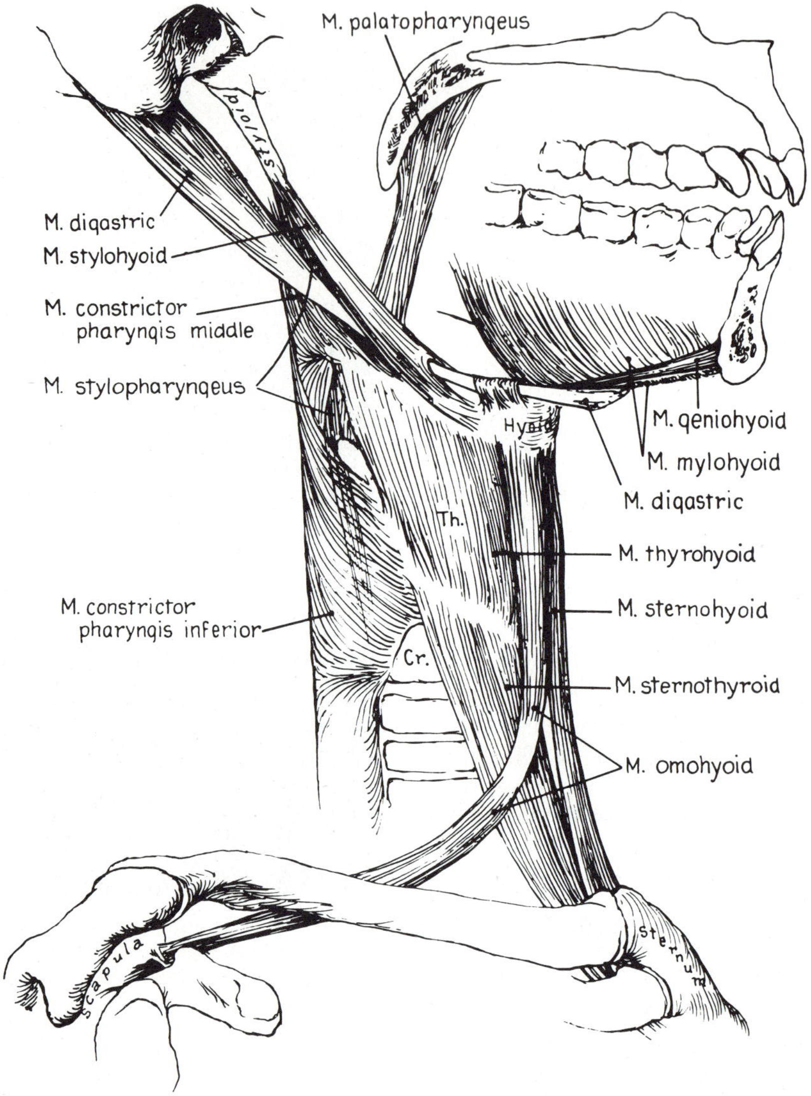

FIG. 1-14. Muscles of the neck, which are involved in movements of the larynx, in relation to neighboring structures. (From Proctor, D. F.[24])

airflow during breathing. In this regard the narrowing of the extrathoracic trachea during inspiration (see p. 18 and Fig. 1-9) must be taken into account as another factor that increases airflow resistance especially when the lumen is compromised by disease. Because of its small size (Table 1-9), the trachea of the newborn and infant is at particular risk to the compromising effects of natural or iatrogenic irritation.

INTRATHORACIC AIRWAYS, LOBES AND SEGMENTS

The intrathoracic trachea bifurcates at the carina (so-called because the separation has a spur-like appearance) into the right and left main bronchi. The course of the right main bronchus is more in line with the trachea than that of the left, the angulation of the left being about two times more acute than that of the right. This fact and the somewhat greater diameter of the right main bronchus (see Table 1-9) make it the favored site for deposition of aspirated material. Airway division continues from the main bronchi by either symmetrical or asymmetrical branching. Using the figures of Weibel for symmetrical branching in the *adult lung* (Table 1-10), *lobar bronchi* may be defined as the nine generations of airways from the trachea in which luminal diameter decreases from about 12.2 mm (main bronchi) to 1.5 mm; *lobular bronchi* as the tenth through sixteenth generations in which luminal diameter decreases to about 0.6 mm; and *respiratory bronchioles* as the seventeenth through nineteenth generations in which luminal diameter decreases to

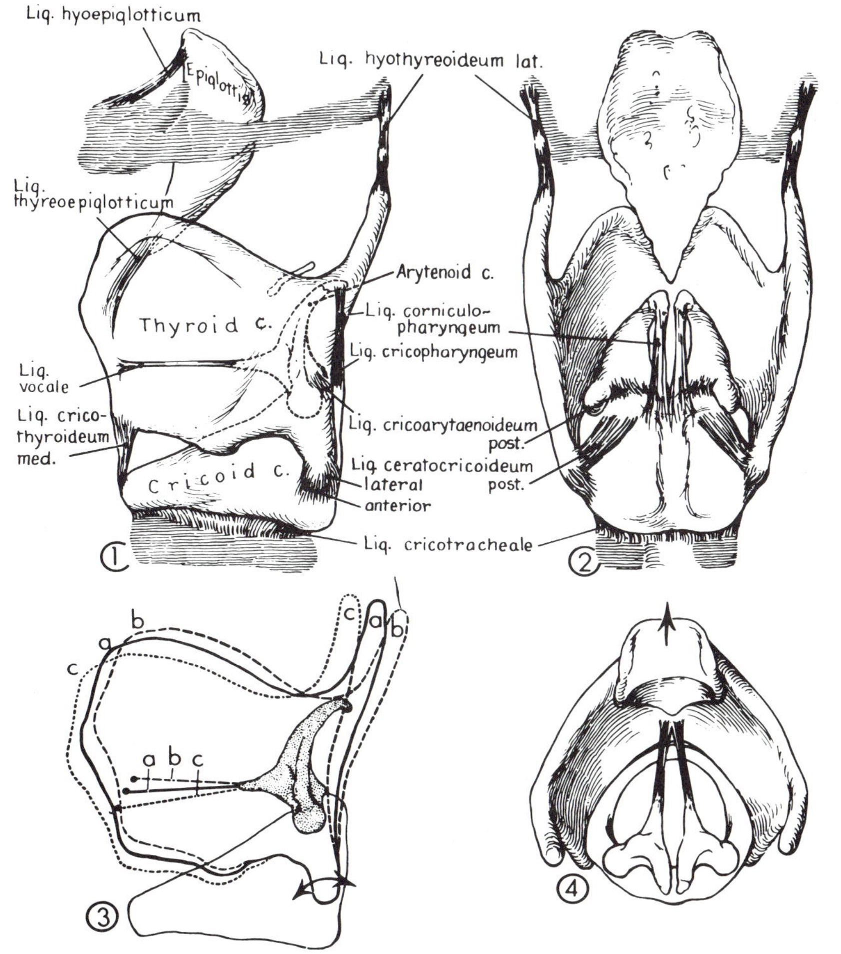

FIG. 1-15. The cartilages and ligaments of the larynx seen from the side (1), from the back (2), and from above (4). Lengthening of the vocal cords resulting from rotation of the thyroid cartilage on its articulation with the cricoid cartilage is shown in (3a, b, c). In (2) and (4) the arytenoids are drawn in a position of relative adduction. (From Proctor, D. F.[24])

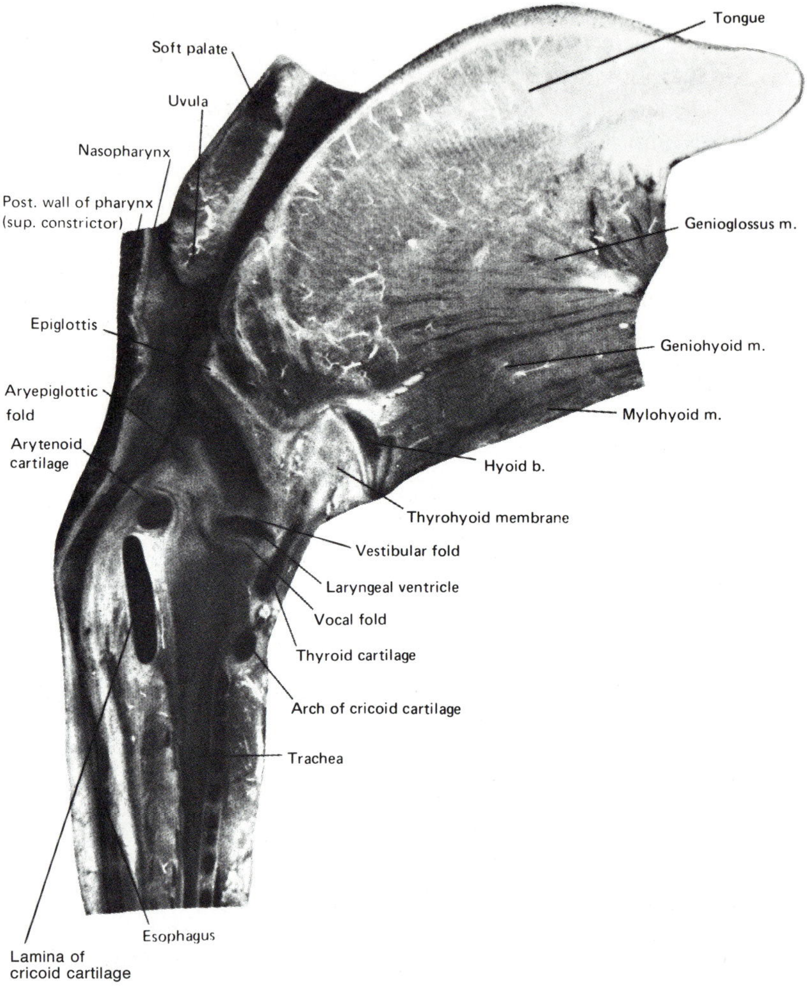

FIG. 1-16. Sagittal section of the tongue, pharynx, and laryngotracheal region of the human fetus. (From Parke, W. W.[21])

about 0.47 mm and alveoli first appear in the walls of these terminal airways. Despite the marked progressive narrowing of individual airways, the total cross-sectional area is greater with each succeeding generation: Thus the total area of the airways of the first generation is 2.3 cm^2, the tenth generation is 13.4 cm^2, the seventeenth generation is 300 cm^2, and the nineteenth generation is 944 cm^2. The twentieth through twenty-third generations constitute the alveolar ducts, sacs, and alveoli.

The lung of the newborn infant is comparable to that of the child or adult in that the right and left main bronchi lead to three and two lobes respectively and the lobes are separated by pleural reflections, which produce the interlobar fissures (Fig. 1-18). Differences between the infant and adult lungs include (1) those that are determined by the conformation of the thorax, i.e., the relatively greater anteroposterior diameter of the infant's lung, which gives it a round rather than flattened appearance (Fig. 1-19) and the rela-

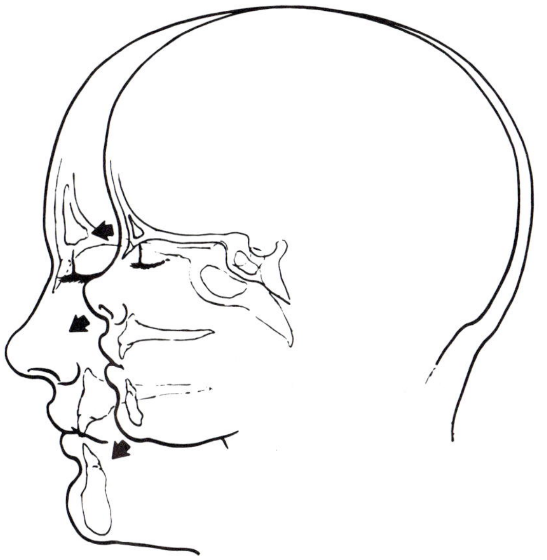

FIG. 1-17. Growth of the head from childhood to adult life. Note that the structures of the face, including the nose, mouth, and paranasal sinuses, increase in size out of proportion to the contents of the cranial cavity. (From Proctor, D. F.[24])

tively greater diaphragmatic than apical transverse diameter, which gives it a somewhat bell-shaped appearance, and (2) those that are determined by the developmental timetable; i.e., the neonatal lung contains less generations of airways and fewer alveoli than the adult lung. Nonetheless, segmentation of the lung is complete at birth, and one may use the conventional diagrams illustrating the various lobar segments (Fig. 1-20) as topographic guides for the examination of the infant. The conventional "adult" diagrams are presented alongside photographs of the fetal lung in Figures 1-21 through 1-24.

ALVEOLI

The lung of the newborn infant has about 10% the number of alveoli (about 24×10^6) and airways (about 1.5×10^6) as does that of

TABLE 1-9. Airway and Alveolar Dimensions from Birth to Adulthood*

	Trachea		Bronchus†		Alveoli		
Age	Length	Diameter (lumen) (frontal/sagittal)	Length	Diameter (frontal/sagittal)	Diameter (μ)	No. $\times 10^6$	S A (m^2)
Birth–1 mo	40.0	5.0/3.6	9.0 (21.0)	5.0/4.6 (4.2/3.9)	50	24	2.8
5–6 mo	42.0	5.8/5.0	8.0-10.0 (21.0)	5.9/6.1 (4.3/4.9)	—	112	8.4
~1 yr‡	44.0	6.9/6.0	11.0 (29.0)	6.3/5.9 (5.1/4.4)	100	129	12.2
~3 yr	50.0	8.8/7.0	13.0 (31.0)	7.3/7.4 (5.5/7.0)	—	257	22.2
5–6 yr‡	55.5	9.6/8.6	13.5 (34.0)	7.5/8.6 (7.0/6.3)	140	280	32.0
10 yr‡	63.0	10.7/9.4	14.0 (35.0)	9.2/8.6 (8.4/7.3)	170	—	—
13–16 yr	72.0	14.0/12.7	22.0 (42.0)	10.9/9.6 (8.5/8.5)	170-200	—	—
Adult	90-150	12.0-18.0/13.0-23.0	20.0 (52.0)	12.7/14.0 (11.1/11.5)	220	296	75.0

*Data derived from tables in Respiration and Circulation (Biological Handbooks), Federation of American Societies for Experimental Biology, Bethesda, Md., 1971.

†Figures for right main bronchus and (in parentheses) for left main bronchus.

‡Tracheal dimensions are averages of several values given.

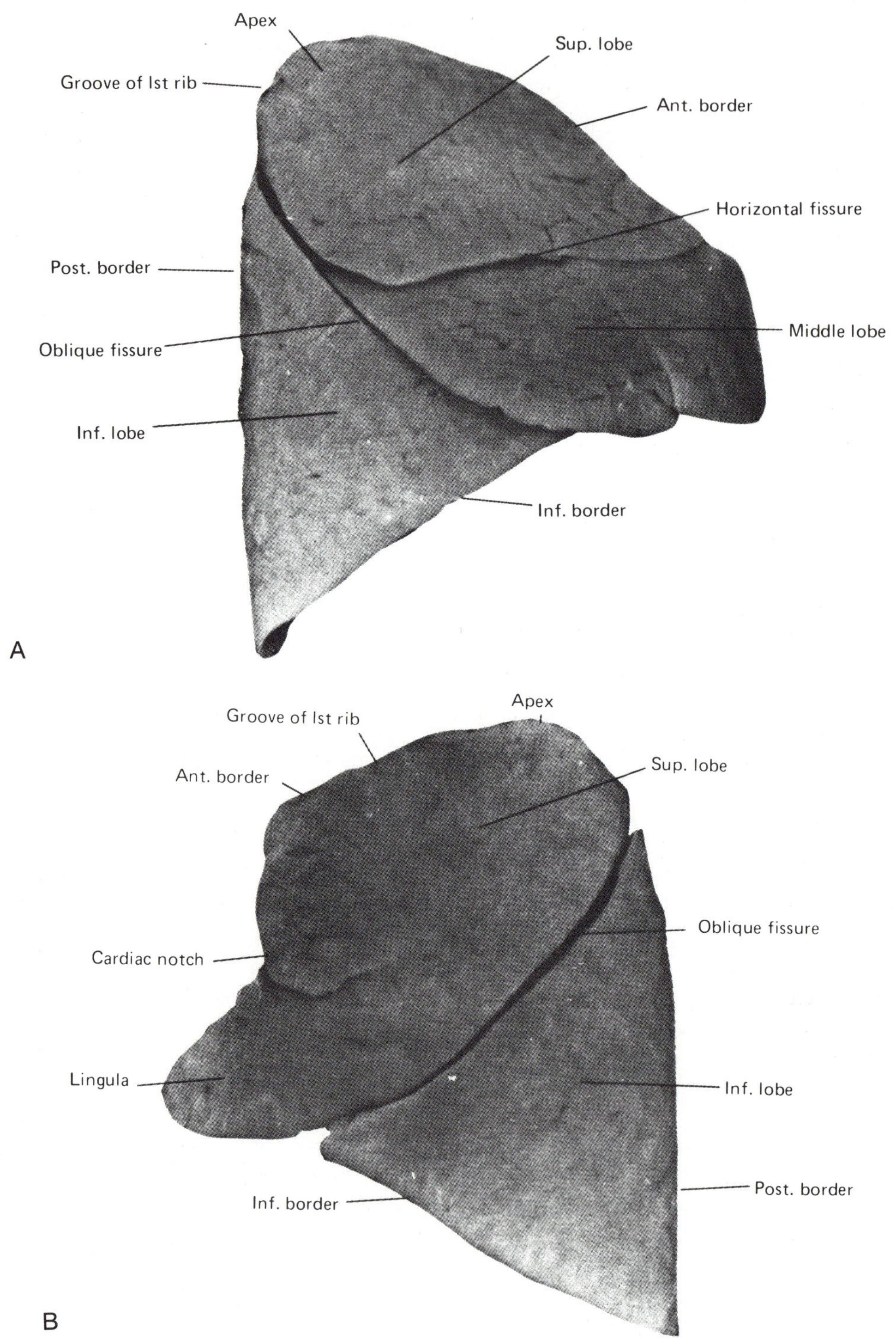

FIG. 1-18. Superficial anatomy, lateral aspect, of the right lung (A) and left lung (B) of a human fetus. (From Parke, W. W.[21])

TABLE 1-10. Generations of Dichotomous Branching and Dimensions*

Generation	No. per Generation	Diameter (cm)	Total Cross Section (cm^2)
0	1	1.8	2.54
1	2	1.22	2.33
2	4	0.83	2.13
3	8	0.56	2.00
4	16	0.45	2.48
5	32	0.35	3.11
6	64	0.28	3.96
7	128	0.23	5.10
8	256	0.186	6.95
9	512	0.154	9.56
10	1,024	0.130	13.4
11	2,048	0.109	19.6
12	4,096	0.095	28.8
13	8,192	0.082	44.5
14	16,384	0.074	69.4
15	32,768	0.066	113.0
16	65,536	0.060	180.0
17	131,072	0.054	300.0
18	262,144	0.050	534.0
19	524,288	0.047	944.0
20	1,048,576	0.045	1,600.0
21	2,097,152	0.043	3,220.0
22	4,194,304	0.041	5,880.0
23	8,388,608	0.041	11,800.0

*Data from Weibel, E. R.[27]

the adult. Because the newborn's alveoli are smaller (Table 1-9), his alveolar surface area is about 3% of the adult's. Since his body surface area is 10% of the adult's, the relatively smaller pulmonary surface for gas exchange indicates that he probably has less "reserve pulmonary function" with which to handle increased metabolic demands or to cope with pulmonary disease. The transitional state of the alveoli of the newborn and the role of the more compliant chest cage, as they may influence the physical examination, were discussed on page 10.

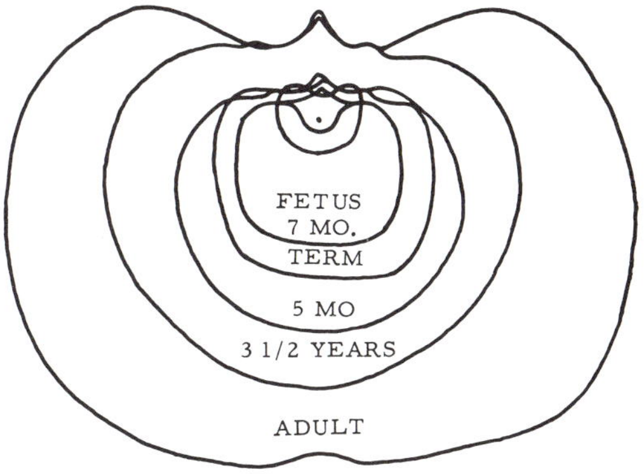

FIG. 1-19. Superimposed outlines of thoracic skeletal contours at various ages to illustrate the transition from the rounded thorax of the fetus to the dorsoventrally flattened thorax of the adult. Alignment is with respect to the center of the vertebral body. (From Krahl, V. E.[15])

BONY THORAX

The thorax is formed posteriorly by the 12 thoracic vertebrae and the posterior parts of the ribs, anteriorly by the sternum and the costal cartilages, and laterally by the ribs,

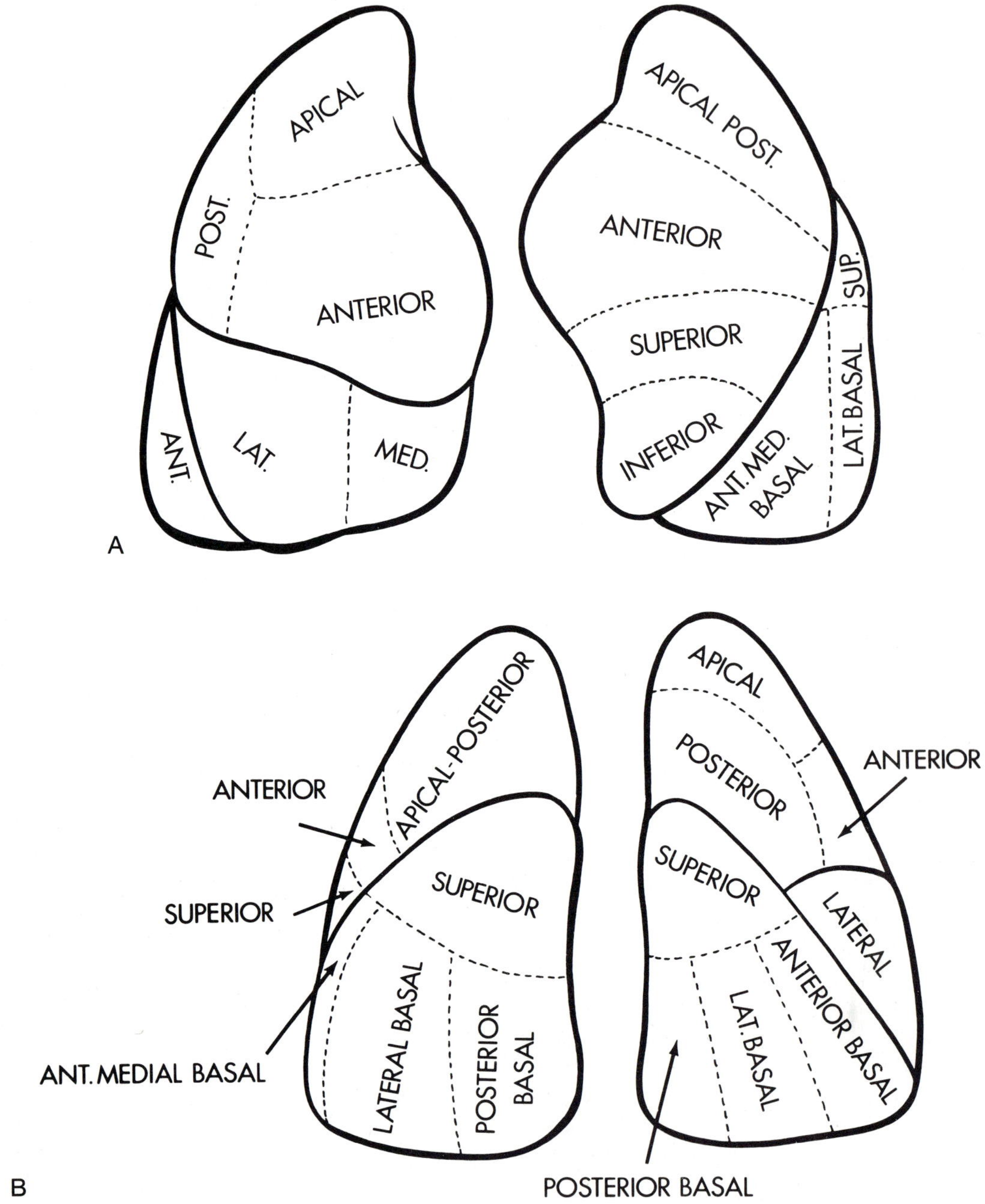

FIG. 1-20. Bronchopulmonary segments of the lung: *A*, anterior aspect; *B*, posterior aspect.

which are separated from each other by the 11 intercostal spaces. The upper end of the sternum supports the clavicles, and its margins articulate with the cartilages of the first seven pairs of ribs (Fig. 1-25). At birth the sternum is cartilaginous; ossification centers (the manubrium and xiphoid have one center each and the body has four centers) first ap-

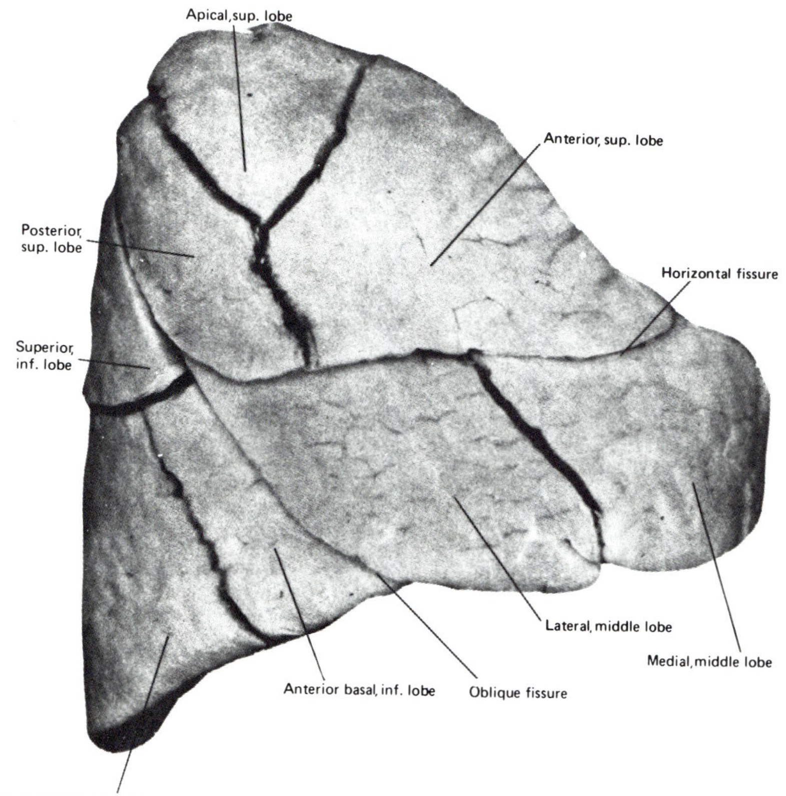

A

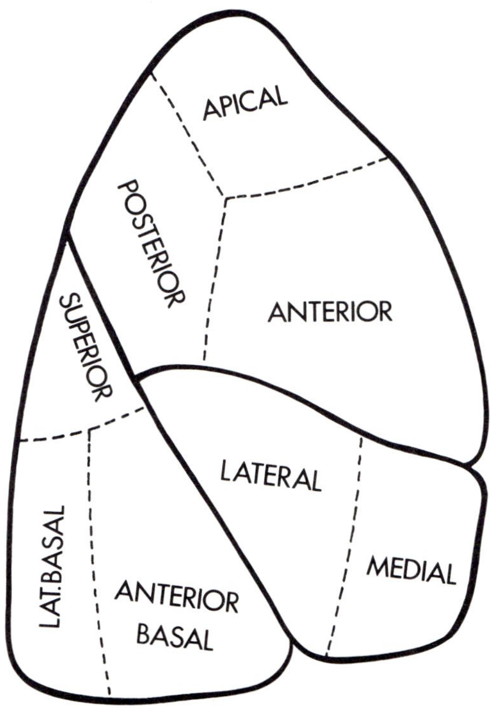

B

FIG. 1-21. Bronchopulmonary segments of right lung, lateral aspect: *A*, Photograph of human fetus (From Parke, W. W.[21]); *B*, Drawing, conventional (adult) model.

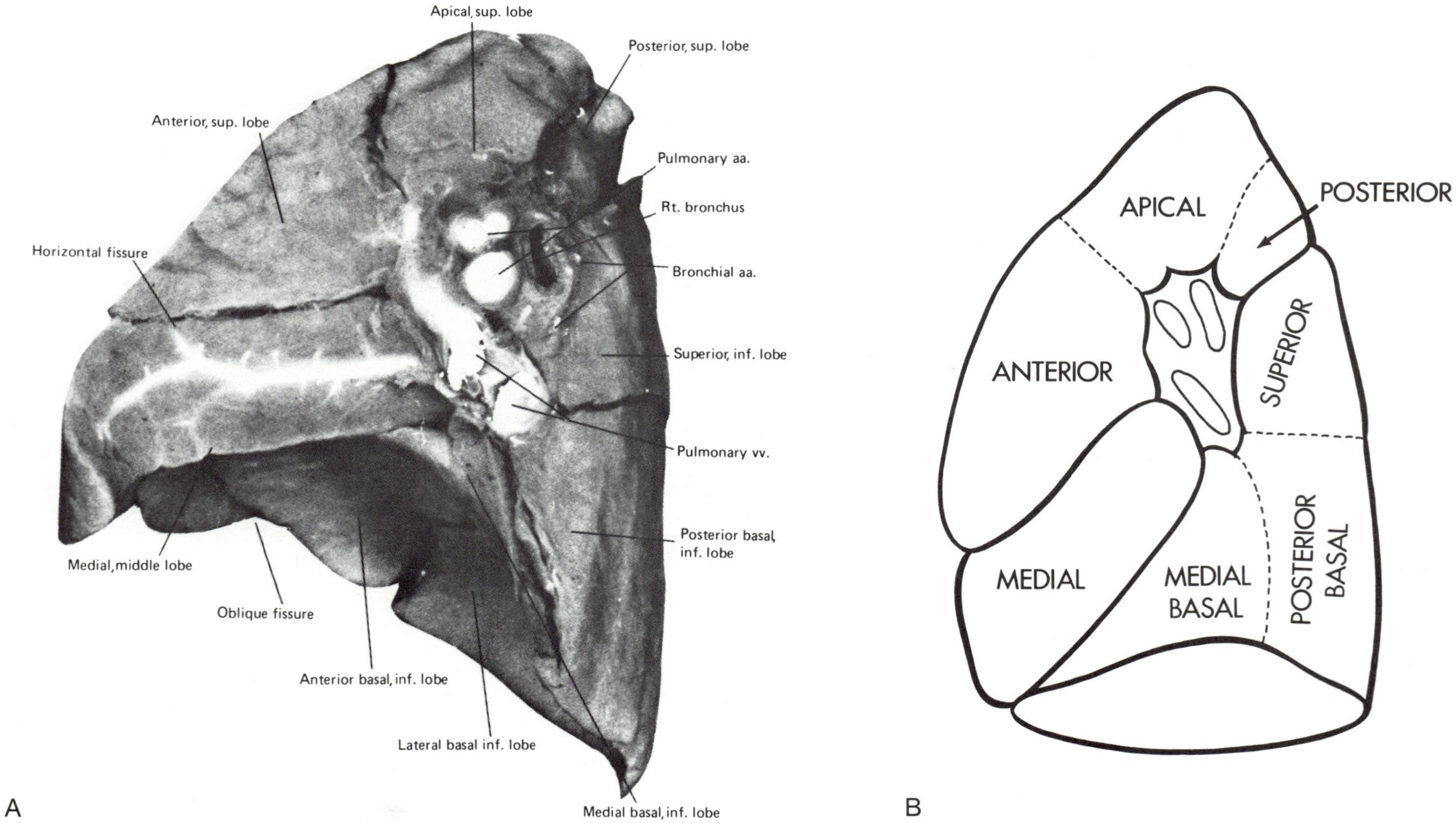

FIG. 1-22. Bronchopulmonary segments of right lung, medial aspect: *A*, Photograph of human fetus after pulmonary vessels have been injected with neoprene (From Parke, W. W.[21]); *B*, Drawing, conventional (adult) model.

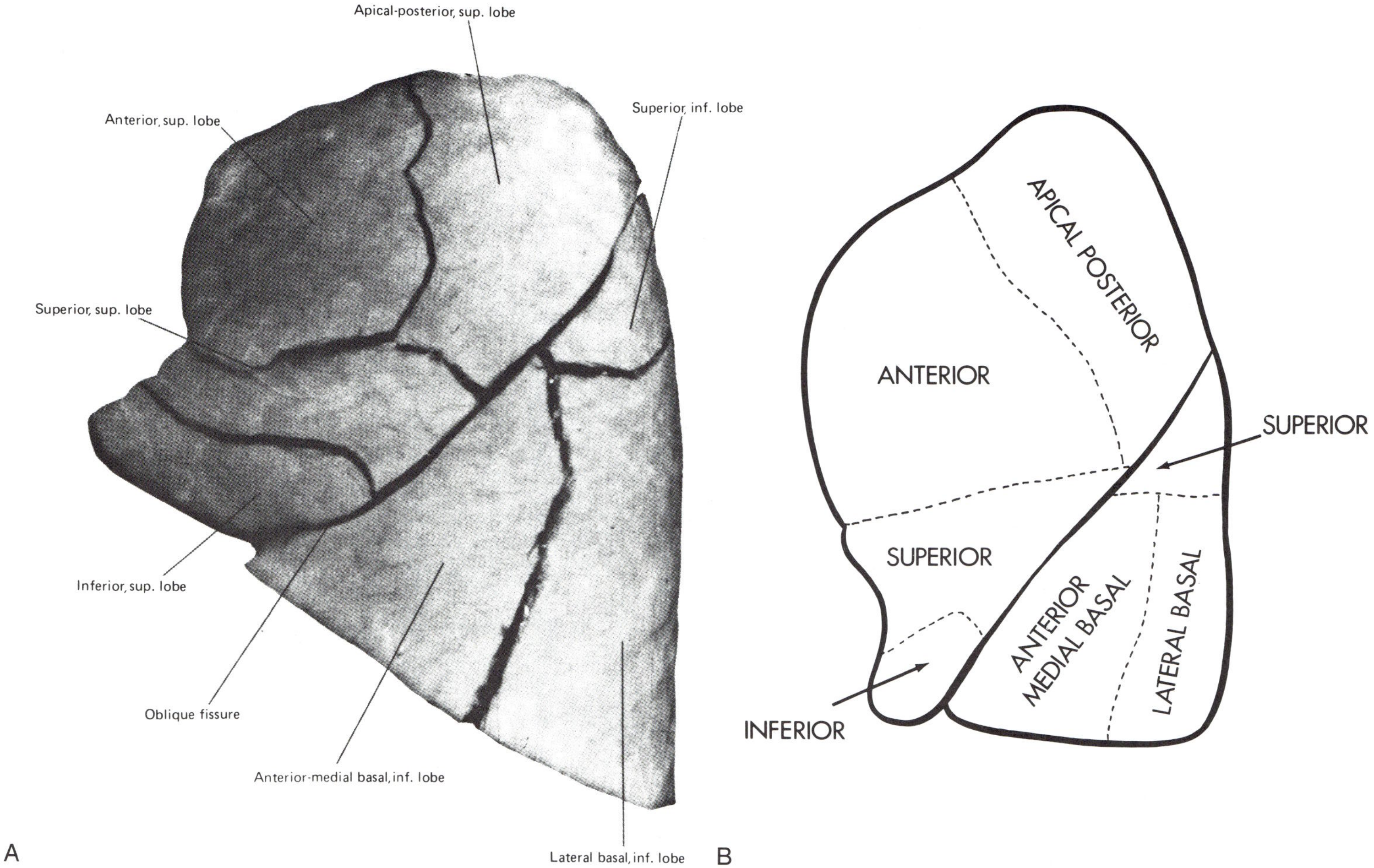

FIG. 1-23. Bronchopulmonary segments of left lung, lateral aspect: *A*, Photograph of human fetus (From Parke, W. W.[21]); *B*, Drawing, conventional (adult) model.

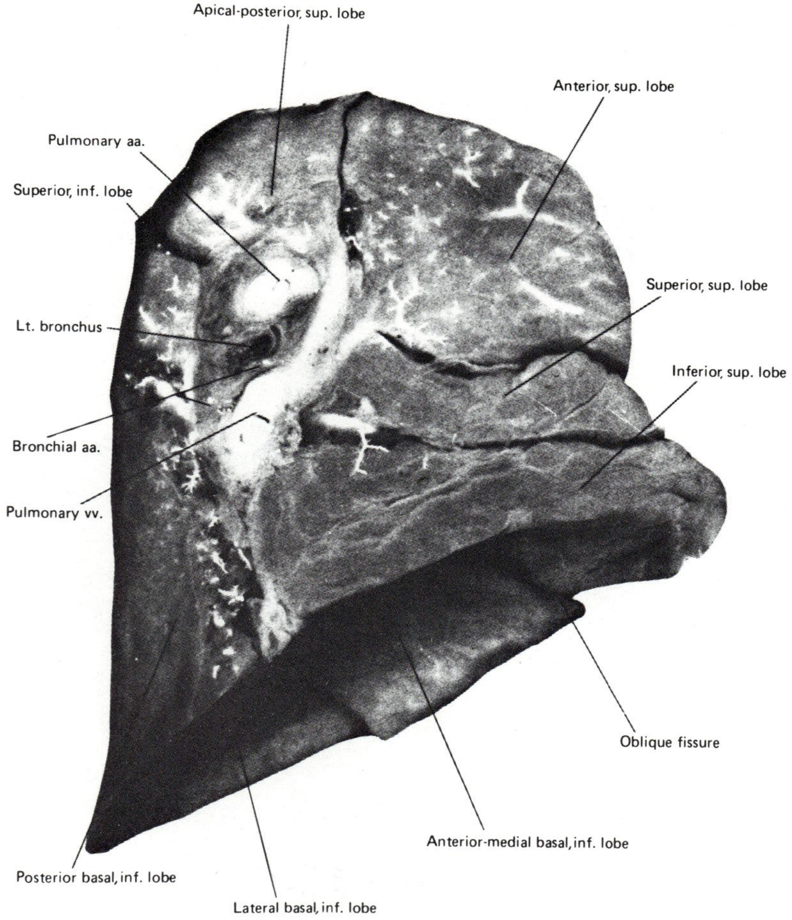

A

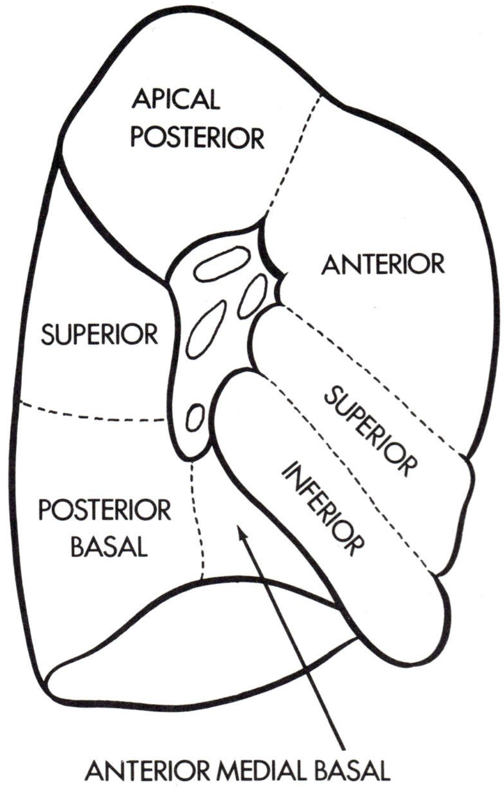

B

FIG. 1-24. Bronchopulmonary segments of left lung, medial aspect: *A*, Photograph of human fetus after pulmonary vessels have been injected with neoprene (From Parke, W. W.[21]); *B*, Drawing, conventional (adult) model.

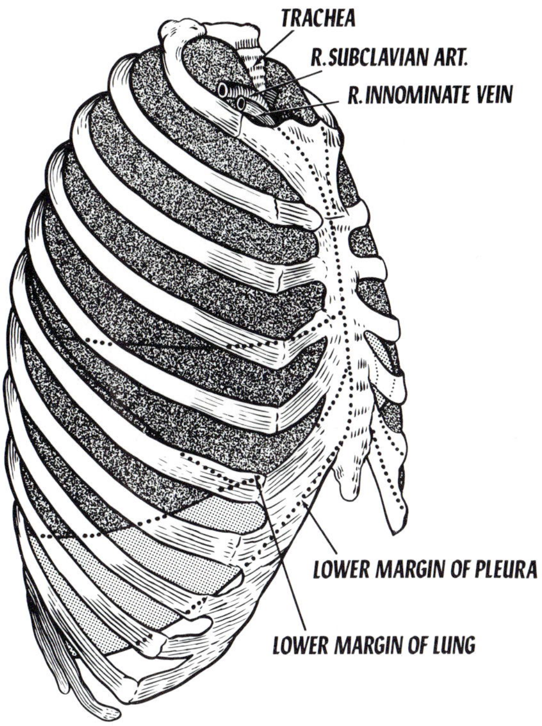

FIG. 1-25. Right oblique view showing the relation of the pleura and lung to the chest wall. (Redrawn after Goss, C. M.: *Gray's Anatomy*. Lea & Febiger, Philadelphia, 1954.)

pear during the sixth to seventh fetal months (manubrium and three body centers), then at about 1 year of age (the fourth body center), and lastly between 5 and 18 years of age (the xiphoid center). The centers of the body fuse between puberty and age 25, whereas the body rarely fuses to the manubrium, and the xiphoid remains partly cartilaginous throughout life.

The first seven ribs have been called "true ribs" because of their articulation with the sternum; the eighth through tenth ribs have their cartilages attached to the cartilage of the rib above; and the last two ribs are free at their anterior extremities. Occasionally a rib of varying length may form from the seventh cervical vertebra (cervical rib); though usually a benign anomaly, this rib may cause symptoms if it puts pressure on the brachial plexus and subclavian artery and vein that may cross over it.

RESPIRATORY MUSCLES

The *diaphragm* is the principal muscle of inspiration; during eupnea in the adult it accounts for about two-thirds the tidal volume when the subject is in the sitting or standing positions and 75% in the supine position. Although diaphragmatic paralysis is followed by marked reduction of vital capacity in adults, the other muscles of respiration are able to sustain normal activity. Vital capacity returns to normal about 6 months after unilateral ablation of the phrenic nerve. In the newborn, unilateral phrenic nerve paralysis causes respiratory distress: Most patients recover as full diaphragmatic activity returns, some may recover even if paralysis persists, and some may die. The muscle fibers of the diaphragm originate (1) from the second and third lumbar vertebrae, the medial arcuate ligaments (psoas) and the lateral arcuate ligaments (quadratus lumborum); (2) from the side and upper margin of the lower six ribs; and (3) from the back of the xiphoid process. The fibers converge at the central tendon. The movement of the adult diaphragm is presented in Figure 1-26. Because of its relatively wider base, the infant's diaphragm may have a mechanical advantage as an inspiratory muscle.

The *external intercostal muscles* extend from the tubercles of the ribs to the costochondral junction where they become continuous with the anterior intercostal membrane; the *internal intercostals* extend from the anterior end of the intercostal space to the angles of the ribs posteriorly where they become continuous with the posterior intercostal membrane. The many theories that attempt to explain the action of the intercostals have been summarized by Campbell, Agostoni, and Davis. These authors favor the conclusion that during inspiration (eupnea) the

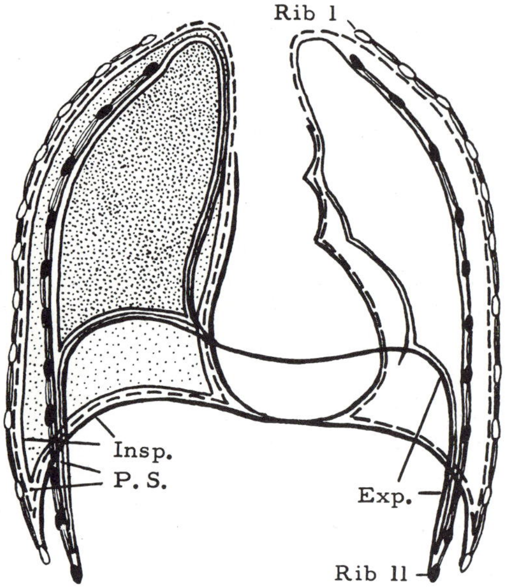

FIG. 1-26. Frontal section of the thorax (adult model) showing changes in size of thorax and position of heart and diaphragm with the phases of respiration: Light stippling = inspiration; heavy stippling = expiration. Note entry of lower lung margin into phrenicocostal sinus (P.S.) on inspiration. (From Braus, H.: *Anatomie des Menschen.* Bd. 2, Aufl. 3. Springer, Berlin, 1956.)

intercartilaginous internal intercostals of the upper three to five spaces (the parasternals) and the external intercostals posteriorly contract to elevate the rib cage and that the interosseous internal intercostals in the lower four spaces laterally contract during expiration (eupnea) to depress the ribs. With increased ventilation all external intercostals (the outer layer), as well as the parasternals, are active during inspiration, and all interosseous internal intercostals (the inner layer) are active during expiration. In addition to producing movements of the ribs, contraction of the intercostals increases tension in the intercostal spaces and prevents them from bulging or receding under the influence of varying intrathoracic pressure, an effect which is not achieved fully in the newborn with his rather meager muscle mass. As muscles of inspiration, the intercostals are of secondary importance to the diaphragm; their contribution to expiration has not been quantified but must be minimal.

The *muscles of the abdominal wall* (external oblique, internal oblique, transversus abdominis, and rectus abdominis) are the most powerful expiratory and expulsive muscles. Although they are subject to rhythmic respiratory activation, their contribution to expiration during eupnea is negligible. As respiratory activity increases, their contribution to expiration increases progressively, more so during nasal breathing than with mouth breathing. The greatest power of the abdominal muscles is not used for respiratory functions, except for coughing wherein it increases the kinetic energy of the airstream. Moreover, obstruction to expiratory airflow during spontaneous breathing is not met primarily by an increase in the activity of abdominal muscles but rather by the recoil of the lung and thoracic cage as end-inspiratory volume is increased (e.g., the hyperaeration that usually accompanies bronchospasm in asthma). However, one can be trained to use his abdominal muscles efficiently for expiration; indeed, such training is often indicated.

Of all the muscles generally regarded as accessory muscles of inspiration, only the *scaleni* and *sternomastoids* exhibit significant respiratory activity in man. The scaleni arise from the transverse processes of the lower five cervical vertebrae and are inserted into the upper surfaces of the first and second ribs. Their action is to elevate or fix these ribs both during quiet breathing and with increased inspiratory movements. Their total contribution is small compared to other inspiratory muscles, and they probably play no role in expiration, except perhaps during coughing. The sternomastoids arise from the manubrium of the sternum and the medial part of the clavicle and are inserted into the mastoid processes and occipital bone. Their action is to elevate the sternum, thus increasing the anteroposterior diameter of the thorax. They are probably the most important accessory muscles of inspiration, as witness their obvious activity in states of dyspnea. The progressively greater activity of the scaleni and sternomastoids as inspiratory efforts increase is shown in Figure 1-27.

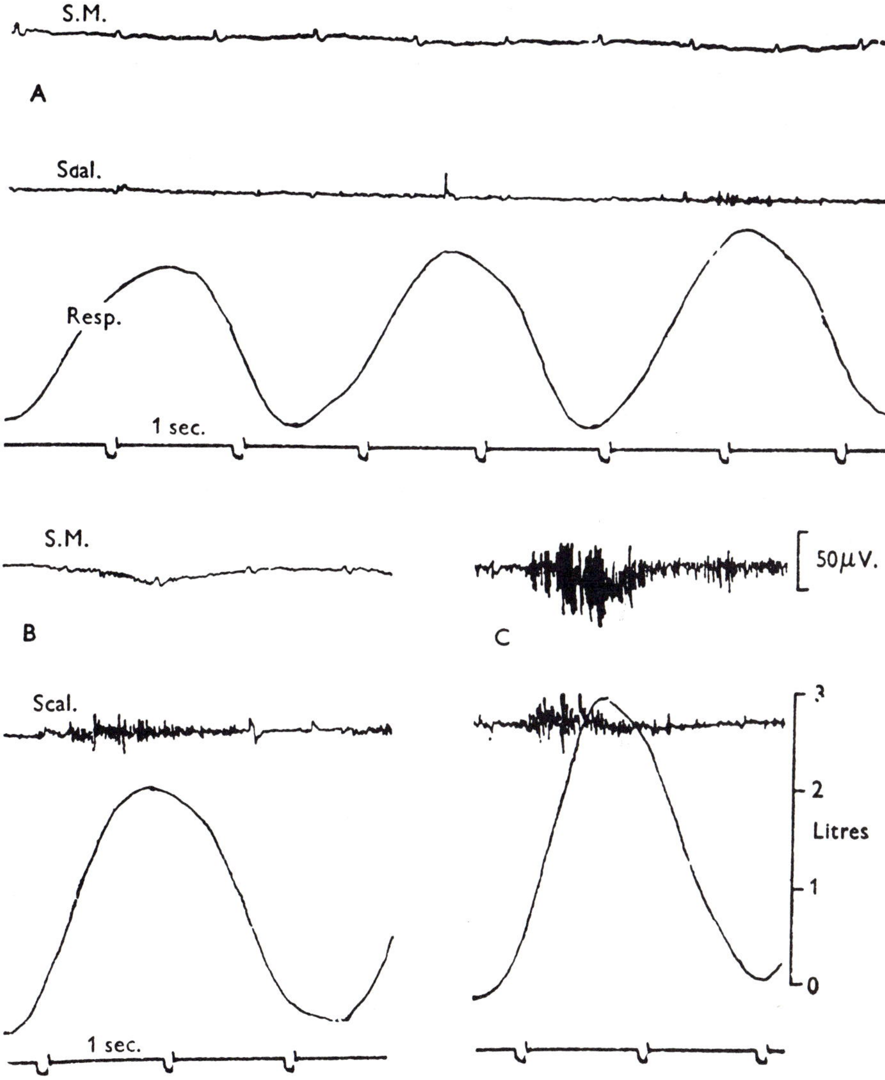

FIG. 1-27. Behavior of sternomastoid and scalene muscles during increased breathing. Healthy young male subject, supine: S.M. = sternomastoid electromyogram; Scal. = scalene electromyogram; Resp. = record of respiration in which upward deflection denotes inspiration. *A*, Onset of inspiratory activity in the scaleni. Ventilation increases from 42 to 52 l/min.; *B*, Development of activity in sternomastoids. Ventilation = 60 l/min.; *C*, Increased sternomastoid and scalene activity. Ventilation = 78 l/min. (From Campbell, E. J. M.: The role of the scalene and sternomastoid muscles in breathing in normal subjects. An electromyographic study. *J. Anat.* (*London*) *89:*378, 1955. Published by Cambridge University Press.)

Physical Examination of the Lung

The following account is presented in the sequence in which the pulmonary examination is usually conducted, i.e., inspection of breathing movements, examination of the larynx and trachea, palpation and percussion of the thorax, and auscultation of the lung.

BREATHING MOVEMENTS

Careful and thorough evaluation of the breathing movements of the patient provides important information about the seriousness of his illness and, with regular reexamination, its course. Ideally, the patient should be resting quietly; particularly for children and infants, a meaningful examination can be made while the patient is asleep.

Breathing Frequency. Normally breathing frequency for any given level of alveolar ventilation is regulated according to the principle of minimum effort; i.e., the spontaneous frequency is that which involves the least energy cost to the subject. Since the mechanical properties of the lung and chest wall determine the work of breathing, optimal frequency is established according to these properties. The relationship to frequency of elastic (compliance) work, viscous and turbulent (airflow resistance) work, and total (compliance plus resistance) work of breathing is shown in Figure 1-28. It is apparent that (1) normal minute ventilation in the adult is achieved with minimal total work when the frequency of breathing is about 13 to 17 breaths/min.; (2) should elastic work increase (lower compliance), the optimal frequency will be higher; and (3) should airflow resistance increase, the optimal frequency will be lower. The mechanical properties of the infant's lung and chest wall are such that its optimal frequency is higher than that of the adult. The change of normal optimal frequency with age is given in Table 1-4.

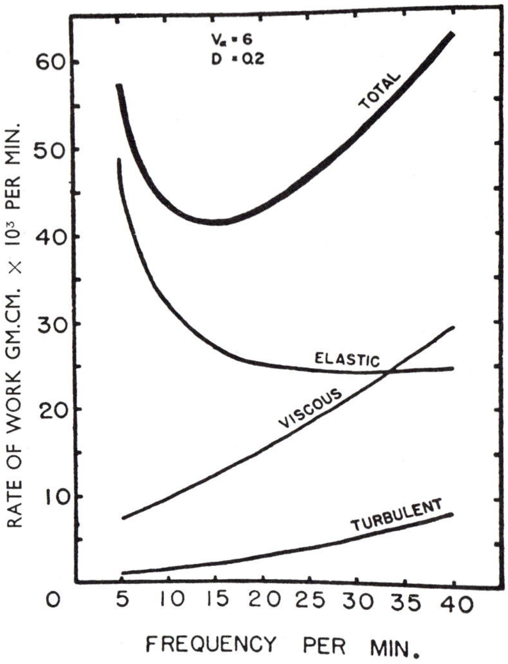

FIG. 1-28. Relationship of elastic, viscous, turbulent, and total work of breathing per minute to frequency of breathing. Alveolar ventilation is 6 l/min. and dead space is 200 ml (adult). (From Otis, A. B. et al.: Mechanics of breathing in man. *J. Appl. Physiol.* 2:592, 1950.)

It is also important to remember that optimal frequency increases as alveolar ventilation increases (Fig. 1-29); thus the need to increase alveolar ventilation in the presence of pulmonary disease (in order to maintain adequate gas exchange at the alveolar-capillary level) results in a higher frequency. In addition, the overriding drive of hypoxemia, which invariably accompanies pulmonary disease, also produces increased breathing frequency, as does hypercapnia when it develops. Thus the earliest sign of pulmonary disease is tachypnea.

The following points are relevant when assaying breathing frequency:

(1) The patient should be at rest or asleep, and breathing movements should be counted for at least 1 minute or longer, e.g., when breathing is irregular or periodic.

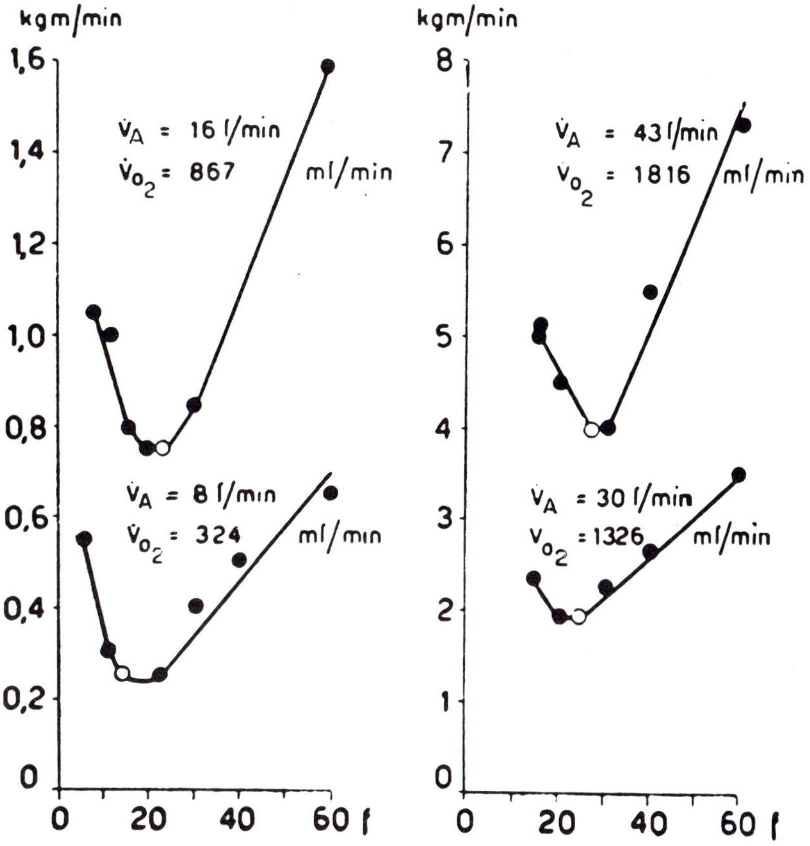

FIG. 1-29. Mechanical work of breathing in kg/min. as a function of frequency of breathing in breaths/min. at several constant rates of alveolar ventilation (V̇A). The open circles indicate the frequencies that were chosen spontaneously by the subject. (From Milic-Emili, G. and J. M. Petit: Il lavoro meccanico della respirazione a varia frequenza respiratoria. *Arch. Sci. Biol. 43*:326, 1959.)

(2) Sleeping frequency is slower than that of the awake subject, and the difference is greater the younger the child (Tables 1-11 and 1-12).

(3) Factors associated with the primary pulmonary disease may augment rapid breathing (e.g., anxiety, fever, acidemia due to diarrhea, pain, medication with salicylates).

(4) One of the first signs of cardiac decompensation or failure is tachypnea, probably in response to reduced lung compliance and/or hypoxemia.

(5) Because optimal breathing frequency decreases as airflow resistance increases (e.g., in diseases producing bronchospasm) and whereas concomitant hypoxemia with or without anxiety results in tachypnea, it is generally in the patient's favor to attempt to regulate his breathing at a slower frequency and higher tidal volume.

(6) Whereas slowing of a previously rapid frequency may be a sign of improvement, one must also keep in mind that rapid slowing or an abnormally slow frequency (bradypnea) may be a sign of deterioration related to hypoxemia, hypercapnia, or reduced cardiac output, each of which may directly depress the central nervous system.

Minute Ventilation. This rate is the product of the depth (tidal volume) and frequency

TABLE 1-11. Respiratory Rates per Minute of Normal Children, Sleeping and Awake*

	Sleeping			Awake			Mean Difference Between Sleeping and Awake
Age	No.	Mean	Range	No.	Mean	Range	
6–12 mo	6	27	22–31	3	64	58–75	37
1–2 yr	6	19	17–23	4	35	30–40	16
2–4 yr	16	19	16–25	15	31	23–42	12
4–6 yr	23	18	14–23	22	26	19–36	8
6–8 yr	27	17	13–23	28	23	15–30	6
8–10 yr	19	18	14–23	19	21	15–31	3
10–12 yr	11	16	13–19	17	21	15–28	5
12–14 yr	6	16	15–18	7	22	18–26	6

*From Kendig, E. L.[14]

(per minute) of breathing. When dead space has not been altered, its estimation provides a reliable assay of alveolar ventilation.

$\dot{V}_A = \dot{V}_E - \dot{V}_D$, where $\dot{V}_A$ is alveolar ventilation (l/min), $\dot{V}_E$ is the product of volume expired per breath (V_E) and frequency (f) per minute, and $\dot{V}_D$ is the product of dead space volume (V_D) and (f).

However, it is often difficult to estimate and certainly impossible to quantify tidal volume by inspection at the bedside. A pocket-sized instrument, the Wright respirometer, is available for measuring minute volume of a cooperative patient. Although a convenient, reliable, and objective method for determining minute volume in all infants and

TABLE 1-12. Slowing of Heart Rate, Cardiac Output, and Respiratory Rate in 15 Subjects (16–34 Years) During Sleep

	Heart Rate (per min.)	Cardiac Output (l/min.)	Respiratory Rate (per min.)
Awake	62 ± 12.2	7.6 ± 1.3	18.1 ± 3.0
Stage I	−3.6 ± 10.2*	−0.94 ± 1.3 (<0.05)	−2.2 ± 2.5 (<0.001)
Stage II	−4.6 ± 8.5 (<0.02)	−0.75 ± 0.54 (<0.001)	−1.8 ± 2.5 (<0.001)
Stages III, IV	−5.1 ± 9.5 (<0.01)	−0.53 ± 1.1 (<0.01)	−1.9 ± 2.4 (<0.001)
Arousal	−0.7 ± 11.6*	−0.37 ± 1.4*	−1.3 ± 2.1*

EEG sleep stages:
I = "drowsy"
II = slow eye movement
III, IV = EEG pattern of large, slow waves (100 μv; 1–2 cycles/sec) occurring more than 2 times/10 sec
* = no significant change from awake state
parenthesis = significance at given level of confidence (P values)
Data from Khatri, I. M. and E. D. Freis: Hemodynamic changes during sleep. *J. Appl. Physiol.* 22:867, 1967.

children would be of value to the examining physician, no such method is available at present.

Alveolar ventilation is to pulmonary function as cardiac output is to cardiac function, i.e., an index of the competency of the organ system. An approximation of normal values of minute ventilation at different ages may be derived from the nomogram of Radford (Fig. 1-30). In the presence of pulmonary disease, alveolar ventilation increases (usually as a result of increased depth and frequency of breathing) in an attempt to return alveolar gas exchange to normal. Whereas compensation may be achieved for carbon dioxide transfer out of the lung, transfer of oxygen into the blood stream is limited by the finite capacity of hemoglobin to bind oxygen. Thus the effectiveness of increased alveolar ventilation is reflected in its ability to sustain a normal arterial carbon dioxide tension in the presence of pulmonary disease, whereas the extent of pulmonary damage is often reflected by the level of hypoxemia. From this point of view, our inability to quantify or reliably estimate alveolar ventilation during the bedside examination is of no serious consequence, provided the other diagnostic methods, including determination of blood gas tensions, are employed.

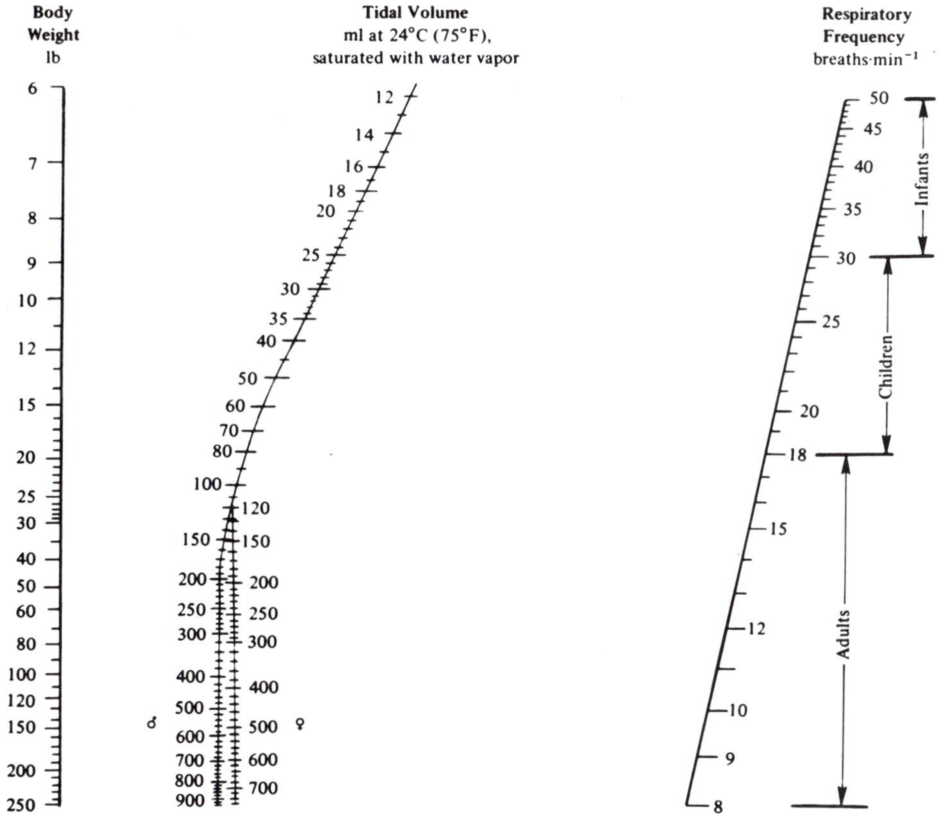

FIG. 1-30. Nomogram for predicting tidal volume. The following correction factors have been suggested: add 10% for daily activity and eating; add 5% for each degree rectal temperature is above 99° F; add 5% for each 2000 feet above sea level; subtract a volume equal to one-half the body weight when patient has had tracheotomy. (From Radford, E. P., Jr.: Ventilation standards for use in artificial respiration. *J. Appl. Physiol.* *7*:451, 1955.)

Still, the examiner is not lost completely. With experience he learns to relate the amplitude of chest wall and diaphragmatic excursions to the normal movements of infants and children of the same size; thus he can judge whether the patient is breathing too deeply (hyperpnea) or too shallowly. Placing the hands on the rib cage and on the abdomen gives a feeling of the depth of breathing compared to the normal patient; subsequent examination with the stethoscope reinforces these impressions. Although we cannot put a number on our impressions, it is important to make a serious attempt at estimating minute ventilation and the depth of breathing by inspection as they may provide the first sign of respiratory muscle weakness, ineffectiveness, or exhaustion, and are thereby the first sign of frank or impending respiratory failure.

Breathing Rhythm. Although breathing movements are generally regular during eupnea, variations in the depth of and interval between individual breaths are not uncommon. Periodic deep breaths or sighs are also normally seen at all ages from the fetus in utero (Fig. 1-31) to the adult, and it has been said—though not proved—that these sighs help sustain or restore the normal surface film of pulmonary surfactants in the alveolar lining layer.

The variable breathing rhythm of the newborn infant and the several distinctive breathing patterns (i.e., periodic breathing, apneic breathing, deep-sighing respiration) that are especially characteristic of the immature neonate were discussed on page 9.

The periodic breathing known as *Cheyne-Stokes* breathing, often seen with cardiac or renal failure, is probably a sign of central nervous system hypoxia and possibly hypercapnia. It is characterized by breathing efforts that are at first weak but become successively stronger until definite hyperpnea is present. This pattern then diminishes to the point of apnea or, more commonly, to very shallow breaths that lead into another crescendo of breathing movements. This rhythmic waxing and waning of the depth of breathing may be accompanied by corresponding changes in consciousness. The mechanism underlying Cheyne-Stokes breathing has not been defined. It is generally thought, however, that the underlying respiratory center depression (due to hypoxia/hypercapnia) is reversed periodically by arousal from impulses originating in peripheral chemoreceptors, which lead to the hyperpneic phase. The resultant increased ventilation and change in gas tensions inhibit the peripheral receptors, the fall of CO_2 reduces chemical stimulation of the respiratory center, and breathing movements decrease once more. Because it is a sign of central nervous system depression, Cheyne-Stokes breathing is ominous.

Kussmaul's breathing, which is loud, deep, sighing breathing at an inconstant rate, was used to describe the breathing pattern associated with severe diabetic acidosis. It is sometimes used to characterize the hyperventilation seen with severe anemia, e.g., from hemorrhage. *Biot's* breathing, which may be characterized by completely irregular cycles of breathing movements and periods of apnea, is an indication of severe compromise to the central mechanisms that control breathing.

The Thorax and Respiratory Muscles. Deformities of the thorax may or may not affect pulmonary function. Those that are related to rickets provide a small lexicon of diagnostic signs that have no direct association with lung disease: The rachitic rosary (bulging at the costochondral junctions) is seen during the active stages of rickets; pigeon breast (also seen with Marfan's syndrome and primary kyphoscoliosis) refers to anterior bulging of the sternum and narrowing of the transverse dimensions of the thorax; Harrison's groove is a transverse indentation along the line of attachment of the diaphragm to the thorax, with outward flaring of the ribs below; and pectus excavatum, which may be produced by rickets, is more often idiopathic. Severe pec-

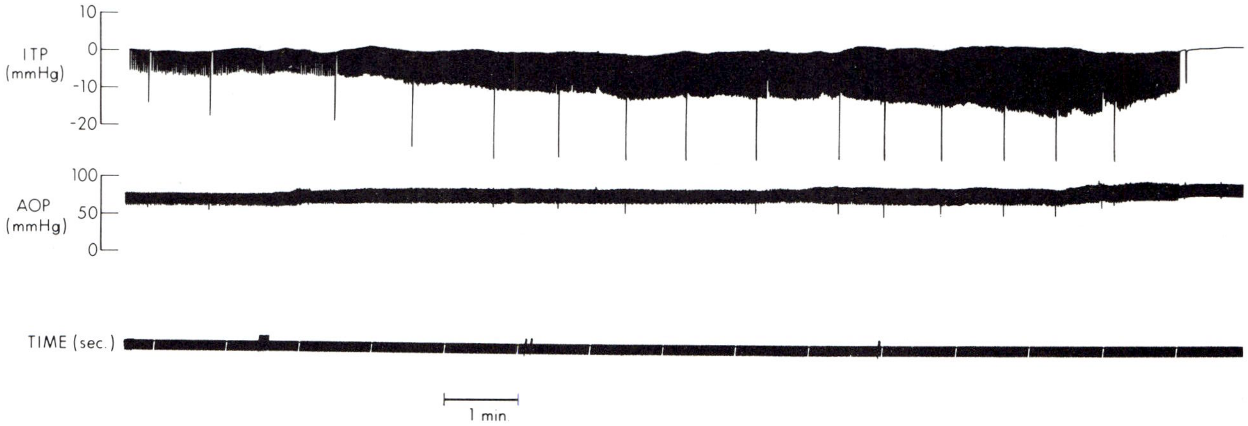

FIG. 1-31. Spontaneous breathing movements of the sheep fetus in utero. Respiratory rate and depth were increased after glucose was administered intravenously to fetus (at first signal on time channel). Periodic deep inspirations ("sighs") are seen both before and after glucose administration: ITP = intratracheal pressure; AOP = thoracic aortic pressure. (From Cosmi, E. V., S. Condorelli, and E. M. Scarpelli; cited in Cosmi, E. V.: Drugs, anesthetics and the fetus.[26])

tus excavatum, with deep inward retraction of the lower sternum and xiphoid, may distort the position of the heart.

The barrel chest, i.e., increased anteroposterior and transverse dimensions of the thorax, usually signals chronic airway obstruction, as may be seen in patients with cystic fibrosis, in which case the deformity may be fixed. The hyperaerated lung of asthmatics may also produce an increase in chest wall size, which however may be evanescent, related to acute episodes of bronchospasm. Patients with kyphoscoliosis generally have some degree of impairment of pulmonary function.

The unusual genetic disorder, Jeune's syndrome or asphyxiating thoracic dystrophy, is characterized by an extremely narrow thorax, which often produces respiratory insufficiency or failure. Mortality is high in infancy and childhood; survival to adolescence or adulthood is rare.

Inspection of the movements of the respiratory muscles may reveal the following actions.

(1) Generalized retractions of the intercostal muscles occur during inspiration due to either high elastic or airflow resistance, such that the chest wall tends to move inward in response to the highly negative pleural pressure developed during inspiration. The chest wall of infants, which is highly compliant, tends to retract more easily, and attempts have been made to grade these retractions in relation to other signs of respiratory distress (see Fig. 1-7).

(2) Generalized flattening or outward bulging of the intercostal muscles may be apparent when expiratory obstruction requires the development of relatively high pleural (positive) pressures during expiration.

(3) Localized bulging or retractions suggest localized disease either on the contralateral side (e.g., with hemidiaphragmatic paralysis) or on the ipsilateral side (e.g., with pleural effusion, tension pneumothorax, and flail chest). Flail chest is seen when the fracture of several ribs or the separation of several contiguous costal cartilages results in paradoxic movement of that region, i.e., local bulging during expiration and retraction during inspiration.

(4) Movements of the diaphragm sometimes may be seen by shining a light in a direction parallel to the side of the thorax. As the patient inhales slowly, a transverse shadow may appear at about the seventh interspace moving downward to the tenth rib during inspiration and upward again during expiration (Litten's phenomenon).

(5) If the diaphragm is flattened, e.g., due to hyperaeration of the lung as occurs with diffuse obstruction of the airways, the lower costal margins anteriorly may move inward during inspiration (subcostal retractions) as some of the force of contraction of the flattened diaphragm is directed toward pulling-in the thoracic wall.

(6) Unilateral phrenic nerve paralysis produces elevation of the hemidiaphragm, decreased movement of the diaphragm on the affected side, and paradoxic diaphragmatic movements. Careful inspection of the chest wall may reveal each of these signs.

(7) Prominent use of the accessory muscles of breathing is generally associated with dyspnea. Flaring of the alae nasa during inspiration (see Fig. 1-7) indicates that accessory muscles are being used. Prominent contraction of the sternomastoid and scaleni muscles during inspiration may be seen when resistance (elastic and/or airflow) to breathing is high; the action of these muscles is to lift or stabilize the rib cage during inhalation. The extent to which these muscles contribute to total ventilation in disease is problematic.

(8) The abdominal muscles are normally passive during eupnea. However, they may be used to assist expiration when there is obstructive disease of the airways and, in adults primarily, when the elastic recoil of the lung is low (e.g., the highly compliant lung of

emphysema). Normally the abdomen protrudes during inspiration, more so in infants. However, inspiratory protrusion of the abdomen may disappear or the abdomen may become scaphoid when there is bilateral paralysis or eventration of the diaphragm.

THE TRACHEA AND LARYNX

The position of the trachea may be assessed by palpating its relationship to the tissues in the suprasternal notch. The examiner directs his forefinger into the notch, and the size of the space between the right and left heads of the clavicle and the respective lateral walls of the trachea is felt. Alternatively, the pronated forefinger may be directed posteriorly over the center of the suprasternal notch and the location of the anterior aspects of the tracheal rings determined. Since the larynx and trachea are midline structures in the neck and are the pivotal axis for shifts in the position of the carina and peripheral lung units, lateral displacement may be produced by shifts of the viscera within the thorax as well as by cervical masses.

Lateral tracheal deviation may be caused by local masses either above (e.g., cervical goiter or enlarged lymph nodes) or below (e.g., retrosternal goiter) the suprasternal notch. The trachea may move laterally to the *ipsilateral* side when there is atelectasis, because local reduction of volume permits increased expansion of the ventilated alveoli, which move into the "vacated space." The diaphragm tends to behave in the same way as the ventilated alveoli and, in the presence of a large area of atelectasis, the ipsilateral hemidiaphragm may tend to move upward. The trachea may move laterally to the *contralateral* side when there is large pleural effusion, pneumothorax, or hydropneumothorax in a hemithorax. The explanation is that the force of the unilateral lesion finds the intrathoracic viscera (the lung primarily) relatively more compliant than the chest wall, although the chest wall may indeed bulge. The intrathoracic causes of tracheal deviation are summarized in Figure 1-32.

PALPATION AND PERCUSSION OF THE THORAX

The topographic boundaries of the lung and its relationship to other thoracic structures are shown in Figures 1-25 and 1-33. The bronchopulmonary segments are outlined in Figures 1-18 and 1-20 through 1-24. The reader is also referred to the discussion of anatomic landmarks of infants (p. 25ff).

Palpation of the thorax is best done with the palmar bases of the fingers, which are most sensitive to vibrations. With phonation, vibrations are conducted throughout the air spaces and to the chest wall where they may be perceived by palpation (*vocal fremitus*) by the examiner. Decreased vocal fremitus may be caused by any lesion that damps conduction of vocal vibrations, e.g., blockade of the airways, air or liquid in the pleural cavity, the presence of lung cysts or bullae, and fibrosis of the pleura. Conversely, increased transmission may occur when the ratio of lung tissue or solid matter to air is increased, provided the bronchus to that particular area is patent, e.g., consolidation of lung parenchyma in pneumonia.

Percussion of the thorax may be done by either the direct or indirect methods (Fig. 1-34). The decision rests on the experience and comfort of the examiner. The sounds produced by percussion (*percussion notes*) vary with the density of the organ and overlying tissue. Certain terms are used to describe these sounds: The percussion note from an air-filled lung is resonant; that from a gas-filled stomach, for example, is tympanitic; the note from the heart is dull; and from a thick muscle mass such as the buttocks the note is flat. Between resonance and tympany would be hyperresonance, the note of the

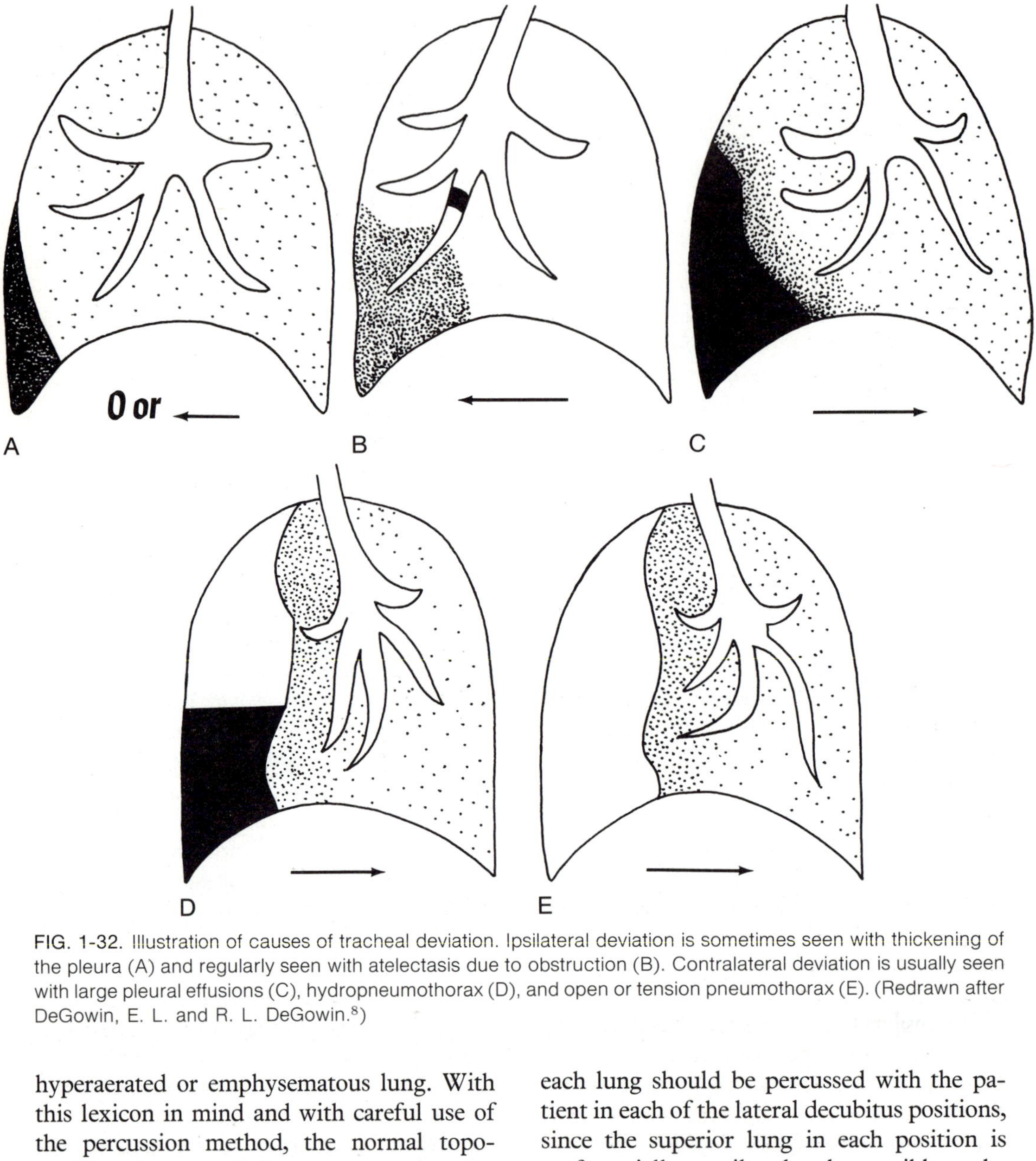

FIG. 1-32. Illustration of causes of tracheal deviation. Ipsilateral deviation is sometimes seen with thickening of the pleura (A) and regularly seen with atelectasis due to obstruction (B). Contralateral deviation is usually seen with large pleural effusions (C), hydropneumothorax (D), and open or tension pneumothorax (E). (Redrawn after DeGowin, E. L. and R. L. DeGowin.[8])

hyperaerated or emphysematous lung. With this lexicon in mind and with careful use of the percussion method, the normal topographic anatomy of the thorax can be outlined and described. Essential points of the examination must include (1) an outline of the boundaries of cardiac, hepatic, and splenic dullness and gastric tympany and (2) an outline of the boundaries of pulmonary resonance. Ideally the patient should be in the sitting position. When he must be recumbent, each lung should be percussed with the patient in each of the lateral decubitus positions, since the superior lung in each position is preferentially ventilated and accessible to the examiner's fingers.

A dull percussion note would suggest the presence of a mass, atelectasis, consolidation, pleural thickening, and (especially at the bases) pleural effusion. Flatness in the thorax almost invariably results from massive pleural effusion, whereas hyperresonance is usu-

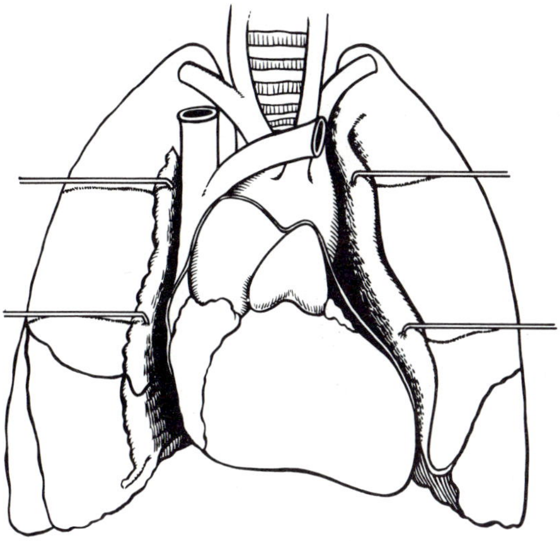

FIG.1-33. Anterior view showing relation of the lung to other thoracic viscera. By means of retractors, the anterior medial border of lung is reflected laterally to show underlying viscera. (Redrawn after Goss, C. M.: *Gray's Anatomy.* Lea & Febiger, Philadelphia, 1954.)

ally associated with hyperaeration, (lobar) emphysema, or pneumothorax. A large pneumothorax or lobar emphysema may give a tympanitic note.

AUSCULTATION OF THE LUNG

Both the bell and diaphragm of the stethoscope should be used, and each lobe and segment of the lung should be examined from all sides. It should be remembered that the bell transmits all sounds from the chest, with the low-pitched sounds transmitted particularly well; and that the diaphragm may exclude the lowest-pitched sounds so that high-pitched sounds appear to be amplified. Pediatric stethoscopes have no acoustic superiority and their only possible advantage is a better fit against the skin of the patient.

The mechanism whereby breath sounds are produced is not known. It has been suggested that the sounds originate at the glottic aperture and are then transmitted along the airways. However, since the sound changes at the periphery of the lung (Fig. 1-35), where inspiration becomes louder than expiration and the quality of the sound is different, the alteration of the original glottic noise has been attributed to the damping effect of the lung parenchyma and the entry of air from terminal bronchioles into acinar units. It could also be suggested that reduction of the expiratory sound at the periphery is analogous to the effect one gets when listening to a

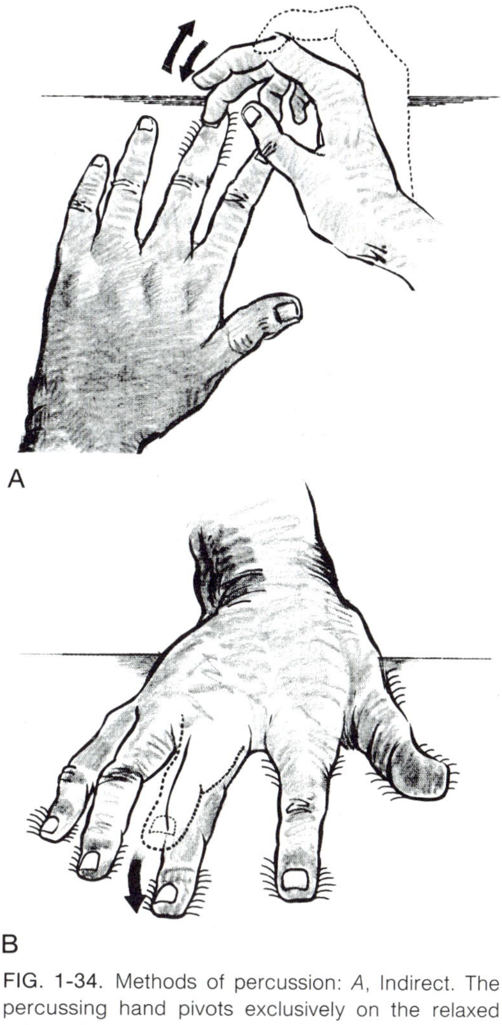

FIG. 1-34. Methods of percussion: *A*, Indirect. The percussing hand pivots exclusively on the relaxed wrist to furnish blows of equal intensity. After striking the blow, the plexor finger is withdrawn rapidly to avoid damping the vibrations; *B*, Direct. The percussing finger strikes the interspace sharply and is then held momentarily in place to damp the vibration. (Redrawn from DeGowin, E. L. and R. L. DeGowin.[8])

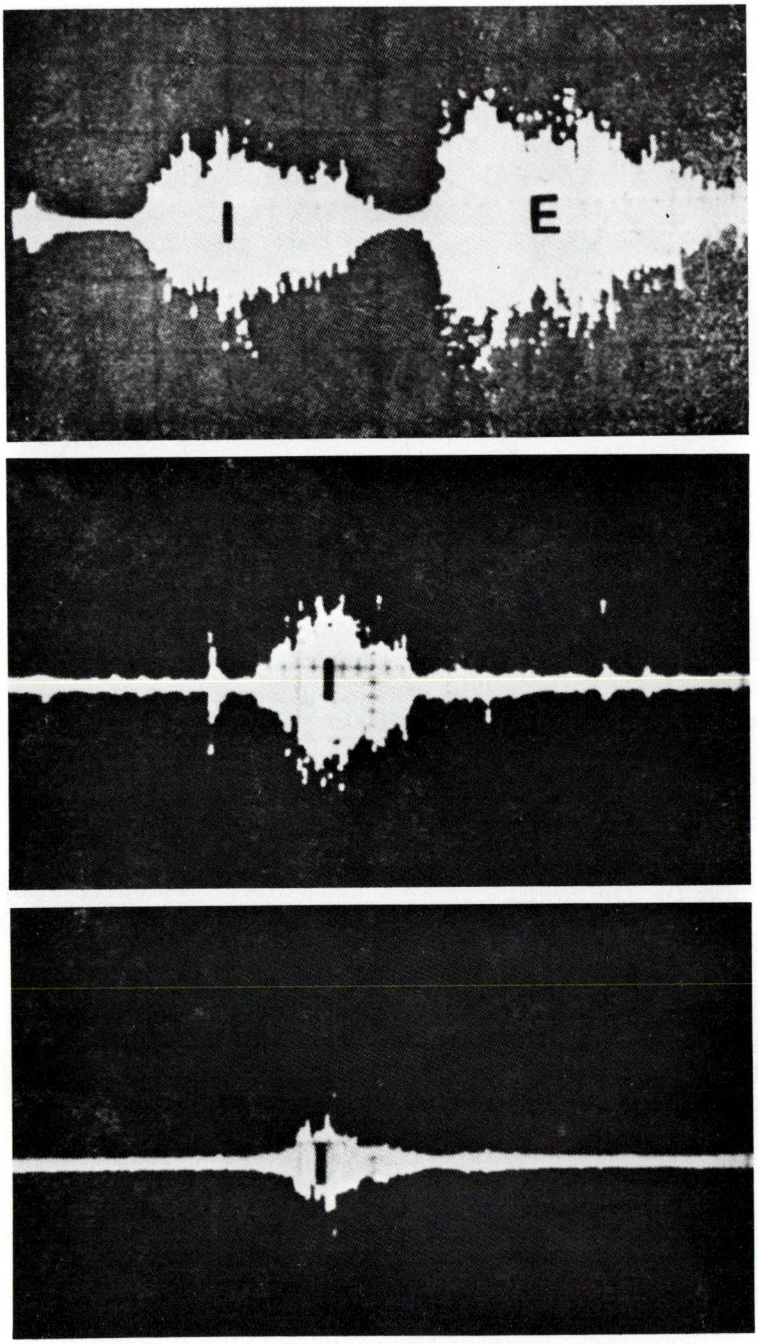

A

B

C

FIG. 1-35. Recordings of normal breath sounds: *A*, Bronchial breathing recorded from the trachea. Expiration is louder, higher pitched, and longer than inspiration; *B*, Bronchovesicular sounds from right middle lobe. Intensity of expiration is markedly reduced; *C*, Vesicular sounds from the base of the lung. I = inspiration; E = expiration. (From Weiss, E. B. and C. J. Carlson: Recording of breath sounds. *Am. Rev. Respir. Dis. 105*:835, 1972.)

trumpet while standing behind the trumpet player.

Normal Breath Sounds and Their Modification. *Bronchial* or tubular sounds have a relatively short inspiratory phase and a longer expiratory phase (see Fig. 1-35*A*). These loud sounds may be heard normally from the stethoscope placed in the suprasternal notch or over the sixth and seventh cervical vertebrae. When heard over the lung parenchyma, bronchial sounds are abnormal, usually resulting from consolidation or compression of pulmonary tissue.

Vesicular sounds are the soft noises that may be heard over the surface of the lung during quiet breathing (see Fig. 1-35*C*). The inspiratory phase is much longer than the expiratory phase. These sounds are usually not heard over the sternum and in the upper interscapular region where they are replaced by bronchovesicular sounds.

Bronchovesicular sounds are intermediate between bronchial and vesicular sounds. The duration of inspiration and expiration is about the same, but the intensity of expiration is markedly reduced (see Fig. 1-35*B*). These sounds are normal in the regions mentioned, but may be abnormal when heard elsewhere in the lung, as they suggest the presence of small areas of consolidation or compression. In the latter case the bronchovesicular sound may be looked upon as a stage in the change from vesicular to bronchial sounds as the disease process progresses.

It should also be noted that on occasion, when a cavity forms in consolidated lung tissue, breath sounds may take on a hollow, reverberating, low-pitched, cavernous quality. Finally, normal breath sounds may become amphoric, i.e., high-pitched and metallic in quality, in the presence of a tension pneumothorax (with or without bronchopleural fistula) over a collapsed lung.

Adventitious Sounds. The terms to describe adventitious bronchopulmonary sounds have, in general, been used loosely by physicians. For us to take a rigid approach to terminology in this text might add to the confusion. Thus we present in Table 1-13 the rather generally or more commonly used classification for historic purposes, while we elect to follow the classification proposed by Forgacs (who has presented a most lucid contemporary analysis of adventitious sounds). In this classification, sounds are either *crackles* or *wheezes*—the former being explosive, nonmusical sounds and the latter being musical—without stress on continuity and pitch, but with more appropriate emphasis on the phase of the respiratory cycle in which they are heard. Thus qualifying words such as crepitant, dry, moist, and high-pitched as-

TABLE 1-13. Classifications of Adventitious Breath Sounds

CONVENTIONAL WITH SYNONYM		
Pulmonary Sounds		
Discontinuous:	Rales (crackles)	
		Fine (crepitations)
		Medium (dry)
		Coarse (moist)
Continuous:	Rhonchi (wheezes)	
		Sibilant (high-pitched; musical)
		Sonorous (low-pitched)
Pleural Sounds		
	Rub (friction rub)	
	Click (crunch)	
AS USED IN THIS CHAPTER*		
*Crackles		
Early inspiratory (usually with obstructive disease)		
Late inspiratory (usually with restrictive disease)		
Expiratory (associated with inspiratory crackles)		
Pleural		
*Wheezes		
Inspiratory (due to critical narrowing of airways)		
End-Inspiratory (usually associated with crackles)		
Expiratory (usually with diffuse airway obstruction)		

*After Forgacs, P.[10,11]

sume minor importance, but the words, rales (from death-rattle) and rhonchi (from wheezes), may be retained as synonyms for crackles and wheezes respectively. The scheme suggested by Forgacs is also presented in Table 1-13.

(1) *Crackles.* All crackles (rales) may be heard during inspiration and expiration. *Inspiratory crackles* are usually heard at the base of the lung, often louder and more profuse on the right side. The repetitive sequence of explosive inspiratory sounds suggests that they are produced by the sudden equalization of transairway pressure that follows the delayed opening of previously collapsed or closed airways. Thus crackles are heard in pulmonary diseases in which compliance and functional residual capacity are low (e.g., diffuse lung disease such as fibrosing alveolitis, atelectasis, fibrosis, interstitial edema, pneumonia) or airway obstruction exists. The contribution of gravity to the genesis of crackling may be ascertained by having the patient change position (Fig. 1-36): Basal crackling may be heard best in the upright position and may disappear when the patient is supine; similarly crackling may be silenced in the upper lung and accentuated in the dependent lung when the patient is in the lateral decubitus position. Inability to reduce or eliminate crackling with position suggests more serious disease.

The electronic recording of crackles indicates that the explosive sounds are produced by opening of previously closed airways and that the difference in timing between early and late inspiratory crackles can be related to the site of airway closure. Thus early inspiratory crackles are related to airway obstruction as seen in asthma, bronchitis, and (in adults) emphysema (Fig. 1-37); they suggest obstruction of relatively larger airways since the sound is frequently well transmitted to the mouth (Fig. 1-37). Late inspiratory crackles are usually more profuse, gravity-dependent, and only rarely transmitted to the mouth (Fig. 1-38 and Table 1-14). They are more often associated with restrictive disorders such as fibrosis, infiltration, or edema.

Isolated *expiratory crackles* are uncommon, but may follow inspiratory crackles (see Fig. 1-37). They may be detected in any of the diseases just mentioned. The mechanism for production of expiratory crackles associated with bronchospastic disease is not known. However, when associated with liquid in the airways, crackles must occur during both phases of the respiratory cycle.

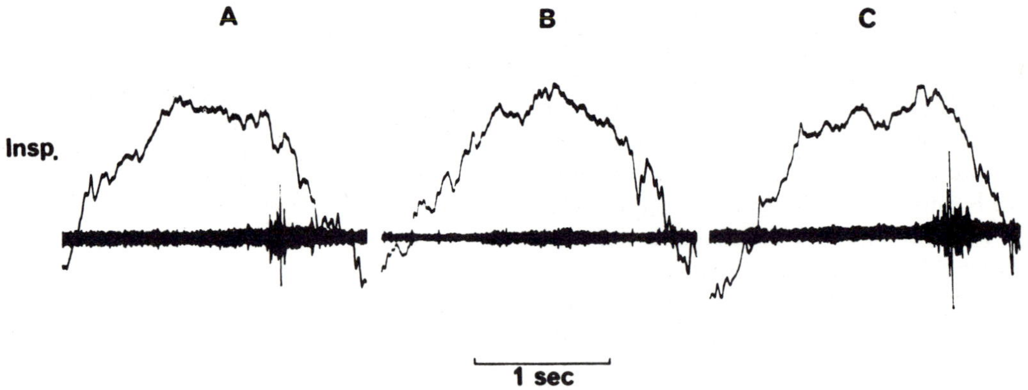

FIG. 1-36. Recordings of breath sounds and inspiratory flow to show effect of change in posture on late inspiratory crackles. Crackles are present when patient is standing (A) and silenced when he bends forward (B). They reappear when he again stands up (C). (From Nath, A. B. and L. H. Capel: Inspiratory crackles—early and late. *Thorax 29*:223, 1974.)

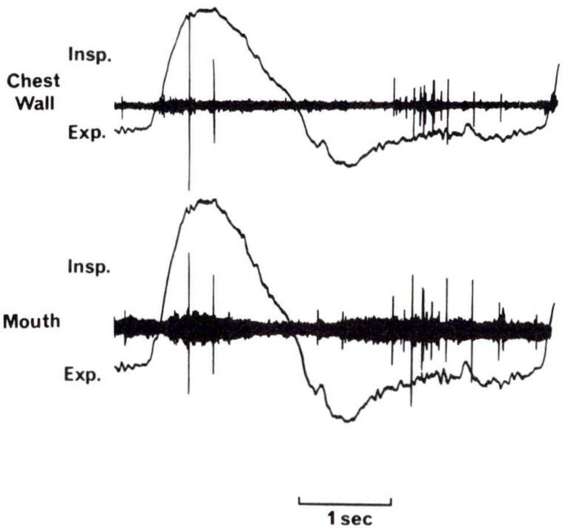

FIG. 1-37. Recordings of inspiratory-expiratory flow and breath sounds from the chest wall (above) and mouth (below). A pair of early inspiratory crackles can be identified at these two sites. Note also expiratory crackles. (From Nath, A. B. and L. H. Capel: Inspiratory crackles—early and late. *Thorax 29*:223, 1974.)

The sound of *pleural crackles* (rubs, clicks) may resemble that produced by the bronchopulmonary system. However, whereas bronchopulmonary sounds are necessarily damped immediately, surface sounds are picked up and maintained for a finite period by the chest wall. Nonetheless, it is often necessary to differentiate the sources of the sound on the basis of clinical judgment.

(2) *Wheezes*. The musical lung sounds called wheezes (rhonchi) may be heard both at a distance from the patient and through the stethoscope. Forgacs believes that the pitch of the sound is related to the velocity of airflow through airways whose walls are in apposition so that their caliber is reduced to the

TABLE 1-14. Clinical Distinction Between Early and Late Inspiratory Crackles*

Early	*Late*
Scanty	Profuse
Lower zones	Lower zones: may extend to mid and upper zones
Gravity independent	Gravity dependent
Usually transmitted to mouth	Rarely transmitted to mouth
Associated with severe airway obstruction	Associated with restrictive disease

*From Nath, A. R. and L. H. Capel: Inspiratory crackles—early and late. *Thorax 29*:223, 1974.

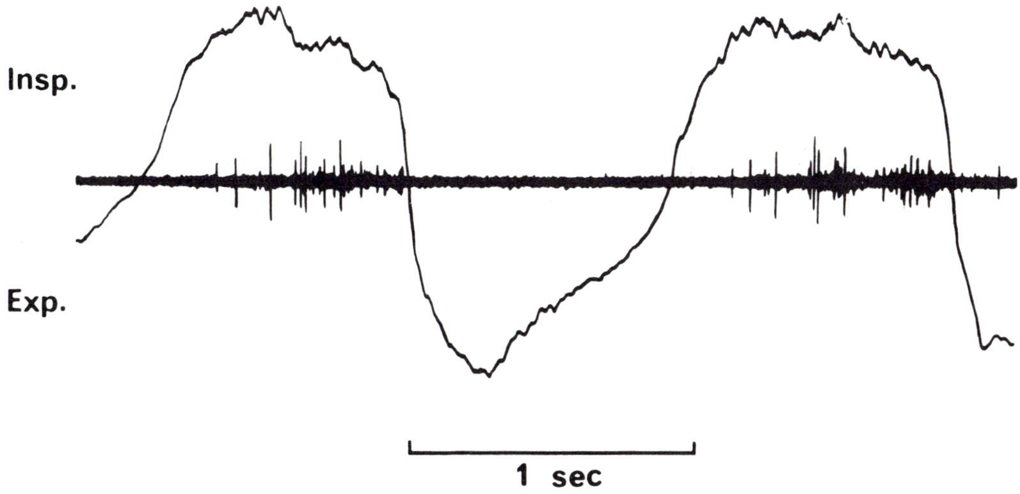

FIG. 1-38. Recordings of inspiratory-expiratory flow and breath sounds showing early, mid, and late inspiratory crackles. (From Nath, A. B. and L. H. Capel: Inspiratory crackles—early and late. *Thorax 29*:223, 1974.)

point of closure. He gives compelling reasons to doubt the classic idea that pitch identifies site of obstruction (i.e., that high-pitched wheezes are from small airways and low-pitched wheezes from large airways).

Inspiratory wheezes are rare as an isolated phenomenon. Rather, they are usually associated with expiratory wheezes, since transmural pressure gradients that may further reduce airway caliber are produced during expiration (see p. 17). The mechanics of inspiratory wheezing or *stridor,* as is heard in diseases of the trachea and glottis, have been discussed (p. 18). End-inspiratory wheezes (short, single noises), often accompanying inspiratory crackles, are produced by the same physical dynamics that account for crackling.

Expiratory wheezes generally consist of a cluster of several musical notes (polyphonic) with a loud hiss in the background. (Thus they have been classified as "continuous" sounds in the older terminology.) They are generally recognized as a sign of diffuse airway obstruction. They may also be induced by forced expiratory efforts in patients with bronchospastic diathesis and by a violent expiratory effort even in healthy subjects. Although they are reflective of diffuse airway disease (indeed because of it), Forgacs presents convincing arguments that the major contribution to the expiratory wheeze takes place at the level of the lobar bronchi. That the polyphonic wheeze is loud and appears to contain only a modest number of individual wheezes supports these arguments. The polyphonic wheeze is often filtered as it passes through lung and chest wall, so that it may be perceived as a monophonic wheeze. The filtration artifact can be demonstrated by listening at the back of the neck (where minimal selective filtration of sound occurs). A truly monophonic sound by this test can be attributed to disease of a single airway, although no conclusion may be drawn as to the size of the obstructed airway.

Clinical Laboratory Tests

Examination of the lung of a patient with pulmonary disease is not complete until blood and sputum are collected for laboratory analysis of certain essential factors that may now be included as part of the routine workup. In addition, the tuberculin skin test with intermediate strength purified protein derivative (PPD), the sweat test by iontophoresis, recording of the electrocardiogram, and administration of selected pulmonary function tests should be considered usual and ordinary laboratory aids to the complete evaluation of pulmonary dysfunction in the patient.

BLOOD TESTS

In addition to the regular examination of blood for hemoglobin concentration, hematocrit, white blood cell count, differential count, glucose concentration, and electrolyte composition (normal values for which are presented in Tables 1-15 and 1-16), the first three of the following blood tests are always indicated.

Arterial Oxygen Pressure (Pa_{O_2}). Oxygen pressure is only meaningful when it is measured in arterial blood that has been collected anaerobically in a syringe previously rinsed with dilute heparin (1000 U/ml). The radial or brachial arteries are the sites of choice for collection in children and with experience may even be used in infants. Some groups prefer the temporal artery in infants and have used it for repeated samplings without difficulty. The arteries mentioned have the additional advantage of providing blood from the preductal region of the aorta and thus, for example, give a more accurate estimate of Pa_{O_2} of blood that perfuses the brain, even in the presence of right-to-left shunt across a patent ductus arteriosus. Pa_{O_2} is determined rapidly with the Po_2 (Clark) electrode (Fig. 1-39), in which the oxygen in blood is brought into contact with a polarized polypropylene membrane, which is permeable to oxygen, and oxygen pressure is read in terms of the electrical potential from a platinum electrode on the opposite side of the membrane. Ordinarily Pa_{O_2} is 10 to 15 mm Hg less than true alveolar Po_2 because of normal venous-to-arterial shunts (e.g., bronchial and coronary) on the left side of the circulation. Normal values are presented in Tables 1-17 and 1-18.

Since Pa_{O_2} does not provide a direct estimate of the oxygen content of the blood, the hemoglobin-oxygen dissociation curve (Figs. 1-40 and 1-41) must be used to determine this value: The dissociation curve provides the percent saturation of hemoglobin with oxygen at a given pressure, and (% saturation) multiplied by (hemoglobin concentration per 100 ml blood) gives the oxygen content in ml/100 ml blood. To the latter value must be added the volume of oxygen dissolved in blood according to the formula:

$$\text{ml dissolved } O_2/100 \text{ ml} = (Pa_{O_2})\ (0.003).$$

When using the hemoglobin-oxygen dissociation curve, one must remember to employ the corrections for body temperature, blood pH (see Fig. 1-40), and hemoglobin type of the patient (see Fig. 1-41). It should also be remembered that normal Pa_{O_2} of the newborn infant may not be the same as that of the adult (Fig. 1-42).

Arterial Carbon Dioxide Pressure (Pa_{CO_2}). Ideally Pco_2 should be measured in arterial blood. However, since Pco_2 may be the only means for direct assessment of pulmonary function under certain circumstances (see p. 43) and since the arteriovenous difference for Pco_2 is normally relatively small (about

TABLE 1-15. Normal Blood Values at Various Ages*

Age	Hemoglobin (g/100 ml) Mean	SD	Red Count (in million RBC/mm³) Mean	SD	Hematocrit (volume of packed cells/100 ml) Mean	SD	Reticulocytes (per 100 RBC) Avg	White Cells (per mm³) Avg	Granulocytes (%) Avg	Lymphocytes (%) Avg	Monocytes (%) Avg	Platelets (per mm³) Avg
Birth (Cord)	17.1	1.5	4.9	0.4	53	5	3.0	20,000	70	20	10	350,000
3 days–2 mo	14.6	2.9	4.2	0.7	43	9	0.3	12,000	31	63	6	300,000
2–4 mo	11.1	1.0	3.9	0.4	34	3	1.5					
4–8 mo	12.3	0.9	4.2	0.3	37	3	0.5	12,000	31	63	6	300,000
8–12 mo	11.8	0.7	4.3	0.2	37	1	0.5	12,000	36	58	6	
1–1½ yr	11.7	0.8	4.3	0.2	36	2	0.5	11,000	40	54	6	
1½–2 yr	12.7	1.0	4.3	0.2	38	2	0.5	10,000	45	49	6	
2–3 yr	12.7	0.8	4.4	0.2	39	2	0.5					
3–4 yr	13.2	0.8	4.4	0.3	40	3	0.5					
4–5 yr	13.4	1.0	4.4	0.2	40	2	0.5	8,000	60	34	6	300,000
5–6 yr	13.3	0.7	4.4	0.2	40	2						
6–7 yr	13.3	0.8	4.4	0.2	40	2						
7–8 yr	13.3	0.7	4.4	0.2	40	2	0.5	8,000	62	32	6	
8–9 yr	13.6	0.7	4.4	0.2	41	2						
9–10 yr	13.9	0.7	4.5	0.2	41	2						
10–11 yr	14.0	0.9	4.5	0.3	42	2						
11–12 yr	14.2	0.8	4.6	0.2	42	2	0.5	8,000	65	29	6	300,000
12–13 yr	14.5	0.9	4.7	0.2	43	2						
Adult men	16.5	0.8	5.4	0.3	48	2	0.5	7,000	65	29	6	300,000
Adult women	14.5	0.7	4.6	0.2	43	2	0.5	7,000	65	29	6	300,000

*Data from Barnett, H. L. and A. H. Einhorn (Eds.). *Pediatrics,* Appleton-Century-Crofts, New York, 1972.

TABLE 1-16. Normal Blood Chemistries*

Determination	Values	
Ammonia (whole blood)		
Newborn	90–150 μg/100 ml	
Later	45–80 μg/100 ml	
Bicarbonate (serum)	24–31 mEq/l	
Bilirubin (serum)		
Cord	Up to 1.8 mg/100 ml	
1–5 days	Mean peak 6 ml/100 ml Range 2–12	
Later	<0.8 mg/100 ml total	
Calcium (serum)	8.8–10.4 mg/100 ml	
Chloride (serum)	100–107 mEq/l	
Cholinesterase	0.56–1.32 pH units/hr/100 ml	
Creatinine (serum)		
Cord blood	0.6–1.8 mg/100 ml	
Newborn	0.6–1.5 mg/100 ml	
Infants	0.8–1.4 mg/100 ml	
Later	0.7–1.7 mg/100 ml	
Fibrinogen (plasma)	200–390 mg/100 ml	
Glucose (fasting)		
Newborn	20–80 mg/100 ml	
Later	75–95 mg/100 ml	
Hydroxycorticoids (plasma)		
Newborn	—	
Later	10–15 μg/100 ml	
Iodine, Protein-Bound		
2–6 days	7.0–11.7 μg/100 ml	
Later	4.0–8.0 μg/100 ml	
Ketones	Up to 1.5 mg/100 ml	
Lactic Acid (fasting)	1.06–1.78 mmol/l	
Lactic Dehydrogenase	200–680 units/ml	
Lead (serum)	<60 μg/100 ml	
Magnesium (serum)	1.6–2.6 mEq/l	
Nonprotein Nitrogen (serum)		
Newborn	20–38 mg/100 ml	
Infants	23–44 mg/100 ml	
Later	25–40 mg/100 ml	
Osmolality (serum)	285–295 mOsm/l	
Phosphatase, Acid	0.5–5.0 King-Armstrong units	
Phosphatase, Alkaline		
Infants	10–20 King-Armstrong units	
Adults	4–13 King-Armstrong units	
Phosphorus, Inorganic (serum)	3.6–5.9 mg/100 ml	
Potassium (serum)		
Newborn	4–7 mEq/l	
Later	4.1–5.9 mEq/l	
Sodium (serum)	133–148 mEq/l	
Transaminases (serum)		
	SGOT units	SGPT units
Infants	<67	<54
Later	<27	<30
Urea Nitrogen (serum)		
Newborn	7–13 mg/100 ml	
Infants	9–16 mg/100 ml	
Later	11–18 mg/100 ml	
Uric Acid (serum)	2–5.7 mg/100 ml	

* Data from Barnett, H. L. and A. H. Einhorn (Eds.). *Pediatrics,* Appleton-Century-Crofts, New York, 1972.

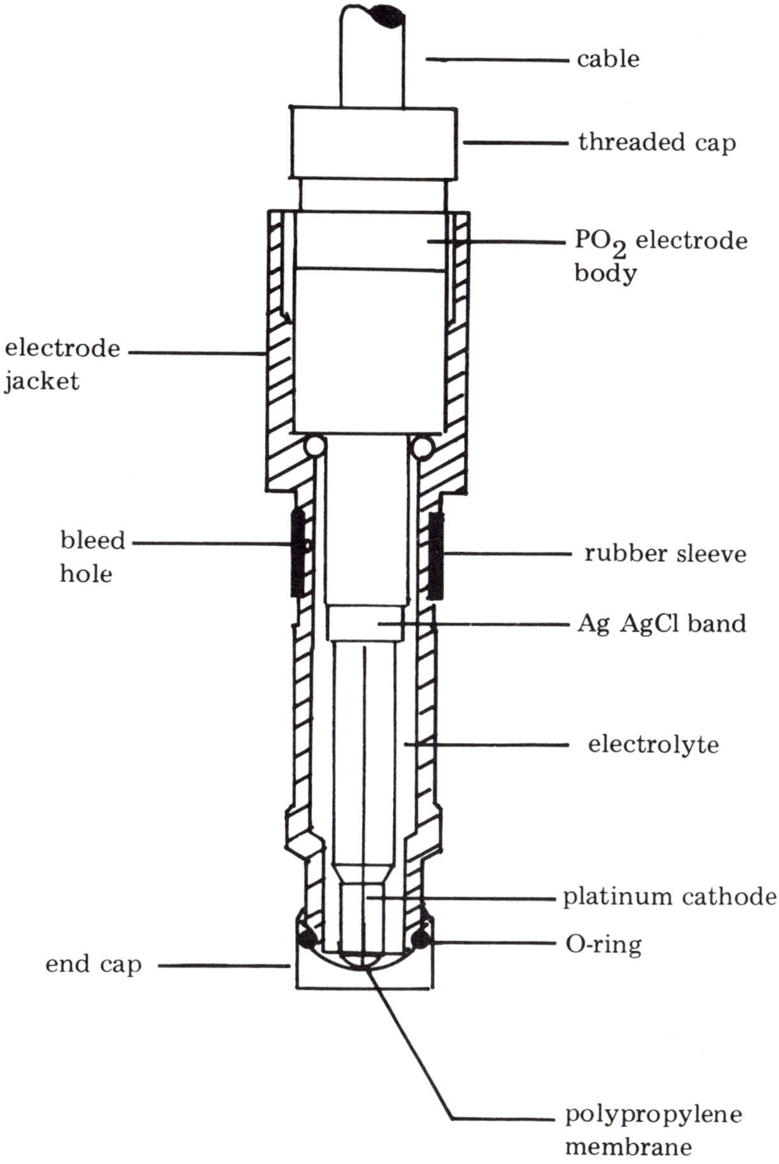

FIG. 1-39. The Po_2 electrode.

6 mm Hg) and does not change markedly with metabolism and perfusion, one may use venous blood to estimate Pa_{CO_2} when repeated arterial punctures are not feasible. (Most contemporary facilities are, or should be, equipped with instruments that measure Po_2, Pco_2, and pH on the same small sample of blood, so that each time arterial Po_2 is obtained, there should also be a report of Pa_{CO_2} and pHa.) Pco_2 is usually determined in an electrode system containing a membrane that is preferentially permeable to CO_2, which then equilibrates with a (bicarbonate) buffer system (Fig. 1-43). The change in pH

TABLE 1-17. Fetal Scalp Blood Po_2, Pco_2, and pH*

	Po_2 (mm Hg)	Pco_2 (mm Hg)	pH
Stage I Labor			
Early	—	—	7.34(7.23–7.40)
Late	25(±7)	—	7.24(±0.09)
Stage II Labor			
Late	20(±5)	48(±5)	7.26(7.14–7.42)

*Data are from accumulated and compiled data from the tables of Respiration and Circulation (Biological Handbooks), Federation of American Societies for Experimental Biology, Bethesda, Md., 1971. Po_2 and Pco_2 values have been rounded off to nearest whole number. All values are indiscriminant averages from all sources available. Figures in parentheses are either range or ±SD.

of the buffer, which is proportional to Pco_2, is read in units of Pco_2. The change in Pa_{CO_2} that normally occurs at birth is given in Figures 1-44 and 1-45.

Arterial pH (pHa). The arteriovenous pH difference is small (normally about 0.02 pH units), so that the same statements regarding the measurement of arterial and venous Pco_2 may be applied to the measurement of pH. A diagram of the pH electrode system in general use is given in Figure 1-46.

The interrelationship between pHa, Pa_{CO_2},

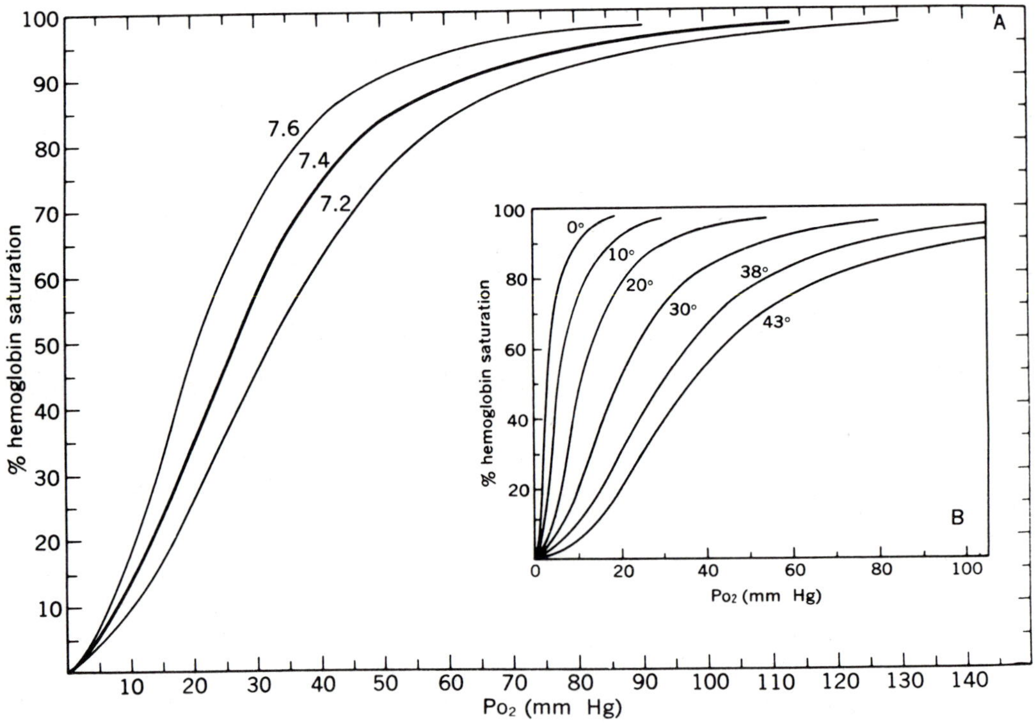

FIG. 1-40. Hemoglobin-oxygen dissociation curves. Effects of pH and temperature. Adult whole blood. (From Lambertsen, C. J.: Transport of oxygen and carbon dioxide by the blood. In *Medical Physiology,* Vol. 2. 13th ed, V. B. Mountcastle, (Ed.). The C. V. Mosby Co., St. Louis, 1974.)

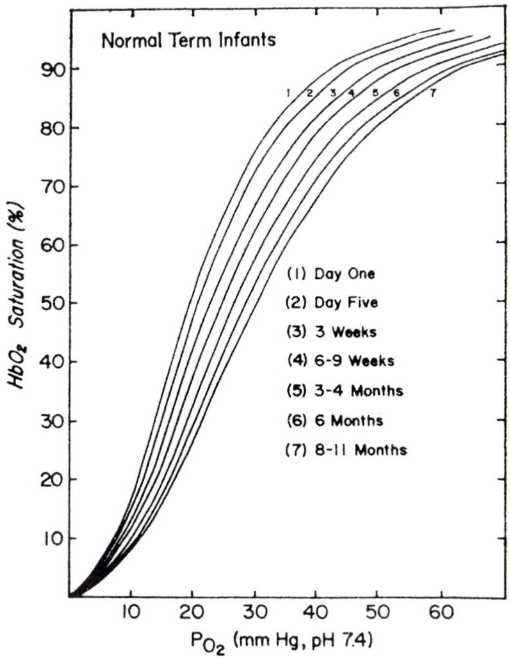

FIG. 1-41. Comparison of curves from blood of infants at different postnatal ages. (From Delivoria-Papadopoulos, M. et al.: Postnatal changes in oxygen transport of term, premature and sick infants: the role of red cell 2,3-diphosphoglycerate and adult hemoglobin. *Pediatr. Res.* 5:235, 1971.)

and plasma bicarbonate concentration is the basis for understanding the nature and extent of pathologic alterations of the acid-base status of the individual (e.g., acidemia of respiratory origin as opposed to metabolic acidemia or combined acidemia) and is incorporated in the classic equation of Henderson and Hasselbalch:

$$pH = pk + \log \frac{[HCO_3^-]}{[H_2CO_3]},$$

where $[H_2CO_3]$ in mEq/1 plasma $= (Pa_{CO_2})\ (0.03)$, and $pk = 6.1$.

Many nomograms have been proposed to present this interrelationship graphically. The nomogram of Siggaard-Andersen, which is convenient and popular, is given in Figure 1-47. Using this nomogram, one needs two of the three unknowns of the equation plus the hemoglobin concentration to derive all other variables.

Special Tests. When indicated, the following blood tests may be useful. *Serum protein* concentration and albumin:globulin ratio may reveal the hyperglobulinemia that often accompanies sarcoidosis or the hypoalbumin-

TABLE 1-18. Blood Gas Tensions and pH of Neonate Following Vaginal Delivery*

	Po_2 (mm Hg)		Pco_2 (mm Hg)		pH	
	UA	UV	UA	UV	UA	UV
Cord intact	19(7–30)	31(14–48)	52(33–70)	42(22–62)	—	—
Cord clamped	16(3–29)	28(12–49)	54(29–100)	42(21–93)	7.25 (6.95–7.39)	7.31 (7.05–7.45)
1-minute Apgar						
0–4	11(1–20)	35(17–49)	70(42–99)	51(34–93)	—	—
5–7	17	23	59(33–92)	45(32–57)	—	—
8–10	17(9–29)	30(19–48)	54(33–78)	44(23–70)	—	—
Meconium-stained	16(4–23)	28(16–23)	51	44	7.20	7.30
Adult	96(86–107)		40(31–46)		7.43(7.37–7.49)	

Adult arterial values are given for comparison. UA = umbilical artery; UV = umbilical vein.

*Data are from accumulated and compiled data from the tables of Respiration and Circulation (Biological Handbooks), Federation of American Societies for Experimental Biology, Bethesda, Md., 1971. Po_2 and Pco_2 values have been rounded off to nearest whole number. All values are indiscriminant averages from all sources available. Figures in parentheses are either range or ± SD.

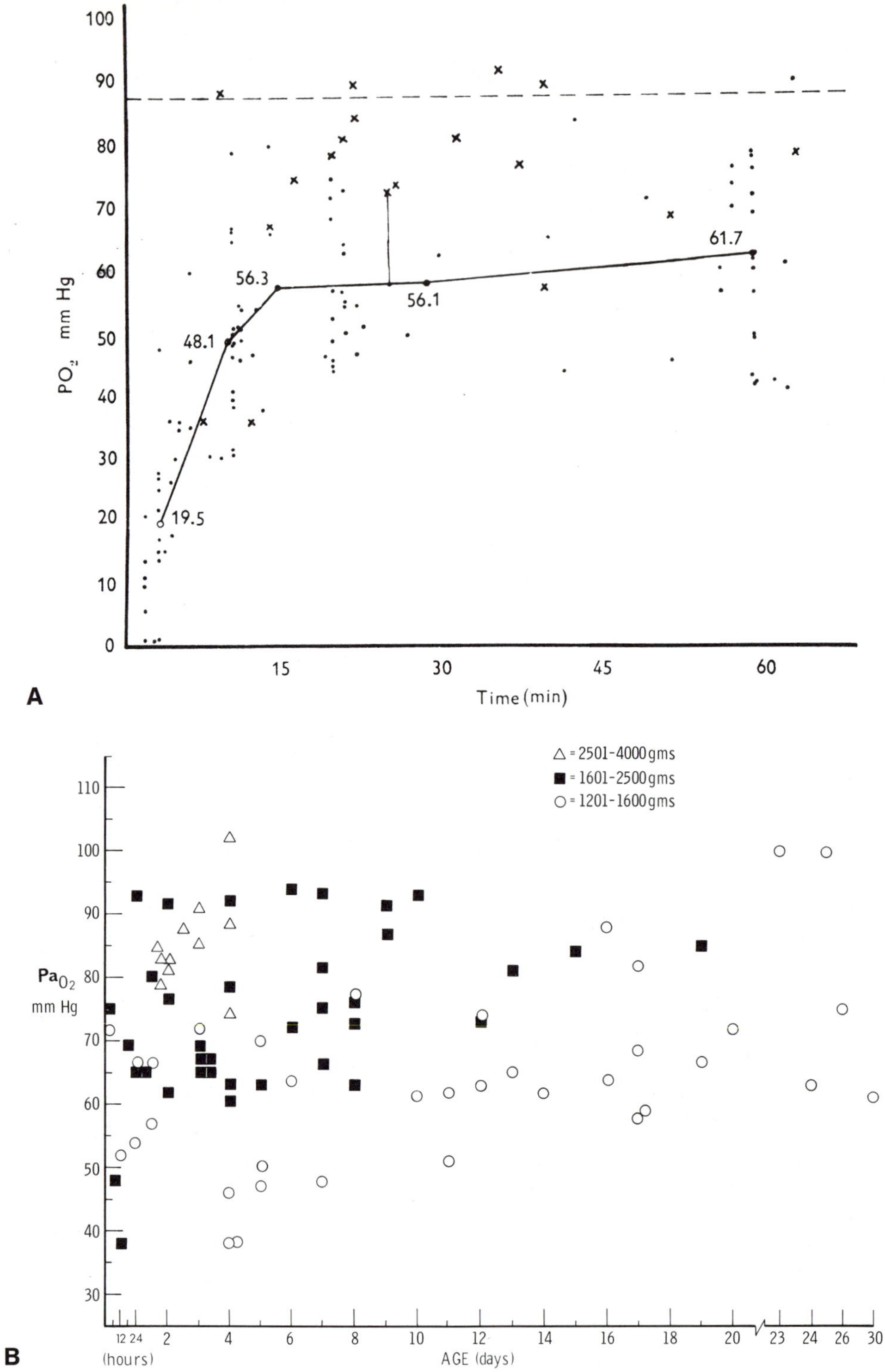

FIG. 1-42. *A*, Pa$_{O_2}$ versus time during the first hour of life. All subjects were mature neonates by weight except for three subjects whose weights were 2.495, 2.407, and 2.280 kg respectively. Numerals in the graph are the means of the five time periods. Dots indicate umbilical arterial samples; crosses indicate left atrial samples. Dashed line is the lower limit of normal Pa$_{O_2}$ for older children and adults (i.e., ~ 88 mm Hg). (From Oliver, T. K., Jr., J. A. Demis and G. D. Bates. Serial blood-gas tensions and acid-base balance during the first hour of life in human infants. *Acta Paediatr.* *50*:346, 1961.)
B, Temporal artery Po$_2$ in infants. (From Auld, P. A. M. Pulmonary physiology of the newborn infant.[25])

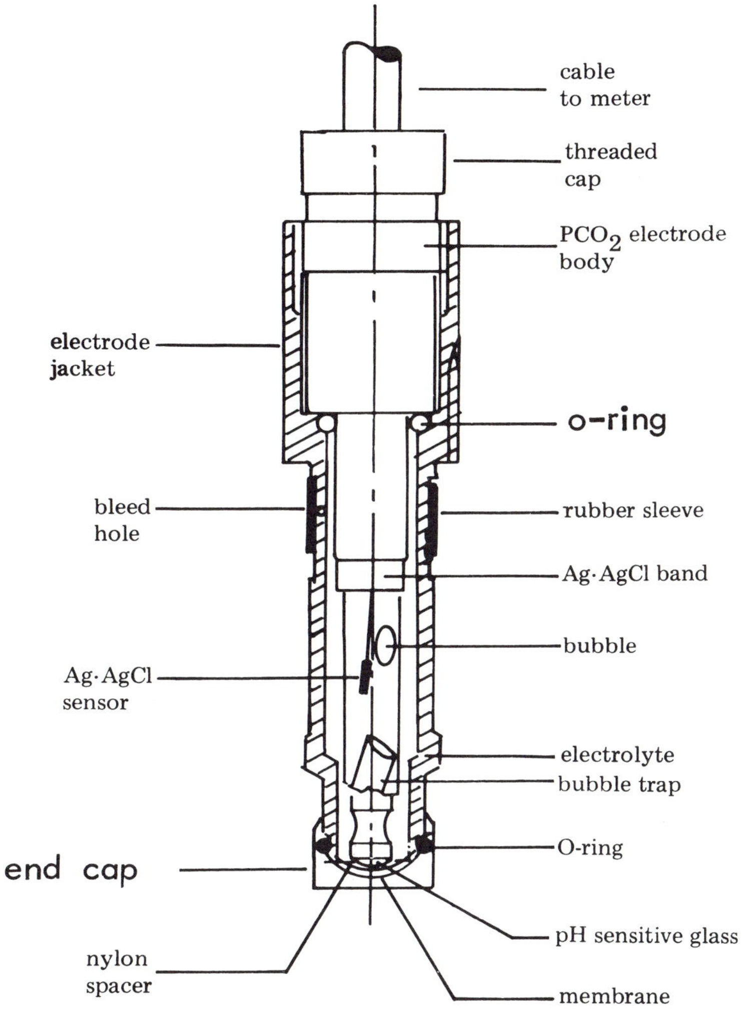

FIG. 1-43. The Pco_2 electrode.

emia that is seen on occasion in respiratory distress syndrome or in association with peripheral edema or in cystic fibrosis. Serum electrophoresis or immunodiffusion for determination of α_1 *antitrypsin* may reveal a deficiency of this protease inhibitor. Although familial pulmonary emphysema (α_1 antitrypsin deficiency) is not associated with obstructive pulmonary disease in the pediatric population, it may be in the young adult. Pulmonary infarction, e.g., in association with pulmonary embolism or lung disease of sickle cell anemia, may be *suggested* by the presence of elevated levels of serum *bilirubin* and *lactic dehydrogenase* with concomitantly normal values of *glutamic oxaloacetic transaminase.* Although disorders of the immunoglobulins are not known to produce pulmonary disease directly, it is sometimes necessary to quantify the *immunoglobulins* when one suspects that dysgammaglobulinemia or hypogammaglobulinemia may be related to pulmonary disease, especially if disease is recurrent. Normal values for the

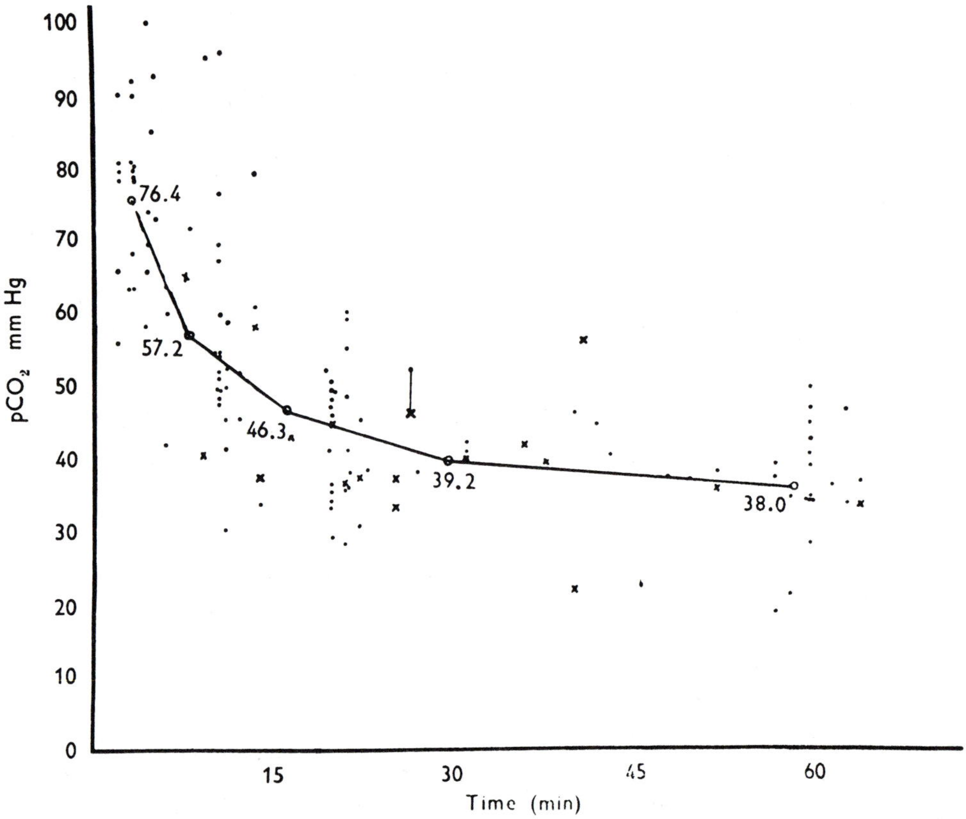

FIG. 1-44. Pa_{CO_2} versus time during the first hour of life. Subjects and symbols same as Figure 1-42A. (From T. K. Oliver, Jr., J. A. Demis and G. D. Bates: Serial blood-gas tensions and acid-base balance during the first hour of life in human subjects. *Acta Paediatr.* *50*:346, 1961.)

immunoglobulins are given in Table 1-19. *Blood cultures* are indicated in acutely ill patients with suspected pulmonary infections. Two or three blood cultures in the first few hours of hospitalization may indicate the severity of the infection and on occasion may provide a pure culture of the organism. *Serologic tests* for infecting microorganisms can also be most valuable: Some of the currently available tests are listed in Table 1-20.

SPUTUM TESTS

Proper collection of sputum is the sine qua non of reliable laboratory examination. Although it is often impossible to meet this criterion when dealing with infants or young children, attempts should be made to obtain sputum, e.g., by aspiration of the posterior pharynx, in all patients with pulmonary disease. Ideally, sputum should be obtained from a deep cough by the patient after he has rinsed his mouth with warm saline solution, and it should be collected in a sterile, disposable receptacle. Tapping the patient's chest in the area of suspected pathology, putting the patient in a position of postural drainage, and using inhalation of warmed hypertonic saline (5 to 10% NaCl) solution are bedside maneuvers that may aid the production and collection of sputum from a cooperative patient. In serious illnesses, when examination of sputum is vital to diagnosis and treatment, transtracheal aspiration (in the hands of experienced physicians) has been used successfully.

Fresh sputum should be smeared immediately and stained. Preliminary screening by the gram-staining technique will permit early categorization of the infecting organism and will usually help differentiate more resistant organisms (e.g., staphylococcal or gram-negative) from the pneumococcal variety.

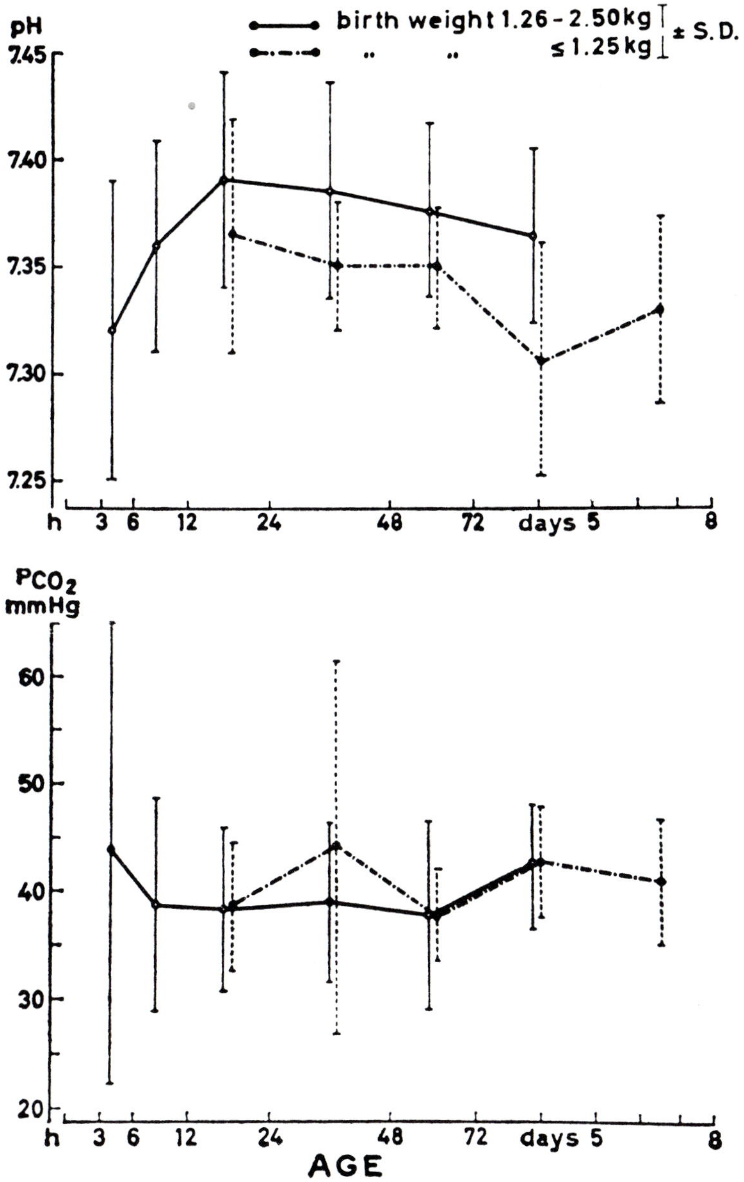

FIG. 1-45. Pa_{CO_2} and pH of "arterialized" capillary blood from normal premature infants during the first week of life. Averages and standard deviations are shown. (From Bucci, G. et al.: Acid-base status of "normal" premature infants in the first week of life. *Biol. Neonate* 8:81, 1965. Published by S. Karger AG, Basel.)

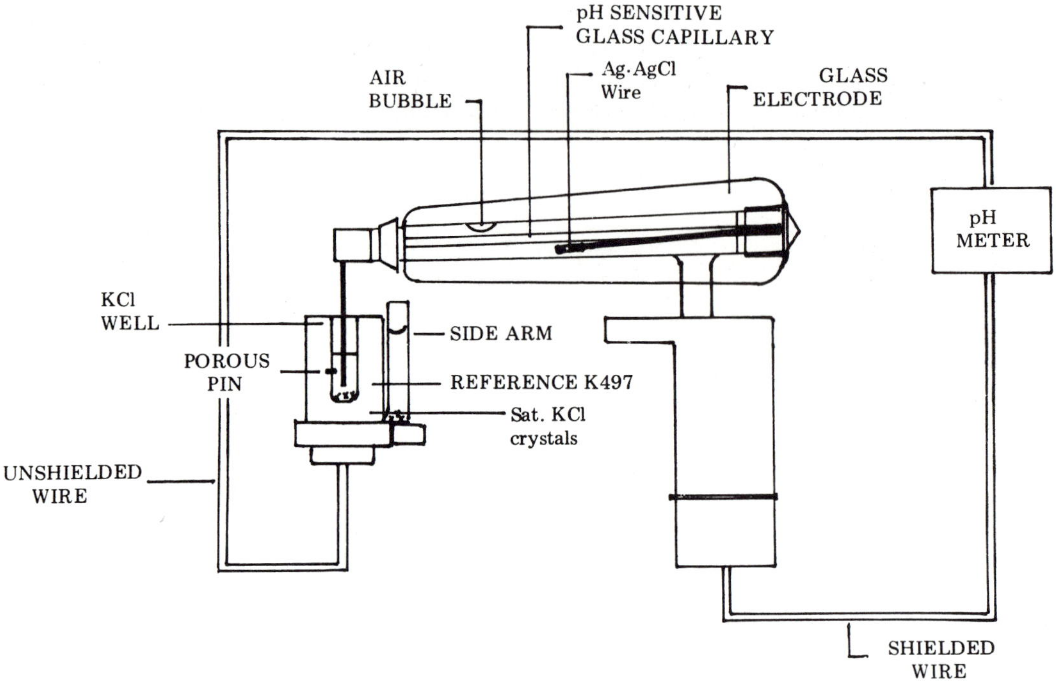

FIG. 1-46. The pH electrode.

Wright's stain is of added help: A high concentration of neutrophils corroborates the impression of purulence, and eosinophils suggest a basic or concurrent allergic component. Curschmann's spirals, first described by von Leyden, often may be seen in association with eosinophils and Charcot-Leyden crystals in patients with chronic asthma. The spirals are mucinous material twisted around a central thread. They are probably casts of small airways containing mucoproteins, cells, and crystals. Spirals may also be observed in chronic bronchitis, pneumonia, and tuberculosis where eosinophils and crystals are usually absent. Crystals are believed to originate from eosinophils and basophils or mast cells.

TABLE 1-19. Plasma Immunoglobulin Concentrations During Normal Development*

	Immunoglobulin Concentrations (mg/100 ml)				
Age	IgM	IgA	IgG	IgD	IgE($\times 10^{-3}$)
Newborn	5–30	0–11	700–1,300	0.01	0
1–3 mo	15–70	6–50	280–750	—	—
4–6 mo	10–90	8–90	200–1,200	—	—
7–12 mo	25–120	16–100	300–1,500	0.5–5	—
13 mo–3 yr	30–120	20–230	400–1,300	0.5–5	—
3–6 yr	22–100	50–150	600–1,500	0.5–5	—
6 yr–adult	50–150	75–400	900–1,900	0.5–50	5–150

*Data from Robbins, J. B.: In *Pediatrics,* H. L. Barnett and A. H. Einhorn (Eds.). Appleton-Century-Crofts, New York, 1972.

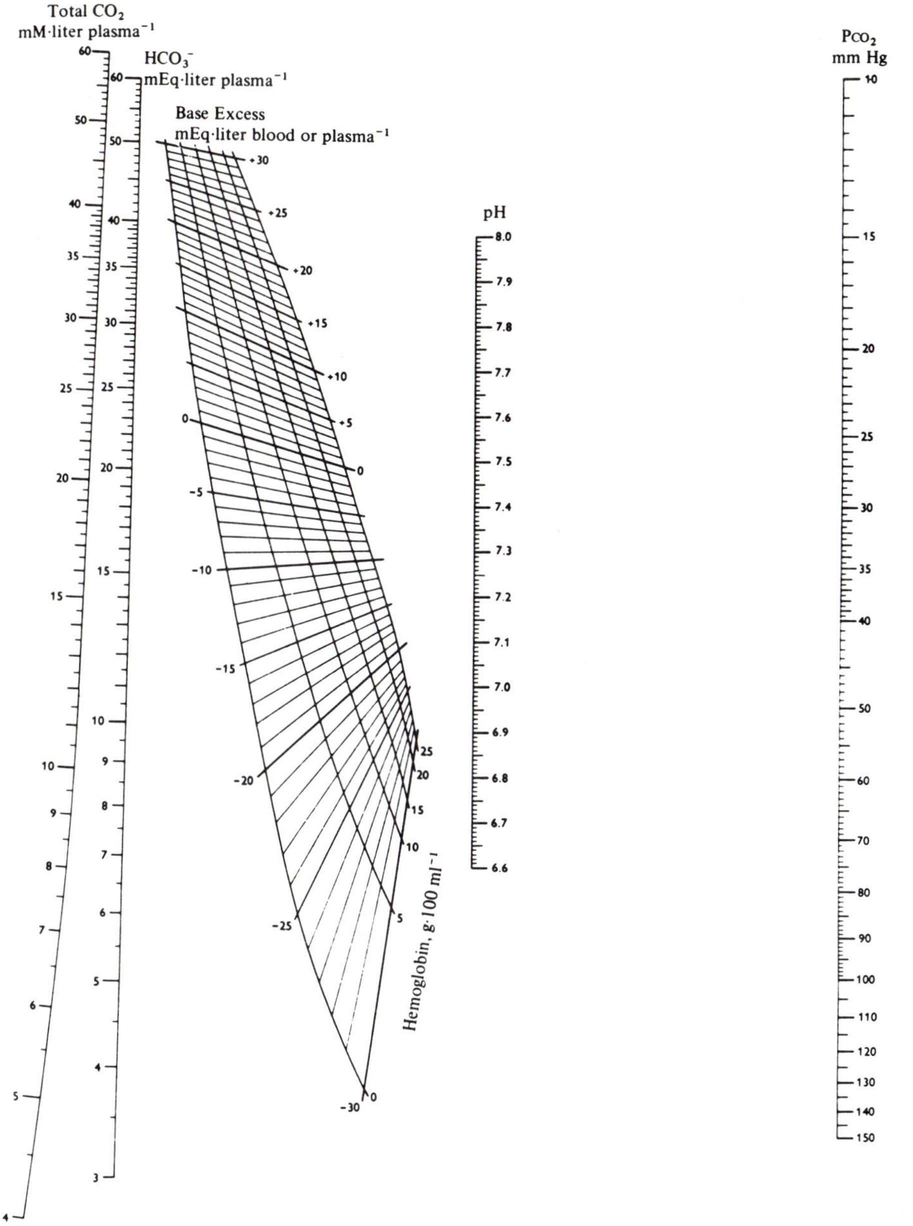

FIG. 1-47. Nomogram that relates plasma and whole blood acid-base parameters. (From Siggaard-Andersen, O.: *The Acid-Base Status of the Blood.* The Williams & Wilkins Co., Baltimore, 1964.)

All sputum specimens should be delivered to the bacteriology laboratory for culture. Suspicion of a viral pneumonia should not dissuade the physician from seeking bacterial pathogens, since pneumonias are often of the mixed variety. It should also be noted that rather accurate diagnosis of pulmonary fungal disease can be made from sputum cul-

TABLE 1-20. Serologic and Skin Tests Available for Specific Bacteria, Rickettsia, Viruses, and Fungi*

Organism (Bacteria, Rickettsia, Viruses)	Serologic Test	Skin Test	Organism (Fungi)	Serologic Test	Skin Test
Adenoviruses	C	−	*Actinomyces israelii*	−	−
Brucella species	A	+	*Allescheria boydii*	−	−
Cat scratch fever	−	+	Aspergillus species	P	+
Coxsackie virus	N	−	*Blastomyces brasiliensis*	C	+
Cytomegalovirus	C;A	−	*Blastomyces dermatitidis*	C	+
Diplococcus pneumoniae	T	−	Candida species	A	+
ECHO viruses	C;N	−	*Coccidioides immitis*	A;C	+
Infectious mononucleosis	HAA	−	*Cryptococcus neoformans*	P	−
Influenza virus	C;H;F;N	−	Geotrichum species	A	+
Klebsiella aerogenes	T	−	*Histoplasma capsulatum*	A;C	+
Lymphocytic choriomeningitis	C	−	Mucormycosis	−	−
Lymphogranuloma venereum	C	+	Nocardia species	−	−
Malleomyces mallei	A;C	+	*Sporotrichum schenckii*	C;A	+
Mycobacterium tuberculosis	D;H	+	*Torulopsis glabrata*	−	−
Mycoplasma pneumoniae	Co;C;F	−			
Parainfluenza virus	C;N;He	−			
Pasteurella pestis	A;C	−			
Pasteurella tularensis	A	−			
Pseudomonas pseudomallei	A	−			
Psittacosis-ornithosis	C	−			
Respiratory syncytial virus	C;N	−			
Salmonella species	A	−			
Varicella-zoster	C;N;F	−			

A = agglutination test; C = complement fixation; Co = cold agglutination; D = agar double diffusion; F = fluorescent antibody; H = hemagglutination; HAA = heterophile antibody agglutination; He = hemabsorption; N = neutralization; P = precipitation; T = specific antiserum to identify type; (+) = skin test available and (−) not available.

*Data from Fraser, R. G., and J. A. P. Paré.[10]

tures if collection is done carefully and the results of the culture are related to serologic tests and skin tests for fungal disease (Table 1-20).

Special features of the sputum examination are summarized in Tables 1-21 through 1-23: The physical characteristics of normal and purulent sputum are given in Table 1-21; the small molecule and protein composition of normal sputum is given in Table 1-22; and the changes in sputum secondary to pulmonary infection in Table 1-23.

TABLE 1-21. Some Characteristics of Mucoid and Purulent Sputum*

	Mucoid	*Purulent*
Total cell population	½ or less of low-power field	⅔ or more of low-power field
Polymorphonuclear leukocytes	<60%	>70%
Dry weight	2–5%	6–10%
Average pH	7.59	7.83
Viscosity	Lower (large range)	Higher (large range)

*Adapted from Dulfano, M. J. (Ed.).[9]

TABLE 1-22. Composition of Normal Tracheobronchial Secretions*

Small Molecules
- In mM/1000 g: sodium 165 ± 42; potassium 13.2 ± 5.4; chloride 162 ± 60; calcium 3.1 ± 1.0.
- In mEq/1000 g: phosphorus 27 ± 16.

Proteins and Probable Activity
- Fucomucins, sialomucins, sulfomucins: form the mucous blanket; blood group activity. Sialomucin also binds virus particles.
- Lysozyme: bactericidal for certain organisms.
- Lactoferrin: bacteriostatic for iron-dependent organisms.
- Secretory IgA: major antibody of secretions.
- IgG: antibody
- Others (specific function not defined): salivary β_1 and α_2 globulins, albumin, transferrin, α_1 antitrypsin, haptoglobin, hemopexin, ceruloplasmin, fibrinogen, α_2 macroglobulin, β_{1AC} and β_{2A} globulins.

*Adapted from Dulfano, M. J. (Ed.).[9]

SKIN TESTS

Skin tests that evoke a wheal and flare response within 15 to 30 min. are tests of hypersensitivity to allergens. In these tests the allergen is administered either by scratching the skin or by injecting the allergen intradermally. They are used commonly to test hypersensitivity in children with asthma or other allergic disorders.

TABLE 1-23. Changes in Tracheobronchial Secretions Secondary to Pulmonary Infections*

Component	*Concentration*
Solids	I
Protein	I
DNA	I
Carbohydrate	I
Lipid	I
K,Ca,P	I
Ash	D
Na,Cl	D

I = increased
D = decreased
*Adapted from Dulfano, M. J. (Ed.).[9]

Intradermal skin tests that are used in the diagnosis of bacterial, fungal, and parasitic diseases usually give a delayed reaction 24 to 72 hours after injection of the antigen. Microbial antigens that are currently available for such tests are listed in Table 1-20.

The Kveim test, which depends in part on the activity of the injected sarcoid tissue and in part on the reactivity of the patient, is of help in making the diagnosis of sarcoidosis. The saline suspension of tissue from the spleen or lymph nodes of patients with sarcoidosis is injected intradermally. A positive reaction consists of the development of a sarcoid granuloma at the site of injection after 2 to 6 weeks. A biopsy of the area must follow, and the tissue is then examined microscopically for typical sarcoid morphology.

Pulmonary Function Tests

The degree of functional abnormality due to pulmonary disease is best assessed by tests of specific parameters of pulmonary function. These tests often do not lead to a causal or anatomic diagnosis, but do give extremely important information regarding the extent to which expected lung function has been compromised. Few tests can be performed by the patient at bedside, and often the patient is best studied in the pulmonary function laboratory. Techniques and significance of pulmonary function testing have been presented in other publications (see Polgar and Promadhat; Scarpelli and Auld (editors)).

Bedside spirometry can be performed reliably in cooperative children. A variety of small, portable spirometers is available for this purpose. The patient is asked to make a maximal forceful expiratory effort starting with the lung in the fully inflated position (Figs. 1-48 and 1-49). The total volume that

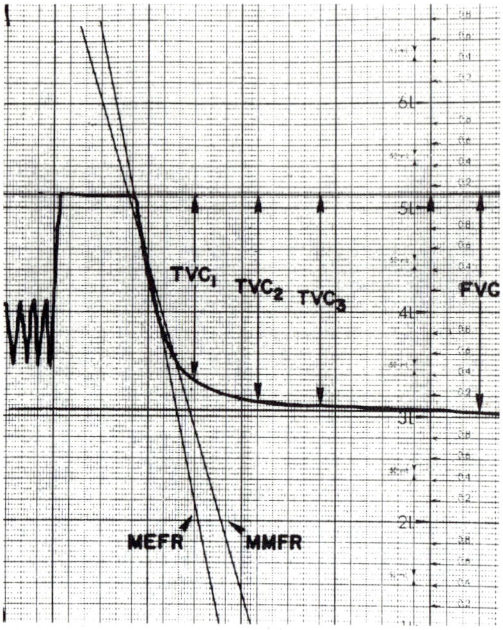

FIG. 1-48. Tracing of forced vital capacity maneuver, i.e., maximal forced exhalation after maximum inhalation; normal subject. TVC_1, TVC_2, TVC_3 are fractions of total forced vital capacity (FVC) during first, second, and third seconds of the maneuver. Slopes of lines drawn give maximum midexpiratory flow rate (MMFR) and maximum expiratory flow rate (MEFR). Note: For routine measurement of VC only, the subject is asked to perform a maximum exhalation at a comfortable (not forced) expiratory rate. (From Clutario, B. C.: Clinical pulmonary function.[25])

can be expelled from the lung by this maneuver is the *forced vital capacity* (FVC), and the volume expelled at various time intervals during this maneuver (e.g., 0.5, 0.75, and 1.0 sec.) is the *forced expiratory volume* (FEV). The slope of the expiratory curve of the spirogram gives the *maximum expiratory flow rate* (MEFR) and the *maximum midexpiratory flow rate* (MMFR). Conventionally, vital capacity (VC) is the volume expired *at a comfortable expiratory rate* after a maximal inspiration.

VC is a useful, though nonspecific determination by which the course of lung disease in general may be followed: Thus a reduced VC often indicates reduction of distensible lung tissue; it also falls when respiratory movements are limited (e.g., by neuromuscular depression), when expansion of the thorax is restricted (e.g., in kyphoscoliosis), when function of the diaphragm is abnormal (e.g., phrenic nerve paralysis), and when lung movement is restricted (e.g., with pneumothorax). In the presence of airway obstructive disease, the forced VC will be reduced as a consequence of the increased closing volume of the lung.

The 1-second FEV ($FEV_{1.0}$), MMFR, and

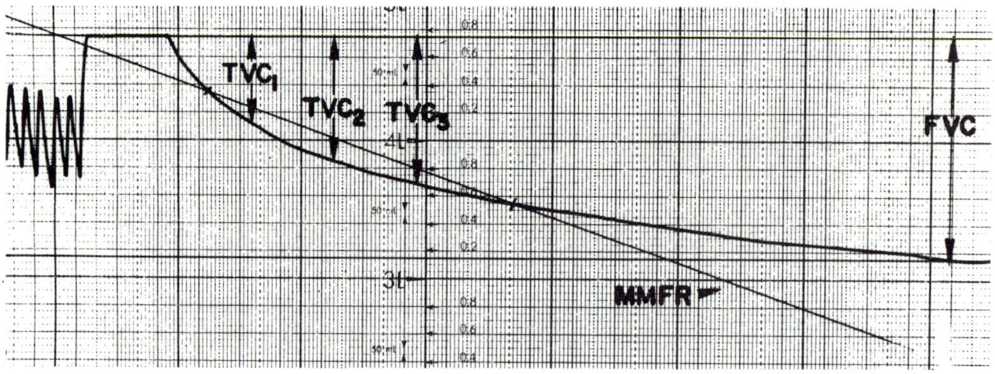

FIG. 1-49. Tracing of forced vital capacity maneuver, i.e., maximal forced exhalation after maximum inhalation; subject with airway obstruction (asthma). TVC_1, TVC_2, TVC_3 are fractions of total forced vital capacity (FVC) during first, second, and third seconds of the maneuver. Slopes of lines drawn give maximum midexpiratory flow rate (MMFR) and maximum expiratory flow rate (MEFR). Note: For routine measurement of VC only, the subject is asked to perform a maximum exhalation at a comfortable (not forced) expiratory rate. (From Clutario, B. C.: Clinical pulmonary function.[25])

MEFR are general tests of the overall mechanical properties of the lung. They are not specific measurements or indices of airway caliber, as has been assumed by some, since the flow rates are as much a function of lung compliance as they are of airway resistance. These tests may be used also to estimate the efficacy of therapy. Thus improvement following inhalation of a bronchodilator suggests that the particular drug may be useful in the management of the patient. One must note that the post-bronchodilator MMEF should be taken from the same level of lung inflation as was the pre-bronchodilator MMEF. The reason is that dilatation of airways may contribute to an increased VC, which—if significant—is accompanied by an increased total expiratory time so that the absolute mid-flow may actually be reduced in conventional calculations.

Other pulmonary function tests, which are better reserved for the patient in the laboratory, are necessary complements of a comprehensive clinical examination of the lung.

SUGGESTED READING AND REFERENCES

1. Abramson, H. (Ed.): *Resuscitation of the Newborn Infant.* 2nd ed. The C. V. Mosby Co., St. Louis, 1966.
2. Avery, M. E. and B. D. Fletcher: *The Lung and Its Disorders in the Newborn Infant.* 2nd ed. W. B. Saunders Co., Philadelphia, 1974.
3. Baum, G. L. (Ed.): *Textbook of Pulmonary Diseases.* 2nd ed. Little, Brown and Co., Boston, 1974.
4. Beerman, H. and B. A. Kirschbaum: Some associated pulmonary and cutaneous diseases: a review of recent literature. *Am. J. Med. Sci. 242*:494, 1961.
5. Burnell, P. A.: Symposium on laboratory diagnosis. *Pediatr. Clin. North Am. 18*:1, 1971.
6. Campbell, E. J. M., E. Agostoni and J. N. Davis: *The Respiratory Muscles. Mechanics and Neural Control.* W. B. Saunders Co., Philadelphia, 1970.
7. Crofton, J. and A. Douglas: *Respiratory Diseases.* Blackwell Scientific Publications, Oxford, 1969.
8. DeGowin, E. L. and R. L. DeGowin: *Bedside Diagnostic Examination.* The Macmillan Co., London, 1969.
9. Dulfano, M. J. (Ed.): *Sputum. Fundamentals and Clinical Pathology.* Charles C Thomas, Publisher, Springfield, Ill., 1973.
10. Forgacs, P.: Crackles and wheezes. *Lancet 2*:203, 1967.
11. Forgacs, P.: Lung sounds. *Br. J. Dis. Chest 63*:1, 1969.
12. Fraser, R. G. and J. A. P. Paré: *Diagnosis of Diseases of the Chest.* (2 vols.) W. B. Saunders Co., Philadelphia, 1970.
13. Gluck, L. (Ed.): *Modern Perinatal Medicine.* Year Book Medical Publishers, Chicago, 1974.
14. Kendig, E. L., Jr. (Ed.): Disorders of the respiratory tract in children. In *Pulmonary Disorders,* Volume. 1, 2nd ed. W. B. Saunders Co., Philadelphia, 1972.
15. Krahl, V. E.: Anatomy of the mammalian lung. In *Handbook of Physiology, Section 3, Respiration,* Volume I, W. O. Fenn and H. Rahn (Eds.). American Physiological Society, Washington, D.C., 1964.
16. Kuhns, L. R., F. J. Bednarek, M. L. Wyman, D. W. Roloff and R. C. Borer: Diagnosis of pneumothorax or pneumomediastinum in the neonate by transillumination. *Pediatrics 56*:355, 1975.
17. Levine, M. I. and A. V. Mascia: *Pulmonary Disease and Anomalies of Infancy and Childhood.* Harper & Row Publishers, New York, 1966.
18. Macleod, J. (Ed.): *Clinical Examination.* Churchill Livingstone, Edinburgh, 1973.
19. Nadas, A. S. and D. C. Fyler: *Pediatric Cardiology,* 3rd ed. W. B. Saunders Co., Philadelphia, 1972.
20. Nagaishi, C.: *Functional Anatomy and Histology of the Lung.* University Park Press, Baltimore, 1972.
21. Parke, W. W.: *Photographic Atlas of Fetal Anatomy.* University Park Press, Baltimore, 1975.
22. Petty, T. L.: *Pulmonary Diagnostic Techniques.* Lea & Febiger, Philadelphia, 1975.
23. Polgar, G. and V. Promadhat: *Pulmonary Function Testing in Children.* W. B. Saunders Co., Philadelphia, 1971.
24. Proctor, D. F.: Physiology of the upper airway. In *Handbook of Physiology, Section 3, Respiration,* Volume I. W. O. Fenn and H. Rahn (Eds.). American Physiological Society, Washington, D.C., 1964.
25. Scarpelli, E. M. and P. A. M. Auld (Eds.): *Pulmonary Physiology of the Fetus, Newborn and Child.* Lea & Febiger, Philadelphia, 1975.
26. Scarpelli, E. M. and E. V. Cosmi (Eds.): *Reviews in Perinatal Medicine,* Volume 1, University Park Press, Baltimore, 1976.
27. Weibel, E. R.: *Morphometry of the Human Lung.* Academic Press, New York, 1963.
28. Winters, R. W. (Ed.): *The Body Fluids in Pediatrics.* Little, Brown and Co., Boston, 1973.

Concepts in Respiratory Pathophysiology

EMILE M. SCARPELLI

2

Disease of the respiratory system may be classified conveniently according to the component of the system that is most affected by the pathologic derangement. Thus the primary target of disease may be:

(1) The peripheral or central nervous system and the centers that control and regulate breathing patterns.

(2) The chest wall (rib cage and diaphragm) and pleural space, which provide the power and power transfer for ventilation.

(3) The airways, from the oronasal cavity to the bronchioles, which are the conduits through which gas is distributed to the exchange surfaces.

(4) The alveolar-capillary units where both gas and liquid exchange are effected and modulated.

(5) The pulmonary interstitium, which is the basic structural support of the lungs.

This categorization, which is incomplete particularly with regard to its exclusion of the so-called nonventilatory functions of the lung,[93] is still useful for developing concepts of pathophysiology and thus a first approach to understanding the clinical manifestations of disease.

Since ventilation is the product of breathing frequency (f) and tidal volume (V_T), a quick estimate of normal ventilation may be obtained from standard tables[79] or from nomograms such as the one provided by Radford et al.[81] (Fig. 1-30). These standards, however, suffer from a basic deficiency: They do not take into account the metabolic requirements of the moment and other mitigating factors, which may in fact dictate that the patient's ventilation must be greater than the predicted normal. Thus corrections must be made, for example, for the level of activity and the acid-base status of the patient if he is not in the basal state.[81] Alterations of dead space also must be taken into account. In addition, when there is impairment of the distribution of ventilation and perfusion to the alveoli, it is practically impossible to quantify the impairment to the extent that proper ventilation ($f \times V_T$) may be predicted with certainty. Nonetheless, the apparent dilemma is rather easily resolved by considering the *adequacy of ventilation.* Ventilation is adequate if it maintains normal Pa_{O_2} and Pa_{CO_2}; it is either inadequate or excessive if it does not.

The essential additional factor which must be taken into account in our considerations of the adequacy of ventilation is whether the lung in question is normal. If the lung is normal, we may assume that the air breathed per unit time is distributed to alveoli in general. If under such circumstances hypocapnia is present, we may assume that alveoli are generally overventilated and thus define the condition as general hyperventilation. Conversely, the presence of hypercapnia would define the condition of general hypoventilation. If, on the other hand, the lung is abnormal, the pathophysiologic mechanisms of right-to-left shunt, diffusion defect, and ventilation-perfusion abnormality dictate the extent to which pulmonary function, and thus the subject, has been compromised. Some distinguishing characteristics, based on gas analyses, of the pathophysiologic processes that are discussed in this chapter are presented in Table 2-1 and Figure 2-1.

General Hyperventilation

Excitation of the central nervous system to produce an increase in ventilation results in an elevation of PA_{O_2} and lowering of PA_{CO_2}.* When the alveolar-capillary exchange surfaces are otherwise normal, Pa_{O_2} and Pa_{CO_2} will change proportionately, and once a steady state is achieved, there will be no significant gradients between alveolar and arterial gas pressures. This general hyperventilation may be voluntary, passive, or spontaneous and, within the latter category, either appropriate or inappropriate.

PASSIVE HYPERVENTILATION

Passive hyperventilation was a relatively common syndrome during the polio era, when paralysis of the respiratory muscles was treated with tank respirators.[101] Passive hyperventilation may be having a mild resurgence in pediatrics as large numbers of ventilators find their way into nurseries and children's intensive care units.[61] Although passive hyperventilation may sometimes be justified to reduce the conscious desire to breathe of selected patients who require prolonged ventilator care,[91] to transiently inhibit spontaneous breathing in certain patients with crushed chest injuries,[6] or to aid in the reversal of life-threatening metabolic acidosis,[2] passive hyperventilation—which is in fact iatrogenic—should be avoided because of its potentially adverse systemic effects.

*The symbol A refers to alveolar gas and a to arterial gas. $PA_{O_2} = (FA_{O_2})(P_T)$ and $PA_{CO_2} = (FA_{CO_2})(P_T)$; i.e., the partial pressure of a gas (PA_{O_2}, PA_{CO_2}) in a mixture of gases is related to the total pressure of the mixed gases (P_T) as the percent concentration of that gas is related to the total amount of gas.

Thus, $\frac{PA_{O_2}}{P_T} = \frac{\%O_2}{100\%}$, where $\frac{\%O_2}{100\%} = FA_{O_2}$,

giving $\frac{PA_{O_2}}{P_T} = FA_{O_2}$.

TABLE 2-1. Some Distinguishing Characteristics of Respiratory Pathophysiologic Processes

Pathophysiologic Condition	Distinguishing Characteristics	
Hyperventilation	Low PA_{CO_2}, Pa_{CO_2}	High PA_{O_2}, Pa_{O_2}
Hypoventilation	High PA_{CO_2}, Pa_{CO_2}	Low PA_{O_2}, Pa_{O_2}
Right-to-Left Shunt	AaD_{O_2} breathing O_2 (shunt on 100% O_2)	Low Pa_{O_2}
Diffusion Defect	AaD_{O_2} especially with exercise (low diffusing capacity)	Low Pa_{O_2}
$\dot{V}A/\dot{Q}$ Abnormality:		
Weighted high	AaD_{O_2}, aAD_{CO_2} breathing air (wasted $\dot{V}$; $VD_{physiol}$-effect)	Low Pa_{O_2}
Weighted low	AaD_{O_2}, aAD_{N_2} breathing air (wasted $\dot{Q}$; shunt-effect)	Low Pa_{O_2}

SPONTANEOUS HYPERVENTILATION

Spontaneous hyperventilation may accompany a variety of conditions. In some it is in a sense appropriate, whereas in others it is not. It may be considered appropriate when it tends to counteract a basic pathologic disorder, as in the following situations:

(1) *Hypoxemia.* The chemoreceptor or baroreceptor-mediated response to hypoxemia is increased ventilation ($f \times V_T$), which results in the lowering of Pa_{CO_2}. Among the causes of hypoxemia in man with normal lungs may be listed exposure to environments that are deficient in oxygen (e.g., decreased ambient pressure and contamination of the air with foreign gases), inadequate transportation and delivery of oxygen (e.g., anemia and hypotension), and extrapulmonary right-to-left shunts (e.g., cyanotic congenital heart disease). The lowering of Pa_{CO_2} that can occur in these conditions may be accompanied by a reciprocal increase of Pa_{O_2}, which however is usually not sufficient to restore Pa_{O_2} to normal.

(2) *Acidemia.* General hyperventilation may be induced by the accumulation of fixed acids (metabolic acidosis) in traumatic and hemorrhagic shock,[24] diabetic or starvation ketosis,[51] renal failure,[74] and extracorporeal circulation.[28] It may occur also when the body's buffer base reserve is depleted in diarrhea. The acidemic stimulus that produces hyperventilation in these cases is probably mediated through the chemoreceptors. The ensuing respiratory activity may have a characteristic pattern, such as the Kussmaul type of breathing that sometimes is associated with diabetic and renal acidemia. Hypocapnia in these conditions tends to compensate in part for the fixed acidemia.

(3) *Hyperthermia.* Increasing the heat content of the body, for example, in febrile states or by exposure to hot environments, may result in hyperventilation. Increased ventilation accelerates the rate of heat dissipation from the lungs.

Spontaneous hyperventilation may occur in other situations in which its appropriateness is difficult to assess:[49]

(1) Psychogenic causes include hysteria, anxiety, and other highly emotional states.

(2) Central neurogenic hyperventilation may occur in association with encephalitis, hypoglycemia, gram-negative sepsis, and cerebral infarction.

(3) Hyperventilation associated with intoxicants (salicylate, paraldehyde, dinitrophenol, ammonium salts, and alcohol) and with the use of respiratory stimulants (nikethamide, ethamivan, doxapram, epi-

		$(A-a)D_{O_2}$ on air	$(A-a)D_{O_2}$ on 100% O_2	$(A-a)D_{O_2}$ on low O_2	$(a-A)D_{CO_2}$	$(a-A)D_{N_2}$
Venous admixture		+ +	+ + + +	+	◌	O
Diffusion limitation		+	◌	+ +	◌	O
Uneven $\dot{V}_A/\dot{Q}$	High $\dot{V}_A/\dot{Q}$	+ +	+	+	+ + + +	+
	Low $\dot{V}_A/\dot{Q}$	+ +	+	+	+	+ + + +

FIG. 2-1. Effect of shunts, diffusion defect, and $\dot{V}_A/\dot{Q}$ abnormalities on alveolar-arterial gas relationships. (From Farhi, L. E.: *Recent Advances in Respiratory Physiology,* C. G. Caro (Ed.) Edward Arnold (Publishers) Ltd., London, 1965.)

nephrine, aminophylline, and progesterone) is mandatory if not appropriate.

(4) Reflex hyperventilation may occur in response to distention of the urinary bladder, sudden cooling of the skin, and pain as a result of general arousal of the respiratory centers by the afferent stimuli. Pulmonary vascular occlusion (e.g., pulmonary embolism) and other conditions in which pulmonary compliance is reduced (e.g., congestive heart failure and pneumothorax) may also produce hyperventilation through stimulation of afferents within the lung parenchyma.

(5) The spontaneous hyperventilation of normal pregnancy seems to be due to an increased irritability of the respiratory center and to be hormone-stimulated.[40] Although it has been suggested that the consequent lowering of Pa_{CO_2} and elevation of maternal Pa_{O_2} may help provide an optimal environment for the fetus, it is also true that hyperventilation during labor and delivery may promote hypoxemia and acidemia in the fetus and newborn and that the alkalosis of hyperventilation may produce equally hazardous effects on the fetus during gestation.[66,67,85]

VOLUNTARY HYPERVENTILATION

Voluntary hyperventilation may be useful. It has been used by physiologists to determine the relative effects of changes in arterial O_2 and CO_2 on the subsequent ability to hold one's breath, that is, to suppress the respiratory center drive.[46] It can also effectively increase the underwater time of swimmers. However, the latter advantage must be weighed against the hazard that hyperventilation before diving has been responsible for a number of drownings.[25,26] The low Pa_{CO_2}

apparently so depresses the respiratory center drive to breathing that severe hypoxic depression may occur without prior warning to return to the surface. Children especially should be warned of this danger.

METABOLIC CONSEQUENCES OF HYPERVENTILATION

The metabolic effects of hyperventilation include respiratory alkalosis, which is characterized by low concentration of hydrogen ions, low P_{CO_2}, and low serum bicarbonate. The degree to which these changes take place is a function of the magnitude and duration of the increased ventilation and the underlying abnormality. At the cellular level the loss of hydrogen is replaced in part by serum sodium and potassium. Concomitantly anions such as lactate in tissue and chloride in erythrocytes leave the cells and displace extracellular bicarbonate that is bound to cations. Thus additional CO_2 is formed for elimination by the lungs. The anion shift, which effectively lowers the bicarbonate level, tends to minimize the change in bicarbonate:CO_2 ratio that would occur from the loss of CO_2 alone. This shift reduces the height to which pH might otherwise rise.

Eventually the shift of hydrogen into the extracellular space may restore the extracellular hydrogen ion concentration to normal or increase it. In the first instance the alkalemia may be termed "compensated" and in the latter "decompensated," in which case a secondary metabolic acidemia is present.[31] At this point diagnosis of the respiratory component rests on the determination of Pa_{CO_2}. If it is low, one may be assured that an underlying abnormality is hyperventilation. Renal mechanisms also tend to compensate for the alkalemia of hyperventilation through conservation of hydrogen and ammonium and excretion of cations and bicarbonate.[95]

Finally the concentration of ionized calcium decreases during hyperventilation,[34] which may explain the similarity between the tetany of hyperventilation and the tetany associated with hypocalcemia in other diseases.

PHYSIOLOGIC CONSEQUENCES OF HYPERVENTILATION

The physiologic consequences of hyperventilation are manifested primarily as pulmonary, cardiovascular, neuromuscular, and psychomotor effects:[49]

(1) *Pulmonary effects.* A decrease of pulmonary and chest wall compliance has been observed during passive hyperventilation.[35] This effect, in addition to the large mechanical workload imposed by the increased ventilation itself, can result in a sharply increased oxygen cost of breathing in the spontaneously breathing subject.[59,64] If underlying pulmonary disease is present or if the subject is obese, the energy cost of hyperventilation may become prohibitive to the point of aggravating symptoms and producing exhaustion. Hyperventilation also produces an increase in the steady-state diffusing capacity,[89] probably as a result of concomitant changes in the distribution of alveolar ventilation in relation to the pulmonary capillary diffusing surface.

(2) *Cardiovascular effects.* Electrocardiographic changes, including S-T segment depression and lowering or inversion of the T wave, often accompany hyperventilation. Such changes may be due to alterations of myocardial potassium, and they may be confused with expressions of the underlying disease, for example, when hyperventilation is associated with congestive heart failure. Regional circulations are also affected during hyperventilation. Thus vasoconstriction occurs in the skin (leading to cold, pale, and moist extremities), intestines, and brain. Cerebral blood flow may fall to half normal,[20,52,102] producing cerebral hypoxia, which is manifested by a slowing of the electroencephalogram[41,63] and clinically by disturbances of consciousness (light-headedness, confusion) and epileptiform seizures.

(3) *Psychomotor and neuromuscular effects.* Anxiety, inability to concentrate, irritability, vertigo, tinnitis, and syncope are all possible symptoms of hyperventilation. In some patients it may be difficult to distinguish cause and effect, and sometimes a self-perpetuating cycle is established. Tetany may occur, usually unilateral and on the same side as the dominant hemisphere (an observation with no convincing explanation). The interaction among altered concentrations of hydrogen and calcium ions and local vasomotor control probably explains the augmented peripheral irritability, including hyperreflexia and sensations of numbness and tingling, that may accompany hyperventilation.

TREATMENT

The treatment of hyperventilation must be directed against the underlying cause. Except for passive and psychogenic types of hyperventilation, "no measure designed specifically to suppress it has any real place in medicine."[2]

General Hypoventilation

Depression of or interference with neural transmission, from the cerebral cortex to the spinal cord and its motor nerves, may depress ventilation (i.e., respiratory frequency and/or tidal volume) so that $P_{A_{O_2}}$ falls and $P_{A_{CO_2}}$ rises in otherwise healthy alveoli. Because alveoli are generally affected and because alveolar-capillary gas exchange is usually not impaired, pulmonary venous and systemic arterial gas pressures change proportionately. Thus Pa_{O_2} falls, Pa_{CO_2} rises, and little difference exists between alveolar and arterial gas pressures (Table 2-1). This condition is general hypoventilation. It may also result from any pathologic process that compromises the power source for ventilation or that obstructs total gas flow to the lungs, including restriction of movement of the thorax (e.g., asphyxiating thoracic dystrophy), restriction of diaphragmatic movements (e.g., eventration of the diaphragm or abdominal distention), and obstruction of the upper airway from the oronasal pharynx to the trachea (e.g., choanal atresia, epiglottitis, or laryngotracheal foreign body).

General hypoventilation, in our discussion, is defined as hypercapnia due to a reduction in total ventilation ($f \times V_T$) in a subject whose lungs are essentially normal. It is characterized by an increase of Pa_{CO_2} and a decrease of Pa_{O_2}. The fall of Pa_{O_2} is usually proportionately greater than the increase of Pa_{CO_2} because the respiratory exchange ratio (R) is usually less than 1.0. General hypoventilation may also be called "concentric" because, presumably, all alveoli are ventilated inadequately. In this section we will distinguish "primary" and "secondary" general hypoventilation.

PRIMARY HYPOVENTILATION

The *primary alveolar hypoventilation syndrome* has been reported in patients whose lungs and cardiovascular system are essentially normal. It is most often associated with obesity,[3,84,94] the Pickwickian syndrome,[16] where the characteristic diagnostic features are hypercapnia in the presence of normal ventilatory capacity, diffusing capacity, and gas distribution in the lungs. The obese hypoventilator is usually somnolent and may appear cyanotic,[10,33,47,73] especially when asleep or in the recumbent position, at which times Pa_{O_2} may be very low.[29] (Since the heart and lungs are essentially normal in these patients, the subject may effectively return Pa_{O_2} and Pa_{CO_2} to normal by voluntarily increasing his ventilatory efforts.) In the chronic hypoventilator, pH may be normal in the presence of hypercapnia. This normalcy is achieved by establishment of a proportionately high serum bicarbonate level, an important diagnostic criterion of chronic hypoventilation, especially in children. Thus, for example, a child may hyperventilate in response to anxiety, agitation, or pain when blood samples are taken or while performing tests of pulmonary function. The transient hyperventilation may lower Pa_{CO_2} acutely, whereas the high bicarbonate level is affected very little. In such cases the elevated bicarbonate indicates that the patient's ventilation is ordinarily not as high as it was during the sampling or testing period. Bates and his colleagues and others feel that the Pickwickian syndrome develops only when obesity is accompanied by poor responsiveness of the respiratory center to carbon dioxide.[10] The decreased responsiveness to carbon dioxide, when added to the effects on pulmonary function of obesity itself (which include an increased O_2 consumption and CO_2 production,[9] a lowering of the compliance of the chest wall,[71] and a reduced functional residual capacity with normal residual volume,[12,29]) results in generalized hypoventilation.

Chronic, apparently primary hypoventilation has been reported also in nonobese subjects. This relatively rare occurrence sometimes is associated with signs of central nervous system disorder and sometimes not,[42,88,98] and it may have respiratory center insensitivity to carbon dioxide as the underlying defect.[86,87] The term, *central alveolar hypoventilation,* has been used to describe the syndrome of hypoxemia and hypercapnia in the absence of both drug ingestion and primary cardiopulmonary, skeletal, or neuromuscular disease and in the presence of the ability to correct the blood gas abnormalities by assisted or voluntary increased ventilation. Recent studies of a 2-year-old child revealed (1) an irregular respiratory rhythm, (2) diminished ventilatory response to inhaled CO_2 (suggesting possibly an abnormality of central control mechanisms), and (3) relatively normal change in breathing with sleep and exercise.[72] These findings may be contrasted with those of another patient[60] in whom (1) respiratory rhythm was regular and (2) there was an abnormal interaction of sleep and ventilation. Thus the syndrome, central alveolar hypoventilation, may reflect a variety of functional abnormalities of the central nervous system control of ventilation.[72]

The syndrome, *apnea of prematurity* (see also Chapter 16), is another example of inappropriate and inadequate central ventilatory control (cause unknown) in which recurrent, sustained periods of apnea become serious clinical problems of therapy and management associated with significant infant mortality. The apparent effectiveness of induced afferent stimuli in reducing the frequency and duration of the periods of apnea suggests that central control mechanisms may be intact but need to be aroused periodically in these infants.[50] These findings are consonant with those obtained from animal experiments which show that sustained fetal breathing can be induced in the apneic fetus in utero by nonspecific somatic sensory stimulation.[22]

SECONDARY HYPOVENTILATION

Concentric hypoventilation may develop in a variety of conditions of known cause in which either the drive to ventilation or the ability to respond to that drive is impaired. Impairment of the ventilatory drive by depression of the respiratory center may be caused by anesthetics, drugs, cerebral trauma or ischemia, increased intracranial pressure, electrocution, metabolic alkalosis, hypercapnia, and hypoxia.[21]

Ventilatory drive may be impaired also by massive or excessive neuronal discharge in the brain that results in tonic and sustained contraction of skeletal muscles, i.e., epilepsy either associated with an underlying disorder, or of idiopathic or genetic origin. Status epilepticus is a true medical emergency in which the hypoventilation or apnea and hypoxemia must be relieved immediately.[32,62]

Voluntary or reflex blockade of the normal drive to respiration may underlie breath-holding spells, i.e., *cyanotic infantile syncope.*[53] This syndrome is seen in nonepileptic children who are usually less than 6 years of age. It is often triggered by a recognizable nociceptive or emotional stimulus. The child may gasp or cry, hold his breath, and then lose consciousness. Occasionally myoclonic activity is associated with this condition. The episode is short-lived (usually less than 1 minute), and the child returns to consciousness without serious sequelae. Lambroso and Lerman stress the importance of differentiating these episodes from others that may be associated with brief periods of ventricular asystole (*pallid infantile syncope*).[53] The former require no specific drug therapy whereas the latter may be helped by treatment with atropine.

Normal ventilatory activity may be impaired also by periods of prolonged or sustained coughing to the point where consciousness is lost (*cough syncope*).[58] As in breathholding spells, the combination of acute hypoventilation or apnea and increased intrathoracic pressure, which may impede the return of blood to the heart, produces cerebral hypoxia and ischemia.

Special mention must be made of the apparent peculiar sensitivity of some newborn infants to hypoxia during the first week of life. It has been shown that the transient excitation of ventilation produced by hypoxia may be followed by respiratory depression and that exposure of the infant to a cool environment may accentuate the depressant effects of hypoxia.[13,18] Conversely, it is probably true that the newborn infant is capable of responding to hypercapnia in much the same way as the adult,[97] despite conflicting reports in the literature,[7,27,96] and that his response to hypercapnia, in contrast to his response to hypoxia, is independent of environmental temperature and postnatal age.[14]

Right-to-Left Shunts

Normally about 1 to 3% of the cardiac output bypasses the pulmonary capillaries and returns to the left side of the heart with relatively deoxygenated blood. Coronary venous return through thebesian veins and in addition, perhaps, bronchial venous blood, as well as direct communications from pulmonary artery to pulmonary vein, probably account for most of this normal right-to-left shunt or venoarterial admixture. With certain diseases right-to-left shunting may become enormous. For a discussion of diseases with intracardiac or extracardiac-extrapulmonary shunts, the reader is referred to contemporary cardiology texts[70,90] and to the discussion of pulmonary arteriovenous fistulas or malformations in Chapter 7. The present section deals with intrapulmonary shunts.

The magnitude of all right-to-left shunts may be estimated rather easily at the bedside by having the patient breathe oxygen* for up to 20 minutes at which time a sample of arterial blood is obtained for Pa_{O_2} and hemoglobin concentration determinations. The ratio of right-to-left shunt flow to total systemic flow (cardiac output), i.e., the *percent shunt*, is obtained by substituting in the equation

$$\frac{C\acute{c}_{O_2} - Ca_{O_2}}{C\acute{c}_{O_2} - C\bar{v}_{O_2}}$$

where C is the oxygen content and ć, a, and v̄ refer to end-pulmonary capillary, systemic arterial, and mixed venous bloods respectively. End-pulmonary capillary O_2 content ($C\acute{c}_{O_2}$) is estimated by assuming that pulmonary capillary P_{O_2} is equal to alveolar P_{O_2} for those capillaries that perfuse ventilated

*Great care must be taken when the "oxygen test" is done to be sure that the subject clears his lungs of 100% oxygen when the test is completed. Since oxygen is absorbed extremely rapidly from the lung, oxygen in poorly ventilated units will be absorbed, leaving atelectasis. (Thus the test may not be indicated in patients in whom intrapulmonary gas trapping is suspected, e.g., patients with severe or diffuse airway obstruction.) The patient must be encouraged or stimulated to ventilate his lungs well with air when the test is done.

alveoli (i.e., nonshunted blood). Since 100% oxygen is breathed, PA_{O_2} = 760-47-40 mm Hg, where 760 is barometric pressure, 47 is water vapor pressure at normal body temperature, and 40 is alveolar PCO_2 (assuming that PA_{CO_2} equals Pa_{CO_2} and that both are normal; if Pa_{CO_2} is not 40 mm Hg, the actual pressure should be substituted). Thus if PA_{O_2} is 673 mm Hg and capillary PO_2 is the same, hemoglobin is fully saturated, and $C\acute{c}_{O_2}$ equals the oxygen capacity of hemoglobin (about 1.34 ml O_2 per g Hb) × (g Hb per 100 ml blood) plus the amount of O_2 dissolved in blood (0.003 ml O_2 per 100 ml blood per mm Hg PO_2). Arterial O_2 content (Ca_{O_2}) is determined in the same way using the measured Pa_{O_2}. Since accurate determination of mixed venous O_2 content ($C\bar{v}_{O_2}$) requires sampling of pulmonary arterial blood, it may be estimated rather reliably by subtracting four volumes percent from the calculated Ca_{O_2}. Tables are available from which percent shunt may be estimated from the measured Pa_{O_2} during oxygen breathing (Figs. 2-2 and 2-3). These tables are based on the equation given previously. Derivation of the equation and its significance have been presented succinctly by McIlroy.[57]

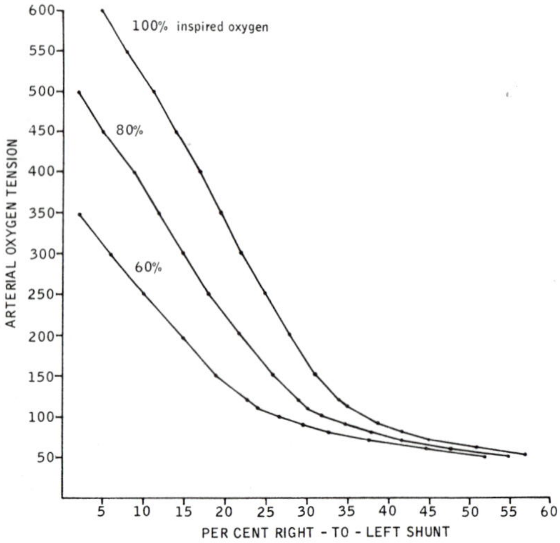

FIG. 2-2. Estimation of magnitude of right-to-left shunt with subject breathing either 100%, 80%, or 60% inspired oxygen. Assumptions made in these calculations: hemoglobin concentration = 16 g/100 ml; arteriovenous O_2 difference = 4 volumes %; respiratory exchange ratio = 0.8, arterial PCO_2 = 40 mm Hg. (From Avery, M. E.: *The Lung and Its Disorders in the Newborn Infant,* 2nd ed. W. B. Saunders Co., Philadelphia, 1968. Courtesy of Dr. Scott Faulkner.)

Intrapulmonary shunts due to pulmonary disease are generally the result of pulmonary capillary perfusion of alveoli that are collapsed (atelectasis) or perfusion of those that are filled with nongaseous fluid (alveolar-filling). The exemplar of atelectasis is respiratory distress syndrome of the newborn infant in which blood flow continues, to some degree, through areas of widespread alveolar collapse.[68] Outside the newborn period, atelectasis most commonly follows complete obstruction of a large airway (e.g., a lobar bronchus), but may or may not follow obstruction of smaller airways since, within each lobe, direct connections between alveolar walls may permit collateral ventilation of the obstructed segment by the adjacent unobstructed segment.[55] Alveoli may also collapse from external pressure (e.g., lung cyst, hemothorax, herniated abdominal viscera) and from lack of surfactant as in respiratory distress syndrome.[8]

Intrapulmonary right-to-left shunts also characterize alveolar occlusive diseases in which the alveolar space is filled with nongaseous fluid. Pulmonary edema, pneumonias, aspiration of bulk liquid, accumulation of alveolar products as in alveolar proteinosis, and hemorrhage are examples of occlusion of alveoli in which gas exchange with capillaries is not possible.

Although blood flow through the capillaries of occluded and collapsed alveoli is reduced, continued flow and widespread involvement may result in significant shunting. Because of compensatory hyperventilation of uninvolved pulmonary segments, Pa_{CO_2} may be normal or low while Pa_{O_2} is low and the hallmark alveolar-arterial oxygen gradient

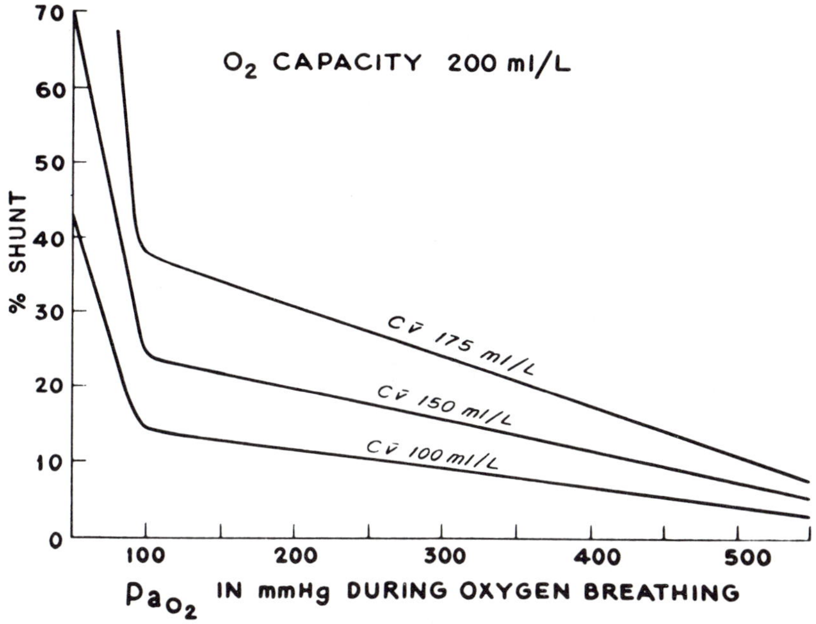

FIG. 2-3. Graph showing level of arterial oxygen pressure during oxygen breathing with different percentages of right-to-left shunt and different levels of mixed venous oxygen content. (From McIlroy, M. B.[57])

(See Fig. 2-1 and Table 2-1) during oxygen breathing is established.

ATELECTASIS

Blood flow through atelectatic areas of the lung may be considerable especially when the pleural space is otherwise undisturbed. It is probably negative pleural pressure that promotes capillary flow through collapsed lung units, since intrapulmonary shunting may be reduced dramatically when pneumothorax and thus elevated pleural pressures accompany atelectasis. In their development of the point that the major roentgenographic difference between atelectasis and "consolidation" (i.e., alveolar-filling) is one of volume,* Fraser and Paré[38] provide a classification of atelectasis based on causal mechanisms. The classification that follows borrows from these authors, although terminology has been changed somewhat. This section identifies four types of atelectasis: resorption, compression, surface, and fibrosis atelectasis (Figs. 2-4 to 2-6).

Resorption Atelectasis. Atelectasis due to resorption (Figs. 2-4B and C), the most common pathogenetic type, follows obstruction—either "intrinsic" or "extrinsic"—of the communication between alveoli and their airway(s). The topic is discussed thoroughly by Fraser and Paré.[38] To appreciate the possible effects of airway obstruction, one must recall the anatomy of terminal lung units and the physics of trapped gas. Alveoli are ventilated principally by the major airways (bronchi, bronchioles) that serve them; in addition, "side channels" permit ventilation of alveoli indirectly, so-called collateral ventilation. These channels include the pores of Kohn

*As would be expected, both atelectasis and alveolar-filling present a roentgenographic picture of airlessness and unit density. Whereas volume is reduced in atelectasis, it may be normal in alveolar-filling.

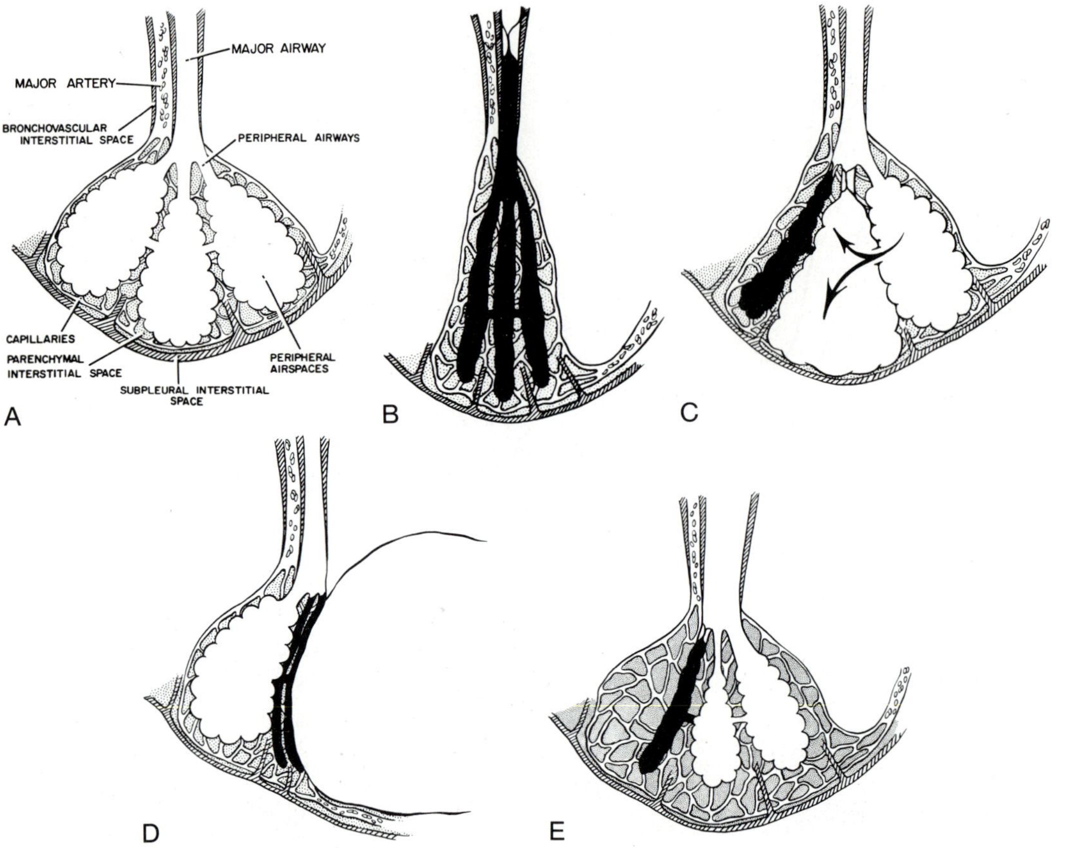

FIG. 2-4. Schematic presentation of some forms of atelectasis.

A, Normal lung units.

B, Resorption atelectasis due to obstruction of a major airway.

C, Resorption atelectasis due to obstruction of small airway and "side channel" (unit on left). Collateral ventilation continues in center air space because of unobstructed "side channel" to unobstructed air space on right.

D, Compression atelectasis from bulla on the right.

E, Fibrosis atelectasis due to fibrosis of the interstitial space, which is increased in amount and density. One air space is collapsed while others show different degrees of loss of volume. The major airway is dilated as is the peripheral airway on the right. (Schematics from Fraser, R. G. and J. A. P. Paré.[38] Nomenclature and legends adapted by present author to conform to discussion in text.)

(discontinuities in the alveolar wall; Fig. 2-5) and the canals of Lambert (epithelium-lined tubules from preterminal bronchioles to adjacent alveoli). The resorption of gas from alveoli that are distal to an obstructed airway (assuming also that the side channels are not patent) would proceed as follows: As oxygen is taken up by the capillaries, volume of the alveoli decreases and pressure of its constituent gases increases to the point where PA_{CO_2} and PA_{N_2} exceed the corresponding pressures in mixed venous blood coming to the capillaries. Thus O_2 continues to be absorbed from the alveoli, as alveolar-capillary gradients for CO_2 and N_2 develop in favor of CO_2 and N_2 transfer *into* the capillaries. Alveolar volume continues to fall and gradients continue to increase until all gas is removed. If alveoli contain O_2 instead of a mixture of gases when obstructed, resorption time is shortened significantly (see footnote, p. 77). For example, an obstructed mixed gas-containing lobe may become atelectatic in 18 to 24 hours, whereas an O_2-containing lobe may collapse in less than 1 hour.

Several factors modify the rate and extent of alveolar collapse following obstruction.

(1) *Site of bronchial obstruction.* Obstruction of a lobar bronchus may produce lobar atelectasis because of the absence of interlobar side channels, whereas segmental or subsegmental bronchial obstruction retains the possibility of collateral ventilation from side channels.

(2) *Collateral ventilation and the check valve mechanism.* If side channels are patent (see Fig. 2-4C), adjacent obstructed alveoli may continue to be ventilated; indeed they may become overinflated.[15] Similarly, if the obstruction produces a check-valve effect, peripheral alveoli may become overinflated.[55]

(3) *Infection* distal to the obstruction,

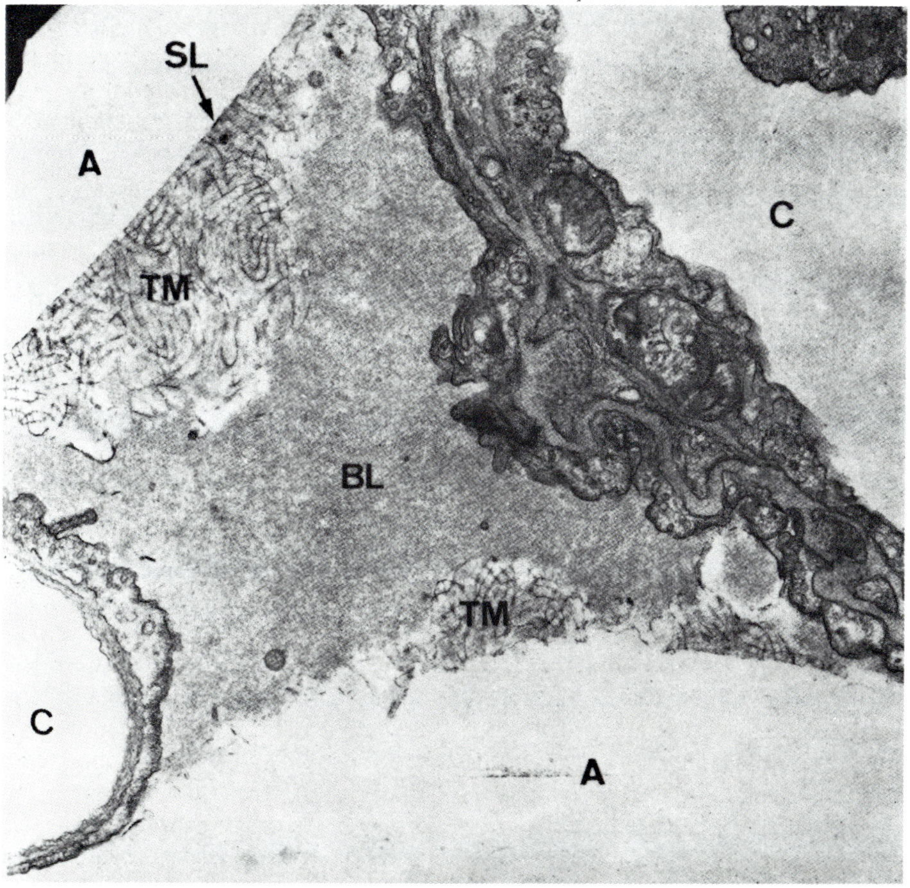

FIG. 2-5. Pore of Kohn containing acellular lining material, which is probably analogous to the normal acellular alveolar lining layer. This lining material is probably no barrier to gas diffusion between alveoli: A = alveolus; SL = interfacial layer of lining material; TM = tubular myelin figure; BL = hypophase or base layer of the lining material; C = capillary. ×21,060 (From Gil, J. and E. R. Weibel: Improvements in demonstration of lining layer of lung alveoli by electron microscopy. *Respir. Physiol. 8*:13, 1969–70.)

which may produce transudates and exudates to occlude side channels and/or produce alveolar-filling.

(4) *Formation of alveolar edema* distal to the obstruction so that, in effect, collapse and alveolar-filling are competitive processes. (Post-obstruction edema may result from the increased negative pressures that develop in the pleural space as alveoli collapse; as the volume of the hemithorax adjusts to the reduced alveolar volume, local pleural pressure may become less negative and the liquid may be resorbed leaving collapsed alveoli.)

Compression Atelectasis. We use the term, compression atelectasis for both passive atelectasis and compression atelectasis as discussed by Fraser and Paré.[38] Compression atelectasis may occur in the presence of pneumothorax, hydrothorax, and tension pneumothorax (passive) or from a space occupying mass within the thorax (see Fig. 2-4D), e.g., cysts, abscesses, enlarged heart, abdominal viscera, and tumors. The mechanism underlying alveolar collapse in these conditions is probably related to the fact that local pleural pressure is increased and thus adjacent alveoli are reduced in size to minimal volume. With sustained compression alveoli collapse completely. Since alveoli are rather stable at minimal volume, the forces responsible for the final collapse are not well understood.

Surface Atelectasis. Surface or adhesive atelectasis may result when surface tension at the alveolar-air interface is abnormally high (see Fig. 2-6). The effect of high surface tension is to produce a force directed centripetally at the alveolar level, resulting in alveolar collapse.[92] Although a great deal has been written about the central role of alveolar surfactant in the maintenance of pulmonary stability, and disruption or deficiency of surfactant has been implicated in the pathogenesis of a number of pulmonary diseases,[92] it seems that only respiratory distress syndrome of newborn infants can be attributed positively to surfactant deficiency. Experimentally, it can be shown that disruption of pulmonary surfactant in situ leads to complete alveolar collapse and that various interventions can produce lung damage pari passu with a reduction of surfactants (e.g., aspiration of hydrocarbons, oxygen toxicity, irradiation of the lung, surgical cardiopulmonary bypass, pulmonary infection in which alveoli adjacent to infected zones become unstable and collapse, and pulmonary edema, lavage, and drowning in which surfactants are washed from the lung thereby rendering the lung unstable when it is reinflated). Nonetheless, respiratory distress syndrome remains the exemplary disease of surfactant deficiency and massive alveolar collapse (see Fig. 16-28).

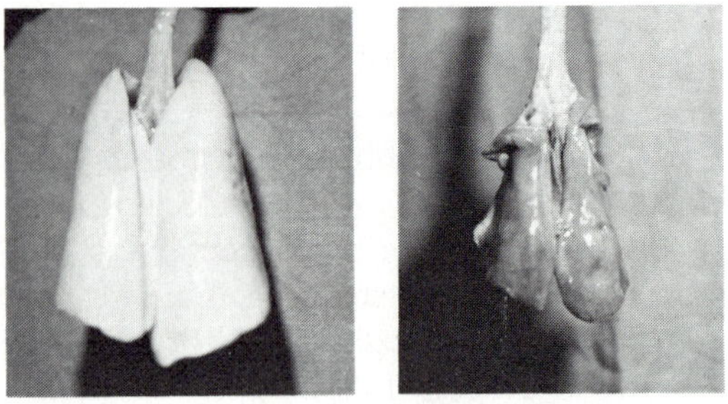

A B

FIG. 2-6. Normal excised rabbit lungs on left (A) contain air. When normal surfactants are displaced from the lungs (B), alveoli become unstable and collapse. (From Scarpelli, E. M.: The pulmonary surfactant system. *Clin. Notes Respir. Dis.* 9:number 3, 1970.)

Fibrosis Atelectasis (see Fig. 2-4E). It is well known that the ratio of air to pulmonary tissue volume is decreased in fibrotic diseases of the lung, due both to the absolute reduction of air volume and to an increase of tissue volume. It is chiefly for this reason that Fraser and Paré[38] have included these diseases in their classification of atelectasis, using the term, cicatrization atelectasis.[38] Fibrotic disease may be localized as with chronic granulomatous infections or it may be generalized as with chronic interstitial fibrosis.[39] The production of fibrosis atelectasis in these diseases is a consequence of the destruction of pulmonary parenchyma followed by fibrosis and cicatrization. Dr. Donald Massaro, of the University of Miami's School of Medicine has informed us recently that alveoli in generalized fibrotic disease of the lung may be unusually labile and tend to collapse upon maximal expiration.

Cardiopulmonary Response. The effects of obstructive atelectasis on cardiopulmonary function have been fairly well documented in the research laboratory by studies in which a major bronchus is occluded by the experimenter. Such studies indicate that acute obstruction produces hyperventilation of the contralateral lung, hypocapnia secondary to hyperventilation, and hypoxemia due mainly to the right-to-left shunt. Compression atelectasis has been studied mainly in humans and animals with spontaneous and induced pneumothoraces.[40] Acute pneumothorax produces lung collapse and an immediate fall in arterial oxygen saturation. Progressively after the acute insult, perfusion of the collapsed lung decreases (perhaps through local vasoconstriction) and arterial Po_2 increases, as hyperventilation of the contralateral lung sustains some degree of hypocapnia. The right-to-left shunt that accompanies surface atelectasis in respiratory distress syndrome is due to flow through the ductus arteriosus, foramen ovale, and pulmonary capillaries of collapsed alveoli. Of the three, ductal flow accounts for less than 15% of the total shunt, whereas atelectasis accounts for most of it.[68] The successful use of continuous positive airway pressure[44] for the treatment of respiratory distress syndrome (Fig. 2-7) is most likely due to reduction of intrapulmonary right-to-left shunts.[44]

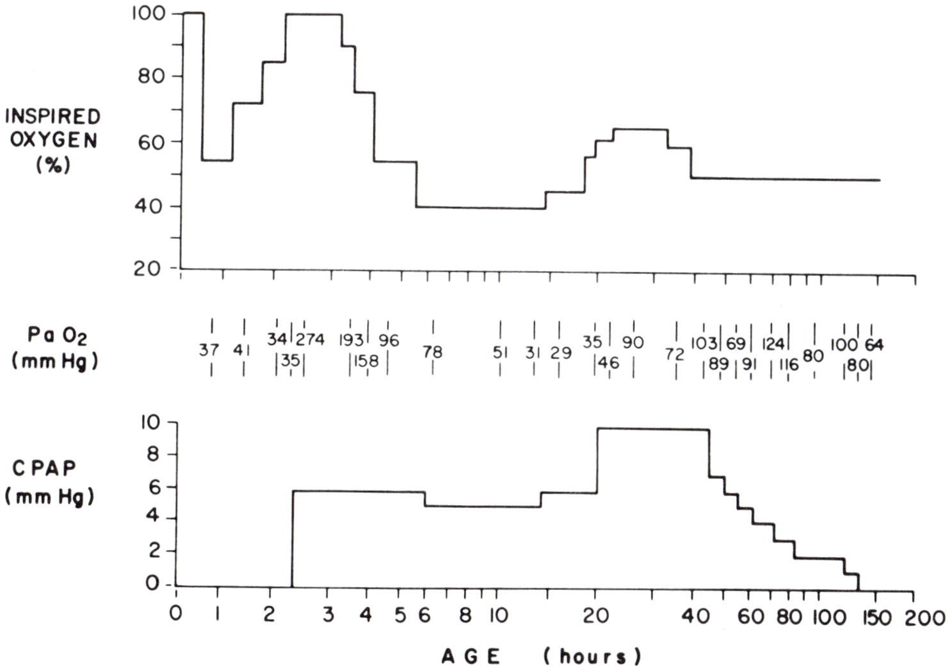

FIG. 2-7. Relationship of inspired oxygen percentage, arterial oxygen pressure (Pa_{O_2}), and continuous positive airway pressure (CPAP) throughout the course of idiopathic respiratory distress syndrome in a 1.94-kg infant. (From Gregory, G. A. et al[44]. Reprinted, by permission, from *N. Engl. J. Med. 284*:1333, 1971.)

ALVEOLAR-FILLING

Blood flow through capillaries of alveoli filled with nongaseous material is a right-to-left shunt. Diseases that can produce this effect are many. A representative listing of such diseases and conditions is given in Table 2-2. It is apparent from inspection of this list that alveolar-filling is just one of several pathogenetic processes that may affect pulmonary function and that the relative importance of alveolar-filling and right-to-left shunt is variable.

Some of the diseases, such as pulmonary edema, pulmonary hemorrhage, alveolar proteinosis, desquamative interstitial pneumonia, and delayed resorption of fetal pulmonary fluid, may be considered examples of conditions in which alveolar-filling is a primary derangement. However, other conditions, including the aspiration syndromes and accidental aspiration of toxic fluids and pathogens, may produce considerable destruction of airway epithelium in addition to the eventual filling of alveoli with cellular debris and exudate. The pathophysiologic derangements resulting from the latter include, within the same lung, $\dot{V}_A/\dot{Q}$ abnormalities (related to airway injury), diffusion defects (related to alveolar-filling and to destruction of alveolar and interstitial tissues), and right-to-left shunts (alveolar-filling).

TABLE 2-2. Some Conditions Associated with Alveolar-Filling

- Delayed Resorption of Fetal Pulmonary Fluid
- Pulmonary Edema (with congestive heart failure or with increased capillary permeability)
- Pulmonary Hemorrhage (idiopathic; traumatic; other)
- Pneumonias (inflammatory exudates)
- Therapeutic Pulmonary Lavage
- Aspiration Syndromes
    - Meconium
    - Swallowing difficulties (local laryngeal; with neurological disease)
    - Fistulas (tracheoesophageal; biliary-bronchial)
    - Gastric aspiration (regurgitation-aspiration)
- Accidental Aspiration
    - Toxic fluids (smoke, acids, alkali, hydrocarbons, alcohol, mineral oil, animal fats)
    - Water (salt or fresh water, often including particulate matter)
    - Bacterial pathogens
- Alveolar Proteinosis; Desquamative Interstitial Pneumonia

The hypoxemia that develops early in the course of most pneumonias is probably the result of shunts from perfusion of exudate-filled alveoli.[103] However, there is always a variable element of airway obstruction and constriction caused by secretions within the bronchi of nonconsolidated areas, and there is always the possibility of collapse of contiguous noninfected areas probably as a result of impairment of production or function of surfactant locally.

Drowning produces a number of pathophysiologic responses. The initial response of a submerged mammal is to hold its breath;[43] within a minute or two some water is inhaled and this action may produce laryngospasm and further breathholding. However, as asphyxia progresses, inhalation is resumed and more water is aspirated resulting in airway obstruction and alveolar-filling. Therefore resuscitation must include immediate gravity drainage of liquid from the lung and reestablishment of respiration by assisted or controlled respiratory therapy. The observation that positive end-expiratory pressure is more effective in reversing hypoxemia after sea water drowning than after fresh water drowning[65] is probably related to the greater stability of surfactant in the latter liquid and thus to greater stability of the alveoli once the liquid is removed.

Mention also should be made of pulmonary lavage for the treatment of alveolar proteinosis,[23,56] desquamative interstitial pneumonia,[45] and other diseases in which alveoli are filled with particulate debris. Although lavage may be of significant benefit, it must be recalled that the post-lavage lung, like the nearly drowned lung, is rather unstable[48] and thus should be monitored carefully, especially for possible development of atelectasis. Although right-to-left shunting is the major problem in conditions in which alveolar-filling with liquid is the principal disorder and one would expect positive airway pressure to be an effective therapeutic adjunct (since it would tend to promote the movement of liquid out of alveoli and help maintain alveolar patency with air), the presence of particulate debris demands that attempts be made first to remove the debris; hence, the rationale for therapeutic pulmonary lavage. Similarly, when airway injury is an associated problem, the airways must be cleared by the most appropriate means before alveoli can be managed rationally.

ADULT RESPIRATORY DISTRESS SYNDROME (SHOCK LUNG)

The term, *adult respiratory distress syndrome,* was applied to the condition in which severe, unexpected, and life-threatening acute respiratory distress occurred in patients with no previous lung disease, after a variety of *unrelated* pulmonary insults, including sepsis, hemorrhagic shock, overwhelming uremia, pancreatitis, thoracic or nonthoracic trauma, fat embolism, aspiration, and diffuse intravascular coagulation.[77,78]

Marked dyspnea, increased respiratory effort, refractory and severe hypoxemia, and diffuse pulmonary densities on chest roentgenograms are the clinical features that characterize the syndrome. Since it may follow a variety of apparently predisposing conditions and since the pathologic morphology is not strictly comparable in all cases (although marked damage of the alveolar-capillary membrane, edema, and atelectasis are a common theme), it has been suggested that the appellation is a practical misnomer, especially since the disease may not in fact be the analogue of respiratory distress syndrome of the newborn infant.[69] The controversy around nomenclature notwithstanding,[69,77] it is important to recognize that the major problem is failure to oxygenate the blood and that this failure is related, to a significant degree, to intrapulmonary shunting.

Diffusion Defects

Except for pulmonary edema, diseases of the pulmonary interstitium, including the alveolar-capillary unit, are relatively rare in children. Fibrotic diseases of the lung involve the capillary and alveolar walls, increasing the distance between alveolar gas and capillary blood. The list of diseases is extensive, ranging from idiopathic pulmonary fibrosis through the pulmonary manifestations of collagen disease to sarcoidosis and the pneumoconioses.[11] Diffusion defect may occur in the early stages of development of pulmonary edema, when there is significant accumulation of liquid in the interstices (including the interstitium between alveolar and capillary walls) before the alveolar space becomes occluded.[54] These diseases are characterized by an alveolar-capillary diffusion defect expressed principally as an inability to transfer sufficient quantities of oxygen to the blood as it traverses the pulmonary capillaries. In addition, since normal diffusion of oxygen requires adequate alveolar-capillary surface area as well as a normal alveolar-capillary cell boundary, any condition (including those mentioned) in which surface area is compromised also manifests itself as a diffusion defect. Because the solubility in pulmonary tissue of CO_2 is about 24 times greater than O_2 and because of concomitant compensatory hyperventilation, diffusion defects are usually associated with some degree of hypoxemia and normal to low Pa_{CO_2}. No appreciable alveolar-arterial gradients occur unless the subject is made to breathe low concentrations of oxygen, which reveal the diffusion defect by a $P_{A_{O_2}}$ greater than the Pa_{O_2}, i.e., by an alveolar-arterial O_2 gradient (see Fig. 2-1 and Table 2-1).

DIFFUSING CAPACITY

The rate at which oxygen diffuses from alveolus to capillary red blood cell (the diffusing capacity of the lung, DL) is a function of (1) its diffusion through the alveolar-capillary cell boundary (the diffusing capacity of the membrane, DM), (2) its diffusion into the red blood cell, and (3) the total alveolar-capillary surface area. Implicit in the clinical measurements of DL and DM are specific factors that determine diffusion and diffusion rate, e.g., solubility of the gas, the alveolar-capillary gas pressure gradient, and the time spent by the red blood cell in the capillary.

Loss of effective alveolar-capillary surface area results in a proportionate reduction of the measured values of DL, DM, and red cell diffusing capacity, since diffusion in general is compromised by removal of all exchange surfaces in affected areas. Clinical diseases that produce a proportionate fall of DL, DM, and red cell diffusing capacity include primary pulmonary vascular disease, pulmonary embolism, large space-occupying lesions, discrete nodular lesions as occur in sarcoidosis and eosinophilic granuloma, and emphysema as seen in adults. Similarly, diffusing capacity is diminished in diseases of alveolar-filling and alveolar collapse in which there is a large right-to-left shunt, since large volumes of blood are diverted from the alveolar-capillary exchange surfaces.

Diffusion defects in which there is also a fall in DM include the many forms of diffuse interstitial pulmonary disease (see following section). With regard to cause and classification of these diseases of the lung, we note with Rankin and Chester[83] that specific cause is known for only a few and is uncertain for many. The classification proposed by these authors, based on the predominant tissue reaction, is given in Table 2-3.

ALVEOLAR-CAPILLARY BLOCK

The term, *alveolar-capillary block syndrome,* was used with reference to diseases, from a variety of causes, in which diffuse interstitial and fibrotic disease of the lung is associated with reduced lung volumes, hyperventilation with high $P_{A_{O_2}}$ and low Pa_{CO_2},

TABLE 2-3. Some Interstitial Diseases of the Lung*

Septal Pneumonias and Fibroses
Hamman-Rich disease
Rheumatoid lung; scleroderma; systemic lupus erythematosis
Idiopathic interstitial pneumonitis and fibrosis
Secondary to long-standing congestion and edema (e.g., uremic lung)
Secondary to damage by infections or toxins
Specific Reactions to Toxins
Inorganic dusts (e.g., silica, asbestos, beryllium, hard metals, talc, graphite, kaolin)
Organic dusts (e.g., bagassosis, farmer's lung)
Fumes and gases (e.g., sulfur dioxide, phosgene, oxides of nitrogen, bauxite)
Radiation
Granulomatoses
Sarcoid
Mycobacterial and fungal
Toxic (e.g., organic dusts)
Allergic (e.g., associated with polyarteritis nodosa or eosinophilia; Wegener's syndrome)
Histiocytic Reticuloses
(Eosinophilic granuloma, Hand-Schüller-Christian syndrome, Letterer-Siwe disease, histiocytosis X)
Neoplasms and Other Diseases
Lymphomas and leukemias
Miliary and lymphangitic metastases
Alveolar proteinosis; hemosiderosis (including Goodpasture's syndrome); alveolar microlithiasis

*Modified from the classification of Rankin, J. and E. H. Chester.[83]

and reduced diffusing capacity of the lung.[5] The term indicated that impairment of diffusion across the thickened alveolar-capillary cell boundary was the principal defect. Recently doubt has been raised regarding the exclusivity of a diffusion defect across the alveolar-capillary cell boundary as the principal pathogenetic mechanism, and it has been suggested that alveolar-capillary block may be a misnomer. The problem is well summarized by Rankin and Chester,[83] so it is only highlighted in this discussion. There is little doubt that the alveolar-capillary cell boundary is thickened and that the effective surface area for gas exchange is reduced in these diseases. Therefore, both factors probably play a pathophysiologic role, but it appears that the surface area defect dominates. However, Finley and his colleagues theorized that the boundary could not become thick enough to cause a decrease in oxygen transport and concluded that reduced surface area and $\dot{V}_A/\dot{Q}$ abnormalities were the basic pathophysiologic mechanisms.[37] Thus the histologic "block" was removed. However, although the final answer is not in yet, it seems safe to conclude on the basis of subsequent speculation and experimentation that there is, in fact, a diffusion defect across the alveolar-capillary cell boundary in patients with hypoxemia and interstitial pulmonary disease. Thus the idea of alveolar-capillary block may be restored, with the understanding that $\dot{V}_A/\dot{Q}$ abnormalities and reduced surface area for gas exchange add to the total picture of hypoxemia and low D_L in these patients.

The extensive infiltration of the lung with cellular or fibrotic tissue explains the physiologic abnormalities encountered in these diseases.

(1) Vital capacity and static lung volumes are reduced.

(2) The lung is stiff; pulmonary compliance is low.

(3) Compensatory hyperventilation may yield apparently normal hemoglobin-oxygen saturation when the patient is resting, but cannot prevent hypoxemia during exertion.

(4) Pulmonary arterial hypertension during exercise, or at rest in severe cases, follows the reduction in size of the pulmonary vascular bed. Since the airways generally are not obstructed, tests of air flow are usually normal: Maximal voluntary ventilation, forced expiratory volumes expressed as a fraction of the forced vital capacity (timed vital capacity), and other indirect measurements of airway resistance are relatively normal.

Ventilation-perfusion Abnormalities

By far the most common functional derangement associated with respiratory diseases is the so-called mismatching of pulmonary ventilation and blood flow, i.e., *$\dot{V}_A/\dot{Q}$ abnormalities.* This derangement operates to some degree in all disease states mentioned thus far and is also the principal functional abnormality of diseases of the bronchi and bronchioles. Thus, any discussion of clinical manifestations and natural history of such conditions, e.g., asthma, bronchiolitis, cystic fibrosis, and toxic inhalation or aspiration syndromes, must rest on an understanding of the underlying $\dot{V}_A/\dot{Q}$ abnormality.[4,100]

$\dot{V}_A/\dot{Q}$: THE CONCEPT

The concentration or amount of any gas in any given alveolar-capillary unit is determined by the balance of processes that, on the one hand, bring that gas to the unit and, on the other hand, remove that gas from the unit. (A unit may be defined as the respiratory bronchiole and the alveolar ducts and sacs that branch from it, e.g., from generations 17 through 23 in the nomenclature for branching within the lung.[99]) Since ventilation of the alveolar-capillary unit ($\dot{V}_A$) is the primary determinant of the rate at which O_2 is added and CO_2 is removed, any increase of $\dot{V}A$ in the ratio $\dot{V}A/\dot{Q}$ results in elevated PA_{O_2} and reduced PA_{CO_2} within the unit. Conversely, reduction of $\dot{V}A$ in the ratio $\dot{V}A/\dot{Q}$ results in reduced PA_{O_2} and elevated PA_{CO_2} within the unit. An analogous conceptual analysis can be given for changes in perfusion ($\dot{Q}$), based on the understanding that perfusion of the alveolar-capillary unit is the primary determinant of the rate at which O_2 is removed from and CO_2 is added to the unit. Thus an increase of $\dot{Q}$ in the ratio $\dot{V}A/\dot{Q}$ leads to reduced PA_{O_2} and increased PA_{CO_2}, whereas a reduction of $\dot{Q}$ leads to increased PA_{O_2} and reduced PA_{CO_2}. If there is no impediment to alveolar-capillary gas exchange within the unit, gas tensions in capillary blood are the same as alveolar gas tensions.

However, the lung is not the single alveolar-capillary unit to which the preceding discussion was directed; rather it is a collection of thousands of such units. The simplest way of looking at the complex total picture is to consider all alveoli collectively in the term $\dot{V}A$ and all capillaries collectively in the term $\dot{Q}$, and to understand that, even in the normal lung, there is a distribution of units within this collective, ranging from units with $\dot{V}A/\dot{Q}$ of about 3.3 (upper lung zones in the upright adult) to those with $\dot{V}A/\dot{Q}$ of about 0.63 (lower zones) (Fig. 2-8). If overall $\dot{V}A/\dot{Q}$ were matched and the total lung behaved as described for single units, arterial and alveolar gas pressures would be the same. However, as overall $\dot{V}A/\dot{Q}$ becomes mismatched (i.e., as overall $\dot{V}A/\dot{Q}$ deviates from 1.0), CO_2

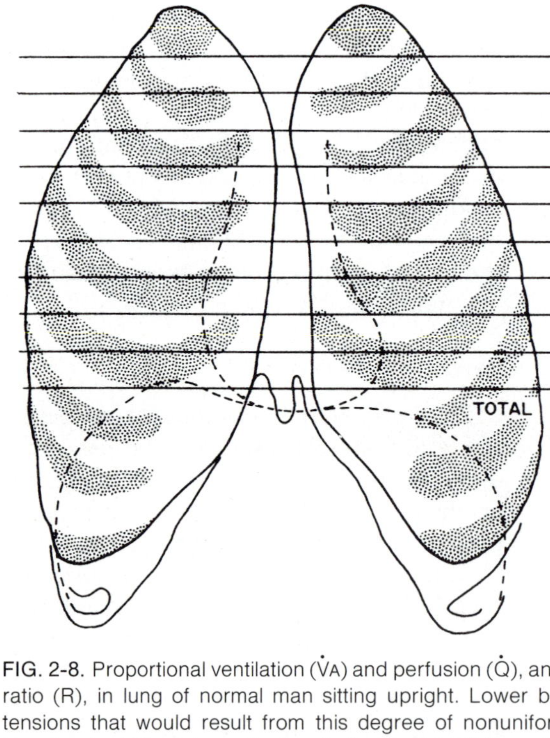

Vol. %	$\dot{V}A$ (liters/min)	$\dot{Q}$ (liters/min)	$\dot{V}A/\dot{Q}$	Po_2 (mm Hg)	Pco_2 (mm Hg)	PN_2 (mm Hg)	R
7	·24	·07	3·3	132	28	553	2·0
8	·33	·19	1·8	121	34	558	1·3
10	·42	·33	1·3	114	37	562	1·1
11	·52	·50	1·0	108	39	566	·92
12	·59	·66	0·90	102	40	571	·85
13	·67	·83	0·80	98	41	574	·78
13	·72	·98	0·73	95	41	577	·73
13	·78	1·15	0·68	92	42	579	·68
13	·82	1·29	0·63	89	42	582	·65
TOTAL 100	5·09	6·00					

	Po_2	Pco_2	PN_2
Mixed Alveolar	101	39	572
Mixed arterial	97	40	575
A-a diff.	4	1	3

FIG. 2-8. Proportional ventilation ($\dot{V}A$) and perfusion ($\dot{Q}$), and consequent gas tensions and respiratory exchange ratio (R), in lung of normal man sitting upright. Lower box: mixed alveolar and mixed systemic arterial gas tensions that would result from this degree of nonuniformity of $\dot{V}A/\dot{Q}$. (From Bates, D. V.: Chapter 57. In *Handbook of Physiology, Section 3: Respiration.* Volume 2. American Physiological Society, Washington, D.C., 1965. Data are from West, J. B.: Regional differences in gas exchange in the lung of erect man. *J. Appl. Physiol.* *17*:893, 1962.)

output and O_2 uptake are compromised (Fig. 2-9), and arterial and alveolar gas pressures* are no longer the same. This change occurs because lung units with high $\dot{V}A/\dot{Q}$ contribute disproportionately more to expired gas from which alveolar gas pressures are determined, whereas units with low $\dot{V}A/\dot{Q}$ contribute disproportionately more to pulmonary venous and systemic arterial blood. This effect is presented graphically in the O_2-CO_2 diagram shown as Figure 2-10.

Because overall $\dot{V}A/\dot{Q}$ of the normal lung is 0.8 to 0.9, arterial and alveolar gas tensions are not the same (see Fig. 2-8): Pa_{O_2} is about 4 mm Hg less than PA_{O_2}, Pa_{CO_2} is about 1 mm Hg greater than PA_{CO_2}, and Pa_{N_2} is about 3 mm Hg greater than PA_{N_2}. These differences are termed gradients or "differences," and are expressed as follows: AaD_{O_2} = 4 mm Hg; aAD_{CO_2} = 1 mm Hg; aAD_{N_2} = 3 mm Hg. When overall $\dot{V}A/\dot{Q}$ mismatching is accentuated by disease, the gradients may increase markedly: The initial effect is a lowering of Pa_{O_2} and elevation of Pa_{CO_2} (see Fig. 2-9) because the disease process tends to produce a disproportionate number of units with low $\dot{V}A/\dot{Q}$. The chemoreceptor response to consequent changes in blood gas pressures is to increase overall ventilation; relatively normal lung units are especially capable of increasing $\dot{V}A$ so that a number of units with high $\dot{V}A/\dot{Q}$ are brought into the overall picture. This response is often effective in returning Pa_{CO_2} to normal or even subnormal levels, whereas Pa_{O_2} is generally not effectively restored to normal.* When a steady state is restored (and this may be defined as the point at which overall respiratory exchange of gases equals overall bodily production and consumption of gases, i.e., $\dot{V}CO_2/\dot{V}O_2$[respiration] = $\dot{V}CO_2/\dot{V}O_2$[metabolism]), the relative proportions of units with high and those with low $\dot{V}A/\dot{Q}$ are reflected in the gradients: Whereas all $\dot{V}A/\dot{Q}$ abnormalities have abnormal AaD_{O_2}, the aAD_{CO_2} is especially high when high $\dot{V}A/\dot{Q}$ units predominate and the aAD_{N_2} is especially high when low $\dot{V}A/\dot{Q}$ units predominate (see Figs. 2-1 and 2-10 and Table 2-1).

*In practice PA_{O_2}, PA_{CO_2}, and PA_{N_2} are the mean pressures for the whole lung (the "collection of units") and are determined by measurement of end-expiratory gas pressures.

*The reason is that PCO_2 and CO_2 content in blood are practically linearly related. Thus as PCO_2 decreases, CO_2 content in blood falls proportionately. Conversely PO_2 and O_2 content are related according to the sigmoid curve of the Hb-O_2 dissociation diagram. At pressures of 100 mm Hg and more, O_2 content is not significantly increased. Thus units of high $\dot{V}A/\dot{Q}$ are limited in the success with which they may deliver O_2 to the blood, whereas there is no practical limitation to the elimination of CO_2.

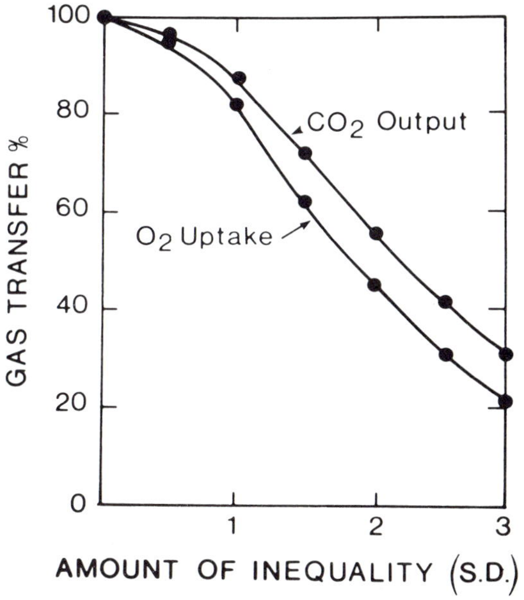

FIG. 2-9. Reduction of O_2 uptake and CO_2 output in a lung model when $\dot{V}A$ and $\dot{Q}$ are mismatched but everything else is unchanged. Note that CO_2 as well as O_2 transfer is interfered with. Log normal distribution of $\dot{V}A/\dot{Q}$ ratios; SD = standard deviation. (From West, J. B.: *Respiratory Physiology.* The Williams & Wilkins Co., Baltimore, 1974, Reprinted, by permission, from *N. Engl. J. Med. 284*:1232, 1971.)

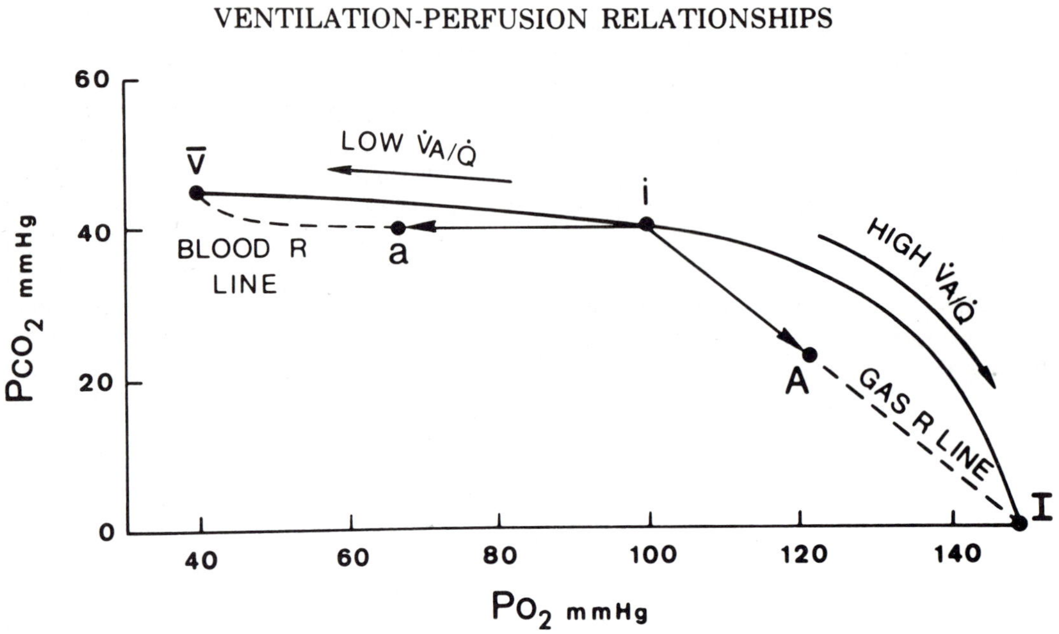

FIG. 2-10. O_2-CO_2 diagram showing the ideal point, i, where, hypothetically, the composition of alveolar gas and end-capillary blood is uniform and no $\dot{V}A/\dot{Q}$ inequality is present ($\dot{V}A/\dot{Q} = 1$). As inequality develops, the arterial (a) and alveolar (A) points diverge along their respective respiratory exchange ratio (R) lines. The mixed alveolar-arterial difference (or "gradient") is the distance between the points. (From West, J. B.: *Respiratory Physiology.* The Williams & Wilkins Co., Baltimore, 1974.)

The limits of the O_2-CO_2 diagram (see Fig. 2-10) should be noted: The point $\bar{v}$ indicates a $\dot{V}A$ of zero; thus $\dot{V}A/\dot{Q} = 0$. At this point blood flows through unventilated alveolar units, e.g., collapsed or occluded alveoli in which right-to-left intrapulmonary shunting therefore occurs. This condition has been discussed previously in the section on shunts. The point I on the O_2-CO_2 diagram indicates a $\dot{Q}$ of zero; thus $\dot{V}A/\dot{Q} = \infty$. Examples include obstruction of blood flow to ventilated alveoli as occurs in pulmonary embolism. Abnormalities of perfusion are discussed in Chapter 7.

SHUNTS, DEAD SPACE, AND $\dot{V}A/\dot{Q}$

The concepts of zero and infinite $\dot{V}A/\dot{Q}$, i.e., of right-to-left shunt and occlusion of blood flow (Fig. 2-11) respectively, can be extended to the discussion of $\dot{V}A/\dot{Q}$ abnormalities (Fig. 2-12) in which these limits are *not* reached. Thus the shunt condition is approached in alveolar-capillary units in which $\dot{V}A/\dot{Q}$ is low, and the vascular-obstructed condition is approached in those units in which $\dot{V}A/\dot{Q}$ is high (Fig. 2-12).

The "wasted" blood flow, as a percentage of total cardiac output, in low $\dot{V}A/\dot{Q}$ may be computed by the same equation used to compute right-to-left shunts (p. 77). Wasted flow and shunt flow may be distinguished by performing the computation for the subject breathing air and then again for the subject breathing oxygen. The computed percent shunt while breathing air provides an estimation of blood flow through alveolar-capillary units with low $\dot{V}A/\dot{Q}$ and also of flow through units with right-to-left shunting. (It is understood that flow through extrapulmonary channels in which there is right-to-left shunting is also included.) On the other hand, the computed percent shunt while breathing oxygen provides an estimation of blood flow only through those alveolar-capillary units (and also extrapulmonary channels) in which right-to-left shunting is present. During oxygen breathing the PA_{O_2} of units with low $\dot{V}A/\dot{Q}$ will increase significantly (it will be less than the PA_{O_2} of normal units only to the extent that PA_{CO_2} is greater than that of the normal units), so that the oxygen content of blood leaving low $\dot{V}A/\dot{Q}$ units is not significantly less than the oxygen content of blood leaving the normal units. (Oxygen content is determined primarily by Hb-O_2 saturation, and saturation is virtually complete when PO_2 is about 100 mm Hg, a condition easily achieved during oxygen breathing even in units with low $\dot{V}A/\dot{Q}$.) Thus the computed percent shunt during air breathing minus the computed percent shunt during oxygen breathing gives the percent shunt or the wasted blood flow through areas of low $\dot{V}A/\dot{Q}$ (see Fig. 2-12).

The "wasted" ventilation in alveolar-cap-

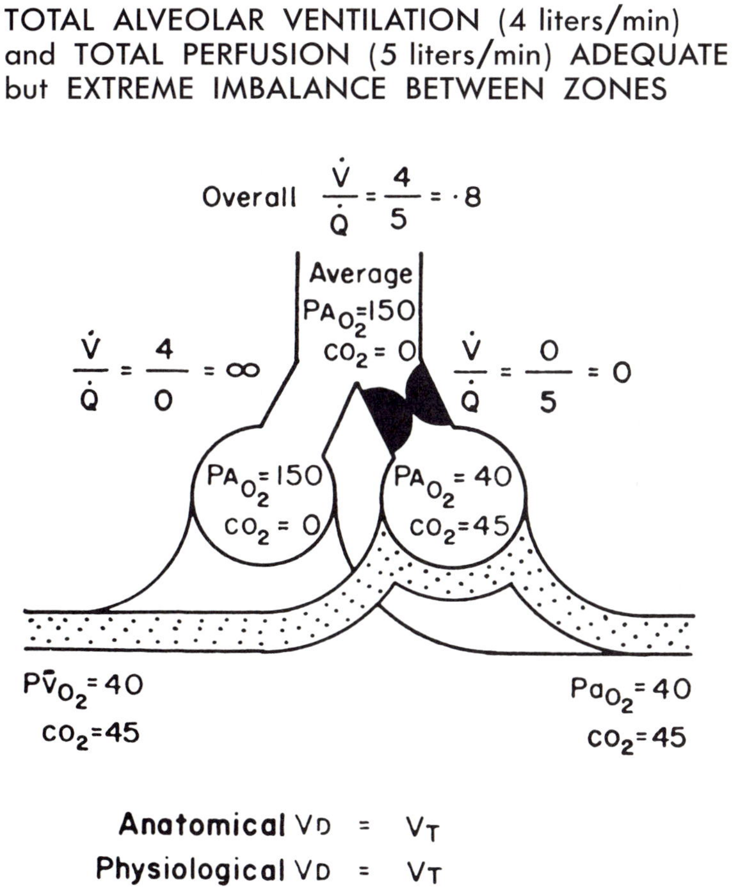

FIG. 2-11. An extreme example in which total ventilation is to one lung and total perfusion is to the other lung. Thus $\dot{V}A/\dot{Q}$ is ∞ in the lung on the left and $\dot{V}A/\dot{Q}$ is zero in the lung on the right, i.e., the limits are vascular obstruction and right-to-left shunt, respectively. Although overall $\dot{V}A$ and $\dot{Q}$ are normal, there is no gas exchange. (From Bates, D. V. et al.[10])

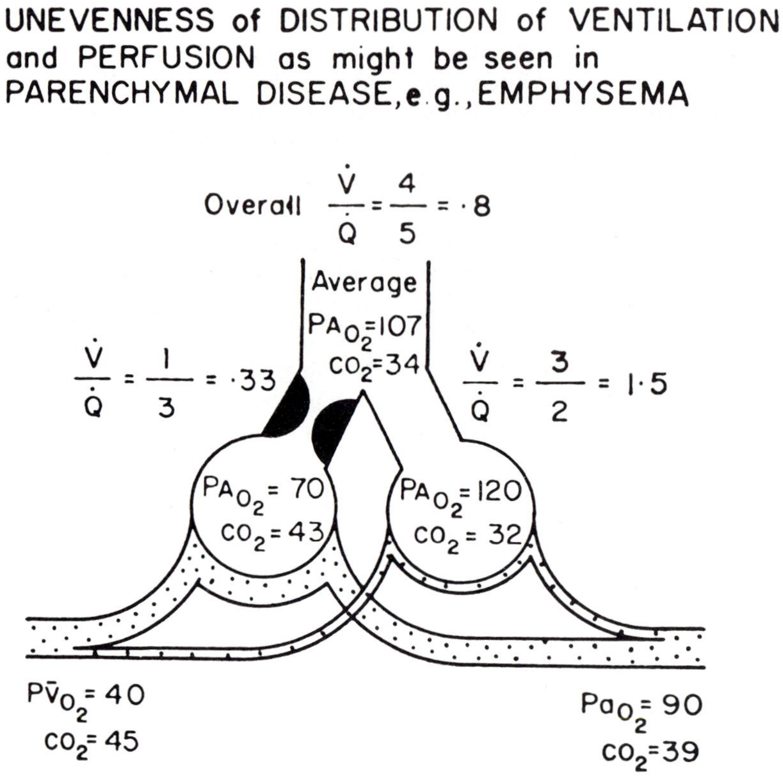

FIG. 2-12. An example of severe inequalities of $\dot{V}_A$ and $\dot{Q}$ within the same lungs as might be encountered clinically, e.g., in obstructive diseases. In this example $V_{D_{anat}}$ is 150 ml, $V_{D_{physiol}}$ is 201 ml, and the difference (alveolar dead space or "wasted" ventilation) is 51 ml. In addition the estimated "wasted" perfusion is about 9% of the total cardiac output, i.e., the shunt-effect. One should also note the abnormal AaD_{O_2} of 17 mm Hg and aAD_{CO_2} of 5 mm Hg. (From Bates, D. V. et al.[10])

illary units with high $\dot{V}_A/\dot{Q}$ may be estimated by computation of the physiologic dead space. Recall that anatomic dead space ($V_{D_{anat}}$) is computed from the Bohr equation in which only alveolar and expired gas are taken into account:[19]

$$V_{D_{anat}} = \frac{(F_{A_{CO_2}} - F_{E_{CO_2}})}{F_{A_{CO_2}}} V_E,$$

where $F_{E_{CO_2}}$ is the CO_2 fraction in expired gas and V_E is the volume of expired gas from a single breath. Physiologic dead space ($V_{D_{physiol}}$) is computed from the same general equation substituting arterial P_{CO_2} for $F_{A_{CO_2}}$ and using units of pressure instead of fractional content:

$$V_{D_{physiol}} = \frac{(Pa_{CO_2} - P_{E_{CO_2}})}{Pa_{CO_2}} V_E.$$

Because the $V_{D_{physiol}}$ equation takes into account the gas *after* exchange within the alveolar capillary units, the numeric figure obtained is an expression of the volume that does not effectively take part in gas exchange, i.e., the volume of wasted ventilation.* Normally

*Analogously, because the $V_{D_{anat}}$ equation takes into account only that gas delivered from the airways and alveoli during expiration, the numeric figure obtained is an expression of the volume that does not come from the alveoli during expiration. Obviously, this volume also does not take part in gas exchange.

VD_{anat} and $VD_{physiol}$ are practically equal. When $VD_{physiol}$ exceeds VD_{anat}, the difference (called alveolar dead space) is due to the additional volume that does not effectively take part in gas exchange, i.e., the wasted ventilation (see Fig. 2-12).

In summary, it is apparent that units with low $\dot{V}A/\dot{Q}$ produce wasted blood flow (the shunt-like effect) and that units with high $\dot{V}A/\dot{Q}$ produce wasted ventilation (the physiologic dead space effect). The combined effects are illustrated in Figure 2-12.

CLINICAL CORRELATES

Ventilation-perfusion abnormalities play a role in virtually all diseases of respiration. In those diseases in which general hypoventilation, right-to-left shunting, or diffusion defects seem to be the primary pathophysiologic process, some degree of $\dot{V}A/\dot{Q}$ abnormality virtually always adds to the hypoxemia and distress of the patient, as mentioned in the previous discussions of these conditions. Similarly, when the basic pathophysiologic problem of disease is production of $\dot{V}A/\dot{Q}$ abnormalities, some degree of right-to-left shunting and diffusion limitation virtually always occurs.[82] The proportional contribution of these three factors may be estimated from the arterial-alveolar gradients shown in Figure 2-1 and Table 2-1. In certain diseases, especially those of the small and medium airways, $\dot{V}A/\dot{Q}$ abnormality is the primary pathophysiologic process. Unfortunately, no simple and reliable method exists for quantifying the abnormality in the clinical setting, especially when dealing with small children. Nonetheless, clinical evaluation of Pa_{O_2}, Pa_{CO_2}, pHa, response to oxygen breathing, physiologic dead space, and measurement of DL when indicated, should permit rather reliable categorization of the relative extent to which the various pathophysiologic processes are operative in a given subject with respiratory disease.

Respiratory Failure

Except for hyperventilation, the usual result of each of the pathophysiologic processes of respiratory disease is some degree of hypoxemia (see Table 2-1). This inability of the respiratory system to maintain normal Pa_{O_2} is indeed—at minimum—the expression of respiratory insufficiency, and it seems unnecessary to attempt strict definitions to distinguish insufficiency from failure. Respiratory disease is respiratory insufficiency; the clinical goal is to prevent respiratory failure and restore respiratory normalcy. The topic, respiratory failure, has been reviewed by a number of authors.[10,30,36,61,75,76,80] Clinical manifestations are outlined in Chapter 1; general principles of recognition and management in Chapters 3, 15, and 16; and relationship to specific diseases in their respective chapters in this text.

It would be most desirable to have firm objective criteria with which to define the point, in the natural history of disease, at which the respiratory system begins to fail. However, this is not possible and one must continue to develop his clinical skills (albeit subjective) in making the signs and symptoms meaningful measures of severity of disease. The use of conventional measurements of pulmonary function for comparison with normal standards is not always practical, especially in the pediatric clinical setting: Techniques are often complicated and require patient cooperation.

However, there are objective measurements of great value that must be employed in the clinical evaluation of every patient admitted to hospital with acute or chronic respiratory disease. These determinations comprise arterial blood buffer base, pH, PCO_2, and PO_2 levels. Without these data clinical evaluation is incomplete and clinical judgment is tenuous.

Estimation of *buffer base* will allow judgment of chronicity of disease and some estimation of the effectiveness of compensatory adaptations to concurrent alterations of pHa, Pa_{CO_2}, and Pa_{O_2}.[95] One must know *pHa* in order to assess the possible influence on the patient's clinical status (especially with regard to the effects of altered hydrogen ion concentration on pulmonary, cardiovascular, and nervous system function and on responsiveness to therapeutic drugs) and to determine the appropriate corrective therapy.

Pa_{CO_2} often is the single "pulmonary function test" of value to the clinician. Many authors have suggested that a Pa_{CO_2} of 50 mm Hg or higher defines the state of respiratory failure in a given patient. As a generalization this concept is valuable; however, there are mitigating factors.

(1) Since the number 50 is based on the understanding that normal Pa_{CO_2} is about 40 mm Hg, it should be recalled that normal Pa_{CO_2} of the infant and very young child is lower (33.8 ± 3.7 mm Hg),[1] so that 50 mm Hg may be too high for this group.

(2) On occasion, progressive deterioration of lung function may not yet have reached the stage at which Pa_{CO_2} is at the upper acceptable limit, e.g., 50 mm Hg, so that a Pa_{CO_2} below the limit may give false reassurance. (The basis for this statement has been established in the previous discussions of shunts, diffusion defects, and $\dot{V}A/\dot{Q}$ abnormalities.) Certainly, if failure has been established, the limit will be reached (and exceeded), but the opportunity to provide early corrective therapy may have been missed.

(3) Since a single determination of Pa_{CO_2} can be misleading, it is imperative (whenever possible) to have two or more determinations, suitably separated in time as the clinical condition of the patient dictates, in order to establish the progression (or resolution) of the pathophysiologic process. For example, elevation of Pa_{CO_2} from 29 to 40 mm Hg in the span of 30 minutes could be a more ominous sign than a change of Pa_{CO_2} from 48 to 50 over a period of 2 hours.

Pa_{O_2} most often provides the first reason for establishing respiratory therapy. Sufficient concentrations of inspired oxygen must be given to maintain Pa_{O_2} above 50 mm Hg, while recognizing that excessive concentration of inspired oxygen can be poisonous to the lung directly with time.[17] Nonetheless, the acceptable minimal Pa_{O_2} must be maintained. (It should be noted that a Pa_{O_2} of 70 mm Hg produces over 90% saturation of normal hemoglobin with oxygen. However, it should also be noted that the total oxygen supply to tissues is determined by both the $Hb\text{-}O_2$ saturation and the hemoglobin content of the blood. Therefore, severe anemia must be corrected in order to provide optimal cardiopulmonary therapy.) Pa_{O_2} is also used as a criterion for establishing the diagnosis of respiratory failure, and it is generally suggested that a Pa_{O_2} below 50 mm Hg indicates failure.

Thus the diagnosis of respiratory failure can stand on solid ground, provided proper use is made of the blood gas and chemistry laboratories, and this information is integrated into the clinical manifestations of disease as discussed in Chapter 1.

REFERENCES

1. Albert, M. S. and R. W. Winters: Acid-base equilibrium of blood in normal infants. *Pediatrics 37*:728, 1966.
2. Auchincloss, J. H., Jr.: Ventilatory disturbances in disease. In *Handbook of Physiology, Section 3, Respiration,* Volume II, W. O. Fenn and H. Rahn (Eds). American Physiological Society, Washington, D.C., 1965.
3. Auchincloss, J. H., Jr., E. Cook and A. D. Renzetti: Clinical and physiological aspects of a case of obesity polycythemia and alveolar hypoventilation. *J. Clin. Invest. 34*:1537, 1955.
4. Auld, P. A. M.: Concepts in pulmonary physiology. In *Pulmonary Physiology of the Fetus, Newborn and Child,* E. M. Scarpelli and P. A. M. Auld (Eds.). Lea & Febiger, Philadelphia, 1975.
5. Austrian, R., J. H. McClement, A. D. Renzetti, Jr., K. W. Donald, R. L. Riley and A. Cournand: Clinical and physiologic features of some types of pulmonary diseases with impairment of alveolar-capillary diffusion. The syndrome of "alveolar-capillary block." *Am. J. Med. 11*:667, 1951.

6. Avery, E. E., E. T. Mörch and D. W. Benson: Critically crushed chests. *J. Thorac. Surg. 32*:291, 1956.
7. Avery, M. E., V. Chernick, R. E. Dutton and S. Permutt: Ventilatory response to inspired carbon dioxide in infants and adults. *J. Appl. Physiol. 18*:895, 1963.
8. Avery, M. E. and J. Mead: Surface properties in relation to atelectasis and hyaline membrane disease. *Am. J. Dis. Child. 97*:517, 1959.
9. Barrera, F., M. M. Reidenberg and W. L. Winters: Pulmonary function in the obese patient. *Am. J. Med. Sci. 254*:785, 1967.
10. Bates, D. V., P. T. Macklem and R. V. Christie: *Respiratory Function in Disease.* W. B. Saunders Co., Philadelphia, 1971.
11. Baum, G. L. (Ed.): *Textbook of Pulmonary Diseases.* Little, Brown and Co., Boston, 1974.
12. Bedell, G. N., W. R. Wilson and P. M. Seebohn: Pulmonary function in obese persons. *J. Clin. Invest. 37*:1049, 1958.
13. Brady, J. P. and E. Ceruti: Chemoreceptor reflexes in the newborn infant: effects of varying degrees of hypoxia on heart rate and ventilation in a warm environment. *J. Physiol. (Lond.) 184*:444, 1966.
14. Brady, J. P. and W. H. Tooley: Cardiovascular and respiratory reflexes in the newborn. *Pediatr. Clin. North Am. 13*:801, 1966.
15. Brown, B. St. J., H. Ma, J. S. Dunbar and D. W. MacEwan: Foreign bodies in the tracheobronchial tree in childhood. *J. Can. Assoc. Radiol. 14*:158, 1963.
16. Burwell, C. S., E. D. Robin, R. D. Whaley and A. G. Bickelmann: Extreme obesity associated with alveolar hypoventilation—a Pickwickian syndrome. *Am. J. Med. 21*:811, 1956.
17. Campbell, E. J. M.: The management of acute respiratory failure in chronic bronchitis and emphysema. *Am. Rev. Respir. Dis. 96*:626, 1967.
18. Ceruti, E.: Chemoreceptor reflexes in the newborn infant: effect of cooling on the response to hypoxia. *Pediatrics 37*:556, 1966.
19. Clutario, B. C.: Clinical pulmonary function. In *Pulmonary Physiology of the Fetus, Newborn and Child,* E. M. Scarpelli and P. A. M. Auld (Eds.). Lea & Febiger, Philadelphia, 1975.
20. Clutton-Brock, J.: The cerebral effects of overventilation. *Br. J. Anaesth. 29*:111, 1957.
21. Comroe, J. H., Jr., R. E. Forster, A. B. DuBois, W. A. Briscoe and E. Carlsen: *The Lung. Clinical Physiology and Pulmonary Function Tests.* Year Book Medical Publishers, Chicago, 1962.
22. Condorelli, S. and E. M. Scarpelli: Fetal breathing: induction in utero and effects of vagotomy and barbiturates. *J. Pediatr. 88*:94, 1976.
23. Costelli, J. F., D. C. Moriarty, M. A. Branthwaite, M. Turner-Warwick and B. Corrin: Diagnosis and management of alveolar proteinosis: the role of electron microscopy. *Thorax 30*:121, 1975.
24. Cournand, A. R., R. L. Riley, S. E. Bradley, E. S. Breed, R. P. Noble, H. D. Lauson, M. I. Gregerson and D. W. Richards, Jr.: Studies of the circulation in clinical shock. *Surgery 13*:964, 1943.
25. Craig, A. B. Underwater swimming and loss of consciousness. *J.A.M.A. 176*:255, 1961.
26. Craig, A.B.: Causes of loss of consciousness during underwater swimming. *J. Appl. Physiol. 16*:583, 1961.
27. Cross, K. W., J. M. D. Hooper and T. E. Oppé.: The effect of inhalation of carbon dioxide in air on the respiration of the full-term and premature infant. *J. Physiol. (Lond.) 122*:264, 1953.
28. Dobell, A. R. C., J. R. Gutelius and D. R. Murphy: Acidosis following respiratory alkalosis in thoracic operations with and without heart-lung bypass. *J. Thorac. Cardiovasc. Surg. 39*:312, 1960.
29. Doll, E., W. Kuhlo, H. Steim and J. Keul: The genesis of cor pulmonale in the Pickwick syndrome. *Dtsch. Med. Wochenschr. 93*:2361, 1968.
30. Downes, J. J., T. Fulgencio and R. C. Raphaely: Acute respiratory failure in infants and children. *Pediatr. Clin. North Am. 19*:423, 1972.
31. Eichenholz, A., R. O. Mulhausen, W. E. Anderson and F. M. MacDonald: Primary hypocapnia: a cause of metabolic acidosis. *J. Appl. Physiol. 17*:383, 1962.
32. Epstein, M. H. and J. S. O'Connor: Destructive effects of prolonged status epilepticus. *J. Neurol. Neurosurg. Psychiatry 29*:251, 1966.
33. Falsetti, H. L., J. S. Hanson and B. S. Tabakin: Obesity-hypoventilation syndrome in siblings. *Am. Rev. Respir. Dis. 90*:105, 1964.
34. Fanconi, A. and G. A. Rose: The ionized, complexed, and protein-bound fractions of calcium in plasma: an investigation of patients with various diseases which affect calcium metabolism, with an additional study of the role of calcium ion in the prevention of tetany. *Q. J. Med. 27*:463, 1958.
35. Fenn, W. O., H. Rahn, A. B. Otis and L. E. Chadwick: Physiologic observations on hyperventilation at altitude with intermittent pressure breathing by the pneumolator. *J. Appl. Physiol. 1*:773, 1949.
36. Filley, G. F.: *Pulmonary Insufficiency and Respiratory Failure.* Lea & Febiger, Philadelphia, 1967.
37. Finley, T. N., E. W. Swenson and J. H. Comroe, Jr.: The cause of arterial hypoxemia at rest in patients with "alveolar-capillary block syndrome." *J. Clin. Invest. 41*:618, 1962.
38. Fraser, R. G. and J. A. P. Paré: *Diagnosis of Diseases of the Chest.* W. B. Saunders Co., Philadelphia, London, Toronto, 1970.

39. Fulmer, J. D. and R. G. Crystal: The biochemical basis of pulmonary function. In *The Biochemical Basis of Pulmonary Function,* R. G. Crystal (Ed.). Dekker, New York, Basel, 1976.
40. Gaensler, E. A.: Lung displacement: abdominal enlargement, pleural space disorders, deformities of the thoracic cage. In *Handbook of Physiology, Section 3: Respiration,* Volume II, W. O. Fenn and H. Rahn (Eds.). American Physiological Society, Washington, D.C., 1965.
41. Gotoh, F., J. S. Meyer and Y. Takagi: Cerebral effects of hyperventilation in man. *Arch. Neurol. (Chicago) 12*:410, 1965.
42. Grant, J. L. and W. Arnold, Jr.: Idiopathic hypoventilation. *J.A.M.A. 194*:119, 1965.
43. Greene, D. G.: Drowning. In *Handbook of Physiology, Section 3, Respiration,* Volume II, W. O. Fenn and H. Rahn (Eds.). American Physiological Society, Washington, D.C., 1965.
44. Gregory, G. A., J. A. Kitterman, R. H. Phibbs, W. H. Tooley and W. K. Hamilton: Treatment of the idiopathic respiratory-distress syndrome with continuous positive airway pressure. *N. Engl. J. Med. 284*:1333, 1971.
45. Harris, J. O., J. R. Castle, E. W. Swenson and A. J. Block: Lobar lavage: therapeutic benefit in pulmonary alveolar filling disorders. *Chest 65*:655, 1974.
46. Hill, L. and M. Flack: The influence of oxygen inhalations on muscular work. *J. Physiol. (Lond.) 40*:347, 1910.
47. Hiroka, M., Y. Inaba and T. Ohno: The Pickwickian syndrome in a child. *Tohoku J. Exp. Med. 98*:363, 1969.
48. Huber, G. L., L. H. Edmunds, Jr. and T. N. Finley: Effect of experimental saline lavage on pulmonary mechanics and morphology. *Am. Rev. Respir. Dis. 104*:337, 1971.
49. Johnson, C. The physiology of hyperventilation. In *Hyperventilation and Hysteria,* T. P. Lowry (Ed.). Charles C Thomas, Springfield, Ill., 1967.
50. Kattwinkel, J., B. S. Nearman, A. A. Fanaroff, P. G. Katona and M. H. Klaus: Apnea of prematurity. *J. Pediatr. 86*:588, 1975.
51. Kety, S., B. D. Polis, P. S. Nadler and C. F. Schmidt: The blood flow and oxygen consumption of the human brain in diabetic acidosis and coma. *J. Clin. Invest. 27*:500, 1948.
52. Kety, S. S. and C. F. Schmidt: The effects of active and passive hyperventilation on cerebral blood flow, cerebral oxygen consumption, cardiac output and blood pressure of normal young men. *J. Clin. Invest. 25*:105, 1946.
53. Lambroso, C. T. and P. Lerman: Breathholding spells (cyanotic and pallid infantile syncope). *Pediatrics 39*:563, 1967.
54. Levine, O. R. and R. B. Mellins: Liquid balance in the lung and pulmonary edema. In *Pulmonary Physiology of the Fetus, Newborn and Child,* E. M. Scarpelli and P. A. M. Auld (Eds.). Lea & Febiger, Philadelphia, 1975.
55. Macklem, P. T.: Airway obstruction and collateral ventilation. *Physiol. Rev. 51*:368, 1971.
56. Mazyck, E. M., J. T. Bonner, H. M. Herd and P. N. Symbas: Pulmonary lavage for childhood pulmonary alveolar proteinosis. *J. Pediatr. 80*:839, 1972.
57. McIlroy, M. B.: Pulmonary shunts. In *Handbook of Physiology, Section 3, Respiration,* Volume II, W. O. Fenn and H. Rahn (Eds.). American Physiological Society, Washington, D.C., 1965.
58. McIntosh, H. E., E. H. Estes and J. V. Warren: The mechanism of cough syncope. *Am. Heart J. 52*:70, 1956.
59. McKerrow, C. and A. B. Otis: Oxygen cost of hyperventilation. *J. Appl. Physiol. 9*:375, 1956.
60. Mellins, R. B., H. H. Balfour, Jr., G. M. Turino and R. W. Winters: Failure of automatic control of ventilation (Ondine's curse). *Medicine 49*:487, 1970.
61. Mellins, R. B., V. Chernick, C. F. Doershuk, J. J. Downes, J. C. Sinclair and W. W. Waring: Respiratory care in infants and children. *Am. Rev. Respir. Dis. 105*:461, 1972.
62. Meyer, A., E. Beck and M. Shepherd: Unusually severe lesions in the brain following status epilepticus. *J. Neurol. Neurosurg. Psychiatry 18*:24, 1955.
63. Meyer J. S. and F. Gotoh: Metabolic and electroencephalographic effects of hyperventilation. *Arch. Neurol. (Chicago) 5*:539, 1960.
64. Miller, W. F., R. L. Johnson, Jr. and I. E. Cushing: Mechanics of breathing. In *Clinical Cardiopulmonary Physiology,* B. G. Gordon (Ed.). Grune & Stratton, New York, 1960.
65. Modell, J. H., H. W. Calderwood, B. C. Ruiz, J. B. Downs and R. Chapman, Jr.: Effects of ventilatory patterns on arterial oxygenation after near-drowning in sea water. *Anesthesiology 40*:376, 1974.
66. Motoyama, E. K., G. Rivard, F. Acheson and C. Cook: Adverse effect of maternal hyperventilation on the fetus. *Lancet 1*:286, 1966.
67. Moya, F., H. Morishima, S. M. Schnider and L. S. James: Influence of maternal hyperventilation on the newborn infant. *Am. J. Obstet. Gynecol. 91*:76, 1965.
68. Murdock, A. I., B. S. L. Kidd, M. A. Lilewellyn, M. McCreid and P. R. Swyer: Intrapulmonary venous admixture in the respiratory distress syndrome. *Biol. Neonate 15*:1, 1970.
69. Murray, J. F.: The adult respiratory distress syndrome (may it rest in peace). *Am. Rev. Respir. Dis. 111*:716, 1975.

70. Nadas, A. S. and D. C. Fyler: Pediatric Cardiology, W. B. Saunders Co., Philadelphia, 1972.
71. Naimark, A. and R. M. Cherniack: Compliance of the respiratory system and its components in health and obesity. *J. Appl. Physiol. 15*:377, 1960.
72. Nattie, E. E., D. Bartlett, Jr. and A. A. Rozycki: Central alveolar hypoventilation in a child: an evaluation using a whole body plethysmograph. *Am. Rev. Respir. Dis. 112*:259, 1975.
73. Nitzan, M., S. Spitzer and E. Elian: Obesity-hypoventilation (Pickwickian) syndrome in a child. *Isr. J. Med. Sci. 4*:264, 1968.
74. Pauli, H. G., H. Reidwil, F. Reubi and W. H. Wegmullar: H^+ and renal failure as factors in uremic hyperventilation. *Clin. Sci. 25*:37, 1963.
75. Petty, T. L.: The clinical spectrum of acute respiratory failure. Management of acute and chronic respiratory insufficiency in chronic airways obstruction. In *Textbook of Pulmonary Diseases,* G. L. Baum (Ed.). Little, Brown and Co., Boston, 1974.
76. Petty, T. L.: *Intensive and Rehabilitative Respiratory Care.* Lea & Febiger, Philadelphia, 1974.
77. Petty, T. L.: The adult respiratory distress syndrome (confessions of a "lumper"). *Am. Rev. Respir. Dis. 111*:713, 1975.
78. Petty, T. L. and L. D. Hudson: Acute pulmonary injury and repair (the adult respiratory distress syndrome): the 16th Aspen Lung Conference. *Chest 66*:supplement, 1974.
79. Polgar, G. and V. Promadhat: *Pulmonary Function Testing in Children.* W. B. Saunders Co., Philadelphia, 1971.
80. Pontoppidan, H., B. Geffin and E. Lowenstein: *Acute Respiratory Failure in the Adult.* Little, Brown and Co., Boston, 1973.
81. Radford, E. P., Jr., B. G. Ferris, Jr. and B. C. Kriete: Clinical use of a nomogram to estimate proper ventilation during artificial respiration. *N. Engl. J. Med. 251*:877, 1954.
82. Rahn, H. and W. O. Fenn: *A Graphical Analysis of the Respiratory Gas Exchange. The O_2-CO_2 Diagram.* The American Physiological Society, Washington, D.C., 1955.
83. Rankin, J. and E. H. Chester: Diffuse interstitial disease of the lung as a cause of pulmonary insufficiency: the alveolar-capillary block syndrome. In *Textbook of Pulmonary Diseases,* G. L. Baum (Ed.). Little, Brown and Co., Boston, 1974.
84. Ratto, O., W. A. Briscoe, J. W. Morton and J. Comroe: Anoxemia secondary to polycythemia and polycythemia secondary to anoxemia. *Am. J. Med. 19*:958, 1955.
85. Reardon, A. S., M. L. Bauman and E. J. Haddad: Respiratory alkalosis; a frequent phenomenon observed in newborn infants. *Am. J. Dis. Child. 88*:371, 1965.
86. Richter, T., J. R. West and A. P. Fishman: The syndrome of alveolar hypoventilation and diminished sensitivity of the respiratory center. *N. Engl. J. Med. 256*:1165, 1957.
87. Rodman, T. and H. P. Close: The primary hypoventilation syndrome. *Am. J. Med. 26*:808, 1959.
88. Rodman, T., M. E. Resnick, R. D. Berkowitz, J. F. Fennelly and J. Olivia: Alveolar hypoventilation due to involvement of the respiratory center by obscure disease of the central nervous system. *Am. J. Med. 32*:208, 1962.
89. Ross, J. C., R. Frayser and J. B. Hickam: A study of the mechanism by which exercise increases the pulmonary diffusing capacity for carbon monoxide. *J. Clin. Invest. 38*:916, 1959.
90. Rudolph, A. M.: *Congenital Diseases of the Heart.* Year Book Medical Publishers, Chicago, 1974.
91. Safar, P., B. Berman, E. Diamond, K. Hoffman, W. Holtley, H. Moore and B. Scoville: Cuffed tracheotomy tube vs. tank respirator for prolonged artificial ventilation. *Arch. Phys. Med. Rehabil. 43*:487, 1962.
92. Scarpelli, E. M.: *The Surfactant System of the Lung.* Lea & Febiger, Philadelphia, 1968.
93. Scarpelli, E. M. and S. Condorelli: Nonventilatory functions of the lung. In *Pulmonary Physiology of the Fetus, Newborn and Child,* E. M. Scarpelli and P. A. M. Auld (Eds.). Lea & Febiger, Philadelphia, 1975.
94. Sieker, H. O., E. H. Estes, Jr., G. A. Kelser and H. D. McIntosh: A cardiopulmonary syndrome associated with extreme obesity. *J. Clin. Invest. 34*:916, 1955.
95. Sinclair, J. C.: Pulmonary-renal relationships in acid-base balance. In *Pulmonary Physiology of the Fetus, Newborn and Child,* E. M. Scarpelli and P. A. M. Auld (Eds.). Lea & Febiger, Philadelphia, 1975.
96. Stahlman, M.: Ventilation control in the newborn. *Am. J. Dis. Child. 101*:216, 1961.
97. Tooley, W. H., M. Klaus, E. C. Costley, W. Way and R. Rock: The lung and acid-base balance in the newborn. *Am. J. Dis. Child. 104*:520, 1962.
98. Tsitouris, G. and A. Fertakis: Alveolar hypoventilation due to respiratory center dysfunction of unknown cause. *Am. J. Med. 39*:173, 1965.
99. Weibel, E. R.: *Morphometry of the Human Lung.* Academic Press, New York, 1963.
100. West, J. B.: *Ventilation/Blood Flow and Gas Exchange.* Blackwell Scientific Publications, Oxford, 1965.
101. Wilson, J. L. and D. G. Dickinson: Prevention of longtime dependence of poliomyelitis patients on tank respirator. *J.A.M.A. 158*:551, 1955.
102. Wollman, H., S. C. Alexander, P. J. Cohen, T. C. Smith, P. E. Chase and R. A. Van Der Molen:

Cerebral circulation during general anesthesia and hyperventilation in man. *Anesthesiology 26*:329, 1965.

103. Wright, G. W. Tuberculosis and pneumonia. In *Handbook of Physiology, Section 3, Respiration,* Volume II, W. O. Fenn and H. Rahn (Eds.). American Physiological Society, Washington, D.C., 1965.

Airway Management, Mechanical Ventilation and Cardiopulmonary Resuscitation

JOHN J. DOWNES
ALLEN I. GOLDBERG

3

. . . A simple child, that lightly draws its breath,
And feels its life in every limb,
What should it know of death? . . .
"We Are Seven"
WILLIAM WORDSWORTH

Clinical medicine is an art rather than a science. Evidence for this statement abounds in those aspects of clinical medicine described in this chapter. A physician does not learn the art of resuscitation and respiratory care from a book, but rather from practice under supervision. However, the physician who reads about his art and its scientific foundations can improve his skill, judge the techniques of others, and advance the art to improve the welfare of many patients.

This chapter deals with the art of maintaining the airway, ventilating the lungs, and resuscitating the heart of the critically ill infant and child. Many of the aspects of anatomy and physiology are presented in the companion volume to this text.[114b] Herein we aim to describe principles as well as techniques, to present our opinions and the bases for them, and to refer the reader to the appropriate literature, especially where controversy exists. We think the principles put forth are sound and widely applicable. The techniques described provide therapeutic guidelines to be used by the physician as he determines best for each patient.

Airway Management

HISTORY

Upper airway obstruction has been recognized as a cause of death for many centuries. The Greek surgeon Antyllus (2nd century, A.D.) describes one of the earliest documented attempts to relieve potentially fatal airway obstruction by means of tracheostomy: "When, therefore, we engage in the operation we slit open a part of the *arteria aspera** (for it is dangerous to divide the whole) below the top of the windpipe, about the third or fourth ring. . . . Wherefore, bending the patient's head backwards, so as to bring the windpipe better into view, we are to make a transverse incision between two of the rings, so that it not be the cartilage which is divided, but the membrane connecting the cartilage."[6]† Andreas Vesalius in his monumental work on human anatomy, *De Humani Corporis Fabrica,* describes the technique of tracheotomy and insufflation of air into the lungs of a newly delivered animal fetus whose heart was fibrillating; ventilation of the lungs resulted in restoration of heart beat and a normal arterial pulse.[133] In 1796, Herholdt and Rafn described a tactile method of orotracheal intubation of victims of near-drowning.[61] Desault in 1801 successfully introduced a catheter through the nose into the trachea in a patient with severe glottic edema.[30] The catheter was left in place for 36 hours, then removed, and the patient recovered. Chaussier in 1806 described a curved metal tube that was introduced by palpation into the larynx of the newborn for resuscitation.[23]

Although numerous reports of tracheal intubation and tracheostomy utilizing a variety of tubes appeared in the literature during the 19th century, the modern era of airway management begins with the report of Trendelenburg in 1871.[132] He described the use of cuffed metal tracheostomy tubes to prevent aspiration during surgical anesthesia, and also provided the first detailed modern account of the surgical technique of tracheotomy in man. In 1878, the Glasgow surgeon, William MacEwen, employed a metallic orotracheal tube in lieu of tracheostomy for the treatment of severe subglottic edema; he later utilized the method for anesthetic management during surgical procedures in the oropharynx.[88,89] In the subsequent decade, O'Dwyer developed a technique for the insertion of a small brass stent, with the aid of a metal introducer, through the mouth and into the glottis and subglottic region for the relief of airway obstruction due to diptheria.[98] This technique became widespread throughout the western world and persisted for nearly 50 years.

Between 1910 and 1925, Chevalier Jackson synthesized the work of the preceding century into a systematic approach to the management of airway obstruction with direct laryngoscopy, bronchoscopy, and tracheostomy.[68,69] Endotracheal anesthesia utilizing flexible rubber tubes was developed by Rowbotham and Magill to meet the requirements of plastic surgery of the head and neck during World War I.[110] By the early 1930's, Jackson's approach to airway management had become universally accepted, and tracheostomy with double-lumen silver tubes for all ages had become the standard method for management of severe airway obstruction. Concurrently, orotracheal intubation for anesthesia in a wide variety of operations was perfected.[50]

**Arteria aspera* is a medieval Latin term for the trachea.

†This quotation appears in the works of Paulus Aegenita (625–690 A.D.), who refers to other less precise descriptions of tracheotomy by various surgeons of antiquity.[6] When the modern vertical tracheal incision (see p. 107) was introduced remains uncertain.

Although sporadic reports on the use of endotracheal tubes for long-term intubation appeared during the 150 years after Desault, it was the report of Brandstater in 1962, describing success with plastic nasotracheal tubes for prolonged airway management in the newborn, that stimulated the resurgence of interest in this technique.[16] In 1965, Allen and Steven,[5] McDonald and Stocks,[93] and others reported their satisfactory long-term results with polyvinylchloride nasotracheal tubes in the treatment of upper airway obstruction and of acute respiratory failure in pediatric patients requiring mechanical ventilation. At the same time, Aberdeen developed an anatomically shaped single-lumen polyvinylchloride tracheostomy tube for infants and small children;[2] it has gradually replaced the metal Jackson tubes. In 1966 and 1967, Striker and Downes[33,123] reported a high incidence of subglottic stenosis associated with nasotracheal intubation for severe laryngotracheitis in infants, and advocated a return to tracheostomy with the use of the Aberdeen tube for that disease.

At present, both tracheostomy and nasotracheal intubation play a major role in the airway management of critically ill infants and children. Development of polyvinylchloride and silastic tubes has greatly reduced the complications and difficulties formerly encountered with rubber endotracheal and metal tracheostomy tubes, especially in the small infant[2,122,127] We can anticipate the eventual development of materials with less tissue reactivity and improvement in the design of artificial airway systems.

DISORDERS REQUIRING INTENSIVE AIRWAY MANAGEMENT

The common disorders that require intensive respiratory care and an artificial tracheal airway are outlined in Table 3-1. Included are disorders of the upper airway (from the nares to the carina), disorders associated with cardiopulmonary failure, disorders of the nervous system that alter respiratory control, and neuromuscular diseases that cause failure of mechanical function of the thoracic wall and diaphragmatic muscles. The diagnosis and estimate of severity of upper airway obstruction can be made readily by using a scoring system (Table 3-2)[36] and measurement of Pa_{CO_2} and Pa_{O_2}.[136] The use of a scoring system facilitates communication. Determining the cause of airway obstruction requires careful examination of the nares, oropharynx, and chest, as well as lateral neck and anteroposterior chest roentgenograms. Radiographic examination identifies most, but not all, aspirated foreign bodies. Patients with airway obstruction should receive high inspired concentrations of oxygen throughout the period of transportation, evaluation, and initial therapy; it is progressive hypoxemia that causes cardiac arrest, brain damage, and death in these patients. Examination of the oropharynx with a tongue blade can be carried out safely if the patient receives oxygen before and after a brief examination.

The criteria for the diagnosis of life-threatening impairment of gas exchange in the lungs (acute respiratory failure) in infants and children with cardiopulmonary disease and neuromuscular disease are presented in Tables 3-3 and 3-4. These patients require an artificial tracheal airway for effective tracheobronchial toilet and mechanical ventilation.

INITIAL TREATMENT OF UPPER AIRWAY OBSTRUCTION

Once the clinical diagnosis of upper airway obstruction has been established, secretions must be aspirated from the nares and oropharynx. *Oxygen* in a concentration of 40 to 60% usually relieves the hypoxemia that inevitably accompanies serious airway obstruction. Oral fluid intake should be prohibited in patients with airway obstruction, and intravenous fluids given to correct existing dehydration and provide for maintenance fluid requirements. In the stuporous or unconscious patient with soft-tissue obstruction, insertion of an oropharyngeal airway ordi-

TABLE 3-1. Disorders of Infants and Children Commonly Requiring an Artificial Tracheal Airway

Upper Airway Obstruction	
Choanal atresia	Tracheal stenosis
Hypertrophied tonsils/adenoids	vascular ring
Epiglottitis	post-tracheotomy
Vocal cord paralysis	Foreign body
Laryngotracheitis	Neoplasm
infectious	cyst, granuloma,
foreign body	lymphangioma
Subglottic edema	Hypoplasia
post intubation	Pierre-Robin syndrome
allergic	congenital laryngotracheal
Subglottic stenosis	Inhalation burns
congenital	
post-intubation	
Cardiopulmonary Failure	
Status asthmaticus	Pneumonitis
Bronchopneumonia (bronchiolitis)	Pulmonary edema
Cystic fibrosis	Pulmonary hemorrhage
Aspiration syndrome	Pulmonary hypertension
Near-drowning	Pulmonary contusion
Inhalation burn	Oxygen toxicity
Nervous System/Neuromuscular Failure	
Head trauma	Polyneuritis
Cerebral hypoxia	(Guillain-Barré syndrome)
Encephalitis	Poliomyelitis
Encephalopathy	Myopathy
Poisoning/drug ingestion	Myasthenia gravis
Status epilepticus	Tetanus

TABLE 3-2. Upper Airway Obstruction Score

	0	1	2
Stridor	None	Inspiratory	Inspiratory and expiratory
Cough	None	Hoarse cry	Bark
Retractions and nasal flaring	None	Flaring and suprasternal retractions	Flaring and suprasternal retractions plus subcostal, intercostal retractions
Cyanosis	None	In air	In 40% O_2
Inspiratory breath sounds	Normal	Harsh with wheezing or rhonchi	Delayed

TABLE 3-3. Criteria for Diagnosis of Respiratory Failure in Infants and Children with Acute Pulmonary Disease*

Clinical	
	Decreased or absent inspiratory breath sounds
	Severe inspiratory retractions and use of accessory muscles
	Cyanosis in 40% ambient oxygen
	Depressed level of consciousness and response to pain
	Poor skeletal muscle tone
Physiologic	
	$Pa_{CO_2} > 75$ mm Hg
	$Pa_{O_2} < 100$ mm Hg in 100% oxygen

*Three clinical plus one physiologic criteria = acute respiratory failure

narily bypasses the obstruction and permits restoration of adequate ventilation.[107a,114] In the conscious patient, an endotracheal tube lubricated with a water-soluble cream and gently inserted through the larger naris into the nasopharynx is well tolerated and provides an adequate nasopharyngeal airway.[107a] The tube should be taped so that the tip lies below the level of the uvula, but well above the epiglottis; this position should be confirmed by oral examination with a tongue blade.

Emergency tracheostomy performed outside the operating room without prior orotracheal intubation and controlled ventilation is rarely, if ever, indicated. Tracheostomy under such conditions has been associated with an appalling mortality and morbidity,[5,99] which is virtually eliminated by orotracheal intubation, general anesthesia, and performance of the procedure in an operating room by a qualified anesthesiologist and surgeon.[5]

TABLE 3-4. Criteria of Respiratory Failure in Infants and Children with Neuromuscular Disease*

Clinical	
	Weak to absent cough reflex
	Weak to absent gag reflex
	Incompetent swallowing mechanism
	Pooled oropharyngeal secretions
Physiologic	
	Vital capacity < 12 ml/kg
	$Pa_{O_2} < 60$ torr (in air)

*Two clinical plus one physiologic criteria = impending respiratory failure

The most common form of upper airway obstruction requiring intensive respiratory care is viral laryngotracheitis with subglottic inflammation and edema (croup). Initial steps in therapy include administration of oxygen with high humidity and intravenous fluids. Humidity and systemic hydration help liquefy the secretions in the larynx and trachea, thereby decreasing the hazard of thick, inspissated secretions producing further obstruction. The efficacy of systemic corticosteroids in this disease remains controversial.[42,71]

An airway obstruction score of 4 or more (see Table 3-2) in croup warrants administration of an aerosolized vasoconstricting drug, which may decrease subglottic edema. The need for an artificial tracheal airway in this disease appears to be reduced by the inhalation of aerosolized vasoconstricting agents such as racemic epinephrine.[4,128]

A dose of approximately 100 μg/kg/min. of racemic epinephrine is usually effective and can be given as follows: (1) A volume of 0.05 ml/kg of 2.25% racemic epinephrine is diluted with sterile saline solution to make 3.0 ml; (2) this solution is nebulized at an oxygen flow of 15 l/min. and delivered by mask for a total of 10 minutes. This procedure has been associated with a remarkable reduction in the upper airway obstruction score, an increase in Pa_{O_2}, and a decrease of an elevated Pa_{CO_2}. Aerosol treatments may be required at 1- to 4-hour intervals for periods as long as 36 hours.[128] Whether aqueous l-epinephrine or other vasoconstricting drugs such as phenylephrine[52] are effective has not been determined.

If a score of 7 or more persists, despite this therapy, consideration must be given to immediate insertion of an artificial tracheal airway. We do not advocate the use of aerosol therapy for croup on an outpatient basis.

Aerosolized epinephrine in the dosage required can produce tachycardia, and the patient's heart rate and electrocardiogram (ECG) should be monitored continuously during and immediately following treatment. Because the improvement may be transient, the patient should be kept in the hospital for at least 24 hours after the last treatment.

Epinephrine aerosol has not been effective in children with acute epiglottitis. In our opinion and that of others,[91] once diagnosis of epiglottitis is made, the patient should have an artificial tracheal airway (nasotracheal tube or tracheostomy) inserted.[3,11] Since many of these patients have systemic *H. influenzae* infection, high doses of appropriate antibiotics should be administered immediately.

In cases of known or suspected foreign body aspiration, bronchoscopy is required. Prior orotracheal intubation should be avoided unless absolutely necessary to prevent fatal asphyxia, since insertion of the tube may produce further tracheal damage or force the foreign body into a more difficult position for removal. However, when the foreign body occludes the trachea and fatal asphyxia seems imminent despite administration of oxygen, insertion of an orotracheal tube may advance the foreign body into a main bronchus and permit ventilation of the opposite lung until bronchoscopy can be performed. Bronchoscopy for removal of a foreign body should be carried out in the operating room by a qualified endoscopist with an anesthesiologist in attendance to support cardiopulmonary function and monitor precordial heart tones and breath sounds, ECG, systemic arterial pressure, and color. General inhalation anesthesia is necessary to provide optimal operating conditions in most patients.

INDICATIONS FOR AN ARTIFICIAL TRACHEAL AIRWAY

The major indications for an artificial tracheal airway are life-threatening upper airway obstruction and acute respiratory failure. High-pitched inspiratory and expiratory stridor, nasal flaring, severe retractions, harsh and delayed inspiratory breath sounds, and cyanosis in air (an upper airway obstruction score equal to or greater than 7) and a rising Pa_{CO_2}[136] constitute signs of life-threatening impairment of gas exchange due to airway obstruction. Immediate administration of 100% oxygen by bag and mask, and aspiration of oropharyngeal secretions, helps relieve hypoxemia and prepares the patient for direct laryngoscopy and insertion of an orotracheal tube by the most experienced available person. A subsequent decision whether long-term management of the airway would be accomplished best with a nasotracheal tube or tracheostomy can be deferred until arrival of qualified personnel and transfer of the child to the operating room or intensive care unit.

In the infant or child with cardiopulmonary or neuromuscular disease who develops acute respiratory failure despite conservative therapy, steps should be taken immediately to improve ventilation. Initially this procedure is accomplished by clearing the upper airway of obstruction and secretions, assisting ventilation with 100% oxygen by bag and mask, establishing an adequate intravenous infusion route with a plastic cannula or cutdown, monitoring precordial heart tones and ECG, and using intravenous sodium bicarbonate to restore arterial pH to 7.20 or higher. Unless a dramatic improvement in ventilation and blood gas tensions occurs as a result of these immediate resuscitative measures, an orotracheal tube should be inserted, and consideration given to the selection of a nasotracheal tube or tracheostomy for prolonged airway management.

In the fasting patient with thick, copious bronchial secretions without respiratory failure, orotracheal intubation under intravenous anesthesia and neuromuscular blockade, followed by tracheobronchial irrigation with saline solution, chest physiotherapy in both lateral positions, and repeated sterile tracheobronchial aspiration, has proven effective in clearing the airways. After these steps, the orotracheal tube may be removed. This procedure can be repeated once or twice daily. Occasionally, bronchoscopy under general anesthesia may be required. Removal of thick secretions from the airways may avert the onset of acute respiratory failure, and obviate the need for a long-term artificial tracheal airway. However, unless ventilation and arterial blood gas tensions show substantial improvement from these measures, the orotracheal tube should remain in place and a decision be made regarding long-term airway management with a nasotracheal tube or tracheostomy.

OROTRACHEAL INTUBATION

Insertion of an orotracheal airway must be undertaken in an orderly, planned sequence such as the following: (1) ventilation with 100% oxygen by bag and mask for approximately 3 minutes; (2) intravenous atropine (0.01 mg/kg) to prevent bradycardia during laryngoscopy; (3) aspiration of nasal and oropharyngeal secretions; (4) oxygenation by bag and mask for at least 1 minute; (5) aspiration of stomach contents; (6) oxygenation by bag and mask for at least 1 minute; (7) direct laryngoscopy with the proper blade (Fig. 3-1); and (8) insertion of the appropriate size tube (Table 3-5). A flexible stylet (Fig. 3-2) facilitates intubation if the tube is highly flexible or the larynx is very anterior.

Because most critically ill patients have retained gastric secretions and food, the stomach should be aspirated with the largest practical size catheter (No. 14 French in the infant, No. 18 French in the child). At the time of emergency tracheal intubation the usual "full stomach" precautions minimize the hazard of regurgitation and pulmonary aspiration of gastric contents. These precautions include: sedation with thiopental or ketamine, neuromuscular blockade with succinylcholine; external cricoid pressure to occlude the esophagus; a stylet in the endotracheal tube; and high-volume suction with a tonsil suction tip. Intravenous sedation and muscle relaxants are required in most conscious and many unconscious patients for atraumatic insertion of the orotracheal tube. However, these agents should be used in these circumstances only by individuals with training in anesthesiology. Most patients with severe airway obstruction or acute respiratory failure can be maintained with 100% oxygen by bag and mask until personnel with anesthesia experience arrive. However, circumstances do arise in which such personnel are not available and tracheal intubation is mandatory; for this reason, all pediatricians should receive training and acquire skill in bag and mask ventilation and orotracheal intubation of all sizes of pediatric patients.

Following orotracheal intubation, auscultation of the chest helps to ensure that both lungs are ventilated. A bite block then must be inserted and the tube properly taped. After ventilation with oxygen and intratracheal instillation of sterile saline solution, secretions in the trachea and bronchi should be aspirated. When the patient's condition permits, chest physiotherapy, tracheobronchial toilet, and hyperinflation of the lungs should be repeated with the patient in both lateral positions. This procedure serves to reinflate atelectatic lung segments and decrease intrapulmonary venoarterial shunting. Then a secure form of tracheal airway can be established by nasotracheal intubation or tracheostomy.

NASOTRACHEAL INTUBATION

If one anticipates that an artificial tracheal airway is going to be required for longer than 12 hours but less than 5 to 7 days, a nasotracheal tube generally is sufficient.[36,59,123] A properly placed nasotracheal tube provides for more stable fixation, less danger of accidental extubation, and better care of the mouth with fewer oropharyngeal secretions than is possible with an orotracheal tube.

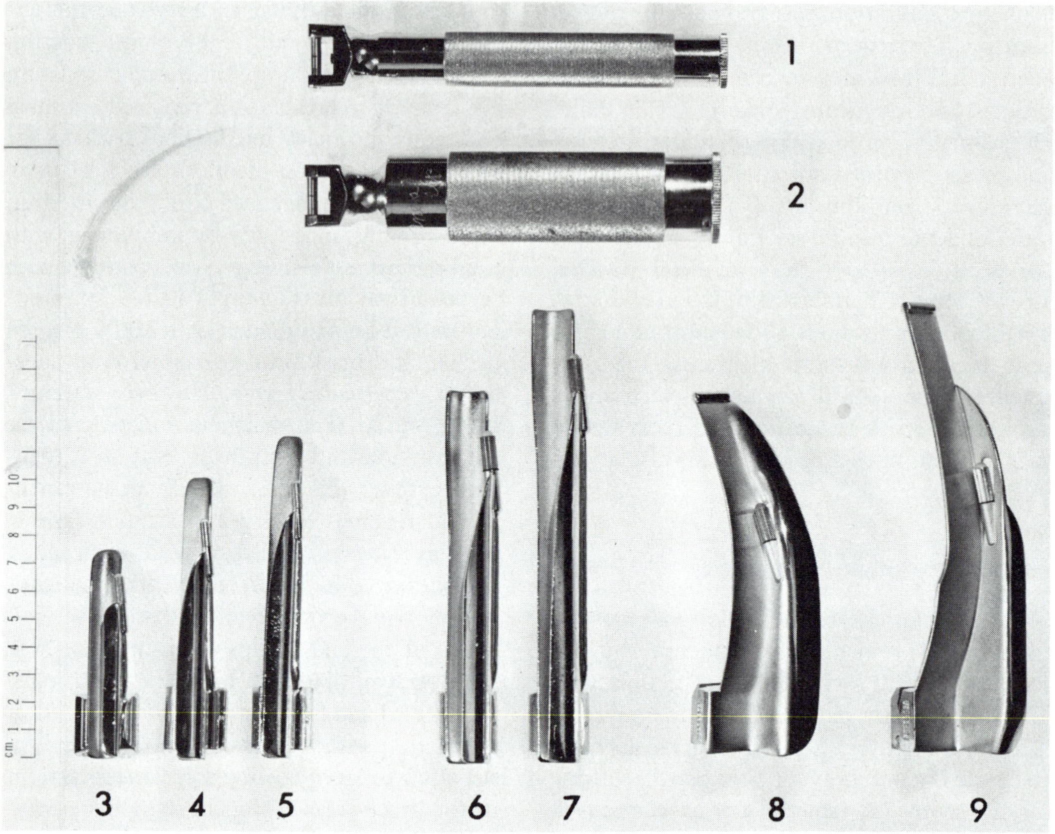

FIG. 3-1. Laryngoscope handles and blades*† *1,* Pediatric handle; *2,* Adult handle; *3,* Miller premature blade (infants < 2 kg); *4,* Wis-Hipple No. 1 blade (infants 2–5 kg); *5,* Wis-Hipple No. 1½ blade (infants 5–12 kg); *6,* Flagg child blade (children 12–30 kg); *7,* Flagg adult blade (children > 30 kg); *8,* Macintosh No. 3 blade (child or adult > 50 kg); *9,* Macintosh No. 4 blade (large adult).

*Handles available from Welch-Allyn Co.
†Blades available from major anesthesia equipment distributors.

Nasotracheal intubation is technically more difficult, especially in the small infant; yet, with rare exceptions, the same diameter tube as that used in the oral route can be inserted nasally.

Prior to nasotracheal intubation, the nares should be aspirated to remove secretions, atropine given intravenously (0.01 mg/kg), the patient's head placed in the "sniffing" position (occiput elevated with extension of the occipitoatlantal joint), and the appropriate size Magill forceps situated at hand (see Fig. 3-2). A stylet should not be used. Cuffed tubes are not necessary in patients under 8 years of age since their narrow subglottic diameter ensures an adequate tracheal seal. Children over the age of 8 years may require a tube with a low-pressure, large-volume cuff[19,20] when high airway pressures are necessary to provide adequate alveolar ventilation, e.g., in status asthmaticus. All tubes should be made of implant-tested plastic material and meet standard specifications (see Table 3-5).

At the time the nasotracheal tube is being inserted, suprasternal palpation of the trachea

TABLE 3-5. Dimensions of Endotracheal Tubes*

Age	Internal Diameter (ID) (mm)	Connector (ID)† (mm)	Minimal Length (Oral)‡ (cm)
Premature	2.5–3.0	3.0	10–11
Full term	3.0–3.5	3.0–4.0	11–12
6 mo	4.0	4.0	13
12 mo	4.5	5.0	14
18–24 mo	5.0	5.0	15
4 yr	5.5	6.0	16
6 yr	6.0	6.0	18
8 yr	6.5	7.0	20
10 yr§	7.0	7.0	21
12 yr§	7.5	8.0	22
14 yr§	8.0	8.0	23
Adult§	8.5–9.5	9.0–10.0	24–26

**Average* size for age. Occasionally a size 0.5-mm ID smaller or larger will be required in normal patients.

†We recommend only connectors with tapered 15-mm male machine end. Size refers to ID of tube end.

‡For nasal tubes, add 2 to 3 cm length.

§Patients age 10 years and older vary widely in size. High-volume, low-pressure cuffs may be required for short-term use (less than 24 hours). When using a cuffed tube, select size 0.5-mm ID smaller.

Note: We recommend thin-wall, uncuffed plastic tubes that conform to ANSI standard Z-79.1 and the USP animal implantation test. Such tubes will be labelled "Z.79 IT" with internal and external diameter in mm.

References: ANSI Standard Z.79.1, "Tracheal Tubes and Cuffs," American National Standards Institute, 1430 Broadway, New York, N.Y. 10018.
Guess, W. L.: Tissue testing of polymers. *Int. Anesthesiol. Clin.* *8*:787, 1970.
United States Pharmacopoeia, Volume 17, p. 905.

may help determine the depth of insertion of the tube in infants.[13] The tube should be secured by careful application of waterproof adhesive tape* following drying and preparation of both the tube and skin with tincture of benzoin. Meticulous attention to the details of fixation (Fig. 3-3) protects the patient against the disaster of accidental extubation. Bilateral auscultation of the chest prior to and following taping of the tube, and a subsequent chest roentgenogram detect bronchial intubation and pneumothorax. The tip of the tube should lie in the middle or lower third of the trachea (opposite the third thoracic vertebra) but remain above the carina when maximally advanced after fixation.

*Waterproof, 1.25-cm (0.5-in.) wide, heavy-duty tape (Curity Wet Proof No. 3063 adhesive tape, Hospital Products Division, The Kendall Company, Chicago, Illinois)

TRACHEOSTOMY

Tracheostomy is preferable to nasotracheal intubation when the tracheal airway is required for more than 7 days, when intrinsic laryngeal disease includes severe congenital or traumatic upper airway disorders, and when very thick tracheal secretions or blood clots are present. The operation should be performed after an orotracheal tube or bronchoscope has been placed in the trachea, preferably under general anesthesia and controlled ventilation.

Preferred surgical techniques for tracheostomy in infants and children call for a horizontal skin incision, a vertical tracheal incision in the third to fifth tracheal rings, and no removal of cartilage.[3,122] Retraction sutures placed in the lateral margins of the tracheal opening so that they emerge through the skin incision provide a means of stabilizing the tracheal stoma for reinsertion of the trache-

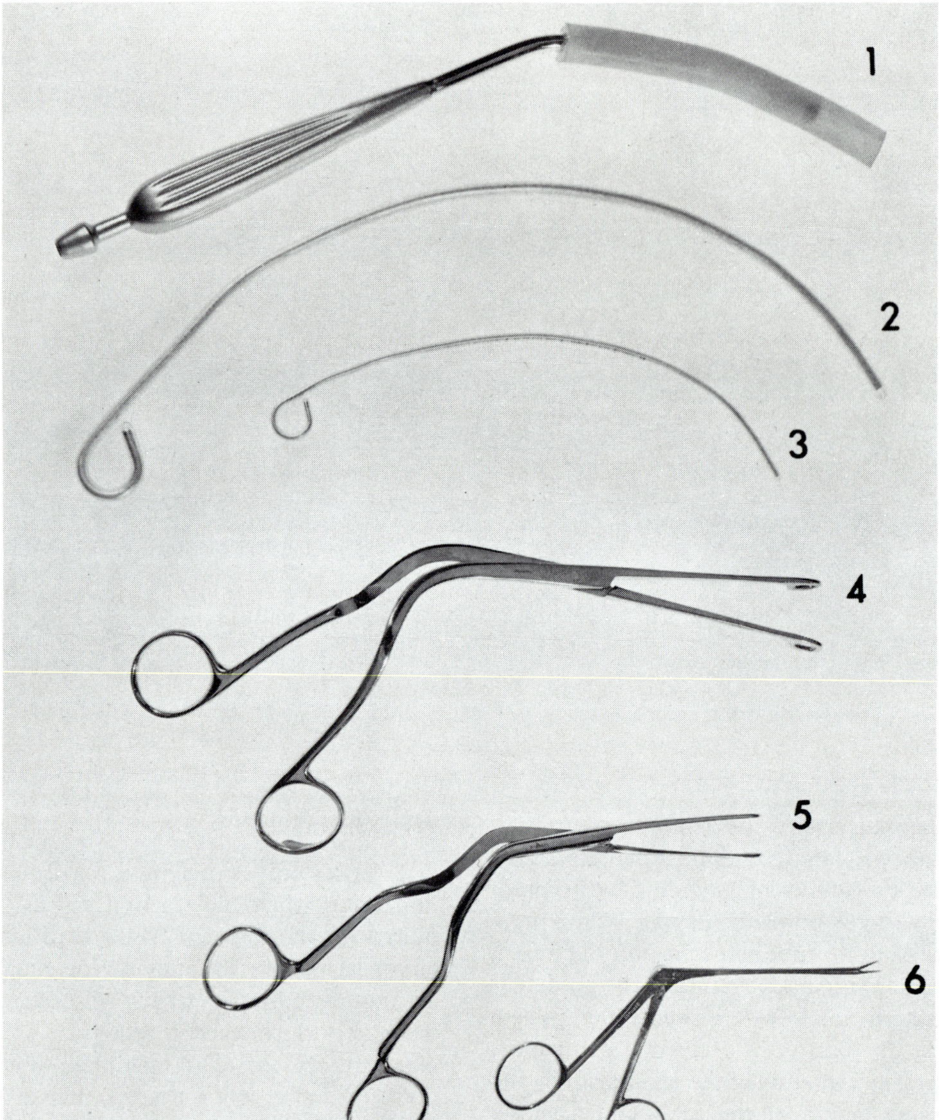

FIG. 3–2. Intubation accessories. *1*, Tonsil aspirator (Yankauer) with metal tip replaced by thick wall latex rubber tubing; *2,* Adult Teflon-coated stylet* for tubes $>$ 5.0 mm ID; *3,* Infant Teflon-coated stylet* for tubes $<$ 4.5 mm ID; *4*, Adult Magill forceps† (children $>$ 50 kg); *5*, Child Magill forceps (children 5–50 kg); *6*, Small alligator forceps‡ (infants $<$ 5 kg).

*National Catheter Co.

†Magill forceps, used in nasotracheal intubation (see text), are available from major anesthesia equipment distributors.

‡Small alligator forceps, used as a Magill forceps in infants, are available from major surgical instrument distributors.

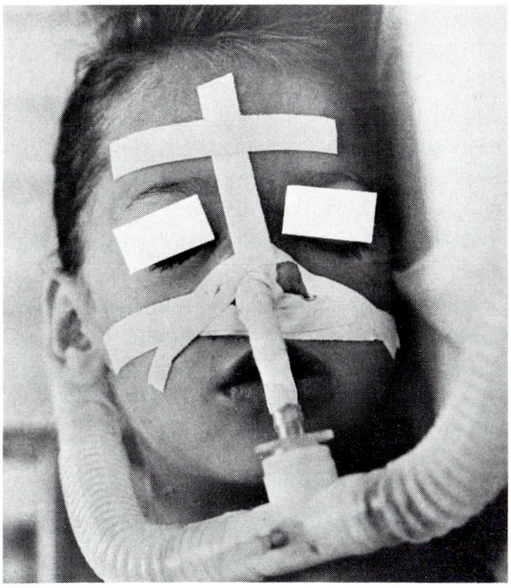

FIG. 3-3. Nasotracheal tube secured with waterproof adhesive tape (see text).

ostomy tube if it becomes dislodged during the first 3 postoperative days.[122] A flexible swivel attachment from the tracheostomy tube to the source of inspired gas or ventilator (Fig. 3-4) minimizes tube motion in the trachea and accidental decannulation. The tracheostomy tube must be secured as meticulously as the nasotracheal tube. The skin of the neck should be cleaned, dried, and painted with tincture of benzoin. New heavy-duty cotton tape (2.5 cm wide) that cannot be broken or torn by hand should be used. Foam rubber with adhesive backing attached to the tape over the entire length that is in direct contact with the skin of the neck helps prevent excoriation and pressure necrosis. The tape should be tied snugly around the neck while the tube is held firmly in the stoma. Since tape inevitably stretches, it should be tied sufficiently tight that the tracheostomy tube can be withdrawn less than 1 cm; this seems excessively tight at the outset, but is necessary to avoid decannulation a day later.

Since experience has been gained with humidification, airway care, and the use of polyvinylchloride and silastic tubes, metal tubes with an inner cannula have become obsolete. Cuffed tracheostomy tubes are rarely required in the care of infants and children. If a cuff must be used, it should be of the low-pressure, high-volume type,[21] with a pilot balloon, inflated to the minimal pressure required to provide a tracheal seal at peak inspiratory airway pressures up to 40 cm H_2O. An air leak should be audible with a stethoscope over the tracheal stoma at peak pressures. Periodic deflation of the cuff for 1- to

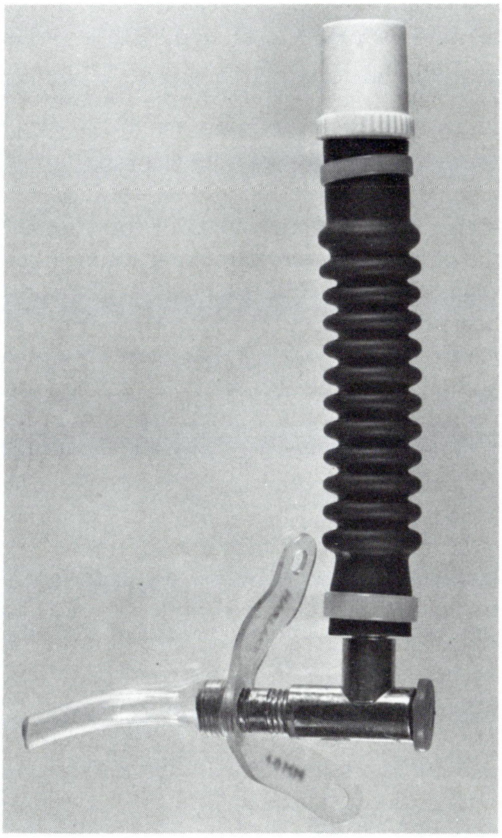

FIG. 3-4. Aberdeen pediatric tracheostomy tube, size 3.5 mm ID and pediatric swivel attachment with 15-mm male connector. Tubes available in sizes 3.5 to 7.0 mm ID from Harris-Lake Co., Cleveland, Ohio; swivel available from Clarence E. Smith Co., Arlington, Mass.

2-minute intervals helps minimize the risk of tracheal ischemia. Cuffed tracheostomy tubes can lead to tracheal stenosis with disastrous sequelae,[27] and their use in infants and children should be discouraged.

CARE OF THE ARTIFICIAL TRACHEAL AIRWAY

Care of the tracheal airway is an art that must be mastered by all of the medical and nursing personnel who care for critically ill children. The three major factors in airway care are: humidification, chest physiotherapy, and tracheobronchial toilet.

Humidification. An artificial tracheal airway permits inspired gas to bypass the normal humidifying mechanisms of the nares and oropharynx, which raise the temperature of the gas to approximately 33° C, and add 44 mg of water vapor per liter of gas (100% relative humidity).[107] Inspired gas ideally should be brought to these same conditions at the point of delivery through a tracheal airway. Commercially available heated humidifiers provide these conditions at the time gas leaves the humidifier,[60] but because of the failure to heat the inspiratory line tubing and the low specific heat of gases, the inspired gas cools and water vapor condenses in the tubing. When the inspired gas is reheated in the trachea and bronchi, it contains less than 40 mg per liter of water vapor (less than 80% relative humidity at 37° C). As inadequately humidified gas is inspired, water is extracted from the mucous carpet and epithelium of the trachea, resulting in increased viscosity of secretions with inhibition of ciliary activity[64] and striking alterations in cell structure.[22] Because most humidifying systems fail to provide adequate water vapor at body temperature, it is necessary to instill saline solution into the trachea at 1- to 2-hour intervals. The volume of saline solution instilled should be proportional to the body size and viscosity of secretions (see Tracheobronchial Toilet).

Chest Physiotherapy. Insertion of an artificial tracheal airway bypasses the glottic sphincter essential to an effective cough and inhibits the normal cephalad ciliary propulsion of the mucous carpet lining the bronchi and trachea. Other maneuvers must be undertaken to raise tracheobronchial secretions to a level where they can be aspirated, i.e., changes in the patient's position to utilize the effects of gravity on secretions, techniques of chest physiotherapy, and artificial coughing.

Placing the patient in a 10-degree head-down or head-up tilt, turning the patient from supine to a 90-degree lateral position, and alternating lateral supine-opposite lateral positions every 2 hours facilitate drainage of many pulmonary segments. The more extreme positions required for draining the remaining segments often are not tolerated by the critically ill infant or child, or are not practical because of equipment attached to the patient.

Chest physiotherapy consists of a series of steps designed to mobilize secretions in smaller peripheral airways, and to move them toward the trachea so they can be aspirated.[94] Chest vibration by manual or mechanical means appears to aid the mobilization of secretions in the smaller peripheral airways. Chest percussion, which is achieved by forceful, rapid, manual "cupping," sets up more explosive forces that propel the mobilized secretions to the carina. Vibration and percussion are done over the entire hemithorax with the patient in a lateral position, followed by tracheobronchial aspiration. The patient is then turned to the opposite lateral position and the maneuvers repeated.

Artificial coughing is a technique used with a patient in the lateral position, and consists of: (1) manual inflation of the lungs to a large volume (near vital capacity), which then is held by maintaining peak airway pressure; (2) subsequent application of manual pressure on the upright hemithorax; and (3) sudden deflation of the lungs by release of airway pressure while manual pressure on the thorax is maintained. This technique has proven useful in bringing thick secretions (previously mobilized by chest vibration and percussion) to the level of the carina where they can be aspirated.

Prior to and following chest physiotherapy, the patient's lung should be hyperinflated with oxygen (see next section). Chest physiotherapy and tracheobronchial toilet should be limited to a 5- to 10-minute period, and repeated at approximately 2-hour intervals or as required, so that the viscosity and volume of secretions remain manageable.

Tracheobronchial Toilet. Tracheobronchial toilet includes those maneuvers involved in the removal, through a tracheal airway, of secretions or other material (clots, aspirated foreign matter, tissue debris) that have been raised to the level of the main bronchi and carina. The first step is the instillation of sterile isotonic saline solution (0.5 ml in the newborn, 1 to 2 ml in older infants, 3 to 5 ml in children) to help liquefy partially dried, viscous secretions or other material, and to provide a medium in which such matter can be suspended for purposes of passage through the suction catheter. This step is followed by tracheal aspiration utilizing a sterile one-glove technique with rapid insertion of the catheter to a maximum depth (into the main bronchi). The catheter should be of the largest practical diameter for easy passage through the tracheal airway, yet should not occlude the lumen of the airway nor impede the entrainment of air through the tracheal tube (which could result in excessive subatmospheric intratracheal pressures). The catheter should be wetted with sterile saline solution prior to insertion, and should be equipped with a molded tip and end hole, but no side hole. Catheters with a side hole can impinge against the wall of the trachea or bronchi when the end hole is occluded, thus applying all of the suction to mucosal surfaces and intensifying the mucosal damage associated with aspiration.

The amount of suction to apply has never been scientifically determined and constitutes another aspect in the art of respiratory care that is achieved mainly through experience. Vacuum pressures of 150 to 300 mm Hg (during occlusion of the suction catheter) usually indicate sufficient suction flow to adequately remove tracheobronchial secretions and debris through catheters varying from 5 Fr. to 14 Fr. in size.

Prior to tracheal aspiration, the patient should be hyperventilated with 100% oxygen for a period of 1 to 2 minutes; this practice raises alveolar oxygen tension, displaces nitrogen and fills the functional residual capacity of the lung with oxygen, and thus provides a longer period of time for tracheal aspiration before hypoxemia occurs. Studies in apneic adult man with normal pulmonary function indicate that prior hyperventilation with oxygen increases the time from 1 to 2 minutes before arterial oxygen saturation falls below 93%.[32] Following chest physiotherapy and tracheobronchial toilet, the lungs should be manually inflated with oxygen several times to a volume near vital capacity, and then hyperventilated at an appropriate tidal volume for approximately 3 minutes prior to reconnection of the tracheal airway to the source of inspired gas or ventilator. This maneuver serves to correct arterial hypoxemia, which may have occurred during aspiration, and helps reexpand atelectatic segments of the lung following removal of secretions.[16a]

CONTINUOUS POSITIVE AIRWAY PRESSURE (CPAP)

Studies in the newborn infant with diffuse alveolar disease indicate that insertion of an artificial tracheal airway results in a decrease in functional residual capacity (FRC) and Pa_{O_2} when the end-expiratory pressure remains at the atmospheric level. Application of CPAP (2.0 cm H_2O) restores FRC and Pa_{O_2} to their previous values.[14] Preliminary data in children and published data in adults[48a] indicate that the same mechanisms operate in older patients. Thus, in all acute conditions involving diffuse alveolar disease, CPAP of at least 2.0 cm H_2O is recommended after insertion of an artificial tracheal airway.

TRACHEAL EXTUBATION AND DECANNULATION

Once the need for a tracheal airway no longer exists, it should be removed in a planned and orderly manner. Provision should be made for reinsertion of the tracheal airway in the event that its removal has proven premature.

Nasotracheal Tube. A nasotracheal tube ought to be removed as soon as possible in order to minimize the incidence and severity of complications. The patient should ingest no solids or milk for at least 12 hours and drink only clear liquids up to 6 hours prior to extubation because the laryngeal sphincter mechanism remains imcompetent for several hours following extubation. Also, reintubation under anesthesia and neuromuscular blockade may be necessary. Sedative drugs should be withheld for at least 4 hours, and narcotics given only in small doses for relief of pain without excessive sedation.

The patient should have the optimal cardiopulmonary and neuromuscular function that can be achieved in his present condition. A chest roentgenogram and arterial blood gas tension measurement obtained within 6 hours prior to extubation are used to determine whether atelectasis or other intrapulmonary complications have occurred. To tolerate extubation, the patients' forced vital capacity determined with a respirometer should exceed 15 ml/kg, and their inspiratory force should exceed 20 cm H_2O negative pressure.[13a] If non-depolarizing muscle relaxants have been used, they must be completely reversed with atropine and neostigmine. The patient should be afebrile, have minimal tracheobronchial secretions, a normal or resolving chest roentgenogram, and optimal arterial blood gas tensions.

Immediately prior to extubation, the following ought to be performed: (1) evacuation of stomach contents; (2) chest physiotherapy and tracheobronchial aspiration; (3) gentle suctioning of secretions from the nares; and (4) manually assisted ventilation for 2 minutes with 100% oxygen, including several large sustained tidal volumes (near vital capacity) during each minute. The tape securing the tube is then detached, the cuff (if in use) deflated, the lungs manually inflated to near vital capacity, and with airway pressure held at peak inflation, the tube removed. This maneuver causes the patient to cough out secretions as the tube leaves the larynx. The naris that contained the tube then should be suctioned with a moistened sterile catheter to remove the residual secretions that surrounded the tube. Oxygen can be given by bag and mask as the patient is placed in a tent or head hood, and the inspired oxygen concentration initially set at least 10% higher than that utilized while the nasotracheal tube was in place.

A program of chest physiotherapy and nasopharyngeal as well as oropharyngeal aspiration every 2 hours should be continued for at least 8 hours, and thereafter three to four times a day for at least 2 additional days. This procedure is necessary because tracheobronchial ciliary function and an effective cough mechanism do not recover immediately upon removal of the tube. The patient should be kept without intake by mouth for at least 8 hours, then given water, and thereafter receive only clear liquids by mouth up to 24 hours following extubation. If cry, voice, and an effective cough have returned to nearly normal by that time, regular feedings can be resumed. It is advisable to obtain a chest roentgenogram and measurement of arterial blood gas tensions within 2 hours following extubation.

Tracheostomy. The indications and prior conditions for decannulation of a tracheostomy are similar to those for removal of a nasotracheal tube. Since the laryngeal sphincter mechanism is more likely to function adequately with a tracheostomy, the hazard of aspiration of stomach contents may be less with decannulation. However, the feeding schedule described under extubation should be followed. In the event the tracheostomy tube cannot be readily inserted, orotracheal intubation may be required to reestablish the airway; regurgitation of solids from the stomach at that time poses a major hazard. If the tracheostomy has been in place for more than 7 days, it is advisable to perform a bronchoscopy under general anesthesia, or with a flexible fiberoptic bronchoscope.[121] When granulation tissue has accumulated at the cephalad margin of the stoma, or at the tracheal end of the tube, it must be removed prior to decannulation.

Chest physiotherapy, tracheobronchial toilet, and hyperventilation with oxygen should be carried out immediately prior to removal of the tube, as described previously. In small infants, intravenous morphine (0.1 mg/kg) may be used prior to decannulation in order to provide quiet ventilation and permit the infant to readjust to the sensation of breathing through the upper airway. Failure to decannulate small infants is most commonly associated with instability of the anterior tracheal wall and granulation tissue at the stoma.

The tracheostomy wound should be covered with a small dressing following decannulation. These wounds close with amazing rapidity in infants and children, often causing inability to reinsert the same tube after a period of less than 1 hour. If reinsertion is necessary, but difficult due to partial closing of the stoma, a small suction catheter can be inserted through the stoma into the trachea, and a sterile moistened tracheostomy tube reinserted over the catheter. This practice helps to ensure placement of the tube in the tracheal lumen rather than in the pretracheal tissue spaces.

Post-decannulation care is similar to that following removal of a nasotracheal tube. If tracheal obstruction occurs over a period of weeks, bronchoscopy is indicated because the most common cause will be development of granulation tissue at the tracheostomy stoma or at a level where the tracheal end of the tube touched the tracheal wall.

COMPLICATIONS

Artificial tracheal airways bypass the normal humidifying and heating mechanism of the upper airway, resulting in dehydration of the tracheobronchial mucous carpet and epithelium. Even the least reactive materials available[120] are foreign bodies, which denude the cilia and superficial mucosal cells, and produce inflammatory tissue reactions.[47a,62,109,135] These sequelae are inevitable in artificial tracheal airway placement. Accidental tracheal extubation or occlusion of the lumen of the tracheal airway by secretions can be prevented by attention to the details of airway fixation, tracheal airway care, and proper humidification of the inspired gas.

Infection poses one of the major risks involved in the treatment of acute respiratory failure and the use of an artificial tracheal airway. Trauma to the tracheal mucosa associated with catheter aspiration and inadvertent breaks in aseptic technique account for the high incidence of tracheitis due to pathogenic bacteria.[111] However, because of the danger of emergence of virulent gram-negative pathogens or antibiotic-resistant strains, we do not advocate the use of antibiotics unless there is evidence of associated bronchopneumonia or other infection. Gram-negative septicemia often occurs in critically ill patients in whom the artificial airway and multiple intravascular catheters represent the probable routes of contamination, and the hands of professional personnel the major vector.[85] The incidence of infection can be substantially reduced by the following practices: (1) for physicians and nurses, careful hand washing with a bactericidal agent initially and between patients; (2) limited handling of the patient by personnel not immediately involved with his care; (3) strict aseptic practice in the handling of the patient's airway and vascular catheters; (4) the use of sterile respiratory therapy equipment, which is changed at least daily; (5) proper care of the patient's skin; and (6) meticulous handling of airway connections.

Prolonged Nasotracheal Intubation. Such prolonged intubation can result in subglottic stenosis, granuloma formation, mucosal ulceration, and fibrotic bands in the larynx and trachea. The incidence of these complications varies considerably with different diseases, with the duration of intubation, and between institutions.[1,5,33,59,83,93,100,123,125] Subglottic narrowing and stenosis have been reported to occur in 3[123] to 5%[59] of infants and children intubated over 24 hours who had cardiopulmonary disease but not intrinsic laryngotracheal disorders. In patients who require an artificial tracheal airway because of laryngotracheitis (croup) or acute epiglottitis, nasotracheal intubation[11] or tracheostomy[3,91] can be selected, and each has its own complications. In children with laryngotracheitis, one group observed subglottic stenosis or granuloma in 5 of 11 cases;[33,123] others reported a much lower incidence of complications: none in 12 cases,[100] and one in 27 cases.[5] The management of 40 children with acute epiglottitis by nasotracheal intubation[11] resulted in only two cases of granuloma and no subglottic stenosis. The reasons for these discrepancies remain unclear, but the use of a nasotracheal tube in the presence of intrinsic laryngeal disease carries the inherent risk of placement of a foreign body in an already inflamed tissue.

Status asthmaticus requiring tracheal intubation and mechanical ventilation has been associated with a higher incidence of post-intubation subglottic stenosis and granulation tissue formation than observed in other cardiopulmonary diseases.[137] This problem may occur because these patients often have an upper respiratory infection; also, the need for an adequate tracheal seal with the increased pressure of the tube or cuff on the tracheal mucosa may contribute to these complications. The occurrence of such sequelae has become less frequent with the use of implant tested tubes, and with neuromuscular blockade to minimize motion of the tube and facilitate coordination of the patient with the mechanical ventilator.

Cuffed tubes can produce mucosal ulceration, necrosis, erosion with tracheoesophageal fistula, and post-extubation tracheal stenosis at the site of the cuff. The incidence and severity of tissue damage appear to be less with high-volume, low-pressure cuffs.[19,20,40,138]

Tracheostomy. At the time of operation, tracheostomy may be associated with severe asphyxia if the tracheal airway is not established with an endotracheal tube or bronchoscope.[5,99] Performance of the operation under endotracheal general anesthesia in an operating room by a trained anesthesiologist and surgeon, as compared with performance of the operation without tracheal intubation by house officers on a hospital ward, reduced the mortality associated with tracheostomy itself from 30% to 0; undoubtedly, delayed recognition of severe asphyxia contributed to the mortality of tracheostomy performed on the ward, but the major factors in the reduced mortality were the presence of an established tracheal airway, controlled ventilation, and experienced personnel.[5]

At the time of operation, tracheostomy may be associated with severe surgical bleeding, pneumothorax from accidental incision of the anterior pleural reflection, and insertion of the tracheostomy tube into the anterior tracheal fascial planes.[99] The postoperative complications of tracheostomy include wound infection, bleeding at the tracheostomy stoma, granulation tissue formation at the stoma and the tracheal end of the tracheostomy tube, and tracheal stenosis.[1,3,27,99] Erosion of metal tubes into the innominate artery with fatal hemorrhage can also occur.[17,78]

Following decannulation, instability of the tracheal wall at the site of the stoma, or airway obstruction due to proliferation of granulation tissue at the cephalad margin of the tracheostomy stoma may occur. When cuffed tracheostomy tubes are utilized, tracheal stenosis secondary to ischemic damage can occur and produce intense airway obstruction requiring tracheal resection[55a] or a prosthesis.[84] The incidence of this disastrous complication apparently can be minimized by the use of a high-volume, low-pressure cuff and monitoring of intracuff pressure with an aneroid gauge.[20,21,90]

Mechanical Ventilation

HISTORY

Since ancient times, man has employed a host of mechanical devices to augment the ventilation of victims of acute respiratory failure. For the interested reader, this subject has been reviewed in detail by W. W. Mushin.[95b] The modern era of mechanical ventilation begins with the experiments of Rudolph Matas in 1903 in the United States,[92] and the clinical work of Läwen and Sievers in Germany.[80] The latter, in 1910, described a volume preset ventilator with a piston-cylinder force generator that delivered a constant tidal volume to patients undergoing thoracic surgery and to victims of tetanus whose seizures were controlled with curare. The importance of these advances was not recognized for nearly half a century until Engström, faced with patients in respiratory failure during the devastating poliomyelitis epidemics of the early 1950's in Scandinavia,[79] developed the modern volume preset ventilator.[44] This mode of mechanical ventilation quickly replaced the "iron lung" cuirass ventilators. During the late 1950's, gas-powered intermittent positive-pressure breathing machines were adapted to serve as pressure preset devices for long-term ventilation; time cycle-constant flow ventilators also were developed. Since 1970, mechanical ventilators have increased in complexity of design and function, and the need for specific criteria of performance and safety has led to the development of an international standard for these devices.[67a]

INDICATIONS

The infant or child who has acute life-threatening impairment of gas exchange (acute respiratory failure) despite establishment of an adequate tracheal airway requires mechanical ventilation. The criteria for the diagnosis of acute respiratory failure in pediatric patients are outlined in Tables 3-3 and 3-4, and are similar to the guidelines for ventilatory support in the adult.[102] If muscular fatigue due to the excessive work of breathing or neuromuscular disease, or central nervous system depression has led to acute respiratory failure, pulmonary gas exchange can be improved substantially with mechanical ventilation. When gas flow patterns and respiratory frequency are adjusted for the patient's airways resistance, total compliance, and cardiac output, mechanical ventilation can alter favorably the distribution of gas within the lung and the matching of alveolar gas with pulmonary blood flow. This adjustment, in turn, results in a decrease in the alveolar-arterial oxygen tension gradient and Pa_{CO_2} level.[103]

THE VENTILATOR

Mechanical ventilators can be classified according to their major method of control: (1) volume preset; (2) pressure preset; and (3) time-flow preset (Table 3-6). The type of ventilator employed is far less important than the skill and experience of the medical and nursing team caring for the patient. However, certain types of ventilators are more effective than others.

The ultimate test of the effectiveness of a

TABLE 3-6. Mechanical Ventilators Used in Infants and Children*

Volume Preset	Pressure Preset
Engstrom†	Bird (MK 7,8,14)†
Emerson†	Baby Bird‡
Bennett MA-1†	Bennett PR-2†
Drager Spiromat†	Time-Flow Preset
Bourns LS 150‡	Loosco‡
Elema-Schonander	Bourns BP-200‡

* Ventilators that were commercially available in the United States in 1977 and have been used in pediatric patients.
† Adult ventilator with pediatric modification.
‡ Infant ventilator.

mechanical ventilator is its ability to provide adequate ventilation under conditions of increased airway resistance and decreased total compliance. In the face of grossly impaired pulmonary mechanics, volume preset ventilators are more effective at maintaining a constant tidal volume than those that are pressure preset.[46] Although pressure preset ventilators can compensate to a limited extent for minor leaks in the tracheal airway, this advantage is of minimal importance when the proper size airway has been inserted.

The assist mode provided with many mechanical ventilators is of little practical value in infants and small children because the volume that must be inspired by the patient in order to trigger the device is usually excessive.[45] The control mode has proven effective and more reliable in pediatric patients. Intermittent mandatory ventilation (IMV) is a technique that has obviated assisted mode ventilation.[38] The gas flow through the ventilator inspiratory system is maintained at a rate that precludes rebreathing when the patient ventilates spontaneously between cycles of the ventilator. Mandatory lung inflations are provided by the ventilator at preset tidal volumes delivered at a frequency from 20 per minute to 1 per four minutes, depending on the patient's ability to maintain an adequate spontaneous, unassisted minute volume.

Most commercially available volume preset ventilators have an internal compliance (compression volume) that is excessive when the ventilator is used in infants and small children. Internal compliance can be defined as the volume of gas compressed in the ventilator system per unit airway pressure; this gas does not participate in the minute ventilation of the patient.[56] For example, if the internal compliance is 4 ml/cm H_2O, and an infant is ventilated with a tidal volume that results in an airway pressure of 20 cm H_2O, 80 ml of gas will be compressed within the ventilator tubing, humidifier, water trap, and alarm system. Thus, a volume setting of 80 ml results in virtually no fresh inspired gas passing through the tracheal tube to the patient's lungs. The ventilator volume setting must be increased to compensate for the internal compliance. Apparatus dead space, i.e., the apparatus volume in which inspired and expired gases mix, has received considerable attention in the past but is seldom of critical importance in clinical care. Apparatus dead space may exceed 10 ml, yet readily be compensated for by a small increase in the ventilator tidal volume.

Humidification of the inspired gas must be assured for any patient receiving mechanical ventilation. However, most ventilators are not equipped with heated inspiratory and expiratory tubing, resulting in condensation of water in the lines, which can obstruct gas flow or cause spillage of large volumes of water into the trachea. Water traps serve to decrease this risk, but must be in a dependent position well below the level of the patient to be effective.

All mechanical ventilators must be equipped with an inspiratory line pressure alarm with high and low limits to detect excessive inspiratory line pressures indicative of airway obstruction, and low pressures indicative of serious leaks or disconnection. It is desirable to have alarm systems that monitor the patient's expired minute volume, the inspired oxygen concentration, the level of water in the humidifier, and the temperature of the inspired gases at the tracheal connection. All mechanical ventilators should be equipped to provide for CPAP during use in the controlled, assisted, or IMV modes.

Additional discussion of the operation of specific ventilators and of their care and maintenance is found in Chapter 4.

VENTILATION OF THE PATIENT

Adjustment of a mechanical ventilator to achieve optimal gas exchange in the patient involves a number of considerations. At the outset, we prefer the controlled mode with or without IMV. The minute volume required[108] is difficult to predict unless the patient's wasted ventilation (dead space/tidal volume or VD/VT ratio) is known. Usually one must rely on visual and auscultatory evidence of ventilation during the initial adjustments. Tidal volume, and respiratory frequency are reset according to sequential Pa_{CO_2} and Pa_{O_2} determinations. The pattern of respiratory gas flow and pressure, the temporal relation of the inspiratory and expiratory cycles (I:E ratio), and the frequency of ventilation must be adjusted for the individual patient. In general, the following prove effective: (1) a relatively slow inspiratory gas flow and gradual rise in pressure to a peak pressure plateau; (2) an I:E ratio of 1:1 to 1:2; (3) tidal volumes between 15 and 20 ml/kg (corrected for internal compliance); and (4) a frequency of approximately two-thirds that appropriate for the patient's age.[26,65a] Patients with peripheral neuromuscular disorders and normal lungs should be ventilated at their normal predicted tidal volumes[108] and frequencies[65a] (see also Chapter 1).

During mechanical ventilation of patients with diffuse alveolar collapse due to cardiopulmonary disease, CPAP at levels in excess of 2 cm H_2O reduces the alveolar-arterial oxygen tension gradient.[8,14,54,55] A balance must be achieved between the inspired oxygen concentration, the level of CPAP, cardiac output, and an acceptable Pa_{O_2}. Thus, achievement of the optimal CPAP level[124] is a complex endeavor, and presently is achieved by trial and error in individual patients in most clinical situations.[37]

Coordination of the patient with the ventilator often can be achieved by providing adequate alveolar ventilation and oxygenation, as well as general physical comfort. In the restless infant or child, diazepam (0.1 mg/kg) or morphine (0.1 mg/kg) in repeated intravenous doses or continuous infusion usually produces adequate sedation and depression of respiratory drive. Patients with intense bronchospasm and air trapping (e.g., status asthmaticus or bronchiolitis), or those with marked tachypnea due to severe pneumonitis may require neuromuscular blockade by continuous infusion of curare or pancuronium.[34,36,137] This blockade provides minimal chest wall resistance to ventilation and appears to reduce the hazards of pneumothorax and pneumomediastinum. When muscle relaxants are used, the patient must be cared for by physicians and other personnel who have considerable experience with these drugs and the handling of apneic, paralyzed infants and children. Continuous intravenous infusions of drugs result in a more uniform effect than intermittent injection, but such infusions should be stopped daily and not restarted until signs of recovery from the pharmacologic effects are evident.

DISCONTINUING MECHANICAL VENTILATION

A program for discontinuing mechanical ventilation can be initiated when the basic disease has come under control, the central nervous system regulation of respiration is intact, the patient's neuromuscular capacity is sufficient to sustain unassisted ventilation, and circulatory stability has been achieved.[13a,48] The Pa_{CO_2} should remain under 50 mm Hg and the Pa_{O_2} over 100 mm Hg at 50% inspired oxygen during mechanical ventilation with peak inflating pressures less than 25 cm H_2O. In children with cyanotic congenital heart disease, a Pa_{O_2} over 35 mm Hg is usually adequate.[35]

Unfortunately, there are no reliable additional physiologic criteria for use in predicting whether ventilator support can be withdrawn. For that reason, and not because of psychic dependence on the ventilator, a program of progressively longer intervals without mechanical ventilation or IMV must be carried out. During this period, frequent determinations of arterial pH and blood gas tensions as well as chest roentgenograms are necessary to confirm clinical observations. Increased use of the accessory muscles of breathing, tachypnea, tachycardia or bradycardia, and a progressive rise in Pa_{CO_2} or fall in Pa_{O_2} indicate that the patient still requires mechanical ventilation. Once the patient maintains adequate spontaneous ventilation for at least 12 hours, removal of the tracheal airway should be considered. Criteria for extubation or decannulation are discussed in detail on page 112.

COMPLICATIONS

Mechanical ventilation, when properly applied to normal lungs, does not result in serious physiologic dysfunction or histologic damage.[81,96] Complications associated with the artificial tracheal airway have been cited on page 113. The major pulmonary complications are: (1) retention of tracheobronchial secretions; (2) contamination of the airways with pathogenic organisms; (3) overdistention of the lungs due to maldistribution of gas at high inflating pressures; (4) excessive pulmonary extravascular water; (5) oxygen toxicity; and (6) pneumothorax. The hazard of pneumothorax appears to be increased when the peak airway pressure exceeds 25 cm H_2O and CPAP exceeds 5 cm H_2O.[77] Sudden deterioration of circulatory status or arterial blood gas tensions of a patient receiving mechanical ventilation requires that a chest roentgenogram be obtained immediately to exclude tension pneumothorax.

In some children undergoing prolonged mechanical ventilation, a decrease in urinary output, a fall in Pa_{O_2} and hematocrit, weight gain, and roentgenographic evidence of interstitial pulmonary edema have been observed; a similar syndrome occurs in adults.[118] Fluid restriction, infusion of 25% salt-poor albumin if oncotic pressure is low, and diuretics such as furosemide often result in a brisk diuresis with weight loss, an increase in Pa_{O_2} and hematocrit, and improvement in the chest roentgenogram. Most of these patients also require large tidal volumes and CPAP to maintain an optimal Pa_{O_2}. The cause of fluid retention in such patients remains obscure, but may involve decreased renal plasma flow[39] and release of antidiuretic hormone.[9] Ultrasonic nebulizers should not be used with mechanical ventilation in infants because they can produce an excessive volume of water as submicronic particles that are absorbed from the lungs, resulting in pulmonary lesions[95a] and fluid overload.[97,117]

Oxygen has the ability to damage alveolar tissue after prolonged exposure at high inspired concentrations. However, inspired concentrations under 50% for many days do not appear to harm normal human lungs,[24] but the effect on diseased lungs remains uncertain. The most sensitive indicator of impaired lung function due to oxygen toxicity is a progressive decrease in Pa_{O_2} at a constant inspired oxygen concentration. However, fear of pulmonary oxygen toxicity should not preclude the use of sufficiently high inspired oxygen concentrations to maintain the Pa_{O_2} at a level compatible with adequate oxygenation of the brain and other major organs. The term, respirator lung, has been incorrectly applied to many cases of fatal pulmonary oxygen toxicity or other pulmonary conditions; it is not mechanical ventilation per se, but the primary disease or oxygen that produces damage to the lungs.[81,96]

Mechanical complications associated with

the use of ventilators include: (1) disconnection at any point in the ventilator system or tracheal attachments; (2) obstruction of the inspiratory or expiratory tubing due to kinking or accumulated condensation; (3) malfunction of the valves; (4) power failure within the ventilator itself; and (5) erratic ventilator cycling due to electrical or gas flow malfunctions. These types of complications can be virtually eliminated by detailed attention on the part of nurses, physicians, and respiratory therapists to the ventilator system itself, and by the use of reliable, tested equipment. Mechanical complications are quite common when a team of physicians and nurses first embark on a program of intensive respiratory care; as they gain experience, such events become much less frequent and the complications associated with the control of infection, oxygen toxicity, fluid retention, and the sequelae of artificial tracheal airways become the most difficult problems to manage.

Cardiopulmonary Resuscitation

HISTORY

Man has attempted to retrieve his fellow man from the claws of sudden death since biblical times. To this end, he has employed a variety of ingenious techniques from flagellating, rectally insufflating smoke, rolling the victim over a barrel, and riding the victim prone on a horse's back, to more reasonable methods including expired air insufflation and closed chest cardiac massage.[7] Although modern cardiopulmonary resuscitation dates from 1960, elements of present-day techniques are to be found in the literature of past centuries.

Elijah (circa 550 B.C.) describes in the Book of Kings the resuscitation of an apparently dead young boy by means of mouth-to-mouth breathing.[73] Although successful expired air resuscitation has been reported sporadically since ancient times, this technique was not perfected and widely employed until the reports of Safar[112,113] and Gordon[53] in 1958. The insertion of an artificial airway for resuscitation was suggested by the experiments of Vesalius in 1543, but was not employed in clinical practice until Herholdt,[61] Desault,[30] and Chaussier[23] inaugurated the technique of orotracheal intubation at the end of the 18th century.

Investigations into the techniques of cardiac resuscitation began in the 1870's with the animal experiments of Boehm,[15] using external cardiac compression, and later of Schiff,[115] who studied open cardiac massage. However, in 1868 Hill had already described the first successful human resuscitations utilizing closed chest massage in an adult and two children undergoing surgery of the extremities with chloroform anesthesia.[63] Since Hill's account appeared in the dental literature, the technique was ignored by physicians for 24 years until 1892 when Maass[87] described successful closed chest massage in a boy under chloroform anesthesia. Similar case reports soon followed.[25,119] Igelsrud, in 1901, successfully described open chest cardiac massage in anesthetized patients.[65] In 1903, G. W. Crile introduced the use of intravenous and intracardiac epinephrine in addition to external cardiac massage with success in animals[28] and later in anesthetized patients.[28a] The eminent Philadelphia surgeon, W. W. Keen,[72] published (in 1904) a classic compilation of case reports of human cardiopulmonary resuscitation performed by himself and numerous others, including Igelsrud and Crile; of the 28 cases, four recovered without apparent sequelae.

The treatment of ventricular fibrillation by electrical shock (defibrillation) began with the experimental work of Prevost and Batelli in 1898,[104,105,106] followed by the more definitive studies in 1932 by Kouwenhoven.[74] Beck[12] reported the first successful open chest cardiac defibrillation in 1947, and successful external defibrillation was described in 1955 by Zoll.[139] The highly successful, systematic modern approach to cardiopulmonary resuscitation in clinical practice began with the work of Safar and others in 1958,[112] proving the superiority of expired air techniques (mouth-to-mouth breathing) over other methods of artificial ventilation, and with the demonstrated effectiveness of closed chest cardiac compression described by Kouwenhoven, Jude, and Knickerbocker in 1960.[75]

DIAGNOSIS OF CARDIOPULMONARY ARREST

The cardinal signs of cessation of *effective* ventilation and circulation are: (1) gasping or apnea; (2) pallor; (3) severely diminished or absent peripheral pulses (carotid and femoral); (4) faint or absent heart tones; and (5) dilatation of the pupils. The appearance of dilated pupils indicates cessation of cerebral circulation for a period of at least 3 minutes; this sign does not imply that resuscitation should not be initiated, especially in infants and children whose central nervous system has a remarkable capacity to recover.

MANAGEMENT OF CARDIOPULMONARY ARREST

The American Heart Association has developed an alphabetic mnemonic utilizing the letters A through F.[7] Basic resuscitation consists of (A) airway management, (B) breathing, and (C) cardiac massage. Advanced resuscitation includes (D) drugs, (E) ECG, endotracheal intubation, evaluation, and (F) fibrillation treatment. A cart with the items outlined in Table 3-7 should be available at all times in emergency rooms, hospital ward treatment rooms, and intensive care units for infants and children. The items outlined should be used in conjunction with a bedside ECG writer and oscilloscope, measurement of systemic arterial pressure, and temperature monitors.

Basic Resuscitation. The patient should be supine on a firm surface with ready access to the head and thorax by the personnel performing resuscitation. Achieving this position may require placement of a board underneath the patient's body.

Ⓐ The airway is cleared by turning the head to one side and aspirating secretions as well as solid material from the oropharynx; if a suction apparatus is not available, the oropharynx should be wiped with a finger. The head is then returned to the face-up position, and the occiput maximally extended while the cervical spine is slightly flexed. The mandible is drawn forward to open the pharyngeal airway and bring the tongue anterior. If attempts to ventilate are unsuccessful because of airway obstruction, an oropharyngeal or nasopharyngeal airway of appropriate size should be inserted (see p. 105).[107a] If a foreign body is lodged in the larynx or trachea, sudden external compression of the epigastrium by the resuscitator may expel the foreign body.[60a]

Ⓑ Breathing by the mouth-to-mouth, mouth-to-nose, or bag and mask[114a] method should be initiated as soon as the airway is cleared. Four large tidal volumes delivered rapidly increase alveolar oxygen tension prior to cardiac massage. Thereafter, the respiratory frequency in infants and children under 3 years of age should be approximately 20 breaths/min., and in older children and adults, 12 to 15 breaths/min. An inspiratory:expiratory ratio of 1:1 is appropriate. The hallmark of effective ventilation is a synchronous rise of the thorax and abdomen during the inspiratory phase. One may also listen for exhaled air through the nose or mouth. A resuscitator's exhaled air contains approximately 17% oxygen, which will raise the alveolar oxygen tension to approximately 80 mm Hg. If supplementary oxygen is available, it should be used in order to further elevate the alveolar oxygen tension and increase the uptake of oxygen from the lungs. The delivered inspired oxygen concentration varies from 30 to 80% with self-inflating

TABLE 3-7. Recommended Contents for a Pediatric Resuscitation Cart

Airway Equipment

1. Bag and masks (infant, child, adult) with nonrebreathing valve that has universal 15-mm female adaptor for male 15-mm endotracheal tube connectors
2. Oropharyngeal airways (Guedel sizes 00, 0, 1, 2, 3, 4)
3. Orotracheal uncuffed tubes (complete sterile set of 2 of each size 2.5 mm ID to 8.0 mm ID) with appropriate size straight 15-mm male connectors; cuffed tubes 6.0 to 8.0 mm ID; lengths cut to oral minimum length plus 2 cm
4. Layrngoscope*
   Adult handle, pediatric handle
   Blades: Miller-premature
   Wis-Hipple 1 and 1½
   Flagg—child
   Macintosh—adult (No. 3,4)
   2 extra batteries
   1 extra light
   1 extra light bulb for each blade
5. Aspiration equipment†
   Metal tonsil aspirator (Yankauer)
   Disposable sterile plastic suction catheters, sizes (Fr.) 5, 8, 10, 14.
6. Magill forceps†
7. Stylets (Teflon coated for tubes size 2.5–8.0 mm ID)†

Drugs

Sodium bicarbonate	Dopamine
Epinephrine	Dextrose (50%)
Isoproterenol	Diazepam
Calcium chloride (10%)	Heparin
Calcium gluconate (10%)	Saline solution (for dilution)

Defibrillator

Direct current with range of 20–400 watt-seconds.
—Saline soaked 4 × 4 gauze pads stored with external paddles.
—Pediatric (5-cm diameter) and adult (10-cm diameter) external paddles.

Miscellaneous

Intracardiac needles: 20 and 22 gauge, 6–8 cm length
Plastic intravenous cannulae (16, 18, 20, and 22 gauge) and scalp vein sets
Sterile cutdown tray with pediatric instruments

Tongue blades	Scissors
Alcohol swabs	Syringes (plastic disposable)
Sterile hemostat	Needles

Sterile 4 × 4 gauze sponges

*See Fig. 3-1.
†See Fig. 3-2.

resuscitator bags at oxygen flows of 5 to 15 liters;[18] when 100% inspired oxygen is needed, a modified "T" piece system[31a] should be used with mask or endotracheal tube.

Ⓒ Cardiac massage is achieved by downward displacement of the sternum and ventricular compression against the thoracic vertebrae at a rate of 100 per minute in infants, and 60 to 80 per minute in children and adults. The middle of the sternum should be depressed 2 to 3 cm in infants, and 5 to 6 cm in adults. The sternum should be held depressed for 0.2 to 0.3 seconds to produce a pulse contour and mean arterial pressure that approach normal.[47] In the infant one can use the two-thumb, chest encircling midsternal method[130,131] (Fig. 3-5). In older infants, two or three fingers, and in a child over 2 years of age, the heel of one hand placed over the midsternum are effective. In children over 6 years of age, the two-hand adult method should be employed. The hallmarks of effective circulation are a palpable carotid or femoral pulse, and a decrease in the size of the pupils.

Advanced Resuscitation. Once the airway has been opened, ventilation of the lungs initiated, and reasonably effective cardiac compression with systemic perfusion achieved, the next phase in cardiopulmonary resuscitation can be undertaken. An intravenous infusion must be established with an indwelling plastic cannula inserted percutaneously or by cutdown in the largest accessible vein. In the event of intense vasoconstriction, a scalp vein needle can be inserted in any peripheral vein until such time as a larger vein can be cannulated. However, a small peripheral scalp vein needle is not a safe lifeline for a patient who requires cardiopulmonary resuscitation. The proper intravenous fluid regimen depends upon the cause of the arrest. The patient's weight, or a reasonable estimate, must be assessed in order to select the appropriate fluid infusion rates and drug dosages.

(D) The fundamental drug administered

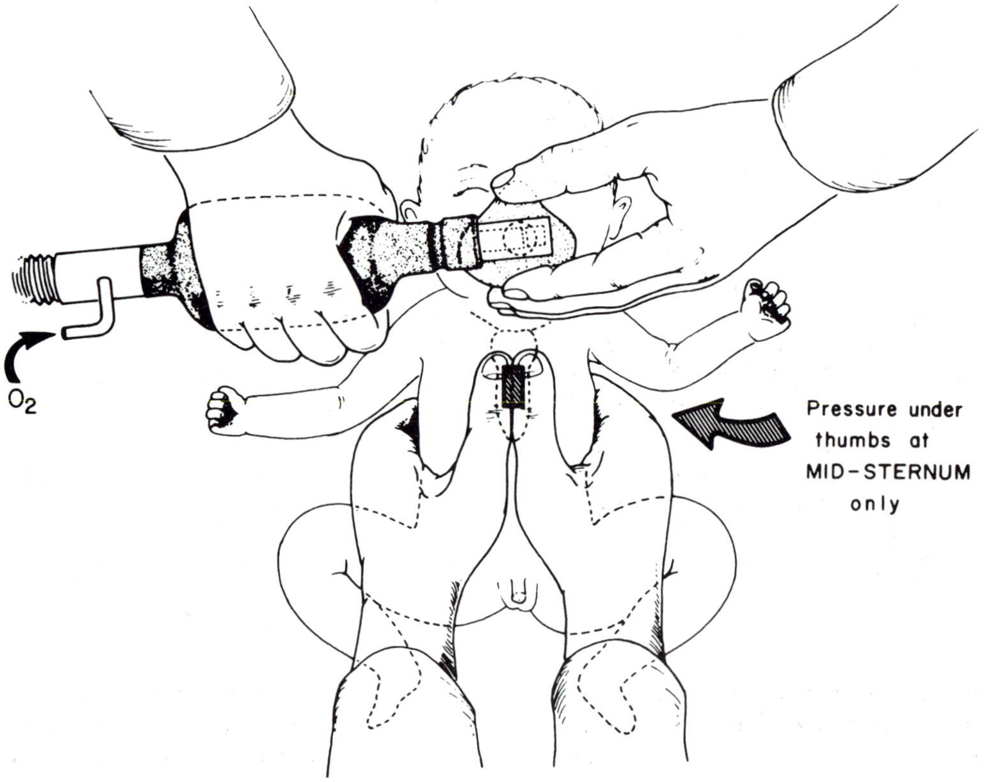

FIG. 3-5. Technique of basic resuscitation in infants using two-thumb sternal compression for closed chest massage, and Rendell-Baker Soucek infant mask with Penlon self-inflating bag-valve system for ventilation (see text). (Reproduced from Todres, D. and M. C. Rogers: Methods of external cardiac massage in the newborn infant. *J. Pediatr. 86*:781, 1975. (With kind permission of authors and publisher, The C. V. Mosby Co., St. Louis.)

in cardiopulmonary resuscitation is *oxygen.* Oxygen (100%) should be given by mask or through an endotracheal tube with controlled ventilation as soon as possible. The other drugs in recommended concentrations and dosages are presented in Table 3-8. Sodium bicarbonate in an initial intravenous dose of 2 to 4 mEq/kg serves to partially correct the inevitable metabolic acidosis associated with the severe tissue hypoxemia that results from ineffective ventilation and circulation. In the presence of cardiac standstill that is refractory to effective ventilation, closed chest massage, and intravenous sodium bicarbonate, intravenous epinephrine should be administered. In the event of failure of an intravenous dose, epinephrine can be given by the intracardiac route. If an intravenous infusion cannot be readily started in cases of cardiac standstill, epinephrine in the same dose as given by the intracardiac route, diluted to a volume of 2 to 5 ml with saline solution (depending on the size of the patient), can be instilled into the trachea. Uptake from the lungs will occur if pulmonary perfusion is maintained by closed cardiac massage. This route is a conservative alternative to intracardiac injection.

Intracardiac injection should be reserved for those instances where repeated intravenous or intratracheal injections of drugs have proven ineffective, a situation that occurs when the circulating blood volume is inadequate or closed chest massage is not effective because of congenital aortic outflow tract

TABLE 3-8. Pediatric Resuscitation Dosages

Drug	Concentration Used	Intravenous Dose	Intracardiac Dose	Frequency of Dose
Sodium bicarbonate	1 mEq/ml	2–4 mEq/kg, up to 200 mEq	½ intravenous	5–10 min.*
Epinephrine	1:10,000 (0.1 mg/ml)	0.01 mg/kg, up to 0.5 mg	Same as intravenous	5–10 min.
	μg/ml numerically equal to wt in kg†	0.2–2.0 μg/kg/min.	—	Continuous infusion
Isoproterenol	1:10,000 (0.1 mg/ml)	0.01 mg/kg up to 0.5 mg	—	Single dose
	μg/ml numerically equal to wt in kg†	0.2–2.0 μg/kg/min.	—	Continuous infusion
Dopamine	μg/ml numerically equal to wt in kg†	2.0–20.0 μg/kg/min.	—	Continuous infusion
Calcium chloride	10% (100 mg/ml)	20 mg/kg	Same as intravenous	10 min.
Calcium gluconate	10% (100 mg/ml)	60 mg/kg	Same as intravenous	10 min.
Defibrillation: 2 to 5 watt-sec/kg initially (external)				

*Obtain arterial sample for pH, PCO_2, base excess as soon as possible to guide alkali therapy.
† See p. 124.

obstruction. Intracardiac injection should be performed with a 10-cm, 22-g needle inserted in the notch between the xiphoid and the left costochondral margin, with the needle aimed at the acromion process of the left shoulder. Advancement of the needle through the diaphragm into the base of the left ventricle then can be performed with slight negative pressure on the syringe until a free flow of blood is obtained. The drug should be rapidly injected and the needle withdrawn. The classic position for intracardiac injection in the fourth intercostal space to the immediate left of the sternum produces a very high incidence of pneumothorax, and less reliable entrance into the left ventricle.

The inhibitory effect of an acidotic pH on the chronotropic and inotropic action of catecholamines should be kept in mind if the initial injection of epinephrine proves ineffective.[116,129] It may be necessary to administer an additional dose of sodium bicarbonate immediately prior to injection of the epinephrine. Atropine (0.01 mg/kg) intravenously can be used for recurring bradycardia, and can be repeated twice in 1 hour.[29,66] Calcium chloride should be reserved for those instances where an increase in myocardial contractility beyond that achieved with epinephrine is required. Intravenous calcium increases the hazard of ventricular arrhythmias in patients who have been receiving digitalis.

Once spontaneous cardiac activity is restored, cardiac output may be insufficient to maintain adequate tissue perfusion. Temporarily, closed chest cardiac massage should be continued and consideration given to a constant infusion of an inotropic drug. Epinephrine increases stroke volume, peripheral vascular resistance, and the cardiac rate even in the presence of a diminished circulating blood volume.[101] If the circulating blood volume is adequate or excessive, and a decrease in systemic vascular resistance is desirable, isoproterenol can provide increased stroke volume and heart rate with a decrease in peripheral vascular resistance.[66a] Dopamine has minimal effects on systemic vascular resistance, increases stroke volume with a small increase in heart rate, and is useful in patients who have tachycardia but require increased cardiac output.[51] The concentration of these drugs should be determined by the following formula:

Concentration = micrograms per ml numerically equivalent to body weight (kg)

Example

20-kg child = concentration of 20 μg/ml

With this concentration, the number of milliliters per mintue equals the micrograms per kilogram per minute (μ/kg/min.) (see Table 3-8).

(E) As soon as possible in cases of cardiopulmonary arrest, a continuous writing ECG and oscilloscope monitor should be attached. The standard lead 2 will usually provide the best assessment of cardiac rhythm. The four common ECG arrhythmias seen are: standstill; ventricular fibrillation; multifocal ventricular tachycardia; and idioventricular rhythm with a wide QRS complex (dying heart). Except for multifocal ventricular tachycardia, the intravenous injection of epinephrine usually facilitates correction of the arrhythmia. Multifocal ventricular tachycardia should be treated with an intravenous injection of lidocaine (Xylocaine) in an initial dose of 1.0 mg/kg.[49]

Tracheal intubation should be performed as soon as basic resuscitation has become effective, or previously if the airway cannot be maintained as described under A. The details of tracheal intubation are presented on page 105.

Evaluation of the cause of the arrest and a written record must be initiated at this point. The few moments spent may ultimately save the patient's life. The record should include: (1) the time that the cardiopulmonary arrest was diagnosed, resuscitation begun, and restoration of breathing and cardiac activity achieved; (2) the drugs, routes and doses employed, as well as other maneuvers performed; and (3) the names of all actively participating personnel.

Inadvertent hypothermia with core temperatures below 36° C can develop during resuscitation, and have disastrous effects: apnea, progressive metabolic acidosis, decreased cardiac output with persistent arterial hypotension, and ventricular arrhythmias. During the period of resuscitation it is important to maintain the patient's core temperature with external heating devices such as water blankets and overhead radiant heaters. Mild hypothermia does little to protect the brain against hypoxemia, and creates conditions that retard or prevent successful resuscitation.

(F) Electrical defibrillation ordinarily is required to convert the heart with ventricular fibrillation to a standstill or regular rhythm. A direct current defibrillator should be utilized with appropriate sized paddles (3- to 4-cm diameter in infants; 4- to 5-cm diameter in the child; 8-cm diameter in the adult). The initial external defibrillation energy dose should be 2 to 5 watt-sec/kg.[126,126a] If this is not successful, the shocks can be gradually increased to 10 watt-sec/kg with a maximum of 400 watt-seconds.[7] The risk of skin burns increases with increasing dosages; saline soaked gauze pads provide a good conductor that minimizes the risk of burns. Severe acidosis, extreme hyperkalemia or hypokalemia, or a Pa_{O_2} less than 30 mm Hg may make the fibrillating ventricle refractory to defibrillation.

POST-RESUSCITATION CARE

Immediately following successful resuscitation, treatment must be directed at two problems: the underlying cause, and the sequelae of the cardiopulmonary arrest. This treatment can be executed best in an intensive care unit. The immediate common sequelae of cardiopulmonary arrest are (1) metabolic acidosis (rebound acidosis) secondary to increased perfusion and removal of lactic acid from peripheral tissues that had been ischemic during the period of inadequate circulation; (2) hyperkalemia secondary to extreme metabolic acidosis; (3) acute renal tubular failure secondary to extreme hypotension; (4) cerebral edema with possible increased intracranial pressure secondary to extreme hypoxemia; and (5) cardiovascular instability with arterial hypotension, arrhythmias, or recurrent arrest if the primary cause is uncorrected.

Treatment of post-resuscitation acidosis should be guided by repeated arterial pH and blood gas tension measurements. Hyperkalemia with serum potassium levels in excess of 6 mEq/l should be treated, during continuous ECG monitoring, by intravenous infusion of (1) calcium gluconate 50 mg/kg (0.5 ml/kg of 10% solution); (2) 2 ml/kg of 25% glucose and insulin; and (3) $NaHCO_3$ 2 mEq/kg (if arterial pH is below 7.30).[31,136a] The treatment of acute renal tubular failure in the early phase involves the rapid infusion of intravenous fluids, followed by a single intravenous injection of mannitol (1.0 g/kg) or furosemide (1 mg/kg) once cardiovascular stability has been achieved. If this treatment fails to produce urine flow, the fluid challenge can be repeated. If urine flow remains less than 0.5 ml/kg/hr for 6 hours, the patient must be considered oliguric or anuric, and be placed on a severely restricted fluid and electrolyte regimen;[31] peritoneal dialysis should also be considered.[10,95]

The key to successful post-resuscitation management is adequate monitoring. The ECG and heart rate must be assessed continuously with high and low rate alarms. The systemic arterial pressure should be continuously measured through a peripheral arterial cannula (radial or dorsalis pedis artery) whenever feasible. Frequent determination of systemic pressure utilizing a conventional cuff with an aneroid manometer and Doppler stethoscope permits some assessment of peripheral perfusion, but is not as reliable as a direct arterial pressure tracing and the continuous use of high and low alarms for systemic arterial pressure. The arterial line also provides an easily accessible means of obtaining blood for arterial pH and blood gas analyses, and determination of electrolytes as well as other biochemical factors.

In patients who have suffered a severe anoxic episode, the continuous monitoring of intracranial pressure with a subdural bolt provides the only effective early warning system of progressive cerebral edema and elevated intracranial pressure.[70,86] When the intracranial pressure exceeds 20 to 30 mm Hg, whether or not decerebrate or decorticate posturing or convulsions occur, the following steps to decrease intracranial pressure should be undertaken immediately:[86] (1) hyperventilation to reduce the Pa_{CO_2} to a level between 25 and 30 mm Hg, which in turn decreases cerebral blood volume; (2) intravenous infusion of mannitol (1.0 g/kg) to decrease brain water content; (3) adrenocorticosteroids (dexamethasone 1.0 mg/kg/6 hr); and rarely (4) deliberate hypothermia (esophageal temperatures between 30 and 32° C) to decrease brain oxygen consumption. In most cases, a hypothermia blanket is needed to prevent hyperthermia and maintain the patient's core temperature between 37 and 38° C.

COMPLICATIONS

The immediate common complications are pneumothorax, skin burns from the defibrillator paddles, and metabolic sequelae (e.g., hypernatremia, hyperosmolality, and alkalosis). Fluid overload from excessive administration of intravenous fluids during resuscitation can manifest itself as pulmonary edema shortly after the resuscitation; this condition is best treated with diuretics such as furosemide, mechanical ventilation with CPAP, and fluid restriction.

Lacerations of the liver as a result of misplaced excessive pressure during closed chest cardiac massage is exceedingly rare.[130a] A portable chest roentgenogram taken as soon as the patient is stable following successful resuscitation is necessary to rule out pneumothorax, to assess the proper placement of a tracheal airway, and to exclude atelectasis or aspiration pneumonitis. The most disastrous late sequelae are acute renal tubular necrosis, and severe, permanent cortical brain injury due to delayed or ineffective therapy.

TERMINATION OF RESUSCITATION

The decision to terminate an unsuccessful resuscitation must be a joint one involving the patient's primary physician or his representative, as well as other participating physicians. This decision usually is based on one or more of the following three criteria: (1) cardiac function cannot be restored; (2) other factors such as massive hemorrhage or massive brain trauma make recovery impossible; or (3) the patient has a known fatal disease that has reached its terminal state. In the last instance, the preferable course is for the primary physician, as well as his consultants and the nurses attending the patient, to reach a decision prior to cardiopulmonary arrest that resuscitation is not indicated. Whether the patient and his parents should participate in this decision depends on many factors beyond the scope of this chapter.

In the post-resuscitation phase of treatment, life support may be withdrawn if the patient meets the specific criteria of brain death: apnea, areflexia, an isoelectric EEG taken at normothermia in the absence of sedatives, and fixed, dilated pupils.[57,58,67] These criteria must persist for 24 hours or more.

RESULTS

Recent data indicate high success rates in cardiopulmonary resuscitation,[41,76,82] especially in infants and children. Ultimate survival of pediatric patients with arrest in a large university hospital with a well-organized pediatric resuscitation team was 47%; 88% of the survivors had no evidence of brain damage.[43] The message seems quite clear: In infants and children who are not afflicted with a terminal disease or anomalies incompatible with conscious, potentially enjoyable life, an all-out effort must be made to restore effective ventilation and circulation, and to support life following resuscitation.

REFERENCES

1. Aass, A. S.: Complications of tracheostomy and long-term intubation: a follow-up study. *Acta Anaesthesiol. Scand. 19*:127, 1975.
2. Aberdeen, E.: Mechanical pulmonary ventilation in infants. Tracheostomy and tracheostomy care in infants. *Proc. R. Soc. Med. 58*:900, 1965.
3. Aberdeen, E. and J. J. Downes: Artificial airways in children. *Surg. Clin. North Am. 54*:1155, 1974.
4. Adair, J. C., W. H. Ring, W. S. Jordan and R. A. Elwyn: Ten years' experience with IPPB in treatment of acute laryngotracheobronchitis. *Anesth. Analg. 50*:649, 1971.
5. Allen, T. H. and I. M. Steven: Prolonged endotracheal intubation in infants and children. *Br. J. Anaesth. 37*:566, 1965.
6. Antyllus (A.D. 117), as cited by Paulus Aegenita (625–690 A.D.) in Adams, F.: *The Seven Books of Paulus Aegenita.* Volume 2, Book 6, Syndenham Society, London, p. 301, 1846.
7. A.M.A.: Standards for cardiopulmonary resuscitation (CPR) and emergency cardiac care (ECC). *J.A.M.A. 227*:165, 1973.
8. Ashbaugh, D. G. and T. L. Petty: Positive end-expiratory pressure. *J. Thorac. Cardiovasc. Surg. 65*:510, 1973.
9. Baratz, R. A., D. M. Philbin and R. W. Patterson: Plasma antidiuretic hormone and urinary output during continuous positive-pressure breathing in dogs. *Anesthesiology 34*:510, 1971.
10. Barry, K. G. and F. D. Schwartz: Peritoneal dialysis—current status and future applications. *Pediatr. Clin. North Am. 11*:593, 1964.
11. Battaglia, J. D. and C. H. Lockhart: Management of acute epiglottitis by nasotracheal intubation. *Am. J. Dis. Child. 129*:334, 1975.
12. Beck, C. S., W. H. Pritchard and H. S. Feil: Ventricular fibrillation of long duration abolished by electric shock. *J.A.M.A. 135*:985, 1947.
13. Bednarek, F. J. and L. R. Kuhns: Endotracheal tube placement in infants determined by suprasternal palpation: A new technique. *Pediatrics 56*:224, 1975.

13a. Bendixen, H. H., L. D. Egbert, J. Hedley-Whyte, M. B. Lauer and H. Pontoppidan: *Respiratory Care.* The C. V. Mosby Co., St. Louis, p. 51, 1965.

14. Berman, L. S., W. W. Fox, R. C. R. Raphaely and J. J. Downes: Optimum levels of CPAP for tracheal extubation of newborn infants. *J. Pediatr. 89*:109, 1976.
15. Boehm, R.: Ueben wiederbelebung nach vergiftungen and asphyxie. *Arch. Exp. Pathol. Pharmacol. 8*:68, 1878.
16. Brandstater, B.: Prolonged intubation: an alternative to tracheostomy in infants. *Paper 106. Proc. First European Congr. Anaesth.,* Vienna, 1962.

16a. Brandstater, B. and M. Muallem: Atelectasis following tracheal suction in infants. *Anesthesiology 31*:468, 1969.

17. Brantigan, C. O.: Delayed major vessel hemorrhage following tracheostomy. *J. Trauma 13*:235, 1973.
18. Carden, E. and M. Bernstein: Investigation of the nine most commonly used resuscitator bags. *J.A.M.A. 212*:589, 1970.
19. Carroll, R. G.: Evaluation of tracheal tube cuff designs. *Crit. Care Med. 1*:45, 1973.
20. Carroll, R. G. and A. Grenvik: Proper use of large diameter, large residual volume cuffs. *Crit. Care Med. 1*:153, 1973.
21. Carroll, R. G., G. E. McGinnis and A. Grenvik: Performance characteristics of tracheal cuffs. *Int. Anesthesiol. Clin. 12*:110, 1974.
22. Chalon, J., D. A. Y. Loew and J. Malebranche: Effects of dry anesthetic gases on tracheobronchial ciliated epithelium. *Anesthesiology 37*:338, 1972.
23. Chaussier, M.: Reflexions sur les moyens propres à determiner la respiration dans les enfants. *Histoire Soc. R. Med. 4*:346, 1780.
24. Clark, J. M. and C. J. Lambertsen: Pulmonary oxygen toxicity: a review. *Pharmacol. Rev. 23*:37, 1971.
25. Cohen, H. M.: Report of a case of combined diaphragmatic or bimanual massage of the heart. *J.A.M.A. 41*:1145, 1903.
26. Cook, C. D. and Motoyama, E.: Respiratory physiology in infants and children. In *Anesthesia for Infants and Children. 3rd ed.,* R. Smith (Ed.). The C. V. Mosby Co., St. Louis, 1968, p. 32.
27. Cooper, J. D. and H. C. Grillo: The evolution of tracheal injury due to ventilatory assistance through cuffed tubes: a pathologic study. *Ann. Surg. 169*:334, 1969.
28. Crile, G. W.: *Blood-Pressure in Surgery.* J. B. Lippincott Co., Philadelphia, p. 411, 1903.

28a. Crile, G. W. (1903–1904): cited in Keen, W. W.[72]

29. Dauchot, P. and J. S. Gravenstein: Effects of atropine on the electrocardiogram in different age groups. *Clin. Pharmacol. Ther. 12*:274, 1971.
30. Desault, P. J.: *Oeuvre Chirurgicales. Exposé de la Doctrine et de la Practique de Desault; par Bichat.* Paris, p. 266, 1801.
31. Dobrin, R. S., C. D. Larsen and M. A. Holliday: Acute renal failure. In *The Critically Ill Child,* C. A. Smith (Ed.). W. B. Saunders Co., Philadelphia, 1972.
31a. Dorsch, J. A. and S. E. Dorsch: *Understanding Anesthesia Equipment.* The Williams & Wilkins Co., Baltimore, p. 159, 1975.
32. Downes, J. J., J. F. Wilson and D. Goodson: Apnea, suction, and hyperventilation: effect on arterial oxygen saturation. *Anesthesiology 22*:29, 1961.
33. Downes, J. J., T. W. Striker and S. Stool: Complications of nasotracheal intubation in children with croup. *N. Engl. J. Med. 274*:226, 1966 (letter).
34. Downes, J. J., D. W. Wood, T. W. Striker and C. Haddad: Acute respiratory failure in infants with bronchiolitis. *Anesthesiology 22*:29, 1961.
35. Downes, J. J., H. F. Nicodemus, W. S. Pierce and J. A. Waldhausen: Acute respiratory failure in infants following cardiovascular surgery. *J. Thorac. Cardiovasc. Surg. 59*:21, 1970.
36. Downes, J. J. and R. C. Raphaely: Pediatric intensive care. *Anesthesiology 43*:238, 1975.
37. Downes, J. J.: CPAP and PEEP—a perspective (editorial). *Anesthesiology 44*:1, 1976.
38. Downs, J. B., E. F. Klein, D. Desautels, J. H. Modell and R. R. Kirby: Intermittent mandatory ventilation. *Chest 64*:331, 1973.
39. Drury, D. R., J. P. Henry and J. Goodman: The effects of continuous pressure breathing on kidney function. *J. Clin. Invest. 26*:945, 1947.
40. Dunn, C. R., D. L. Dunn and K. M. Moser: Determinants of tracheal injury by cuffed tracheostomy tubes. *Chest 65*:128, 1974.
41. Dupont, B., E. Flensted-Jensen and E. Sandoe: The long-term prognosis for patients resuscitated after cardiac arrest. A follow-up study. *Am. Heart J. 78*:444, 1969.
42. Eden, A. N., A. Kaufman and R. Yu: Corticosteroids and croup. *J.A.M.A. 200*:403, 1967.
43. Ehrlich, R., S. M. Emmet and R. Rodriguez-Torres: Pediatric cardiac resuscitation team: a 6 year study. *J. Pediatr. 84*:152, 1974.
44. Engström, C. G.: Treatment of severe cases of respiratory paralysis by the Engström universal respirator. *Br. J. Med. 2*:666, 1954.
45. Epstein, R. A.: Sensitivities and response times of ventilatory assistors. *Anesthesiology 34*:321, 1971.
46. Fairley, H. B. and D. D. Hunter: The performance of respirators used in treatment of respiratory insufficiency. *Can. Med. Assoc. J. 90*:1397, 1964.
47. Falsetti, H. L. and D. G. Greene: Technique of compression in closed-chest cardiac massage. *J.A.M.A. 200*:793, 1967.
47a. Farmati, O., J. R. Quinn and R. H. Fennell, Jr.: Exfoliative cytology of the intubated larynx in children. *Can. Anaesth. Soc. J. 14*:321, 1967.
48. Feeley, T. W. and J. Hedley-Whyte: Weaning from controlled ventilation and supplemental oxygen. *N. Engl. J. Med. 292*:903, 1975.
48a. Feeley, T. W., R. Saumarez, J. M. Klick, T. G. McNabb and J. J. Skillman: Positive end-expiratory pressure in weaning patients from controlled ventilation—a prospective randomised trial. *Lancet 2*:725, 1975.
49. Gelband, H. and M. R. Rosen: Pharmacologic basis for the treatment of cardiac arrhythmias. *Pediatrics 55*:59, 1975.
50. Gillespie, N. A.: *Endotracheal anesthesia* (3rd ed.). University of Wisconsin Press, Madison, p. 6, 1963.
51. Goldberg, L. I.: Dopamine—Clinical uses of an endogenous catecholamine. *N. Engl. J. Med. 291*:707, 1974.
52. Goodman, L. S. and A. Gilman (Ed.): The Pharmacological Basis of Therapeutics. (5th ed.) Macmillan Co., Inc., New York, p. 502, 1975.
53. Gordon, A. S., C. W. Frye, L. Gittelson, M. S. Sadove and E. J. Beattie, Jr.: Mouth-to-mouth versus manual artificial respiration for children and adults. *J.A.M.A. 167*:320, 1958.
54. Gregory, G. A., J. A. Kitterman, R. H. Phibbs and W. H. Tooley: Treatment of the idiopathic respiratory-distress syndrome with continuous positive airway pressure. *N. Engl. J. Med. 284*:1333, 1971.
55. Gregory, G. A., L. H. Edmunds, Jr., J. A. Kitterman, R. H. Phibbs and W. H. Tooley: Continuous positive airway pressure and pulmonary and circulatory function after cardiac surgery in infants less than three months of age. *Anesthesiology 43*:426, 1975.
55a. Grillo, H. C.: The management of tracheal stenosis following assisted respiration. *J. Thorac. Cardiovasc. Surg. 57*:52, 1969.
56. Haddad, C. and C. C. Richards: Mechanical ventilation of infants: significance and elimination of ventilator compression volume. *Anesthesiology 29*:365, 1968.
57. Harp, J. R.: Criteria for the determination of death. *Anesthesiology 40*:391, 1974.
58. Harvard Medical School: A definition of irreversible coma—report of the ad hoc committee to examine the definition of brain death. *J.A.M.A. 205*:337, 1968.
59. Hatch, D. J.: Prolonged nasotracheal intubation in infants and children. *Lancet 1*:1272, 1968.
60. Hayes, B. and J. S. Robinson: An assessment of methods of humidification of inspired gas. *Br. J. Anaesth. 42*:94, 1970.

60a. Heimlich, H. J.: A life-saving maneuver to prevent food-choking. *J.A.M.A. 234*:398, 1975.

61. Herholdt, J. D. and C. E. Rafn: Life Saving Measures for Drowning Persons. H. Tikiob, Copenhagen, p. 52, 1796; cited by Gillespie, N. A.[50]

62. Hilding, A. C.: Laryngotracheal damage during intratracheal anesthesia. Demonstration by staining the unfixed specimen with methylene blue. *Ann. Otol. Rhinol. Laryngol. 80*:565, 1971.

63. Hill, J. D.: Observations on some of the dangers of chloroform in surgical practice, and a successful mode of treatment. *Br. J. Dent. Sci. 2*:355, 1868.

64. Hirsch, J. A., J. L. Tokayer, M. J. Robinson and M. A. Sackner: Effects of dry air and subsequent humidification on tracheal mucous velocity in dogs. *J. Appl. Physiol. 39*(2):242, 1975.

65. Igelsrud, K. (1901): cited by Keen, W. W. (1904).[72]

65a. Iliff A. and V. A. Lee: Pulse rate, respiratory rate, and body temperature of children between two months and eighteen years of age. *Child Dev. 23*:237, 1952.

66. Innes, J. R. and M. Nickerson: Atropine, scopolamine, and related antimuscarinic drugs. In *The Pharmacological Basis of Therapeutics,* 5th ed., L. S. Goodman, and A. Gilman (Eds.) Macmillan Publishing Co., New York, p. 518, 1975.

66a. *Ibid.,* p.493.

67. Institute of Society, Ethics, and the Life Sciences: Refinements in criteria for the determination of death: an appraisal. A report by the task force on death and dying. *J.A.M.A. 221*:48, 1972.

67a. International Standards Organization (I.S.O.) Technical Committee 121, Subcommittee 3 (Chairman, M. Saklad): Breathing Machines for Medical Use (1972). To be published by the I.S.O., Geneva, Switzerland, 1978.

68. Jackson, C.: Laryngeal, bronchial, and esophageal endoscopy. *Laryngoscope 21*:1183, 1911.

69. Jackson, C.: The technique of insertion of intratracheal insufflator tubes. *Surg. Gynecol. Obstet. 17*:507, 1913.

70. James, H. E., L. Bruno and L. Schut: Intracranial subarachnoid pressure monitoring in children. *Surg. Neurol. 3*:313, 1975.

71. James, J. A.: Dexamethasone in croup. A controlled study. *Am. J. Dis. Child., 117*:511, 1969.

72. Keen, W. W.: A case of total laryngectomy (unsuccessful) and a case of abdominal hysterectomy (successful) in both of which massage of the heart for chloroform collapse was employed, with notes of 25 other cases of cardiac massage. *Ther. Gaz. 28*:217, 1904.

73. Kings II, Chapter 4, verses 32–37, *Holy Bible, Douay-Rheims Version,* Benzinger Brothers, New York, 1941.

74. Kouwenhoven, W. B., R. Hooker and O. R. Langworthy: The current flowing through the heart under conditions of electric shock. *Am. J. Physiol. 100*:344, 1932.

75. Kouwenhoven, W. B., J. R. Jude and G. G. Knickerbocker: Closed-chest cardiac massage. *J.A.M.A. 173*:1064, 1960.

76. Kravitz, A. E. and T. Killip: Cardiopulmonary resuscitation: status report. *N. Engl. J. Med. 286*:1000, 1972.

77. Kumar, A., H. Pontoppidan, K. J. Falke et al.: Pulmonary barotrauma during mechanical ventilation. *Crit. Care Med. 1*:181, 1973.

78. Lane, E. E., G. D. Temes and W. H. Anderson: Tracheal-innominate artery fistula due to tracheostomy. *Chest 68*:678, 1975.

79. Lassen, H. C. A.: A preliminary report on the 1952 epidemic of poliomyelitis in Copenhagen with special reference to the treatment of acute respiratory insufficiency. *Lancet 1*:37, 1953.

80. Läwen, A. and R. Sievers: Zur praktischer Anwendung der instrumentellen kunstilchen Respiration am Menschen. *Munch. Med. Wochenschr. 57*:2221, 1910.

81. Lee, C. J., J. H. Lyons, S. Konisberg, F. Morgan and F. D. Moore: Effects of spontaneous and positive-pressure breathing of ambient air and pure oxygen at one atmosphere on pulmonary surface characteristics. *J. Thorac. Cardiovasc. Surg. 53*:759, 1967.

82. Lemire, J. G. and A. L. Johnson: Is cardiac resuscitation worthwhile? A decade of experience. *N. Engl. J. Med. 286*:970, 1972.

83. Lindholm, C. E.: Prolonged endotracheal intubation. *Acta Anaesthesiol. Scand.,* Suppl. 23, 1969.

84. Louhimo, I., B. Grahne, M. Pasila and T. Suutarinen: Acquired laryngotracheal stenosis in children. *J. Pediatr. Surg. 6*:730, 1971.

85. Lowbury, E. J. L., B. T. Thom, H. A. Lilly, J. R. Babb and K. Whittall: Sources of infection with Pseudomonas aeruginosa in patients with tracheostomy. *J. Med. Microbiol. 3*:39, 1970.

86. Lundberg, N., A. Kjällquist, G. Kullberg, U. Pontén and G. Sundbärg: Non-operative management of intracranial hypertension. In *Advances and Technical Standards in Neurosurgery,* Volume 1, Springer-Verlag, New York, 1974.

87. Maass: Die method der wiederbelebung bei herztod nach chloroformeinathmung *Berl. Klin. Wochenschrift 29*:265, 1892.

88. MacEwen, W.: Clinical observations on the introduction of tracheal tubes by the mouth instead of performing tracheotomy or laryngotomy. *Br. Med. J. 2*:122, 1880.

89. MacEwen, W.: The surgical treatment of croup and diphtheria by the introduction of tubes into the trachea through the mouth. *Br. Med. J. 2*:523, 1881.

90. Magovern, G. J., J. G. Shively, D. Fecht and

F. Thevoz: The clinical and experimental evaluation of a controlled-pressure intratracheal cuff. *J. Thorac. Cardiovasc. Surg. 64*:747, 1972.

91. Margolis, C. L., D. L. Ingram and J. H. Meyer: Routine tracheotomy in *Hemophilis influenzae* type b epiglottitis. *J. Pediatr. 81*:1150, 1972.
92. Matas, R.: Artificial respiration by direct intralaryngeal intubation with a modified O'Dwyer tube and a new graduated air-pump, in its applications to medical and surgical practice. *Am. J. Med. 3*:97, 1902.
93. McDonald, I. H. and J. G. Stocks: Prolonged nasotracheal intubation. A review of its development in a paediatric hospital. *Br. J. Anaesth. 37*:161, 1965.
94. Mellins, R. B.: Pulmonary physiotherapy in the pediatric age group. *Am. Rev. Respir. Dis. 110*:137, 1974.
95. Miller, R. B. and C. R. Tassistro: Peritoneal dialysis. *N. Engl. J. Med. 281*:945, 1969.

95a. Modell, J. H., S. T. Giammona and J. H. Davis: Effect of chronic exposure to ultrasonic aerosols on the lung. *Anesthesiology 28*:680, 1967.

95b. Mushin, W. W., L. Rendell-Baker, P. W. Thompson and W. W. Mapleson: *Automatic Ventilation of the Lung* (2nd ed.), F. A. Davis Co., Philadelphia, 1969.

96. Nash, G., J. A. Bowen and P. C. Langlinais: Respirator lung: a misnomer. *Arch. Pathol. 91*:234, 1971.
97. Norlander, O. P. and C. G. Engstrom: Volume-controlled respirators. *Ann. N.Y. Acad. Sci. 121*:766, 1965.
98. O'Dwyer, J: Fifty cases of croup in private practice treated by intubation of the larynx. *Med. Record 32*:557, 1887.
99. Oliver, P., J. R. Richardson, R. W. Clubb and C. G. Flake: Tracheotomy in children. *N. Engl. J. Med. 267*:631, 1962.
100. Owen-Thomas, J. B.: A follow-up of children treated by prolonged nasal intubation. *Can. Anaesth. Soc. J. 14*:543, 1967.
101. Pearson, J. W. and J. S. Redding: Epinephrine in cardiac resuscitation. *Am. Heart J. 66*:210, 1963.
102. Pontoppidan, H., B. Geffin and E. Lowenstein: Acute respiratory failure in the adult. *N. Engl. J. Med. 287*:690; 743; 799, 1972.
103. *Ibid.,* p. 801.
104. Prevost, J. L. and F. Batelli: La mort par les courants électriques: courants alternatifs à haute tension. *J. Physiol. Pathol. Gen. 1*:427, 1899.
105. Prevost, J. L. and F. Batelli: La mort par les déscharges électrique. *J. Physiol Pathol. Gen. 1*:1114, 1899.
106. Prevost, J. L. and F. Batelli: Quelques effects des déscharges électriques sur le coeur des mammifères. *J. Physiol. Pathol. Gen. 2*:40, 1900.
107. Proctor, D. F.: Physiology of the upper airway. In *Handbook of Physiology, Section 3, Respiration,* Volume 1, W. O. Fenn and H. Rahn (Eds.). American Physiological Society, Washington, p. 323, 1964.

107a. Proctor, D. F. and P. Safar: Management of airway obstruction. In *Respiratory Therapy,* P. Safar (Ed.). F. A. Davis, Philadelphia, p. 30, 1965.

108. Radford, E. P., Jr., B. G. Ferris, Jr. and B. C. Kriete: Clinical use of a nomogram to estimate proper ventilation during artificial respiration. *N. Engl. J. Med. 251*:877, 1954.
109. Rasche, R. F. H. and Lawrence R. Kuhns: Histopathologic changes in airway mucosa of infants after endotracheal intubation. *Pediatrics 50*:632, 1972.
110. Rowbotham, E. S. and J. W. Magill: Anesthetics in plastic surgery of the face and jaws. *Proc. R. Soc. Med. 14*:17, 1921.
111. Sackner, M. A., J. F. Landa, N. Greeneltch and M. J. Robinson: Pathogenesis and prevention of tracheobronchial damage with suction procedures. *Chest 64*:284, 1973.
112. Safar, P., L. A. Escarraga, and J. O. Elam: A comparison of the mouth-to-mouth and mouth-to-airway methods of artificial respiration with the chest-pressure arm-lift methods. *N. Engl. J. Med. 258*:671, 1958.
113. Safar, P.: Ventilatory efficacy of mouth-to-mouth artificial respiration. Airway obstruction during manual and mouth-to-mouth artificial respiration. *J.A.M.A. 167*:335, 1958.
114. Safar, P.: Recognition and management of airway obstruction. *J.A.M.A. 208*:1008, 1969.

114a. Safar, P. (Ed.): *Respiratory Therapy.* F. A. Davis, Philadelphia, p. 82, 1965.

114b. Scarpelli, E. M. and P. A. M. Auld: *Pulmonary Physiology of the Fetus, Newborn, and Child.* Lea & Febiger, Philadelphia, 1975.

115. Schiff, M.: *Receuil des Memoires Physiologiques,* Volume 3, 1896. Cited in Pearson, J. W.: *Historical and Experimental Approaches to Modern Resuscitation.* Charles C Thomas, Springfield, Ill., 1965.
116. Schroeder, J. S., S. C. Robison, H. A. Miller and D. C. Harrison: Effects of respiratory acidosis on circulatory response to isoproterenol. *Am. J. Physiol. 218*:448, 1970.
117. Shakoor, M. A., J. Sabean, K. M. Wilson, H. H. Hurt and V. D. Graff: High-density water environment by ultrasonic humidification: pulmonary and systemic effects. *Anesth. Analg. 47*:638, 1968.
118. Sladen, A., M. B. Laver and H. Pontoppidan: Pulmonary complications and water retention in

prolonged mechanical ventilation. *N. Engl. J. Med. 279*:448, 1968.

119. Starling, E. A. and W. A. Lane: Reflex inhibition of the heart during administration of ether. *Lancet 2*:1397, 1902.
120. Stetson, J. B. and W. L. Guess: Causes of damage to tissues by polymers and elastomers used in the fabrication of tracheal devices. *Anesthesiology 33*:635, 1970.
121. Stiles, C. M.: A flexible fiberoptic bronchoscope for endotracheal intubation of infants. *Anesth. Analg. 53*:1017, 1974.
122. Stool, S. E., J. R. Campbell and D. G. Johnson: Tracheostomy in children: the use of plastic tubes. *Pediatr. Surg. 3*:402, 1968.
123. Striker, T. W., S. Stool and J. J. Downes: Prolonged nasotracheal intubation in infants and children. *Arch. Otolaryngol. 85*:210, 1967.
124. Suter, P. M., H. B. Fairley and M. D. Isenberg: Optimum end-expiratory airway pressure in patients with acute pulmonary failure. *N. Engl. J. Med. 292*:284, 1975.
125. Symchych, P. S. and M. Cadotte: Squamous metaplasia and necrosis of the trachea complicating prolonged nasotracheal intubation of small newborn infants. An autopsy study. *J. Pediatr. 71*:534, 1967.
126. Tacker, W. A., F. M. Galioto, E. Giuliani, L. A. Geddes and D. G. McNamara: Energy dosage for human transchest electrical ventricular defibrillation. *N. Engl. J. Med. 290*:214, 1974.

126a. Gutgesell, H. P., W. A. Tacker, L. A. Geddes, J. S. Davis, J. T. Lie and D. G. McNamara: Energy dose for ventricular fibrillation in children. *Pediatrics 58*:898, 1976.

127. Talbert, J. L. and J. A. Haller: Improved silastic tracheostomy tubes for infants and young children. *J. Pediatr. Surg. 3*:408, 1968.
128. Taussig, L. M., O. Castro, P. H. Beaudry, W. W. Fox and M. Bureau: Treatment of laryngotracheobronchitis (croup). Use of intermittent positive-pressure breathing and racemic epinephrine. *Am. J. Dis. Child. 129*:790, 1975.
129. Tenney, S. M.: Sympatho-adrenal stimulation by carbon dioxide inhalation and inhibitory effect of carbonic acid on epinephrine response. *Am. J. Physiol. 187*:341, 1956.
130. Thaler, M. M. and G. H. C. Stobie: An improved technic of external cardiac compression in infants and young children. *N. Engl. J. Med. 269*:606, 1963.

130a. Thaler, M. M. and V. W. Krause: Serious trauma in children after external cardiac massage. *N. Engl. J. Med. 267*:500, 1962.

131. Todres, I. D. and M. C. Rogers: Methods of external cardiac massage in the newborn infant. *J. Pediatr. 86*:781, 1975.
132. Trendelenberg, F.: Tamponade de trachea. *Arch. Klin. Chir. 12*:121, 1871.
133. Vesalius, A.: *De Humani Corporis Fabrica, Book* 7, Oporinus, Basel, p. 662 (incorrectly numbered p. 658), 1543.
134. Waters, R. M., E. A. Rovenstein and A. E. Guedel: Endotracheal anesthesia and its historical development. *Anesth. Analg. 12*:196, 1933.
135. Way, W. L. and F. A. Sooy: Histologic changes produced by endotracheal intubation. *Ann. Otol. Rhinol. Laryngol. 74*:799, 1965.
136. Wesley, A. G.: Interpretation of arterial carbon dioxide tension in laryngotracheobronchitis. *S. Afr. Med. J. 48*:1152, 1974.

136a. Williams, G. S., E. L. Klenk and R. W. Winters: Acute renal failure in pediatrics. In *The Body Fluids in Pediatrics,* R. W. Winters (Ed.) Little, Brown and Co., Boston, p. 523, 1973.

137. Wood, D. W., J. J. Downes and H. I. Lecks: The management of respiratory failure in childhood status asthmaticus. Experience with 30 episodes and evolution of a technique. *J. Allergy 42*:261, 1968.
138. Wu, W., I. Lim, F. A. Simpson, Jr. and H. Turndorf: Pressure dynamics of endotracheal and tracheostomy cuffs. 1. Use of a tracheal model to evaluate performance. *Crit. Care Med. 1*:197, 1973.
139. Zoll, P. M., A. J. Linenthal, W. Gibson, M. H. Paul and L. R. Norman: Termination of ventricular fibrillation in man by externally applied electrical countershock. *N. Engl. J. Med. 254*:727, 1956.

Inhalation Therapy

CARL F. DOERSHUK, MARVIN D. LOUGH,
AND LEROY W. MATTHEWS

4

Several textbooks have discussed the many aspects of inhalation therapy.[7,11,16,42] The purpose of this chapter is to emphasize areas of importance to the pediatrician and to pediatric patients. A pediatric respiratory text[28] provides additional details.

General Considerations

If the respiratory or inhalation therapy department has a separate pediatric section, that unit should have as its medical director a pediatrician versed in all aspects of the specialty. If, however, pediatric service is provided as part of the overall obligation of the department to the hospital, a pediatrician interested and experienced in respiratory therapy should be a member of the directing group of physicians. All of the therapists should be aware of the special needs of the pediatric patient. The department should be responsible for using, providing, cleaning, and sterilizing all of the equipment and for supervising the maintenance of such equipment. The department should have at least one registered therapist who is especially skilled in pediatrics and a technical director who supervises the day-to-day activities of the department.

The respiratory therapist provides the equipment and responds to all emergency calls for ventilatory assistance. This service must be available on a 24-hour, 7-day-a-week basis. Since blood gas analysis is an integral part of successful ventilatory assistance, this facility is also needed around the clock. Best results are obtained when the technicians themselves perform the analyses.

Two factors of primary concern with regard to inhalation therapy of infants and children are the size of the infant or child and the psychologic preparation required for treatment.

SIZE OF PATIENT

The first considerations are related to body size of the patient. These aspects include size of face masks and resuscitation bags, oral airways, laryngoscope blades, and the length and diameter of endotracheal tubes. Appropriately sized connectors and adaptors must be immediately available for the successful support of ventilation or resuscitation for any size patient from the smallest premature infant to the largest child or adolescent.

For example, as recently as 1967, Fearon and Whalen reported the disagreement concerning the optimal and safe lengths of the tracheal portion of endotracheal tubes and presented the results of measurements of tracheal length in 100 living infants from birth to 18 months of age.[20] Table 4-1 gives the results for their living subjects and, for contrast, the measurements obtained at autopsy by Engel.[17]

TABLE 4-1. Tracheal Length in Living and Autopsied Infants

Age (mo)	Mean Length Living (cm)	Mean Length Autopsy (cm)
Birth–3	5.7 (5.0–7.5)	4.0
3–6	6.7 (5.5–8.0)	4.2
6–12	7.2 (5.0–9.0)	4.3
12–18	8.1 (7.0–9.0)	4.5

Body surface area, tidal volume, lung volumes, and anatomic dead space are reported to be similar on a weight basis throughout life. Radford et al.[38] constructed a nomogram for predicting the optimal tidal volume based on body weight, sex, and breathing frequency[38] (see Fig. 1-30). This nomogram provides a useful first approximation for initiating ventilatory support until subsequent blood gas determinations are available to guide the selection of appropriate tidal and minute volumes.

PSYCHOLOGIC PREPARATION

A thorough and understandable explanation appropriate to the age of the child should be provided, with opportunity for the child to verbalize fears and ask questions about each type of therapy planned. Where appropriate, the child should be permitted to handle or inspect the equipment, and every effort should be made to alleviate fear by dispelling erroneous ideas. Often the opportunity to observe successful treatment of another child ensures acceptance of therapy. Parents also require an explanation, and often this discussion helps the child to accept the therapy.

A calm attitude and continuing reassurance should always be a part of the approach to any child and actually to patients of any age. Repeated brief explanations facilitate therapy. All patients should be warned before a painful procedure is performed; reassurances, followed by unexpected pain, are counterproductive. It is particularly helpful to establish some physical contact. With younger children this factor is perhaps easiest to accomplish because they can be held on the therapist's lap during treatment, in a natural position and in a comforting way. The therapy period should be supervised throughout by a respiratory therapist or a similarly trained person known to the child.

Oxygen Administration

Correct administration of oxygen is an important aspect of inhalation therapy, whether for adults or for pediatric patients. Excessive amounts of oxygen can destroy living cells and produce permanent damage to vision in premature infants and to the respiratory tract of patients of any age.

OXYGEN ANALYZERS

An oxygen analyzer is one of the most important tools available to the pediatric inhalation therapist. The three types of oxygen analyzers or monitors most commonly used are (1) thermal conductivity, (2) paramagnetic susceptibility (Pauling type), and (3) electrode sensor (see also Fig. 1-39).

The thermal conductivity analyzer cannot detect oxygen concentrations in gases other than oxygen-nitrogen mixtures, and should never be used to analyze mixtures that contain a flammable gas, such as those encountered in anesthesia. The analyzer should be checked frequently by testing with a known oxygen-nitrogen mixture.

The advantage of the paramagnetic analyzer is its ability to analyze oxygen concentrations in any mixture of gases. Although its calibration is generally reliable, it is somewhat fragile.

The electrode sensing analyzer (Clark electrode) is a reliable unit that can be plugged into a monitor so that an oxygen percentage reading with a high-low limit alarm can be supplied continuously. This dual capability makes it more useful.

NASAL ADMINISTRATION

The *oxygen nasal cannula* is used to deliver low to moderate concentrations of oxygen (up to 40%). The usual flow rate is 6 to 8 l/min. The oxygen must be well humidified to prevent nasal irritation. Care is required with this technique, since the oxygen cannula usually is not well tolerated by children. The tendency of children to breathe through their mouth when there is associated upper respiratory disease decreases the effectiveness of this therapy. The cannula is also easily dislodged and thus requires close observation.

The *oxygen nasal catheter* is placed through the nose so that the tip is in the oropharynx. This technique of administering oxygen is suitable for moderate concentrations of 40 to 50% oxygen at a flow rate of 6 to 8 l/min. Adequate humidification is very important.

The nasal catheter, like the cannula, is usually not tolerated well by children. When used, the catheter should be changed every 8 hours using alternate nostrils. Humidification must be adequate in order to prevent irritation of the nasal and pharyngeal mucosa. Abdominal distention may occur if there is an impaired epiglottic reflex. The catheter may be partially removed because of faulty fixation or patient motion and thus requires close observation. Nonallergenic adhesive tape should be used to secure the catheter and prevent skin irritation.

ORONASAL ADMINISTRATION

Oxygen masks are of varying sizes, shapes, and forms. Not long ago, a common household funnel was a substitute for an oxygen mask. Only recently have oxygen masks designed specifically for children become available. Use of the new soft vinyl masks prevent the pressure necrosis and skin irritation produced by the more rigid plastic masks. Head straps used to hold the mask in place are often uncomfortable. Small pieces of cotton placed above the ear help relieve the pressure and discomfort caused by the strap. The mask should be removed frequently and dried. The patient's face should be dried and lightly powdered to prevent the accumulation of moisture, which softens the skin.

Sufficient flow of gas (6 to 7 l/min.) must enter the mask to prevent carbon dioxide buildup since the space under the mask and around the face is added dead space. For this reason, an adult mask should not be used to administer oxygen to children.

It is recommended that an oxygen tent rather than an oxygen mask be used for infants and children in coma because of the increased risk of aspiration if the patient vomits during mask therapy.

Several oxygen masks meet specific needs. The medium concentration mask (Fig. 4-1) can provide oxygen concentrations from 35 to 60% depending on gas flow (Table 4-2). The partial rebreathing mask utilizes a reservoir bag and, when close fitting, oxygen concentrations up to 95% can be obtained (Table 4-2).

Venturi mixing masks such as the Mix-O-Mask (see Fig. 4-1) are designed to deliver low to moderate concentrations of oxygen (24, 28, 35, or 40%) over extended periods of time. The concentration of oxygen is determined by the diameter of the jet orifice that is used to limit the amount of air being pulled into the large-bore tube just before entering the face mask.

Because of its shape and construction, the Ventimask should not be used for children. The diameter of the face piece is unnecessarily large, covers the child's whole face, and obscures vision. The plastic material is rigid and has pointed edges, which can cause skin irritation.

OXYGEN TENTS

Currently tents are used as the most common, but not most efficient, method for administering moderate concentrations (30 to 50%) of oxygen to the pediatric patient. Pediatric tents also provide some control of humidity and temperature, and elimination of carbon dioxide. The tent most frequently

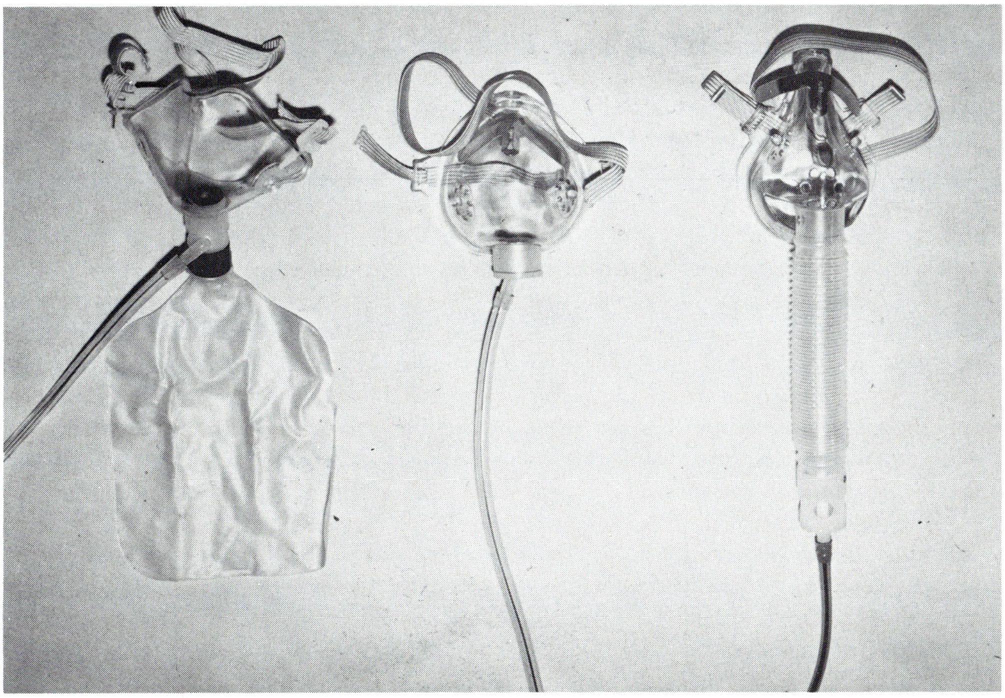

FIG. 4-1. Three soft vinyl masks commonly used for pediatric oxygen therapy showing the medium concentration mask in the middle, the partial rebreathing mask on the left, and the Venturi-type mask on the right.

TABLE 4-2. Oxygen Flow Required to Achieve Desired Oxygen Concentration in Mask Therapy*

Oxygen Flow Required (l/min.)	Mask Therapy Oxygen Concentration Desired (%)	
	Partial rebreathing oxygen mask	Pediatric medium-concentration oxygen mask
6–8	40–50	35–45
8–10	50–60	45–55
10–12	90–95	55–60

* Approximate figures.

used is referred to as a croup tent. These tents are designed to be placed in a crib or hung at the head of a youth bed. A cool environmental temperature (6 to 8° F below ambient) can be achieved by circulating the tent atmosphere through an ice chamber, and care must be taken not to overcool the patient. High levels of humidity may be attained by means of the nebulizer, which produces relatively large liquid particles. A tightly fitting canopy must be maintained to minimize oxygen leakage, but a tight fit may be very difficult to achieve with a restless or uncooperative child. At this point, the repetition of a complete explanation of the prescribed therapy to the child and parents may prove beneficial. Permitting the mother to hold the child's hand through a small opening in the zipper of the canopy is sometimes helpful in calming the fearful child.

The fewer times the tent atmosphere is disrupted by opening the canopy, the better therapy the patient receives. The smallest practical tent should be used in order to achieve the desired concentration of oxygen, while maintaining patient comfort, which is also of concern. If the ice in the cooling chamber is allowed to melt without being replenished, the tent temperature may increase 8 to 10° F or more.

The disadvantage of the tent is that the child cannot be easily observed for vital signs and cyanosis in a tent.

OXYGEN HOODS

If a small plastic hood is placed over an infant's head, better control of the oxygen atmosphere can be achieved, since the incubator can be entered repeatedly without disturbing the inner hood. Mestayan et al. demonstrated that cold oxygen blown on an infant's face increases oxygen consumption.[30] To avoid this stimulus, the oxygen must be warmed to the infant's neutral thermal temperature or to the environmental temperature of the incubator. The oxygen also must be humidified in order to minimize water loss and prevent drying of secretions in the respiratory tract. An all-purpose nebulizer with an adjustable heater permits hood temperature control and provides adequate humidification. The hood oxygen concentration should be recorded at regular intervals. The hood temperature should also be checked frequently until stable, and then hourly to prevent overheating or cooling of the infant and to keep the oxygen consumption at a basal level. An oxygen ratio controller can also be used to provide precise concentrations of oxygen. By adjusting the flow of each gas independently, an exact mixture of oxygen and air can be obtained. A total flow of 7 l/min. is required to remove carbon dioxide from the infant hood.

Careful monitoring of arterial oxygen partial pressure and saturation is mandatory when using an oxygen enriched atmosphere, whether above or below 40%. Direct sampling of arterial blood is ideal. In small infants, the two sites commonly used are the umbilical or temporal artery. Later in life the brachial or radial artery is used.

INCUBATORS

Newborn infants with respiratory disease require isolation, warming, and humidity. Precise control of temperature, oxygen, humidity, and isolation is made possible by the design of the incubator. One of the important features of an incubator provides for isolation of the infant from the surrounding, potentially hostile environment. Air is passed through a microfilter before entering the incubator. The microfilter is effective in removing airborne contaminants down to 0.5 μ in diameter. Due to a slight positive pressure maintained inside the hood by the air circulation system, there is always a tendency for the air inside the unit to flow to the outside thus assuring a higher degree of isolation.

The circulating air passes through a heating coil to achieve the desired incubator temperature. The infant is warmed by convection; however, because the temperature of the plastic wall cannot be controlled, it is often difficult to control the infant's temperature. The heat loss of the infant to the walls of the incubator varies with room temperature. If the incubator is placed near a cold window or wall, the infant loses heat to the cold incubator walls and it is almost impossible to maintain a neutral thermal environment. A plastic heat shield may be placed over the infant inside the single-walled incubator. The warm incubator air heats the plastic wall of the shield to the same temperature as the air within the incubator; the infant radiates only to the warm inner plastic wall, since the radiant waves from the infant (2 to 9 μ) cannot penetrate the plastic wall.

High relative humidity is achieved by the warm air passing over water in the humidity reservoir. This humidity (75 to 90%) helps in preventing water loss from the skin and respiratory tract. It also prevents drying of secretions in the respiratory tract by decreasing the amount of water for humidification that must come from the infant's respiratory tract.

An enriched oxygen atmosphere can be attained whenever necessary. An oxygen limiter prevents the oxygen concentration inside the incubator from exceeding 40% (Table 4-3). Higher concentration for respiratory emergencies can be obtained by placing the Red Reminder Flag in a vertical position. The vertical position reduces the air intake and results in oxygen concentrations up to 85% (Table 4-3).

A different approach to temperature control is obtained by attaching a highly sensitive temperature-sensing thermistor to the infant's

TABLE 4-3. Incubator Oxygen Therapy

Red Reminder Flag in Horizontal Position				
Flow of oxygen (l/min.)	4	6	8	
Concentration of oxygen	28–31%	32–36%	37–40%	
Red Reminder Flag in Vertical Position				
Flow of oxygen (l/min.)	4–6	8	10	12
Concentration of oxygen	Flow not sufficient for high concentration	70–75%	75–80%	80–85%

abdomen. This thermistor activates the heating unit to provide modulating heat according to the needs of the infant. A disadvantage of such a unit is that it eliminates the use of body temperature as an index of disease.

Radiant heat panels may be used when one is prepared to exchange isolation and precise temperature control for easy access to the patient. Without a complete enclosure, changes in environmental temperature make it difficult to locate the infant's neutral thermal environment and to maintain this temperature. Radiant heat panels are used for short-term warming in the delivery room and for procedures that require complete access to the infant.

TRANSPORT INCUBATOR

The transport incubator is designed to provide a controlled environment under adverse ambient conditions. It is used primarily for transporting sick infants from an outside location or between departments within a hospital complex. A three-way power system permits its operation on 115 volts A.C., in motor vehicles with a 12-volt D.C. power supply, and on the 12-volt D.C. powerpack housed within the unit itself. The design is essentially the same as for the regular incubator with the addition of double-walled construction to minimize radiant heat loss from the infant. When not in transit, the unit should be plugged into an A.C. power source to insure a warm stable environment and a fully charged D.C. power pack. A "D" or "E" cylinder of oxygen should be mounted to the support module in order to provide an oxygen enriched environment while in transit.

Aerosol Therapy

Aerosol therapy consists of the administration of medication in droplet form directly into the respiratory tract. Aerosols may be administered in one of two ways: (1) by spontaneous inhalation from a nebulizer at atmospheric pressure or (2) through a positive pressure respirator. In either case the quantities of solution used are small, usually 2 to 5 ml, nebulized over a 10- to 15-minute period. *It is important to recognize that inhalation of any aerosol can produce irritation or other undesirable side effects, and that such therapy must be employed with care.*

The volume of solution and the nebulization rate employed are not adequate to permit the effective bulk delivery of water to the tracheobronchial tree. However, deposition of useful quantities of potent pharmacologic agents such as bronchodilators can be achieved. In general, it is felt that the smaller the particle (within limits), the deeper its penetration before deposition occurs. Larger particles deposit preferentially in the nasopharynx and upper airways. With nasal breathing a large percentage of the particles never reaches the trachea. For this reason delivery of aerosol by a mouthpiece is usually preferred to the use of a mask. In infants and young children, however, mouth breathing cannot be assured, and nose clips are often not tolerated. Therefore a mask is usually employed for such situations.

MEDICATIONS

The types of medication used in aerosol therapy can be classified into at least five groups: decongestants, bronchodilators, antibiotics, mucolytics, and steroids. Aerosol therapy can be used for immediate relief or for extended periods in the home care of children with chronic or recurrent conditions.

For the routine administration of aerosol therapy, we use a small hand-held nebulizer driven by compressed air at 10 to 12 p.s.i. A small oil-free compressor is used for home therapy. The Bennett twin-jet or Mead-Johnson Maximist nebulizers generate a small particle mist, deliver approximately 2 ml in 10 minutes, and are very convenient.

Most children with a recurring or chronic

pulmonary problem for whom aerosol therapy would be prescribed have cystic fibrosis, asthma, or some form of bronchitis. These conditions are all associated with irritation and/or inflammation and edema of the bronchial mucosa. This factor has led us to use a *simple decongestant* (⅛% phenylephrine HCl) in 10% USP propylene glycol as our basic aerosol solution. Phenylephrine has some bronchodilating activity in addition to its action as a decongestant. Rebound phenomena to phenylephrine have rarely been encountered, except in small infants. This characteristic is perhaps due to the dilution employed (⅛%) and/or to the fact that the tracheobronchial mucosa is less vascular than nasal mucosa. This solution has been inhaled daily for periods of up to 15 years without the development of rebound or other harmful effects.

In the clinical situations described previously, aerosol therapy should be used in conjunction with other forms of respiratory care. Segmental postural drainage is especially important to aid in the removal of secretions from the respiratory tract. Other forms of bronchial toilet, such as suctioning, may be required in very young, weak, or very ill patients.

Bronchodilators may be administered to patients with bronchospasm. One of the commonly used preparations is isoproterenol (Isuprel), 0.05 to 0.5 ml of a 1:200 solution, depending on the age and size of the patient and the response to the initial dose. Newer, and preferred, agents such as isoetherine (Bronkosol)[10] have the theoretic advantage of selectively acting on the beta-2 receptors (bronchial smooth muscle) and avoiding cardiac stimulation with tachycardia and palpitations. The routine use of bronchodilators in patients without documented bronchospasm has been criticized on the grounds that relaxation of bronchial muscle tone might interfere with effective cough. On the other hand, recent, as yet experimental data suggest that the rate of mucociliary transport may be increased by beta-adrenergic agents in patients with chronic bronchitis and cystic fibrosis. These studies may eventually lead to the use of pharmacologic agents for the promotion of mucociliary clearance.

Isoproterenol solution has been inhaled for 10 to 15 minutes one to four times daily for up to 10 years by asthmatic children and adolescents using a compressor-driven nebulizer. Significant side effects have not been observed with this mode of treatment provided that the treatments are not used too frequently. This method seems much more effective in children than one or two uncoordinated sprays from a pressurized cartridge inhaler, and overuse is much more easily controlled. *In England, an increasing death rate in asthmatic patients has been associated with the increasing use of the pocket-sized cartridge inhaler.* Patient overdosage has been implicated in many deaths. Stolley reviewed the mortality statistics and medication usage in 14 countries from 1959 to 1968 and concluded that a pressurized inhaler containing a highly concentrated (5X) isoproterenol solution contributed to the increased mortality from asthma reported in certain countries.[46]

All cartridge nebulizers use fluorohydrocarbon propellants. Repeated inhalations of such chemicals in the presence of hypoxemia can be cardiotoxic[47] and may be involved in the increased mortality. The pressurized units may also aggravate asthmatic symptoms,[24] in contrast with our experience with the compressor-driven nebulizer. Two recent reviews include those by Sheldon on nebulized bronchodilators[44] and those by Aviado on toxicity.[2]

Antibiotics were first administered by aerosol in the 1940's to treat pneumonia. It remains unclear whether their effectiveness stems from systemic absorption or local effects, but the latter seems more likely in view of the amounts of drug involved. Because of the poor penetration of antibiotics into bronchial secretions after parenteral administration, aerosolized antibiotics have been employed especially in the treatment of cystic fibrosis. Antibiotics are often administered prior to postural drainage, but might be more effective following treatment with a decongestant aerosol and postural drainage, thus allowing deposition in more diseased areas. Treatment at bedtime may be helpful, as decreased activity and cough may promote longer retention.

Aerosolized antibiotics can produce irritation of the nasal and/or tracheobronchial mucosa. Systemic absorption may also occur, with toxic side effects, most notably hearing loss due to neomycin. This problem is not necessarily dose-related; it may involve an idiosyncratic reaction, as the hearing loss tends to occur also in neomycin-treated siblings of the index cases.

Mucolytic agents may be nebulized separately or added to the basic solutions. We use these agents selectively for 2- to 4-week periods. They may cause bronchospasm, especially in asthmatic patients. N-acetyl cysteine is the mucolytic agent used most often in the treatment of patients with cystic fibrosis. Criteria for selection of patients for such treatment remain to be established.

Corticosteroids are sometimes needed in the treatment of patients with severe allergy and bronchospasm who are uncontrolled by the usual therapeutic methods. To avoid the side effects of oral steroids, 0.5 to 0.10 ml of a solution of dexamethasone (4 mg/ml) may be added to the aerosol b.i.d. or t.i.d. This treatment has frequently enabled patients to reduce or stop oral steroids if other forms of therapy are continued. In contrast to the experience of others who have used steroid aerosol delivered from pressurized cartridge inhalers, we have seen no steroid side effects when using a compressor-driven nebulizer on a b.i.d.-t.i.d. basis.

INTERMITTENT POSITIVE PRESSURE BREATHING (IPPB)

This therapy may improve the penetration of nebulized medications into smaller airways, to the extent that it improves the depth of inspiration; *however, it has no advantage over other forms of aerosol therapy for the patient capable of voluntarily inhaling deeply.*

IPPB therapy is rarely necessary in home therapy during childhood, and is frequently overused in the hospital. The pressure treatment alone produces a significant increase in airway resistance in chronic asthmatic and normal children, while a water aerosol does not.[35] The IPPB unit should not be driven by oxygen unless the patient requires additional oxygen. Compressed air alone is sufficient for most patients. In addition, at low flows the 40% oxygen control may be inaccurate, and much higher oxygen concentrations may be given to the patient unintentionally.

When IPPB therapy is used, complete orders should be written by the responsible physician and this prescription includes the gas and pressure (usually 10 to 20 cm water) to be used, the frequency (usually b.i.d. to q.i.d.), the duration of each treatment (usually 10 to 15 minutes), the solution to be nebulized, and any precautions to be observed. Physicians should not abdicate their responsibility in this important area.

IPPB therapy should not be used for patients with pulmonary disease without a mainstream humidifier, preferably a heated mainstream humidifier. Nebulization from the sidearm medication nebulizer is considerably diluted by the large volume of dry therapeutic gas and does not provide adequate humidification of the inspired air, especially for the patient breathing through a mouthpiece, and particularly when oxygen is being used. The cascade-type humidifier, which passes minute bubbles of gas through heated water, is particularly efficient and only infrequently becomes contaminated.[43]

IPPB therapy is especially useful in children with compromised ventilation, such as scoliosis patients who have just undergone spinal fusion. When they are introduced to IPPB therapy preoperatively, they accept it well postoperatively. This therapy helps assure better ventilation of all areas of the lungs when used intermittently every day, particularly when pain is still severe and when corrective devices may restrict chest wall and abdominal movement.

Childhood patients with atelectasis may benefit from IPPB therapy, particularly when it is accompanied by segmental postural drainage, oral bronchodilation, and antimicrobials, for example. We have found that it usually is unnecessary in patients with asthma or asthmatic bronchitis and that it may produce more overinflation of the lungs in patients with cystic fibrosis. In the latter patients, the incidence of pneumothorax may be increased when IPPB is used.[25] For cystic fibrosis patients, we use IPPB only in the hospital, for limited periods of 10 to 14 days and only for a specific indication such as atelectasis.

The other complications of IPPB appear to stem largely from the child's adverse reaction to the injudicious use of the equipment. Careful orientation and conditioning of the child are necessary for best results. The child should be permitted to touch the equipment and become aware of its limitations. Observing another child receiving successful IPPB therapy is also helpful. The coordination required to operate the manual Venturi apparatus (Hand-E-Vent, Bennett TA-1) makes this equipment unsuitable for small or very sick children.

Initial treatment should be given at low pressures and for short periods until the child has adapted to this new experience. Reflex glottic closure occurs in the child who has been improperly exposed to high initial pressures (10 to 15 cm) but can be overcome by temporarily lowering the mask pressure (5 to 6 cm) and by reassuring the child and instructing him to "relax and let the machine do the breathing." Pressures can then be gradually increased to the desired level. Slow, deep breathing is desirable in order to prevent hyperventilation and to assure penetration and deposition of the aerosols.

Patients above 4 years of age usually cooperate. Younger patients often do not cooperate until they realize that no pain or discomfort is associated with the apparatus. For best results the child should be seated upright in a straight chair. The small child or infant should be held in a sitting position. The child's back and head are supported by the therapist's chest and shoulders if he holds the child or stands behind him. This technique provides excellent control of head movement. A safeguard against possible aspiration subsequent to IPPB is achieved by removing the mask and tilting the head forward with the supporting shoulder. The child may be rocked during the treatment, thus reducing fear and giving assurance that the therapist does not want to harm him.

PROLONGED MIST THERAPY

This therapy has two general purposes. One is to achieve full humidification of inspired air. The other is to add water to pulmonary secretions in an attempt to increase mucociliary transport and/or cough transport of secretions. The success with which these goals are achieved depends to a great extent on the equipment and techniques used, and the clinical settings in which such therapy is employed.

Principles. The water content of ambient air at room temperature is not sufficient for saturation at body temperature. At least 20 mg of water must be added to each liter of saturated air at 25° C to achieve saturation at 37° C (water content 44 mg/l). This function is normally performed by the nose and upper respiratory tract. If the upper airway is ineffective or has been bypassed, as in patients with a tracheostomy, the inspired air must be supersaturated at room temperature to achieve saturation upon reaching the lung.

The penetration of aerosol particles into the respiratory tract is determined at least in part by particle size. Larger particles are effectively removed by the nose, and only those 5 μ or less effectively reach the lower respiratory tract. Thus the goal of therapy determines to some extent the choice of equipment. If simple humidification is desired, the size of the particles is less important, and simple jet nebulizers may suffice. To achieve deposition of particles in the lung, a small-particle nebulizer must be used or the nose must be bypassed, as by a large-bore mouthpiece. Because the fallout of particles in the equipment itself may be insignificant, the tubing connecting the nebulizer to the patient should be as short as practical.

Any nebulized substance can be irritating to the respiratory epithelium. Patients with bronchial asthma and small infants may demonstrate intolerance to inhalation therapy measures. Sterile distilled water, rather than tap water, should be used in the preparation of solutions. Various solutions are used in therapy, including 5 to 10% propylene glycol and $\frac{1}{4}$ to $\frac{1}{2}$ N saline. Distilled water alone and N saline solution are often irritating, and most patients tolerate dilute saline solution better. Propylene glycol inhibits the rate of bacterial growth in tents, and it may alter hydrogen bonding between molecules of mucus glycoproteins, thus reducing sputum viscosity. Some claim that the addition of solutes reduces or prevents the evaporation of water from the particles, thus stabilizing the mist.

Effective therapy is possible only when adequate equipment is used, and when it is kept clean and in good working order. For home therapy, specific and detailed instructions for cleaning should be given and care taken to see that they are followed. Contaminated equipment may harm patients. In our experience, pneumatic nebulizers are infrequently contaminated. The major contaminants of ultrasonic nebulizers are the gram-negative organisms, chiefly the Pseudomonas.

Practice. Direct inhalation of mist from a nebulizer is most often used in patients with an endotracheal tube or a tracheostomy or for sputum induction. In the first few days after tracheostomy, full humidification, as from a heated jet nebulizer, at relatively high output is necessary to prevent inspissation of secretions and possible plugging of the tube. After the tracheostomy is established and the airway adjusted, an unheated jet nebulizer may provide sufficient humidification. (See also Chapter 3 for additional discussion of tracheostomy and endotracheal tube care.)

Deposition of water in the airways is felt to be enhanced by mouth breathing. Direct inhalations can be used two to four times a day for 20 to 30 minutes preceding segmental postural drainage in an effort to enhance mobilization of secretions.

In some clinical situations sputum is desired for cytology or TB testing in patients without productive cough. Saline inhalation for 15 minutes followed by direct inhalation of distilled water from an ultrasonic nebulizer results in a cough that usually produces sputum in adults and is often effective in children.

Inhalation of mist from a closed compartment (mist tent) is often used for prolonged mist therapy. Effective use of the nebulizer output is enhanced by using a relatively small (24 × 24 × 26 inch) tent. Because water is lost by evaporation and condensation, the density of the mist in the tent is less than that at the outlet from the nebulizer. The best jet nebulizer can produce a mist density of only 26 to 30 mg/l, whereas an ultrasonic nebulizer can produce tent mist densities much greater than the 44 mg/l required for saturation at body temperature. For jet nebulizer therapy it is necessary to use two Mist O_2 Gen MG II C nebulizers in each tent or one Ohio Medical pneumatic nebulizer. The latter is harder on compressors because of the extreme back pressure created. The characteristics of pneumatic nebulizers, air compressors, and the three major ultrasonic nebulizers have been described in detail.[27]

The interior of a mist tent tends to be warmer than the surrounding environment. Cooling of the tent or the room is important for patient comfort and acceptance. In small infants enclosure in a mist tent may alter body temperature regulation. In the small infant, it is possible that overhydration can result from the intensive use of an ultrasonic nebulizer, especially if a saline solution is nebulized. In patients with considerable retention of secretions, rapid mobilization of secretions may follow initiation of mist tent therapy. Use of postural drainage and suctioning is needed to help the patient clear these secretions. In any of the respiratory disorders, adequate hydration of the patient by oral or parenteral route is also important and should not be overlooked. Conversely, overhydration must be guarded against.

Mist tents are used for both acute and chronic (home) treatment. Even in times of acute illness, however, patients should not remain in a tent longer than 18 hours a day. Without this limitation the skin may become macerated, and some patients may develop an acute emotional stress reaction from the isolation.

Mist tent therapy has been used empirically as part of a comprehensive treatment program for patients with cystic fibrosis.[12,13] In our laboratory, improvement in pulmonary function was noted in cystic fibrosis patients during periods of tent therapy. Other investigators have not confirmed this finding, but significant methodologic differences between the studies preclude definitive conclusions. We employ mist tent therapy in many of our patients with cystic fibrosis, but feel the final answer regarding efficacy is yet to come. In any event we feel that mist tent therapy should not be used alone, but as one part of a comprehensive program including intermittent aerosol therapy, segmental postural drainage, antimicrobial therapy, and ongoing care at a specialized center.

Mist tent therapy with small-particle mist is often used in treatment of other obstructive airway conditions, such as bronchitis, asthma, bronchiolitis, and staphylococcal pneumonia. *Neither criteria for patient selection nor the effectiveness of such therapy has been established.* Mist may be useful in providing 100% humidity, particularly in mouth-breathing patients, but care must be exercised, as some patients with asthma may develop more severe bronchospasm when exposed to mist.

In patients with croup and epiglottitis, full humidification and deposition of large mist particles in the affected area have been recommended for years. Although this approach may seem rational, especially if mucociliary transport in the upper airway is impaired, *definite evidence of efficacy is lacking.* Mist tents may produce anxiety and further symptoms in some patients with croup. These problems have been avoided in some hospitals by the use of a cold mist room in which the humidity is kept at 100% and the temperature at 21 to 22° C. In such a room parents and child are not separated, nursing care and patient observation are easier, and several patients may be treated at once. It is important that the humidity be produced in a way that avoids air contamination.[3,48]

In recent years some authors have attacked the theoretic basis for mist tent therapy on grounds of the possibly small amount of water delivered to the lower airways. Wolfsdorf et al. used a technetium-labelled water aerosol delivered into an airtight box by either a croupette (large-particle) nebulizer or an ultrasonic nebulizer with an altered airflow, to observe the deposition of radioactivity in the respiratory tract.[49] Under these conditions and with a slow scanning device, little radioactivity was detected. In a similar study, Bau et al. found a 25% or greater retention of radioactivity in patients with cystic fibrosis as compared to normals.[6] They calculated sufficient water deposition to decrease the viscosity of 50 ml of cystic fibrosis sputum by 50%, as shown by Lifschitz and Denning.[26] Alderson et al. found that 10 to 46% of the radioactivity retained by the subject was deposited in the lungs while over 75% of the original radioactive material remained in the nebulizer and tubing.[1] Yeates et al.[50] in contrast to Wolfsdorf et al.[49] found sufficient technetium aerosol deposition and relatively rapid clearance from the lungs, probably via the pulmonary and bronchial circulation. The assumption that radioactive deposition is directly related to water deposition in the airways has not been substantiated. On the other hand, even small amounts of particulate water have been shown to decrease significantly the viscoelasticity of sputum,[14,26] while an increase in viscosity is observed when humidity is lowered.[41]

There is a continued need for well-designed studies to verify and improve our knowledge in this area.

Manual and Mechanical Ventilation

Most of the mechanical ventilators that are currently commercially available are not completely satisfactory for pediatric care. (See also discussion in Chapter 3.) Only two or three are specifically designed for pediatric use. Because of the special problems presented by infants and small children, the requirements for a pediatric ventilator are quite challenging, since infants cannot be regarded simply as small adults. Infants have a higher metabolic rate, a larger surface area in relation to weight, airways of greater relative diameter, much smaller tidal volume, a higher respiratory rate, and considerably lower tidal and peak flow rates.

At least three major manufacturers of mechanical ventilators have prototypes of respirators to better meet the specific needs of the pediatric patient. Thus, improved ventilators for infants and children may become available in the near future. The indications for mechanical ventilation are covered in Chapter 3.

The resuscitation tray is one of several essential items for the delivery room and newborn nursery. Numerous devices can be used for the application of positive pressure by bag and mask. Figure 4-2 shows equipment used in our delivery room and premature nursery. The mask is applied to the infant's face making sure there is a small, but definite, leak around the mask to act as a "pop off" and prevent carbon dioxide accumulation. Hustead and Avery suggested that pressures of 35 cm of water for intervals of 1 to 2 seconds are safe and may be required.[23] Gruber and Klaus used pressures as high as 65 cm of water when "bagging" infants with respiratory distress syndrome.[22]

Bag and mask resuscitation is frequently underrated as an effective means of treating respiratory failure in both children and adults. Although its use is common as an immediate resuscitative measure, this function is all too often its only role. This technique has definite advantages in many circumstances. Conditions frequently exist where an infant or child requires only intermittent supportive assistance for respiratory insufficiency. Endotracheal intubation and/or tracheostomy are considered by many in pediatrics to be measures taken only when continuous supportive measures are likely to be necessary. The trauma associated with these procedures can often be avoided by a trained therapist intermittently assisting with a bag and mask. The ultimate factor determining the choice of ventilatory support is the frequency with which assistance is needed. The bag and mask obviates the need for a tube in the airway, thereby helping the normal clearance of pulmonary secretions.

Bag and mask resuscitation is useful only when one can establish and maintain an adequate airway. When prolonged assisted or controlled ventilation becomes necessary, a tracheal airway must be established.

MASK AND BAG EQUIPMENT

Flow-Inflating Bags. Anesthesia equipment manufacturers provide a variety of 0.5 to 1.0 liter thin-rubber anesthesia bags suitable for use in children. This type of bag usually utilizes oxygen but may also be used with compressed air. Inflation of the bag is varied by either adjusting the flow of gas or adjust-

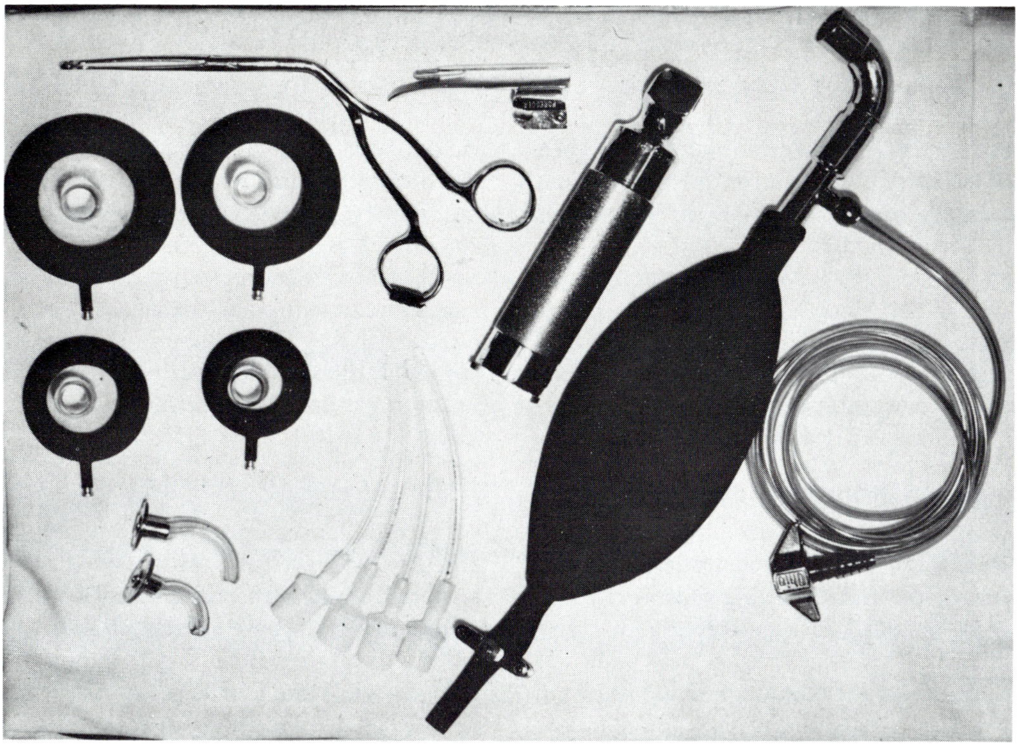

FIG. 4-2. Minimum apparatus required for emergency ventilation of the newborn infant. A tray of sterile equipment provided by the respiratory therapy service is immediately available in all newborn areas.

ing the screw attached to the open tail of the bag.

Self-Inflating Bags. Unlike the flow-inflating bags just discussed, the self-inflating bag does not require a source of gas. The recoil characteristics of this bag allow for reinflation with room air following manual deflation. The advantage is that a source of gas may not always be available wherever an emergency occurs. This bag also may be useful for transporting a patient from one location to another.

Use of the self-inflating bag is limited by certain therapeutic drawbacks. Because of the bag's recoil characteristics, varying and unknown concentrations of oxygen are obtained when it is used with a supplementary flow of oxygen. Concentrations of oxygen at the mask vary anywhere from 35 to 90%. Among the self-inflating bags, the 500-ml Hope Infant Resuscitator is most commonly used for infants and children. This bag has a safety valve and can deliver up to 55% oxygen with a flow of 15 l/min. Because of the recoil characteristics, one drawback to any self-inflating bag is that the "feel" for bagging is lost. This characteristic is particularly important in resuscitation of small infants and children. Except for transport or emergencies, the self-inflating bag is inferior to flow-inflating bags for pediatric use.

POSITIVE PRESSURE VENTILATORS

The basic principles of most of the ventilators commercially available and the details of their construction and function have been provided by Mushin and co-workers.[35] Several ventilators are more commonly used in pediatric practice and deserve some comment.

The *Bird Mark XIV ventilator* is of the pressure generator type and can provide a high inspiratory flow (up to 200 l/min.), high pressure (approaching 100 cm water), and a leak-compensating terminal flow. An oxygen blender is required to control the oxygen percentage because the Mark XIV does not provide for air dilution. The Mark VI Minute Volume ventilator attachment may be added to the Mark XIV whenever a preset minute volume is desired. The infant "J" circuit may be employed when there is a need for instantaneous inspiratory flow, small volumes, minimized dead space, and rapid respiratory rate.

The *Bennett PR-2 ventilator* is also of the pressure generator type and also may be used as an assistor as well as a controller. This unit is one of the mixed cycling type devices. It may be pressure- or time-cycled and is flow sensitive. This unit has a peak flow of 80 l/min. and a maximum pressure of 60 cm water. It does have an air mix feature, but the percentage of oxygen delivered is variable. Therefore, a ventilator oxygen controller is recommended for precise oxygen therapy. For minimum dead space, the tracheostomy circle with a 15-mm adapter should be used.

The *Bourns volume generator type respirator* is designed specifically for pediatric use. At the present time the Bourns respirator is the most sophisticated and versatile unit available for pediatric patients. It is a preset, constant-flow generator, volume and time cycle and pressure-limited ventilator. The unit may be used with a nasal mask or with endotracheal intubation. The Bourns assist mode is triggered with an inspiratory effort producing only a 0.05 cm water negative pressure. In the control mode, breathing rates up to 100 per minute can be maintained. The volume of gas (oxygen or oxygen-air mix) can be regulated between 5 and 150 ml per breath, making it suitable for newborns and young children.

Most adult ventilators are not readily adaptable for pediatric use because of the large internal compliance (compression volume) and the mechanical dead space in the patient circuit. The volume of the adult ventilator circuit can be up to 10 times the capacity of the child's lungs. Therefore, up to 90% of the generated work of the adult respirator may be expended in ventilating itself. A considerable reduction in internal compliance can be achieved by replacing the adult size patient circuit with small-diameter (½-in. ID) low-compliance Tygon tubing. Keeping the humidifier filled with water will also cut down on gas compression.

OTHER MODES OF VENTILATION

Recently, constant positive airway pressure (CPAP) using pressures up to 16 cm water delivered through an endotracheal tube has been shown to improve ventilation in spontaneously breathing infants with respiratory distress syndrome.[21] CPAP or a version thereof has been added to many mechanical ventilators for infants requiring assistance. Barrie discussed CPAP therapy and the design of a simple method of applying this therapy in respiratory distress syndrome, utilizing a plastic bag.[5]

Chernick and Vidyasagar reported good results when using constant negative pressure (CNP) applied to the infant's thorax.[9] They made a modification of the Isolette incubator-respirator so that continuous rather than intermittent negative pressure was provided. This method was considered desirable because it did not require endotracheal intubation, but the unit is expensive and requires alterations and frequent maintenance.[45] Martinez et al. have designed a small, relatively inexpensive plastic chamber that fits inside the infant incubator and provides CNP.[29]

PRACTICAL POINTS

Artificial humidification *must* be provided for *any* patient who is being mechanically ventilated. A cascade-type heated humidifier is preferred to a nebulizer since bacteria may be carried by particles of water and may be transmitted to the patient. The cascade humidifier is efficient and infrequently contaminated.[43]

When oxygen is used, the enriched oxygen atmosphere should always be kept to the minimal concentration possible. All ventilators must have a means of providing oxygen in any concentration from 21 to 100%. Oxygen-air ratio controllers now available can accurately mix and deliver the desired concentration to the ventilator at 50 p.s.i. pressure. The percent of inspired oxygen concentration should be checked every 2 to 4 hours by one of the analyzers previously described.

The adequacy of ventilation is best determined by blood gas studies. In adult care, measurement of exhaled tidal volumes breath by breath provides an additional means of monitoring. However, in small children the airflows are too low to accurately drive the commonly available spirometers. For example, although the vanes of the Wright spirometer are lightweight and very sensitive to airflow, they still do not accurately measure airflows at low flow rates.

Equipment change and cleaning and sterilizing of equipment are important aspects of complete respiratory care. The patient circuit, including the mainstream humidifier, should be changed on every ventilator every 24 hours. Equipment should be disassembled, physically cleaned, and sterilized before being used again. Routine cultures prior to use should be taken to check the effectiveness of the sterilization and storage procedures.

Contamination and Sterilization

Contamination of inhalation therapy equipment occurs readily from airborne infectious agents, from the patient, from unclean practices, from contaminated solutions, and from inadequate cleaning and sterilizing procedures. Because of the threat of spread of contamination of nebulized solutions from the equipment to the patient, the respiratory therapy department should be responsible for cleaning and sterilizing equipment before it is used again for another patient.

CONTAMINATION

Among the contaminants, some organisms are classified as normal human flora. *P. aeruginosa* is one important organism that at times may be part of the normal human flora, but it can also produce serious infections and readily contaminates inhalation therapy equipment.[32] *E. coli, S. aureus,* and *K. pneumoniae* are also in the group of human organisms. Table 4-4 lists the organisms found in dust that rarely cause human disease and the water organisms that are most commonly found in contaminated distilled water in inhalation therapy equipment.

TABLE 4-4. Classification and Examples of Microorganisms

Human Organisms
E. coli
S. aureus
P. aeruginosa
K. pneumoniae
Dust Organisms
Bacillus species
Fungi (e.g., Penicillium species)
S. epidermidis (albus)
Neisseria species
Diphtheroids
Clostridia species
Alpha-hemolytic streptococci
Candida species
Hartmannella species (amoebae)
Water Organisms
Flavobacterium
Nonpigmented Pseudomonas
Alcaligenes species
Acinetobacter species
Achromobacter

The bacteria most frequently recovered from distilled water are the nonpigmented Pseudomonas species (water organism, nonhuman group) as differentiated from the human pathogen, *P. aeruginosa.* The water organisms are normal inhabitants of stagnant water but are not part of the normal human flora and rarely cause human infection. However, the introduction of large numbers of organisms, especially into already compromised patients, may cause serious disease. The organisms in the human flora group, especially *P. aeruginosa,* carry the greatest risk.

Factors in Sterility Control. Moffet found that under test conditions, sterility of the ultrasonic or the Venturi nebulizer system could be maintained for up to 5 days.[33] Contamination with a new organism occurred less frequently in the ultrasonic compared to the Venturi nebulizer. Refilling the nebulizer with sterile water tended to reduce bacteria to low concentrations (Fig. 4-3). Refilling with fresh, nonsterile, distilled water resulted in rapid increases to high concentrations of bacteria. *S. aureus* did not survive in distilled water. Evaporative humidifiers are not considered sources of airborne contamination.[32,33,39]

Distilled water supplies should be heat

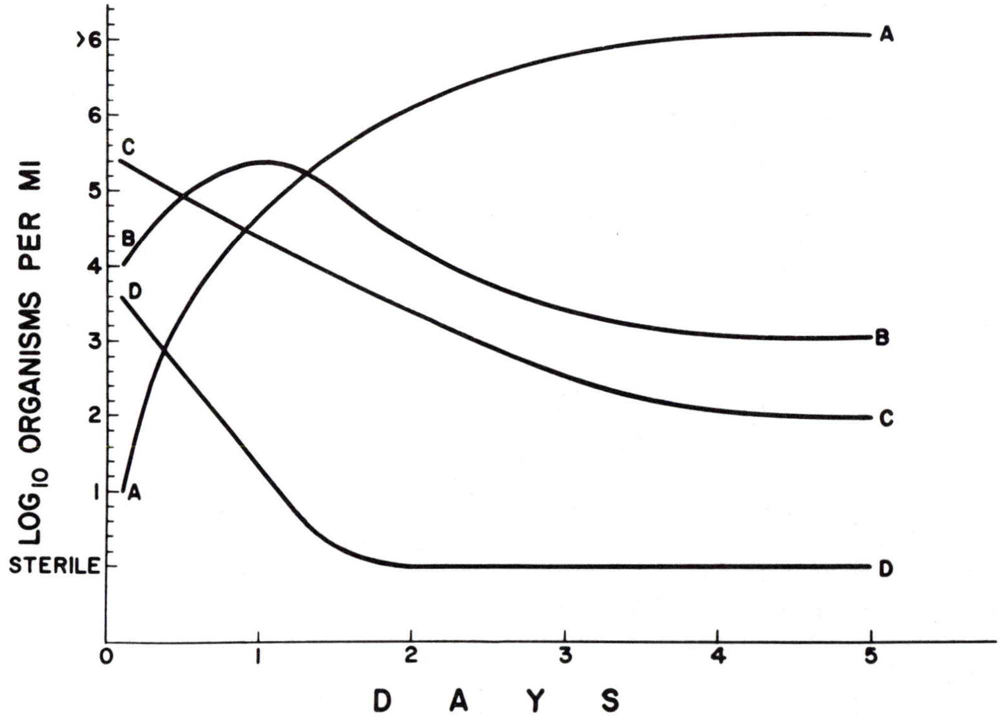

FIG. 4-3. Patterns of survival of bacteria in two types of nebulizers.

A, Venturi nebulizer without initial inoculum. The unit was refilled daily with fresh unsterile water containing Flavobacterium species.

B, Ultrasonic nebulizer inoculated at 0 time with Pseudomonas-Alcaligenes and refilled daily with sterile water.

C, Venturi inoculated at 0 time with Klebsiella and refilled with sterile water.

D, Ultrasonic nebulizer inoculated with *S. aureus* at 0 time and refilled with sterile water (From Moffet, H. L., D. Allan and T. Williams: Survival and dissemination of bacteria in nebulizers and incubators. *Am. J. Dis. Child. 114:*13, 1967. Copyright 1967, American Medical Association.)

sterilized in individual containers prior to delivery to hospital divisions by carefully following the instructions provided by the sterilizer manufacturer. Other factors in sterility control include ionic concentrations, organic nutrients, and moisture control. *P. aeruginosa* survives least well in distilled water, and it does not multiply in distilled water unless organic nutrients are present. Distilled water is usually free of ionic salts and organic material but deionized water is not. The presence of high concentrations of human flora organisms in water reservoirs implies that the water or container is contaminated by organic nutrients and ionic salts.[32] Thus, the physical cleaning of equipment and the cleanliness of the container and water are important (Fig. 4-4). Pettit and Lowbury found that 24 hours after drying, *P. aeruginosa* usually had less than 0.1% survivors while gram-positive cocci had 32 to 87% survivors.[36] Thorough drying of equipment helps decrease the numbers of gram-negative bacteria even if sterilization is not carried out.

Favero et al. reported that *P. aeruginosa* grows at a rapid rate in distilled water of poor quality that has been allowed to stand for a few days.[19] They found that frequent cleaning, disinfecting, drying of glassware, and the use of sterile distilled water and aseptic technique in filling water reservoirs can virtually eliminate the *P. aeruginosa* contamination of inhalation therapy equipment.

Sampling for Contamination. The respiratory therapy department should take responsibility for setting up a surveillance program

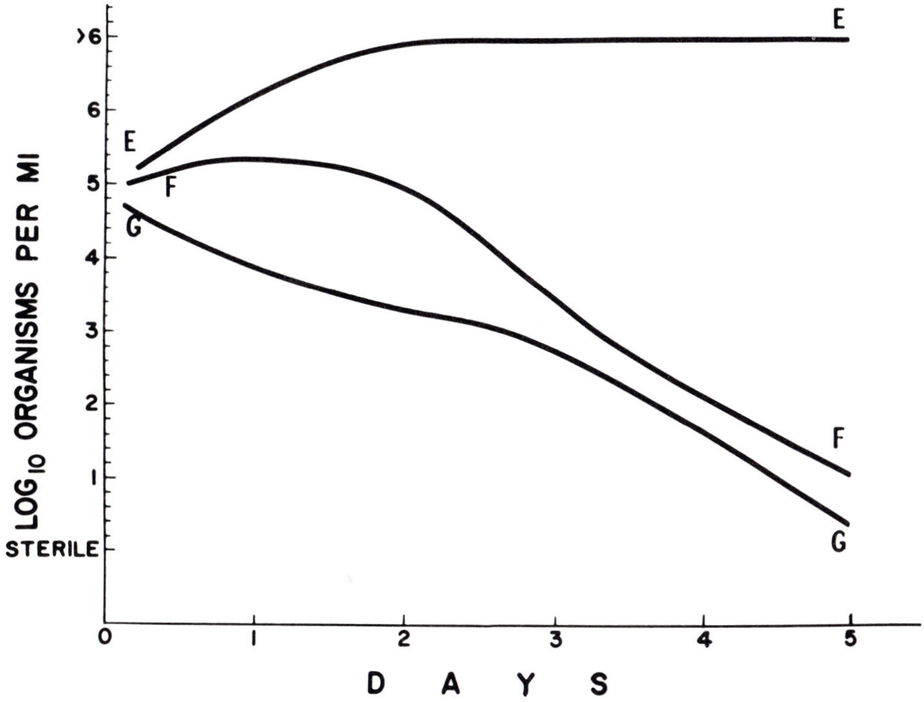

FIG. 4-4. Survival of *P. aeruginosa* or *F. meningosepticum* type C in incubator water at 30° C with and without nutrient added. Curve E represents the mean bacterial concentrations for two experiments with each organism with 1% broth; curve F with 0.1% broth; and curve G with no broth (From Moffet, H. L., D. Allan and T. Williams: Survival and dissemination of bacteria in nebulizers and incubators. *Am. J. Dis. Child. 114:*13, 1967. Copyright 1967, American Medical Association.)

for the sampling of solutions and of the aerosols produced. Edmondson and Sanford discussed sampling directly from nebulizers and within nebulization tents.[15] Rhoades et al. used a slit air sampler, which was simple and seemed reliable for checking gross contamination.[40] The sampling procedures to be used and the frequency of their employment should be determined in each department and reviewed periodically.

Frequency of Change of Hospital Equipment. Moffet found that in an experimental setting, sterility could be maintained on all equipment for 5 days.[33] Miller et al. found frequent contamination of hospital ultrasonic nebulizers by Pseudomonas within 3 days in an in-use type study.[31]

The frequency with which cleaning and sterilizing of equipment should be carried out is still not clear. This policy should be determined locally based on the results of sampling and the effectiveness of the sterilization procedures available. The frequency of change may vary for different pieces of equipment and may also depend on whether disinfecting procedures[37,40] are also being used.

We change nebulizer and oxygen humidifiers every second day. The patient circuit, including humidifier, tubing, and sidearm nebulizer of all ventilators, is changed every 24 hours. The intermittent aerosol nebulizers are changed daily. Equipment that can withstand autoclaving is sterilized in this manner. The remainder is gas sterilized and aired. In addition, all equipment is again disassembled, washed, and sterilized between patients. It may be more convenient to use disposable parts when they are available.

CLEANING AND STERILIZATION

One of the most important aspects of the care of respiratory equipment concerns the physical cleaning that is required. This phase cannot be overemphasized since physical cleaning removes the inorganic salts and organic nutrients that support bacterial growth. It includes detergent and water soaking followed by a thorough scrubbing, particularly making an effort to reach remote areas with a variety of brushes to remove any residues. The cleaning should be followed by a thorough rinse. Nebulizers and other equipment should be disassembled as much as possible before the cleaning. Defective or worn equipment, especially nebulizer jets with burrs or irregular surfaces, should be replaced.[37]

Sterilizing. Following rinsing, the equipment should be allowed to dry completely. It is then ready for reassembly and packaging in plastic bags prior to steam autoclaving or to ethylene oxide gas sterilization. Sterilized equipment should be dated. Some equipment cannot withstand the 120 to 140° C temperatures of the steam autoclave. Most equipment can be gas sterilized; however, some clear plastics may be damaged by the gas. Ethylene oxide provides the most effective sterilizing process, but it is also more expensive and the equipment must be thoroughly dry.[18] Larger equipment inventories are needed since thorough airing is required to permit the gas to escape from the equipment for up to 72 hours before use. This airing is particularly important for equipment that will be in direct contact with the skin or mucous membranes. An aeration chamber can reduce the time required for aeration to only 8 to 12 total hours.[4]

Disinfecting in Hospital. When equipment cannot be autoclaved, and when a gas sterilizer is not available, the alternative to sterilization is disinfection. Care must be taken that harmful residues of disinfectants do not remain to later be in contact with patient tissues. If soaking with a phenol or a 2% glutaraldehyde solution (Cidex) is employed, care must be taken that all surfaces come in contact with the solution and that adequate time, usually at least 30 minutes, is allowed. A thorough rinse with sterile water and complete air drying should follow.

Pierce et al. reported on the long-term use of daily aerosolization of 0.25% acetic acid for 10 minutes for the decontamination of gas-driven reservoir nebulizers and found the method to be practical and effective in routine hospital use.[37] The incidence of contamination was reduced from 84% to less than 10%, and residual contamination was felt to be due to personnel error or corrosion of nebulizer jets.

From a study of ultrasonic nebulizer contamination, Rhoades et al. recommended a 2% acetic acid nebulization for 30 minutes to ensure decontamination of even heavily contaminated units.[40] A sterile saline rinse and 30-minute nebulization followed.

Disinfecting in Home. Miller et al. studied contamination of pneumatic and ultrasonic nebulizers in the home care of patients with cystic fibrosis.[31] Home cleaning had been recommended twice weekly. Contamination with staphylococci was not found in either type of nebulizer. The intermittent aerosol units and tent canopies were free of contamination. Pneumatic nebulizers showed minimal or no growth of contaminating organisms when 10% propylene glycol in distilled water was nebulized, whereas ultrasonic units nebulizing half normal saline solution were frequently contaminated with gram-negative organisms, including *P. aeruginosa.* An every other day cleaning program including nebulizing of 2% acetic acid decreased the incidence of organisms, including the *P. aeruginosa.*

A program of cleaning and disinfecting every other day is recommended for all home care patients. The instructions should be provided in writing and with additional oral explanation. Our routine can be briefly summarized; however, details are available.[8] After the equipment is disassembled and thoroughly washed, scrubbed, and rinsed, all parts to be disinfected are placed in a clean container with a solution of one part vinegar to three parts of distilled water or boiled cooled tap water, making sure all parts are submerged and that the parts are sufficiently agitated to remove air bubbles and permit surface contact by the solution for 15 minutes. This step is followed by rinsing with sterilized water and thorough drying. For ultrasonic nebulizers, the vinegar solution can be nebulized for 15 minutes and followed by disassembly, rinsing, and drying.

REFERENCES

1. Alderson, P. O., R. H. Seaker-Walker, D. B. Strominger, J. Markham and R. L. Hill: Pulmonary deposition of aerosols in children with cystic fibrosis. *J. Pediatr. 84*:479, 1974.
2. Aviado, D. M.: Toxicity of aerosols. *J. Clin. Pharmacol. 15*:86, 1975.
3. Baker, H.: Five years' experience with a high humidity room. *Can. Med. Assoc. J. 72*:914, 1955.
4. Baker, L. R. and R. B. Roberts: Safe use of ethylene oxide sterilization in hospitals. *Respir. Care 16*:37, 1971.
5. Barrie, H.: Simple method of applying continuous positive airway pressure in respiratory distress syndrome. *Lancet 1*:776, 1972.
6. Bau, S. K., R. Aspin, D. E. Wood and H. Levison: The measurement of fluid deposition in humans following mist tent therapy. *Pediatrics 48*:605, 1971.
7. Bendixin, H. H., L. D. Egbert, J. Hedley-White, M. B. Laver and H. Pontoppidan: *Respiratory Care.* The C. V. Mosby Co., St. Louis, 1965.
8. Bolek, J. and M. D. Lough: Care of inhalation therapy equipment. In *Pediatric Respiratory Therapy,* Lough, Doershuk and Stern (Eds.). Year Book Medical Publishers, Chicago, p. 181, 1974.
9. Chernick, V., and D. Vidyasagar: Continuous negative chestwall pressure in hyaline membrane disease. *Pediatrics 49*:753, 1972.
10. Chervinsky, P. and Herstoff, R.: IPPB therapy with Bronkospray or isoproterenol—a comparison. *J. Asthma Res. 4*:197, 1967.
11. Crocker, D., and J. Young: *Inhalation Therapy Procedures.* Year Book Medical Publishers, Chicago, 1970.
12. Doershuk, C. F. and L. W. Matthews: Cystic fibrosis and obstructive pulmonary disease. In *Ambulatory Pediatrics,* M. Green and R. J. Haggerty (Eds.), W. B. Saunders Co., Philadelphia, p. 707, 1968.
13. Doershuk, C. F., L. W. Matthews, C. T. Gillespie,

M. D. Lough and S. Spector: Evaluation of jet-type and ultrasonic nebulizers in mist tent therapy for cystic fibrosis. *Pediatrics 41*:723, 1968.

14. Dulfano, M. J., Adler, K. and Wooten, O.: Physical properties of sputum. IV. Effects of 100 percent humidity and water mist. *Am. Rev. Respir. Dis. 107*:130, 1972.
15. Edmondson, E. B. and Sanford, J. P.: Simple methods of bacteriologic sampling of nebulization equipment. *Am. Rev. Respir. Dis. 94*:450, 1966.
16. Egan, D. F.: *Fundamentals of Inhalation Therapy.* The C. V. Mosby Co., St. Louis, 1969.
17. Engel, S.: *Lung Structure.* Charles C Thomas, Springfield, Ill., 1962.
18. Engley, F. B. and M. T. Metzgar: Ethylene oxide sterilization. *Inhalation Ther. 15*:9, 1970.
19. Favero, M. S., L. A. Carson, W. W. Bond and N. J. Patterson: Pseudomonas aeruginosa: growth in distilled water from hospitals. *Science 173*:836, 1971.
20. Fearon, B. and J. S. Whalen: Tracheal dimensions in the living infant. *Ann. Otol. Rhinol. Laryngol. 76*:964, 1967.
21. Gregory, G. A., J. A. Kitterman, R. H. Phibbs, W. H. Tooley and W. K. Hamilton: Treatment of idiopathic respiratory distress syndrome with continuous positive airway pressure. *N. Engl. J. Med. 284*:1333, 1970.
22. Gruber, H. and M. Klaus: Intermittent mask and bag therapy. *J. Pediatr. 76*:194, 1970.
23. Hustead, R. F., and M. E. Avery: Observations of mask pressure achieved with the Kreiselman infant resuscitator. *N. Engl. J. Med. 265*:939, 1961.
24. Keighley, J. H.: Iatrogenic asthma associated with adrenergic aerosols. *Ann. Intern. Med. 65*:985, 1966.
25. Lifschitz, M. I., F. O. Bowman, C. R. Denning and R. H. Wylie: Pneumothorax as a complication of cystic fibrosis. *Am. J. Dis. Child. 116*:633, 1968.
26. Lifschitz, M. I. and C. R. Denning: Quantitative interaction of water and cystic fibrosis sputum. *Am. Rev. Respir. Dis. 102*:456, 1970.
27. Lough, M. D., C. F. Doershuk and L. W. Matthews: Characteristics of commercial nebulizers and air compressors for mist tent therapy. *Respir. Care 17*:49, 1972.
28. Lough, M. D., C. F. Doershuk and R. C. Stern (Eds.): *Pediatric Respiratory Therapy,* Year Book Medical Publishers, Chicago, 1974.
29. Martinez, A., M. D. Lough and C. F. Doershuk: A new negative-pressure device for treating infants with the respiratory distress syndrome. *Respir. Care, 17*:565, 1972.
30. Mestayan, J., I. Jarai, G. Bata, and M. Fekete: The significance of facial skin temperature in the chemical heat regulation of premature infants. *Biol. Neonate. 7*:243, 1974.
31. Miller, S. T., B. Boxerbaum, C. F. Doershuk, L. Vana and L. W. Matthews: Bacterial contamination of inhalation therapy equipment in hospital and home. Abstract. National Cystic Fibrosis Research Foundation, Eighth Annual Meeting, Atlantic City, p. 28, April 26, 1967.
32. Moffet, H. L.: Sterility control. *Int. Anesthesiol. Clin. 8*:543, 1970.
33. Moffet, H. L., D. Allan and T. Williams: Survival and dissemination of bacteria in nebulizers and incubators. *Am. J. Dis. Child. 114*:13, 1967.
34. Moore, R. B. and E. K. Cotton: The effect of intermittent positive-pressure breathing on airway resistance in normal and asthmatic children. *J. Allergy Clin. Immunol. 49*:137, 1972.
35. Mushin, W. W., L. Rendell-Baker, P. W. Thompson and W. W. Mapleson: *Automatic Ventilation of the Lungs,* F. A. Davis Co., Philadelphia, 1969.
36. Pettit, F. and E. J. L. Lowbury: Survival of normal pathogens under different environmental conditions. *J. Hyg. 66*:393, 1968.
37. Pierce, A. K., J. P. Sanford, G. D. Thomas and J. S. Leonard: Long-term evaluation of decontamination of inhalation therapy equipment and the occurrence of necrotizing pneumonia. *N. Engl. J. Med. 282*:528, 1970.
38. Radford, E. P., B. G. Ferris, Jr. and B. C. Kriete: Clinical use of a nomogram to estimate proper ventilation during artificial respiration. *N. Engl. J. Med. 251*:877, 1954.
39. Reinarz, J. A., A. K. Pierce, B. B. Mays and J. P. Sanford: The potential role of inhalation therapy equipment in nosocomial pulmonary infection. *J. Clin. Invest. 44*:831, 1965.
40. Rhoades, E. R., R. Ringrose, J. A. Mohr, L. Brooks, B. A. McKown and F. Felton: Contamination of ultrasonic nebulization equipment with gram negative bacteria. *Arch. Intern. Med. 127*:228, 1971.
41. Richards, J. H. and C. Marriott: Effect of relative humidity on the rheologic properties of bronchial mucus. *Am. Rev. Respir. Dis. 109*:484, 1974.
42. Safar, P., *Respiratory Therapy.* F. A. Davis Co., Philadelphia, 1965.
43. Schulze, T., E. B. Edmondson, A. K. Pierce and J. P. Sanford: Studies of a new humidifying device as a potential source of bacterial aerosols. *Am. Rev. Respir. Dis. 96*:517, 1967.
44. Sheldon, G. P.: Nebulized bronchodilators in obstructive lung disease. *Ann. Allergy 30*:24, 69, 1972.
45. Somerwill, L., E. G. Brown and A. Y. Sweet: The incubator-respirator: method for improving its reliability. *Pediatrics 49*:761, 1972.
46. Stolley, P. D.: Asthma mortality: why the United States was spared an epidemic of deaths due to asthma. *Am. Rev. Respir. Dis. 105*:883, 1972.
47. Taylor, G. J. IV, and W. S. Harris: Cardiac toxicity of aerosol propellants. *J.A.M.A. 214*:81, 1970.

48. Towell, R. M. and D. M. Little, Jr.: The utilization of fog as a therapeutic agent. *Anesthesiology 18*:470, 1957.
49. Wolfsdorf, J., D. L. Swift and M. E. Avery: Mist tent reconsidered: an evaluation of the respiratory deposition of labelled water aerosols produced by jet and ultrasonic nebulizers. *Pediatrics 43*:799, 1969.
50. Yeates, D. B., N. Aspin, A. C. Bryan and H. Levison: Regional clearance of ions from the airways of the lungs. *Am. Rev. Respir. Dis. 107*:602, 1973.

Anesthetic Drugs and Techniques

H. I. A. NISBET AND D. J. STEWARD

5

Anesthesiologists have a special interest in the respiratory system. They use the lung as a route to administer potent volatile drugs, and following anesthesia and surgical procedure, the lung is the most common site for complications that are a major cause of morbidity and mortality, especially in the newborn.

Pediatric patients span a wide age range, so that the anesthetic drugs and techniques used may have effects upon the central and peripheral control of respiration and upon the lung itself. These effects vary with the maturity of the respiratory system. Present knowledge of the degree and nature of the changes in respiratory function produced by anesthesia in infants and children is still incomplete.

This chapter considers anesthetic techniques for young patients and the known effects of these techniques upon respiratory function, relating them to the clinical conduct of anesthesia under the headings: premedication, induction of anesthesia, maintenance of anesthesia, endotracheal intubation and airway resistance, and artificial ventilation.

Agents Used in Premedication

The objectives of premedication are to provide sedation, interrupt undesirable autonomic reflex responses, prevent the accumulation of excessive secretions in the airway, and minimize the requirements for general anesthetic agents. Narcotic drugs, barbiturates, and tranquilizers quieten the patient, allay fear, and help to smooth the induction of anesthesia. Except in special circumstances such as in cyanotic heart disease, they are usually given only to patients over 18 months old. Atropine or hyoscine is also prescribed to block the cardiac vagus and diminish secretions in the mouth and respiratory tract.

SEDATIVES

Most of these drugs produce some degree of central respiratory depression, which tends to be greater in the newborn than in the adult.[81] The greatest depression is caused by the narcotic analgesics, and in infants morphine causes a greater shift than meperidine in the carbon dioxide (CO_2) response curve (to the right and downward). Since this effect occurs with doses that in adults are equianalgesic and cause equal changes in CO_2 response, infants appear to have an increased sensitivity to morphine.[91] This greater sensitivity may be due to enhanced sensitivity of central nervous system (CNS) receptors, increased permeability of the blood brain barrier, and changes in the distribution and elimination of the drug. Both morphine and meperidine decrease the frequency of sighing,[91] increasing the possible risk of atelectasis and hypoxemia. Premedication is followed by a reduction in functional residual capacity (FRC). Airway closure may then occur during normal tidal breathing, and further increase the likelihood of hypoxemia.

Barbiturates, although they cause considerably less central depression than do the narcotics,[82] are used with caution in the newborn, for in infants under 1 month of age the enzymes responsible for oxidation and conjugation of barbiturates are of low activity.[16,22] Also, in newborn animals the LD_{50} of barbiturates is less than in the adult.[29] Many pediatric anesthesiologists consider it prudent to assume that the newborn has less ability to detoxify barbiturates.

Tranquilizers such as diazepam are widely used to produce preoperative sedation in older children: The doses commonly used cause less central depression of ventilation than do narcotics and barbiturates.[51]

In addition to its central effects, morphine may have more direct effects on the lung. Bronchoconstriction might be expected to occur either from an anticholinesterase effect or from histamine release,[46] though direct evidence to confirm this theory is lacking. Meperidine, in contrast, has a direct relaxing effect on bronchiolar smooth muscle plus an atropine-like effect in that bronchodilation occurs, resulting in decreased airway resistance and increased dead space.

ANTICHOLINERGIC AGENTS

These agents are used in premedication primarily to prevent bradycardia, excessive salivation, and bronchial secretions. Atropine is reputed to give better protection against cardiac arrhythmias in infants than does hyoscine.[6] Hyoscine produces a smoother induction of anesthesia, a sedative effect, and less laryngospasm,[25] and causes a greater drying effect on salivation and mucus secretions.[24]

As the anesthesiologist is principally concerned with avoiding cardiac arrhythmias and does not wish to produce excessive drying of secretions, atropine is considered to be the anticholinergic drug of choice, although the drugs have not been compared in equipotent doses.[73]

Central Actions of Atropine. Atropine is not a respiratory stimulant,[84] although its administration is followed by an increase in minute volume ($\dot{V}_E$) secondary to an increase in physiologic dead space.[80] Atropine does not reduce and may even potentiate the respiratory depression induced by narcotics.[84] A narcotic effect of atropine has been reported in newborn animals under 1 week old.[79]

Direct Effects of Atropine on the Lung. The principal effect is bronchodilation, leading to decreased airway resistance and increased dead space.[24] In man anatomic dead space is increased by 30% after administration of 0.5 mg atropine;[80] airway conductance is increased[8] and the flow volume curve shifted sharply to the left.[14]

Atropine has been reported to cause hypoxemia[88] although other investigators have been unable to confirm this effect.[35] A fall in FRC of up to 13% has been described.[80,89] Closing volume (CV) may be slightly increased in some subjects by therapeutic doses of atropine.[14] This fall in FRC with increase in CV might lead to airway closure in the tidal volume (V_T) range and hence to arterial hypoxemia. If such an effect occurs, small children will be more liable to hypoxemia after atropine since their susceptibility to airway closure in the V_T range is greater than that of adolescents and young adults.[49] Increased alveolar to arterial oxygen tension gradients (AaD_{O_2}) have also been observed after premedication with Pantopon and Hyoscine[70] and with meperidine and promethazine.[67]

The drying effect of atropine might be expected to produce thicker bronchial secretions and delay mucociliary clearance; the tracheal clearance of radioactively tagged particles appears to be significantly delayed.[97] Atropine is used cautiously in patients in whom such an effect may be detrimental, such as those with cystic fibrosis.

Agents Used to Induce and Maintain Anesthesia

Anesthesia is induced in children either by intravenous drugs such as thiopentone, or by the inhalation of one or more of the potent anesthetic vapors or gases. Each method has advantages and disadvantages. Laryngospasm may occur during induction with barbiturates and certain volatile agents, especially those with irritant properties, such as diethyl ether.

During inhalational induction in children the special characteristics of their cardiovascular and respiratory systems may influence the uptake of the agent. The high cardiac output in infants might be expected to delay the rise in alveolar concentration of the agent, yet alveolar concentrations of both nitrous oxide and halothane have been found to rise faster than in the adult.[78] This difference is probably due to the higher level of alveolar ventilation and the greater total body proportion of "vessel-rich" tissues in the child.

Anesthesia in infants and children is commonly maintained with nitrous oxide, supplemented with volatile agents such as halothane, methoxyflurane, diethyl ether, cyclopropane, or trichloroethylene, newer agents such as enflurane and isoflurane, or intravenous narcotics such as meperidine or fentanyl. These agents may be used in conjunction with muscle relaxants and assisted or controlled ventilation.

Anesthetic circuits used in pediatric practice are designed to minimize apparatus resistance and dead space. Modifications of the T-piece are extensively used in the small infant where the valveless design and very low apparatus dead-space are major advantages, but it is difficult to humidify the gases in this circuit. Circle systems incorporating a CO_2 absorber and specially designed valves of low resistance and dead space overcome this disadvantage to some extent but tend to be cumbersome when used in very small patients.[72]

CENTRAL CONTROL OF VENTILATION

Since in most aspects the central control of ventilation in older infants and children is similar to that in adults,[12] the effects of anesthetics are likely to be similar in both age groups. These effects have been measured by means of the CO_2 response curve, which equates minute ventilation with a given CO_2 level. This method ignores the possible depressant effect of anesthesia upon the action of respiratory muscles, which is known to occur with many different agents.

Concentrations of 50% nitrous oxide have no effect on the response to CO_2. However, after intravenous thiopentone the addition of nitrous oxide does cause a decrease in the response.[23] Diethyl ether decreases the ventilatory response to CO_2,[44] and of the other agents methoxyflurane and fluroxene produce more depression than cyclopropane.[54] In deeper halothane anesthesia the response to CO_2 is progressively lost.[54] In animals 2% trichloroethylene decreases the ventilatory response to CO_2, but this agent has not been studied in humans.[56]

During anesthesia with halothane, trichloroethylene, and several other agents, ventilation is characteristically rapid and shallow. Thus a fall in oxygen saturation and an increase in arterial carbon dioxide tension (Pa_{CO_2}) may result because more ventilation is wasted in the dead space, an effect particularly undesirable in infants where apparatus dead space is large in relation to the size of the child. This tachypnea has been attributed to sensitization of deflation and inflation receptors in the lung.[64,93] However, vagotomy merely delays the onset of the tachypnea, which must therefore be central in origin.[56] The tachypnea is diminished by central depressants such as meperidine.

The main effect of the deflation reflex is a maintained contraction of the diaphragm, but an increase in respiratory rate may also occur.[92] In trichloroethylene anesthesia some diaphragmatic contraction persists throughout expiration, and this contraction is accompanied by an increase in FRC, an effect not reported with any other agent. Cyclopropane[92] and methoxyflurane[56] do not usually reduce V_T but respiratory rate decreases. During halothane anesthesia, V_T in children is about half that measured in the recovery phase but rises during surgical stimulation so that minute ventilation ($\dot{V}_E$) closely approaches that measured during recovery.[94] Respiratory rate varies more during surgical stimulus in infants 3 months or younger than in 3- to 5-year-old children. The high respiratory rates in the infants exaggerate the effect of apparatus dead space, and the unsteady state resulting from intermittent surgical stimulation makes it difficult to predict requirements for anesthetic gas flows. This difficulty is a further reason for preferring controlled ventilation during anesthesia in infants.

CAROTID CHEMORECEPTORS

The rate of carotid body chemoreceptor discharge is increased by certain anesthetics, such as diethyl ether and chloroform.[43] In animals, none of the inhalation anesthetics seem to depress the chemoreceptor response to severe degrees of hypoxemia and hypercarbia.[7] Hypoxemia produces a striking increase in ventilation even during deep anesthesia with methoxyflurane.[38] Lesser changes in Pa_{O_2} and Pa_{CO_2} stimulate the chemoreceptors when cyclopropane and diethyl ether are used but halothane appears to depress the discharge. The effects of hypoxemia during anesthesia result from a combination of central, chemoreceptor, and humoral effects, which are subject to so many variables that the end result is difficult to predict.

THE LUNG

During anesthesia with spontaneous or controlled ventilation, pulmonary compliance (C_L) falls progressively. The initial rapid fall is largely due to anesthesia rather than artificial ventilation,[2] and some changes may even occur prior to induction of anesthesia since premedication with barbiturates and atropine reduces C_L and causes a fall in FRC.[31]

Children have high CV values. The difference between FRC and CV decreases in supine children to such a degree that airway closure may be present during normal tidal breathing in the younger children. In infants chest wall compliance is high and provides little support to maintain FRC, though the static elastic recoil of the lung is reduced.[49] These considerations all suggest that the fall in C_L and FRC is greater in young children and infants than in adults.

Neonates are likely to have a considerable degree of gas trapping.[55] The volume of trapped gas early in anesthesia is greater than the volume after 1 hour.[20] The fall in C_L and FRC seen early in anesthesia could be due to gas trapping; later absorption of this trapped gas leads to atelectasis. The normal Pa_{O_2} is low in these infants, and because of the mechanisms outlined previously, it may fall further during anesthesia; hence inspired oxygen concentrations should be increased during anesthesia.

PULMONARY BLOOD FLOW

Anesthetic agents differ in their effect upon pulmonary vascular resistance. In man cyclopropane increases resistance, probably by constricting pulmonary arterioles, while halothane, alone or with nitrous oxide, does not have this effect. Neither agent prevents the reduction in pulmonary vascular resistance that results from inspiring high concentrations of oxygen.[69] High concentrations of diethyl ether, halothane, and trichloroethylene, however, modify the pulmonary vascular response to hypoxia in animals,[86] and may diminish regional vasoconstriction, which prevents perfusion of poorly ventilated areas.

AIRWAY RESISTANCE

Resistance to gas flow varies indirectly with airway diameter. Since airway diameter varies directly with lung volume, reduced FRC during anesthesia results in increased airway resistance.

During anesthesia, the resistance of the apparatus is added to the resistance of that part of the natural airway not bypassed by instrumentation. Endotracheal tubes for small children are designed with a thin wall, allowing maximal internal diameter for a given external size. Trauma to the subglottic area from an excessively large tube is a potentially serious complication in infants and must be avoided.

The Cole tube,[11] in which the narrow portion is limited to that distal part which passes through the glottis, has only 50% of the resistance of a comparable uniform-bore tube.[36] However, it may cause damage to the glottic region and is not universally favored by pediatric anesthesiologists.

Measurements indicate that endotracheal intubation with an optimal-size tube does not usually increase total air-flow resistance significantly in adults.[96] Similar measurements in children, in whom values for airway resistance vary greatly in the conscious state,[13] demonstrate that in infants intubation generally decreases total flow resistance, but in older children resistance may increase.

Selection of the correct tube is most important. A decrease in internal diameter of an endotracheal tube from 3 to 2.5 mm at a flow of 5 l/min. triples the driving pressure required for gas flow.[63] In anesthetized infants intubated with a small tube, inspiratory resistance may be much greater than in the conscious infant,[76] causing a considerable increase in the work of breathing. Many anesthesiologists prefer to assist or control ventilation in the intubated infant.

In the unintubated child, during anesthesia the structures adjacent to the upper airway, particularly the tongue, may cause significant obstruction. In the conscious subject, an increase in airway resistance causes a decrease in respiratory frequency and an increase in V_T. Studies have been made of the respiratory response of infants under light halothane anesthesia to acute increases in airway resistance.[37] When the endotracheal tube was replaced with one of much smaller internal diameter, respiratory rate decreased as did flow rates and minute ventilation, V_T increased, and work of respiration rose by 200%. Since these responses were immediate, they were not due to change in Pa_{CO_2}, but were attributed to sensory elements in respiratory muscles. Thus, the reflex compensation for increased airway resistance is maintained in infants under halothane anesthesia. This compensation is the result of an increase in muscular effort, however, and when the muscle fatigues, respiratory failure occurs.

Changes in alveolar gas tensions during anesthesia may cause changes in airway resistance. Assisted or controlled ventilation frequently leads to hypocapnia and causes bronchoconstriction. Of the relaxant drugs d-tubocurarine chloride but not pancuronium bromide may cause an increase in airway resistance in subjects who have obstructive lung disease.[15]

The effects of anesthetic drugs on airway resistance in children have not been investigated.

Artificial Ventilation

Two principal questions arise when we assume the responsibility for ventilating a patient—how much ventilation is required and what pattern of ventilation shall we use?

The required minute ventilation is dictated by the predicted oxygen consumption ($\dot{V}O_2$) and the required Pa_{CO_2}.[60] Prediction of $\dot{V}O_2$ is reasonable only if the nature of the anesthetic agents used is taken into account. Under light general anesthesia, such as with nitrous oxide and meperidine, $\dot{V}O_2$ is probably close to the basal values used in construction of the Engstrom nomograms.[27,28,61] Under deeper anesthesia and controlled ventilation the metabolic rate in children 5 to 19 years is below the basal values of Robertson and Reid[77] by about 22%.[57] The North American Standard values are about 15% higher than the values of Robertson and Reid. Thus the nature of the anesthetic used must be taken into consideration in predicting $\dot{V}O_2$ and minute ventilation required.

Deciding upon an optimal level of arterial PCO_2 is also difficult. Overventilation has been considered by many anesthesiologists safer than underventilation in that the patient remains apneic and control of ventilation is easier. A low Pa_{CO_2} may favorably influence the distribution of drugs in the body and the cardiac rhythm.[60] However, low Pa_{CO_2} values are associated with lower cardiac outputs during anesthesia,[71] increases in $\dot{V}O_2$[9,42] and AaD_{O_2},[66,71] and unfavorable changes in the oxyhemoglobin dissociation curve. These effects are related to the degree to which the Pa_{CO_2} is decreased from normal levels, so that ventilation to approximately normal Pa_{CO_2} levels is preferred except in special cases where a low Pa_{CO_2} may help surgical or radiographic techniques.

DISTRIBUTION OF VENTILATION AND PERFUSION

The vertical gradient of transpulmonary pressure is affected differently when lungs are expanded by intermittent positive pressure ventilation (IPPV) from when they are expanded by the action of the respiratory muscles.[1] The distribution of ventilation in anesthetized paralyzed man differs from the awake values and is more even.[75] Some of these changes may be explained by the supine position, when breathing from low lung volumes results in redistribution of inspired gas to the nondependent areas of the lung.[41] The mechanics of the diaphragm are very different in the paralyzed and artificially ventilated patient; maximal excursion occurs in the superior portion instead of the most dependent part.[34] The distribution of pulmonary blood flow is affected by postural changes, by changes in lung volumes, and by the pharmacologic effects of anesthetic agents.

The effects of anesthesia and artificial ventilation upon ventilation-perfusion relationships in the lung have commonly been investigated using changes in the dead space/tidal volume ratio (V_D/V_T) to measure overventilation of underperfused areas, and AaD_{O_2} to indicate overperfusion of underventilated areas. Different anesthetics and patterns of ventilation may produce varying changes in these measurements of pulmonary gas exchange. VD/VT frequently rises significantly above 0.30 during anesthesia. This rise may occur without an increase in AaD_{O_2} in patients ventilated with air to normal Pa_{CO_2} values.[10] This rise has also been demonstrated in dogs,[3] if volatile agents, which may impair the mechanisms normally diverting blood away from areas of alveolar collapse and airway closure, are avoided.[86] The AaD_{O_2} is usually increased during anesthesia and artificial ventilation, however. This increase cannot be interpreted as simply due to a change in the ventilation-perfusion ratio however, since changes in cardiac output, oxygen uptake, and CO_2 tension may all have occurred. In anesthetized ventilated patients the AaD_{O_2} does not, however, invariably rise, and shunting can be minimal when a type of ventilation that maintains lung volume is used.[85]

VD/VT may progressively increase during artificial ventilation with halothane or cyclopropane anesthesia,[4] or remain constant under thiopentone, nitrous oxide, and meperidine.[62] In animals under Nembutal anesthesia, values close to normal have been maintained for many hours using a prolonged inspiratory period. With this type of ventilation no increase in VD/VT may follow the switch from spontaneous respiration to artificial ventilation.[19] In anesthetized man the increased physiologic dead space has been reported to be similar during spontaneous and artificial ventilation.[62]

In summary, the evidence indicates that the disturbances in ventilation-perfusion relationships that occur during anesthesia and artificial ventilation are variable and to some extent may be minimized. Not enough evidence exists to show precisely how best to minimize this effect in children.

LUNG MECHANICS AND FRC

An early fall in dynamic C_L is usual in anesthetized subjects who are artificially ventilated, and may be in part due to a change in posture, since C_L and FRC fall equally when a subject assumes the supine posture.[47] The fall in C_L is apparently not due to a change in lung parenchyma itself since static compliance in both adults[33] and children[58] remains essentially normal after induction of anesthesia and artificial ventilation. Halothane[65] and the muscle relaxant d-Tubocurarine chloride[59] produce little immediate effect upon static compliance.

In adults FRC falls during anesthesia[21] and artificial ventilation.[45,50] The reduction in FRC in anesthetized ventilated children is greater than that reported in adults and is inversely proportional to the size of the child. C_L in these children falls similarly to FRC since specific compliance is close to normal soon after the induction of anesthesia.[18] These changes are probably the result of changes in thoracic and abdominal muscle tone due to anesthesia. IPPB does not alter compliance and FRC in conscious subjects.[26]

Measurements of compliance and FRC during anesthesia may be the best way of demonstrating atelectasis.[2] In normal children a progressive fall in compliance without a fall in FRC may occur in the course of anesthesia and artificial ventilation.[18] It would be ideal if a pattern of ventilation could be discovered to prevent this problem. Watson showed that, in the short term, compliance in artificially ventilated subjects is increased if inspiration lasts more than 1 second;[90] Lyager increased compliance by ventilating with a prolonged no-flow interval at the end of inspiration.[48] Most of our experimental work in animals, however, indicates that it is not easy to prevent the progressive fall in compliance during artificial ventilation over a long period. In young children, who have less collateral ventilation, the difficulties may be greater than in adults.

SURFACTANT

Although lipid-soluble anesthetics such as chloroform and halothane may alter the surfactant in excised lungs at room temperature, these changes are reversed by incubation at 37° C.[95] Sequential lung biopsies during surgical procedure under diethyl ether, halothane, and methoxyflurane have demonstrated normal surface tension.[52] It appears that these agents themselves do not alter the normal surface properties of the lung. Artificial ventilation, however, may alter these properties in various ways.

Repeated expansion and compression of a layer of extracted pulmonary surfactant cause the most surface-active molecules to concentrate at the surface.[87] The effect of a reduction in lung volume such as occurs in anesthetized ventilated children is to decrease the availability of the phospholipids, which help prevent alveolar collapse by reducing surface tension.[18] To prevent this reduction of lung volume, large VT ventilation may be maintained by the anesthesiologist. Large VT, however, may merely further increase the ventilation of poorly perfused areas in the upper zones of the lung and result in regional overexpansion of a layer of pulmonary surfactant. Hyperventilation, or repeated overinflation of the lungs, promotes alveolar atelectasis.[32] Faridy has shown that absence of pulmonary blood flow in lungs ventilated at large VT increases the retractive force of dogs' lungs.[30] Furthermore, in dogs severe overinflation of the lung results in absence of surfactant after a latent period,[39] and assisted ventilation for over 24 hours decreases surfactant.[40] This effect occurs soon after operation in patients with cardiac disease in whom specific compliance may already be low[17] and alveolar surface tension elevated.[40]

Artificial Ventilation in the Newborn

Newborns are under many disadvantages when submitted to anesthesia. We have already mentioned their sensitivity to drugs that depress central control of respiration. They fatigue easily and their response to anesthetics shows wide individual variation. Their breathing is diaphragmatic and easily hindered by abdominal contents.[73] They also have a relatively high true shunt value for the first few days of life,[55] up to 15% of cardiac output, and their pH is normal only because they reduce Pa_{CO_2} sufficiently to counter a deficit in bicarbonate and buffering power. There is doubt as to reputed resistance to hypoxemia of the newborn,[81] which may be characteristic only of animals born in an immature state, such as cats and rabbits. Fluid retention and gas trapping in the lung are considerable at birth, and specific C_L increases 3 to 8 hours after birth. Although ventilation and perfusion become evenly matched soon after birth, the foramen ovale and ductus arteriosus may reopen in up to 11 days if the infant becomes hypoxemic.[55]

The high chest-wall compliance of infants and young children provides a relatively weak expansile force to maintain FRC. The large decrease in FRC seen in anesthetized ventilated children may well be related to the lower elastic recoil of their lungs and the greater tendency for airway closure to occur.[49]

Although specific airway conductance in the neonate is similar to that of the adult[55] and the size of the airways is not reduced in proportion to body size,[5] the small absolute size of the airways means they can easily be blocked by secretions. Similarly, although VD/VT is similar to that in adults, the small absolute size of the neonate's dead space makes the addition of any apparatus dead space much more significant than in adults.

Infants have a shorter time constant (total compliance × total resistance) than adults (0.33 compared to 0.64) and, therefore, need shorter, more rapid breaths.[55]

All these factors, together with an apparently increased liability for laryngospasm to occur in young subjects under light anesthesia, have led some anesthetists to use controlled ventilation for virtually all surgical procedures in newborns and young children.[83] The modified T-piece introduced by Jackson Rees is used with a fast rate of ventilation, and positive end-expiratory pressure (*PEEP*) is applied by controlling the expiratory flow of gases.[74]

The use of PEEP and the rapid rate of ventilation may help to minimize the falls in C_L that have been reported by maintaining FRC.[68,76] Newborns appear to tolerate raised mean intrathoracic pressure well during nitrous oxide anesthesia with muscle relaxant, possibly because they have a relatively high pulmonary artery pressure.[53]

REFERENCES

1. Agostoni, E., E. D'Angelo and M. V. Bonanni: Topography of pleural surface pressure above resting volume in relaxed animals. *J. Appl. Physiol. 29*:297, 1970.
2. Arthur, D. A., A. K. Mathur and H. I. A. Nisbet: Unpublished observations.
3. Arthur, D. A., A. K. Mathur, H. I. A. Nisbet and G. Volgyesi: Unpublished observations.
4. Askrog, V. F., J. W. Pender, T. C. Smith and J. E. Eckenhoff: Changes in respiratory dead space during halothane, cyclopropane, and nitrous oxide anesthesia. *Anesthesiology 25*:342, 1964.
5. Avery, M. E.: *The Lung and Its Disorders in the Newborn Infant,* 2nd ed. W. B. Saunders Co., Philadelphia, 1968.
6. Bachman, L., and A. Freeman: The cardiac rate and rhythm in infants during induction of anesthesia with cyclopropane. *J. Pediatr. 59*:922, 1961.
7. Biscoe, T. J. and R. A. Millar: Effects of inhalation anaesthetics on carotid body chemoreceptor activity. *Br. J. Anaesth. 40*:2, 1968.
8. Butler, J., C. G. Caro, R. Alcala and A. B. Dubois: Physiological factors affecting airway resistance in normal subjects and in patients with obstructive respiratory disease. *J. Clin. Invest. 39*:584, 1960.
9. Cain, S. M.: Increased oxygen uptake with passive hyperventilation of dogs. *J. Appl. Physiol. 28*:4, 1970.
10. Campbell, E. J. M., J. F. Nunn and B. W. Peckett: A comparison of artificial ventilation and spontaneous respiration with particular reference to ventilation-bloodflow relationships. *Br. J. Anaesth. 30*:166, 1958.
11. Cole, F.: A new endotracheal tube for infants. *Anesthesiology 6*:87, 1945.
12. Cook, C. D.: Respiratory physiology in infants and children. In *Anesthesia for Infants and Children,* R. M. Smith (Ed.). The C. V. Mosby Co., St. Louis, 1959.
13. Cook, C. D., J. M. Sutherland, S. Segal, R. B. Cherry, J. Mead, M. B. McIlroy and C. A. Smith: Studies of respiratory physiology in the newborn infant. III. Measurements of mechanics of respiration. *J. Clin. Invest. 36*:440, 1957.
14. Cooper, D. M., H. I. A. Nisbet, D. J. Stewart, A. C. Bryan and H. Levison: Unpublished observations.
15. Crago, R. R., A. C. Bryan, A. K. Laws and A. E. Winestock: Respiratory flow resistance after curare and pancuronium, measured by forced oscillations. *Can. Anaesth. Soc. J. 19*:607, 1972.
16. Dawkins, M. J. R.: Biochemical aspects of developing function in new-born mammalian liver. *Br. Med. Bull. 22*:27, 1966.
17. Dobbinson, T. L., I. G. Gray, H. I. A. Nisbet, D. A. Pelton, H. Levison and G. Volgyesi: Thoracic compliance and lung volumes in children with heart disease. *Acta Anaesthesiol. Scand. 17*:50, 1973.
18. Dobbinson, T. L., H. I. A. Nisbet, D. A. Pelton and H. Levison: Functional residual capacity (FRC) and compliance in anaesthetized paralyzed children. II. Clinical results. *Can. Anaesth. Soc. J. 20*:322, 1973.
19. Dobbinson, T. L., H. I. A. Nisbet and G. Volgyesi: Unpublished observations.
20. Don, H. F., W. M. Wahba and D. B. Craig: Airway closure, gas trapping, and the functional residual capacity during anesthesia. *Anesthesiology 36*:533, 1972.
21. Don, H. F., W. M. Wahba, L. Cuadrado and K. Kelkar: The effects of anesthesia and 100 percent oxygen on the functional residual capacity of the lungs. *Anesthesiology 32*:521, 1970.
22. Done, A. K.: Developmental pharmacology. *Clin. Pharmacol. Ther. 5*:432, 1964.
23. Eckenhoff, J. E., and M. Helrich: The effect of narcotics, thiopental and nitrous oxide upon respiration and respiratory response to hypercapnia. *Anesthesiology 19*:240, 1958.
24. Eger, E. I.: Atropine, scopolamine and related compounds. *Anesthesiology 23*:365, 1962.
25. Eger, E. I., I. D. Kraft and H. H. Keasling: A comparison of atropine, or scopolamine, plus pentobarbital, meperidine or morphine as pediatric preanesthetic medication. *Anesthesiology 22*:962, 1961.
26. Emerson, P. A., G. E. Torres and H. A. Lyons: The effect of intermittent positive pressure breathing on the lung compliance and intrapulmonary mixing of gases. *Thorax 15*:124, 1960.
27. Engstrom, C. G. and P. Herzob: Ventilation nomogram for practical use with the Engstrom respirator. *Acta Chir. Scand. Suppl. 245*:37, 1959.
28. Engstrom, C. G., P. Herzog, O. P. Norlander and S. A. Swensson: Ventilation nomogram for the newborn and small children to be used with the Engstrom respirator. *Acta Anaesthesiol. Scand. 6*:175, 1962.

29. Etsten, B., F. A. D. Alexander and H. E. Himwich: Comparative toxicity of pentobarbital in newborn and adult rat. *J. Lab. Clin. Med. 28*:706, 1943.
30. Fariday, E. E.: Effect of alterations in Po_2, Pco_2, pH, and blood flow on elastic behaviour of dogs' lungs. *J. Appl. Physiol. 27*:342, 1969.
31. Finley, T. N.: Editorial views. Anesthesia and atelectasis. *Anesthesiology 29*:863, 1968.
32. Forrest, J. B.: The effect of hyperventilation on the size and shape of alveoli. *Br. J. Anaesth. 42*:810, 1970.
33. Foster, C. A., P. J. D. Heaf and S. J. G. Semple: Compliance of the lung in anesthetized paralyzed subjects. *J. Appl. Physiol. 11*:383, 1957.
34. Froese, A. and A. C. Bryan: The effects of anesthesia and muscle paralysis on diaphragm mechanics in man. *Anesthesiology 41*:242, 1974.
35. Gardiner, A. J. S., K. N. V. Palmer and M. H. McGregor: Effect of premedication and general anaesthesia on arterial blood gases. *Br. Med. J. 2*:1433, 1964.
36. Glauser, E. M., C. D. Cook and T. P. Bougas: Pressure-flow characteristics and dead spaces of endotracheal tubes used in infants. *Anesthesiology 22*:339, 1961.
37. Graff, T. D., K. Sewall, H. S. Lim, O. Kantt, R. E. Morris, Jr. and D. W. Benson: The ventilatory response of infants to airway resistance. *Anesthesiology 27*:168, 1966.
38. Gray, I. G., H. I. A. Nisbet, P. M. Olley, B. E. Welsh and A. E. Johnston: Cardiovascular and respiratory responses to severe hypoxaemia under anaesthesia. II. Spontaneous and controlled ventilation during methoxyflurane anaesthesia. *Can. Anaesth. Soc. J. 20*:637, 1973.
39. Greenfield, L. J., P. A. Ebert and D. W. Benson: Effect of positive pressure ventilation on surface tension properties of lung extracts. *Anesthesiology 25*:312, 1964.
40. Iyomasa, Y., T. Shimizu and E. Okamura: Postoperative pulmonary insufficiency after open heart surgery and changes in pulmonary surface activity. *Jpn. Circ. J. 36*:153, 1972.
41. Kaneko, K., J. Milic-Emili, M. B. Dolovich, A. Dawson and D. V. Bates: Regional distribution of ventilation and perfusion as a function of body position. *J. Appl. Physiol. 21*:767, 1966.
42. Khambatta, H. J. and S. F. Sullivan: Effects of respiratory alkalosis on oxygen consumption and oxygenation. *Anesthesiology 38*:53, 1973.
43. Landgren, S., G. Liljestrand, Y. Zotterman and A. Wirkung von Alkohol:Äther und chloroform auf die chemoceptoren des glomus caroticum. *Arch. Exp. Pathol. Pharmakol.* (*Berl.*) *219*:185, 1953.
44. Larson, C. P. Jr., E. I. Eger II, M. Muallem, D. R. Buechel, E. S. Munson and Eisele, J. H.: The effects of diethyl ether and methoxyflurane on ventilation:II. A comparative study in man. *Anesthesiology 30*:174, 1969.
45. Laws, A. K.: Effects of induction of anaesthesia and muscle paralysis on functional residual capacity of the lungs. *Can. Anaesth. Soc. J. 15*:325, 1968.
46. Lee, J. A.: The pharmacology of drugs used for pre-operative and post-operative medication. Morphine. In *A Synopsis of Anesthesia*, 6th ed., J. A. Lee and R. S. Atkinson (Eds.). J. Wright, Bristol, 1968.
47. Lim, T. P. K. and U. C. Luft: Alterations in lung compliance and functional residual capacity with posture. *J. Appl. Physiol. 14*:164, 1959.
48. Lyager, S.: Ventilation/perfusion ratio during intermittent positive-pressure ventilation. *Acta Anaesthesiol. Scand. 14*:211, 1970.
49. Mansell, A., C. Bryan and H. Levison: Airway closure in children. *J. Appl. Physiol. 33*:711, 1972.
50. Marsh, H. M., K. Rehder, A. D. Sessler and W. S. Fowler: Effect of posture, muscle paralysis and mechanical ventilation on ventilation-perfusion relation in anesthetized man. *Fed. Proc. 30*:217, 1971 (Abstract).
51. McGarry, P. M. F.: A double-blind study of diazepam, droperidol, and meperidine as premedication in children. *Can. Anaesth. Soc. J. 17*:157, 1970.
52. Miller, R. N. and P. A. Thomas: Pulmonary surfactant:determinations from lung extracts of patients receiving diethyl ether or halothane. *Anesthesiology 28*:1089, 1967.
53. Mott, J. C.: Cardiovascular function in newborn mammals. *Br. Med. Bull. 22*:66, 1966.
54. Munson, E. S., C. P. Larson, Jr., A. A. Babad, M. J. Regan, D. R. Buechel and E. I. Eger, II: The effects of halothane, fluroxene and cyclopropane on ventilation: a comparative study in man. *Anesthesiology 27*:716, 1966.
55. Nelson, N. M.: Neonatal pulmonary function. *Pediatr. Clin. North Am. 13*:769, 1966.
56. Ngai, S. H., R. L. Katz and D. C. Brody: Effect of trichloroethylene and methoxyflurane on central respiratory mechanisms. *Anesthesiology 24*:136, 1963.
57. Nisbet, H. I. A., T. L. Dobbinson, T. A. Thomas and D. A. Pelton: Oxygen uptake in ventilated children during methoxyflurane anaesthesia. *Can. Anaesth. Soc. J. 20*:334, 1973.
58. Nisbet, H. I. A., H. Levison and D. A. Pelton: Static thoracic compliance in normal children under general anaesthesia. *Acta Anaesth. Scand. 15*:179, 1971.
59. Nisbet, H. I. A., D. A. Pelton, J. E. S. Relton and H. Levison: The effect of d-tubocurarine upon the static elastic recoil of the thorax. *Can. Anaesth. Soc. J. 18*:304, 1971.
60. Nunn, J. F.: *Applied Respiratory Physiology with Special Reference to Anaesthesia.* Butterworth and Co., London, pp. 145 and 148, 1969.
61. Nunn, J. F., N. A. Bergman and A. J. Colemen:

Factors influencing the arterial oxygen tension during anaesthesia with artificial ventilation. *Br. J. Anaesth. 37*:898, 1965.
62. Nunn, J. F. and D. W. Hill: Respiratory dead space and arterial to end-tidal CO_2 tension difference in anesthetized man. *J. Appl. Pharmacol. 15*:383, 1960.
63. Orkin, L. R., M. Siegel and E. A. Rovenstine: Resistance to breathing by apparatus used in anesthesia. I. Endotracheal equipment. *Anesth. Analg. 33*:217, 1954.
64. Paintal, A. S.: The location and excitation of pulmonary deflation receptors by chemical substances. *Q. J. Exp. Physiol. 42*:56, 1957.
65. Patterson, R. W., S. F. Sullivan, J. R. Malm, F. O. Bowman, Jr. and E. M. Papper: The effect of halothane on human airway mechanics. *Anesthesiology 29*:900, 1968.
66. Pichotka, J. P., H. Krekeler, J. Schotte and K. Muysers: Die alveolär-arterielle O_2-druckdifferenz bei hyperventilation. *Pfluegers Arch. 327*:53, 1971.
67. Pierce, J. A. and M. L. Garofalo: Preoperative medication and its effect on blood gases. *J.A.M.A., 194*:487, 1965.
68. Podlesch, I. and D. Schettler: Der einfluss der narkose auf die lungenfunktion und den säurebasen-haushalt des säuglings. I. compliance und alveolo-arterielle sauerstoffdruckdifferenz. *Anaesthesist 22*:86, 1973.
69. Price, H. L., L. H. Cooperman, J. C. Warden, J. J. Morris and T. C. Smith: Pulmonary hemodynamics during general anesthesia in man. *Anesthesiology 30*:629, 1969.
70. Prys-Roberts, C.: Applied human pharmacology of analgesic and neuroleptic drugs. *Proceedings Second British Symposium on the Use of Neuroleptanalgesia in Anesthetic Practice,* 1966.
71. Prys-Roberts, C., G. R. Kelman, R. Greenbaum, M. L. Kain and J. Bay: Hemodynamics and alveolar-arterial Po_2 differences at varying Pa_{CO_2} in anesthetised man. *J. Appl. Physiol. 25*:80, 1968.
72. Rackow, H. and E. Salanitre: A new pediatric circle valve. *Anesthesiology 29*:833, 1968.
73. Rackow, H., and E. Salanitre: Modern concepts in pediatric anesthesiology. *Anesthesiology 30*:208, 1969.
74. Rees, G. J.: Anaesthesia in the newborn. *Br. Med. J. 2*:1419, 1950.
75. Rehder, K., D. J. Hatch, A. D. Sessler, H. M. Marsh and W. S. Fowler: Effects of general anesthesia, muscle paralysis, and mechanical ventilation on pulmonary nitrogen clearance. *Anesthesiology 35*:591, 1971.
76. Reynolds, R. N. and B. E. Etsten: Mechanics of respiration in apneic anesthetised infants. *Anesthesiology 27*:13, 1966.
77. Robertson, J. D. and D. D. Reid: Standards for the basal metabolism of normal people in Britain. *Lancet I*:940, 1952.
78. Salanitre, E. and H. Rackow: The pulmonary exchange of nitrous oxide and halothane in infants and children. *Anesthesiology 30*:388, 1969.
79. Schlossmann, H. A.: The relationship between age and the action of atropine and morphine. *J. Pharmacol. Exp. Ther. 60*:14, 1937.
80. Severinghaus, J. W., and M. Stupfel: Respiratory dead space increase following atropine in man, and atropine, vagal or ganglionic blockage and hypothermia in dogs. *J. Appl. Physiol. 8*:81, 1955.
81. Smith, B. E. and F. Moya: Resuscitation of the depressed newborn. *Anesthesiology 26*:549, 1965.
82. Smith, R. M. and M. Jeffries: The evaluation of sedative agents for preoperative use in children. *Anesth. Analg. 38*:166, 1959.
83. Stead, A. L. and D. A. Nightingale: *Anesthesia for the Newborn in Neonatal Surgery,* P. P. Rickham and J. H. Johnston (Eds.). Butterworths, London, p. 87, 1969.
84. Steinberg, S. S., J. W. Bellville and J. C. Seed: The effect of atropine and morphine on respiration. *J. Pharmacol. Exp. Ther. 121*:71, 1957.
85. Stone, J. G. and S. F. Sullivan: Failure of shallow ventilation to produce pulmonary shunting in the anesthetized dog. *Anesthesiology 32*:338, 1970.
86. Sykes, M. K., D. M. Davies, M. K. Chakrabarti and L. Loh: The effects of halothane, trichloroethylene and ether on the hypoxic pressor response and pulmonary vascular resistance in the isolated, perfused cat lung. *Br. J. Anaesth. 45*:655, 1973.
87. Tierney, D. F. and R. P.: Johnson: Altered surface tension of lung extracts and lung mechanics. *J. Appl. Physiol. 20*:1253, 1965.
88. Tomlin, P. J., C. M. Conway and J. P. Payne: Hypoxaemia due to atropine. *Lancet I*:14, 1964.
89. von Czike, A.: Lungenvolumenuntersuchungen unter Einwirkung von Atropin, Adrenalin und Strophantin. *Z. Gesamte Inn. Med. 74*:20, 1930.
90. Watson, W. E.: Some observations on dynamic lung compliance during intermittent positive pressure respiration. *Br. J. Anaesth. 34*:153, 1962.
91. Way, W. L., E. C. Costley and E. L. Way: Respiratory sensitivity of the newborn infant to meperidine and morphine. *Clin. Pharmacol. Ther. 6*:454, 1965.
92. Whitteridge, D.: Effect of anesthetics on mechanical receptors. *Br. Med. Bull. 14*:5, 1958.
93. Whitteridge, D., and E. Bulbring: Changes in activity of pulmonary receptors in anaesthesia and their influence on respiratory behaviour. *J. Pharmacol. 81*:340, 1944.
94. Wilson, L. A., and G. A. Harrison: Pulmonary ventilation in children during halothane anesthesia. *Anesthesiology 25*:613, 1964.
95. Woo, S. W., D. Berlin and J. Hedley-Whyte: Sur-

factant function and anesthetic agents. *J. Appl. Physiol.* *26*:571, 1969.
96. Wu, N., W. F. Miller and N. R. Luhn: Studies of breathing in anesthesia. *Anesthesiology* *17*:696, 1956.
97. Yates, D.: Unpublished observations.

Pediatric Thoracic Surgery

W. HARDY HENDREN AND SAMUEL H. KIM

6

Many conditions of surgical importance can cause reduced pulmonary function and respiratory distress in infants and children. It is pertinent to consider many problems in addition to primary lung conditions; these other disorders include malformations of the chest wall and diaphragm that can embarrass ventilation, space-occupying lesions that can compress the lungs, correctable problems that encroach upon the airway, those infections that can cause surgical complications, and trauma. In the pediatric age group nearly all patients with surgical problems are seen first by a primary care physician. If the physician is not well versed in the spectrum of surgical disease, indications for surgical procedure, and current therapy, the child may suffer. For example, a neglected foreign body in the tracheobronchial tree may result in a destroyed lobe. The risk incurred from diagnostic bronchoscopy in competent hands is relatively small by comparison. On the other hand, children with funnel chest are referred for surgery "to improve lung function," although, except in severe cases, the principal indication for operation is the desire to improve the child's appearance.

In the first part of this chapter, a wide range of respiratory problems of childhood is presented in order to illustrate the gamut of surgically correctable problems. Cardiac anomalies are not included since they deserve separate consideration. It should be mentioned, however, that the infant in congestive heart failure with no audible murmurs is frequently believed to have a primary respiratory disorder. For example, surgically correctable cor triatriatum can masquerade as hyaline membrane disease.

Part I: *Thoracic Surgical Diseases*

Disorders that may lend themselves to treatment by thoracic surgical means include chest wall deformities, tumors, aortic arch anomalies, foreign bodies, diaphragmatic hernia, esophageal atresia and fistula, lobar emphysema, empyema, caustic esophageal burns, hiatus hernia, middle lobe syndrome, pneumothorax, chylothorax, lung cyst, lung abscess, bronchogenic cyst, pulmonary sequestration, bronchiectasis, enteric duplications, and thoracic trauma.

Chest Wall Abnormalities

Pectus excavatum or funnel chest is the most common chest wall deformity. The cause of funnel chest is not known. It is sometimes seen in father and son, or in two siblings, but more often there is no positive family history. The defect varies in extent and severity, but usually consists of an inward depression of the lower sternum and four to five pairs of costal cartilages, which are abnormally long and curve inward to meet the sternum. In some cases the defect is asymmetrical, with rotation of the sternum toward the right or left. Occasionally it appears as a unilateral deformity.

In most patients no physiologic problem is present. However, in a severe case where the sternum almost touches the spine, displacing the heart to the left, some cardiorespiratory compromise can exist due to compression of the right ventricular outflow tract. It is common for parents to state that a child with funnel chest seems to tire easily, or have shortness of breath when exercising. Cardiac catheterization of a group of these youngsters before and after repair showed no significant cardiac defect.[35] Study of pulmonary function in some cases showed no abnormality despite marked deformity.[95] In a larger series of 27 children who had pulmonary function studies, five were found with some decrease in function.[39] Three of those had surgical procedure, but no measurable change in pulmonary function occurred. Although objective data are lacking, these youngsters often claim better exercise tolerance after surgical repair. However, *the principal indication for repair in most cases is cosmetic.* Figure 6-1 shows such a case. Operation on this 16-year-old girl had a remarkably good effect on her self-image. She had been withdrawn and asocial.

The timing of surgical correction should vary according to the severity of the defect and the wishes of the family. Technically it is easier to perform the operation from about age 2 to 6 years, and it can be a difficult operation in older patients. The defect does *not* tend to improve in time. In a young child with funnel chest, it can be predicted that with growth the depression will remain the same or become deeper. A family should strongly desire operative correction before surgical procedure is advised. In the case of

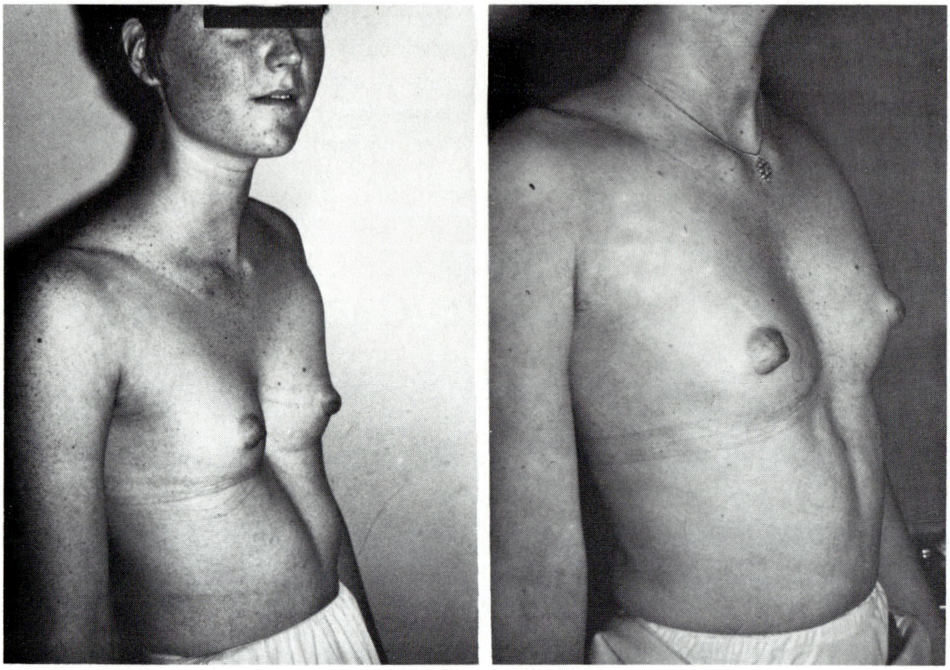

FIG. 6-1. 16-year-old girl before and after repair of moderately severe defect.

older children, it should be desired by the patient himself. We generally defer repair until at least 2 years of age, or longer if the parents have any uncertainties. Operative correction consists of removing the depressed costal cartilages but preserving the perichondrium, from which new cartilages regenerate in a few weeks.[101,135] The anterior periosteum of the sternum is transected at the junction where depressed sternum meets normal sternum, permitting the depressed segment to hinge forward. The pectoral muscles are then reattached to the sternum. *A transverse skin incision is always used,* for it is cosmetically much preferred to a vertical incision over the sternum, which commonly results in a hypertrophied scar. Although infection is rare, its occurrence can result in mediastinitis; therefore, antibiotics are given prophylactically. We prefer to use a metal strut to stabilize the sternum postoperatively.[65,104] Figure 6-2 shows the Rehbein struts used in repairing a severe defect. The two metal struts are thrust into the marrow cavity of the fifth rib on each side, forming an arch to which the sternum is wired. Postoperatively the patient can ambulate in a few days. A protective device is worn for several weeks to guard against accidental trauma (Fig. 6-3). Figures 6-1 and 6-4 show two children before and after repair of moderately severe defects. Recurrence is unusual and results are gratifying to patient, parent, and physician. The physician should never urge a patient with pectus excavatum to be operated upon; the patient and his family should be strongly motivated toward this procedure.

Pectus carinatum, or pigeon breast, is the opposite of funnel chest; the sternum protrudes forward. It is much less common than pectus excavatum. Indications for surgical procedure and details of repair are similar to those for funnel chest.[109]

Other rare chest wall deformities include bifid sternum,[8,31] absent lower sternum associated with a defect in the diaphragm, peri-

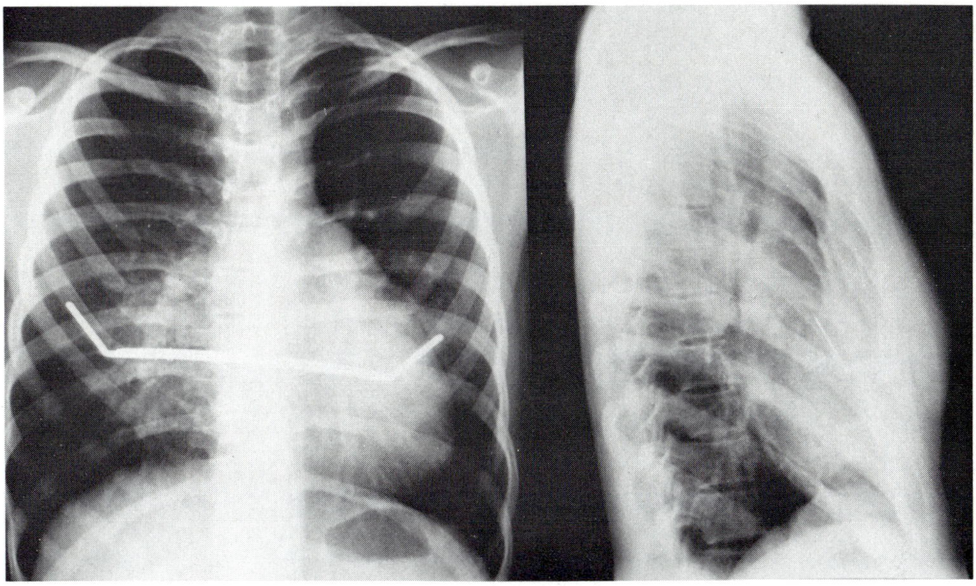

FIG. 6-2. Rehbein metal struts, one of the types used in the repair of funnel chest. These thin, flexible, steel strips are thrust into the end of a rib cavity on each side; when wired together, they form an arch to which the sternum can be sutured forward after resecting the depressed costal cartilages.

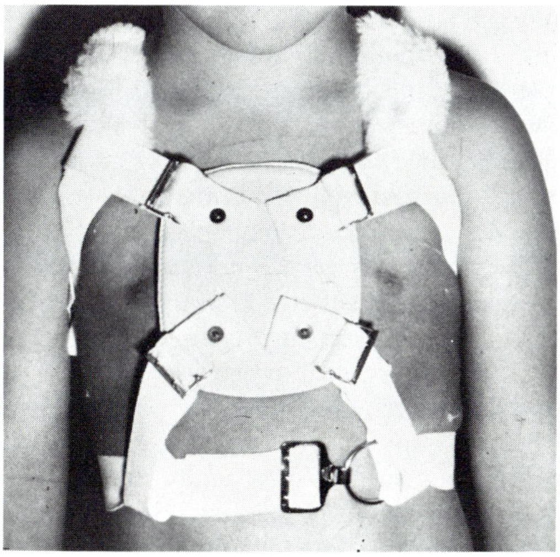

FIG. 6-3. Protective device used after funnel chest repair. This thin metal plate, covered with soft leather, covers the operative area. The figure-of-8 arrangement of the upper straps holds the shoulders back, in a position of good posture, during healing. Children usually have improved posture following repair.

cardium, and omphalocele,[46,90] and segmental absence of ribs.[108] All of these can be corrected surgically.

Tumors

Tumors of the chest wall are seen occasionally in children; the spectrum includes the same types of benign and malignant neoplasms that can arise from bone, cartilage, and soft tissue elsewhere in the body.[94,125] Any unexplained swelling of soft tissue or bony thorax should be regarded with suspicion and a biopsy performed. We have resected neurofibrosarcoma and reticulum cell sarcoma of the chest wall during the first week of life.

Children tolerate extensive resection of the chest wall when required. Sizable defects, spanning several ribs, can be closed with prosthetic mesh. For primary malignant neoplasms arising in ribs, the involved ribs

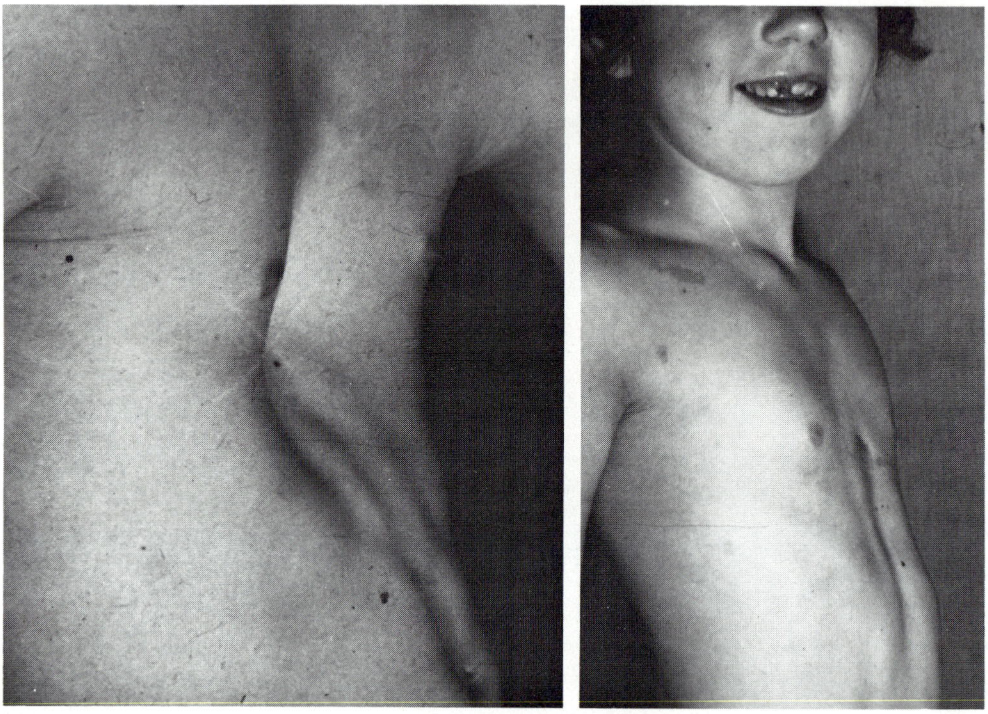

FIG. 6-4. 6-year-old youngster before and after repair of a moderately severe defect. The transverse submammary incision can be seen.

should be taken entirely, with disarticulation of both ends, together with an adjacent normal rib above and below. It is desirable to plan incisions so that the skin closure does not lie directly over an anticipated defect, especially if a prosthetic closure may be used; this practice reduces the likelihood of infection involving the prosthesis. In certain instances it is possible to fill a sizable defect with a muscle flap of latissimus dorsi, by detaching it from the iliac crest and rotating the muscle forward.

Primary lung tumors are exceedingly rare in childhood, but most of the lesions that occur in adults have been reported in children[61,102,131]

Secondary metastatic tumor of the lung is, on the other hand, not unusual in childhood. Wilms' tumor is the most common. It is sensitive to treatment by irradiation and systemic chemotherapy with actinomycin D. Figure 6-5 is the chest roentgenograms of a 4-year-old child with Wilms' tumor, before and 1 month after combined treatment; complete clearing occurred. Figure 6-6 demonstrates massive metastatic involvement by Wilms' tumor seen at the time of admission of a 3-year-old boy with hematuria. Ordinarily the presence of lung metastases from Wilms' tumor is *not* a contraindication to an aggressive surgical attack on the primary lesion. The rate of cure is high with triple attack, using surgical procedure, radiation in selected cases, and prolonged postoperative chemotherapy.[72] When even a single lung nodule is seen in Wilms' tumor, it is best to assume that multiple metastases are present and to give low-dose (about 1000 rads in 7 to 10 days) treatment to both lung fields, together with systemic actinomycin D, which potentiates the effect of ionizing radiation.[25,36] If an isolated metastasis reappears following this treatment and cannot be controlled by selective irradiation, surgical exci-

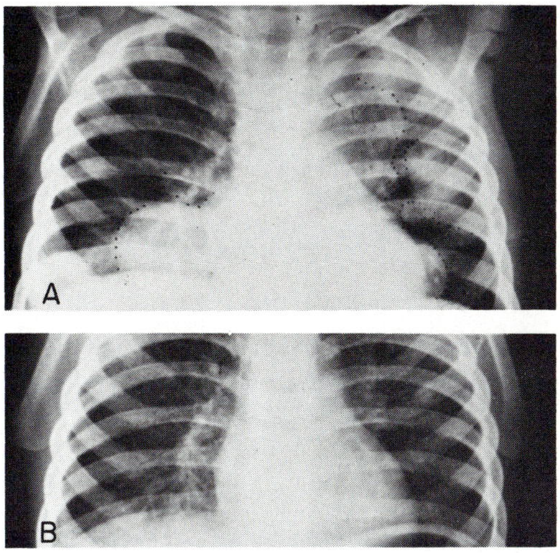

FIG. 6-5. Wilms' tumor with bilateral pulmonary metastases in a 3-year-old boy.

A, Chest roentgenogram on admission. Dots outline multiple nodules. Treatment consisted of radical nephrectomy, with postoperative chemotherapy and radiation therapy of the lungs, to a dose of 1200 rads.

B, Film 1 month later showing complete clearing of metastases. This child is well now, more than 10 years postoperatively.

sion should be considered. Wedge excision is possible, but lobectomy is needed in certain cases. Rarely an extensive extrapleural resection may be necessary when a metastasis recurs in lung and adjacent pleural space.

Other tumors that metastasize to the lungs include rhabdomyosarcoma and osteogenic sarcoma. If one or even several pulmonary metastases exist more than 6 months after initial treatment for osteogenic sarcoma, excision should be considered. A patient we treated 18 years ago by this approach is alive and well. His left leg had been removed for osteogenic sarcoma. Later, right lower lobectomy was performed for a large single metastasis. Four small nodules then appeared in the left lung and were excised by wedge resection. Others have reported success also in selected cases with this type of unconventional and aggressive approach.[81]

Mediastinal tumors can appear with respiratory symptoms in children, due to tracheal

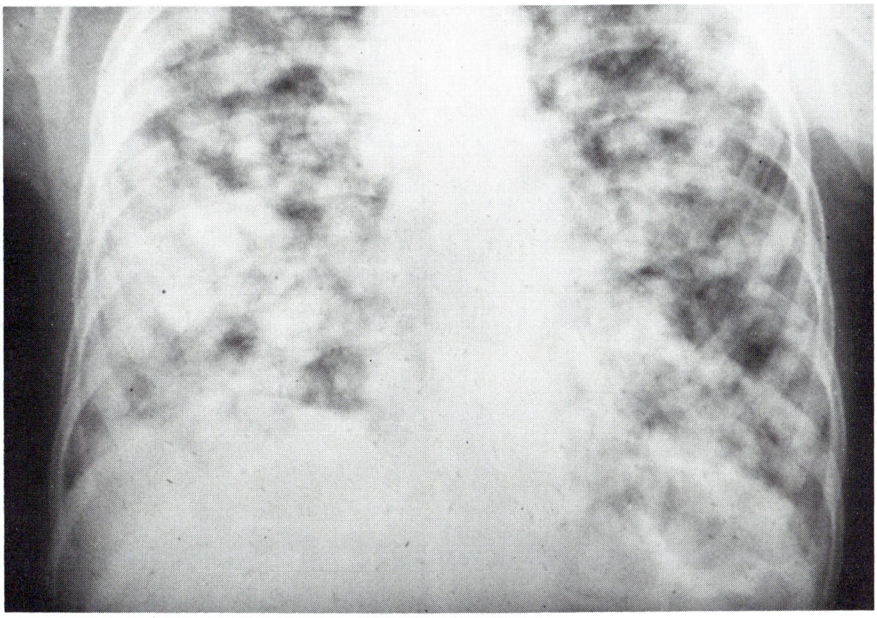

FIG. 6-6. Wilms' tumor with diffuse metastatic pulmonary involvement. This 3-year-old child was admitted with acute respiratory distress from these metastases. The primary kidney tumor had not been symptomatic. With such extensive involvement, initial treatment was directed at the lungs, which temporarily cleared remarkably. The primary tumor was removed subsequently. The child eventually succumbed from regrowth of pulmonary disease despite continuing prolonged chemotherapy.

compression or displacement of the lung if the mass attains very large size. Most common are those of neural origin, arising from the sympathetic chain in the posterior mediastinum. Curiously the prognosis is better in children with intrathoracic neuroblastoma as compared to those with tumors arising in the abdomen.[38,71,97] A typical case of mediastinal neuroblastoma is shown in Figure 6-7. This child came to the clinic with a nonspecific respiratory complaint. Chest film disclosed the mass. Figure 6-8 shows a small paraspinal ganglioneuroma arising from the sympathetic chain just above the diaphragm. These tumors can extend along nerve trunks into the spinal canal. Occasionally a patient initially has symptoms of spinal cord compression. Surgical excision, which is sometimes incomplete, together with radiotherapy and chemotherapy, can produce long-term survival in about 75% of these children. Chemotherapy has proven less effective, however, than in other types of tumors. About 40% of intrathoracic neural tumors are malignant.

Two special types of tumors of neural origin are plexiform neurofibroma and pheochromocytoma. Plexiform neurofibroma can arise in the upper mediastinum and neck and encroach upon the trachea, causing respiratory symptoms.[99] They are histologically benign but troublesome to remove because they infiltrate locally and frequently involve nerve trunks that cannot be removed, such as the brachial plexus. Pheochromocytoma, as shown in Figure 6-66, is seen in the thorax often enough that careful screening films of the chest are mandatory in any patient with pheochromocytoma in other locations. They can be multiple.

Other types of mediastinal tumors in children include thymoma, lymphoma, teratoma, hygroma, hemangioma, lymphangioma, and lipoma.[50,64,89,91,127] About 50% of these mediastinal masses prove malignant. All should be explored unless the physician has strong reason to suspect lymphoma, which is not best treated by surgical procedure. Figures 6-9 through 6-12 illustrate four large mediastinal tumors, all in conjunction with respiratory symptoms. It should be emphasized that *size and operability are not necessarily related.* Sometimes a mass can fill a hemithorax but prove to be resectable. Two examples are shown in Figures 6-11 and 6-12.

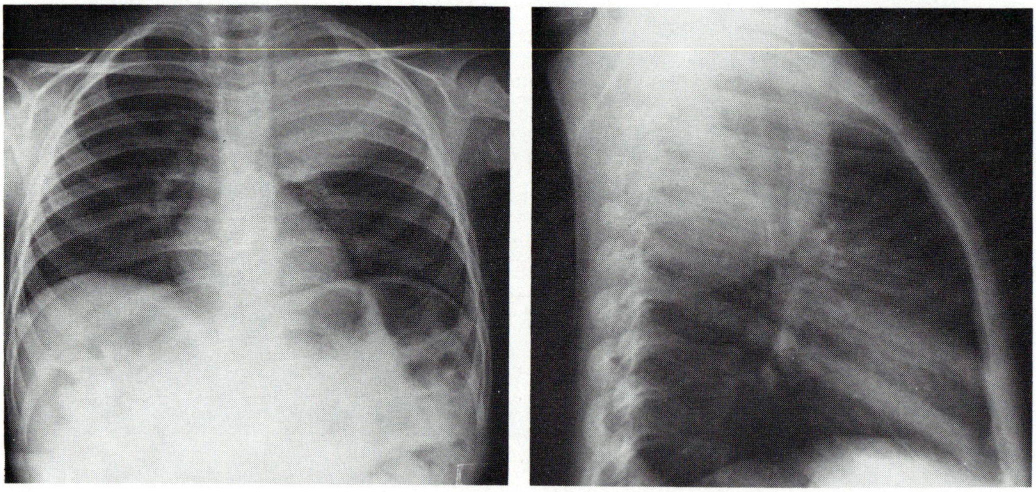

FIG. 6-7. Thoracic neuroblastoma in a 3-year-old girl. This roentgenogram was taken during an upper respiratory infection, and the mass was noted. Compression erosion involved two ribs. The tumor was resectable, and the patient is well 10 years postoperatively.

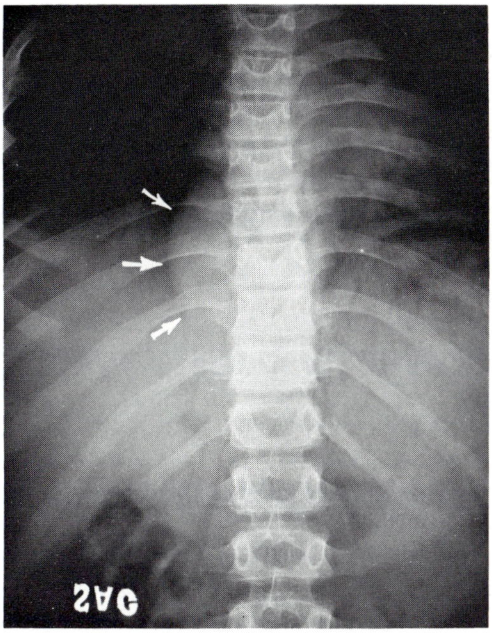

FIG. 6-8. Paraspinal ganglioneuroma arising from the right thoracic sympathetic chain. Frequently pseudopods extend from these neural tumors into the spinal foramina, which can cause cord compression and require laminectomy to remove an intraspinal extension. Paraplegia can be the initial clinical symptom.

Both were huge tumors originating in the thymus, but they were well encapsulated and not invasive. If metastatic survey is negative, one cannot assume a mass is inoperable except by surgical exploration. This statement is underscored poignantly by Figure 6-10, which shows the roentgenogram of a youngster who died with a tumor that might have been removed.

In children with very rapid onset of symptoms, whose roentgen examination is strongly suggestive of lymphoma (see Fig. 6-9), we use a brief course of treatment by steroids and radiation therapy. A prompt response confirms the diagnosis of lymphoma, while simultaneously alleviating the respiratory distress. We consider this therapy safer than insisting on having a tissue diagnosis first. We have seen two such patients asphyxiate during a simple biopsy procedure. Therefore, in a patient with airway compression by suspected lymphoma we begin treatment, await a response, and then secure histologic confirmation.

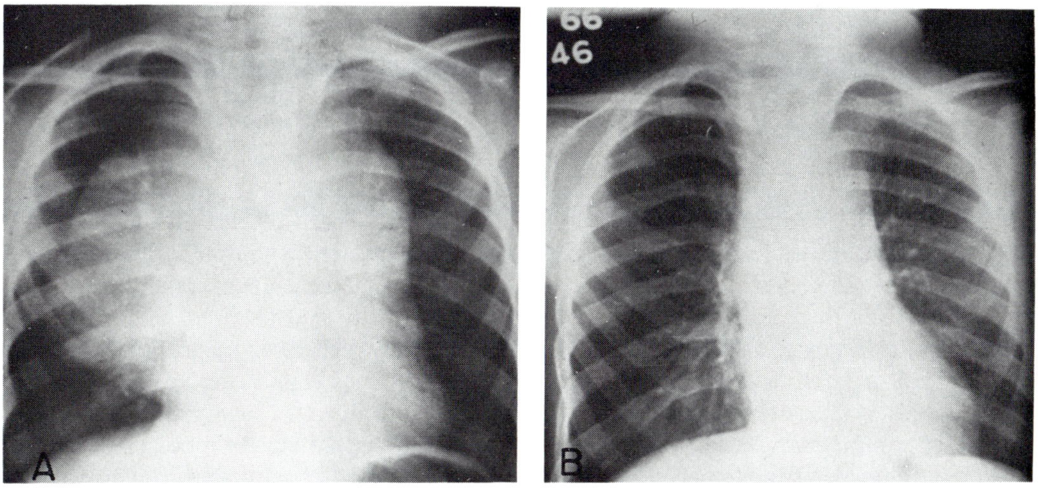

FIG. 6-9. Mediastinal lymphoma. This child entered with acute respiratory distress and the superior mediastinal syndrome, which included distended neck veins, facial suffusion, and a bull neck. A prominent venous pattern covered the anterior chest wall. After the presumptive diagnosis of lymphoma, treatment was begun immediately with Prednisone and radiotherapy, followed by prompt relief of symptoms.

A, Thoracic roentgenogram on admission.

B, Repeat film 3 days after admission. This youngster had a remission for several months, but succumbed eventually with acute leukemia.

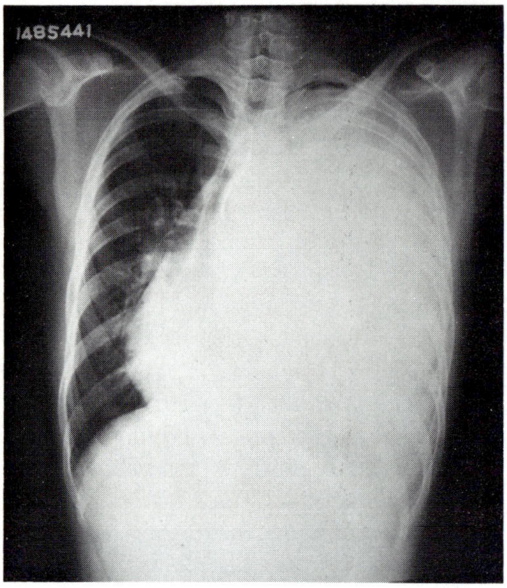

FIG. 6-10. Large mediastinal tumor filling left chest. Unfortunately a needle biopsy was performed on this mass; the report was malignant tumor. Surgical consultation was not requested. At postmortem examination the mass was found to be a very large, but encapsulated and noninfiltrating tumor, which could probably have been removed if exploration had been performed. *Unless disseminated disease indicates incurability, most large masses deserve exploration to determine resectability.* It is not possible to make this judgment by radiographic evaluation alone.

Aortic Arch Anomalies

Vascular malformations that compress the trachea are among the most interesting surgically correctable causes for respiratory distress in infants and children. During embryonic development there are six pairs of aortic arches, corresponding to the branchial clefts. The third pair forms the carotid arteries. The fourth becomes the aortic arch. The sixth produces the pulmonary artery and ductus. Later, the right side of the fourth arch disappears, thus forming the normal course of aorta arching to the left and descending to the left of the spine. If the left fourth arch disappears and the right persists, the individual has a right aortic arch. This anomaly is common. If both arches persist, they form a double arch or vascular ring encircling trachea and esophagus. Since Gross first described the operative correction of this problem in an infant,[43] excellent accounts of large series have been reported.[32,37,44,76] Although many anatomic variations exist,[123] the most important and common types are shown in Figures 6-13 through 6-18. Some of the anomalies may not cause symptoms. In others there can be very tight compression of the airway, with severe symptoms starting at birth. Most impressive are those patients whose trachea and esophagus are completely encircled by a true ring, producing respiratory obstruction, often aggravated during feeding. Sometimes symptoms are intermittent. Others have a history of "noisy breathing" but no actual distress until they develop an upper respiratory infection. These infants commonly lie in a hyperextended position, which stretches the trachea taut, thereby reducing the constricting effect of a compressing vessel. Flexing the head forward in one of these infants can shut off the airway totally.

The diagnosis of a vascular compressive anomaly is often suggested by appropriate plain films of the chest, with views to show the trachea air column (see Fig. 6-65). The addition of a barium swallow, showing esophageal indentation, is of further help. When the barium swallow is normal, and plain films of the trachea are inconclusive, endoscopy should be performed, looking for tracheal indentation just above the level of the carina. Tracheogram can prove helpful but is usually not necessary. That examination can be performed by passing a soft plastic catheter through the larynx, without anesthesia, introducing a small amount of contrast medium, and obtaining appropriate films.

The sine qua non of surgical correction in all of these anomalies begins with accurate and complete identification of the vascular anatomy in the mediastinum before dividing any structures. We prefer a left thoracotomy, through the third or fourth intercostal space.

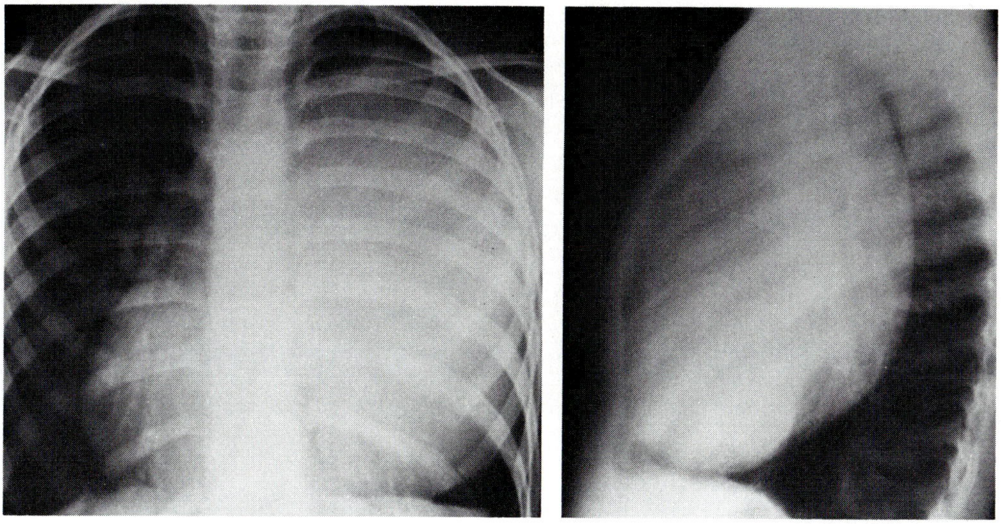

FIG. 6-11. Large mediastinal tumor in 6-year-old boy discovered when x-ray examination was performed for a persisting cough. It was well encapsulated and easily removable through a left thoracotomy, and proved to be thymolipoma.

Most of the thymus is removed to permit exposure of the aortic arch and its branches. Subtotal thymectomy after birth has resulted in no clinically evident problems. The most common of the ring anomalies is shown in Figure 6-13; the *large arch lies posteriorly,* and the smaller is in front. The ring is divided at an appropriate point, usually between the left carotid and left subclavian artery. Division of the ligamentum arteriosum may further open the constricting ring. It is important to dissect the segment of trachea and esophagus previously constricted to make certain that they are liberated thoroughly. Hasty decision and inadequate dissection can be catastrophic. We treated an infant in serious distress 5 days after "correction" elsewhere. The ligamentum arteriosum had been divided, but a true double arch anomaly had not been appreciated because a thorough dissection had not been performed. The ring was divided, with relief of tracheal compression.

Figure 6-14 shows that type of double arch in which the *smaller limb lies in back;* it lies deep in the mediastinum and is frequently very short. It can slip away when divided, resulting in fatal hemorrhage. It is best to ligate the far end of this vessel securely, leaving an ample cuff of vessel beyond the ligature before surgically dividing it. A clamp is used to control the end of the vessel nearer the operator, oversewing it flush with the descending aorta rather than relying on a ligature.

Right aortic arch (see Fig. 6-15) is a common variant. In association with a left ligamentum arteriosum, or patent ductus arteriosus, it can entrap the trachea and esophagus causing the same clinical picture as seen with double arch.

Anomalous innominate artery is one of the most difficult of the compressive anomalies to diagnose with certainty.[34] As shown in Figure 6-16, the trachea is compressed by impingement in a crotch formed by the innominate and left common carotid artery. Several variations are possible; for example, the innominate can be displaced far to the left and actually cross the tracheal wall. Conversely the left carotid can originate more proximally on the arch than normal and can be the principal cause for compression. The thymus

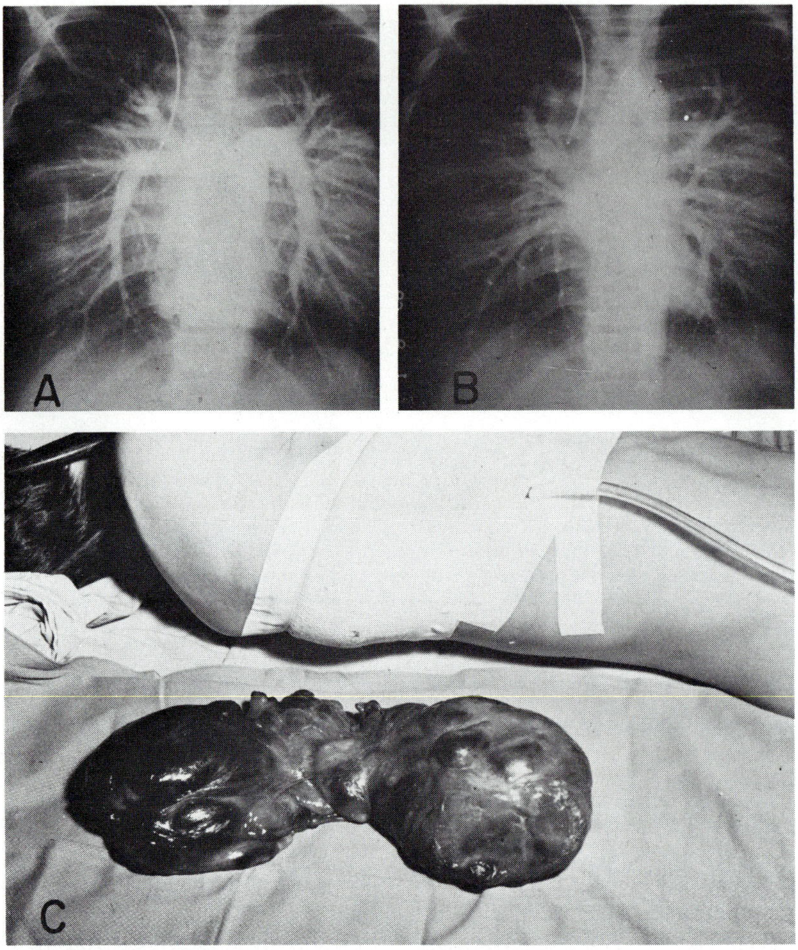

FIG. 6-12. Mediastinal tumor in a 13-year-old boy who complained of shortness of breath. Plain film of the chest showed a huge, saddlebag-shaped mass surrounding the heart.

A, and *B*, Cardiac angiograms showing the right heart and pulmonary arteries (A) and the left heart and aorta (B) to be separate from the very large overlying mass.

C, The operative specimen, which proved completely resectable using a bilateral thoracotomy approach with transection of the sternum. This mass was a cystic thymoma; the patient is well now, 6 years later.

often appears to be slightly enlarged, and may contribute to the problem by "crowding" the superior mediastinum.

The barium swallow is completely normal in these infants, in contrast to the true vascular ring anomalies. The plain film of the chest may be inconclusive. Tracheography can prove of definite value (see Chapter 19 for additional discussion). Bronchoscopy should be performed looking for a pulsating vessel that indents the anterior wall of the trachea. *It is best to be prepared for thoracotomy straightway* because the examination can aggravate the infant's respiratory distress if something therapeutic is not done also. Through a left thoracotomy, the thymus is subtotally removed. A few sutures are placed in the adventitia of the vessels, suspending them forward to the sternum (see Fig. 6-16). This procedure can give dramatic results in some infants even when tracheal compression appears equivocal preoperatively.

Aberrant subclavian artery (see Fig. 6-17) is a common malformation, which occurs in about 1% of subjects at postmortem examination; it causes no symptoms in most. It was described as an entity almost two centuries ago.[5] The right subclavian originates in an anomalous position, far to the left on the aortic arch, beyond the origin of the left subclavian artery. Often a pseudodiverticulum of the aorta is present at its origin. The artery sweeps posteriorly, traversing the mediastinum behind the esophagus, in most instances, and emerging at the right thoracic inlet to go to the arm. In an occasional case it causes enough esophageal compression to partially occlude the lumen, causing difficulty with swallowing, particularly a solid bolus. Barium swallow in the anteroposterior projection shows an oblique indentation of the barium column. The clinical state is usually that of difficulty in swallowing, often with regurgitation and aspiration when the upper

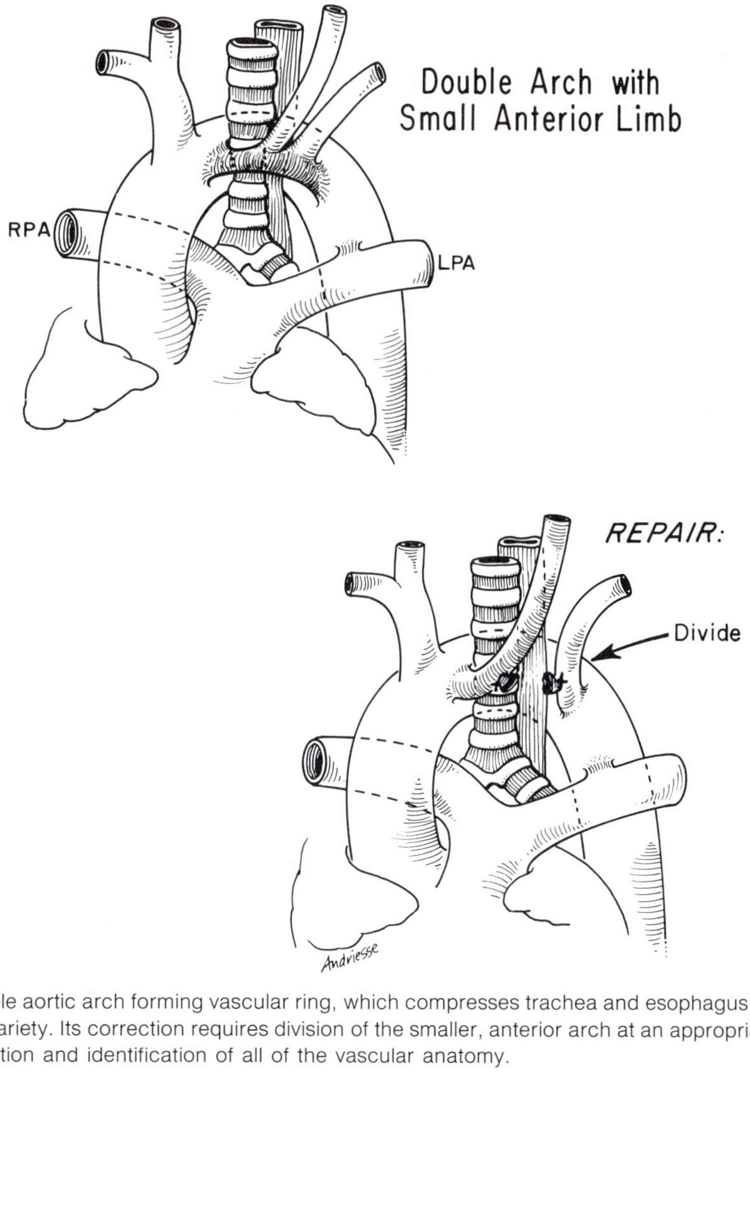

FIG. 6-13. Double aortic arch forming vascular ring, which compresses trachea and esophagus. This ring is the most common variety. Its correction requires division of the smaller, anterior arch at an appropriate point after a thorough dissection and identification of all of the vascular anatomy.

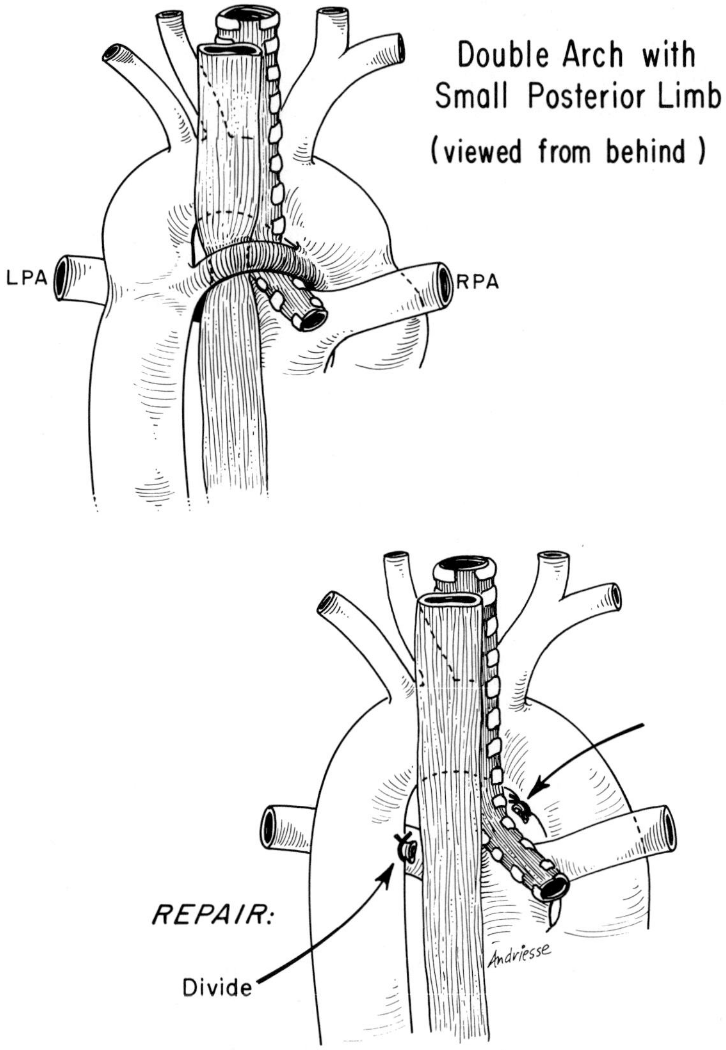

FIG. 6-14. Vascular ring formed by double aortic arch, with the smaller component lying behind the esophagus. The smaller arch is usually short; accurate ligation and positive control of the proximal end are imperative before dividing the short arch, lest it slip into the depths of the wound when it is cut.

esophagus fills and spills over into the trachea. This picture is similar to that in patients with esophageal stricture or diverticulum of the esophagus. Diagnosis by barium swallow examination is usually easy. Esophagoscopy shows narrowing of the lumen by a pulsating vessel. Surgical correction, when indicated, is performed through a left thoracotomy. The artery is divided; its distal end is allowed to retract into the mediastinum. There is no difficulty with blood supply to the right arm when the subclavian is divided at this proximal point; collateral circulation at the shoulder suffices.

Anomalous left pulmonary artery, shown in Figure 6-18, is a rare but interesting cause of vascular compression of the trachea. The vessel may cross anterior to the trachea, but also can be located between the trachea and esophagus. In two of three cases right upper lobe collapse occurred due to compression of the bronchus.[76] Angiography can be helpful in making the diagnosis. Surgical correction is accomplished by moving the origin of the left pulmonary artery to an appropriate location and dividing the ligamentum arteriosum. Anesthetic management in all of these anomalies must allow for the constriction in the lower trachea. The endotracheal tube must pass beyond this to maintain effective ventilation.

Postoperatively residual symptoms may be

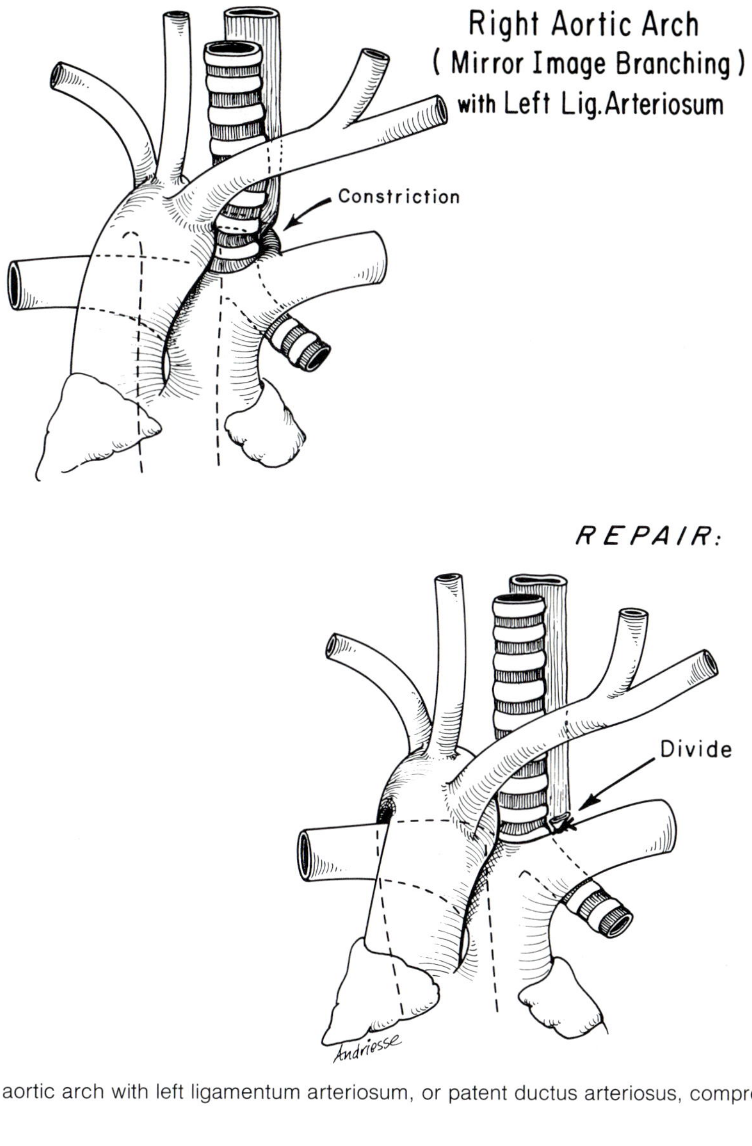

FIG. 6-15. Right aortic arch with left ligamentum arteriosum, or patent ductus arteriosus, compressing trachea and esophagus.

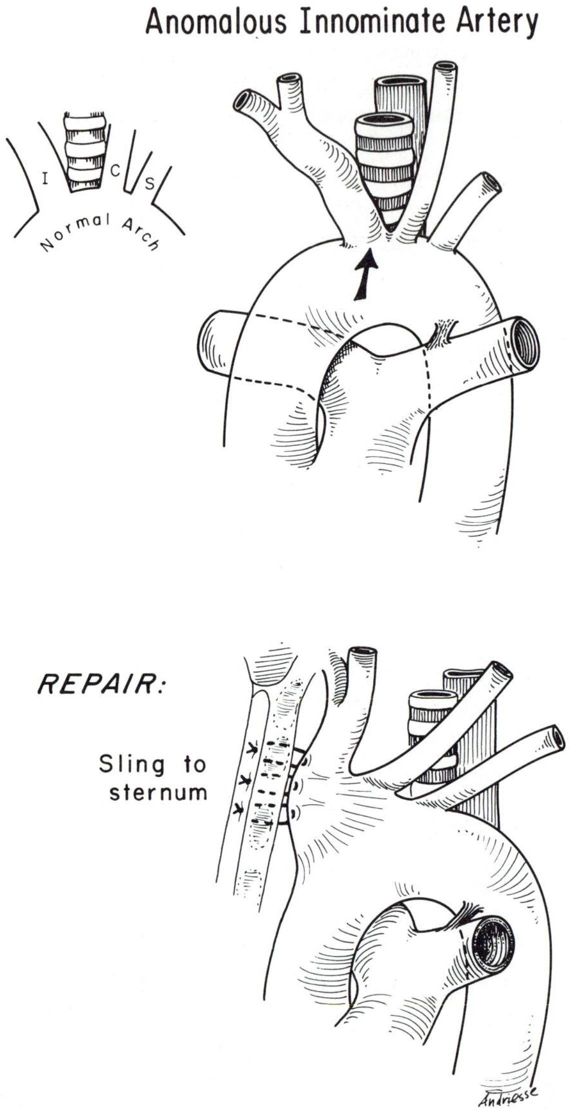

FIG. 6-16. Anomalous innominate artery. The origin of the innominate artery is closer than usual to the left common carotid, so that the trachea is caught in the crotch between these vessels. This problem can be accentuated by a large thymus gland in the neonate. This most common type of vascular compression of the trachea is also the most difficult to diagnose.

present for a time despite relief of obstruction, due to deformity of that segment of trachea previously compressed. Respiratory assistance postoperatively for several days is often needed. Oral feedings should not be attempted in these infants until they are free from respiratory distress.

Foreign Bodies

Inhaled foreign body is a commonly misdiagnosed problem. With a history of sudden onset of coughing, foreign body should be suspected even if the physical examination is negative and the chest film, including fluoroscopy, is normal. If the proper facilities are available, bronchoscopy should be performed. In trained hands it does not carry risk, and it can avert the serious complications of a retained foreign body.

Only with a high index of suspicion can occult foreign bodies be suspected. The following brief accounts serve to illustrate this situation.

(1) A 4-month-old baby with a bizarre respiratory picture was seen, but foreign body was not suspected in so young a child. Later, bronchoscopy disclosed an inhaled popcorn kernel given to him by an older sibling.

(2) A child was seen whose mother insisted he had swallowed a large wooden bead, such as the type strung on the side of a playpen. Initially trouble swallowing was noted by the

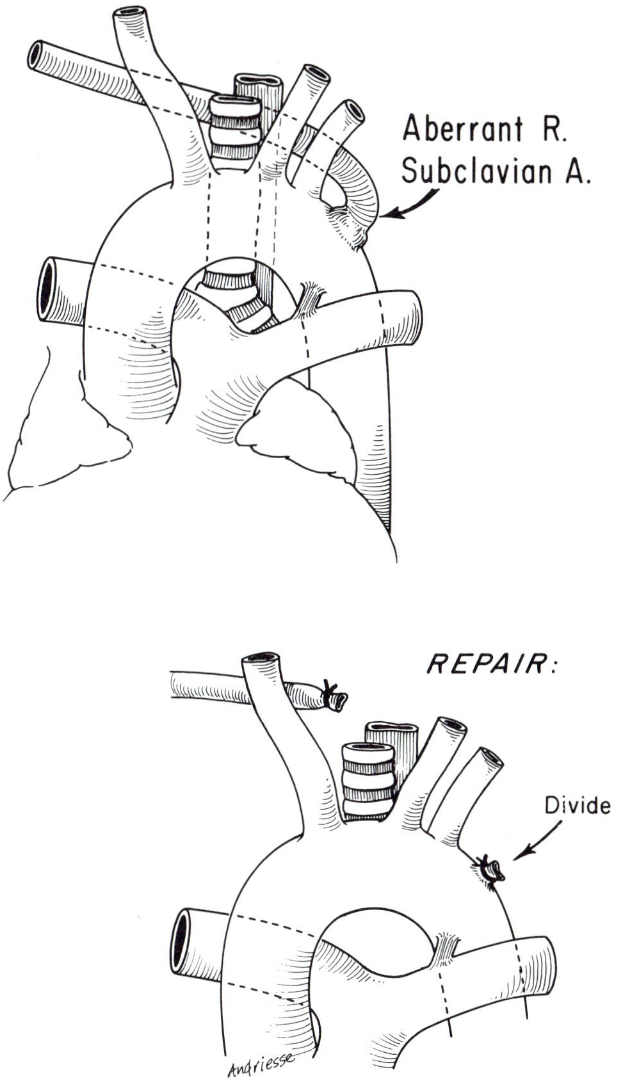

FIG. 6-17. Aberrant right subclavian artery originating distal to the origin of the left subclavian, and crossing through the mediastinum posterior to the esophagus.

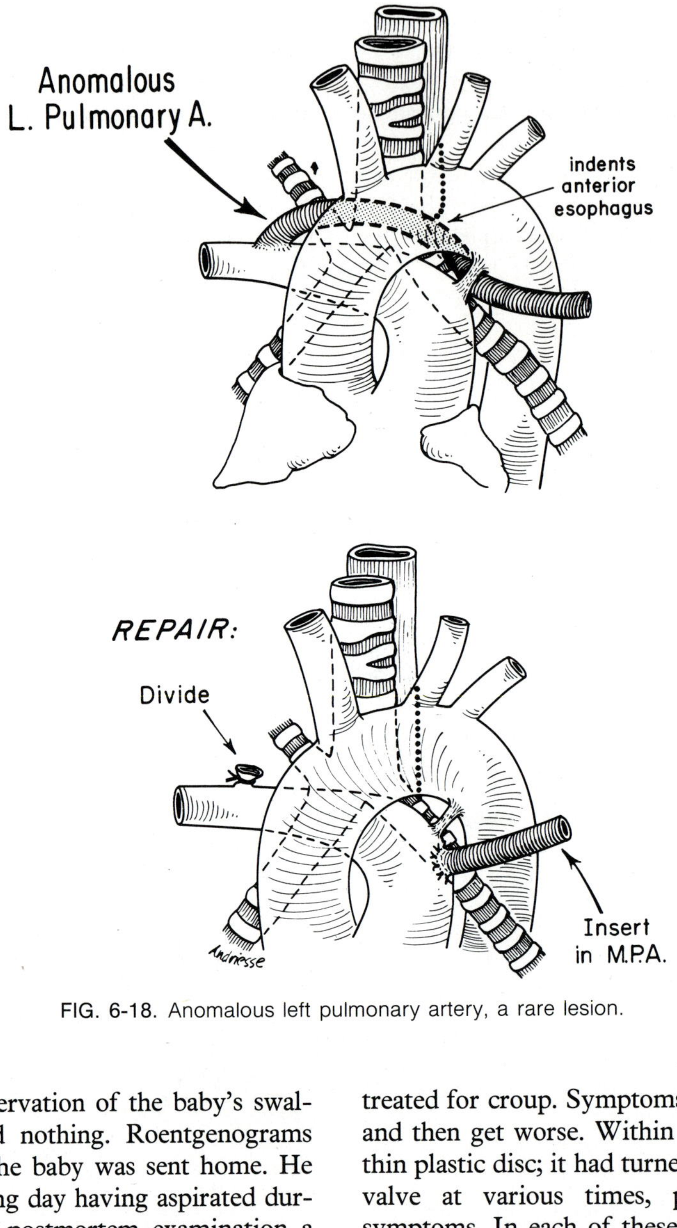

FIG. 6-18. Anomalous left pulmonary artery, a rare lesion.

mother, but observation of the baby's swallowing disclosed nothing. Roentgenograms were negative; the baby was sent home. He died the following day having aspirated during feeding. At postmortem examination a large wooden bead was found in the cervical esophagus. Evidently for a time the lumen of the bead had been properly aligned to permit feeding, but turned subsequently to occlude the esophagus.

(3) An infant with intermittent respiratory distress was not laryngoscoped until 4 weeks after admission to the hospital, where he was treated for croup. Symptoms would improve and then get worse. Within the larynx lay a thin plastic disc; it had turned like a butterfly valve at various times, producing these symptoms. In each of these three cases foreign body had not been suspected strongly enough. Weston reported a high incidence of fatalities with airway foreign bodies in children.[136] Great morbidity occurs when they are not recognized.[26,122]

Figure 6-19 shows the chest roentgenogram of a child with a foreign body lodged in the left main stem bronchus, causing hyper-

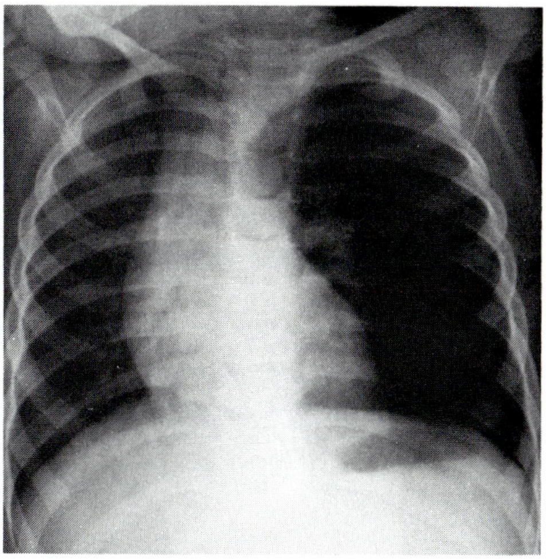

FIG. 6-19. Foreign body in left main stem bronchus of a toddler. Air trapping appears in the left lung, with mediastinal shift to the right.

inflation of that lung and slight shift of the mediastinum toward the right. When such an obvious picture is present, diagnosis offers little problem. *In its absence, however, suspicion should be no less keen.* Fluoroscopy can show subtle degrees of air trapping in different phases of inspiration and expiration, not evident by a plain film of the chest. Little reliance should be placed on a negative fluoroscopy report.

Many of the foreign bodies are not opaque, such as peanuts, pieces of vegetable, plastic objects, and wood. They must be searched for endoscopically using endoscopic equipment suitable for infants and children. Further, a complete set of foreign body instruments should be available. To remove a piece of soft, crumbly peanut intact requires a particularly gentle foreign body forceps which grasps without crushing. The Fogarty arterial embolectomy balloon catheter is of great help in extracting some foreign bodies. It can be passed through even small bronchoscopes without occluding the view; when the tip is beyond the object, the balloon is inflated and the catheter withdrawn to remove the foreign body. If a child has aspirated a plastic cone-shaped object, such as the screw cap for a tube of toothpaste, its removal requires a very special forceps that will insert into the open end of the cone and expand, gripping it from the inside. Being prepared with special forceps for special foreign bodies can prevent needless thoracotomies for transbronchial extraction of these objects.

Figure 6-20 shows the chest film of a youngster whose history was consistent with aspirating a peanut. Bronchoscopy was not performed because the initial chest film was negative. Pneumonia occurred; this condition improved temporarily on antibiotic therapy, but recurred with total consolidation of the right lower lobe. Bronchoscopy at this point was unavailing. The peanut was lodged firmly, beyond view, in a bronchus filled with pus and granulation tissue. Lobectomy was required. The destroyed lower lobe is shown in Figure 6-21. Another foreign body not uncommon in childhood is an aspirated timothy grass head (Fig. 6-22).

Swallowed foreign bodies in the esophagus

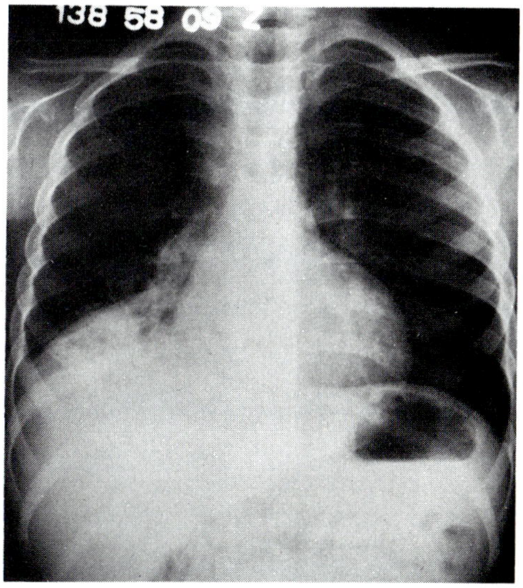

FIG. 6-20. Destroyed right lower lobe caused by a neglected foreign body (peanut). Despite a positive history consistent with aspiration of a peanut, bronchoscopy was not requested. The result, 2 months later, was thoracotomy with pulmonary resection.

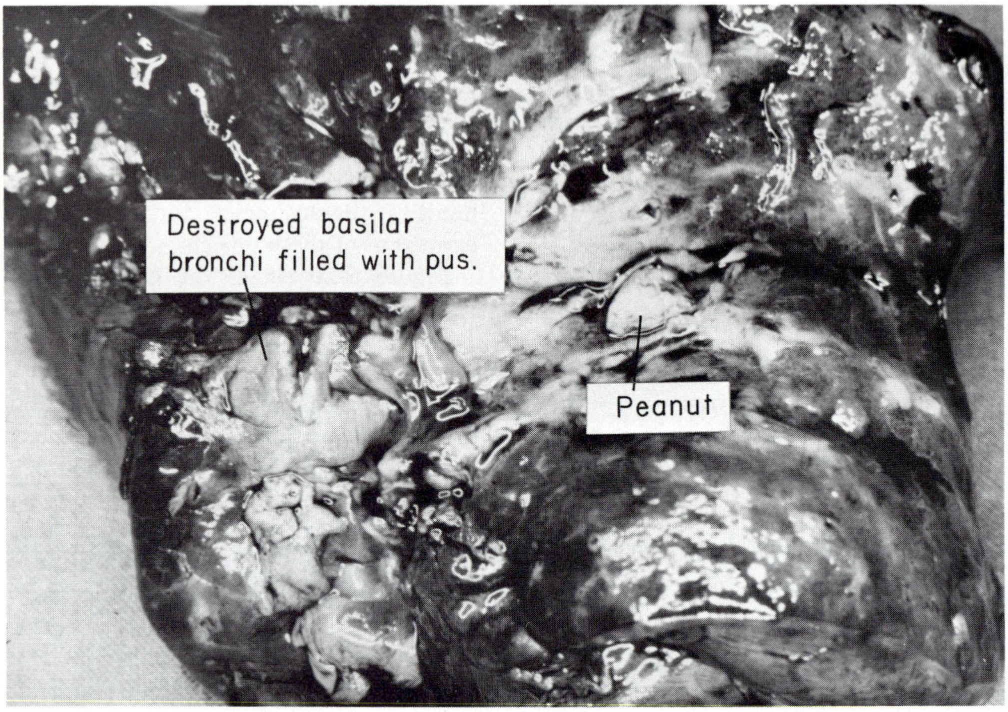

FIG. 6-21. Destroyed right lower lobe in another child with a story and roentgenogram similar to those shown in Fig. 6-20. The peanut, a piece of which is visible, was wedged in the lower lobe bronchus, causing massive sepsis in the lobe and its destruction.

can also cause respiratory symptoms.[40] They usually lodge just below the level of the cricopharyngeus, behind the larynx, or at the level of the cervical trachea. Some, such as a coin, can be retrieved by passing a Foley catheter beyond the foreign body, inflating the balloon with contrast medium, and extracting balloon and coin together during fluoroscopy with the child in prone position. Burrington has reported considerable success in removal of airway foreign bodies by vigorous physiotherapy.[14] Unquestionably the most important single point in avoiding death or serious morbidity from foreign bodies is not in the method used for retrieving them, but for the clinician to have a high index of suspicion and to be willing to recommend endoscopic examination without apology if it proves negative.

Diaphragmatic Hernia

Congenital hernia of the diaphragm occurs about once in every 2500 births. It can be one of the most urgent causes for respiratory distress in the newborn. In the most common type a free communication exists between the peritoneal and pleural cavities without a sac; the defect is located posteriorly in the diaphragm. In addition, the primitive pleuroperitoneal canal normally present in the early embryo persists. The other common variety is anatomically slightly different. The central tendon of the diaphragm shows marked thinning. These patients have a thin sac, which is pleura on its upper surface and peritoneum on its lower surface. Physiologically both defects can cause great respiratory distress, permitting herniation of abdominal contents

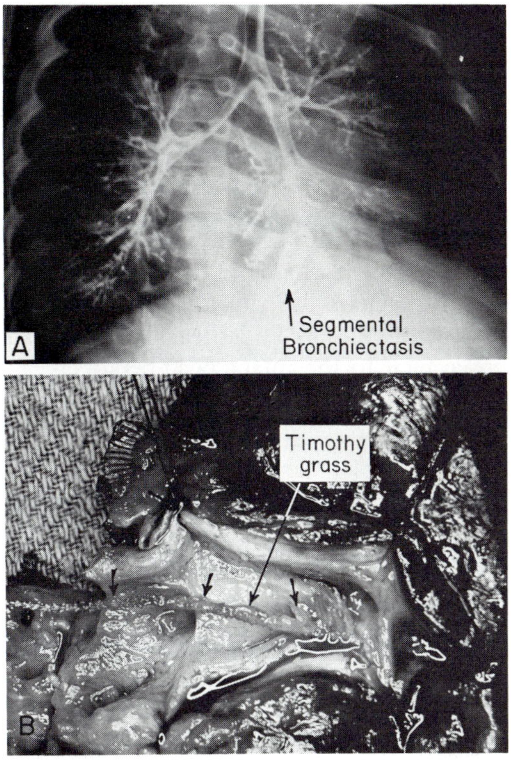

FIG. 6-22. Timothy grass (foreign body) in basal segment of right lower lobe.

A, Bronchogram; *B*, Specimen showing blade of grass impacted in bronchus. Note arrowhead-like barbs, which cause distal migration of this special foreign body and prevent its expulsion by coughing.

into the chest. Eighty percent occur on the left side (Fig. 6-23), presumably because the liver, on the right side, helps partition the chest from the peritoneal cavity. About one in five cases occurs on the right side (Fig. 6-24); very rarely they are bilateral. In a typical case on the left side the viscera that herniate into the chest include spleen, stomach, left lobe of the liver, and most of the intestine. Often malrotation occurs.

A plain film of the chest should be obtained immediately in any infant with respiratory distress; the diagnosis of diaphragmatic hernia is usually obvious. The infant should be transferred immediately to a center where surgical correction can be performed. *Respiratory support of the baby en route* can be life saving. A nasogastric tube can help decompress the stomach and prevents further swallowing of air and increasing intestinal distention. Positioning with the affected side down can, by gravity, prevent further shift of the mediastinum toward the good side. *It is important not to disturb the baby* by sticking him with a needle for blood samples or using other procedures that can cause crying and further distress. Oxygen is mandatory. The infant must be kept warm. A qualified person should accompany the infant, ready to pass an endotracheal tube for gentle positive pressure ventilation if needed.

Although the diagnosis is being made earlier these days, the survival statistics have not improved much. Mortality remains relatively high in those who are symptomatic in the first 24 hours of life, obviously the worst affected

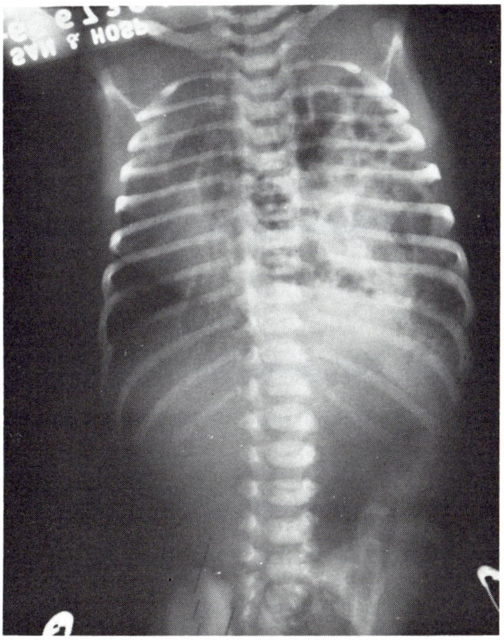

FIG. 6-23. Left diaphragmatic hernia in newborn with respiratory distress. Note intestine herniated into the left chest through Bochdalek defect, with shift of the mediastinum to the right and moderate compression of the right side. The left side is involved in about 80% of cases.

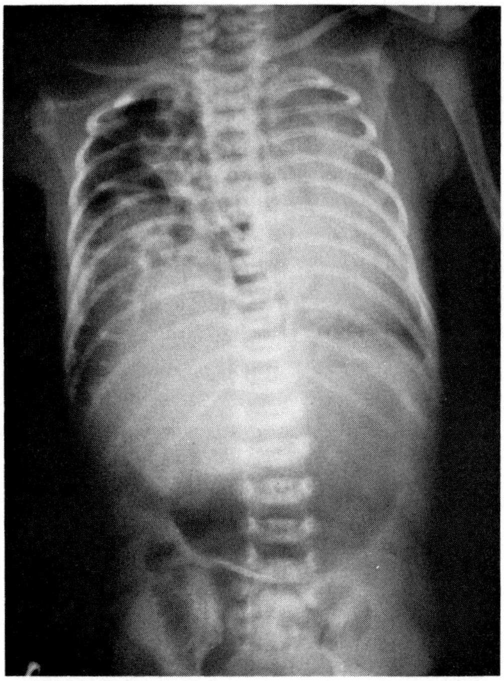

FIG. 6-24. Right-sided diaphragmatic hernia with severe respiratory distress caused by massive shift of the mediastinum toward the left, almost totally compressing the opposite lung also. This infant had corrective surgery and survived.

babies.[83] Those whose distress occurs after age 2 days usually do well. Rarely, a child attains several months or even years of age before onset of symptoms from a congenital diaphragmatic hernia. Figure 6-25 is a roentgenogram from a 3-year-old girl who came to the clinic with intestinal obstruction, heralded by green vomitus, caused by loops of bowel kinked within a previously unsuspected diaphragmatic hernia. The smooth dome over the herniated bowel suggested that it was a congenital eventration with a sac, rather than a posterolateral defect.

Strangulation of bowel within the chest has been reported, but is rare.[107] A transthoracic approach has been advocated by some,[66] but most surgeons prefer a transabdominal approach. Upon opening the belly, one can gently extract the herniated viscera and then repair the defect from below, averting a struggle with distended loops of bowel. Another advantage of the transabdominal approach is the possibility of performing a decompressive gastrostomy; the bowel can be deflated by milking its gas and fluid up to the gastrostomy tube, which facilitates closure. Malrotation can be repaired if duodenal obstruction is present. The belly may be too small to contain the gut. Rather than struggling with a closure under tension, which can prove fatal to the infant postoperatively, in

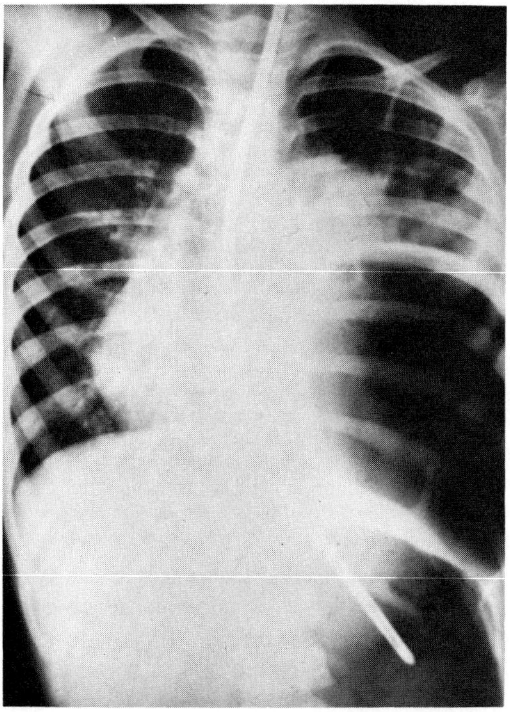

FIG. 6-25. Diaphragmatic hernia in an older child who was first seen for vomiting at age 3 years when she developed intestinal obstruction from loops of gut caught in the defect. These cases are rare beyond the neonatal period, when most are symptomatic. The rounded smooth contour over the herniated intestine suggested the presence of a peritoneal sac, which indicated that the defect was an eventration, or thinning, of the central tendon of the diaphragm. The more common defect of a posterolateral foramen of Bochdalek hernia has no sac; instead a free communication exists between the peritoneal cavity and the pleural space.

some it is best to close only the skin, leaving a generous hernia defect in the abdominal wall.[85] Several days later a definitive repair of the abdominal wall can be done. Alternatively, a temporary prosthetic pouch has been used to cover the abdominal wall defect as another method of avoiding tension.[118] It is then removed in stages several days later. It is important to avoid excessive positive pressure ventilation and in particular to resist the temptation of inflating the atelectatic lobes on the affected side. The pressure required for inflation can cause rupture of the good lung on the other side and possibly fatal tension pneumothorax. A catheter is placed in the pleural cavity, and it is connected to very gentle suction (2 to 3 cm of water). The atelectatic, hypoplastic lung will inflate gradually in the following few days. In critically ill cases we place a pleural catheter prophylactically on the opposite side as well, having seen several instances of fatal pneumothorax with collapse of the contralateral lung.

If no posterior rim of diaphragm exists for joining to the anterior leaf, sutures are placed around the tenth and eleventh rib to facilitate closure of the defect. In the rare instance where not enough diaphragm is present, one can create a flap of muscle from the transversalis layer of the abdominal wall. This layer is anatomically contiguous with the diaphragm. The flap can be used to accomplish closure. Rarely an extralobar pulmonary sequestration is seen in association with congenital diaphragmatic defect[111] (see Fig. 6-35).

Occasionally a small eventration of the diaphragm occurs with minimal or no symptoms; in some it is discovered as an incidental finding. *If clinically indicated,* repair can be accomplished easily through a small, low-placed thoracotomy, reefing up the defect by plication.[126]

Paralysis of the diaphragm in the newborn can result from birth trauma, with stretching of the phrenic nerve in the neck.[11] An associated Erb's palsy is usually present. The respiratory problem is physiologically similar to that in diaphragmatic hernia. In extreme cases, where marked parodoxic motion occurs during inspiration, plication of the diaphragm can prove helpful. Since positive pressure pulmonary ventilation techniques are so reliable nowadays, however, plication should seldom be necessary as an urgent measure in a neonate.

The previously described diaphragmatic hernias constitute the majority of those seen in childhood; rarely one encounters a hernia at the retrosternal foramen of Morgagni. In a series of 134 Morgagni hernias at the Mayo Clinic, only eight were in children.[4] Three of these children had no symptoms. The others had symptoms of gastrointestinal dysfunction or mild respiratory complaints. These defects should be repaired because of the danger of bowel strangulation.

Esophageal Atresia and Tracheoesophageal Fistula

Esophageal atresia is one of the most exciting chapters in the development of pediatric surgery. Just three decades ago all of these infants died. Today the vast majority survive and are normal youngsters. Many refinements in management of this complicated anomaly have occurred since the initial reports of treating these youngsters by staged repair,[73] and soon thereafter by primary repair.[45] The various types of esophageal atresia with and without tracheoesophageal fistula are shown in Figure 6-26.

DIAGNOSIS AND PREOPERATIVE MANAGEMENT

The diagnosis should be suspected in an infant who appears to have excessive mucus; this secretion is in fact saliva that cannot be swallowed. Often parents report a history of the infant choking and turning blue when first fed. Usually abdominal distention occurs in the most common variety, from air being

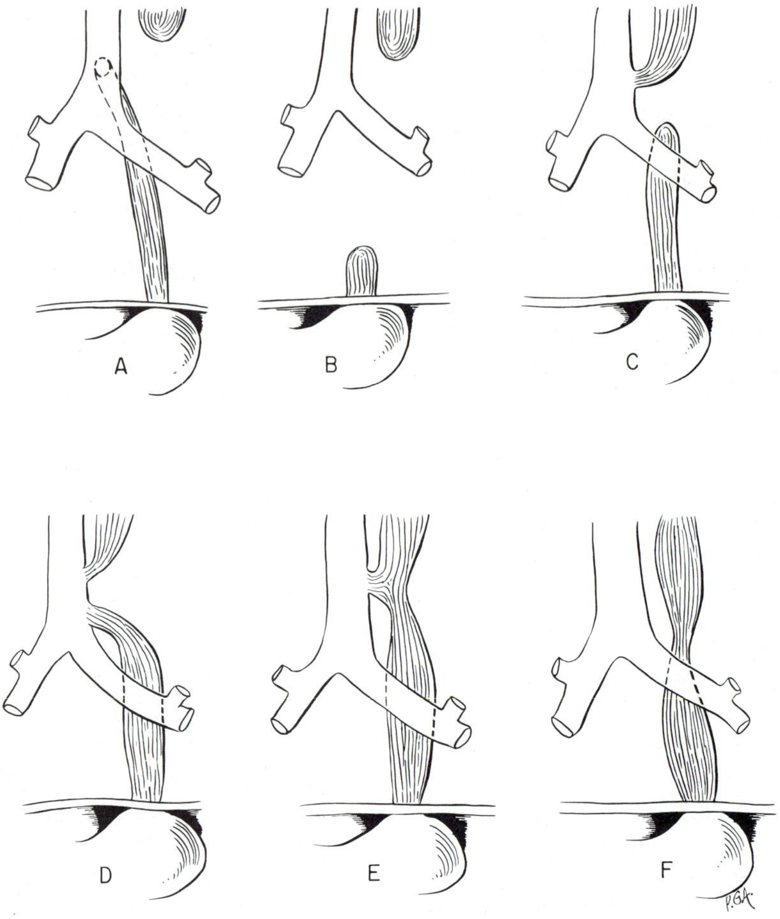

FIG. 6-26. Types of esophageal atresia and tracheoesophageal fistula: *A*, The most common (about 85% of cases); *B*, The second most common (about 8%). The other types, *C* through *F*, are rare.

blown via the tracheoesophageal fistula into the stomach. A normal fetus swallows in utero. In these babies, inability to swallow amniotic fluid upsets the equilibrium of fluid exchange between mother, infant, and amniotic sac. Polyhydramnios results and often causes premature delivery.

To make the diagnosis a No. 8 or 10 French *moderately stiff* catheter should be inserted through the nose to determine whether it will pass to the stomach. In esophageal atresia it meets a point of obstruction about 4 inches from the nostril. If the catheter is too small or too soft, it can curl up in the esophageal pouch, giving an impression of passing to the stomach. Confirmation can be obtained by injecting through the catheter a small amount (1 to 2 ml) of contrast material to outline the blindly ending upper pouch (see also Chapter 19 for details of the radiographic procedure). A typical case is shown in Figure 6-27. The contrast material should then be aspirated from the upper pouch to avoid its spilling over into the trachea, which can cause further pulmonary complications. These infants should never be sent to the radiology department for injection of contrast medium without adequate supervision. Hap-

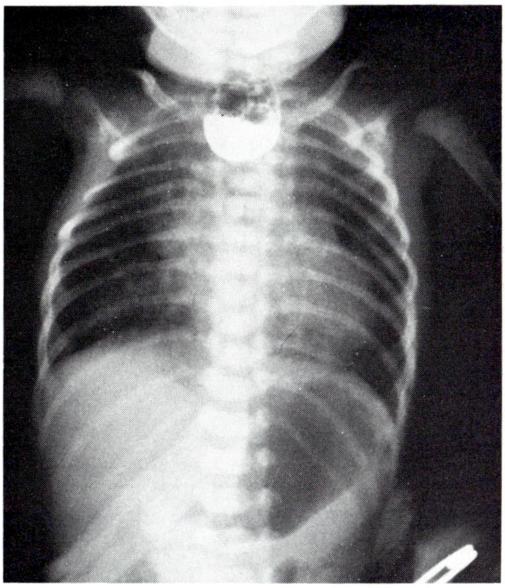

FIG. 6-27. Radiographic method for demonstrating esophageal atresia. A moderately stiff, opaque catheter is introduced through the nose into the upper pouch, and taped in place. A *small amount* of thin contrast medium is introduced through the tube during fluoroscopy, using just enough to produce a meniscus of contrast material at the lower end of the pouch. A spot film is taken to document this, and the radiopaque material is then removed by aspiration.

hazard injection of too much contrast medium without fluoroscopic guidance can overfill the pouch, spilling over into the larynx and causing aspiration (Fig. 6-28). Occasionally the contrast medium spills over into the trachea even when the proximal pouch is not overfilled. This occurrence should lead to suspicion of a fistula from the upper pouch to the trachea. One should obtain a lateral or oblique view when fluoroscoping the blindly ending pouch, to prevent overlooking a proximal fistula. Figure 6-29 is an example of an upper pouch tracheoesophageal fistula.

Absence of intestinal gas in esophageal atresia generally indicates that no tracheoesophageal fistula is present. In these babies the distal esophagus is *usually* rudimentary; these cases must be handled in a special manner, as described later. Figure 6-30 depicts a gasless abdomen and the typical right upper lobe pneumonia so often seen in infants with esophageal atresia.

When the diagnosis of esophageal atresia with tracheoesophageal fistula is not made promptly, these infants usually develop severe pneumonia. One factor is spillover of saliva from the upper esophagus into the trachea. A second is the regurgitation of gastric juice up the distal esophagus into the lungs. (Gastric juice is very high in acid content in the first day or two of life.) A decade or two ago esophageal atresia was considered an emergency, and surgical procedure was undertaken straightway. Analysis of results, however, disclosed many deaths from pulmonary complications. Accordingly if pneumonia is present, most surgeons delay operation until the lungs have improved. As soon

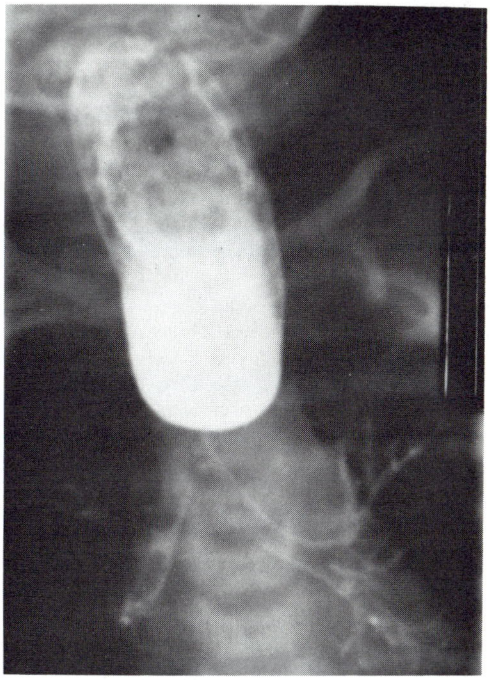

FIG. 6-28. An unsupervised examination in esophageal atresia. The blindly ending upper pouch was overfilled with barium, which spilled into the tracheobronchial tree and caused additional pulmonary distress.

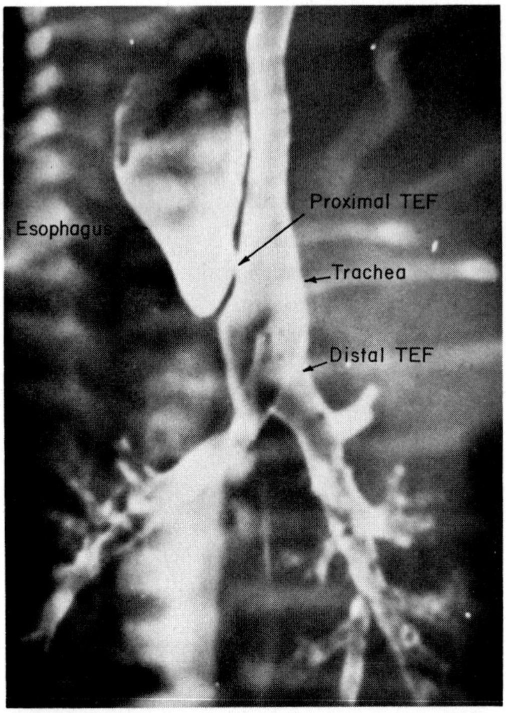

FIG. 6-29. Esophageal atresia with two tracheoesophageal fistulas. Besides the usual fistula between the trachea and the distal esophageal pouch, a more proximal fistula is located between the upper pouch and the back wall of the trachea. A lateral or oblique film when introducing contrast into the upper pouch will help exclude a proximal fistula. Another clue to the presence of a proximal fistula is an abnormally small upper pouch, indicating that it has been decompressed in utero through a fistula. Inflation of the upper pouch by air at thoracotomy, coincident with positive pressure ventilation of the endotracheal tube by the anesthesiologist, is a third diagnostic sign. Repair of esophageal atresia, with failure to identify the presence of a proximal fistula, can be catastrophic.

as the diagnosis of esophageal atresia is made, a suction catheter should be placed in the upper pouch to aspirate the saliva.

A *sump suction catheter* is much more efficient than a simple catheter. It can be made in a few minutes by inserting a small plastic catheter, such as is used for venous cutdown, into a larger catheter, made from a piece of soft, plastic intravenous tubing.[52] Sump catheters are also available commercially. If the infant has considerable pneumonia, a Stamm gastrostomy is performed under local anesthesia; it takes only about 20 to 30 minutes. The gastrostomy tube evacuates air from the tracheoesophageal fistula, decompressing the gut. Even more important it prevents further reflux of gastric juice to the lungs. With a sump suction catheter in place in the upper pouch, and gastrostomy tube in the stomach, pneumonia clears rapidly with appropriate treatment. The infant then becomes a far more fit candidate to undergo thoracotomy for repair of the defect.

SURGICAL MANAGEMENT

Details of surgical management of these children should vary according to the size of the infant and the presence of other anoma-

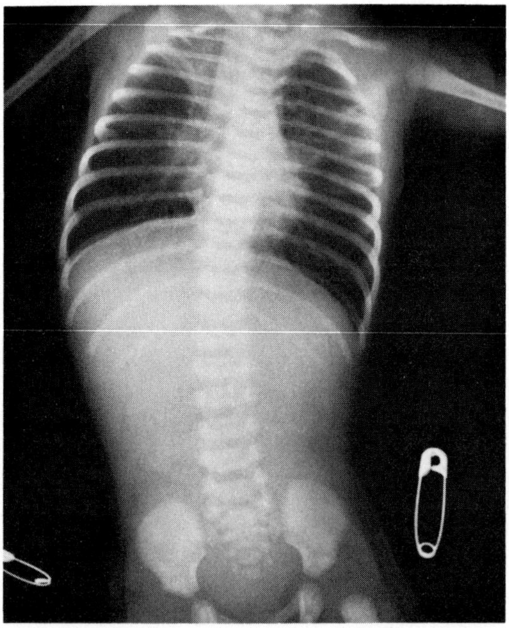

FIG. 6-30. Esophageal atresia without tracheoesophageal fistula. Note the right upper lobe pneumonitis, characteristic in esophageal atresia. Absence of gastrointestinal air denotes probable lack of a communication between the trachea and distal esophagus. This condition in turn signifies that the distal esophagus is usually rudimentary, obviating a primary esophageal repair.

lies. The current salvage rate for uncomplicated cases is in the range of 90%.[56,60] Generally a right thoracotomy is employed, entering through the fourth intercostal space. One can go directly through the pleural space to approach the esophagus, but it is better to do the operation in a *retropleural manner.* This procedure involves spending a few extra minutes separating the delicate pleura from the chest wall, and then retracting it. Its great advantage is that it prevents complete collapse of the lung during operation, so that fewer postoperative respiratory complications appear. Even more important, should an anastomotic leak occur postoperatively, which is not uncommon, it is confined to the extrapleural gutter, rather than becoming a generalized empyema, which can prove fatal.[57]

The upper esophageal pouch is mobilized far up into the neck. The distal esophageal connection with the trachea is divided. Next the two ends are brought together end to end. In certain cases the ends do not reach. In this unhappy circumstance the surgeon should not try the impossible, attempting to join them under undue tension. This attempted joining usually disrupts in about a week, with a possibly fatal outcome. It is better to abandon the goal of primary repair in this circumstance. Instead the tracheoesophageal fistula is divided, closing over the distal esophageal end and bringing the upper esophagus out into the neck as a fistula. The infant can be then maintained on gastrostomy feedings. Later, at 6 to 12 months of age, reconstruction is accomplished using a segment of colon. The colonic segment can be placed beneath the sternum to bridge the gap;[78] this method is the one most often used to bypass inoperable carcinoma in poor risk adults. Alternatively the colon conduit can be placed in the left chest, by the technique of Waterston.[3] We prefer this method in children, although it is a more difficult operative procedure. The postoperative barium swallow in one of these youngsters is shown in Figure 6-31.

Another method consists of making a tube

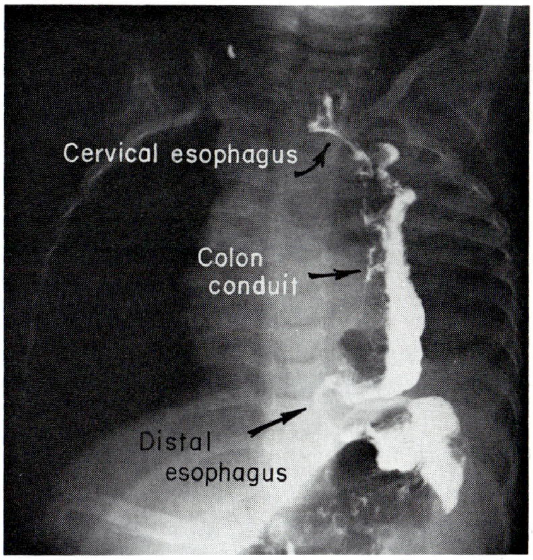

FIG. 6-31. Colon "esophagus." This youngster was born with esophageal atresia without tracheoesophageal fistula, and a primary repair was impossible. The upper esophagus was marsupialized to the neck, and a gastrostomy was inserted for feeding. At 1 year of age the gap between the cervical esophagus and the rudimentary nubbin of the distal esophagus was bridged using a segment of transverse colon placed in the left chest according to the technique of Mr. David Waterston of London.[3]

from the greater curvature of the stomach, rotating it upward to bridge a gap in the esophagus.[13] We have been reluctant to use this procedure because it imposes some risk in losing a part of the stomach, which is of nutritional importance in a growing child. Also peptic esophagitis at the upper anastomotic line may become a problem in later years.

Direct repair of esophageal atresia can carry a high risk in the premature infant, or in the full-term infant with other severe anomalies. The most common associated anomalies are imperforate anus and congenital heart disease. This risk has led to a staged approach in selected cases.[55,70] A sump suction catheter is inserted and gastrostomy is performed; this procedure stops further pulmonary insult. Under local anesthesia in the next day or two a small incision is made in the chest, approaching the tracheoesophageal fistula extrapleurally and dividing it. Simple ligation can result in a recurrent fistula, so it is best to completely divide it. Then gastrostomy feedings can be started without danger of reflux of milk into the tracheobronchial tree. Sump suction can be maintained to the upper pouch for several weeks, with expert nursing care. When the infant becomes a satisfactory size, an attempt can be made to anastomose the upper pouch to the lower pouch previously disconnected from the trachea.

A special approach is required in infants with esophageal atresia in whom no gas is evident in the abdominal film. This lack of gas usually means absence of a tracheoesophageal fistula to the distal pouch. Most of those infants have a rudimentary nubbin in place of the distal esophagus. Occasionally one has a suitable distal esophagus that can be anastomosed to the upper pouch. It is not necessary to perform a thoracotomy to determine this point. Instead gastrostomy is performed, inserting a small Malecot catheter into the stomach, which is usually tiny, since it has not been used in utero. After securing the catheter in the stomach, a few milliliters of contrast material are injected, while gently occluding the pylorus with a noncrushing clamp. This procedure causes the radiopaque material to reflux into whatever esophagus is present, showing whether it is rudimentary or longer. When only a rudimentary distal esophagus is present, which is most often the case, we have chosen the course of marsupializing the upper esophageal pouch through the left neck, avoiding thoracotomy. The infant's swallowed saliva then spills out onto the skin just above the clavicle. Feedings are continued by gastrostomy. A substitute esophagus from colon is made at 6 to 12 months of age.

An alternative method is the intermittent stretching of the upper pouch by bougienage, attempting to elongate it enough to anastomose with the distal esophagus.[138] Some surgeons have used this method successfully; others have not. Rehbein reported slowly pulling the two ends of esophagus together with a traction device.[62] It consists of a metal olive in each pouch, brought together by heavy threads, which emerge through the mouth and the gastrostomy site. Simultaneous electromagnetic stretching of both esophageal ends has proven successful in elongating the esophageal segments to allow delayed primary anastomosis.[105,117]

Swallowing function is not always normal in children who have had successful primary anastomosis for esophageal atresia. Fluroscopic and manometric studies have shown an appreciable incidence of dyskinesia of the distal esophagus. Uncoordinated peristaltic activity and gastroesophageal reflux occur.[19] Some of these youngsters have a sliding hiatus hernia, possibly caused by the mobilization of the distal esophagus required to anastomose the two ends of the esophagus.

Swallowing function in postoperative colonic conduits is not like the vigorous, coordinated propulsive activity of a normal esophagus. The bolus goes down slowly, more by gravity than from peristaltic activity of the colon. In fact, we have not observed much difference when the colon segment was placed in an antiperistaltic manner, as has been done in a few patients for technical reasons. Although some of these children are small and underweight, the majority seem to get along reasonably well.[79,115]

ISOLATED TRACHEOESOPHAGEAL (H-TYPE) FISTULA

Isolated tracheoesophageal fistula is an uncommon anomaly. Its diagnosis depends on the index of suspicion of the physician who treats an infant with recurrent pneumonitis. The fistula is usually located in the neck. It runs in an oblique downward direction from the esophagus to the trachea. A typical example is shown in Figure 6-32. The esophagogram needs to be done carefully and with certain techniques that tend to maximize the ability to make the diagnosis. The correct

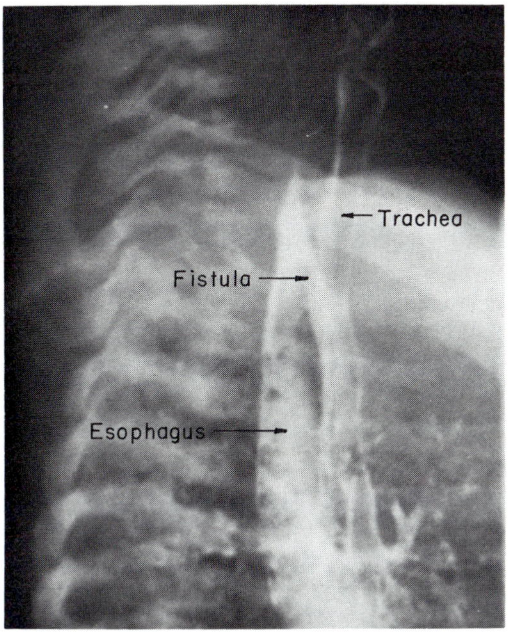

FIG. 6-32. Isolated tracheoesophageal fistula. Note oblique course of connection, typical in these fistulas, which are usually accessible through a neck incision.

manner for visualizing one of these fistulas by roentgenographic means involves first placing a small tube into the cervical esophagus. With the infant in a prone position, a small amount of thin contrast medium is injected, and the surgeon looks carefully for a small communication with the trachea. (A detailed description of radiographic methods is given in Chapter 19.) If these methods fail, endoscopy should be performed (Fig. 6-33).

Under general anesthesia, the back wall of the trachea is then searched with a fore-oblique telescope to visualize the opening in the back wall of the trachea. Should that fail, a tightly fitting endotracheal tube can be passed just through the vocal cords, inflating the trachea intermittently with positive pressure, and an esophagoscope passed into the upper esophagus. An intermittent whistling of air passing from the trachea into the esophagus can be heard distinctly through the esophagoscope, and the odor of anesthetic gas can be detected. Methylene blue can be in-

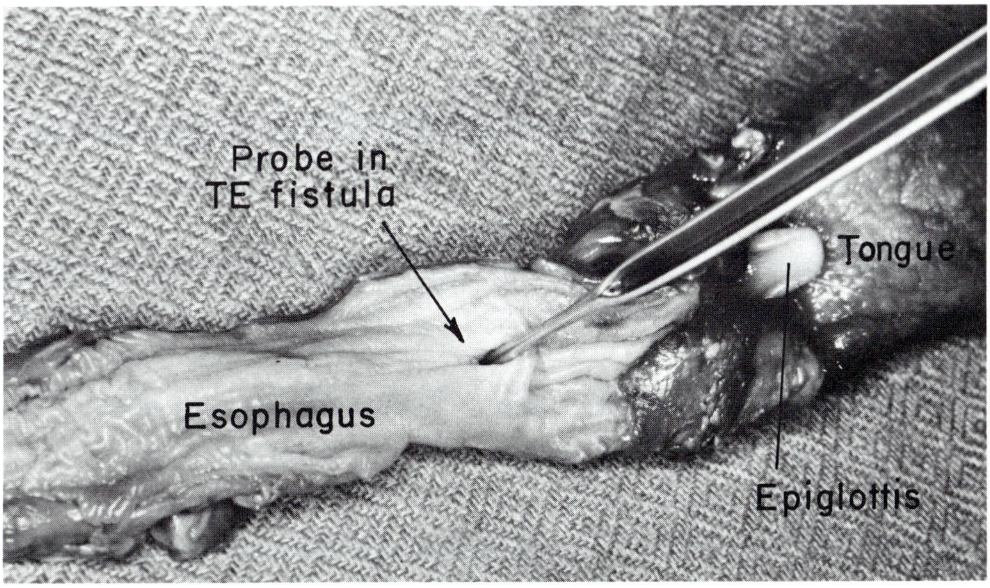

FIG. 6-33. Isolated tracheoesophageal fistula. Autopsy specimen of infant who died with recurrent aspiration pneumonia from isolated H-type tracheoesophageal fistula. This condition was not diagnosed during life because appropriate diagnostic studies were not performed. Only a routine barium swallow in the erect position had been used to exclude this diagnosis.

jected into the endotracheal tube, confirming its appearance on the anterior wall of the esophagus. We prefer to operate on these fistulas through the right neck. During surgical division of these fistulas special care should be taken to avoid injury to the recurrent laryngeal nerve. Passing a Fogarty catheter through the fistula and inflating its balloon makes fistula identification especially easy with minimal dissection.

Lobar Emphysema

Since lobar emphysema is an uncommon cause of respiratory distress in infancy, infants with this disorder are seldom referred with the correct diagnosis, even though the diagnosis is usually evident from the plain film of the chest. As shown in Figure 6-34, respiratory symptoms occur usually in early infancy. Usually one lobe is overinflated, with air trapping, causing compression atelectasis in the adjacent lobe or lobes, and shift of the mediastinum to the other side. The affected lobe can herniate across the anterior mediastinum toward the opposite thorax. Most often involved is the left upper lobe (Fig. 6-35) and next most frequently the right middle lobe. A lower lobe is involved only rarely.[53,74,77] The causes of lobar emphysema are depicted in Figure 6-36. Among those cases of unknown cause, some may have bronchial cartilagenous dysplasia. The surgeon must leave a bronchial stump for surgical closure; it may contain the actual site of pathology, which would not be available for pathologic examination.

The diagnosis of lobar emphysema can

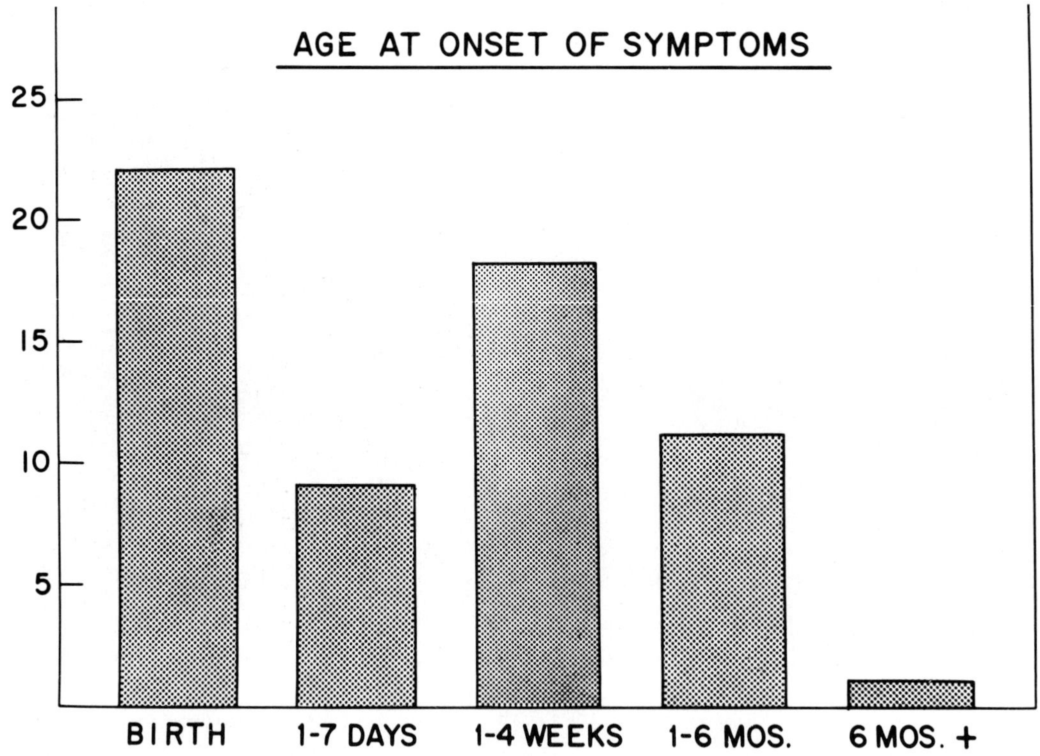

FIG. 6-34. Age of presentation in lobar emphysema.

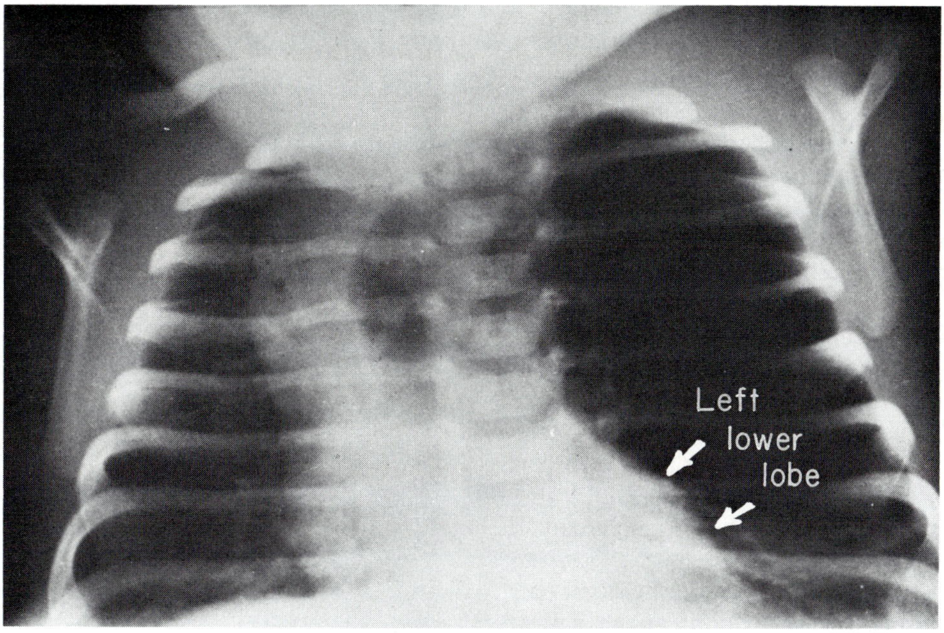

FIG. 6-35. Lobar emphysema, left upper lobe, in 1-day-old infant who had severe respiratory distress. Note herniation of the upper lobe across the midline, marked displacement of the mediastinum to the right, and collapse of the left lower lobe, which is seen as a triangular density behind the heart. This infant also had a large patent ductus arteriosus, which was palpated and ligated at the time of emergency left upper lobectomy. About 10% of these infants have an associated cardiac defect.

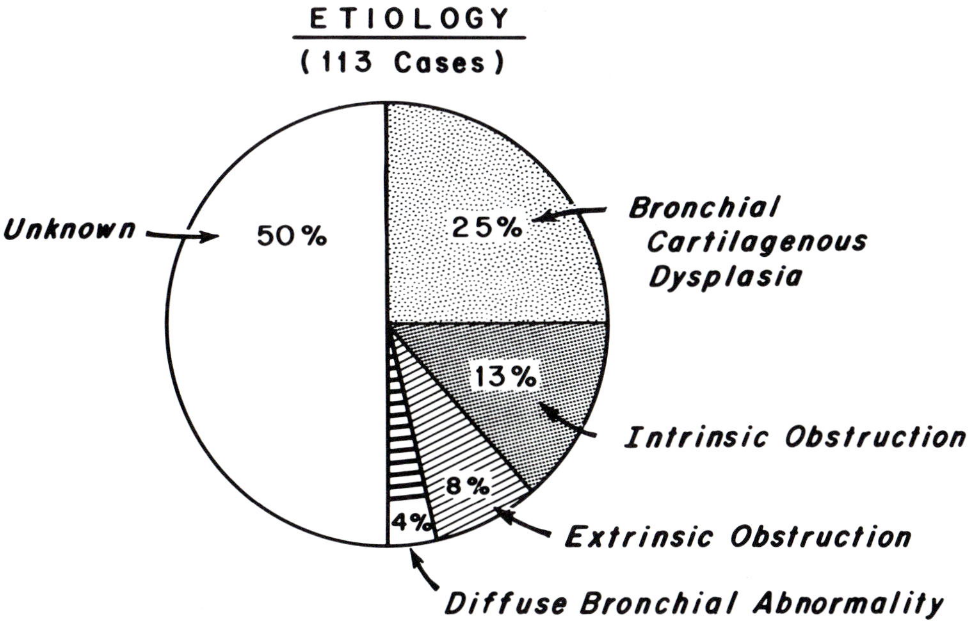

FIG. 6-36. Causes of lobar emphysema.

usually be made by examination of the plain roentgenogram of the chest. The emphysematous lobe can fill a hemithorax, as seen in Figure 6-35, crowding the noninvolved lobe into the corner of the hemithorax where it can be easily missed. Bronchovascular markings are present in the emphysematous area, although they are abnormally far apart. These findings and other radiographic landmarks (see Chapter 19) help rule out other diagnoses such as congenital lung cyst, pneumatocele, or pneumothorax. Bronchography (Fig. 6-37) can confirm the diagnosis, but *ordinarily should not be done in the newborn period.* Pulmonary scanning[82] is an additional diagnostic aid.

The treatment for lobar emphysema is prompt removal of the involved lobe—and occasionally this procedure must be performed immediately. In one of our patients respiratory distress was too great to permit induction of anesthesia; the infant was intubated, and the chest was opened quickly without general anesthesia, delivering the emphysematous lobe, then proceeding with induction of general anesthesia and lobectomy. The pathology is usually striking. When the chest is opened, the greatly distended lobe pops out; it remains somewhat distended when removed from the patient. The collapsed adjacent lobes reexpand to fill the chest.

Review of the literature discloses low mortality in those treated by lobectomy. A considerably higher mortality occurs in those treated by nonoperative means, such as a misguided attempt to needle the lobe; this practice is not only ineffective, but also dangerous. Occasionally more than one lobe is involved. The majority of these children have no subsequent pulmonary problems although later a few may have a picture of bronchial asthma that may have some relation to the original problem of lobar emphysema. In one of our cases the child has a problem of diffuse bronchial dysplasia that has resulted in severe and disabling pulmonary symptoms.

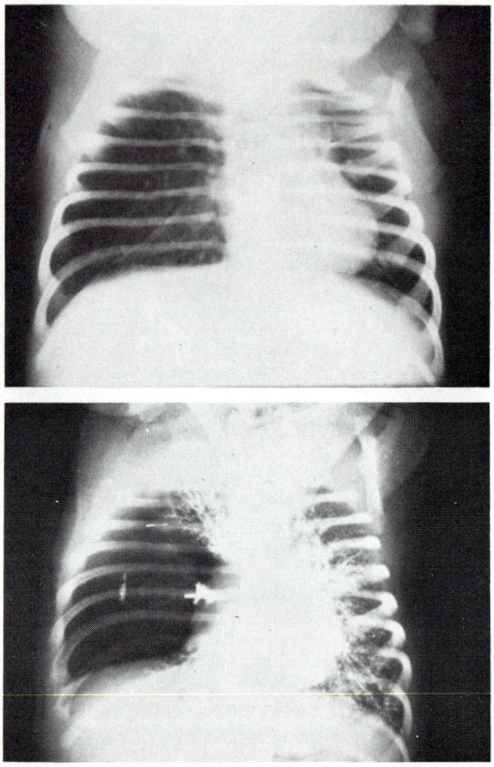

FIG. 6-37. Lobar emphysema, right middle lobe, the second most often affected area.

A, Despite relative radiolucency of the right mid lung field, bronchovascular markings are perceptible. It is typical to see this spreading-out of bronchovascular markings in an emphysematous lobe. Note relative compression of markings of the right lower lobe, displaced downward and medially, and the right upper lobe, which is collapsed in the apex of the chest. There is slight shift of the mediastinum to the opposite side.

B, Bronchogram outlining the compressed bronchial anatomy of the normal lobes, in contrast to the hyperinflated right middle lobe, in which there is no contrast medium. Although bronchography was performed in this particular infant, it is *generally not needed to make the diagnosis.*

Empyema

Empyema, now uncommonly seen, was a frequent diagnosis among hospitalized children in the pre-antibiotic era.[51,124] Frequently Streptococcus and Pneumococcus were the offending organisms. Today the vast majority of cases of empyema in childhood are caused by *S. aureus.* Despite changing organisms and incidence of empyema, the principles of present-day management do not differ from those of several decades ago.[113] Early and total evacuation of empyema is the physician's goal.

The patients most often affected are infants in the first 6 months of life, although an occasional case is seen in older children. A common situation is an antecedent exposure to a known source, such as a breast abscess in the mother. Figure 6-38 shows sequential films from an infant with some of the characteristic features of staphylococcal empyema. Usually a high fever is followed soon by respiratory symptoms. Rapid progression to a bronchopleural fistula with tension pyopneumothorax may occur. The baby may become moribund within hours from this combination of sepsis and reduced lung capacity. Closed tube drainage of the pleural space should be performed immediately using a tube of adequate caliber, as shown in Figure 6-39. Tube drainage of the pleural space at the outset usually evacuates pus and allows the lung to reexpand. This drainage, together with appropriate antibiotics to control infection, has reduced the mortality from empyema to about 2%.

Frequently pneumatoceles form, and this paradox may occur as the patient's clinical course is improving. It is not unusual to see

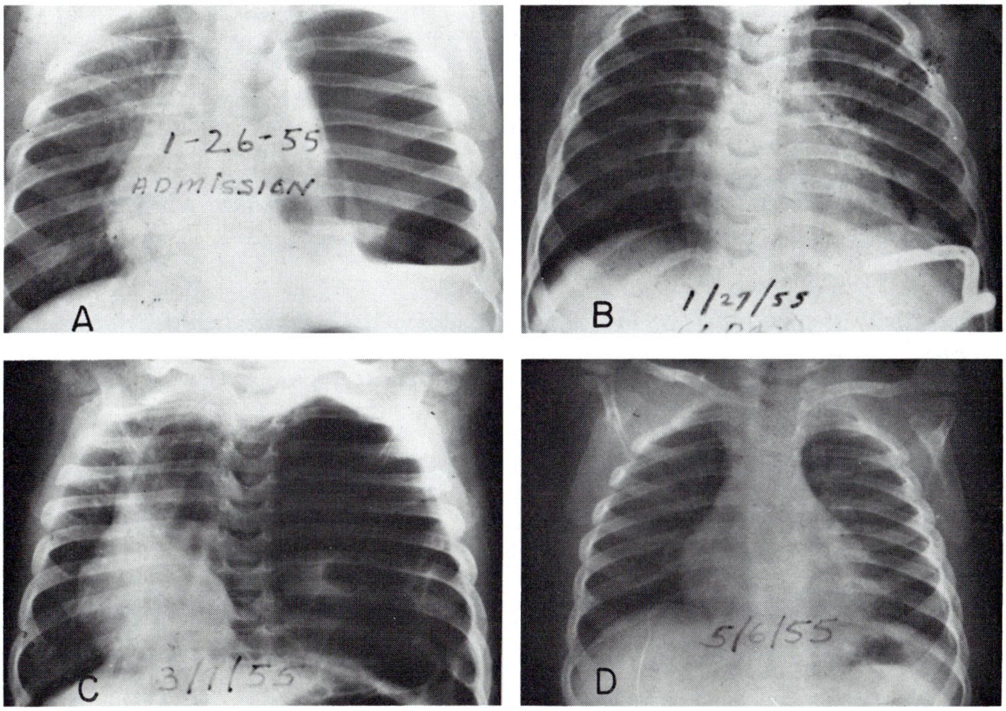

FIG. 6-38. Staphylococcal pneumonia in 6-month-old infant.

A, On admission, desperately ill with tension pyopneumothorax, which was relieved immediately by inserting large-bore intercostal catheter to evacuate air under tension and pus. The child improved dramatically.

B, 24 hours later, re-expansion of lung is evident.

C, 2 months later, massive pneumatocele has formed in the left lung, but the child is clinically well and afebrile. Prolonged antibacterial treatment was maintained.

D, 4 months later, pneumatoceles have been spontaneously resolved. Slight pleural thickening remains.

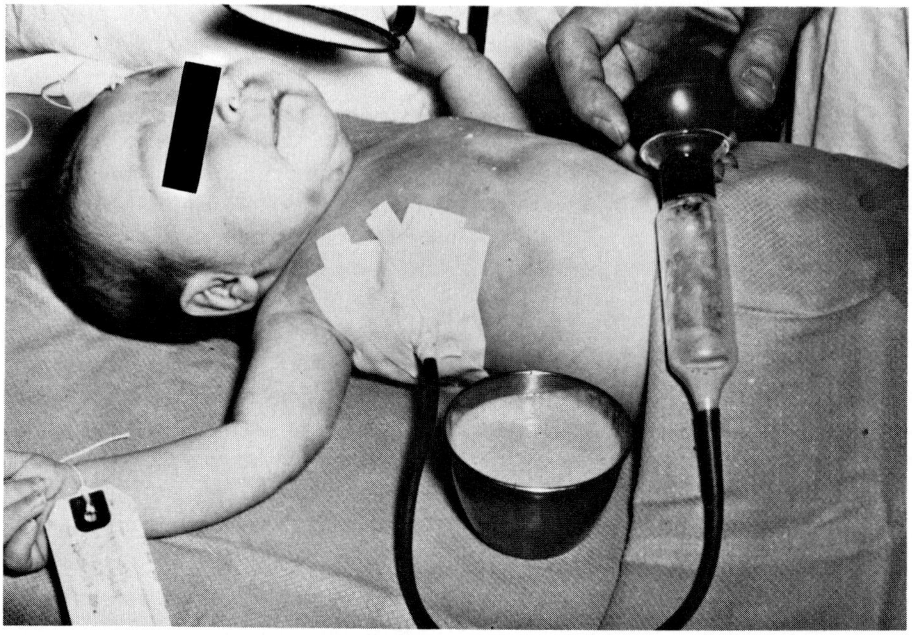

FIG. 6-39. Staphylococcal pneumonia with empyema. This 2-month-old infant entered with severe respiratory distress with massive right-sided empyema evident by chest roentgenogram. A large-bore rubber intercostal catheter was inserted into the right pleural space under local anesthesia in the treatment room soon after hospital admission. When approximately 300 cc of thick yellow pus had been evacuated, much of the baby's respiratory distress was relieved. Note oxygen funnel over infant's face during procedure. The baby did well following continued treatment with prolonged antibiotic therapy, high humidity, blood transfusion, and continuing tube drainage of the affected pleural space. Occasionally bilateral pleural space complications occur in these children.

an apparently worsening chest film in a clinically improving patient. It is important to appreciate that nearly all pneumatoceles resolve with nonoperative treatment. One should not be pushed toward thoracotomy in a child who appears well simply because large pneumatoceles are present. A pneumatocele that has ruptured into the pleural space may have an air leak for several days, or weeks. After tube drainage of the pleural space it eventually stops leaking. Occasionally it is desirable to insert an intercostal catheter directly into a large pneumatocele if it is expanding rapidly or causing undue distress. In some cases it may be necessary to employ more than one intercostal suction catheter.

It is rarely necessary to perform pulmonary decortication when adequate drainage of empyema has been instituted early. Among those children we have treated, decortication was required in only five. In each instance early drainage had not been employed because the patients had been referred late in the course of their disease (Fig. 6-40). This child's empyema did not respond to insertion of chest tubes, and instillation of proteolytic enzymes; decortication was elected. This procedure released the entrapped lung, which reexpanded well.

A child with a cystic lesion of the lung poses the differential diagnosis of congenital lung cyst versus post-inflammatory pneumatocele. The latter would be suggested by an antecedent history of infection, the presence of pleural changes, or the presence of several "cysts" of varying size. If one is in doubt, and the patient's condition permits, it is prudent to wait several weeks for possible

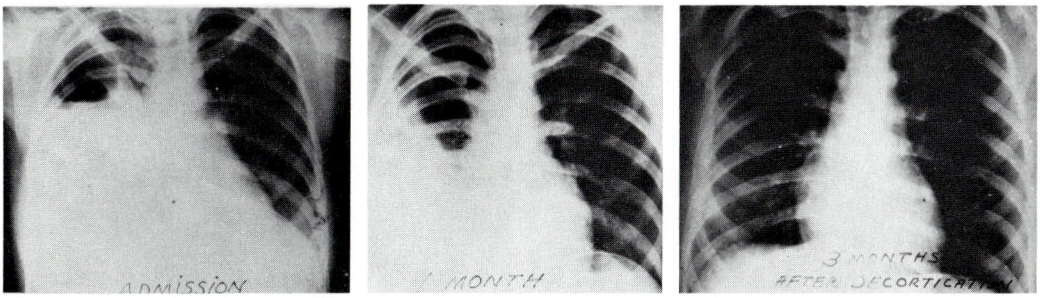

FIG. 6-40. Staphylococcal penumonia requiring pulmonary decortication. This youngster, age 10 years, developed pneumonia with empyema treated initially elsewhere by multiple needle aspirations of the chest. When referred 2 weeks later, with loculated empyema, the right pleural space collection could not be evacuated by closed means of inserting a chest tube and use of proteolytic enzymes.

A, Film on admission showing extensive collection of pus in the right pleural space.

B, 1 month later after only partial removal by closed drainage and continued antibiotic therapy. Decortication was elected.

C, 3 months following right pulmonary decortication. In our experience decortication has been avoided in all cases where closed intercostal drainage was initiated early in the treatment of empyema. Those requiring decortication, like this child, were uniformly cases in which needle aspiration had been employed instead of more effective intercostal tube drainage.

resolution of an inflammatory pneumatocele, rather than proceeding to thoracotomy for a lesion that might well resolve spontaneously.[96]

Corrosive Burns of the Esophagus

Nearly every household has some corrosive substance to unstop drains or toilets; easy accessibility to these products sets the stage for the pediatric accident to be described next. In an experimental study in rabbits, contact with a 22% solution of sodium hydroxide for 10 seconds produced necrosis of the entire esophageal wall, extending into the mediastinum; most household solutions are much stronger, in the range of 50 to 90% sodium hydroxide![10]

When a child is seen with possible caustic ingestion, one cannot rely on the presence of burns about the month as a guide to whether the esophagus has been burned. Some children with obvious burns of the lips and mouth have spit out the substance without swallowing any; curiously, others may have no evidence of mouth burns, but have extensive esophageal burns that if untreated can result in severe stricture. It is our inflexible policy to admit to the hospital any child who may have swallowed a corrosive substance.

A barium swallow does not adequately determine whether the esophagus has been burned. Figure 6-41 shows the films from a 2 year old whose initial swallow 2 days after alleged ingestion was interpreted as normal. Repeat examination 2 weeks later showed a high degree of involvement of the mid-esophagus. Esophagoscopy is done in all of these children to determine by direct inspection whether a burn has occurred at any level of the esophagus. This procedure is usually performed within 48 hours of admission, depending on the general condition of the child. If the burns of the pharynx are severe and the epiglottis is swollen, endoscopy should be delayed until this condition has improved, treating the child meanwhile as if a burn had been sustained. If the youngster is in good condition, we would perform esophagoscopy a few hours after admission.

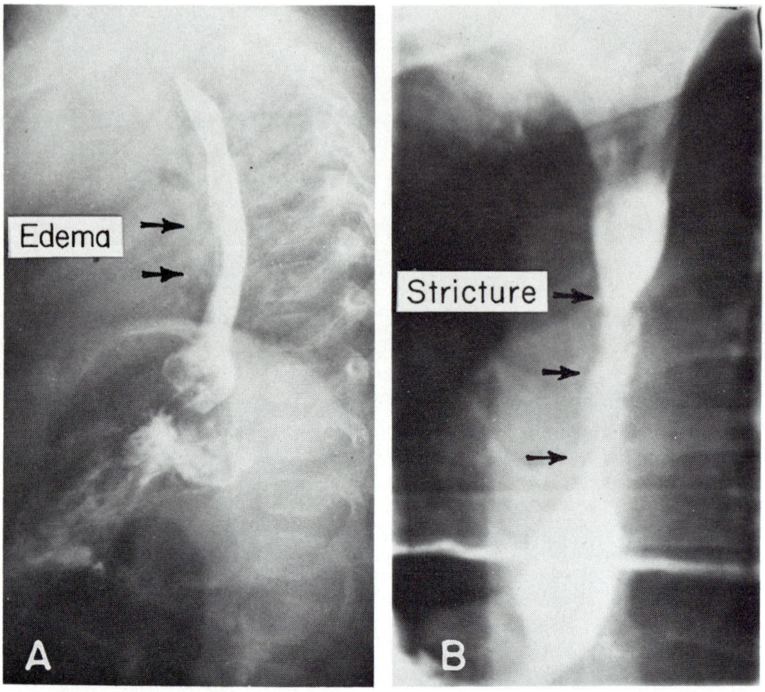

FIG. 6-41. Lye burn of the esophagus.

A, Barium swallow 2 days after ingestion of corrosive material, showing an apparently normal esophagus. It was therefore erroneously assumed that the child had no significant problem. One week thereafter she began to have difficulty swallowing.

B, Esophagogram 2 weeks after ingestion, showing severe involvement of the middle third of the esophagus.

Various combinations of antibiotics, bougienage, and steroids have been used in experimentally produced burns of the esophagus in animals. A combination of all three seems most effective,[69] and this treatment has been confirmed clinically in children.[48,87,129]

Our policy is to admit all of these children on the assumption that a burn exists, and to begin treatment immediately. This treatment includes close observation, a broad-spectrum antibiotic such as ampicillin or prednisone (2 to 3 mg/kg/24 hr), and then diagnostic endoscopy as soon as feasible. At esophagoscopy many children have a perfectly normal esophagus. If so, treatment is discontinued and they are discharged. However an esophagogram is done after several weeks to be absolutely certain that all is well. If esophagoscopy is positive, no attempt should be made to pass the esophagoscope all the way through the burned area to the stomach as it may perforate the esophagus. Treatment with steroids and antibiotics is continued for about 2 weeks, in combination with a program of bougienage. In an occasional child, pharyngeal burns are so severe as to require early tracheotomy for respiratory distress. In this same situation a feeding gastrostomy is usually desirable.

Techniques for dilating a child's esophagus to prevent stenosis include:

(1) Blind passage of stiff dilators to the stomach, the least safe method.

(2) Passing of olive-tipped metal bougies over a string guide that has been swallowed, a safer method.

(3) Endoscopic passing of filiform guides to which are attached following dilators of graduated sizes.

(4) Retrograde passing of bougies upward

from below, utilizing a gastrostomy site. (A swallowed string, or endoscopically passed filiform catheter, is fished from the stomach by probing with a clamp. The dilators are tied to this string and pulled upward to the pharynx.)

(5) Swallowing of soft-rubber mercury-weighted bougies.

All of these methods can produce perforation if used inexpertly. Even the most safe technique of retrograde dilatation can cause esophageal perforation if too large a dilator is pulled through the esophagus, as it may split its wall longitudinally.

The esophagus is dilated several times, under anesthesia, in the first 2 to 3 weeks. Then the mother is taught to pass a mercury-weighted bougie of appropriate caliber. She can then continue treatment at home for an indefinite time depending on the severity of the burns. The majority of those cases treated early and vigorously regain satisfactory esophageal function.

Esophagectomy and colon replacement is the unhappy aftermath of too many who have been neglected. Figure 6-42 is the films of a 3-year-old girl in whom dilatations were started late, and continued for 2 years. The stricture had already developed and did not respond well to dilatation. She required almost total esophagectomy with colon replacement, a procedure of great magnitude. If colon replacement is required, the esophagus can be left in place, and bypassed. In less extensive burn cases it may be reasonable to remove the scarred esophagus simultaneously. Removing a badly burned esophagus can be a difficult dissection. It is best deferred rather than performed at the same time as a colon conduit is constructed. The question of late development of carcinoma of the esophagus shoud be borne in mind in any patient who has sustained a caustic burn years before.

Recently, direct injection of steroids into localized, benign esophageal strictures, together with dilatation, has proven remarkably effective.[59,86] Through a long needle, which can be passed under direct vision through the esophagoscope, triamcinolone is injected into the area of stricture, and the narrowing is dilated. Stenosis of marked degree can soften and result in a normal esophagogram.

Hiatus Hernia and Chalasia

The term, hiatus hernia, describes protrusion of the stomach through an abnormally wide esophageal hiatus. A common problem in adults, hiatus hernia occurs also in children more often than generally realized. An experience with 755 cases was reported from the Hospital for Sick Children, Great Ormond Street, London; 102 of these cases required surgical procedure.[15] No comparable series has been reported in America. Possibly an actual difference exists in the incidence of this condition on opposite sides of the Atlantic Ocean, but more likely, this disparity relates to a difference in the degree of clinical awareness of the problem.

In a study of 100 newborns, barium swallow showed gastroesophageal reflux in 38%.[68] In newborns with regurgitation, gastroesophageal regurgitation is often demonstrable. Berenberg and Neuhauser termed this chalasia and found that it disappears in the majority of instances.[7] Figure 6-43 is a typical case of free gastroesophageal reflux in association with pyloric stenosis. Evidently the esophageal hiatus becomes relatively smaller with growth of the infant, just as is commonly observed at the navel of the neonate with small umbilical hernia, which tends to disappear as the infant grows older.

DIAGNOSIS

Infants with hiatus hernias are brought to the clinic with a variety of admitting diagnoses, e.g., feeding problem, milk allergy, recurrent pneumonia (due to regurgitation and aspiration), pyloric stenosis, and anemia (from peptic esophagitis).[75,84,110,130] This diagnosis should be considered in any infant with vomiting, failure to thrive, recurrent

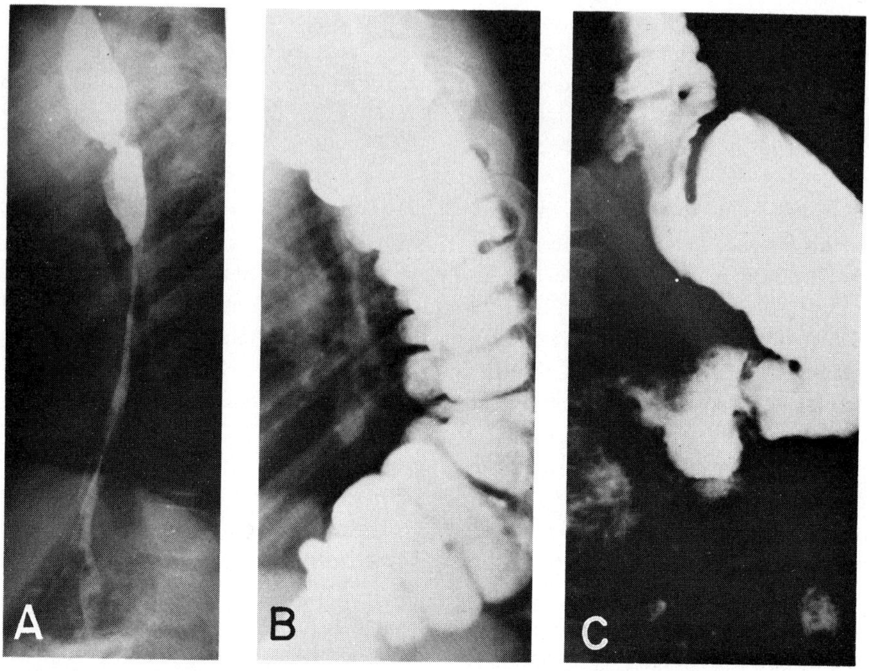

FIG. 6-42. Severe, extensive caustic burn of the esophagus, which did not improve with multiple dilatations for 2 years, and required colon replacement of the esophagus.

A, Preoperative esophagogram showing stenosis at the thoracic inlet and level of the aortic arch, and a long stricture from there to the diaphragm.

B, 2 weeks after esophagectomy and replacement by a segment of transverse colon, based on blood supply of the left colic artery. The upper end of the conduit was anastomosed to the cervical esophagus. In some, this anastomosis must be as high as the pharynx. The lower end of the conduit was anastomosed directly to the stomach, for there was no usable distal esophagus.

C, Anastomosis of lower end of colon conduit to posterior wall of the stomach, after resection and closure of original esophagogastric junction.

pneumonia, or unexplained anemia. A routine barium swallow may fail to provide the diagnosis. Special maneuvers of compressing the epigastrium, tilting the child into Trendelenburg position, and even using a continuous recording system, e.g., magnetic tape or cine, may be necessary to show a small hernia. A typical sliding hiatal hernia is shown in Figure 6-44, with much of the gastric fundus in the mediastinum. Other films from this series looked perfectly normal. Esophagoscopy can be of value;[54] the trained eye can recognize an incompetent cardia, and also a minimal degree of esophagitis not visible by roentgen examination. Some infants, and older children, may have symptoms of esophageal obstruction caused by stricture from reflux esophagitis, a very serious complication. Not infrequently they require esophagectomy and colon interposition. *This dire consequence can be prevented if physicians look for this entity and institute appropriate early treatment.*

TREATMENT

The early treatment for an infant with hiatus hernia includes propping the infant upright, thickening his feedings, and giving antispasmodics plus an antacid for any suggestion of esophagitis. On this program many of these infants improve. Others do not, however, and the physician should not hesi-

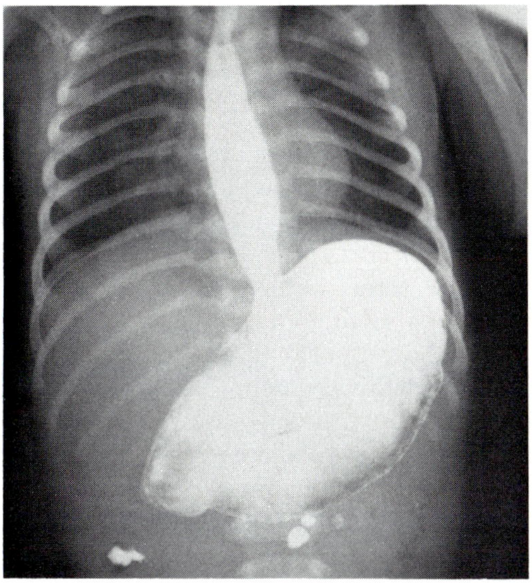

FIG. 6-43. Chalasia or free gastroesophageal reflux. This infant also had pyloric stenosis; note the large stomach. Pyloromyotomy relieved the vomiting; chalasia disappeared.

tate to recommend surgical repair. The operation can be done safely and with excellent results in experienced hands. Various techniques are available for repairing hiatus hernias, some through the chest, others through the abdomen, and occasionally via a thoracoabdominal approach.[137] In general, repair involves reducing the stomach and terminal esophagus into the abdominal cavity, anchoring it there so that it cannot slide up into the mediastinum, together with making the hiatus smaller. A temporary gastrostomy may be of value in a small underweight infant postoperatively, particularly if a lot of aspiration pneumonitis has occurred preoperatively. Vagotomy and pyloroplasty are useful additional adjuncts in those who have peptic esophagitis.[22] If a stricture is present, dilatation is often done simultaneously with hiatus hernia repair. It may be necessary postoperatively also. Scarring of the esophagus from hiatus hernia can be as severe as in untreated lye burns. It is one of the most frequent indications for colon esophageal replacement in children.

It should be noted that after successful hiatus hernia repair the youngster may be unable to vomit normally. Should the child develop a gastrointestinal upset, with gastric dilatation, a tube should be passed to empty stomach contents in order to prevent serious gastric dilatation.

In summary, hiatus hernia is much more common than appreciated. The majority do not require surgery, but some do. In some, severe complications can result, particularly if an early diagnosis is not made.

Achalasia

Achalasia of the esophagus occurs rarely in children[21] and gives symptoms of obstruction, regurgitation, and pulmonary complications. The pathology in the lower esophagus is similar to Hirschsprung's disease of the rectum, with absence of intramural ganglion cells. The terminal esophagus appears narrow radiographically, with dilatation above,

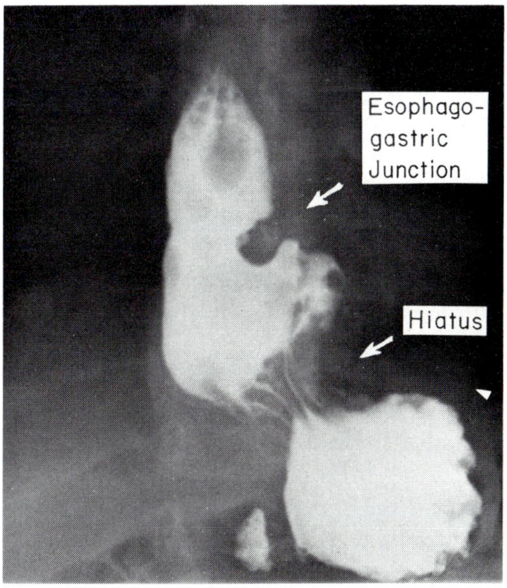

FIG. 6-44. Large sliding hiatus hernia in a child with vomiting and failure to thrive. About half of the stomach is herniated into the mediastinum.

sometimes to a great degree. Methods of treatment have included dilatations, esophageal resection, and various plastic procedures to the involved segment. Most surgeons have found the Heller operation satisfactory. This simple esophagomyotomy is similar to that done in hypertrophic pyloric stenosis. A longitudinal incision is made through the muscle of the narrow segment, allowing the esophageal mucosa to protrude into the defect. It is a technically simple procedure, with very low morbidity, and relieves the functional obstruction in most cases. Simultaneous fundoplication prevents gastric reflux.

Middle Lobe Syndrome

Recurrent pneumonitis of the right middle lobe, with atelectasis, is a familiar clinical picture, termed middle lobe syndrome. It was associated with pulmonary tuberculosis formerly.[27,49]

The typical case is an infant, 1 to 2 years of age, with recurrent episodes of infection in the right middle lobe. Usually, clearing of the pneumonic process is slow or incomplete after each episode. Bronchoscopy may reveal compression of the middle lobe orifice. Bronchography may show nonfilling of the middle lobe, or collapse, as seen in Figure 6-45. When pathology is localized to the middle lobe, with repeated episodes of involvement, lobectomy is indicated. At operation it is usual to find a pancake-like lobe (Fig. 6-45), with large inflammatory lymph nodes in the lung hilum compressing the relatively small middle lobe bronchus. We treated one youngster with Kartagener's syndrome, who had situs inversus, sinusitis, and recurrent pulmonary infection and atelectasis in the *left* middle lobe.

Decision regarding lobectomy should be made in terms of whether pneumonia is frequent and severe and whether the lung clears between episodes. Certainly surgical procedure should not be advised after one or two episodes in a well child, but would be indicated after repeated episodes with persistent collapse of a lobe.

Occasionally the middle lobe syndrome is seen in children with cystic fibrosis. The surgeon should be cautious in considering pulmonary resection in a child with diffuse disease, but it can provide great benefit when one lobe seems particularly involved as a continuing septic focus.

Bronchoscopy should precede pulmonary resection in this age group, to rule out foreign body. We have found unsuspected foreign bodies in several children referred for pulmonary resection. In one, a fragment of peanut had been lodged in the lower lobe bronchus for 1 year. In another a piece of upholsterer's foam rubber was extracted from the bronchus; it had been inhaled 3 years earlier.

Pneumothorax

Air in the pleural space, especially when under tension, is a serious emergency that can be encountered in anyone from a premature infant to a teenaged athlete. The incidence in neonates is higher than in previous years, due to the more common use of positive pressure ventilation of the newborn with respiratory difficulty. In a recent study pneumothorax was noted in: 1% of infants born by routine vaginal delivery, in 1% of 100 premature infants, in 2% of 100 cesarean section babies, and in 6% of infants who required intubation at birth.[121] Other reports have called attention to the role of positive pressure ventilation in producing tension pneumothorax.[92,120] A typical example is shown in Figure 6-46. It can be bilateral.[17]

Beyond the neonatal period pneumothorax is rare, until the teen years. Then it is seen in the healthy youngster who suddenly develops acute distress, sometimes with pain in the chest. The pathology is generally rupture of a small apical air bleb. A striking example,

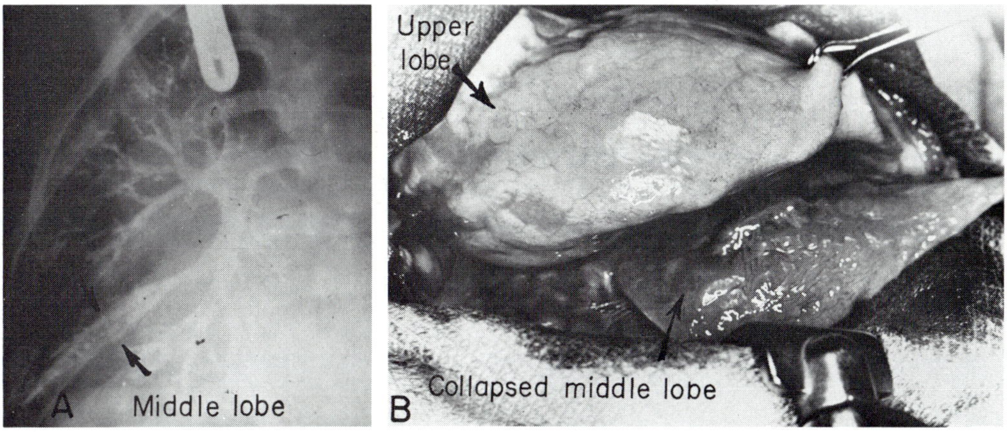

FIG. 6-45. Middle lobe syndrome. 4-year-old child with recurrent right middle lobe pneumonia.
A, Bronchogram showing collapse of right middle lobe.
B, Operative photograph showing air-filled upper lobe, and pancake-like airless middle lobe, which could not be inflated with positive pressure.

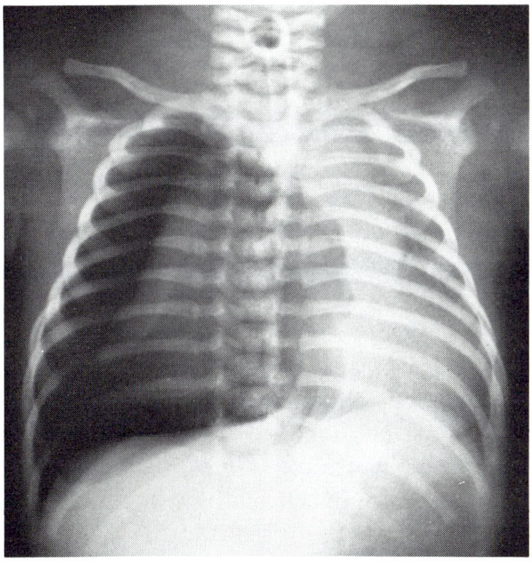

FIG. 6-46. Tension pneumothorax in an infant caused by too vigorous positive pressure ventilation through a tracheotomy tube. The infant had laryngeal obstruction from an endolaryngeal hemangioma. Tracheotomy had been performed previously, uneventfully. Some days later during tracheotomy aspiration and bag insufflation of the lungs, the right lung was blown out, resulting in this tension pneumothorax. It was treated initially by percutaneous insertion of a small plastic catheter, and later insertion of an intercostal chest tube.

unusual because it was bilateral, is shown in Figure 6-47. Occasionally pneumothorax is seen in unfortunate children with pulmonary metastases, especially osteogenic sarcoma.

Pneumothorax can occur in nonpenetrating trauma, from compression which ruptures the trachea or a smaller bronchus. Air dissects beneath the visceral pleura, rupturing into the pleural space. Pneumothorax can result from puncture of the lung by the end of a fractured rib.

In the circumstances just described, and particularly in the neonate, air may accumulate by interstitial dissection into the mediastinum. It can also dissect below the diaphragm retroperitoneally, rupturing into the peritoneal cavity and appearing clinically as a massive pneumoperitoneum.[29] Pneumopericardium has been noted also.[42]

Treatment of pneumothorax should be guided by the amount of air, determination of whether it is under tension, and the clinical status of the patient. In a neonate, or older child, with minimal difficulty, and a small amount of air over the lung, it is feasible to observe the patient, aspirating the air only if the size of the pneumothorax should increase. Compared with multiple needle aspirations,

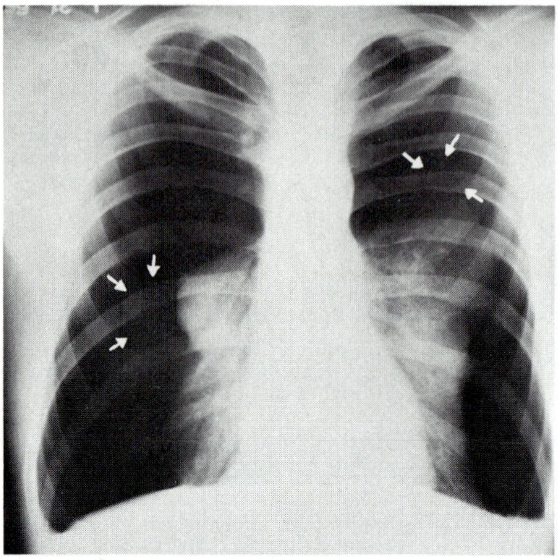

FIG. 6-47. Bilateral severe pneumothorax. This teenaged boy entered with severe respiratory distress. This film was obtained, although likely the diagnosis could have been made clinically and treatment begun immediately. A large-bore needle was thrust into each pleural space, with simple underwater seal, giving immediate relief of tension. Chest tubes were placed soon thereafter. Later staged thoracotomies were performed with resection of bilateral apical blebs (see arrows).

the insertion of a catheter is a safer and more efficient method for the continuous aspiration of a large air collection in a patient with limited respiratory reserve. For active air leaks, suction is necessary to assure reexpansion of the lung. Thereafter a period of water-seal drainage should precede removal of the tube. Positive pressure ventilation can be required, despite an active leak, in youngsters with limited pulmonary function. Most of these leaks seal spontaneously, but occasionally thoracotomy is required to suture the leaking point.

In older children with spontaneous pneumothorax, the recurrence rate is about 50%. The patient and his family must be warned of this high incidence. Should the lung fail to reexpand during the first episode, or should a second occur, thoracotomy is performed with suturing of the bleb. No longer is talcum powder dusted into the pleural space, as was once done, to promote adhesions between the visceral and parietal pleural surfaces. It suffices to rub the lung and chest wall briskly with a dry gauze sponge to promote adherence between the two postoperatively, thus preventing the possibility of a recurrent pneumothorax. In apical bleb disease it can help further to strip away the parietal pleura at the dome of the chest, as an additional measure to promote adherence postoperatively.

Chylothorax

Chylothorax is a rare condition causing respiratory distress from accumulation of lymph in the pleural space, more often on the right side. Spontaneous chylothorax in the newborn probably relates in most instances to birth trauma. High venous pressure can rupture intrathoracic lymphatics.[9] The most common cause for chylothorax is a recent operation with mediastinal dissection, as shown in Figure 6-48.

The treatment for chylothorax, whether it is spontaneous, appears after thoracotomy, or occurs in chest trauma, should be initial removal of the accumulated chyle by needle aspiration or chest tube. We prefer the latter. If the leak does not diminish, and the lung does not reexpand in a few days,[100] operative intervention should follow. The leaking source can be identified by injecting Evan's Blue Dye beneath the skin of the thigh a few minutes before operation; from the thigh, the dye flows into the lymphatics. A dissecting microscope provides additional help in identifying the leaking point. It is oversewn with nonabsorbable sutures.

These children should not have exploratory surgical procedures immediately because many of these leaks seal. On the other hand they should not be maintained on protracted aspiration or intercostal drainage, because a continuing loss of chyle can lead to severe nutritional depletion. Swenson advocated a

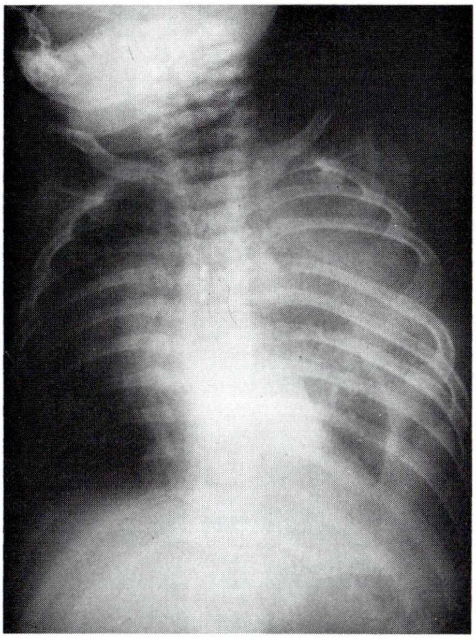

FIG. 6-48. Chylothorax in 4-month-old baby following surgical correction of aortic arch anomaly. After initial nonoperative treatment, and persistent reaccumulation of chyle, the chest was re-explored. A small lymphatic in the mediastinum, not the thoracic duct, was identified with the help of vital contrast material injected subcutaneously into the thigh. The leaking duct was suture ligated. Note also the wide fourth interspace.

period of intravenous reinfusion of aspirated chyle.[30] In the newborn chylothorax may at first seem like a pleural effusion, yielding straw-colored fluid. When the infant begins to feed, the fluid acquires the typical milky appearance of fat-laden mesenteric lymph.[139]

Lung Cyst

In the older literature it was held that all cysts of the lung in childhood are acquired, like the post-inflammatory pneumatoceles in staphylococcal pneumonia. Supporting that view is the rarity of lung cysts in large autopsy series of stillborns. Possibly the rarity in stillborns occurs because epithelial clefts that exist are not obvious until dilated in vivo by air or until mucus accumulates in them in life.[103] Lung cysts have been seen in very young infants, in the absence of infection, and found lined with tall, ciliated, columnar epithelium appropriate for the respiratory tract. They are seen also in association with other lung malformations and with arterial blood flow from the aorta instead of the pulmonary arterial tree. In some hamartomatous development is evident, with abnormal epithelial formation.

They can be unilocular or multilocular. When there is superimposed infection, which is common, they can be confused with loculated empyema, lung abscess, or even resolving staphylococcic pneumonia with multiple pneumatoceles. Figure 6-49 shows a large, unilocular, uninfected lung cyst in the right upper lobe of a 3-year-old girl. The clinician must be suspicious that a cystic malformation is present in a case of pneumonia that does not resolve completely. If post-inflammatory pneumatocele is suspected, operation should be delayed for several weeks to see whether it resolves.

The abnormal proliferation of mucous secreting glands or respiratory epithelium in association with cystic disease has been termed congenital cystic adenomatoid malformation of the lung.[6,23,58,88] An example is seen in Figure 6-50. A spectrum of congenital cystic disease is present, with varying amounts of cyst and adenoma. Children do extremely well after resection of lung with localized pathology when the remaining lobes are normal; this generally applies to children with congenital lung cysts.[24,63,67] A special type of lung cyst is encountered in children in those parts of the world where Echinococcus disease is prevalent, for example, in the Mediterranean area, the Orient, Australia, and South America.[119,128] Hydatid cysts require careful surgical handling lest cyst contents spill, with myriads of daughter scolices that can implant and grow. This disease is seen seldom in America, except in an occasional immigrant from an endemic region. Saidi

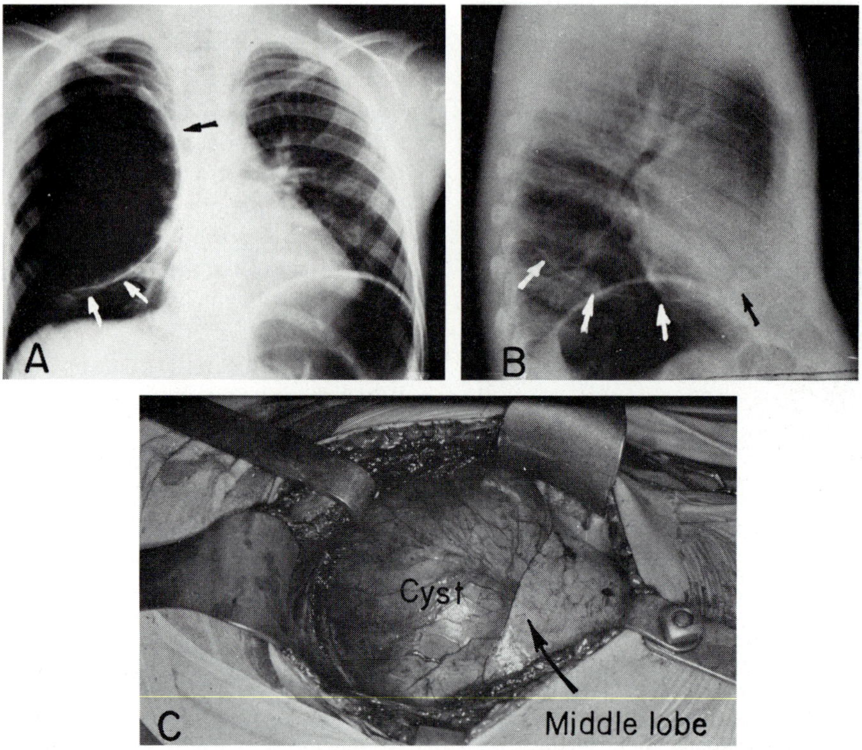

FIG. 6-49. Large lung cyst, right upper lobe, 3-year-old girl. She had acute respiratory distress, with some right chest pain.

A and *B*, Chest roentgenograms showing large lucent area in right thorax. The rounded configuration and total lack of bronchovascular markings distinguish this from lobar emphysema or pneumothorax.

C, Operative view of cyst filling the right hemithorax. It involved most of the right upper lobe. Lobectomy-cystectomy permitted the middle and the lower lobe to expand normally and fill the right hemithorax.

described an ingenious method of safe removal by temporarily freezing a metal funnel to the chest wall with liquid nitrogen and evacuating the cyst fluid and lining through the protective funnel.[112]

Lung Abscess

Lung abscess in childhood can have several causes, which include: (1) aspiration, particularly of a foreign body; (2) pulmonary infections like Staphylococcus, *K. pneumoniae,* tuberculosis, *Entamoeba histolytica,* Salmonella, fungi, and Echinococcus; (3) secondary infection in congenital lung cysts; (4) septic infarction in congenital heart disease; and (5) diffuse lung disease such as cystic fibrosis.[134] In pre-antibiotic days lung abscess carried a mortality approaching 50%. Although the incidence has been reduced greatly, principles of management must include measures from previous generations, if antibiotic therapy does not clear the process entirely.

Initial treatment is antibiotic therapy for the specific organism involved. Usually pneumonitis is present, with consolidation, in which tissue destruction and abscess formation occur. If this abscess erodes into a bronchus, a productive cough and sometimes hemoptysis appear. Bronchoscopy can help

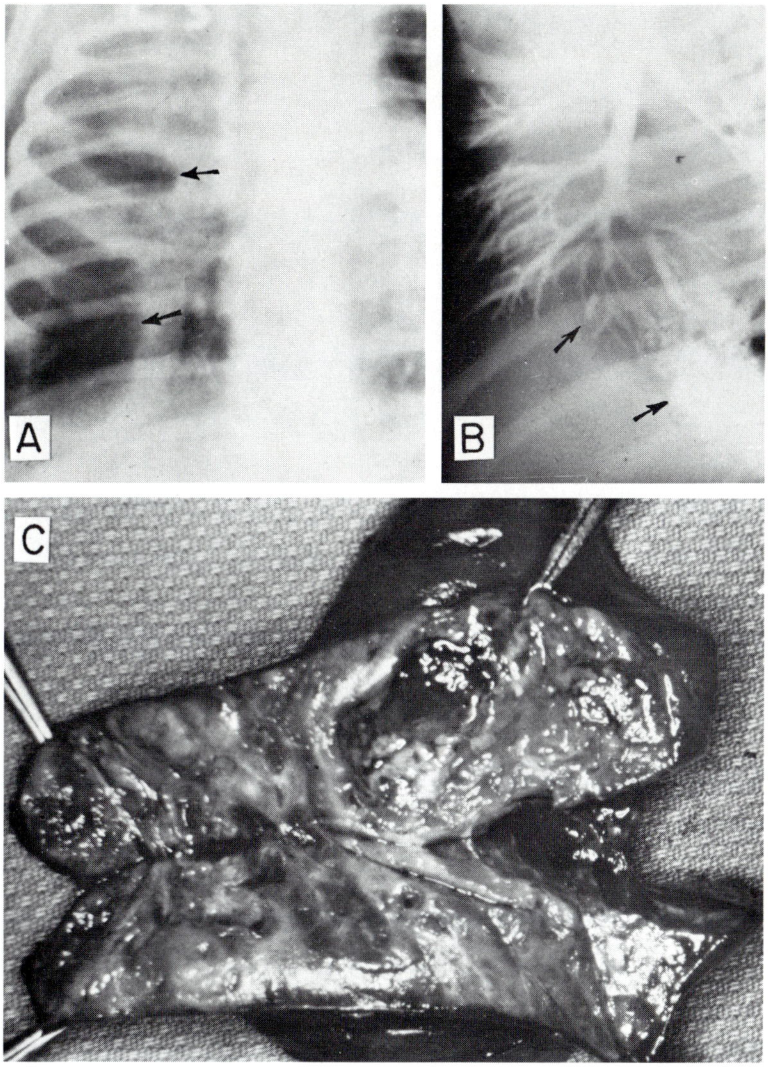

FIG. 6-50. Cystic hamartomatous malformation of right lower lobe.
A, Plain film showing cysts.
B, Bronchogram showing communication.
C, The surgical specimen, which was an admixture of cysts and solid adenomatous tissue.

suction away some of the material that is draining. While hoping for complete resolution on antibiotics, the clinician must appreciate the possibility of an underlying problem such as a foreign body or previously existing disease in the lung, which may require resection. Figure 6-51 depicts a large lung abscess, involving most of the right upper lobe in a 3-year-old girl. It failed to improve during 2 months of antibiotic treatment. Lobectomy revealed a completely destroyed right upper lobe, but no apparent underlying cause for the abscess.

Occasionally surgical drainage of an intrapulmonary abscess is necessary when it does not spontaneously drain into a bronchus.

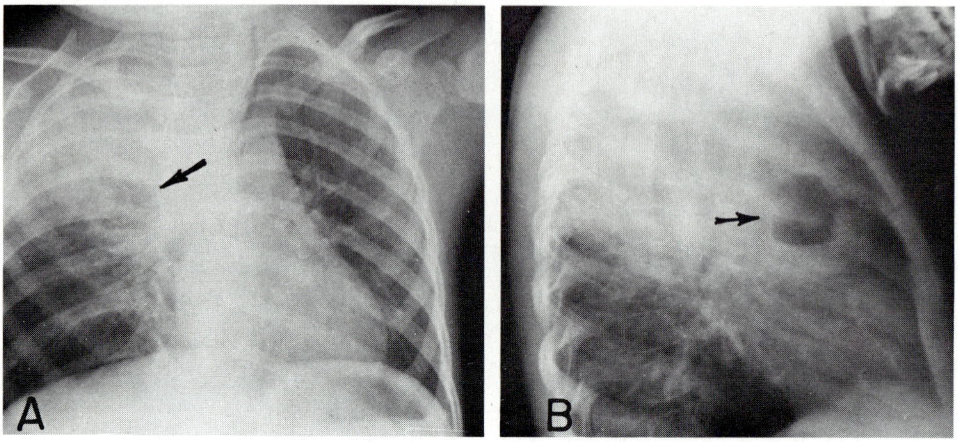

FIG. 6-51. *A*, Right upper lobe lung abscess in 3-year-old girl. She had been treated with antibiotics for 2 months for right upper lobe consolidation, which did not clear. Bronchoscopy excluded a foreign body. *B*, Lobectomy was performed, revealing a totally destroyed right upper lobe containing a thick walled, chronic abscess cavity.

Figure 6-52 shows films from a 1-year-old infant with a large abscess in the superior segment of the right lower lobe. His course was toxic, and the abscess continued to enlarge. Monaldi drainage was employed, a method used widely several decades ago. An incision was made down to the pleura overlying the abscess cavity, and the wound was packed with gauze. The inflammatory reaction in the pleura from the gauze promotes adherence of the lung to the chest wall. One week later a tube was placed directly into the abscess cavity through this area of adherence. This staged procedure permits drainage without causing empyema or pneumothorax. Indications for surgical resection of a lung abscess include failure to resolve with long-term drug therapy, life-threatening hemorrhage, and bronchial obstruction with failure to drain.[132]

Bronchogenic Cyst

Bronchogenic cysts can occur at any age; these unilocular cysts are lined with respiratory epithelium. They do not usually communicate with the tracheobronchial tree. In a review of 31 cases, 25 had symptoms.[93] Figure 6-53 shows a sizable bronchogenic cyst that lay adjacent to the trachea, causing no symptoms, but discovered on a routine chest roentgenogram. In contrast, Figure 6-54 shows films from a newborn with severe respiratory distress caused by a small bronchogenic cyst located beneath the carina and compressing the left main stem bronchus. Bronchogenic cyst in the mediastinum can be diagnosed by roentgenographic means if it is large enough. In some, displacement of the esophagus is noted on barium swallow, or compression of the tracheobronchial tree is evident on plain films of the chest. Bronchography does not fill the cyst, but may show bronchial indentation, as evident in Figure 6-54. Surgical excision is indicated.[33,41]

Pulmonary Sequestration

Sequestration is a term for lung tissue that does not communicate with the tracheobronchial tree and derives its blood supply di-

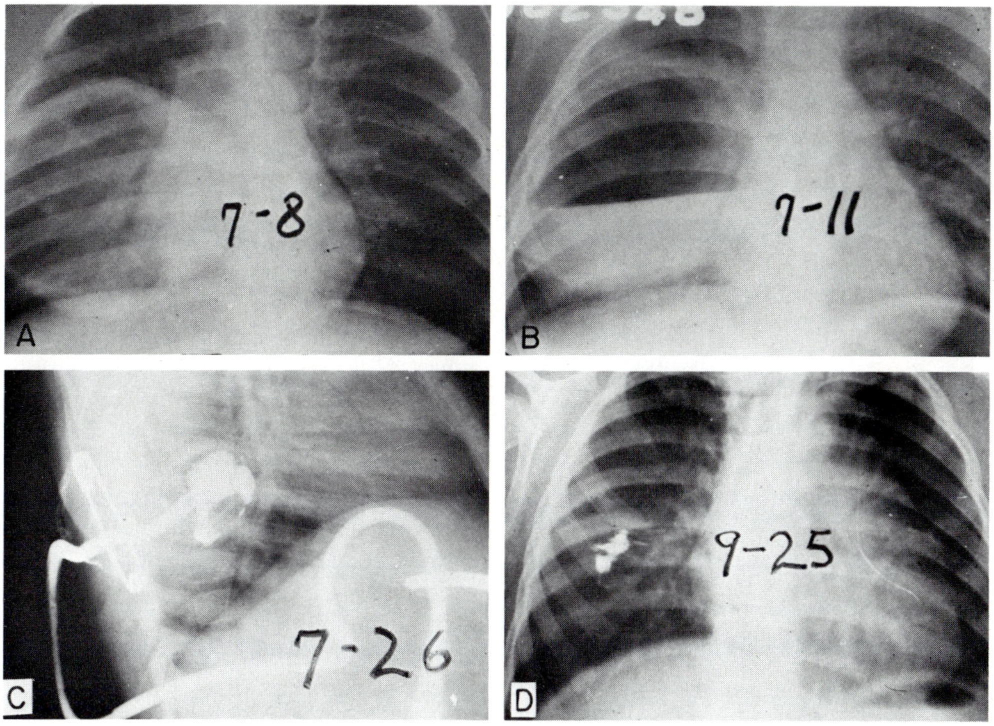

FIG. 6-52. Lung abscess treated by Monaldi drainage in 1-year-old child.

A, On admission.

B, 3 days later. Child toxic despite antibiotics. An incision was made to the pleura overlying the abscess and the wound packed, stimulating adherence of the lung to the parietal pleura. Five days later, a tube was inserted through this point of adherence into the abscess.

C, Contrast study of shrinking lung abscess 1 week after tube drainage.

D, Film 2 months later. Well child. Small amount of contrast still present. No sequelae.

rectly from the aorta, not the pulmonary artery. Venous drainage can be into systemic or pulmonary veins. In a recent report 80 cases in childhood were reviewed.[28]

Extralobar sequestration (Fig. 6-55) occurs on the left side, in the lower thorax, often in association with congenital diaphragmatic hernia. There may be a rudimentary connection to esophagus or stomach, but anatomically the sequestrated tissue is separate from the lower lobe. In older patients the tissue may be mistakenly diagnosed as a mediastinal tumor.

Intralobar sequestration is more common. It usually appears as pulmonary infection in older children. A typical example is shown in Figure 6-56. Pathologically an area of cystic degeneration is present within a lobe, usually the lower lobe, left more commonly than the right. Sometimes a communication does exist with the bronchial system of the surrounding normal lung parenchyma. The arterial blood supply comes from the aorta, sometimes below the diaphragm.

Intralobar sequestration can mimic other lung pathology, such as cystic disease, localized bronchiectasis, and lung abscess. A sharply localized nonsegmental involvement within a lobe may suggest the true diagnosis. It can be confirmed by aortography, demon-

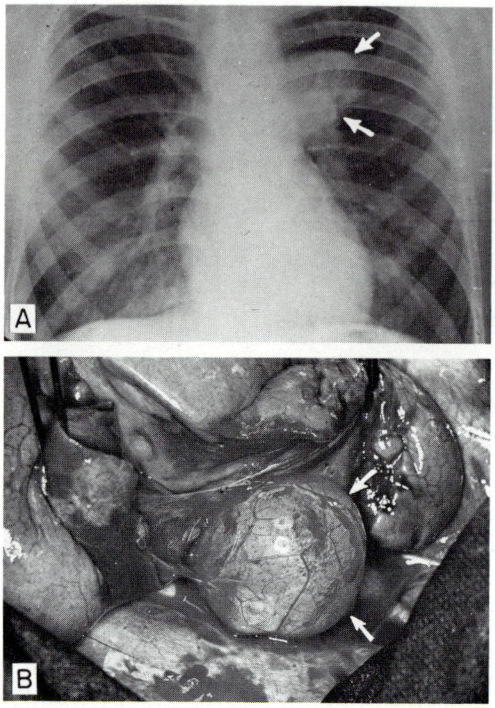

FIG. 6-53. Paratracheal bronchogenic cyst discovered by chance in a 12-year-old boy.
A, Plain film.
B, Operative view.

strating an anomalous blood supply. Lobectomy in this condition does not differ from other cases except that the surgeon must ligate the anomalous arterial blood supply arising from the aorta.[12]

Bronchiectasis

Like lung abscess, bronchiectasis has decreased greatly in frequency since the advent of antibiotics, which have reduced the postpneumonic form by early arrest of pneumonia. Bronchography was introduced 50 years ago, permitting anatomic delineation of this disease. Forty years ago segmental pulmonary resection was developed by Churchill, largely to deal with bronchiectasis in young individuals.[20] In a review of 287 cases treated at the Boston Children's Hospital from 1940 to 1968, Welch emphasized that, although the absolute number of patients with bronchiectasis is much reduced, the relative incidence of bronchiectasis due to underlying lung disease is higher.[133] Bronchiectasis was seen in the following clinical situations: (1) secondary to infections like pneumonia, pertussis, tuberculosis, measles, scarlet fever, and nonspecific infection; (2) with *cystic fibrosis;* (3) secondary to pulmonary anomalies, agammaglobulinemia, cardiovascular anomalies, pulmonary vascular anomalies, and thymic aplasia; (4) following aspiration of a foreign body, blood, or feeding.

Symptoms of bronchiectasis are those of chronic pulmonary infection, often with a cough that is either dry or productive. Although a plain film of the chest is often not diagnostic, it may show increased markings, or contraction of segments or lobes. Bronchography can accurately delineate the extent of disease. The areas of lung most often involved are basilar segments, the right middle lobe, and the lingular segment of the left upper lobe. The decision for surgical procedure depends on whether the disease is severe and sharply localized and refractory to medical therapy. Early cylindrical changes may be reversed by appropriate antibacterial therapy and physiotherapy. On the other hand if advanced, saccular changes are evident, resection of localized disease is desirable (Fig. 6-57 and 6-58). (See also Chapter 19 for discussion of the role of bronchography.)

For the child with diffuse bronchiectasis, usually with an underlying medical problem, the decision is much more difficult. Nonoperative therapy is pursued unless there is an area of particularly severe involvement in which removal of a functionless, chronically infected area of the lung may greatly help the child.[116]

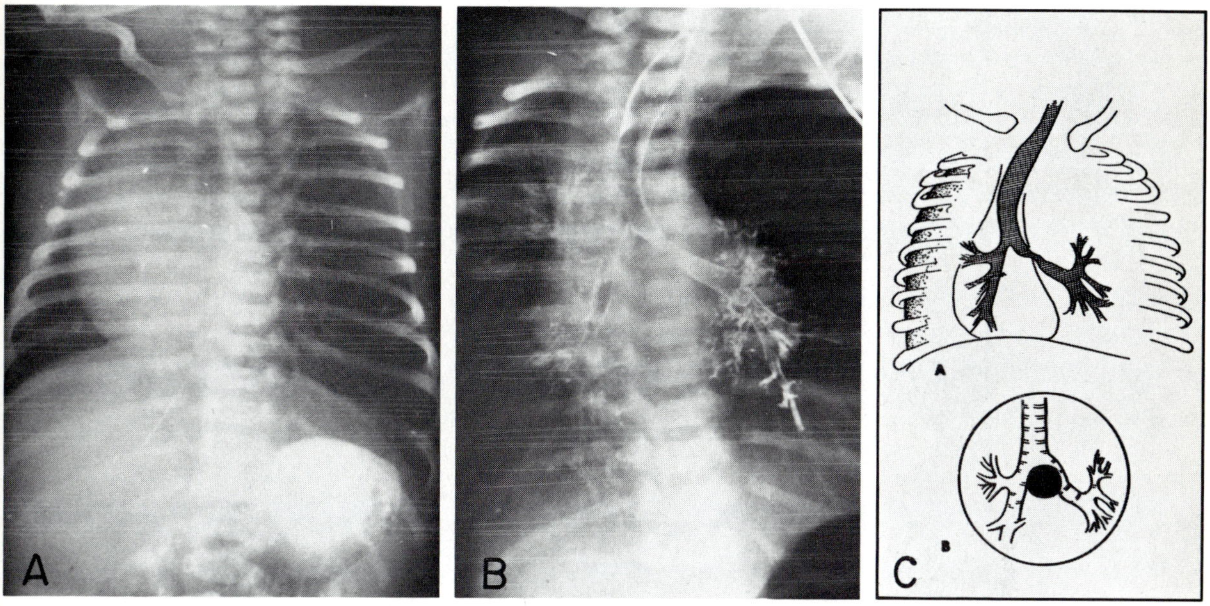

FIG. 6-54. Bronchial compression by mediastinal cyst, in a 1-week-old infant.

A, Plain film of the chest showing emphysematous left lung with shift of mediastinum to the right and slight compression atelectasis of the right lung.

B, Bronchography, through a bronchoscope, disclosing coarctation-like narrowing of the left main stem bronchus 2 centimeters from the carina.

C, Diagram of operative findings. A small bronchogenic cyst in the mediastinum compressed the left main stem bronchus; its excision cured the problem.

Duplications

Two principal types of duplications occur in the thorax. Each can cause respiratory symptoms. The first type is simple esophageal duplication; the second is the giant duplication of foregut origin, which generally connects below the diaphragm and extends upward into the chest.

Esophageal duplications, the more common variety, lie next to the esophagus, more often on the right than on the left, and rarely in the neck. During early embryonic development the gut is a solid cord, which becomes vacuolated. The vacuoles subsequently coalesce to form a lumen. It is thought that this type of duplication represents a pinching off of a vacuole from the gut, so that it is excluded from continuity with the gastrointestinal tract. The majority of esophageal duplications do not communicate with the adjacent esophageal lumen. They frequently have gastrointestinal mucosa inappropriate for the level at which they are found, and commonly are lined by gastric mucosa, which can cause them to ulcerate, bleed, and perforate into the mediastinum or lung.[18] Aspirating one of these "cysts" at the operating table and finding an acid pH can be a clue to the presence of gastric mucosa. These duplications can cause respiratory distress by compression of adjacent bronchi. The differential diagnosis includes lung cyst and mediastinal tumor. In excising one of these unilocular esophageal duplications, the surgeon must bear in mind that they have a common muscular wall with the esophagus, which should be preserved. They should be dissected free,

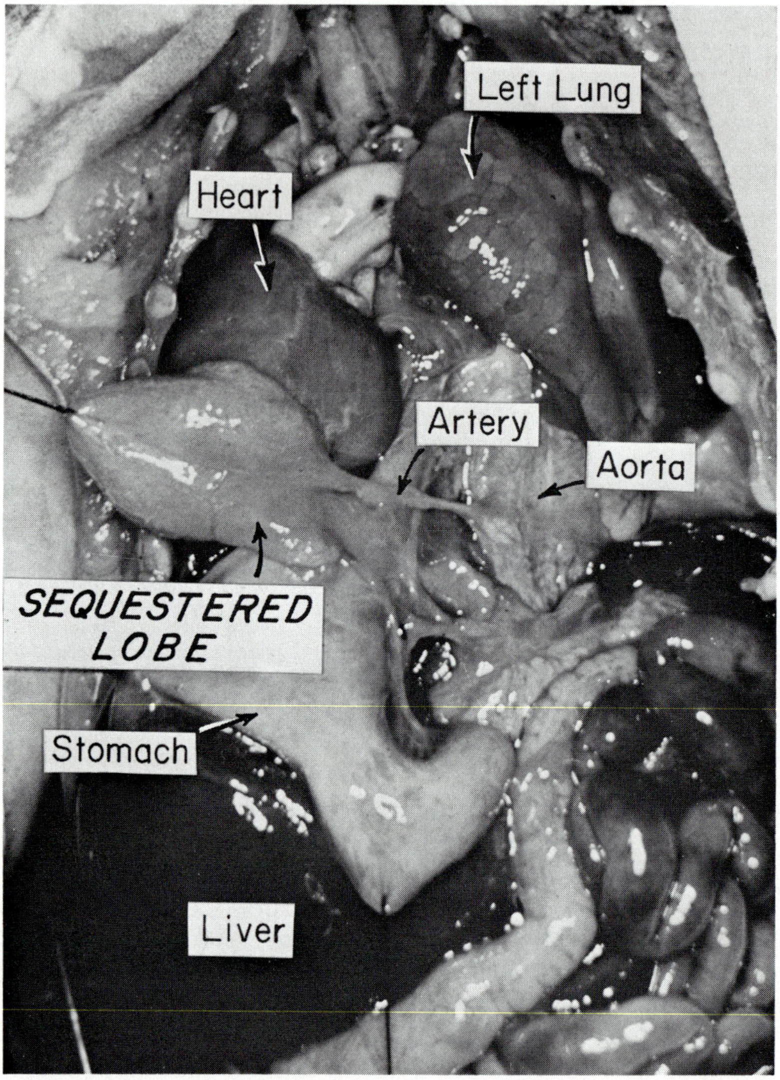

FIG. 6-55. Autopsy specimen of extralobar sequestration below diaphragm in newborn with congenital diaphragmatic hernia. Note its arterial blood supply from the aorta.

avoiding entry into the esophageal mucosa, and enough of the esophageal wall should be preserved to repair it without narrowing. An alternative method is the complete removal of the cyst lining.

The second type of duplication is rare but fascinating. At an early stage in development, the neural canal and enteric canal lie adjacent to one another. Later they are separated by ingrowth of mesoderm, which surrounds the neural canal, forming vertebra. If incomplete separation occurs, a communication may remain between the neural canal and the gastrointestinal tract. Commonly a vertebral defect is associated, a helpful diagnostic clue.[106] This defect is most often seen in the lower neck, but sometimes lower in the spinal canal. As the gut elongates, coming to lie below the

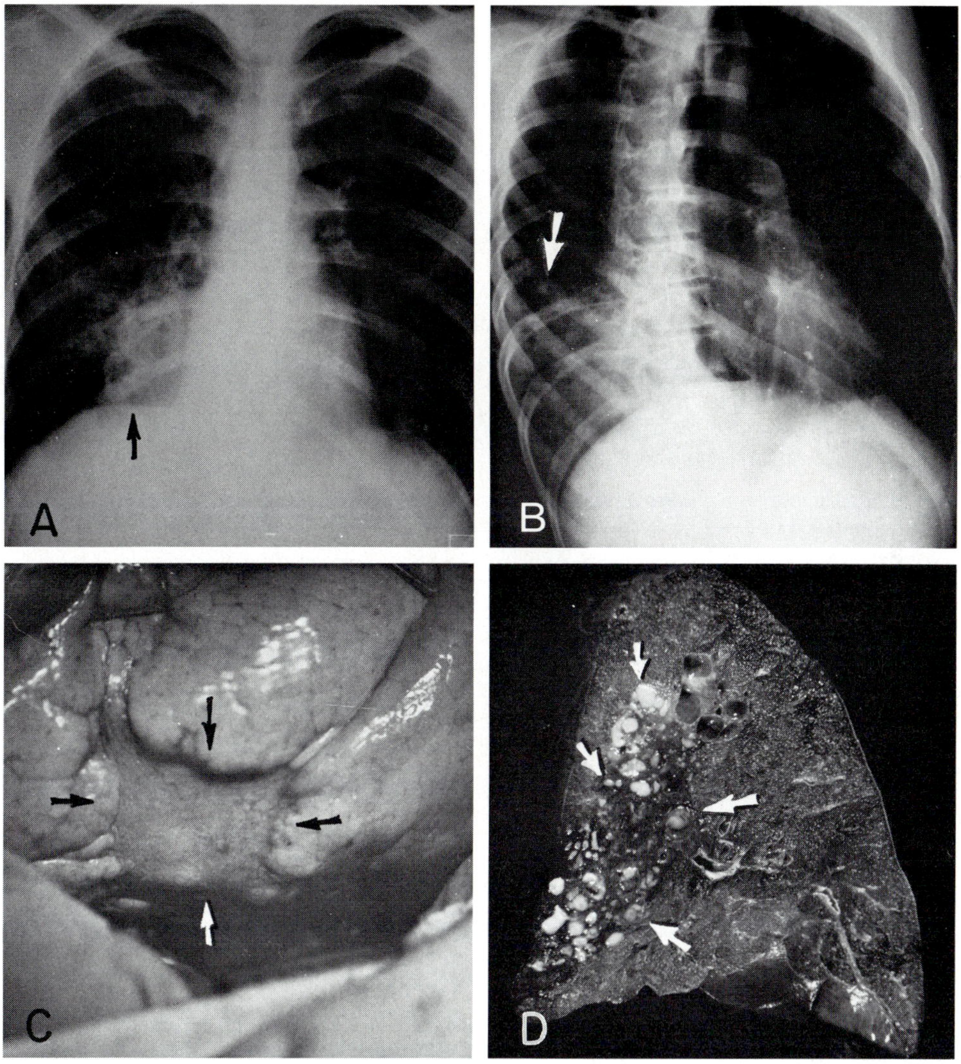

FIG. 6-56. Intralobar sequestration, right lower lobe.

A, and *B*, Plain films of the chest in posteroanterior and oblique views, showing involved area of the right lower lobe in 13-year-old boy. An episode of pneumonia had occurred 1 year before with incomplete clearing, followed by a second acute infection when these films were obtained. Bronchography showed no communication of the lower lobe bronchial tree with this area of lung tissue, suggesting an intralobar sequestration.

C, The right lower lobe at thoracotomy, showing a solid, airless, chronically infected area; lobectomy was performed.

D, Surgical specimen hemisected after preliminary inflation with formalin, showing sequestrated pulmonary tissue surrounded by more normal lung. No bronchial communication existed between the two; the sequestrated portion was filled with multiple abscesses. Latex injection of the blood supply to the lobe showed the two independent arterial systems.

diaphragm in the abdomen, the enteric communication is pulled downward, often retaining its attachment to the cervical vertebral region, traversing the thorax, and communicating with the gut at the level of jejunum or duodenum. A typical case is shown in Fig-

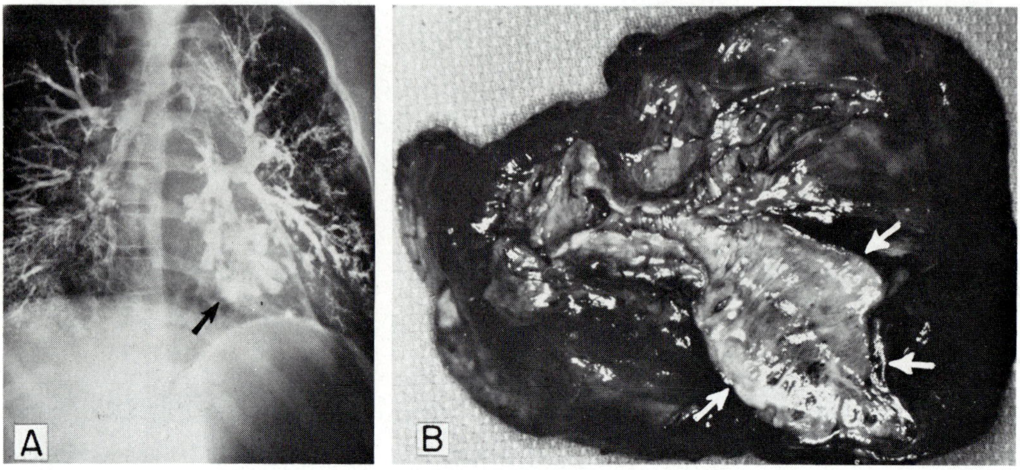

FIG. 6-57. Bronchiectasis in left lower lobe of 8-year-old girl.
A, Bronchogram showing extensive saccular bronchiectasis in the left lower lobe, which is contracted.
B, The surgical specimen with a segmental bronchus laid open to demonstrate the destructive changes and dilatation.

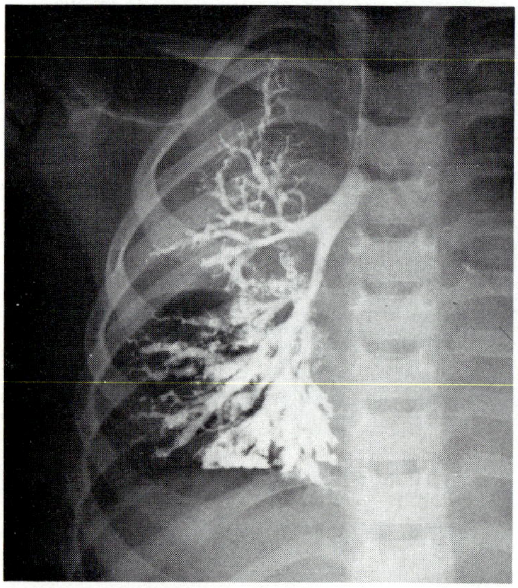

FIG. 6-58. Right lower lobe bronchiectasis. This 4-year-old child had aspirated a peanut at some uncertain time in the past. Pneumonia resulted. The peanut was removed endoscopically, but permanent damage had occurred. This bronchogram was done 2 months later, confirming the presence of progressive severe saccular bronchiectasis, as compared to previous films. Right lower lobectomy was performed. This selective right-sided bronchogram was performed under anesthesia with fluoroscopic control by introduction of contrast material through a bronchoscope.

ure 6-59, a newborn with respiratory distress. An air- and fluid-filled structure was present in the right hemithorax, with a defect in the lower cervical spine. A previous barium swallow had demonstrated its communication with the gastrointestinal tract. Another especially interesting one of these duplications extending into the chest is shown in Figure 6-60. Details of this case have been reported previously.[16] This diagnostic problem of recurrent aspiration pneumonitis was due to constant regurgitation of duodenal contents into the tracheobronchial tree. The occurrence of a congenital enteric communication between the biliary tree and the tracheobronchial tree has also been reported.[114]

Trauma

Penetrating trauma to the thorax is unusual in children, as compared to the adult population where wounds with guns and knives are common. It should be appreciated, however, that a child who has been hit by an automobile or has fallen from a tree can have serious

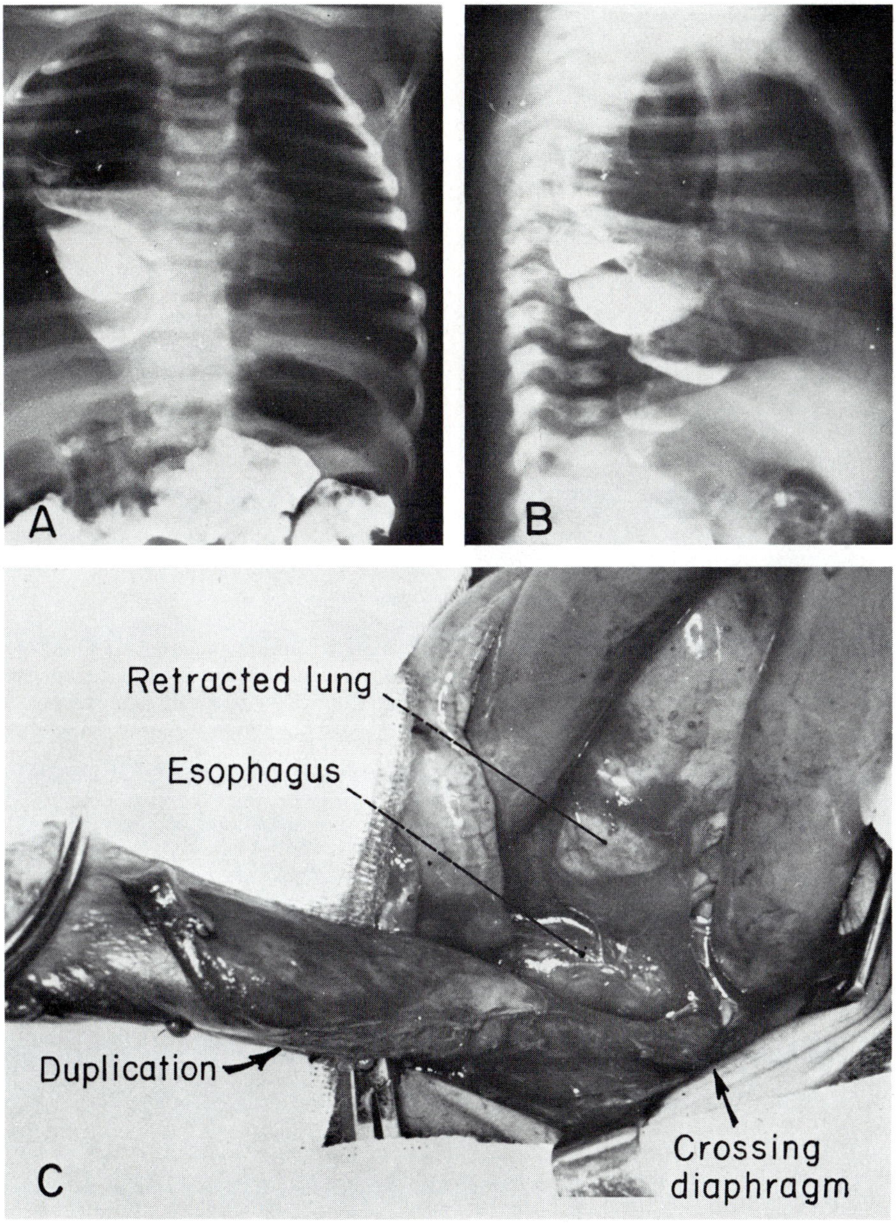

FIG. 6-59. Giant intrathoracic enteric duplication originating below the diaphragm, in a 2-day-old infant who suffered respiratory distress. Abnormality of the lower cervical vertebra raised suspicion of enteric duplication.

A and *B*, Chest roentgenograms after barium swallow showing entry of contrast into the giant diverticulum extending from the proximal jejunum up through the lesser sac into the right pleural space.

C, Operative photograph showing the thoracic component. It had the appearance of a thick-walled segment of colon, but proved to have gastric mucosa as its lining. It was resected down through the diaphragm, and closed at that point. At a second procedure the lower segment in the abdomen was removed. In some cases complete removal can be accomplished in one stage.

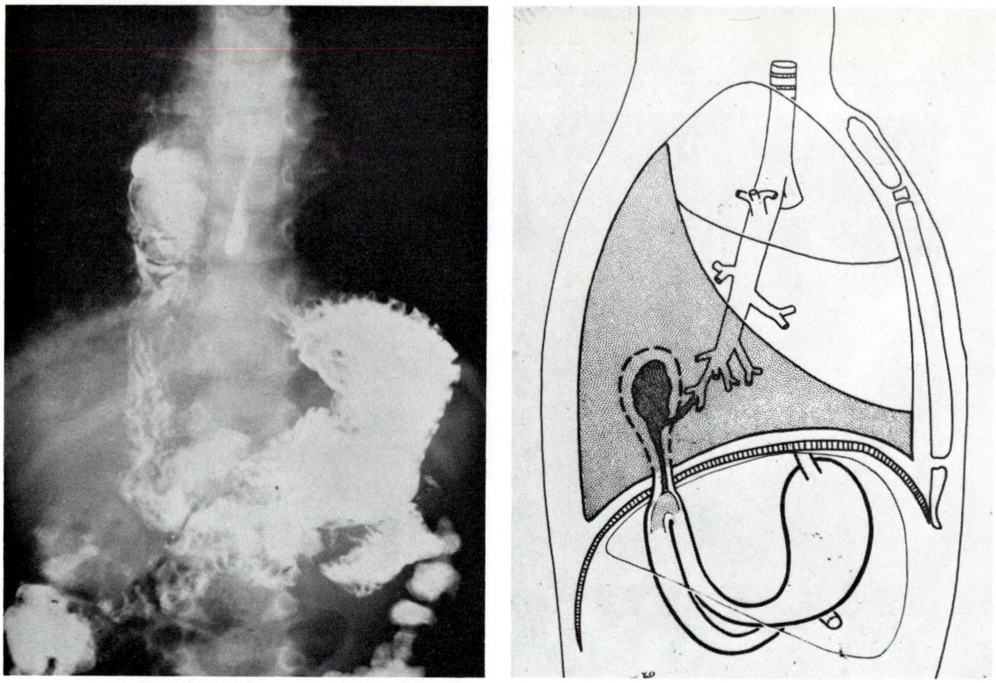

FIG. 6-60. Enteric duplication communicating with right lower lobe.

A, Barium examination showing communication from below diaphragm into right lung.

B, Drawing of anatomy discovered when operation was performed. This consisted of right lower lobectomy and excision of the enteric diverticulum. This 5-year-old boy had been treated for a persistent cough since age 1 year. After extensive previous investigation, including bronchoscopy, diagnosis had been made of recurring infection of unknown cause. Subsequent barium examination revealed the true nature of his difficulty.

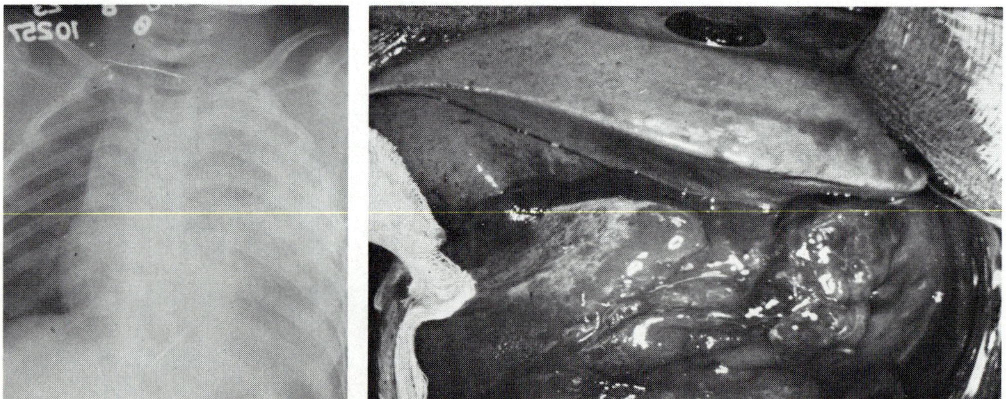

FIG. 6-61. Closed chest trauma with massive left hemothorax and avulsion injury to the lung. This 5-year-old boy was struck by a car, and sustained multiple left rib fractures. Observation and thoracentesis showed continuing bleeding.

A, Preoperative roentgenogram, showing left hemothorax.

B, Operative view showing severely lacerated superior segment of the left lower lobe, treated by segmental resection.

intrathoracic trauma and serious respiratory difficulty. A severe blow to the chest that breaks ribs can lacerate intercostal vessels, causing hemothorax (Fig. 6-61), or a broken rib end can puncture the lung. Serious pulmonary contusion can result from an external force that strikes the chest wall but does not injure the bony thorax. An example is shown in Figure 6-62. This lad was "body slammed" to the floor by his older brother, a wrestling enthusiast, and developed severe pulmonary contusion. Occasionally a sudden compressive injury can rupture the diaphragm, giving the same physiologic consequences as congenital diaphragmatic hernia.[1,2,98] An example is shown in Fig. 6-63.

Any child with signs or symptoms of chest injury should have a chest film as part of the initial evaluation. Fractures of the lower ribs are a good indication of the degree of trauma a child has sustained, and can also be helpful as regards the possibility of rupture of the spleen or liver. Rib fractures are unusual in small children, whose chest cages are more flexible than they will be later. The child in Figure 6-63 had tire marks of a truck passing across the chest, with no rib fractures!

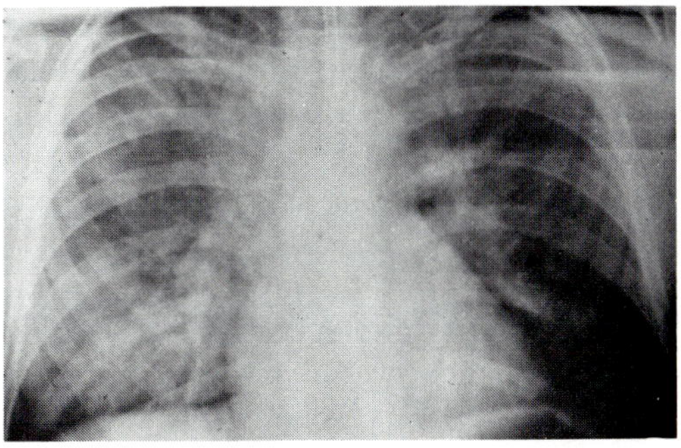

FIG. 6-62. Pulmonary contusion from blunt trauma. This 12-year-old boy was body-slammed flat on his back to the floor by his older brother, a wrestling enthusiast. This diffuse, blunt trauma resulted in the marked bilateral intrapulmonary contusion evident on the roentgenogram. With temporary ventilatory support, he recovered.

The presence of blood in the chest does not necessarily indicate a need for thoracotomy. Closed tube drainage should be employed. Thoracotomy should be considered if the bleeding continues. An air leak may indicate

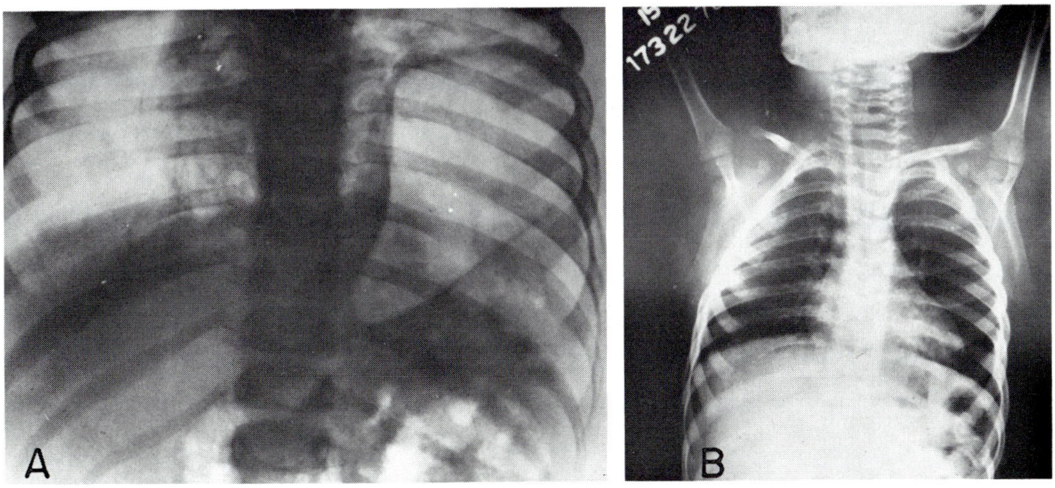

FIG. 6-63. Traumatic rupture of the diaphragm. This 18-month-old boy was run over by a truck. Although there were tire tread marks across the upper abdomen and lower chest, there were no broken bones or other injuries than rupture of the central tendinous part of the diaphragm and laceration of the spleen, both repaired transabdominally.

A, Absence of left diaphragm shadow, with herniation of gastric fundus into lower chest.

B, 2 weeks postoperatively.

rupture of a bronchus and would prompt exploration only if persisting. Caudal displacement of a collapsed lung in the mediastinum should suggest transection of a major bronchus,[80] which can be repaired if done before the onset of mediastinitis. Bronchoscopy would confirm this suspected diagnosis.

Many patients died in previous years from pulmonary contusion and flail chest, formerly treated by external traction devices. Today respiratory support with prolonged endotracheal intubation and ventilatory assistance can sustain many of those patients whose pulmonary contusion and edema formerly proved fatal. These contusions can clear dramatically with the use of ventilatory support and moderate positive end-expiratory pressure.

REFERENCES: PART I

1. Andrus, C. H. and J. H. Morton: Rupture of diaphragm after blunt trauma. *Am. J. Surg. 119*:686, 1970.
2. Asbury, G. F.: Rupture of the diaphragm from blunt trauma. *Arch. Surg. 97*:801, 1968.
3. Azar, H., A. R. Chrispin and D. J. Waterston: Esophageal replacement with transverse colon in infants and children. *J. Pediatr. Surg. 6*:3, 1971.
4. Baran, E. M., H. E. Houston, H. B. Lynn and E. J. O'Connell: Foramen of Morgagni hernias in children. *Surgery 62*:1076, 1967.
5. Bayford, D.: An account of a singular case of deglutition. *Mem. Med. Soc. (Lond.) 2*:275, 1789.
6. Belanger, R., L. LaFleche and J. L. Picard: Congenital cystic adenomatoid malformation of the lung. *Thorax 19*:1, 1964.
7. Berenberg, W. and E. B. D. Neuhauser: Cardioesophageal relaxation (chalasia) as a cause of vomiting in infants. *Pediatrics 5*:414, 1950.
8. Bernhardt, L. C., T. Meyer and W. P. Young: Bifid sternum: case report and surgical management. *J. Thorac. Cardiovasc. Surg. 55*:758, 1968.
9. Blalock, A., R. S. Cunningham and C. S. Robinson: Experimental production of chylothorax by occlusion of superior vena cava. *Ann. Surg. 104*:359, 1936.
10. Borja, A. R., H. T. Ramsdell, Jr., T. V. Thomas and W. Johnson: Lye injuries of the esophagus. *J. Thorac. Cardiovasc. Surg. 57*:533, 1969.
11. Brigham, J. A. W.: Two cases of unilateral paralysis of the diaphragm in the newborn treated surgically. *Thorax 9*:248, 1954.
12. Burford, T. H. and T. B. Ferguson: Congenital lesions of the lungs and emphysema. In *Surgery of the Chest.* J. H. Gibbons, Jr. (Ed.). W. B. Saunders Co., Philadelphia, London, p. 326, 1962.
13. Burrington, J. D. and C. A. Stephens: Esophageal replacement with a gastric tube in infants and children. *J. Pediatr. Surg. 3*:246, 1968.
14. Burrington, J. D. and E. K. Cotton: Removal of foreign bodies from the tracheobronchial tree. *J. Pediatr. Surg. 7*:119, 1972.
15. Cahill, J. L., E. Aberdeen and D. J. Waterston: Results of surgical treatment of esophageal hiatus hernia in infants and children. *Surgery 66*:596, 1969.
16. Case records of the Massachusetts General Hospital, case 32-1961. *N. Engl. J. Med. 264*:936, 1961.
17. Chernick, V. and M. H. Reed: Pneumothorax and chylothorax in the neonatal period. *J. Pediatr. 76*:624, 1970.
18. Chitale, A. R.: Gastric cyst of the mediastinum. *J. Pediatr. 75*:104, 1969.
19. Chrispin, A. R., G. W. Friedland and D. J. Waterston: Aspiration pneumonia and dysphagia after technically successful repair of esophageal atresia. *Thorax 21*:104, 1966.
20. Churchill, E. D. and R. Belsey: Segmental pneumonectomy in bronchiectasis: the lingula segment of the left upper lobe. *Ann. Surg. 109*:481, 1939.
21. Cloud, D. T., Jr., R. F. White, L. M. Linkner and L. C. Taylor: Surgical treatment of esophageal achalasia in children. *J. Pediatr. Surg. 1*:137, 1966.
22. Coupland, G. A. E. and P. P. Rickham: Vagotomy and pyloroplasty in the surgical treatment of hiatus hernia in children. *Aust. N. Z. J. Surg. 37*:121, 1968.
23. Craig, J. M., J. Kirkpatrick and E. B. D. Neuhauser: Congenital cystic adenomatoid malformation of the lung in infants. *Am. J. Roentgenol. 76*:516, 1956.
24. Crawford, T. J. and J. L. Cahill: The surgical treatment of pulmonary cystic disorders in infancy and childhood. *J. Pediatr. Surg. 6*:251, 1971.
25. D'Angio, G. J., S. Farber and C. L. Maddock: Potentiation of x-ray effects of actinomycin D. *Radiology 73*:175, 1959.
26. Davis, C. M.: Inhaled foreign bodies in children, an analysis of 40 cases. *Arch. Dis. Child. 41*:402, 1966.
27. Dees, S. C. and A. Spock: Right middle lobe syndrome in children. *J.A.M.A. 197*:8, 1966.
28. DeParedes, C. G., W. S. Pierce, D. G. Johnson and J. A. Waldhausen: Pulmonary sequestration in infants and children: a 20-year experience and

review of the literature. *J. Pediatr. Surg. 5*:136, 1970.

29. Donahoe, P. K., D. R. Stewart, J. D. Osmond and W. H. Hendren: Pneumoperitoneum secondary to pulmonary air leak. *J. Pediatr. 81:*:797, 1972.
30. Donnellan, W. L.: Respiratory emergencies in the newborn. In *Pediatric Surgery,* 3rd ed., O. Swenson (Ed.) Appleton-Century-Crofts, New York, p. 376, 1969.
31. Eijgelaar, A. and J. H. Bijtel: Congenital cleft sternum, *Thorax 25*:490, 1970.
32. Eklöf, O., G. Ekström, D. O. Eriksson, M. Michaëlsson, O. Stephensen, S. Söderlund, C. Thorén and G. Wallgren: Arterial anomalies causing compression of the trachea and/or the oesophagus. *Acta Paediatr. Scand. 60*:81, 1971.
33. Eraklis, A. J., N. T. Griscom and J. B. McGovern: Bronchogenic cysts of the mediastinum in infancy. *N. Engl. J. Med. 281*:1150, 1969.
34. Ericsson, N. O. and S. Söderlund: Compression of the trachea by an anomalous innominate artery. *J. Pediatr. Surg. 4*:424, 1969.
35. Fabricius, J., H. G. Davidsen and A. T. Hansen: Cardiac function in funnel chest: 26 patients investigated by cardiac catheterization. *Dan. Med. Bull. 4*:251, 1957.
36. Farber, S.: Chemotherapy in the treatment of leukemia and Wilm's tumor. *J.A.M.A. 198*:626, 1966.
37. Fearon, B. and R. Shortreed: Tracheobronchial compression by congenital cardiovascular anomalies in children. *Ann. Otol. Rhinol. Laryngol. 72*:949, 1963.
38. Filler, R. M., D. G. Traggis, N. Jaffe and G. F. Vawter: Favorable outlook for children with mediastinal neuroblastoma. *J. Pediatr. Surg. 7*:136, 1972.
39. Fink, A., A. Rivin and J. F. Murray: Pectus excavatum: an analysis of 27 cases. *Arch. Intern. Med. 108*:427, 1961.
40. Glass, W. M. and M. Goodman: Unsuspected foreign bodies in the young child's esophagus presenting with respiratory problems. *Laryngoscope 76*:605, 1966.
41. Grafe, W. F., E. I. Goldsmith and S. F. Redo: Bronchogenic cysts of the mediastinum in children. *J. Pediatr. Surg. 1*:384, 1966.
42. Grosfeld, J. L., J. W. Kilman and T. R. Frye: Spontaneous pneumopericardium in the newborn infant. *J. Pediatr. 76*:614, 1970.
43. Gross, R. E.: Surgical relief for tracheal obstruction from a vascular ring. *N. Engl. J. Med. 233*:586, 1945.
44. Gross, R. E.: Arterial malformations which cause compression of the trachea or esophagus. *Circulation 11*:124, 1955.
45. Haight, C.: Congenital atresia of the esophagus with tracheoesophageal fistula: reconstruction of esophageal continuity by primary anastomosis. *Ann. Surg. 120*:623, 1944.
46. Haller, J. A. and J. R. Cantrell: Diagnosis and surgical correction of combined congenital defects of supraumbilical abdominal wall, lower sternum and diaphragm. *J. Thorac. Cardiovasc. Surg. 51*:286, 1966.
47. Haller, J. A., Jr., D. O. Majur and W. W. Morgan, Jr.: Diagnosis and management of mediastinal masses in children. *J. Thorac. Cardiovasc. Surg. 58*:385, 1969.
48. Haller, J. A., Jr., H. G. Andrews, J. J. White, M. A. Tamer and W. W. Cleveland: Pathophysiology and management of acute corrosive burns of the esophagus: results of treatment in 285 children. *J. Pediatr. Surg. 6*:578, 1971.
49. Hatch, H. B. and B. C. Buchtel: Roentgenography of the middle lobe syndrome in children. *Am. Rev. Tuberc. 76*:291, 1957.
50. Heimberger, I. L. and J. S. Battersby: Primary mediastinal tumors of childhood. *J. Thorac. Cardiovasc. Surg. 50*:92, 1965.
51. Hendren, W. H. and R. J. Haggerty: Staphylococcal pneumonia in infancy and childhood: analysis of 75 cases. *J.A.M.A. 168*:6, 1958.
52. Hendren, W. H.: Esophageal atresia and tracheoesophageal fistula: principles of management. *Clin. Pediatr. 3*:330, 1964.
53. Hendren, W. H. and D. M. McKee: Lobar emphysema of infancy. *J. Pediatr. Surg. 1*:24, 1966.
54. Hiebert, C. A.: Primary incompetence of the gastric cardia. *Am. J. Surg. 119*:365, 1971.
55. Holder, T. M., V. M. McDonald and M. J. Woolley: The premature or critically ill infant with esophageal atresia: increased success with a staged approach. *J. Thorac. Cardiovasc. Surg. 44*:344, 1962.
56. Holder, T. M., D. T. Cloud, J. E. Lewis, Jr. and G. P. Pilling IV: Esophageal atresia and tracheoesophageal fistula: a survey of its members by the surgical section of the American Academy of Pediatrics. *Pediatrics 34*:542, 1964.
57. Holder, T. M.: Transpleural vs. retropleural approach for repair of tracheoesophageal fistula. *Surg. Clin. North Am. 44*:1433, 1964.
58. Holder, T. M. and M. G. Christy: Cystic adenomatoid malformation of the lung. *J. Thorac. Cardiovasc. Surg. 47*:590, 1964.
59. Holder, T. M., K. W. Ashcraft and L. L. Leape: The treatment of patients with esophageal stricture by local steroid injections. *J. Pediatr. Surg. 4*:646, 1969.
60. Holder, T. M. and K. W. Ashcraft: Esophageal atresia and tracheoesophageal fistula. *Ann. Thorac. Surg. 9*:445, 1970.

61. Holinger, P. H., K. C. Johnston, N. Gossweiler and E. C. Hirsch: Primary fibrosarcoma of the bronchus. *Dis. Chest 37*:137, 1960.
62. Howard, R. and N. A. Myers: Esophageal atresia: a technique for elongating the upper pouch. *Surgery 58*:725, 1965.
63. Izzo, C. and P. P. Rickham: Neonatal pulmonary hamartomas. *J. Pediatr. Surg. 3*:77, 1968.
64. Jaubert de Beaujeu, M., P. Mollard and A. Campo-Paysaa: Surgical tumors of the mediastinum in children. *Ann. Chir. Infants 9*:177, 1968.
65. Jensen, N. R., W. R. Schmidt, J. J. Garamella and M. F. Lynch: Pectus excavatum: the how, when and why of surgical correction. *J. Pediatr. Surg. 5*:4, 1970.
66. Johnson, D. G., R. M. Deaner and C. E. Koop: Diaphragmatic hernia in infancy: factors affecting the mortality rate. *Surgery 62*:1082, 1967.
67. Jones, J. C., C. H. Almond, H. M. Snyder and B. W. Meyer: Congenital pulmonary cysts in infants and children. *Ann. Thorac. Surg. 3*:297, 1967.
68. Keitel, H. G. and S. R. Ziegra: Regurgitation in the full term infant: a controlled clinical study. *Am. J. Dis. Child. 102*:749, 1961.
69. Knox, W. G., J. R. Scott, H. A. Zintel, R. Guthrie and R. E. McCabe: Bouginage and steroids used singly or in combination in experimental corrosive esophagitis. *Ann. Surg. 116*:930, 1967.
70. Koop, C. E. and J. P. Hamilton: Atresia of the esophagus: increased survival with staged procedures in the poor-risk infant. *Ann. Surg. 162*:389, 1965.
71. Koop, C. E.: The role of surgery in resectable, nonresectable and metastatic neuroblastoma. *J.A.M.A. 205*:157, 1968.
72. Koop, C. E., J. W. Hope and E. Abir: Management of nephroblastoma (Wilms' tumor) and abdominal neuroblastoma. *Cancer 14*:178, 1964.
73. Ladd, W. E.: The surgical treatment of esophageal atresia and tracheoesophageal fistula. *N. Engl. J. Med. 230*:625, 1944.
74. Leape, L. L. and L. A. Longino: Infantile lobar emphysema. *Pediatrics 34*:246, 1964.
75. Lilly, J. R. and J. G. Randolph: Hiatal hernia and gastroesophageal reflux in infants and children. *J. Thorac. Cardiovasc. Surg. 55*:42, 1968.
76. Lincoln, J. C. R., P. B. Deverall, J. Stark, E. Aberdeen and D. J. Waterston: Vascular anomalies compressing the oesophagus and trachea. *Thorax 24*:295, 1969.
77. Lincoln, J. C. R., J. Stark, S. Subramanian, E. Aberdeen, R. E. Bonham-Carter, C. L. Berry and D. J. Waterston: Congenital lobar emphysema. *Ann. Surg. 173*:55, 1971.
78. Longino, L. A., M. J. Woolley and R. E. Gross: Esophageal replacement in infants and children with the use of a segment of colon. *J.A.M.A. 171*:1187, 1959.
79. Louhimo, I., M. Pasila and J. K. Visakorpi: Late gastrointestinal complications in patients with colonic replacement of the esophagus. *J. Pediatr. Surg. 4*:663, 1969.
80. Mahour, G. H., H. B. Lynn and D. R. Sanderson: Rupture of the bronchus. *J. Pediatr. Surg. 2*:263, 1967.
81. Martini, N., A. G. Huvos, V. Miké, R. C. Marcove and E. J. Beattie: Multiple pulmonary resections in the treatment of osteogenic sarcoma. *Ann. Thorac. Surg. 12*:271, 1971.
82. Mauney, F. M., Jr., and D. C. Sabiston, Jr.: The role of pulmonary scanning in the diagnosis of congenital lobar emphysema. *Am. Surg. 36*:20, 1970.
83. McNamara, J. J., A. J. Eraklis and R. E. Gross: Congenital posterolateral diaphragmatic hernia in the newborn. *J. Thorac. Cardiovasc. Surg. 55*:55, 1968.
84. McNamara, J. J., D. L. Paulson and H. C. Urschel: Hiatal hernia and gastroesophageal reflux in children. *Pediatrics 43*:527, 1969.
85. Meeker, I. A. and W. H. Snyder, Jr.: Surgical management of diaphragmatic defects in the newborn infant. *Am. J. Surg. 104*:196, 1962.
86. Mendelsohn, H. J. and W. H. Maloney: Treatment of benign strictures of the esophagus with steroid injection. *Ann. Otol. Rhinol. Laryngol. 79*:900, 1970.
87. Middelkamp, J. N., T. B. Ferguson, C. L. Roper and F. D. Hoffman: Management and problems of caustic burns in children. *J. Thorac. Cardiovasc. Surg. 57*:341, 1969.
88. Moncrieff, M. W., A. H. Cameron, R. Astley, K. D. Roberts, L. D. Abrams and J. R. Mann: Congenital cystic adenomatoid malformation of the lung. *Thorax 24*:276, 1969.
89. Munnell, E. R.: Current concepts of thoracic surgery in the management of lymphoma. *Ann. Thorac. Surg. 11*:151, 1971.
90. Murphy, D. A., E. Aberdeen, R. H. Dobbs and D. J. Waterston: The surgical treatment of a syndrome consisting of thoracoabdominal wall; diaphragmatic, pericardial and ventricular septal defects; and a left ventricular diverticulum. Ann. Thorac. Surg. 6:528, 1968.
91. Nanson, E. M.: Lymphangioma of the mediastinum. *J. Cardiovasc. Surg. 9*:447, 1968.
92. Nichols, M. M. and N. J. Hopwood: Alveolar rupture in the newborn. *South. Med. J. 61*:342, 1968.
93. Opsahl, T. and E. J. Berman: Bronchogenic mediastinal cysts in infants. *Pediatrics 30*:376, 1962.
94. Pascuzzi, C.A., D. C. Dahlin and O. T. Clagett:

Primary rib tumors. *Surg. Gynecol. Obstet. 194*:390, 1957.
95. Polgar, G. and C. E. Koop: Pulmonary function in pectus excavatum. *Pediatrics 32*:209, 1963.
96. Potts, W. J. and W. L. Riker: Differentiation of congenital cysts of the lung and those following staphylococcic pneumonia. *Arch. Surg. 61*:68, 1950.
97. Priebe, C. J., Jr. and H. W. Clatworthy: Neuroblastoma. *Arch. Surg. 95*:538, 1967.
98. Radhakrishna, C., S. J. Dickinson and A. Shaw: Acute diaphragmatic hernia from blunt trauma in children. *J. Pediatr. Surg. 4*:553, 1969.
99. Raffensperger, J. and R. Cohen: Plexiform neurofibromas in childhood. *J. Pediatr. Surg. 7*:144, 1972.
100. Randolph, J. G. and R. E. Gross: Congenital chylothorax. *Arch. Surg. 74*:405, 1957.
101. Ravitch, M. M.: The operative treatment of pectus excavatum. *Am. Surg. 129*:429, 1949.
102. Ravitch, M. M.: Tumors of the lung. In *Pediatric Surgery,* Volume 1, 2nd ed., W. T. Mustard, M. M. Ravitch, W. H. Snyder, Jr., K. J. Welch and C. D. Benson (Eds.). Year Book Medical Publishers, Chicago, p. 503, 1969.
103. Ravitch, M. M.: Congenital cystic disease of the lung. In *Pediatric Surgery,* Volume 1, 2nd ed., W. T. Mustard, M. M. Ravitch, W. H. Snyder, Jr., K. J. Welch and C. D. Benson (Eds.). Year Book Medical Publishers, Chicago, p. 452, 1969.
104. Rehbein, F.: The use of internal steel struts in the operative correction of funnel chest. *J. Pediatr. Surg. 1*:80, 1966.
105. Rehbein, F. and N. Schweder: Reconstruction of the esophagus without colon transplantation in casee of esophageal atresia. *J. Pediatr. Surg. 6*:746, 1971.
106. Rhaney, K. and G. P. T. Barclay: Enterogenous cysts and congenital diverticula of the alimentary canal with abnormalities of the vertebral column and spinal cord. *J. Pathol. Bacteriol. 77*:457, 1959.
107. Rickham, P. P.: Strangulated diaphragmatic hernia in the neonatal period. *Thorax 10*:104, 1955.
108. Rickham, P. P.: Lung hernia secondary to congenital absence of ribs. *Arch. Dis. Child. 34*:14, 1959.
109. Robicsek, F., P. W. Sanger, F. H. Taylor and M. J. Thomas: Surgical treatment of costosternal prominence (pectus carinatum). *J. Thorac. Cardiovasc. Surg. 45*:691, 1963.
110. Rohatgi, M., B. Shandling and C. A. Stephens: Hiatus hernia in infants and children: results of surgical treatment. *Surgery 69*:456, 1971.
111. Sabga, G. A., W. E. Neville and L. R. M. DelGuercio: Anomalies of the lung associated with congenital diaphragmatic hernia. *Surgery 50*:547, 1961.
112. Saidi, F. and I. Nazarian: Surgical treatment of hydatid cysts by freezing of cyst wall and instillation of 0.5% silver nitrate solution. *N. Engl. J. Med. 284*:1346, 1971.
113. Samson, P. C.: Empyema thoracis: essentials of present-day management. *Ann. Thorac. Surg. 11*:210, 1971.
114. Sane, S. M., W. K. Sieber and B. R. Girdany: Congenital bronchobiliary fistula. *Surgery 69*:599, 1971.
115. Schiller, M., T. R. Frye and E. T. Boles, Jr.: Evaluation of colonic replacement of the esophagus in children. *J. Pediatr. Surg. 6*:753, 1971.
116. Schuster, S. R., H. Shwachman, G. B. C. Harris and K. Khaw: Pulmonary surgery for cystic fibrosis. *J. Thorac. Cardiovasc. Surg. 48*:750, 1964.
117. Shepard, R., S. Fenn and W. R. Sieber: Evaluation of esophageal function in postoperative esophageal atresia and tracheoesophageal fistula. *Surgery 59*:608, 1966.
118. Simpson, J. S.: Ventral silon pouch: method of repairing congenital diaphragmatic hernias in newborns without increasing intra-abdominal pressure. Surgery 66:798, 1969.
119. Slim, M. S., G. Khayat, A. T. Nasr and Y. D. Jidejian: Hydatid disease in childhood. *J. Pediatr. Surg. 6*:440, 1971.
120. Srouji, M. N.: Pneumothorax and pneumomediastinum in the first 3 days of life. *J. Pediatr. Surg. 2*:410, 1967.
121. Steele, R. W., J. R. Metz, J. W. Bass and J. J. DuBois: Pneumothorax and pneumomediastinum in the newborn. *Radiology 98*:629, 1971.
122. Steelquist, J. H.: Transpleural bronchotomy in treatment of intractable foreign bodies in children. *Am. J. Surg. 118*:188, 1969.
123. Stewart, J. R., O. W. Kincaid and J. E. Edwards: *An Atlas of Vascular Rings and Related Malformations of the Aortic Arch System.* Charles C Thomas, Springfield, Ill., 1964.
124. Stiles, Q. R., G. G. Lindesmith, B. L. Tucker, B. W. Meyer and J. C. Jones: Pleural emphysema in children. *Ann. Thorac. Surg. 10*:37, 1970.
125. Teitelbaum, S. L.: Tumors of the chest wall. *Surg. Gynecol. Obstet. 129*:1059, 1969.
126. Thomas, T. V.: Congenital eventration of the diaphragm. *Ann. Thorac. Surg. 10*:180, 1970.
127. Thompson, D. P. and T. C. Moore: Acute thoracic distress due to spontaneous rupture of a large mediastinal teratoma. *J. Pediatr. Surg. 4*:416, 1969.
128. Tsalyiannis, E., C. Pappis and G. Moussatos: Late results of conservative surgical procedures in hydatid disease of the lung in children. *Surgery 68*:379, 1970.
129. Viscomi, G. J., G. J. Beekhuis and C. F. Whitten: An evaluation of early esophagoscopy and cortico-

steroid therapy in the management of corrosive injury of the esophagus. *J. Pediatr. 59*:356, 1961.
130. Vos, A. and I. Boerema: Surgical treatment of gastroesophageal reflux in infants and children: long-term results in 28 cases. *J. Pediatr. Surg. 6*:101, 1971.
131. Ward, D. E., Jr., H. H. Bradshaw and T. C. Prince, Jr.; Bronchial adenoma in children. *J. Thorac. Cardiovasc. Surg. 27*:295, 1954.
132. Waterman, D. H., S. E. Domm and W. K. Rodgers: Lung abscess—a medicosurgical problem. *Am. J. Surg. 89*:995, 1965.
133. Welch, K. J.: Bronchiectasis. In *Pediatric Surgery,* 2nd ed. W. T. Mustard, M. M. Ravitch, W. H. Snyder, Jr., K. J. Welch and C. D. Benson (Eds.). Year Book Medical Publishers, Chicago, p. 466, 1969.
134. Welch, K. J.: Lung abscess. In *Pediatric Surgery,* Volume 1, 2nd ed. W. T. Mustard, M. M. Ravitch, W. H. Snyder, Jr., K. J. Welch and C. D. Benson. (Eds.). Year Book Medical Publishers, Chicago, p. 482, 1969.
135. Welch, K. N.: Satisfactory surgical correction of pectus excavatum deformity in childhood. *J. Thorac. Surg. 36*:397, 1958.
136. Weston, J. T.: Airway foreign body fatalities in children. *Ann. Otol. Rhinol. Laryngol. 74*:1144, 1965.
137. Woodward, E. R., J. E. Raye and J. M. Clarke: Esophageal hiatus hernia. *Curr. Probl. Surg.,* December, 1970.
138. Woolley, M. M., F. Leix, P. W. Johnston and D. M. Hays: Esophageal atresia types A and B: upper pouch elongation and delayed anatomic reconstruction. *J. Pediatr. Surg. 4*:148, 1969.
139. Yancey, W. S. and A. Spock: Spontaneous neonatal pleural effusion. *J. Pediatr. Surg. 2*:313, 1967.

Part II. *Thoracic Surgical Techniques*

This section is set aside for comment on certain procedures that are important in the evaluation of both medical and surgical thoracic problems. Endoscopy receives major emphasis, and brief comments are made on those radiographic procedures that the surgeon finds most useful. Therapeutic measures, including closed thoracotomy and tracheostomy, are discussed as well.

Diagnostic Techniques

ENDOSCOPY

The newer fiberoptic instruments, with sophisticated lens systems,[3] have made endoscopy practical and useful in children. To care adequately for a toddler who has aspirated a peanut, one must have available the appropriate miniaturized equipment, including special foreign body forceps. It is useless, and possibly hazardous, to attempt treating a child with oversized adult equipment. We believe that the physicians in charge of administrative planning for pediatrics must see to it that the hospital has appropriate endoscopic equipment for neonates, toddlers, and older children; one size does not suit all patients. Although this statement on equipment seems almost too obvious to mention, we have encountered many patients referred from hospitals in which no suitable endoscopic equipment was available.

Laryngoscopy. *Every physician,* regardless of specialty, should be thoroughly acquainted with the equipment and technique for direct laryngoscopy to establish an emergency airway in case time does not allow him to summon an anesthesiologist, otorhinolaryngologist, or general surgeon. This experience can be gained first in the postmortem room as a medical student. The most common error in visualization of the larynx is to hyperextend the head; this positioning throws the larynx forward and out of sight. The larynx is best seen in the "sniffing position,"—a slight forward extension of the head and neck, which one assumes to better sniff a rose held a little in front of and above one's nose. If the child is lying on his back, a small pillow under the head achieves this position.

Clinical circumstances dictate details of the procedure. For example, in a newborn with respiratory distress, laryngoscopic examination can reveal an obstructing cyst or tumor, an abnormality of the epiglottis or the vocal cords, or cord paralysis. Figure 6-64 shows a postmortem specimen from an otherwise healthy newborn who died from asphyxia by a simple mucous-filled cyst at the laryngeal inlet. Immediate laryngoscopy, with passage of an appropriate endotracheal tube beyond the cyst, would have assured a good airway; then it would have been an easy matter to unroof the cyst to cure the infant. Every emergency room should be equipped with pediatric laryngoscopes and all sizes of endotracheal tubes. The new plastic or silicone tubes are most appropriate, for they cause minimal foreign body reaction of the delicate endolaryngeal mucosa.

Laryngoscopy is indicated in some children as an elective study. A general anesthetic is usually administered by mask to an appropriate depth; then a detailed examination can be made of the larynx. The *anterior commissure laryngoscope,* which is shaped to fit into the aperture of the larynx separating the arytenoid cartilages, is particularly useful. With appropriate miniature electrodes one may be able to endoscopically incise a laryngeal web, unroof an endolaryngeal cyst, or electrocoagulate a small hemangioma.

A word of caution is in order with regard to the child who enters with partial respiratory obstruction from acute epiglottitis or acute laryngotracheobronchitis. If the clinical picture suggests that problem rather than a foreign body, an immediate laryngoscopy can

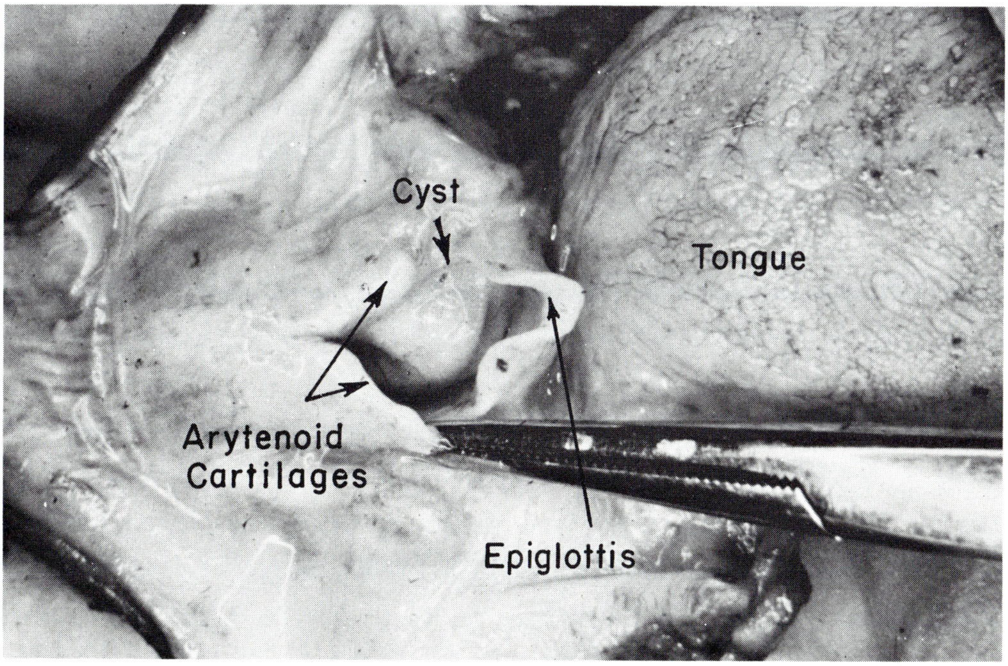

FIG. 6-64. Autopsy specimen of larynx in an otherwise normal newborn who died from airway obstruction caused by a simple cyst at the base of the epiglottis.

precipitate complete respiratory obstruction and cardiac arrest. We would favor first providing high humidity and oxygen as the child is transferred to the operating room where all is in readiness to deal with respiratory obstruction, with equipment for bronchoscopy and tracheostomy and adequate personnel to assist. In many major medical centers, radiographic examination of the neck is used to diagnose epiglottitis, thereby obviating the need for direct laryngoscopy (see Chapter 19).

In adults insertion of a large-bore needle into the trachea has been used by some as an immediate measure to deal with laryngeal obstruction. We would discourage the use of this technique in children because the child's trachea is soft and often not easily palpable. Air exchange through a relatively small needle is not adequate. The use of an endotracheal tube is preferred in an emergency.

In extreme circumstances, when a child is limp, pale and on the verge of hypoxic cardiac arrest, it is usually best to first inflate the lungs with oxygen by positive pressure before attempting insertion of a tube. Mouth-to-mouth ventilation may be the only technique possible; if an oxygen hose is available, the physician can hold it in the corner of his mouth, to deliver a high oxygen concentration. We have resuscitated many infants in this manner while more sophisticated equipment was being fetched. Of course a mask and ventilating bag are best. If the heart is not beating, closed precordial cardiac massage by a second person must accompany the ventilatory assistance. After the patient's oxygenation is improved and heart beat is assured, time can be taken to pass an endotracheal tube to overcome the upper airway obstruction. We have witnessed several tragedies when precious moments were spent trying to intubate the already hypoxic child instead of first pressure-ventilating the patient. (Cardiopulmonary resuscitation is discussed in further detail in Chapter 3.)

Bronchoscopy. This procedure was formerly not very satisfactory in small patients. However, with the new miniaturized fiberoptic instruments, a very clear view can be obtained of endobronchial anatomy. The need for bronchoscopy, like laryngoscopy, varies according to circumstances. It may be indicated in a postoperative child with a mucous plug that is not raised by physiotherapy. Sometimes this procedure may be repeated one or more times. More often bronchoscopy is used to exclude a lesion or distortion of the trachea or bronchi, sometimes with bronchography. In children these diagnostic procedures are best carried out under a general anesthetic in most instances. Halothane anesthesia is administered by mask, and the bronchoscope is introduced. Anesthetic control is maintained by ventilating through a sidearm of the bronchoscope. This practice assures complete and safe control during the examination, which can be performed in an unhurried manner, with close cooperation of anesthesiologist and surgeon. An intravenous line should always be established; electrocardiographic monitoring is essential during these examinations in a darkened operating room.

Mediastinoscopy. This examination is done frequently in adults for biopsy of paratracheal or suprahilar lymph nodes as an aid to diagnosis in cancer, sarcoidosis, and other disorders. Occasionally it can be useful in children. Under a general endotracheal anesthesia a small incision is made above the suprasternal notch, dissecting into the superior mediastinum, just anterolateral to the trachea, taking care not to injure the recurrent laryngeal nerve or adjacent great vessels. When a sterile laryngoscope has been inserted into the wound, next to the trachea, one can visualize down as far as the tracheal bifurcation to secure an appropriate biopsy. One avoids entering the pleural space.

Esophagoscopy. Visualization of the esophagus in children should be performed always under a general endotracheal anesthetic with the same type of monitoring used for bronchoscopy. Much information can be obtained in the appropriate patient. For example, in a child with recurrent aspiration pneumonitis from an isolated tracheoesophageal fistula, introduction of methylene blue through the endotracheal tube, with simultaneous visualization of the cervical esophagus, may show contrast material passing through the fistula in cases where usual radiographic techniques have failed to disclose the communication. Another technique to see these fistulas is visualization of the back wall of the trachea with a fore-oblique telescope.

Those swallowed foreign bodies that lodge in the esophagus and cannot be retrieved by the Foley catheter balloon technique may be removed in most instances with foreign body forceps. In a child with a history of possible ingestion of a corrosive substance, esophagoscopy is of value to determine whether the esophagus has been burned. This technique is a useful guide to further management by steroids, antibiotics, and dilatation. Esophagoscopy is often used in postoperative infants with esophageal atresia, in whom anastomotic stenosis is common. It affords direct visualization of the anastomosis, and introduction of appropriate dilators. More recently injection of triamcinolone into these strictures, using a long endoscopic needle, has proven of value in association with dilatation.[5] This technique has averted segmental esophageal resection in certain cases. In the distal esophagus, direct visualization can confirm the presence of esophageal varices or peptic esophagitis. It can also be of help in the diagnosis of hiatus hernia.[4]

RADIOLOGY

As surgeons we would not presume to describe in detail the radiologic evaluation of pediatric thoracic disease. Nevertheless it is pertinent to underscore those examinations that the surgeon has found most useful in evaluating problems in his area of interest.

The Plain Film of the Chest. Both frontal and lateral views should be routine. Much more information can be obtained if the physician indicates clearly to the radiologist specifically what he is trying to find. For example, if a baby appears to have vascular compression of the trachea, the physician's request for a view with technique to show the tracheal air column, as in Figure 6-65, may provide the basis for diagnosis. If a patient is suspected of having pheochromocytoma, a request for oblique films of the thorax may disclose a small paravertebral tumor not apparent on conventional anteroposterior and lateral films (Fig. 6-66).

If the film is too dark, careful scrutiny of the lung pattern using a bright light can be helpful in making a differential diagnosis of pneumothorax, lobar emphysema, lung cysts, or post-inflammatory pneumatocele. In lobar emphysema all of the bronchovascular markings are present, but splayed out in the emphysematous lobe.

Barium Swallow. Barium examination of the esophagus is essential in diagnosing a number of surgically correctable problems outlined in Part I of this chapter. In the small infant with respiratory distress, the examination should be performed with a soft tube introduced into the upper esophagus. The responsible physician should be present in case aspiration occurs during the examination. Again, close communication between clinician and radiologist is essential. For example, a "routine" barium swallow in erect position may appear perfectly normal in a patient with hiatus hernia; a study in the supine position, or with head down, together with gentle compression of the epigastrium may show the hernia. Barium swallow together with soft tissue films of the trachea can be of great value in the diagnosis of vascular ring malformation, as seen in Figure 6-65. In that particular child a mistaken diagnosis of anomalous subclavian artery had been entertained because posterior compression of the esophagus existed; the narrowed tracheal air column was not noted, a finding that indicated complete encirclement of esophagus and trachea.

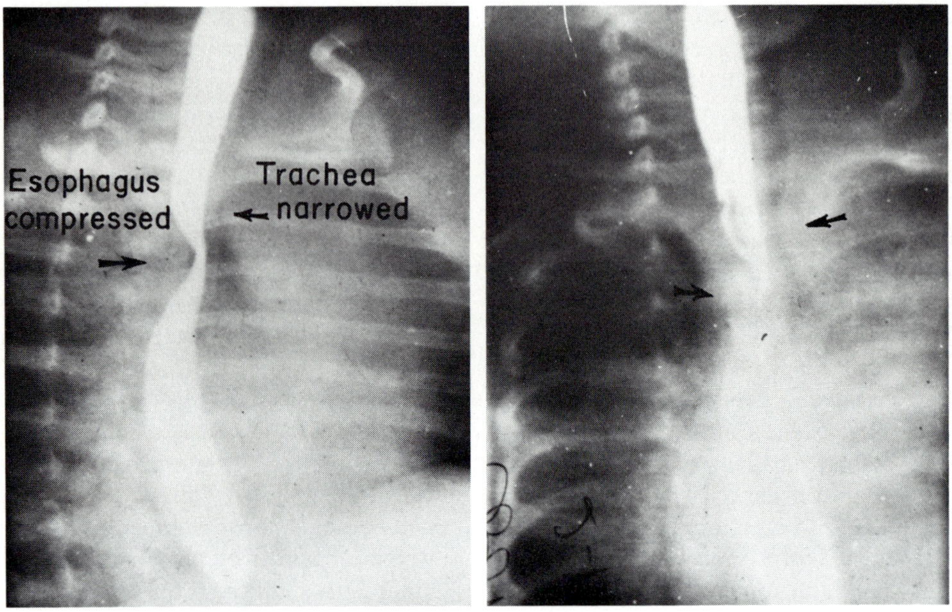

FIG. 6-65. Vascular ring compressing esophagus and trachea in a neonate, with respiratory distress accentuated during feeding. Note obvious indentation of esophagus by the posterior arch, but more subtle "white out" of tracheal air column by anterior aortic arch.

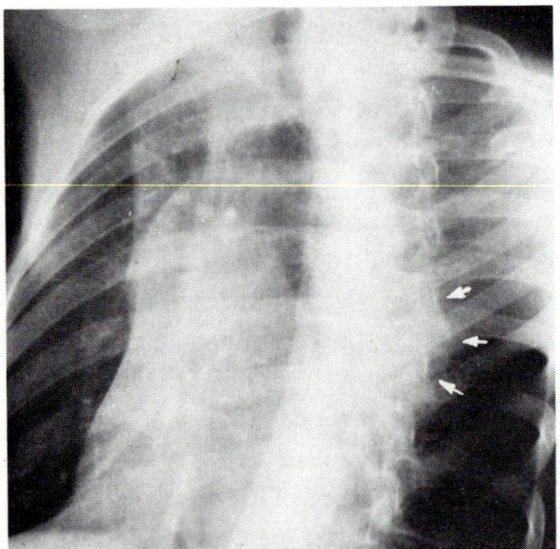

FIG. 6-66. Oblique film of chest showing a small paraspinal pheochromocytoma not evident on conventional anteroposterior and lateral views.

Bronchography. In the adult who will cooperate and agree to remain awake, bronchography can usually be performed by passing an opaque catheter into the tracheobronchial tree after suitable topical spray. This technique can also be done on older children. More often, however, the patient is an infant or a frightened youngster in whom a general anesthetic is necessary. We prefer to do the examination together with bronchoscopy under anesthesia in the department of roentgenology, with the same type of monitoring as used in the operating room. Blindly instilling contrast material through the bronchoscope does not result in good quality films. It is better to have fluoroscopic guidance while injecting the opaque medium, and to obtain appropriate films in various positions when the tracheobronchial tree is suitably filled. Skilled anesthetic control is imperative for, if the youngster coughs, the contrast material is blown into the alveoli, and a poor study results. Topical application of Xylocaine can reduce the likelihood of coughing. Bronchography is of great value in assessing a variety

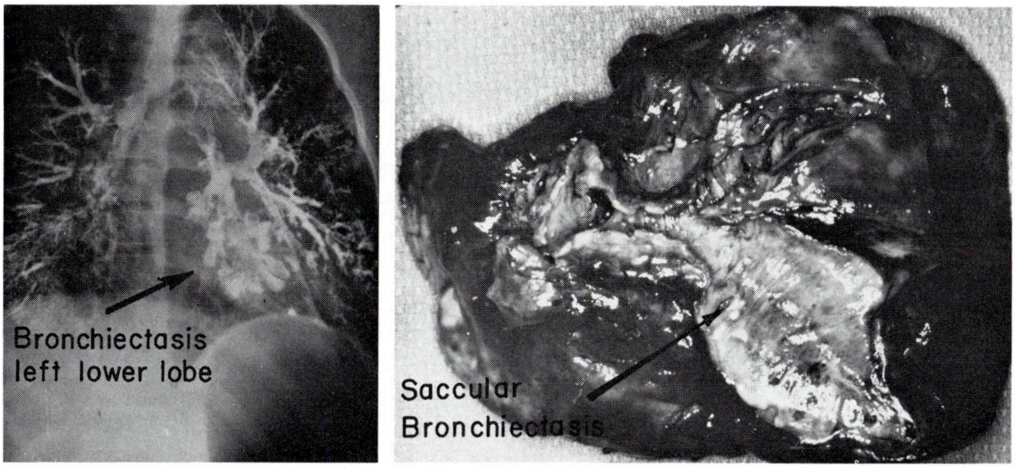

FIG. 6-67. Localized left lower lobe bronchiectasis.
A, Bronchogram showing disease confined to the left lower lobe; remainder of tracheobronchial tree normal.
B, Surgically resected lower lobe, in which one of the diseased bronchi has been laid open to demonstrate its saccular configuration.

of surgically correctable problems. Figure 6-67 is an example of bronchiectasis confined to the left lower lobe. By excluding disease in other lobes, this examination guided the therapy, which was quite properly surgical resection.

Laminography. This technique has proven of value in our experience, both in better defining the borders of an isolated lesion, such as shown in Figure 6-68, and in defining multiple intraparenchymal nodules, for instance, in a youngster with metastatic Wilms' tumor.

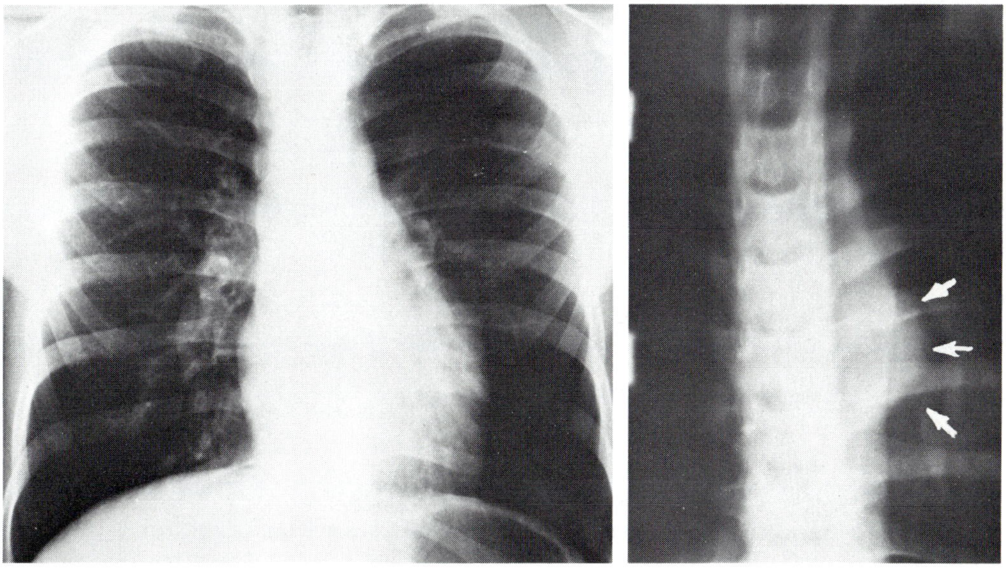

FIG. 6-68. Tomography to better delineate small paraspinal pheochromocytoma of same child shown in Figure 6-66.
A, Anteroposterior view in which mass was completely inapparent.
B, A tomogram "cut" at the level of the vertebra, clearly defining the mass.

Angiography. Modern angiographic techniques have proven of great value in precise delineation of pathology in the abdomen and thorax of infants and children. Figure 6-69 shows a case in which a one-injection venous angiogram proved quickly the absence of a left lung in an infant referred with mild respiratory distress and the diagnosis of left-sided pulmonary pathology. Aside from the obvious value of angiography in defining cardiac anatomy, these studies in selected cases can be useful to better delineate arteriovenous malformations, sequestrated pulmonary lobes, mediastinal masses, and other diagnostic problems. In skilled hands these techniques are generally safe.

Radioscintigraphy. Radioscintigraphy is often a useful adjunct to the establishment of pathophysiologic mechanisms in infants and children with pulmonary disease.[1,8] These methods are discussed in Chapter 19.

Surgical Procedures

THORACENTESIS

The insertion of a needle into the thorax can be life saving in a patient who enters the emergency room with an extreme degree of tension pneumothorax. It can also be of great help diagnostically in many circumstances. Usually plain films of the chest should be obtained first to guide the insertion of a needle; one must keep in mind the structures that lie beneath the point of entry. In the small child who will not cooperate, it is mandatory to have enough nursing assistance to immobilize the patient. With local anesthetic in the skin and chest wall, the needle should be inserted slowly through an interspace on the top of the lower rib, avoiding the neurovascular bundle of the upper rib. Specimens can be obtained for cytology and bacteriology,

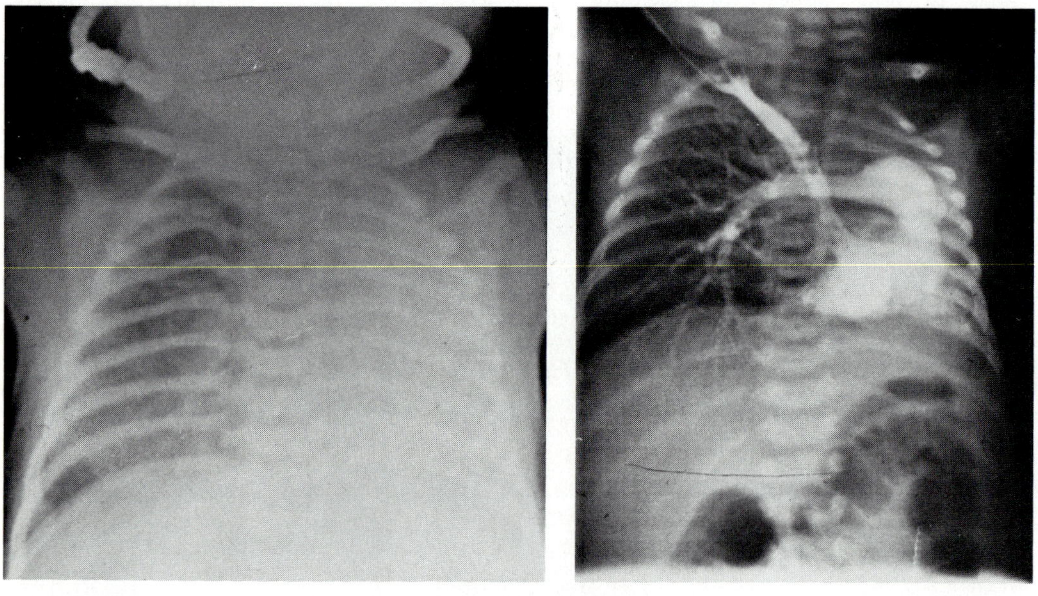

FIG. 6-69. Angiography in a newborn referred with respiratory distress.

A, Plain film of chest (with opaque left thorax) for which the infant was referred with a diagnosis of pulmonary atelectasis or pleural fluid collection. Absence of a mediastinal shadow overlying the spine raised the possibility of no left lung.

B, Angiographic confirmation of agenesis of the left lung. Needle aspiration of this newborn's chest might have been disastrous!

and the procedure may be therapeutic for small fluid or air collections. When there is a large quantity of fluid, such as in empyema, or if an active air leak is present, we would prefer inserting a chest tube as a safer, more effective, and *more conservative* course.

CLOSED THORACOTOMY

The insertion of a chest tube is a simple procedure that can provide great help in a number of thoracic problems of childhood. Like thoracentesis it must be done correctly. Although trocars are available with which to pierce the chest wall and through which catheters can be inserted, we much prefer the following technique, which is safer: A small incision about 4 to 5 mm long is made in the skin at an appropriate point. Using a hemostatic clamp, the surgeon tunnels through to the underlying interspace and into the pleural space. By spreading thc jaws of the clamp, he can hear the rush of air, which signals entry to the pleural space. An appropriate catheter can be introduced through this tract using some hand forceps, followed by withdrawal of the clamp. This technique is safe, does not lacerate the intercostal vessels, and does not risk plunging into the heart or great vessels. It can be accomplished in a moment with minimal equipment.

For a drainage catheter in children an ordinary plastic or rubber urethral catheter suffices. Before the procedure, extra holes are cut along the end of the catheter for better drainage. Also a marking ligature is tied at a point that looks like the proper length of tube to thrust into the chest cavity; otherwise one cannot be certain whether too much or too little tube has been inserted except by x-ray examination. The tube must be firmly anchored with adhesive tape. It is not satisfactory to rely on a single fixation stitch, particularly in a child. Connecting tubing must be thoroughly fastened with adhesive tape, and all drainage bottle connections must be similarly taped to prevent a catastrophic leak. Each hospital has its own system of one-, two-, or three-bottle chest drainage. The clinician and all nurses in attendance must familiarize themselves with the intricacies of the equipment at hand.

When there is a sizeable accumulation of pleural fluid, such as in staphylococcal empyema, the insertion of a tube is more effective and safer than multiple needle aspirations. Likewise, in an infant with severe respiratory distress and a large pneumothorax, we believe that insertion of a chest tube is a more conservative procedure than needle aspiration of the chest. In removing a closed thoracostomy tube, suction is maintained as the tube is extracted, and the hole is quickly covered with vaseline gauze to prevent ingress of air. The hole generally seals in a few hours. When only air, not fluid, must be aspirated from the pleural space, it is often satisfactory to use a percutaneous needle to insert a small plastic catheter such as commonly used for intravenous fluid administration. (If it proves ineffective, a larger tube should be substituted.) Care must be exercised to avoid transecting these small catheters upon withdrawing the introducing needle.

LUNG BIOPSY

Closed needle aspiration of lung parenchyma is an excellent source of material for smear and culture when an adequate sputum specimen cannot be obtained. For microscopic tissue diagnosis, the procedure is rarely indicated in children except in widespread thoracic tumor where a tissue diagnosis is desired. Even then, one must be careful. We recall a child with a large chest mass that was assumed to be inoperable, diagnosed as a malignant teratoma by closed needle biopsy. He died, and at autopsy the tumor was large, but encapsulated, not invasive, and could likely have been removed.

Open lung biopsy is best used when pulmonary histology is needed to make a definite diagnosis in such conditions as sarcoidosis, histiocytosis, tumors, or primary pulmonary vascular disease. It entails a small thoracotomy through an interspace under general anesthesia. The edge of a lobe is grasped with atraumatic lung forceps; a small wedge of tissue is removed and the edge is oversewn. The procedure is short and morbidity is low.

TRACHEOSTOMY[6]

The concept of an emergency tracheostomy should be entirely discarded. What should be substituted is the concept of emergency establishment of an airway by inserting an endotracheal tube or a bronchoscope. This procedure serves to relieve respiratory obstruction and makes possible an *elective tracheostomy* under controlled, safe circumstances.

When a child needs tracheostomy, positive pressure ventilation with 100% oxygen may be needed first, as mentioned earlier in this chapter. Then an endotracheal tube should be passed and secured firmly with adhesive tape, and the child should then be transported to the operating room where the procedure can be performed under optimal circumstances. We customarily administer a brief anesthetic of halothane. The endotracheal tube is then removed and a pediatric bronchoscope is inserted; through it the tracheobronchial tree can be suctioned and anesthetic insufflation maintained. After the child's head has been extended, the tip of the bronchoscope is positioned in the lower cervical trachea and tipped forward, which brings the trachea just beneath the skin where it can be identified easily with minimal dissection (Fig. 6-70).

A short transverse skin incision, only a centimeter or more in length, is made at a point about halfway between the suprasternal notch and the cricoid cartilage. The cricoid cartilage can be palpated readily when a rigid bronchoscope is inserted within the trachea. Satisfactory performance of this operation through a small incision requires adequate assistance. Using four small retractors, the physician can carry the dissection bluntly down to the anterior wall of the trachea. Palpating over the bronchoscope, which is holding the trachea forward, one can count accurately the tracheal rings, making a vertical incision through the second, third, and fourth rings. *No tracheal wall should be resected.* If the surgeon incises through the cricoid cartilage by error and places the tracheostomy tube too high, stenosis of the lower larynx may result.[7] If the tube is placed too low, when the neck is subsequently flexed, the tracheal opening may retract down into the mediastinum, permitting the tube to slip out, and the child may asphyxiate. When the head is extended backward, the upper mediastinal trachea slides up into the neck. Careless placement of the tube, without accurately counting the tracheal rings, can result in placing the tube in a segment of trachea that will retract downward when the neck is subsequently flexed. A suture is placed in the tracheal wall on each side of the opening, and tied over a button, which is fastened to the neck with adhesive. Then two handles are available in case the tracheostomy tube should become dislodged and facilitates replacement of a tube in the immediate postoperative period before a mature sinus tract is established.

For a tracheostomy device, we much prefer the new soft plastic tubes shown in Figure 6-71. Silicone tubes, which are even less reactive, have been made available recently. Metal tracheostomy tubes with inner cannulas are still used in many institutions, but we believe them to be dangerous. They are stiff, can erode the trachea, and do not adapt to changes of position; we think *they should be made obsolete.* The plastic catheters, if kept suitably moist by high humidity, do not tend to encrust with secretions, thus obviating the need for an inner, removable cannula.[9,10]

Postoperative care for a child with a tracheostomy is of great importance.[2] The rate of complications is related to the experience

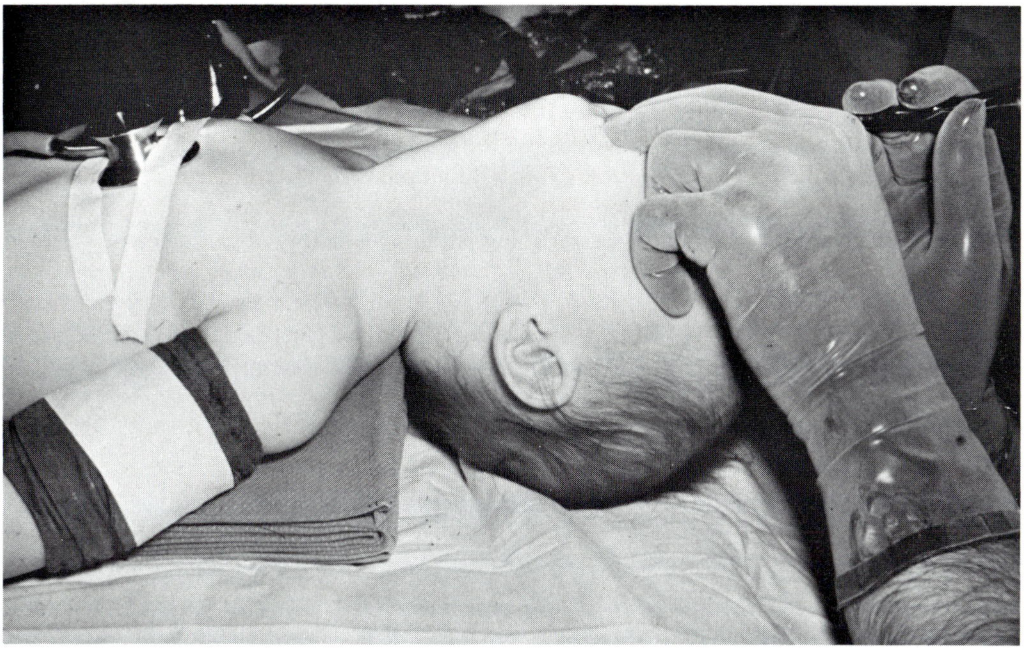

FIG. 6-70. Positioning for tracheotomy. Using a bronchoscope and a brief general anesthetic, the physician can elevate the trachea into a subcutaneous position, facilitating its easy exposure with minimal dissection, and permitting accurate counting of the tracheal rings for insertion of the tracheotomy tube. This procedure is much more reliable than palpating the trachea over a relatively soft pediatric endotracheal tube.

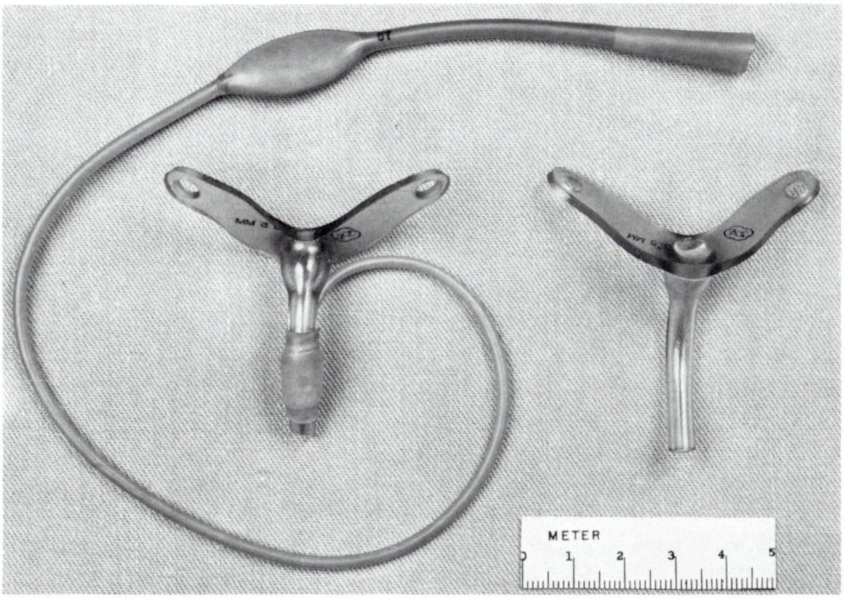

FIG. 6-71. Plastic tracheotomy tubes of Great Ormond Street design. On the left is a tube with an inflatable cuff, which is seldom necessary in children. It is preferable to insert a tube that approximates the internal diameter of the trachea, accepting a small air leak. *Prolonged localized pressure with a cuffed tube can cause tracheal necrosis and subsequent stenosis, a formidable complication of tracheotomy.*

and the diligence of personnel involved. If a child with a new tracheostomy suddenly begins to have respiratory distress, only a moment should be spent suctioning the tube. If suctioning does not relieve the problem immediately, *the tube should be immediately extracted,* assuming that it has become dislodged. An endotracheal tube can be passed, if necessary, and with the previously placed sutures on the wall of the trachea, another tracheostomy tube can be reinserted. Each new group of house officers must be warned of this problem so that they will not fear to extract a tracheostomy tube when the circumstances warrant.

Another extremely important concept is the maintenance of high humidity. If the child breathes dry air through a tube, it will encrust and plug. *Adequate humidity prevents this complication.*

Extubating a child with a tracheostomy can be a formidable undertaking. Several factors make this statement true, particularly for small infants. One is that the infant larynx may be relatively small, and hypoplastic if it has not been used for several weeks or months. Dr. Peter Wurnig of Vienna has devised a clever one-way valve to place in the infant's tracheostomy tube; it permits inhalation through the tube, but exhalation through the larynx. Another important consideration is that granulation tissue can accumulate at the tracheostomy site and may project into the lumen of the trachea like a polyp, causing partial obstruction. This tissue can be seen through a bronchoscope, and can be treated by curettage or cauterization. Localized tracheomalacia seems to develop in some infants who have had a tracheostomy tube in place for a long time.

In most cases where a tube has been used for only a short time, extubation can be accomplished by sedating the child, quietly removing the tube, and observing the baby closely for the succeeding several hours. If one attempts extubating a small infant who is fully awake, he often struggles, begins to cry, and sucks in the tracheostomy opening, completely obstructing the trachea. *A tracheostomy tube should never be removed in the evening.* It should be done only early in the day, with a full staff present, and with close attendance by personnel who are thoroughly versed in resuscitation and airway management.

REFERENCES: PART II

1. Ball, W. C., P. B. Stewart, L. G. S. Newsham and D. V. Bates: Regional pulmonary function studies with xenon-133. *J. Clin. Invest. 41*:519, 1962.
2. Crocker, D.: The critically ill child: management of tracheostomy. *Pediatrics 46*:286, 1970.
3. Gans, S. L. and G. Berci: Advances in endoscopy of infants and children. *J. Pediatr. Surg. 6*:199, 1971.
4. Heibert, C. A.: Primary incompetence of the gastric cardia. *Am. J. Surg. 119*:365, 1971.
5. Holder, T. M., K. W. Ashcraft and L. L. Leape: The treatment of patients with esophageal stricture by local steroid injections. *J. Pediatr. Surg. 4*:646, 1969.
6. Hollinger, P. H., W. T. Brown and D. G. Maurizi: Tracheotomy in the newborn. *Am. J. Surg. 109*:771, 1965.
7. Louhimo, I., B. Grahne, M. Pasila and T. Suutarinen: Acquired laryngotracheal stenosis in children. *J. Pediatr. Surg. 6*:730, 1971.
8. Shannon, D. S., E. J. Riseborough and H. Kazemi: Ventilation-perfusion relationships following correction of kyphoscoliosis. *J.A.M.A. 217*:579, 1971.
9. Stool, S. E., J. R. Campbell and D. G. Johnson: Tracheostomy in children: the use of plastic tubes. *J. Pediatr. Surg. 3*:402, 1968.
10. Talbert, J. L. and J. A. Haller, Jr.: Improved silastic tracheostomy tubes for infants and young children. *J. Pediatr. Surg. 3*:408, 1968.

The Abnormal Pulmonary Circulation

JULIEN I. E. HOFFMAN

7

General Pathophysiologic Mechanisms

(1) *Increased pulmonary vascular resistance.* This abnormality is the most common. By itself it does not interfere with gas exchange and its major effect is on the heart. If there is a sudden and marked rise in pulmonary vascular resistance, as in pulmonary embolism, there will be acute right heart dilatation and failure. Recent studies indicate that one factor in failure of the right ventricle is the high right ventricular systolic pressure, which impairs coronary flow to the right ventricular wall and makes it ischemic.[33] As a result of the acute right ventricular failure, cardiac output and systemic blood pressure fall, the latter further impairing coronary blood flow. Whatever other treatment is given, measures to raise systemic arterial blood pressure may help to restore right ventricular function.[92,103]

If the increased pulmonary vascular resistance is of long standing, pulmonary arterial and right ventricular hypertension occur, and the right ventricle dilates a little and hypertrophies markedly. This phase, which can last for many years, may end with acute right ventricular failure or arrhythmias. It is seen frequently in certain types of congenital heart disease and in cystic fibrosis.

If intracardiac shunt or a patent ductus arteriosus is present, the raised pulmonary vascular resistance has a profound influence on the size and direction of the shunt. With an initial left-to-right shunt, as in a ventricular septal defect, the raised resistance reduces the left-to-right shunt; then, if the resistance rises still further, it may produce a right-to-left shunt with arterial desaturation. Even if there are no septal defects, there may be a right-to-left shunt through a previously closed foramen ovale.

Finally, if the raised resistance continues for a long time, secondary arterial thromboses and hemorrhages may occur in the lung tissue.[46] This complication is relatively uncommon. When it occurs, there may be patchy reduction in flow to parts of the lung, impaired gas transfer, and perhaps an increase in wasted ventilation.

(2) *Decreased pulmonary vascular resistance.* This condition does not occur as an isolated entity, but when a communication exists at atrial, ventricular, or great arterial levels, an abnormally low pulmonary vascular resistance allows a large left-to-right shunt to occur. The huge venous return to the left atrium and ventricle may then cause left ventricular failure and pulmonary edema. If a low resistance communication exists between pulmonary arteries and veins (a fistula), a right-to-left shunt occurs and causes arterial desaturation.

(3) *Low ventilation-perfusion ratios.* When ventilation to a region is reduced and flow to that region is either normal or not reduced as much as the ventilation is, oxygenation will be inadequate and arterial desaturation results. Typically this pattern is seen with regional atelectasis or airway obstruction. Carbon dioxide does not usually accumulate because it can be eliminated in the remaining normally ventilated areas. However, if ventilation is lowered to many regions because of extensive consolidation or airway obstruction, the work of breathing may increase and this problem, with the decreased ability to ventilate, may lead to carbon dioxide retention.

(4) *High ventilation-perfusion ratios.* Ventilation to these regions is normal but perfusion is reduced or absent, as in pulmonary embolism. Oxygenation of blood is adequate, and carbon dioxide elimination is performed adequately in other regions unless the work of breathing is excessively increased. Some alveoli have no carbon dioxide in them because no blood reaches them so that the mixed expired carbon dioxide is unusually low and therefore arterial and end-expired carbon dioxide tensions differ. This gradient was once suggested as a test for pulmonary embolism,[87] but unfortunately cannot be relied on since airways with no carbon dioxide in them tend to constrict to reduce local ventilation and minimize the ventilation-perfusion imbalance.[96,107]

(5) *Increased pulmonary venous pressure.* This pressure stiffens the lungs so that their compliance falls and respiration becomes more rapid and shallow. It also increases transudation of fluid through the capillaries, thus increasing interstitial fluid and adding to the stiffness of the lungs. If these changes are marked, carbon dioxide retention may occur, as is seen frequently in premature babies with congestive heart failure. If the fluid is not removed adequately by the lymphatics, there will be overt pulmonary edema, which, if marked, interferes with oxygenation.

(6) *Increased bronchial flow.* When pulmonary arterial pressures and flows are abnormally low, as in many forms of cyanotic congenital heart disease, bronchial arterial flow increases greatly. Some of this flow enters the pulmonary circulation before the alveoli and helps to bring more oxygen into the systemic circulation. Bronchial flow also increases in bronchiectasis.

Specific Abnormalities

INCREASED PULMONARY VASCULAR RESISTANCE

Six basic mechanisms cause pulmonary vascular resistance to increase.[50] More than one of these mechanisms may coexist.

Increased Viscosity. Polycythemia causes a greater than normal resistance to flow through the pulmonary circulation even if no alteration in vascular geometry is present.[1,76] The exact increase in resistance varies with left atrial pressure and the flows that occur but, as a rough guide, a hematocrit of 70% in patients with normal pulmonary blood flows might double pulmonary vascular resistance when compared with the same flows at a hematocrit of 40%.

Polycythemia is seen in the newborn infant who has an intrapartum and immediate postpartum increased blood volume after transfusion from a twin, the mother, or its own placenta; [21,39,77] when the plasma volume is reduced by diuresis, the high hematocrit remains. The high viscosity blood causes marked pulmonary hypertension with right-to-left shunting at atrial and ductal levels and may cause congestive heart failure. In the lung, channels offering the lowest vascular resistances would be perfused preferentially and so exaggerate the ventilation-perfusion abnormality. As a result these infants have low arterial oxygen tensions and often raised carbon dioxide tensions—changes that can be reversed by decreasing the hematocrit.

Polycythemia also occurs in some varieties of cyanotic congenital heart disease, e.g., tetralogy of Fallot or tricuspid atresia, in which the raised hematocrit is associated with a reduced pulmonary blood flow and pressure because of the basic lesion. The resistance might be slightly elevated but this rise is of no clinical importance. However, in transposition of the great arteries the high hematocrit is accompanied by an increased pulmonary blood flow even in the absence of a ventricular septal defect or patent ductus arteriosus. Some of these children have normal pulmonary arterial pressures and resistances (perhaps because of recruitment of new channels), but many have moderately increased pressures and resistances. We have frequently seen children under 12 months of age with simple transpositions of the great arteries and systolic pressures in the pulmonary artery that are about 50% of the aortic systolic pressure. In these the raised hematocrit might have accounted for at least part of the increased vascular resistance.

In 1966 Ferencz described the postmortem examination of pulmonary vessels in children with transposition of the great arteries, and observed that some of these children had advanced intimal changes (see p. 244) under 1 year of age.[31] These intimal changes could also cause a raised resistance, but we do not know how to separate the effects of hematocrit, vasoconstriction, and intimal changes in producing the raised pulmonary vascular resistance in these children. If the hematocrit remains high for many years, the pulmonary vessels may change due to gradual thrombotic occlusion.[83] For this reason a correctable cyanotic lesion should not be left uncorrected for too long.

While a high hematocrit is the commonest cause of an increased blood viscosity, other causes exist. In sickle cell disease, the formation of sickle cells increases viscosity,[45] which may account for some of the thrombotic episodes that occur in this disease. This explanation is true for the lungs too although the increased resistance seldom is enough in itself to cause acute right heart failure. Viscosity also rises in macroglobulinemia,[72] but complications from the raised pulmonary vascular resistance have not been reported.

Decreased Total Number of Vessels. The total number of vessels may be decreased in congenital lesions like aplasia or hypoplasia of one lung or replacement of some of the lung by congenital cystic changes. More commonly the normal number of arteries is originally present but is reduced by removal of lung tissue (lobectomy or pneumonectomy), by destruction of lungs as in emphysema or cystic fibrosis; following fibrosis due to severe irritation by toxic gases or dusts, or by interstitial pneumonitis; or by occlusion of vessels by thrombi or emboli.[18] Recently, Reid and her colleagues[48d] have shown that in some young children with large ventricular septal defects their increased pulmonary vascular resistance is associated with a decreased number of small acinar pulmonary arteries. There is some suggestion that this decrease in vessel number is postnatal and progressive.

The number of vessels that needs to be removed to cause a noticeable rise in pulmonary vascular resistance depends to some extent upon age. In general, one lung can be removed in an adult without a rise in pressure at rest, although the pressure may rise abnormally on exercise.[9,65] Removal of 60 to 80% of the lungs in animals is necessary to produce an increased pulmonary vascular resistance.[24] In newborn animals, however, removal of one lung may lead to a rise in pulmonary arterial pressure,[81,90] perhaps because at this age all the vessels are perfused even at rest. Thus, it is impossible to recruit new vessels and the existing vessels have thicker walls and narrower lumens than are found at older ages.

While pneumonectomy at older ages is usually well tolerated, this reported success occurs only if the other lung is completely normal. If any doubt exists, it is advisable to study the cardiovascular effects of removal of one lung by passing (at catheterization) a balloon catheter into the pulmonary artery of the lung to be removed and then inflating the balloon to occlude completely the blood flow to that lung. The pressure is then measured in the main pulmonary artery or right ventricle, and flows are measured. This maneuver permits evaluation of the acute effects of removing half of the vascular bed of the lungs and ensures against an excessive rise in pulmonary arterial pressure.[102,107] If the patient is old enough, it is also advisable to study the effects of exercise and make sure that no excessive pressure rise occurs when blood flow through one lung increases.

An effect equivalent to reducing the number of vessels occurs when the total cardiac output is forced to pass through one lung because only one pulmonary artery is present. Pool et al. reviewed the literature on unilateral absence of one pulmonary artery and found pulmonary hypertension in 19% of the patients with no other lesions and in 88% of patients with associated cardiac lesions.[82] That all the patients do not get pulmonary hypertension probably reflects differences either of vascular distensibility or of the number of vessels in the normally perfused lung.

Pulmonary Embolism or Thrombosis. Acute occlusion of the pulmonary arteries may be due to embolism of fat, air, amniotic fluid, tumor cells, or blood clot, or to thrombosis in situ. Fat embolism occurs most often after extensive trauma with bone fractures and is often seen following closed chest cardiac massage.[116] It produces protean symptoms and may cause death, which is usually due to systemic rather than pulmonary embolism.[95,97] However, oil droplet emboli after lymphangiography may decrease pulmonary function in older people.[40] Air embolism is rare but dramatic and can produce an acute obstruction to blood flow through the lungs.

Tumor cell embolism does not have acute effects. It is frequent in Wilms' tumors and sarcomas, but disability is usually due to the malignant process rather than to any effect on pulmonary vascular resistance; however, pulmonary hypertension has been caused by embolism from a right atrial myxoma.[19,47] With one tumor, however, pulmonary hypertension is common and may even be the presenting feature, namely a choriocarcinoma.[3] This tumor usually manifests itself in mid or late pregnancy or after birth, but it may also follow an abortion or even appear before any signs and symptoms of pregnancy exist. The finding of pulmonary hypertension (loud pulmonic component of the second heart sound, forceful right ventricular pulsation, right ventricular hypertrophy on the electrocardiogram) in females of child-bearing age, including adolescents, should always lead to consideration of this disease. Even if no metastases are seen on chest roentgenogram, the patient should be tested for high gonadotropin levels, which are indicative of this tumor. It is most important to make the diagnosis because even the metastases are curable by chemotherapy with methotrexate if treatment is begun early enough.

Most occlusion of the pulmonary arteries is by blood thrombi or emboli. Acute thrombosis of the pulmonary arteries is uncommon at any age but does occur.[4,22,26] It is most likely to happen in infants with dehydration or sepsis and is usually associated with thrombosis of other vessels, notably renal and cerebral veins. At times, however, it may be isolated and simulate an acute pulmonary infection. Diagnosis in life is rare. More common is thrombosis of small arteries in sickle cell disease. Patients with this complication may mention episodes of chest pain and have diffuse infiltrates on chest roentgenogram. Hemoptysis may occur, vital capacity and diffusing capacity may fall, and wasted ventilation may increase. Pulmonary hypertension is seldom a major feature of these thrombi.

Chronic pulmonary embolism may be of two main types. The commoner type is secondary to deep vein thrombosis of varicose veins of long standing, so that the syndrome is commoner in women and rare in children. The second type of chronic embolism is seen in children with ventriculoatrial shunts for decompression of hydrocephalus.[28,36,79] Fibrin and blood thrombi are frequently found along and at the end of the tube; these thrombi break off and produce small or large pulmonary emboli. Usually these emboli are infected so that mycotic aneurysms and infected infarcts occur, but at other times pulmonary arteries gradually occlude with the development of marked pulmonary hypertension. Any child with these shunts should be examined at intervals for fever and for signs of pulmonary hypertension; if these are found, the lesion should be confirmed by cardiac catheterization and blood cultures. If an infected shunt exists, it must be removed and a new one inserted elsewhere.

Acute pulmonary embolism may be of two types—multiple small emboli and fewer large ones. The multiple small emboli may occur in traumatic shock, and evidence exists that part of the shock lung syndrome is due to these emboli or to thrombosis in situ.[104] Treatment with heparin or filtering out of the small emboli before they reach the lung have prevented the shock lung syndrome on an experimental basis.

By far the most important type of acute pulmonary embolism is the sudden large embolus; in many large general hospitals it is the commonest form of acute pulmonary pathology in adults.[43] Emboli are particularly apt to occur in those with slowed circulations, as in congestive heart failure or after a myocardial infarction; after abdominal surgery; after extensive trauma and immobilization of the legs, or after hemiplegia;[59] and in patients with homocystinuria. It is important to note that Sevitt and Gallagher found deep vein thrombosis in 31% of autopsies done on children under 15 years of age.[98] Although many of these causes occur in children, pulmonary embolism is uncommon in them but has been reported.[11,22,27,63,94,117] As a rule, these emboli are either minor or terminal events in a severe illness with sepsis or wasting, but occasionally they may be postoperative or follow acute infections as in adults.

The clinical syndromes associated with acute pulmonary embolism depend mainly on the amount of circulation that is occluded. At one extreme is the massive pulmonary embolus, which usually arises in the leg veins where large thrombi can form and is most commonly seen in the second week after a surgical procedure. Sudden death may occur or else a syndrome characterized by sweating, tachycardia, tachypnea, low blood pressure, cyanosis, anginal pain, and collapse. Acute right heart failure may occur.

The possibility of massive embolism may be anticipated by finding tenderness and induration in the calves or an unexplained fever early in the postoperative course. Unfortunately, venous thrombosis may often be present in an apparently unaffected leg.[58,98] It can be prevented in part by early ambulation and leg and breathing exercises[34] or, if these are not possible, by prophylactic anticoagulant therapy in susceptible patients. Recent studies in adults have shown good protection by 5000 units of heparin subcutaneously two or three times daily even though the clotting time is not changed by this small dose.[57,100] Confirmation of the diagnosis may be obtained from scanning the lung fields with ^{133}Xenon or ^{99}Technetium; macroaggregates of radioiodinated albumin are also used, and angiography gives the most precise information about the sites of obstruction. Treatment consists initially of raising systemic blood pressure with pressor agents; fluid overloading must be avoided because of the risk of pulmonary edema and congestive heart failure, but it is important to maintain blood volume and hence blood pressure. Heparin should be started as soon as possible. If the patient is desperately ill, some form of artificial cardiac assist device can be used (balloon counterpulsation, membrane oxygenator), or an attempt may be made to remove the embolus surgically; these heroic measures should be attempted only in centers with experience in these techniques. Urokinase has been used to help lyse the clots; a controlled clinical trial is still underway.[112]

Less massive embolism may be more difficult to diagnose. While most emboli probably come from the legs, they may also come from cranial or pelvic veins or from the right atrium or ventricle so that signs of a local venous thrombosis may be absent. Furthermore, absence of swelling, tenderness, or induration in the calves or thighs does not eliminate them as the source of emboli.[58,98] The emboli, being smaller, may lodge in more peripheral arteries. Tachypnea and tachycardia usually occur, with a little fever and some leukocytosis. Pleural pain and a small pleural effusion, often hemorrhagic, are also common. Hemoptysis occurs in about 50% of adults. Radiologically no abnormality may be present if the emboli are small. If bigger, there may be an oligemic region, a round or linear opacity, perhaps some pleural effusion, and at times a raised diaphragm on the side of the lesion, due to basal atelectasis.[32,35] The treatment of these smaller emboli is anticoagulation to prevent further and more massive embolization.

Vascular Compression. Marked lung inflation from a raised airway pressure narrows pulmonary vessels directly by compressing them, by raising transpulmonary pressure, and by stretching the vessels in the alveolar septa; it may stop flow completely in zone I.[15,88] These changes are not significant during normal breathing or with moderate inflation but may occur when high negative or positive pressures are used during artificial ventilation or when airway obstruction causes air trapping and local hyperinflation. These effects of inflation are noticeable only in lungs that have high compliance and can be stretched excessively.

When the changes are localized, they probably cause blood to deviate from the inflated regions so that there is better matching of perfusion and ventilation and little effect on the heart or gas exchange. If the lung inflation is marked and extensive, there is pulmonary hypertension with its effects on the right ventricle. In this instance, pulmonary hypertension does not produce much compensation by recruitment of new channels because these channels themselves will be compressed and stretched. An added effect of hyperinflation is seen if the lung compliance is high enough to allow much of the raised alveolar pressure to be transmitted to the pleural space. If this occurs, systemic venous return to the thoracic cavity is reduced and cardiac output falls; the fall in output is temporary since venous congestion and changes in venous tone tend to elevate venous pressure and restore venous return to normal.

The small pulmonary vessels can also be compressed by perivascular fluid. When excessive fluid transudation into interstitial spaces occurs, lymphatic drainage can increase to remove it, but the new equilibrium is achieved with a slight increase in total interstitial fluid. More transudation, as occurs with progressive rises in pulmonary venous pressure, causes more interstitial fluid to accumulate even though with time lymphatic hypertrophy appears.[110,111] Because of gravity this excess interstitial fluid is mainly at the lung bases, where the fluid surrounds the small pulmonary vessels and airways[53,55,114] and compresses them so that resistance to flow of blood and air increases at the bases. As a result, flow and ventilation to the apices (which are usually relatively underperfused and underventilated) increase, and flow through the lung becomes more homogeneous or even predominates in the upper lung zones. The matching of changes in flow and ventilation tends to minimize ventilation-perfusion abnormalities. This redistribution of flow was first shown for adults with mitral stenosis[23] but has more recently been demonstrated in children with pulmonary venous hypertension.[37] The mechanism of redistribution of flow may be more complex than just compression of small vessels by perivascular fluid. Staub et al. showed that, as pulmonary edema developed, fluid first accumulated around small vessels and then appeared in the alveoli.[106] The same group demonstrated that flow redistribution occurred only after alveolar fluid had accumulated.[85] This finding was confirmed by Muir et al., who believed that the mechanism of flow redistribution was in some way related to the associated reduction in basal lung volume.[75]

Vasoconstriction. This topic has been discussed in Chapter 12 of the companion volume in normal physiology.[93a] No evidence exists that circulating chemicals are responsible for sustained, clinically important pulmonary hypertension, but they probably are liberated locally as mediators of many of the responses of the pulmonary vessels. More significant factors are hypoxia and acidemia, which occur in many diseases and are often associated with hypoventilation.

Hypoventilation may be due to many diseases or syndromes[17] (see also Chapter 2):

(1) Central nervous system damage of many types (e.g., encephalitis, tumor, raised intracranial pressure, anoxia, trauma, overse-dation) or else a decreased respiratory drive to carbon dioxide as seen in the preterm neonate.[84]

(2) Neuromuscular diseases of the thorax, e.g., poliomyelitis, muscular dystrophies, myasthenia gravis.

(3) Limitation of thoracic movement—achondroplasia, Jeune's syndrome, massive obesity,[14] kyphoscoliosis,[7,10] elevation of the diaphragm.

(4) Limitation of lung movement by pneumothorax or pleural effusion.

(5) Lung and airway disease—airway obstruction from tumors, laryngeal paralysis, tonsillar hypertrophy;[71] severe interstitial pneumonia; chronic emphysema, cystic fibrosis.[41]

Alveolar hypoxia and some carbon dioxide retention occur; whether there is significant acidemia depends on the adequacy of renal excretion of acid. Hypoxia causes diffuse vasoconstriction, probably of the small pulmonary arteries, so that pulmonary hypertension occurs and, in time, right ventricular hypertrophy and congestive heart failure.[14,71] The vasoconstriction can be partly or completely reversed by raising alveolar oxygen tension, by increasing ventilation or the oxygen tension of inspired gas, as well as by giving an alpha-receptor blocker like tolazoline (Priscoline) to cause vasodilatation and reduce pulmonary hypertension.[60]

Localized regions of hypoxia occur in many conditions. There may be localized airway obstruction due to abnormally large and hypertensive pulmonary arteries;[105] distortion by a patent ductus arteriosus pulling on the left pulmonary artery; congenitally misplaced arteries; or a variety of congenital or acquired obstructions of airways. If the obstruction is complete, the lung distal to it collapses; if incomplete, local hyperinflation may occur. In either event, the arteries passing through that region will be vasoconstricted;[5] this response helps to divert blood to better ventilated areas and also minimizes the arterial desaturation that occurs when blood passes through underventilated areas. Tai and Read have shown that in asthmatic subjects aminophylline or isoproterenol can at times produce regional vasodilatation without relieving local alveolar hypoxia, thereby causing a fall of arterial oxygen tension; these agents have thus overcome the protective local effect of hypoxia.[108] If the atelectatic or hyperinflated areas are not extensive, no pulmonary hypertension occurs, but enough regions of vasoconstriction would ultimately raise pulmonary vascular resistance and increase pulmonary arterial pressure.

If marked hypoxemia exists, a metabolic acidemia due to anaerobic metabolism often occurs. These two changes, hypoxia and acidemia, potentiate each other in causing severe pulmonary vasoconstriction,[29,91] and it is difficult to decide how important each is in any patient. In some diseases, however, acidemia and hypoxemia occur without alveolar hypoxia, namely various forms of cyanotic heart disease with massive right-to-left shunting (tricuspid atresia, pulmonary atresia, severe tetralogy of Fallot) or inadequate flow of oxygenated pulmonary venous blood to the systemic circuit, as in transposition of the great arteries. In these lesions the severe hypoxemia causes a profound metabolic acidemia that, by producing pulmonary vasoconstriction, further reduces pulmonary blood flow.[42] In the treatment of these lesions oxygen plays a minor part, though it should be given to increase the amount of dissolved oxygen and so bring a little more oxygen into the body, and the major form of palliative therapy prior to anatomic correction is to correct the acidemia with adequate amounts of sodium bicarbonate or tromethamine (THAM). Rapid restoration to normal blood pH should be the aim of therapy if the child is to have any chance of survival. Recently the infusion of prostaglandin E_1 or E_2 has been found to dilate the ductus arteriosus in cyanotic infants with ductus dependent pulmonary blood flow.[48b] As a result pulmonary blood flow increases, arterial oxygen saturation rises, aerobic metabolism is restored, and the infant can be sent to surgery with a much better chance of survival.

Recently a syndrome of persistent pulmonary hypertension in the newborn has been described.[68] The infants are brought to hospital with tachypnea and cyanosis that are due to right-to-left shunting through the ductus arteriosus and sometimes the foramen ovale. The lungs appear normal radiologically, and the major differential diagnosis is cyanotic heart disease. Evidence of right-to-left ductal shunting can be obtained by finding lower arterial oxygen tensions of blood in the umbilical artery than in the right radial or temporal arteries; the difference is usually more marked if the infants are breathing 100% oxygen. Sometimes the raised pulmonary vascular resistance can be lowered by bolus injection or continuous infusion of tolazoline (Priscoline) with resultant increase in arterial oxygen tension above and below the ductus arteriosus. Most of these infants gradually return to normal and have no residual cardiac or pulmonary lesions. The syndrome may have many causes, all of which produce pulmonary vasoconstriction in the newborn infant.

Medial Thickening. Any medial muscular hypertrophy narrows the lumen and causes some increase in vascular resistance of that vessel. As far as is known, medial hypertrophy of the arteries is always a response to an increased pulmonary arterial pressure, no matter what caused the pressure to rise; in the absence of pulmonary hypertension, medial hypertrophy does not occur. It is thus found in people who live at high altitude,[2] in those who have chronic hypoxia,[78] and in all the other lesions that feature pulmonary hypertension. What is of particular importance is that whenever pulmonary arterial pressure is elevated from birth because of a large ventricular septal defect or patent ductus arteriosus, incomplete involution of the medial muscle of the arteries occurs.[20,113] Therefore some of the increased pulmonary vascular resistance in these congenital heart diseases is due to narrowing of the lumen by medial hypertrophy.

The medial muscle of the pulmonary arteries is also responsible for some distinctive temporal patterns of response to congenital heart diseases. A progressive increase of vasoconstrictor responsiveness of medial muscle occurs during the latter half of pregnancy. Therefore, a child born very prematurely has less resistance after birth than one born at term and more rapidly achieves a low pulmonary vascular resistance. As a result, if a premature baby has a large ventricular septal defect, a large left-to-right shunt could be present at an early age; in fact, premature infants with this lesion usually develop a large left-to-right shunt within the first 2 months of life in contrast to full-term babies, who usually develop their large left-to-right shunts after 2 months of age.[51,52]

A much commoner application of this finding exists. Premature babies, especially those under 1750 g birth weight, have a high incidence (in the vicinity of 35%) of patent ductus arteriosus,[62] probably due to the inadequate musculature of the premature ductus as well as to its inadequate response to oxygen.[74] Now it is just these small premature babies who are likely to have idiopathic respiratory distress syndrome (IRDS), and formerly many of these died. Today with more effective therapy most of these babies survive.[44] As their lung disease improves and alveolar hypoxia decreases, the hypoxic vasoconstriction is relieved so that the small pulmonary arteries come to have a low vascular resistance. If the patent ductus arteriosus is big, a large left-to-right shunt develops and can cause congestive heart failure and death within a few days unless adequate medical or surgical treatment is given.[48a]

Two points are worthy of note about this sequence of events. One is that we see it more often—perhaps because of the greater salvage of the small premature baby or because of therapy being given now, e.g., fluids, antibiotics, or alkalis. The second is that the initial symptoms of the left-to-right ductal shunt are often misdiagnosed. When the large shunt develops, interstitial edema occurs and the infant may have tachypnea, tachycardia, apneic spells, and carbon dioxide retention, all of which may be taken as evidence of return or persistence of the lung disease. However, the cardinal signs of a large patent ductus arteriosus are also present—wide pulse pressure, hyperactive heart, continuous murmur maximal usually under the left clavicle; on chest roentgenogram evidence of an increased pulmonary blood flow appears, although the pattern may resemble that seen in IRDS. This sequence of events calls for careful observation and restriction of fluids. If congestive heart failure occurs, the infant should be digitalized and diuretics may be needed. If the lesion is severe and medical treatment fails to help, surgical closure of the ductus may be life saving.

The low pulmonary vascular resistance that occurs in preterm infants despite the thick muscular walls of their small pulmonary arteries is due in part to a relatively poor response of these arteries to vasoconstrictor stimuli like hypoxia.[68a] The reasons for this poor vasoconstrictor response are uncertain, but they include immature responsiveness of the smooth muscle as well as a decrease in its peripheral extension.[48c] In term infants there is muscle in the small pulmonary arteries almost as far out as the ends of the terminal bronchioles, but at 28 weeks muscle has extended into pulmonary arteries only as far as the level of the beginning of the terminal bronchioles.

In the full-term child with a large communication between the ventricles or the great arteries, the pulmonary arterial pressure remains at systemic levels, and the medial muscle of the small arteries does not involute completely or rapidly. Therefore for a few weeks after birth a large left-to-right shunt may not appear even with a large defect; in fact children with these defects may not have enough shunting immediately after birth to produce a characteristic murmur.[51] Subsequently, as the pulmonary vascular resistance falls, the left-to-right shunt increases progressively until eventually the volume overload of the left atrium and ventricle causes left-sided heart failure.

Intimal Thickening. Intimal thickening in the small pulmonary arteries may occur in many diseases; it may be of minor importance or it may dominate the clinical picture. Sometimes the pulmonary hypertension is due more to destruction and distortion of lung parenchyma than to the intimal obstruction (see also Chapter 18).

Arteritis is common in the collagen group of diseases: rheumatoid arthritis, polyarteritis nodosa, Wegener's granulomatosis, systemic lupus erythematosus, scleroderma, and dermatomyositis.[18] In these diseases, hemoptysis may occur due to acute necrotizing arteritis or pulmonary hypertension, but these conditions are seldom the major features of the disease. However, the vascular lesions are more important in what some think are a related group of diseases—diffuse interstitial fibrosis (Hamman-Rich syndrome) and desquamative interstitial pneumonitis. These diseases may run acute, subacute, or chronic courses, and the functional manifestations are those of restrictive lung disease (rapid shallow breathing), marked cyanosis due to ventilation-perfusion imbalance, and pulmonary hypertension due to intimal thickening and also destruction of vessels.

Intimal changes are also part of several unrelated diseases in which cor pulmonale occurs rarely; when it does, it is in part due to the intimal changes and in part due to destruction of lung parenchyma. These diseases include tuberous sclerosis, neurofibromatosis, histiocytosis X, amyloidosis, idiopathic hemosiderosis, Gaucher's disease, and Goodpasture's syndrome.[18] However, one disease that is common in the tropics does produce cor pulmonale from vascular obstruction, namely schistosomiasis. Even in children and adolescents the ova that have embolized to the lungs produce a severe endarteritis and periarteritis, and cyanosis and congestive heart failure are frequently seen.[6,13,54,56,109]

Pulmonary Vascular Disease in Congenital Heart Lesions. None of the diseases mentioned in the previous paragraphs are common in the United States or Europe, and in most of them the vascular changes are of minor importance. However, intimal changes are of major importance in many congenital heart diseases all over the world. The pathology of this type of pulmonary vascular disease has been worked out by Dammann and Ferencz,[20] and Heath et al.[46] Grade I changes are medial hypertrophy, as may occur in many cardiac and pulmonary diseases. Grade II implies increased cellularity and thickening of the intima, with resultant narrowing of the lumen. Later the thick intima becomes acellular and hyaline, may become even thicker, and may be associated with partial or complete thrombotic occlusion of the lumen (grade III). Recanalization may occur, producing narrow, tortuous channels. At this stage portions of the artery may be seen to have thin muscle and a dilated lumen; these changes are probably poststenotic dilatations beyond a markedly narrow segment. Grade III lesions are probably irreversible, and all three grades of lesion are associated with an increased pulmonary vascular resistance. Grade I is probably uniform throughout the vascular bed, but grades II and III are notably patchy; as a result, the vascular resistance depends upon how many arteries are involved in the changes.[50] Grades IV to VI have also been described; IV and V display curious plexiform and angiomatoid lesions, while VI is reserved for an acute arteritis that seems to occur mainly in conjunction with a sudden added rise of pulmonary arterial pressure.

The congenital heart lesions most frequently associated with pulmonary vascular intimal proliferation are those in which increased pulmonary arterial blood pressures and flows occur from birth. These lesions include large ventricular septal defects or patent ductus arteriosus, with or without transposition of the great arteries or tricuspid atresia. Some children with these lesions do not have high flows and pressures in the pulmonary artery because of obstructions at the right ventricular outflow or pulmonary artery, and they do not develop pulmonary vascular disease.

In all the preceding lesions the pulmonary arteries communicate with a high pressure ventricle. Immediately after birth pulmonary arterial flow is normal or only slightly increased, but as pulmonary vascular resistance falls, flow increases and pressure remains high. The increased pulmonary flow is thus dependent on changes in pulmonary vascular resistance, and the resultant left-to-right shunt is therefore termed a dependent shunt.[89] When the shunt is large enough to impose a large volume load on the left atrium and ventricle, left and often right ventricular heart failure may occur. As mentioned before, in full-term infants at sea level, congestive heart failure seldom begins before 2 months of age; in addition, it commonly occurs before 6 months of age if it is going to occur at all.[51,52] The dependence of the shunt on vascular resistance is well shown by the lesser incidence of high pulmonary blood flows and congestive heart failure in infants with large ventricular septal defects at Denver where, because of the hypoxia due to an altitude of one mile above sea level, pulmonary vascular resistance does not fall as low as it does at sea level.[61]

If the child who develops heart failure due to an excessive pulmonary blood flow responds to medical treatment and if high pulmonary arterial pressure and flow are not reduced by spontaneous diminution in size of the ventricular septal defect or the development of right ventricular outflow tract obstruction, it is usually only a matter of time until pulmonary vascular disease occurs. Grade I has been shown to be present as early as 2 months of age,[113] and grade II usually begins after 9 to 12 months of age. However, in occasional patients severe pulmonary vascular disease is delayed for several years.[52]

A second group of lesions in which pulmonary vascular disease occurs has, as a common feature, an obligatory shunt, i.e., one independent of changes in pulmonary vascular resistance.[89] Typically this type of shunt is found in endocardial cushion defects with a predominant left ventricular-right atrial shunt; large systemic arteriovenous fistulas in the brain, liver, or limbs are also found in this group, but if the shunt is large, these children may not live long enough to get pulmonary vascular disease. What these lesions have in common is a shunt between a high pressure region (left ventricle or aorta) and a low pressure system (systemic veins or right atrium). As a result, the amount of shunt depends only on the size of the communication and does not depend on the pulmonary vascular resistance. For this reason these infants may show a large left-to-right shunt and congestive heart failure within the first few weeks of life. Furthermore, although the pulmonary artery is not connected directly to the high pressure source, the high obligatory pulmonary blood flow in conjunction with the high pulmonary vascular resistance found immediately after birth keeps pulmonary arterial pressures high. Therefore, involution of the muscle of the pulmonary arteries is incomplete and delayed, and the pulmonary vascular resistance does not usually fall to its normal low level. The combination of high pulmonary arterial pressures and flows produces high risk of early pulmonary vascular disease.

An uncommon but important subgroup of these obligatory large pulmonary blood flows consists of children with one lung supplied by a single pulmonary artery and the other lung supplied only by bronchial arteries or a pulmonary artery coming off the aorta. As a result, the whole cardiac output from the right ventricle passes into the lung connected to the normal pulmonary artery. In adults, doubling the flow to one lung would not raise pulmonary arterial pressure, but in the newborn infant with a high pulmonary vascular resistance, the increased pulmonary blood flow maintains a high pulmonary arterial pressure, and this situation in turn retards the involution of the medial muscle and the fall of pulmonary vascular resistance. In later years many of these children have pulmonary vascular disease,[12,81,82] which is either confined to the normally connected lung or else more severe in it, the abnormally connected lung being protected by the small size of its arteries or by stenoses at their origin.

Finally, two other major congenital heart diseases may lead to pulmonary vascular disease but do not fall within the groups already discussed, namely, large atrial septal defects and transposition of the great arteries without a ventricular septal defect. Both of these have unusual time courses for the vascular disease; those with large atrial septal defects get their vascular disease usually after the age of 20 years, while those with transpositions may get severe pulmonary vascular disease under 1 year of age, earlier than it usually appears in patients with large left-to-right shunts through ventricular septal defects.

While the mechanisms of the vascular changes are not proven, adequate theories do exist to explain them. The medial hypertrophy of grade I is due to increased pressure work while the intimal changes of later grades may be the result of continued wear and tear from increased shearing forces exerted by rapidly moving blood against the endothelial lining of the arteries. These shearing forces have been measured by Fry, who showed that, in dogs, a threefold increase in shearing force would damage the intima; endothelial cells were either torn loose, became necrotic, or became unusually permeable to lipoproteins.[38] It is reasonable to extend this information to what happens when a prolonged increase in pulmonary blood flow occurs. With a large pulmonary flow, more than three times normal (and it is these that seem to be the precursors of pulmonary vascular disease when large ventricular septal defects are present), the shearing forces on the intima may be increased to levels that cause damage. At first there will be repair but ultimately there may be abnormal reparative changes, as occur in other organs, e.g., cartilaginous overgrowth in rickets, and the intimal changes of pulmonary vascular disease will be set in motion. This theory fits most of the high flow, high pressure lesions mentioned but has to be modified to explain the time course of pulmonary vascular disease occurring in atrial septal defects and in transposition of the great arteries. Children with large atrial septal defects may have very large pulmonary blood flows but low pulmonary arterial pressures. They therefore lack hypertrophy of the medial muscle of the small pulmonary arteries, which are in fact more widely dilated than normal; it is usual to calculate a lower than normal pulmonary vascular resistance in this lesion. Therefore even if the pulmonary arterial flows are similarly increased in ventricular and atrial septal defects, the velocity of flow and hence the shearing forces are less through the dilated arteries of the latter, which therefore have less intimal trauma and much later onset of or no pulmonary vascular disease.[50]

Children with transpositions of the great arteries with ventricular septal defects get vascular disease much like their counterparts without the transposition. However, those with no ventricular septal defects may also get early pulmonary vascular disease despite pulmonary blood flows that may be only about twice normal. The same mechanism of intimal damage from shearing forces may still be involved because, when polycythemia is present, the viscosity of blood is raised and the shearing forces are increased at any given flow rate. It is also possible that in these polycythemic children there may be gradual deposition of platelets with narrowing of the arteries. Finally, an increased bronchial arterial inflow may in some way facilitate the development of pulmonary vascular disease.

The effect of pulmonary vascular disease on the circulation is that of producing pulmonary hypertension, right ventricular hypertrophy, and eventually congestive heart failure or sudden death from arrhythmias. The abnormal vascular lesions may also give rise to troublesome hemoptyses. Finally, the patients are usually cyanotic and therefore limited in activity. The degree of increased resistance is probably more related to how many arteries are narrowed than to the grade of pathology, although this does have some effect in itself.

Grade I disease is reversible if the pressure can be lowered, but less is known about the reversibility of higher grades. Many children with grade II and grade III disease improve after surgical correction of the congenital heart lesion, but this improvement may merely indicate that not all the arteries were abnormal.[50] Clearly the problem can be prevented by careful assessment of these children, if necessary by repeated cardiac catheterizations, and surgical correction before irreversible pulmonary vascular disease begins.[25]

A similar histologic picture may be seen in the absence of any of these congenital cardiac lesions, and this relatively rare disease is then termed idiopathic or primary pulmonary hypertension. While seen most often in young women, it does occur in children and may be familial.[80] Some evidence exists that, even in children, the severe pulmonary hypertension is acquired.[30,86] No known treatment is available so that exclusion of all other possible remedial causes of pulmonary hypertension is mandatory.

DECREASED PULMONARY VASCULAR RESISTANCE

This disorder has already been discussed in premature infants with big patent ductus arteriosi and is the only major example of a generalized fall of vascular resistance in the lungs. However, localized regions of low resistance do occur when congenital arteriovenous fistulas are present. These regions are usually abnormal dilated channels with thin walls that bypass alveoli and therefore lead to arterial desaturation that can be marked. Occasionally the arterial supply to the fistula comes from bronchial or intercostal arteries so that no arterial desaturation occurs.[49] The lesions may take the form of a large, solitary mass that replaces a large part of the lung, they may be moderately large and multiple in about 20% of patients and bilateral in 10% of them,[66,67] or they may be multiple and detectable only on histologic examination. In fact, these microscopic lesions may be present even when large lesions exist, and at times the microscopic fistulas have enlarged after resection of the macroscopic lesions.

About 50% of these fistulas are associated with other vascular lesions of hereditary hemorrhagic telangiectasia (Rendu-Osler-Weber disease) so that these patients should always be examined carefully for telangiectases.[49] If the fistulas are small, minimal arterial desaturation and little clinical difficulty may occur. If much arterial desaturation exists, the patients are limited on effort. There can also be complications due to hemothorax, hemoptysis, and polycythemia, and as with any right-to-left shunt, there can be a brain abscess. Infectious endarteritis has rarely occurred.

Occasionally pulmonary arteriovenous fistulas may be associated with marked pulmonary vascular disease in which intimal thickening and medial hypertrophy are extensive.[93] The mechanism is unexplained, but the effect of the raised pulmonary vascular resistance is to divert more blood through the low resistance fistulas and thus further decrease systemic arterial saturation.

Acquired pulmonary arteriovenous fistulas are uncommon at any age. They have been described in a young girl with schistosomiasis and normal pulmonary arterial pressures.[70] In this patient, the lung biopsy showed arteriovenous anastomoses caused by necrosis of adjacent vessel walls as well as possible new formation of fistulas. Probably a commoner cause of multiple small pulmonary arteriovenous fistulas is chronic liver disease.[64,99,101] These fistulas represent regions of infinitely low ventilation-perfusion ratio and thus may produce marked arterial desaturation with polycythemia and its attendant dangers and discomforts. These fistulas are to be distinguished from portal vein-pulmonary vein anastomoses that also occur in cirrhosis of the liver;[115] since portal vein blood is nearly fully saturated, these fistulas do not cause significant lowering of systemic arterial saturation. Finally, extensive arteriovenous fistulas have been found in bronchiectasis[16,69,73] (see also Chapter 18).

INCREASED PULMONARY VENOUS PRESSURE

In adults the commonest cause of an isolated increase in pulmonary venous pressure is mitral stenosis, and this statement may be true for children in Africa and India where severe mitral stenosis is often seen under the age of 10 years. Pulmonary venous pressure is also elevated in left ventricular failure of any cause, and it contributes to the symptoms of that syndrome.

Certain congenital cardiac lesions may also show an increased pulmonary venous pressure. When there is cor triatriatum or stenosis of one or more pulmonary veins, total anomalous pulmonary venous connection with some obstruction to the venous return, or mitral atresia with a small foramen ovale, the pulmonary venous pressure rises and its effect may dominate the clinical picture. There will be tachypnea with retractions, tachycardia, rales, and perhaps some wheezing. The heart is usually not enlarged and has no pathognomonic murmurs, so that frequently the patient is misdiagnosed as having some form of lung disease. An ECG will probably show right ventricular hypertrophy, but this condition does not separate lung from heart disease. On chest roentgenogram there will usually be the picture of chronic pulmonary edema. The clinical and radiologic features do not really mimic any particular lung disease, and it is always wise to be suspicious of one of these cardiac lesions, most of which are correctable. Digitalization is not indicated and does not help, but powerful diuretics may produce marked improvement, which helps to suggest the diagnosis.

Narrowing and fibrosis of the small pulmonary veins of some patients with pulmonary hypertension have been found on autopsy examination.[8,48] These obstructive lesions cause pulmonary hypertension without there necessarily being evident pulmonary edema; a similar protective effect of pulmonary arterial vasoconstriction is sometimes seen in mitral stenosis with high pulmonary venous pressures. The lesion is diagnosable only by careful histologic examination, and Heath et al. report that in this condition pulmonary arterial wedge pressure may be normal. It is possible that some patients thought to have idiopathic pulmonary arterial disease actually have pulmonary veno-occlusive disease.

INCREASED BRONCHIAL FLOW

Normally the bronchial flow is about 1% of the cardiac output but may increase markedly in two types of lesions. One is cyanotic heart disease with a low pulmonary blood flow and pressure, e.g., tetralogy of Fallot, pulmonary atresia, and tricuspid atresia. The flow through the bronchial arteries is in part prealveolar and thus helps to bring oxygen to the body; at times the bronchial vessels are the only source of blood supply to the lung. They are therefore of great use to the patient but may cause much difficulty during surgical correction of the lesion because of the torrential pulmonary venous return, which impairs visibility.

The other type of lesion in which bronchial arterial flow is increased is chronic suppurative lung disease, e.g., bronchiectasis. In these diseases the pulmonary arterial inflow to the abnormal region may be partly or completely occluded, and the bronchial arteries can increase to supply the region.[16,69,73] Some workers have suggested that bronchial flow might increase so much that left ventricular failure could occur, but this event is probably rare.

REFERENCES

1. Agarwal, J. B., R. Paltoo and W. H. Palmer: Relative viscosity of blood at varying hematocrits in pulmonary circulation. *J. Appl. Physiol. 29*:866, 1970.
2. Arias-Stella, J. and M. Saldaña: The muscular pulmonary arteries in people native to high altitude. *Med. Thorac. 19*:484, 1962.
3. Bagshawe, K. D. and M. I. M. Noble: Cardiorespiratory aspects of trophoblastic tumours. *Q. J. Med. 35*:39, 1966.
4. Ball, K. P., J. F. Goodwin and C. V. Harrison: Massive thrombotic occlusion of the large pulmonary arteries. *Circulation 14*:766, 1956.
5. Barer, G. R., P. Howard, J. R. McCurrie and J. W. Shaw: Changes in the pulmonary circulation after bronchial occlusion in anesthetized dogs and cats. *Circ. Res. 25*:747, 1969.
6. Bedford, D. E., S. M. Aidaros and B. Girgis: Bilharzial disease in Egypt. *Br. Heart J. 8*:87, 1946.
7. Bergofsky, E. H., G. M. Turino and A. P. Fishman: Cardiorespiratory failure in kyphoscoliosis. *Medicine 39*:263, 1959.
8. Brown, C. H. and C. V. Harrison: Pulmonary veno-occlusive disease. *Lancet 2*:61, 1966.
9. Burrows, B., R. W. Harrison, W. E. Adams, E. M. Humphreys, E.T. Long and A. F. Reimann: The postpneumonectomy state. *Am. J. Med. 28*:281, 1960.
10. Caro, C. G. and A. B. DuBois: Pulmonary function in kyphoscoliosis. *Thorax 16*:282, 1961.
11. Cashman, M: Massive pulmonary embolism in a boy aged 9. *Arch. Dis. Child. 31*:474, 1956.
12. Caudill, D. R., J. A. Helmsworth, G. Daoud and S. Kaplan: Anomalous origin of left pulmonary artery from ascending aorta. *J. Thorac. Cardiovasc. Surg. 57*:493, 1969.
13. Cavalcanti, I., G. Tompson, N. de Souza and F. S. Barbosa: Pulmonary hypertension in schistosomiasis. *Br. Heart J. 24*:363, 1962.
14. Cayler, G. G., J. Mayes and H. D. Riley, Jr.: Cardiorespiratory syndrome of obesity (Pickwickian syndrome) in children. *Pediatrics 27*:237, 1961.
15. Charlier, A. A.: Beat to beat hemodynamic effects of lung inflation and normal respiration in anesthetized and conscious dogs. (Thèse: Université Catholique de Louvain, Faculté de Médecine, Louvain, Belgium) 1967.
16. Cockett, F. B. and C. C. N. Vass: A comparison of the role of the bronchial arteries in bronchiectasis and in experimental ligation of the pulmonary artery. *Thorax 6*:268, 1951.
17. Comroe, J. H. Jr., R. E. Forster, A. B. DuBois, W. A. Briscoe and E. Carlsen: *The Lung.* Year Book Medical Publishers, Chicago, p. 44, 1962.
18. Crofton, J. W. and A. Douglas: *Respiratory Diseases.* Blackwell Scientific Publications, Oxford, 1969.
19. Cumming, G. R. and K. Finkel: Intracardiac myxoma involving the right and left atria in a young patient. J. Pediatr. *58*:559, 1961.
20. Dammann, J. F. Jr., and C. Ferencz: The significance of the pulmonary vascular bed in congenital heart disease. III. Defects between the ventricles or great vessels in which both increased pressure and blood flow may act upon the lungs and in which there is a common ejectile force. *Am. Heart J. 52*:210, 1956.
21. Danks, D. M. and L. H. Stevens: Neonatal respiratory distress associated with a high haematocrit reading. *Lancet 2*:488, 1964.
22. DeCamp, P. T., A. Ochsner and M. DeBakey: Thrombo-embolism in children. *Ann. Surg. 133*:611, 1951.
23. Dollery, C. T. and J. B. West: Regional uptake of radioactive oxygen, carbon monoxide and carbon dioxide in the lungs of patients with mitral stenosis. *Circ. Res. 8*:765, 1960.
24. Downing, S. E., S. E. Pursel, R. A. Vidone, H. M. Brandt and A. A. Liebow: Studies on pulmonary hypertension with special reference to pressure-flow relationships in chronically distended and undistended lobes. *Med. Thorac. 19*:268, 1962.
25. DuShane, J. W., W. H. Weidman and D. G. Ritter: Influence of the natural history of large ventricu-

lar septal defects on management of patients. In *Congenital Cardiac Defects—Recent Advances,* D. Bergsma (Ed.). In National Foundation-Birth Defects-Original Article Series. Published for the National Foundation—March of Dimes. The Williams & Wilkins Co., Baltimore, *8*:63, 1972.

26. Emery, J. L.: Pulmonary thrombosis and its association with unexpected death in childhood. *Arch. Dis. Child. 28*:187, 1953.
27. Emery, J. L.: Pulmonary embolism in children. *Arch. Dis. Child. 37*:591, 1962.
28. Emery, J. L. and H. B. Hilton: Lung and heart complications of the treatment of hydrocephalus by ventriculo-auriculostomy. *Surgery 50*:309, 1961.
29. Enson, Y., C. Giuntini, M. I. Lewis, T. Q. Morris, M. I. Ferrer, and R. M. Harvey: The influence of hydrogen ion concentration and hypoxia on the pulmonary circulation. *J. Clin. Invest. 43*:1146, 1964.
30. Farrar, J. R., R. D. K. Reye and D. Stuckey: Primary pulmonary hypertension in childhood. *Br. Heart J. 23*:605, 1961.
31. Ferencz, C.: Transposition of the great vessels. Pathophysiologic considerations based upon a study of the lungs. *Circulation 33*:232, 1966.
32. Finley, T. N., W. H. Tooley, E. W. Swenson, R. E. Gardner and J. A. Clements: Pulmonary surface tension in experimental atelectasis. *Am. Rev. Respir. Dis. 89*:372, 1964.
33. Fixler, D. E., J. P. Archie, D. J. Ullyot, G. D. Buckberg and J. I. E. Hoffman: Effects of acute right ventricular systolic hypertension on regional myocardial blood flow in anesthetized dogs. *Am. Heart J. 85*:491, 1973.
34. Flanc, D., V. V. Kakkar and M. B. Clarke: Postoperative deep-vein thrombosis. Effect of intensive prophylaxis. *Lancet 1*:477, 1966.
35. Fleischner, F. G.: Observations on the radiologic changes in pulmonary embolism. In *Pulmonary Embolic Disease,* A. A. Sasahara and M. Stein (Eds.). Grune & Stratton, New York, 1965.
36. Friedman, S., C. Zita-Gozuma and J. Chatten: Pulmonary vascular changes complicating ventriculovascular shunting for hydrocephalus. *J. Pediatr. 64*:305, 1964.
37. Friedman, W. F., E. Braunwald and A. G. Morrow: Alterations in regional pulmonary blood flow in patients with congenital heart disease studied by radioisotope scanning. *Circulation 37*:747, 1968.
38. Fry, D. L.: Acute vascular endothelial changes associated with increased blood velocity gradients. *Circ. Res. 22*:165, 1968.
39. Gatti, R. A., A. J. Muster, R. B. Cole and M. H. Paul: Neonatal polycythemia with transient cyanosis and cardiorespiratory abnormalities. *J. Pediatr. 69*:1063, 1966.
40. Gold, W. M., J. Youker, S. Anderson, and J. A. Nadel: Pulmonary-function abnormalities after lymphangiography. *N. Engl. J. Med. 273*:519, 1965.
41. Goldring, R. M., A. P. Fishman, G. M. Turino, H. I. Cohen, C. R. Denning, and D. H. Andersen: Pulmonary hypertension and cor pulmonale in cystic fibrosis of the pancreas. *J. Pediatr. 65*:501, 1964.
42. Gootman, N. L., E. M. Scarpelli and A. M. Rudolph: Metabolic acidosis in children with severe cyanotic congenital heart disease. *Pediatrics 31*:251, 1963.
43. Gray, F. D., Jr.: *Pulmonary Embolism,* Lea & Febiger, Philadelphia, 1966.
44. Gregory, G. A., J. A. Kitterman and R. H. Phibbs: Treatment of the idiopathic respiratory-distress syndrome with continuous positive airway pressure. *N. Engl. J. Med. 284*:1333, 1971.
45. Harris, J. W. and R. W. Kellermeyer: *The Red Cell.* Harvard University Press, Cambridge, Mass., 1970.
46. Heath, D. and J. E. Edwards: The pathology of hypertensive pulmonary vascular disease. A description of six grades of structural changes in the pulmonary arteries with special reference to congenital cardiac septal defects. *Circulation 18*:533, 1958.
47. Heath, D. and J. Mackinnon: Pulmonary hypertension due to myxoma of the right atrium. *Am. Heart J. 68*:227, 1964.
48. Heath, D., N. Segel and J. Bishop: Pulmonary veno-occlusive disease. *Circulation 34*:242, 1966.

48a. Heymann, M. A.: The ductus arteriosus. In *Heart Disease in Infants, Children, and Adolescents.* A. J. Moss, F. H. Adams and G. C. Emmanouilides (Eds.). The Williams & Wilkins Co., Baltimore, p. 553 ff, 1977.

48b. Heymann, M. A. and A. M. Rudolph: Ductus arteriosus dilatation by prostaglandin E_1 in infants with pulmonary atresia. *Pediatrics 59*:325, 1977.

48c. Hislop, A.: The non-muscular phase of the pulmonary circulation in the child. In 5th International Cystic Fibrosis Conference, D. Lawson (Ed.). C. Nicholls and Co., Ltd., London, p. 340 ff, 1969.

48d. Hislop, A., S. G. Haworth, E. A. Shinebourne and L. Reid: Quantitative structural analysis of pulmonary vessels in isolated ventricular septal defect in infancy. *Br. Heart J. 37*:1014, 1975.

49. Hodgson, C. H., H. B. Burchell, C. A. Good and O. T. Clagett: Hereditary hemorrhagic telangiectasia and pulmonary arteriovenous fistula. *N. Engl. J. Med. 261*:625, 1959.
50. Hoffman, J. I. E.: Diagnosis and treatment of pulmonary vascular disease. In *Congenital Cardiac*

Defects—Recent Advances, D. Bergsma (Ed.). In National Foundation-Birth Defects-Original Article Series. Published for the National Foundation—March of Dimes. The Williams & Wilkins Co., Baltimore, *8*:9, 1972.
51. Hoffman, J. I. E. and A. M. Rudolph: The natural history of ventricular septal defects in infancy. *Am. J. Cardiol. 16*:634, 1965.
52. Hoffman, J. I. E. and A. M. Rudolph: The natural history of isolated ventricular septal defect with special reference to selection of patients for surgery. *Adv. Pediatr. 17*:57, 1970.
53. Hogg, J. C., J. B. Agarwal, A. J. S. Gardiner, W. H. Palmer and P. T. Macklem: Distribution of airway resistance with developing pulmonary edema in dogs. *J. Appl. Physiol. 32*:20, 1972.
54. Ibrahim, M. and B. Girgis: Bilharzial cor pulmonale. *J. Trop. Med. Hyg. 63*:55, 1960.
55. Iliff, L. D., R. E. Greene and J. M. B. Hughes: Effect of interstitial edema on distribution of ventilation and perfusion in isolated lung. *J. Appl. Physiol. 33*:462, 1972.
56. Jongco, A. P. and F. Flaminiano: Chronic cor pulmonale in children. *J. Philipp. Med. Assoc. 37*:734, 1961.
57. Kakkar, V. V., E. S. Field, A. N. Nicolaides, P. T. Flute, S. Wessler, and E. T. Yin: Low doses of heparin in prevention of deep-vein thrombosis. *Lancet 2*:669, 1971.
58. Kakkar, V. V., C. T. Howe, C. Flanc and M. B. Clarke: Natural history of postoperative deep-vein thrombosis. *Lancet 2*:230, 1969.
59. Kakkar, V. V., C. T. Howe, A. N. Nicolaides, J. T. G. Renney and M. B. Clarke: Deep vein thrombosis of the leg. Is there a "high risk" group? *Am. J. Surg. 120*:527, 1970.
60. Kelminson, L. L., E. K. Cotton and J. H. K. Vogel: The reversibility of pulmonary hypertension in patients with cystic fibrosis. *Pediatrics 39*:24, 1967.
61. Kelminson, L. L. and J. H. K. Vogel: Observations of patients with ventricular septal defects (VSD) residing at high altitudes. In *Congenital Cardiac Defects—Recent Advances,* D. Bergsma (Ed.). In National Foundation-Birth Defects-Original Article Series. Published for the National Foundation—March of Dimes, The Williams & Wilkins Co., Baltimore, *8*:69, 1972.
62. Kitterman, J. A., L. H. Edmunds, Jr., G. A. Gregory, M. A. Heymann, W. H. Tooley and A. M. Rudolph: Patent ductus arteriosus in premature infants. *N. Engl. J. Med. 287*:473, 1972.
63. Komrower, G. M. and V. K. Wilson: Homocystinuria. *Proc. R. Soc. Med. 56*:996, 1963.
64. Kravath, R. E., E. M. Scarpelli and J. Bernstein: Hepatogenic cyanosis: arteriovenous shunts in chronic active hepatitis. *J. Pediatr. 78*:238, 1971.
65. Lategola, M. T.: Pressure-flow relationships in the dog lung during acute, subtotal pulmonary vascular occlusion. *Am. J. Physiol. 192*:613, 1958.
66. LeRoux, B. T.: Pulmonary arteriovenous fistulae. *Q. J. Med. 28*:1, 1959.
67. LeRoux, B. T.: Pulmonary "hamartomata." *Thorax 19*:236, 1964.
68. Levin, D. L., M. A. Heymann, J. A. Kitterman, G. A. Gregory, R. H. Phibbs and A. M. Rudolph: Persistent pulmonary hypertension of the newborn infant. *J. Pediatr. 89*:626, 1976.
68a. Lewis, A. B., M. A. Heymann and A. M. Rudolph: Gestational changes in pulmonary vascular responses in fetal lambs in utero. *Circ. Res. 39*:536, 1976.
69. Liebow, A. A., M. R. Hales and G. E. Lindskog: Enlargement of the bronchial arteries, and their anastomoses with the pulmonary arteries in bronchiectasis. *Am. J. Pathol. 25*:211, 1949.
70. Lopes de Faria, J. L., J. V. Barbas, T. Fujioka, M. F. Lion, U. de Andradre e Silva and L. V. Décourt: Pulmonary schistosomatic arteriovenous fistulas producing a new cyanotic syndrome in Manson's schistosomiasis. *Am. Heart J. 58*:556, 1959.
71. Luke, M. J., A. Mehrizi, G. M. Folger, Jr. and R. D. Rowe: Chronic nasopharyngeal obstruction as a cause of cardiomegaly, cor pulmonale and pulmonary edema. *Pediatrics 37*:762, 1966.
72. MacKenzie, M. R., E. Brown, H. H. Fudenberg and L. Goodenday: Waldenström's macroglobulinemia:correlation between expanded plasma volume and increased serum viscosity. *Blood 35*:394, 1970.
73. Marchand, P., J. C. Gilroy and V. H. Wilson: An anatomical study of the bronchial vascular system and its variations in disease. *Thorax 5*:207, 1950.
74. McMurphy, D. M., M. A. Heymann, A. M. Rudolph and K. L. Melmon: Developmental changes in constriction of the ductus arteriosus: responses to oxygen and vasoactive agents in the isolated ductus arteriosus of the fetal lamb. *Pediatr. Res. 6*:231, 1972.
75. Muir, A. L., D. L. Hall, P. Despas and J. C. Hogg: Distribution of blood flow in the lungs in acute pulmonary edema in dogs. *J. Appl. Physiol. 33*:763, 1972.
76. Murray, J. F., R. B. Karp and J. A. Nadel: Viscosity effects on pressure-flow relations and vascular resistance in dogs' lungs. *J. Appl. Physiol. 27*:336, 1969.
77. Naeye, R. L.: Human intrauterine parabiotic syndrome and its complications. *N. Engl. J. Med. 268*:804, 1963.
78. Naeye, R. L. and H. W. Letts: The effects of

prolonged neonatal hypoxemia on the pulmonary vascular bed and the heart. *Pediatrics 30*:902, 1962.
79. Noonan, J. A. and D. A. Ehmke: Complications of ventriculovenous shunts for control of hydrocephalus. *N. Engl. J. Med. 269*:70, 1963.
80. Parry, W. R. and D. Verel: Familial primary pulmonary hypertension. *Br. Heart J. 28*:193, 1966.
81. Pool, P. E., K. H. Averill and J. H. K. Vogel: Effect of ligation of left pulmonary artery at birth on maturation of pulmonary vascular bed. *Med. Thorac. 19*:362, 1962.
82. Pool, P. E., J. H. K. Vogel and S. G. Blount, Jr.: Congenital unilateral absence of a pulmonary artery. *Am. J. Cardiol. 10*:706, 1962.
83. Rich, A. R.: A hitherto unrecognized tendency to the development of widespread pulmonary vascular obstruction in patients with congenital pulmonary stenosis (tetralogy of Fallot) *Bull. Johns Hopkins Hosp. 82*:389, 1948.
84. Rigatto, H. and J. P. Brady: Periodic breathing and apnea in preterm infants. I. Evidence for hypoventilation possibly due to central respiratory depression. *Pediatrics 50*:202, 1972.
85. Ritchie, B. C., G. Schauberger and N. C. Staub: Adequacy of perivascular edema hypothesis to account for distribution of pulmonary blood flow in lung edema. *Circ. Res. 24*:807, 1969.
86. Roberts, W. C.: The histologic structure of the pulmonary trunk in patients with "primary" pulmonary hypertension. *Am. Heart J. 65*:230, 1963.
87. Robin, E. D., C. E. Forkner Jr., P. A. Bromberg, J. R. Croteau and D. M. Travis: Alveolar gas exchange in clinical pulmonary embolism. *N. Engl. J. Med. 262*:283, 1960.
88. Roos, A., L. J. Thomas, Jr., E. L. Nagel and D. C. Prommas: Pulmonary vascular resistance as determined by lung inflation and vascular pressures. *J. Appl. Physiol. 16*:77, 1961.
89. Rudolph, A. M.: The changes in the circulation after birth. Their importance in congenital heart disease. *Circulation 41*:343, 1970.
90. Rudolph, A. M., E. D. B. Neuhauser, R. J. Golinko, and P. A. M. Auld: Effects of pneumonectomy on pulmonary circulation in adult and young animals. *Circ. Res. 9*:856, 1961.
91. Rudolph, A. M. and S. Yuan: Response of the pulmonary vasculature to hypoxia and H^+ ion concentration changes. *J. Clin. Invest. 45*:399, 1966.
92. Salisbury, P. F.: Coronary artery pressure and strength of right ventricular contraction. *Circ. Res. 3*:633, 1955.
93. Sapru, R. P., D. C. S. Hutchison and J. I. Hall: Pulmonary hypertension in patients with pulmonary arteriovenous fistulae. *Br. Heart J. 31*:559, 1969.
93a. Scarpelli, E. M. and P. A. M. Auld. *Pulmonary Physiology of the Fetus, Newborn and Child.* Lea & Febiger, Philadelphia, 1975.
94. Schimke, R. N., V. A. McCusick, T. Huang and A. D. Pollack: Homocystinuria. *J.A.M.A. 193*:711, 1965.
95. Scully, R. E.: Fat embolism in Korean battle casualties. Its incidence, clinical significance, and pathologic aspects. *Am. J. Pathol. 32*:379, 1956.
96. Severinghaus, J. W., E. W. Swenson, T. N. Finley, M. T. Lategola and J. Williams: Unilateral hypoventilation produced in dogs by occluding one pulmonary artery. *J. Appl. Physiol. 16*:53, 1961.
97. Sevitt, S.: The significance and classification of fat-embolism. *Lancet 2*:825, 1960.
98. Sevitt, S. and N. Gallagher: Venous thrombosis and pulmonary embolism. *Br. J. Surg. 48*:475, 1961.
99. Shaldon, S., J. Caesar, L. Chiandussi, H. S. Williams, E. Sheville and S. Sherlock: The demonstration of porta-pulmonary anastomoses in portal cirrhosis with the use of radioactive krypton (Kr^{85}). *N. Engl. J. Med. 265*:410, 1961.
100. Sharnoff, J. G. and G. DeBlasio: Prevention of fatal postoperative thromboembolism by heparin prophylaxis. *Lancet 2*:1006, 1970.
101. Silverman, A., M. D. Cooper, J. H. Moller and R. A. Good: Syndrome of cyanosis, digital clubbing and hepatic disease in siblings. *J. Pediatr. 72*:70, 1968.
102. Söderholm, B.: The hemodynamics of the lesser circulation in pulmonary tuberculosis. *Scand. J. Clin. Lab. Invest. Suppl. 26*:9:1, 1957.
103. Spotnitz, H. M., M. A. Berman and S. E. Epstein: Pathophysiology and experimental treatment of acute pulmonary embolism. *Am. Heart J. 82*:511, 1971.
104. Stallone, R. J., H. Herbst, F. W. Blaisdell, and J. F. Murray: Pulmonary changes following ischemia of the lower extremities and their treatment. *Am. Rev. Respir. Dis. 100*:813, 1969.
105. Stanger, P., R. V. Lucas, Jr. and J. E. Edwards: Anatomic factors causing respiratory distress in acyanotic congenital cardiac disease. *Pediatrics 43*:760, 1969.
106. Staub, N. C., H. Nagano and M. L. Pearce: Pulmonary edema in dogs, especially the sequence of fluid accumulation in lungs. *J. Appl. Physiol. 22*:227, 1967.
107. Swenson, E. W., T. N. Finley and S. V. Guzman: Unilateral hypoventilation in man during temporary occlusion of one pulmonary artery. *J. Clin. Invest. 40*:828, 1961.
108. Tai, E. and J. Read: Response of blood gas tensions to aminophylline and isoprenaline in patients with asthma. *Thorax 22*:543, 1967.

109. Turner, P. P.: Schistosomal pulmonary arterial hypertension in East Africa. *Br. Heart J. 26*:821, 1964.
110. Uhley, H. N., S. E. Leeds, J. J. Sampson and M. Friedman: Role of pulmonary lymphatics in chronic pulmonary edema. *Circ. Res. 11*:966, 1962.
111. Uhley, H. N., S. E. Leeds, J. J. Sampson and M. Friedman: Right duct lymph flow in experimental heart failure following acute elevation of left atrial pressure. *Circ. Res. 20*:306, 1967.
112. Urokinase Pulmonary Embolism Trial Study Group. Phase I Results. *J.A.M.A. 214*:2163, 1970.
113. Wagenvoort, C. A., H. N. Neufeld, J. W. DuShane and J. E. Edwards: The pulmonary arterial tree in ventricular septal defect. A quantitative study of anatomic features in fetuses, infants and children. *Circulation 23*:740, 1961.
114. West, J. R., C. T. Dollery and B. E. Heard: Increased pulmonary vascular resistance in the dependent zone of the isolated dog lung caused by perivascular edema. *Circ. Res. 17*:191, 1965.
115. Williams, J. H. Jr. and W. H. Abelmann: Portopulmonary shunts in patients with portal hypertension. *J. Lab. Clin. Med. 62*:715, 1963.
116. Yarnoff, M.: Incidence of bone-marrow embolism due to closed-chest cardiac massage. *N. Engl. J. Med. 269*:837, 1963.
117. Zuschlag, E.: Infarction of the lung in children. *Am. J. Dis. Child. 74*:399, 1947.

Diseases of the Upper Airways

W. SHAIN SCHLEY AND ALFRED N. KRAUSS

8

Embryology of the Upper Respiratory Tract

Differentiation of the structures of the upper respiratory tract begins during the first half of the first month of gestation. As the early embryo grows and develops, the cranial end folds forward on the rest of the body. At this stage, a portion of the yolk sac is included within the embryo as a tubelike endodermal structure dorsal to the developing heart. This structure becomes lined with mesoderm, and is termed the foregut.[5,17] The foregut grows forward and meets a shallow surface depression on what will become the face of the developing embryo, the stomatodeum. Cranial portions of the foregut, in association with mesoderm derived from the branchial clefts, give rise to the endodermal parts of the mouth, the pharynx, and the endodermal portion of the respiratory system (Fig. 8-1). The caudal portions of the foregut give rise to the esophagus, stomach, upper half of the descending part of the duodenum, and portions of the liver and pancreas.

During the next 3 to 4 weeks of gestation, the facial structures related to breathing undergo differentiation. Four "processes" develop at the side of the head: medial and lateral nasal processes, maxillary process, and mandibular process (Fig. 8-2). Simultaneously, the nasal placodes appear on the surface ectoderm near the stomatodeal orifice. The placodes deepen, form pits, and continue

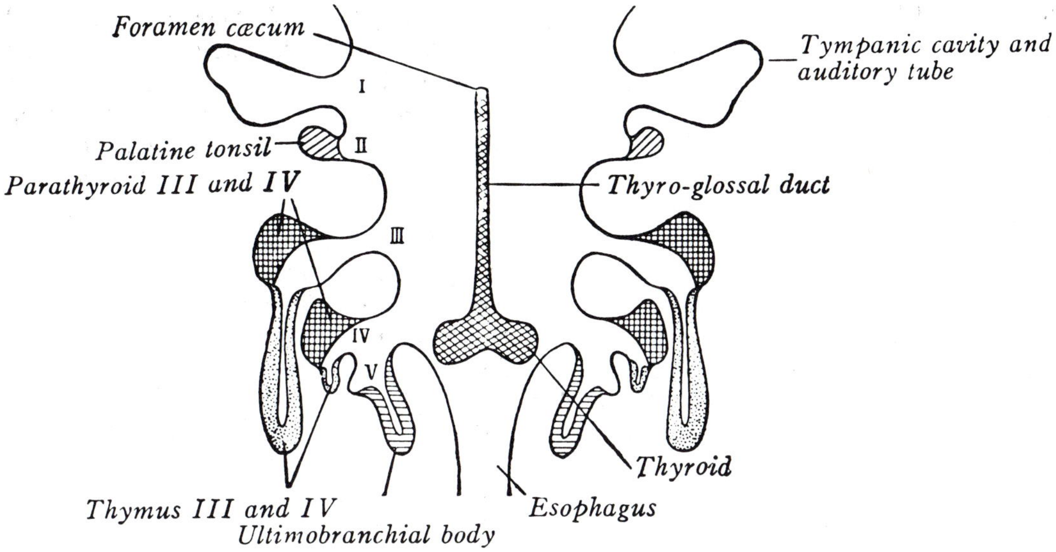

FIG. 8-1. Pharyngeal derivatives. (From Bremer.[5])

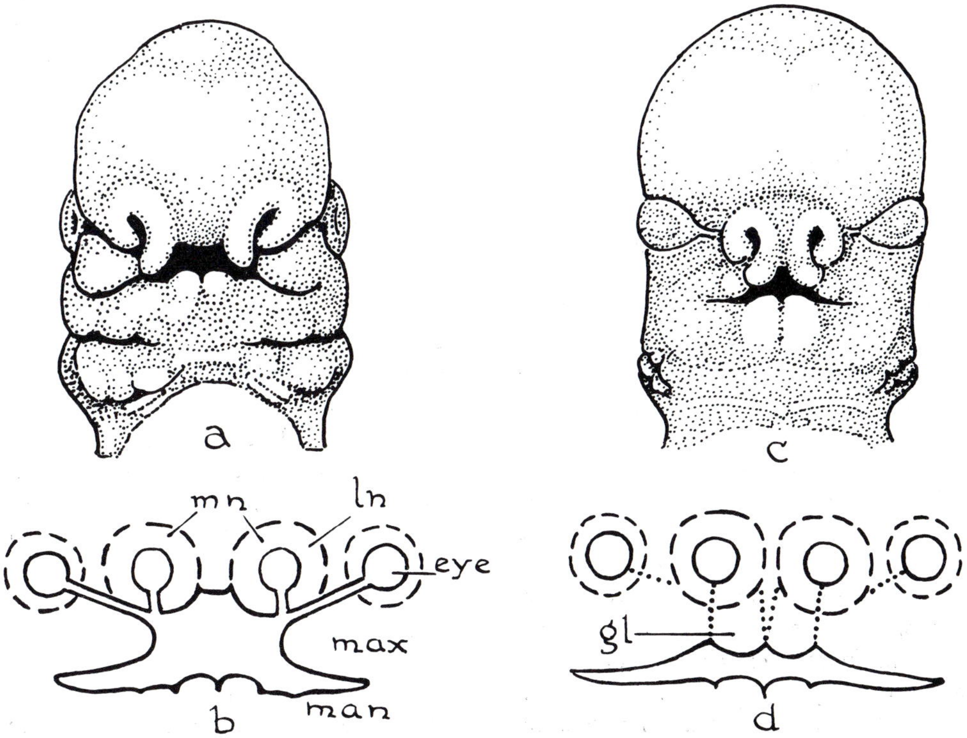

FIG. 8-2. Development of the face: mn = medial nasal; ln = lateral nasal; max = maxillary; man = mandibular. (From Bremer.[5])

to grow caudally opening out onto the surface of the embryo at a point later to be included in the mouth, thus forming the nasal passages. The medial nasal processes grow together and fuse in the midline to form the processus globularis. The lateral nasal processes remain short; thus it is the maxillary processes that grow down and fuse with the processus globularis to form the upper lip. The mandibular processes grow toward the midline, fusing together to form the lower jaw and joining with the maxillary processes to form the cheek. By the fourth month of gestation these maneuvers have resulted in a protruding nose. Elevations developing in the lateral nasal wall result in the conchae, while the maxillary and sphenoidal sinuses appear as diverticula of the lateral nasal wall. The other sinuses develop after birth.

The palate develops from the oral surface of the processus globularis (the product of the fusion of the two medial nasal processes) and the maxillary processes. Abnormal fusion of these processes results in the anomalies of harelip—nonunion of the globular and maxillary processes—or cleft palate—nonunion of the maxillary processes. Maldevelopment of the medial and lateral nasal processes can result in the malformation known as proboscis. Failure of the mandibular processes to unite can result in clefts of the lower lip or mandible. Choanal atresia, a congenital obstruction of the internal nares, results from a failure of resolution of the epithelial plug present at this location from the second to sixth month.

At the thirtieth day of gestation, swellings appear in the floor of the embryonic mouth. Slightly caudal to the region of the first two pharyngeal arches, the tuberculum impar appears. It gives rise to the anterior two-thirds of the tongue. More caudally, in the region of the third and fourth arches, the hypobranchial eminence develops. It gives rise to the remainder of the tongue. The complexity of the innervation of the tongue (fifth, seventh, ninth, tenth, and twelfth cranial nerves) is accounted for by the complexity of embryonic development.[4] The epiglottis is derived from the hypobranchial eminence. During the fifth month of gestation, connective tissue that develops in association with the second pharyngeal arch shows lymphoid aggregations. These aggregations develop into the tonsils and adenoids.

At about 4 weeks another important respiratory structure makes its first appearance. A median ventral diverticulum of the foregut, the tracheobronchial groove, is first noted. The tracheal portion of this structure develops rapidly. Cartilage appears, and by the eleventh or twelfth week the cartilage has reached lobar and segmental bronchi. As described earlier, the hypobranchial eminence forms the epiglottis, while lateral structures, the arytenoid swellings and aryepiglottic folds, form the walls of the larynx. Failure of the trachea to completely separate from the foregut results in tracheoesophageal fistula, and may occur at any level below the larynx[5] (Fig. 8-3). Absence of cartilage in the bronchi has been associated with congenital lobar emphysema.[17]

Clinical Manifestations

The upper airways serve to conduct air from the atmosphere to the patient's lungs. In carrying out this task, the upper airways warm, filter, humidify, and distribute the air. Disease of the upper airways creates symptoms that interfere with these functions. This interference with function should be borne in mind when taking a history or performing a physical examination on a patient suspected of having disease of this portion of the respiratory tract.

SYMPTOMS

Inflammation of the mucosal lining of the respiratory tract structures often results in production of mucus. In an adult or older child this condition may be apparent as sputum. In such an individual, the quantity, vis-

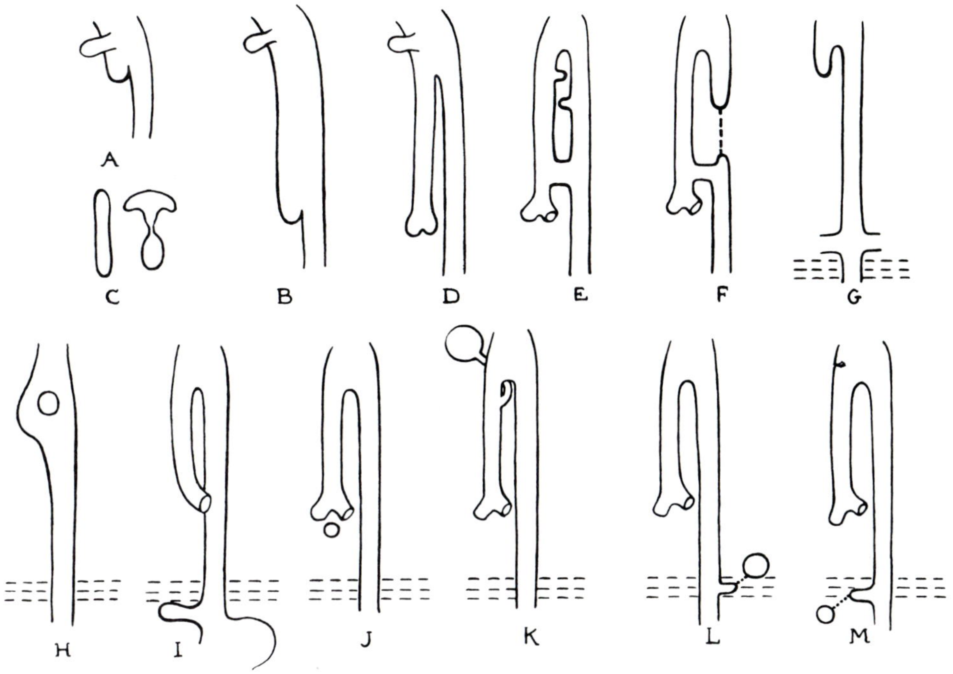

FIG. 8-3. Development of the trachea and its anomalies: (A-D) development of trachea; (E) traction diverticula; (F) tracheoesophageal fistula; (G, H) agenesis of trachea; (G, I-M) misplaced or supernumerary bronchi; (K) tracheocele. (From Bremer.[5])

cosity, and color of the sputum should be sought. The presence of blood should also be noted. In younger children large amounts of sputum may not be coughed out. However, these patients may cough or sneeze as a result of sputum lodging in the posterior pharynx. Similarly, the runny nose is an example of production of mucus in the nasal airways, and often indicates a disease process in this region. The production of large amounts of mucus in the sinuses may result in painful swelling due to blockage of these structures.

Swelling of the mucous membranes is also a result of inflammatory processes involving the upper airways. This swelling can interfere with the distribution of air, as in the case of epiglottitis or rhinitis, where various portions of the airways become obstructed. Obstruction due to extrathoracic interference usually impedes the inspiratory phases of respiration, while intrathoracic obstruction interferes with expiration. Obstruction may also occur because of foreign bodies, tumors, or congenital anomalies. In all cases, the level of the obstruction determines its time, mode, and manner of onset. A tumor, for example, slowly interferes with the distribution of air, while choanal atresia or laryngeal web usually is acute soon after birth.

Pain is an important symptom of disease in the upper respiratory tract, especially a disease of such structures as the sinuses, nose, and larynx. The larynx also contains the vocal structures. Inflammation, obstruction, trauma, or paralysis may all affect the motion of the vocal cords and therefore cause voice changes or stridor. These sources should be sought in the history. In infants, alterations of the cry signify laryngeal problems in the same way that aphonia or hoarseness does in older children or adults.

To summarize, upper airway disease may manifest itself by interference with vocalization; obstruction to airflow; production of mucus, evident as a runny nose or sputum; and localized pain. These factors should be sought in a history of a patient with respiratory disease, and will help direct attention to various regions of the respiratory tract.

PHYSICAL EXAMINATION

Initially the external appearance of the patient should be noted. In a newborn infant anomalies should be sought. Cleft lip and palate should be noted if present. A soft polyvinyl catheter may be passed through both nares. Its appearance in the oropharynx signifies that both nares are patent. The ability to introduce this catheter into the stomach rules out esophageal atresia, frequently associated with tracheoesophageal fistula. The external position of the trachea should always be noted, with special attention paid to any lateral deviations. Hoarseness or aphonia should be noted. Inspection of the patient's external appearance should conclude by observing any external masses, swellings, or inflammations.

Palpation of the patient is the next step. Beginning with the head, the sinuses may be palpated for tenderness. Examination of the mandibular and cervical structures should include palpation for masses, localization of the trachea, and palpation for any painful structures.

Inspection of the patient's internal structures is the next step in examination of the upper respiratory structures. The nares should be carefully inspected for obstruction. The color of the nasal mucosa and the character of its secretions, if any, should be noted. Redness may indicate inflammation, while a pale bluish coloration has been associated with nasal allergies. Inspection of the oropharynx should include observation of the patency of the oropharynx, the size and color of the tonsils, the presence of a cleft palate, the presence of any webs or retropharyngeal masses, and the state of the patient's dentition. The odor of the patient's breath may also be of significance, particularly when chronic infection is suspected. Hoarseness or aphonia indicates that the vocal cords should be examined, by either direct or indirect laryngoscopy. The size and state of the epiglottis should be noted if it is visualized.

Auscultation is of great value in the examination of the upper respiratory tract. A foreign body may result in absent breath sounds on one side of the patient's chest. Obstruction due to webbing, a foreign body, or other tumor may result in a whistle or stridor.[10] Therefore the trachea should be auscultated as well as the lungs when such a lesion is suspected.

Physiologic Principles

The upper airways serve not only as a connection between the external world and the lung, but also as a means of processing the inspired and expired air. This function involves heat and water exchange, removal of particulate matter from the inspired air, and evacuation of mucus from the lower respiratory tract.

Air from the lower respiratory tract is saturated with water vapor at body temperature (37° C). Bouhuys has calculated that a human adult inspiring dry air at 0° C would have to evaporate 420 g of water every 24 hours in order to fully saturate this air with water at body temperature.[4] This process would expend 2200 calories, an amount equal to the normal total metabolic rate of a healthy person. The upper airways are capable not only of adding this volume of water vapor to the inspired air, but also of recovering much of the heat and water vapor added during inspiration. In a cold environment the temperature of the expired air falls as it approaches the nostrils. As this temperature drop happens, the water vapor contained in the expired air condenses and is retained within the body, thus conserving both water and the energy used in its evaporation at a lower level within the respiratory tract. Because cool air contains less water vapor than warm air, any inspired air, even when fully saturated, has a drying effect at any temperature below 53° F.[32] In a warm environment expired gas is not cooled as it reaches the nares. The water vapor contained in the expired gas, therefore, largely remains in the expirate, and thus contributes to the heat loss of the body in a warm environment.

These factors are of clinical importance in dealing with the small premature infant. Addition of water vapor to warm air in an incubator prevents the loss of water through the respiratory tract and therefore conserves energy. This factor may account for the lower mortality rate observed in premature infants nursed in conditions of high humidity.[36] Similarly, release of compressed gas from a tank or wall outlet cools the gas and therefore dries it. Thus a patient breathing this gas, by face mask, nasal cannula, or mechanical ventilator, is breathing an unsaturated gas. Unless this gas is rewarmed and resaturated, the patient may lose both calories and water vapor through the respiratory tract.

A second major role of the upper airways in processing inspired air is the removal of particulate matter. Proctor has pointed out that the filtration of inspired air and removal of suspended matter depends on several factors: area of the airway exposed to the stream of inspired air, turbulence and distribution of the inspired air, character of the fluid coating the surface of the airway mucosa and the ability of the body to remove and replenish this fluid, and the character and quantity of the hairs and cilia lining the airways.

The turbinates of the nose create turbulence in the stream of inspired air; at the same time they increase the area of the mucous membrane available for filtration. This area has been estimated as 158 cm^2 in the adult human. With the aid of the sticky nasal mucus and the hairs lining the anterior aspect of the nasal cavity, the nose removes 95 to 99% of inspired particles greater than 15 μ in diameter.[32] Smaller particles are gradually removed by impaction in the mucus lining of the conducting airways, although some small particles may also be removed by the nose. Particles in the size range from 0.5 to 3 μ in diameter, a range which includes most bacteria, may penetrate to the respiratory spaces of the lung. Particles below this size range are generally exhaled, but may be retained within the lung. Particles remaining within the airways after exhalation are removed by means of the mucus lining the respiratory tract and propelled by means of the cilia lining the respiratory mucosa.

Particles within the nose are easily expelled. Those deposited within the lungs have a longer path. They are floated out by means of a 0.2-μ layer of fluid propelled by cilia lining the respiratory epithelium. Eventually these particles reach the pharynx and are either expelled by coughing or are swallowed. Particles that penetrate the respiratory epithelium despite these defense mechanisms are trapped by phagocytes and deposited in local lymphoid structures. In addition, secretory immunoglobulin A (IgA) is produced by the plasma cells in the submucosal tissue of the respiratory tract and appears in the secretions of the respiratory tract. This IgA takes part in the destruction and neutralization of various viruses and bacteria that invade the respiratory tract.

Factors that affect the processing of air by the respiratory tract include temperature, hydration, and various hormonal and psychologic factors. Dehydration, and prolonged breathing of dry air decrease production of respiratory tract secretions and slow mucus flow and ciliary action. Prolonged exposure to high oxygen concentrations also causes injury to the respiratory mucosa. Hypothyroidism has been associated with chronic nasal congestion, and during pregnancy the nasal mucosa frequently has the appearance of nasal rhinitis. Changes in the vaginal mucosa associated with the menstrual cycle are also found in the mucosa of the nose. Air pollutants, notably sulfur dioxide and ammonia, are well-known irritants of the respiratory mucosa. Morphine, codeine, and local anesthetics are inhibitory to ciliary action. Loss of nasal breathing, either because of nasal obstruction, as in a cold or allergic rhinitis, or because of surgical procedure, as in a tracheostomy, means that increased amounts of water will be lost through the respiratory tract because the nose is a much more efficient organ of water exchange than the lower respiratory tract. As discussed in the section on tracheostomy care, the increased viscosity of the mucosa resulting from this increased loss of water can result in a dry, viscous mucus and seriously complicate care.

Congenital Malformations

CHOANAL ATRESIA

Infants with choanal atresia have a partition that separates the nasal cavity from the nasopharynx. The atresia may be unilateral or bilateral. Since the newborn will not open the mouth to breathe, bilateral atresia always produces severe respiratory distress. Only when he opens his mouth to cry is the infant able to breathe. Respiratory distress secondary to unilateral atresia usually is not as severe. Insertion of an oral airway can be life saving at birth for a newborn with choanal atresia.

This diagnostic possibility can be eliminated if a catheter passed through the nose is visualized in the oropharynx. If the catheter seems to pass but is not seen in the oropharynx, it may be curled in the nose. If a catheter cannot be passed, contrast radiography may be diagnostic. The nasal cavity should be suctioned clear just before the study. Associated congenital anomalies may be found in the cardiovascular system and the facial skeleton (Fig. 8-4).

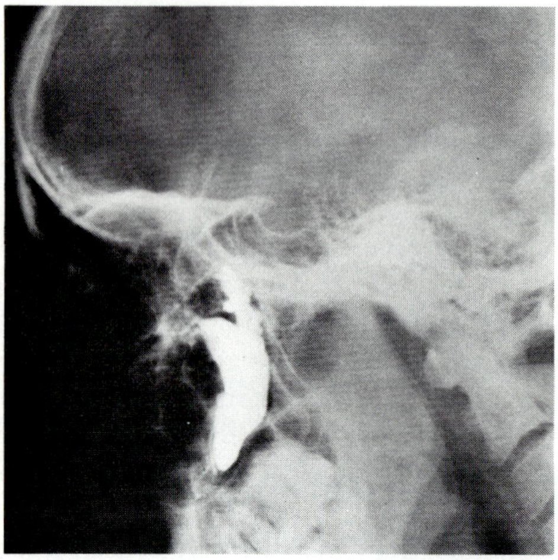

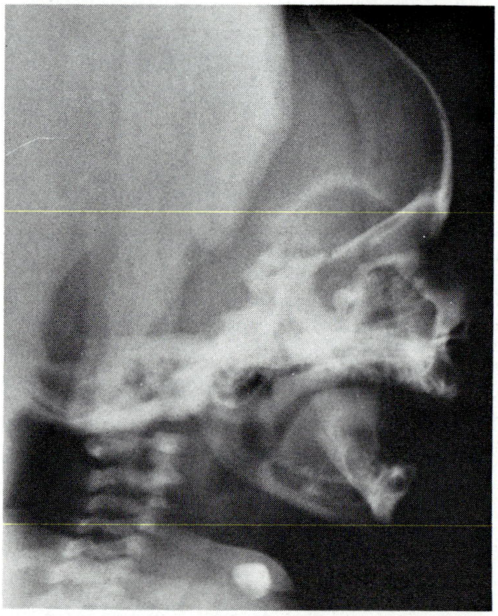

FIG. 8-4. *A*, Lateral roentgenogram with barium contrast demonstrating a right unilateral choanal atresia in a 24-year-old man.

B, Nasal contrast study in a 3-day-old female infant with left unilateral choanal atresia. An anterior filling defect due to retained mucus is seen in the nasal cavity.

Infants with choanal atresia require constant observation and are best followed in an intensive care unit since an oral airway must be maintained and tube feedings are necessary. Early surgical correction reduces management problems. The atresia may be approached through the nasal cavity after general anesthesia has been administered. The operating microscope and an ear speculum are used to visualize the atresia. Nasal secretions are suctioned clear and the membranes constricted. The atresia is usually located 1 $\frac{1}{4}$ in. from the rim of the nostril.[1] Flaps may be devised from the nasal and nasopharyngeal mucous membranes. The bony portion of the atresia is removed with a diamond burr.[37]

The new airway is stented with silastic tubing. This tubing may initially be brought out through the nose and secured with a safety pin. Once the situation has stabilized, the tubing may be trimmed and allowed to rest inside the nose. If the tubing is too long, fluid regurgitates through it during feeding. The tubing may be rinsed with normal saline solution and suctioned clean if it becomes obstructed. The tubing should be left in place for 6 weeks. After removal, some stricturing may occur at the operative site. If the airway becomes inadequate, the tubing should be replaced. Another surgical approach to the atresia is through the palate.[26,31]

MANDIBULOFACIAL DYSOSTOSIS (TREACHER-COLLINS SYNDROME)

Treacher-Collins in 1900 reported two cases of congenital symmetrical notching of the lower lids with underdevelopment of the maxillae. Franceschetti and Klein in 1949 reviewed all available literature and clinical material relating to mandibulofacial dysostoses.[15] Prominent features of this disorder include palpebral fissures sloping downward laterally (antimongoloid) with a coloboma in the outer portion of the lower lids, hypoplasia of the facial bones, and malformation of the ears. A conductive hearing loss occurs in many of the cases. Mental retardation has also been reported in this condition, and may be related to the hearing loss (Fig. 8-5).

Males and females are equally affected. Many of the cases arise as fresh mutations.

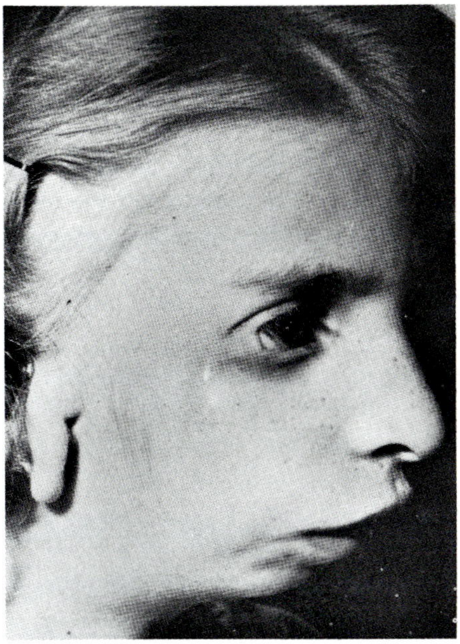

FIG. 8-5. Preadolescent girl with Treacher Collins syndrome, including malar hypoplasia and defect of lower lid. (From Smith, D. W., *Recognizable Patterns of Human Malformation.* Philadelphia, W. B. Saunders Co., 1970. p. 111.)

The risk of recurrence is, therefore, low in such families. If one of the parents is affected, the risk of recurrence is 50% since autosomal dominance is the suspected mode of transmission.

This condition is usually recognized at birth. Speech and hearing should be evaluated at an early age in order to detect the conductive hearing loss associated with this disorder. Patients with Treacher-Collins syndrome usually live a normal span of years unless severe congenital heart disease is found. This disease has been reported in occasional cases of mandibulofacial dysostosis.

PIERRE ROBIN SYNDROME

This syndrome is characterized by micrognathia, cleft palate, and glossoptosis.[11,38] The primary developmental anomaly is micrognathia (Fig. 8-6). The post-alveolar

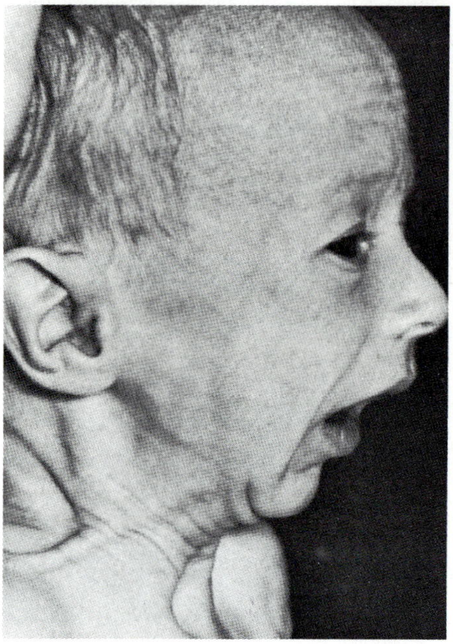

FIG. 8-6. 3-week-old infant with Pierre Robin syndrome. (From Denison, W. M. The Pierre Robin syndrome. *Pediatrics 36*:336, 1965.)

cleft of the hard and soft palate is a common but not constant feature of the syndrome. It is sometimes replaced by a "high-arched" palate. The glossoptosis is brought about by relaxation of the effective anchorage of the tongue due to the posterior displaced attachment of the genioglossus muscles to the hypoplastic mandible. With the influence of gravity, the tongue falls backward and downward, obstructing the oropharynx. Infants with the fully developed Pierre Robin syndrome have a history of respiratory distress dating from birth. The attacks are most marked when the infant is placed on his back or during feeding. Associated anomalies of the eyes, ears, heart, and extremities are common. This syndrome is uncommon, its occurrence estimated as 1 : 30,000 live births. Males and females are affected in equal numbers, but the inheritance of Pierre-Robin syndrome is uncertain.

Feeding may be difficult and the infant may aspirate. Caloric intake may be poor and should be maintained. Skillful nursing is necessary during early infancy if these infants are to survive. Surgical measures employed in this syndrome include suturing the tongue to the lower lip to prevent obstruction of the airway by the tongue; tracheostomy, to prevent asphyxial attacks; and gastrostomy for feeding. When cyanosis persists after airway patency is ensured, cyanotic congenital heart disease should be considered. If the infants survive early infancy, normal growth of the mandible will correct the child's profile. Plastic surgery is therefore not necessary during infancy.

CLEFT PALATE

This disorder is one of the most frequently occurring serious congenital malformations of the oropharynx.[2] Its incidence varies from 1:1500 among Japanese, 1:2700 among white Americans, and 1:5200 among black Americans. As related earlier, the palate is formed by a process of fusion of the bilateral processes forming the embryonic mouth and facial structures. Failure of this fusion results in clefts of the lips and palate.

Palatal clefts are often evident at birth on inspection of the newborn infant's mouth. Submucous clefts may not be evident at birth unless careful examination is made. Transillumination of the oral structures may be necessary to detect this malformation. The association of cleft palate with other anomalies runs from 30% to 50% in various series. Many of these anomalies occur as part of syndromes that are not compatible with life, such as trisomy 18. Among patients who are candidates for surgical procedure, the incidence of associated anomalies is between 13 and 25%.

Surgical closure of the cleft palate is usually carried out between the ages of 24 and 36 months. Cleft lip may be repaired during early infancy when it occurs in association with a cleft palate. Frequently an early cosmetic repair of the infant's lip is an important consideration in establishing a normal parent-child relationship between the mother and her baby. The mother must be instructed in the feeding of an infant with cleft palate, since dropper or syringe feedings may be necessary. Children with cleft palate frequently have serious otitis media, which may produce a conductive hearing loss. This condition may be corrected by myringotomy and ventilating tube. Because of the abnormalities of the palatal structures as well as the possible chronic otitis that may accompany this syndrome, speech and hearing evaluation should be part of the treatment plan of every child with cleft palate.

TRACHEOESOPHAGEAL FISTULA AND ESOPHAGEAL ATRESIA

In a survey taken in 1964, tracheoesophageal fistula and esophageal atresia were reported in 1058 patients.[18,19] The most frequent anomaly was esophageal atresia with tracheoesophageal fistula to the distal segment (86.5%). Esophageal atresia without tracheoesophageal fistula was present in 7.7% of the cases. Tracheoesophageal fistula without esophageal atresia was present in 4.2% of the cases. The remainder had esophageal atresia with tracheoesophageal fistula to the proximal esophageal segment (0.8%), or to both proximal and distal esophageal segments (0.7%). The distal tracheoesophageal fistula allows air to pass from the trachea into the stomach and gastric contents to pass through the esophagus into the trachea. This dysfunction results in chemical and bacterial pneumonia. Esophageal atresia without fistula results in a dilated proximal pouch that compresses the trachea. The contents of the pouch may be aspirated through the larynx. A fistula from the proximal pouch results in direct drainage of saliva into the trachea.

Tracheoesophageal fistula with atresia usually produces symptoms minutes to hours after birth. With feedings, the infant chokes, coughs, and becomes cyanotic. When a distal fistula is present, the abdomen becomes distended and ventilation is impaired. If a fistula is present without atresia, the infant can usually swallow but will frequently aspirate. This aspiration leads to recurrent pneumonitis.

Tracheoesophageal fistula and esophageal atresia are best diagnosed by contrast radiography. A cine-esophagogram study may help to find the fistula. Endoscopic investigation may help locate an isolated fistula (Fig. 8-7).

These infants are best managed on a pediatric surgical service with a pediatric intensive care unit. If a distal fistula is present, a gastrostomy may be done under local anesthesia to decompress the stomach. When the infant is able to withstand general anesthesia, the fistula is divided. Several weeks later the

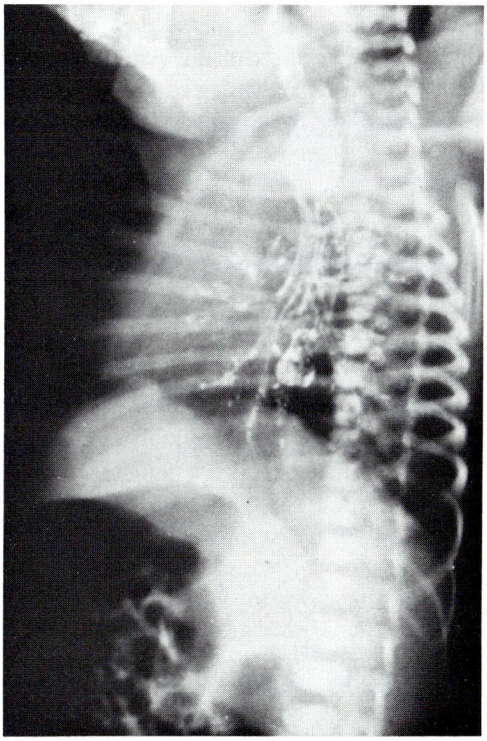

FIG. 8-7. Lateral chest roentgenogram of a newborn infant with esophageal atresia and tracheoesophageal fistula.

esophageal anastomosis can be done. Esophageal atresia without a fistula may be managed by gastrostomy feedings and by stretching of the proximal and distal segments until a direct anastomosis can be performed. If the anastomosis is not possible, a colonic interposition may be done at about 1 year of age. A fistula without atresia may be divided through a cervical incision if the fistula is above the second thoracic vertebra. Fistulas below this level are divided through a thoracotomy incision. A proximal fistula is managed by gastrostomy, cervical esophagostomy, and later colon interposition. If proximal and distal fistulas are present, the gastrostomy should be followed promptly with the definitive repair.

A 1964 survey revealed a 61% overall survival rate.[18] Patients without associated anomalies had a survival rate of 78%. Tracheoesophageal fistula is associated with congenital heart disease in 25 to 50% of all cases. The type and severity of the associated heart disease are important determinants of survival in these children. VATER syndrome has recently been proposed as the acronym for the association of *t*racheo*e*sophageal fistula with *v*ertebral, *a*nal, *a*rm, *r*ectal, and *r*enal anomalies.

KARTAGENER'S SYNDROME

In 1933, Kartagener first described four cases of situs inversus and bronchiectasis.[23] Two years later, he described seven more cases, and all had chronic sinusitis as well. Since that time the triad of situs inversus, bronchiectasis, and sinusitis has been ascribed to Kartagener.[34] Patients with Kartagener's syndrome have recurrent respiratory infections from childhood, recurrent pneumonia, otitis media, productive cough, hemoptysis, and eventual respiratory and cardiac failure. Kartagener's syndrome is probably a congenital defect with the genetic anomaly carried as an autosomal recessive. The complete syndrome has a high familial incidence. It usually appears only in one generation, and multiple siblings may have various combinations of its components.[27]

Pharynx, Larynx, and Trachea

INFECTIOUS DISEASE

The frequent *upper respiratory infections* in children are caused by viruses.[39] Since children lack acquired immunity to these agents, the resulting infection may be severe. Symptoms may include fever, sneezing, thin nasal discharge, nasal obstructions, and malaise. Treatment may include rest, fluids, decongestants, aspirin, and nose drops. Secondary bacterial infections should be suspected if the nasal discharge becomes purulent. Antibiotic therapy should be given at this time. Cultures should be taken to help determine the most effective antibiotics.

The *paranasal sinuses* communicate with the nasal cavities through their ostia, so sinus inflammation may recur with each episode of rhinitis. As the infection clears, any accumulated secretions in the sinuses usually drain spontaneously. If the infection persists in the nose and sinuses, serious complications may develop. Complications tend to occur more often in children who have nasal allergy or who have been swimming during their acute infection. These complications include orbital cellulitis, cavernous sinus thrombosis, endocranial abscesses, and meningitis.[35]

Tonsils, Adenoids, Peritonsillar Tissue. In acute pharyngitis the tonsils and adenoids are usually inflamed. When this inflammation is primarily located in the tonsils and adenoids, it may be called *adenotonsillitis or tonsillitis.* The causes of adenotonsillitis may be viral, bacterial, or both.[40] The nasopharyngeal and oropharyngeal flora of patients with recurrent adenotonsillitis is characterized by the presence of bacterial species usually associated with clinical infections in the head and neck.

These organisms include *S. pyogenes, S. aureus, H. influenzae, Corynebacterium diphtheriae,* pneumococcus, *C. albicans,* and the enteric gram-negative aerobes and anaerobes. Viruses present include adenoviruses and Epstein-Barr viruses. Immunologically, patients with recurrent adenotonsillitis typically have hypergammaglobulinemia. The elevated IgA contains antibodies to viruses, and the elevated IgG contains antibodies to the gram-positive bacteria.

The symptoms of acute tonsillitis include sore throat and dysphagia. Otalgia may be secondary to referred pain from the pharynx. Children may complain only of headache and abdominal pain with vomiting. On examination the tonsils are enlarged and red. The crypts may appear prominent. A purulent exudate may also be present. Enlargement and tenderness of the superior deep cervical lymph nodes located behind the angle of the mandible may also be present. The temperature is elevated and may be as high as 40° C. The white blood cell count is usually elevated. When a membrane is present, diphtheria should be considered and airway obstruction should be guarded against. Infectious mononucleosis may also be associated with a posterior pharyngeal membrane. Exudates present on the tonsils, and any membranes present in the pharynx, should be cultured. Tonsillitis in association with scarlatina is often streptococcal in origin.

Patients with tonsillitis should be put to bed and encouraged to drink fluids. Aspirin may be given for fever or discomfort. A throat culture may be helpful in identifying the infecting organism. Throat irrigations with normal saline solution and sodium bicarbonate help clear any exudate. If patients do not respond promptly to symptomatic treatment, antibiotic therapy should be started. Penicillin is usually a satisfactory choice and may be given orally or parenterally. If the patient is allergic to penicillin, erythromycin may be given. If staphylococcal infection is suspected, a penicillinase-resistant antibiotic should be used. Once antibiotic therapy has been started, it should be continued for 7 to 10 days. Culture and sensitivity tests may be helpful in directing antibiotic choices.

Peritonsillar cellulitis usually accompanies acute tonsillitis. The inflammation usually responds to the therapy for tonsillitis. The inflammation may organize into a peritonsillar abscess, which will require surgical drainage unless it spontaneously drains. The cervical lymph nodes may become suppurative and require drainage. Acute otitis media may develop secondary to adenotonsillitis. Systemic complications in association with group A streptococcal infections may include rheumatic fever and acute glomerulonephritis.

Once the tonsils have been infected, they may not return to their original state of health. The crypts become blocked, resulting in a collection of debris in which bacteria multiply. Small abscesses may become walled off in the tonsil parenchyma. This state of chronic tonsillitis may result in chronic sore throat, halitosis, dysphagia, respiratory distress, persistent cervical adenitis, and recurrent acute tonsillitis.

Conclusive studies of the indications for and the results of tonsillectomy and adenoidectomy are lacking.[29] Understandably then, conscientious physicians maintain divergent attitudes and preferences on the matter. Some guidelines may be helpful in deciding when to seek surgical consultation.[30,33] Adenoidectomy and tonsillectomy are separate procedures and may be helpful in separate situations. Children with recurrent suppurative otitis media, recurrent middle ear effusions, or serous otitis media with hearing loss are often helped by adenoidectomy. If the adenoids are hypertrophied to the extent that they interfere with nasal breathing, adenoidectomy should correct this condition. Rarely, cor pulmonale may result from airway obstruction by enlarged tonsils and adenoids. Occasionally, children fail to gain weight because they are unable to take an adequate diet when the tonsils and adenoids obstruct the pharynx.

A *peritonsillar abscess* may form in the space between the tonsil capsule and the tonsil bed. This condition is painful and may result in serious complications. A tonsillectomy should be performed several weeks after the inflammation has resolved. In selected cases, a tonsillectomy may be helpful in management of an acute peritonsillar abscess. Some children may have convulsions or flare-ups of streptococcal-related entities with acute tonsillitis. Recurrent tonsillitis may occur despite continuous antibiotic therapy. Some children may have recurrent episodes of tonsillitis that respond satisfactorily to antibiotics but result in missed school days and development of allergy to useful antibiotics. In these situations, the clinician must consider the potential surgical risk, psychologic risk, and possible immunologic risk and then reach a decision regarding surgical consultation.

The parapharyngeal space is separated from the peritonsillar space by the superior constrictor muscle and its fascia. Infection may be introduced into the parapharyngeal space through vascular or lymph channels from the tonsils or pharynx. This deep cervical infection may result in thrombosis of the jugular veins or mediastinitis. It also results in marked swelling in the neck below the angle of the mandible. The lateral pharyngeal wall is usually displaced medially. Initial treatment should include bedrest, local heat, and parenteral antibiotics. If an abscess bulges into the pharynx, drainage may be accomplished by an incision through the superior constrictor muscle. If the abscess points externally, local incision and drainage are possible. If the location of the abscess remains obscure, exploration of the neck may be necessary for adequate drainage.

A *retropharyngeal abscess* may develop in the space between the prevertebral fascia and the superior constrictor muscle. This abscess is usually confined above the second cervical vertebra. Such infection may be secondary to inflammation in the retropharyngeal lymph nodes or perforation by a foreign body. Enlargement of the abscess may result in airway obstruction. Spontaneous rupture may be followed by aspiration of pus. Retropharyngeal inflammation may respond promptly to antibiotics. When pus collects in the retropharyngeal space, drainage can be accomplished through the mouth.

Croup and Epiglottitis. One of the most important clinical syndromes involving the upper airway of children is *croup*. Croup is characterized by varying degrees of inspiratory stridor, hoarseness, and coughing. These symptoms may occur in association with a low-grade fever, malaise, and loss of appetite. The causes of croup include viral infection, bacterial infection, and allergic reactions.

The most serious symptoms of the croup syndrome are those related to the degree of airway obstruction.[28] Obstruction in the croup syndrome is due to swelling and edema of the tissues of the upper airways (e.g., larynx, trachea, bronchi). Since the larynx and trachea are extrathoracic, the obstruction to breathing occurs during the inspiratory part of the respiratory cycle. When laryngitis is present alone, the amount of airway obstruction is usually minimal. Swelling of the vocal cords may produce hoarseness, however. As swelling of the lower airways progresses, airway obstruction increases, and the resulting underventilation gives way to signs of air hunger. Suprasternal retractions may appear on inspiration, the accessory muscles of respiration are used, and restlessness may be present if hypoxemia develops. Severe obstruction, associated with marked lower airway swelling, is accompanied by severe retractions, by cyanosis, and, especially in the presence of thickened mucous secretions, by cyanosis, shock, and death. The typical cough of croup is described as brassy or barking.

Epiglottitis is a specific form of croup associated with inflammation of the epiglottis.

Epiglottitis is due to *H. influenzae* type B. The illness is characterized by a rapid onset of sore throat, hoarseness, barking cough, and high fever. Drooling and difficulty in swallowing are prominent symptoms. The rapid onset, the severity of the systemic manifestation, and the presence of drooling and dysphagia serve to differentiate epiglottitis from other forms of croup.

Physical examination of the child with laryngitis or laryngotracheobronchitis generally reveals the presence of malaise and mild fever in an acutely ill child. The pharynx may reveal slight inflammation. The epiglottis should appear normal, if seen. Retractions may be present, but examination of the chest is generally normal. Rhonchi may be present if production of mucus is an important part of the illness. As mentioned, a barking, brassy cough is often present. The presence of air hunger, cyanosis, restlessness, or lethargy, as indications of hypoxemia, should all be carefully sought. Mediastinal emphysema and pneumothorax are serious complications of croup. Subcutaneous emphysema may be present under these circumstances. This condition is often apparent on physical examination, and the patient may draw attention to it by complaining of pain in the neck or shoulder area. Distant heart tones, displacement of the heart, or absent breath sounds on one side of the chest may alert the clinician to the presence of a pneumothorax.

The child with epiglottitis comes to the clinic with a swollen, beefy red epiglottis. This characteristic is often seen on routine examination of the pharynx without resort to the use of tongue blades. If epiglottitis is suspected on the basis of clinical history and physical appearance on examination, great care should be taken to avoid gagging the patient. Gagging may cause a sudden closure of the epiglottis and prevent insertion of an oro- or nasotracheal airway. If possible, it is often best to carry out this part of the examination with an otolaryngologist present, so that an emergency airway may be inserted promptly if required. Lateral radiographs of the neck provide a safe means of diagnosis (Fig. 8-8).

Unlike the syndromes of infectious croup, allergic or spasmodic croup is frequently unaccompanied by general systemic symptoms.[9] Signs of inflammation are usually lacking, although several well-documented cases have occurred in association with acute viral infections. Like other croup syndromes, spasmodic croup often has a nocturnal onset and is associated with a barking cough. Recurrence is a frequent phenomenon in spasmodic croup.

The list of differential diagnoses of croup is small. It is important to consider foreign bodies in any infant or young child with the sudden onset of coughing, choking, and air hunger. A retropharyngeal abscess must also be considered when symptoms of upper airway obstruction are present.

The prognosis of croup due to laryngitis or laryngotracheobronchitis is generally excellent. The principles of treatment are those of maintaining the patient's oxygenation and providing sufficient fluids and calories during the acute phase of the illness. Because of the patient's increased respiratory rate, fatigue is often a problem in croup. Therefore the patient should be allowed to rest as quietly as possible. Restlessness, however, may be an

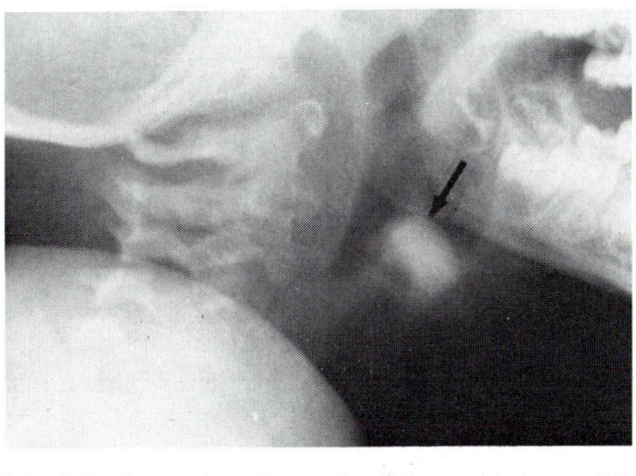

FIG. 8-8. Lateral radiograph of the neck in a child with epiglottitis. Arrow indicates swollen epiglottis virtually occluding the larynx, which may be seen below.

early sign of hypoxemia. Oxygen is often the best sedative for the restless patient with croup. This treatment may be provided by a mist tent. Patients who cannot maintain an adequate oral intake should be supplemented intravenously. If a patient is maintained in a fully saturated environment, insensible water loss is considerably reduced. This consideration should be taken into account when providing intravenous fluids for a hospitalized patient. Specific antibiotic therapy is indicated only for *H. influenzae* type B illness, since nearly all other croup is of viral or allergic cause. Ampicillin or chloramphenicol, in age and weight appropriate doses, is the antibiotic of choice. Steroids have been said to be beneficial in croup.[22] Although many clinicians report dramatic relief of symptoms following administration of steroids, it should be remembered that viral croup is self-limited, and that the studies in support of the use of steroids are not based on sophisticated measurements of physiologic parameters, such as airway resistance. Racemic epinephrine has also been said to be beneficial in relieving the symptoms of croup.[16] Again, results are controversial; additionally, a rebound phenomenon may be present with the use of this drug. Adequate oxygenation, sufficient fluids, rest, and close observation are the cornerstones of the treatment of croup, and should not be neglected in attempts to use pharmacotherapy.

Because of the high likelihood of sudden airway closure in epiglottitis, the most conservative therapy in this illness is to provide an artificial airway at the time of diagnosis. It may take the form of an orotracheal airway, an endotracheal airway, or a tracheostomy. This procedure is best performed in an operating room with direct tracheal observation by a skilled otolaryngologist. Extubation can usually be accomplished within 48 to 72 hours. Specific chemotherapy aids in controlling the infection, especially with regard to its systemic manifestations. However, the use of either steroids or antibiotics should not delay the insertion of an artificial airway. Delay may result in needless death.[24,25]

CONGENITAL ANOMALIES

Infants with *congenital laryngeal anomalies* may utter a weak cry or no cry at all. They may show signs of dyspnea, stridor, or cyanosis. They may have constant fluid in the pharynx and trachea complicated by aspiration pneumonia. The final diagnosis of congenital laryngeal anomaly is made by direct visual examination of the larynx through the laryngoscope. If severe dyspnea is present, direct laryngoscopy may precipitate complete airway obstruction. Facilities for intubation and tracheotomy should always be at hand before direct laryngoscopy is performed. Visualization of the motility of the true vocal cords may be determined best by first inserting the blade of the laryngoscope in the vallecula prior to dipping it under the epiglottis tip to visualize the glottis and the anterior commissure.

Laryngomalacia is a common cause of respiratory obstruction in infants. The laryngeal cartilages are abnormally soft and flaccid. Typically, stridor is present from birth and is at first audible only on inspiration. The stridor is usually louder when the infant is on its back. The partial respiratory obstruction may cause retractions. Laryngoscopy is necessary to confirm the diagnosis of laryngomalacia and to rule out obstruction due to neurogenic causes or to other congenital anomalies. At laryngoscopy the epiglottis is noted to be curled, and the supraglottic structures partially occlude the airway on inspiration. Generally symptoms subside gradually after 1 to 1 ½ years and rarely is tracheotomy necessary.

Laryngotracheal-esophageal cleft is a rare condition in which the cricoid cartilage fails to fuse dorsally.[3] The clinical picture is similar to tracheoesophageal fistula with the addition of an absent or weak cry. A dehiscence between the arytenoids extends inferiorly through the cricoid cartilage and involves the party wall between the trachea and esophagus for varying distances. Surgical correction through a lateral pharyngotomy is recommended. This severe anomaly is often associated with extensive anomalies of other organ systems.

Congenital laryngeal cysts originate from the ventricular appendix. They may cause respiratory obstruction by enlargement over the supraglottic airway. Congenital laryngoceles communicate with the interior of the larynx. These cysts are noticed clinically only when swollen by air forced into them or when filled with a collection of fluid. Glottic cysts have their origin in the true or false cords. Internal thyroglossal duct cysts are found at the base of the tongue. They may cause dyspnea by pushing the epiglottis posteriorly over the larynx.

Laryngeal webs may be found at the glottic level between the true cords or more rarely in the supraglottic areas between the false cords. Congenital subglottic stenosis may cause respiratory obstruction 2 to 3 mm below the level of the superior surface of the true cords. Stridor may be present from birth. Progressive respiratory distress necessitates a tracheotomy.

Vocal cord paralysis may be unilateral or bilateral. In bilateral paralysis, the cry is clear but dyspnea is severe. This lesion is most frequently part of a generalized central nervous system disorder, and the prognosis is relatively poor. Dysphagia with aspiration of food is a common phenomenon because of the frequency of an associated pharyngeal paralysis. A tracheotomy is frequently required. In unilateral vocal cord paralysis, the infant's cry is usually weak or absent. Tracheotomy is usually not required. Unilateral paralysis on the left is frequently associated with congenital cardiovascular lesions.

Subglottic hemangiomas are usually found in infants with obvious skin hemangiomas. Changes in the larynx are progressive, similar to progressive changes noted in the skin lesions. Tracheotomy may be required. Spontaneous involution occurs so therapy is to be avoided if possible. Irradiation probably has little effect on subglottic hemangiomas. Surgical excision by laryngofissure may be utilized for hemangiomas that have not undergone significant natural regression after 1 year.[7]

Congenital vascular anomalies may cause stridor by compression of the trachea or tracheobronchial tree. The commonest anomaly is tracheal compression by an anomalous innominate artery. This diagnosis is readily made at bronchoscopy. Bronchoscopy as well as laryngoscopy may be required as part of the investigation of stridor or wheeze in the infant.[13]

NEOPLASMS

Vocal nodules may develop at the junction of the anterior and middle third of the vocal cords. They result in poor voice quality. The diagnosis may be established by mirror examination or direct laryngoscopy. These lesions are caused by vocal abuse. Voice therapy is the preferred method of treatment. If surgically removed, they promptly recur without proper vocal hygiene.

The cause of *laryngeal papillomas* is uncertain. These tumors may result in poor voice and airway obstruction. Frequently they undergo spontaneous regression. Repeated conservative surgical removal is the preferred therapy. Care should be taken not to damage normal tissue. Tracheotomy may be necessary for airway obstructions.

A series of 210 children with *head and neck cancer* was reported in 1974.[41] The malignant conditions showing the highest incidence were lymphoma (25%), rhabdomyosarcoma and other soft tissue sarcomas (22%), retinoblastoma (16%), brain tumors (15%), and carcinoma of the thyroid (7%). Retinoblastomas are usually found in infancy; lymphomas and thyroid cancer are usually found in older children. Carcinoma of the thyroid is more frequently found in females. Other tumor types more frequently affect boys.

FOREIGN BODIES

These items are most frequently introduced into the air and food passages through carelessness.[6,20,21] Children may aspirate peanuts, nuts, carrots, and bacon if these foods are included in their diet before the age of 4. In fact, children may put any small objects in their mouth and attempt to swallow them. Care must be taken in preparation of their food to exclude seeds, shells, and bones. To establish the diagnosis, the physician must be suspicious and consider the possibility of a foreign body.

Larynx. The initial symptoms brought on by foreign body enlargement in the larynx are choking, gagging, and coughing. Patients may become cyanotic or dyspneic or develop wheezing. These symptoms may be unnoticed in a child, or they may be forgotten. There usually follows a symptomless interval lasting from a few hours to many years. Asphyxia may immediately follow occlusion of the larynx or may develop later from laryngeal edema. If a foreign body has safely passed the larynx into the trachea, impaction in the conus elasticus and asphyxia may occur if the child is held up by the ankles. Once suspected, laryngeal foreign bodies may be diagnosed by indirect mirror examination, direct laryngoscopy, or x-ray examination (Fig. 8-9).

Tracheobronchial Tree. Tracheal foreign bodies usually cause violent paroxysmal cough. When they are forced up and arrested in the conus elasticus, a slap may be heard. Once they become fixed in the trachea or a large bronchus, a wheeze may be noted at the open mouth. Once a foreign body becomes fixed in a bronchus, a symptomless interval practically always occurs. Vegetal objects then cause an exudate resulting in a productive cough. If a bronchus is completely obstructed, the affected pulmonary segment will collapse. Obstructive emphysema may occur behind a foreign body with a valvular action.

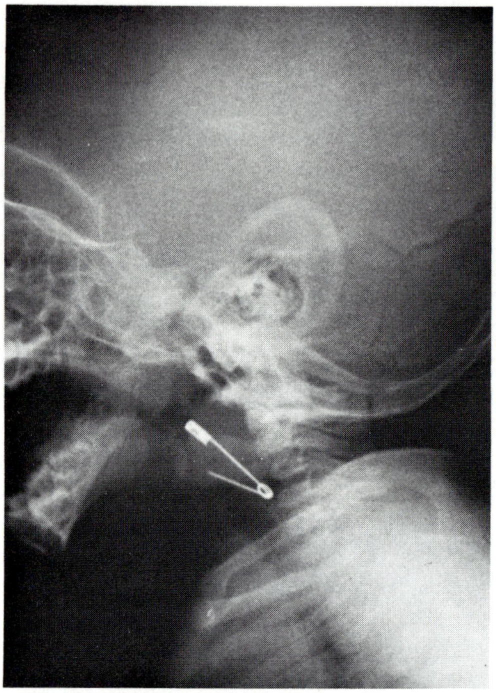

FIG. 8-9. Open safety pin in the hypopharynx of a 7-month-old child.

Esophagus. Esophageal foreign bodies usually produce dysphagia. Compression of the air passages may produce dyspnea, cough, or wheezing. Penetrating objects may produce subcutaneous emphysema (Fig. 8-10A and B).

Nose. Nasal foreign bodies may initially produce airway obstruction. Later, they may cause unilateral mucopurulent discharge. This discharge may be bloody and have a foul odor. Nasal foreign bodies can usually be grasped and removed, or removed with a loop placed behind them. In uncooperative children general anesthesia may be required.

X-ray examination for a foreign body must include all regions from the roof of the nasal cavities to the pelvis. Care must be taken not to overlook multiple foreign bodies. Tracheotomy may be life saving when a child's respiration is obstructed by a foreign body.

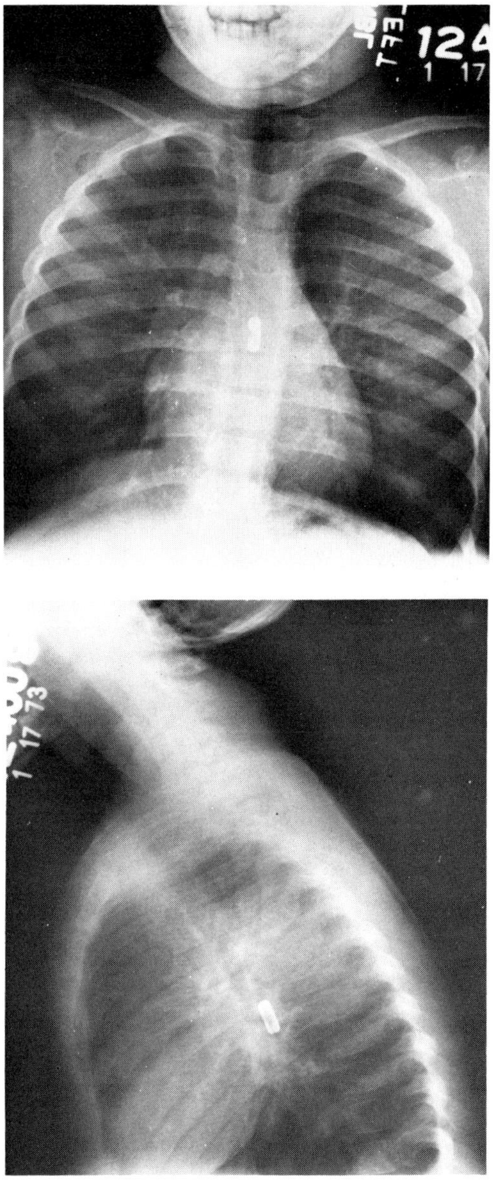

FIG. 8-10. Posteroanterior and lateral views of a key-chain clasp lodged in the esophagus of a child.

The physician should avoid impacting a foreign body by attempting removal with his finger. If the child is not in respiratory distress, an attempt may be made to visualize the foreign body with a mirror. If no foreign body is found, roentgenograms should be taken in anteroposterior and lateral projections. Special training is required for competence in endoscopic removal of foreign bodies. This procedure is best performed in an operating room equipped solely for this purpose. In preparation for endoscopy, the patient should be kept comfortable. The chest, head, and shoulders should be slightly dependent. Do not give emetics. It is helpful if food can be withheld for 6 hours before administration of general anesthesia. A duplicate of the foreign body is helpful in planning the operative procedure.

TRAUMA

Nose and Face. Fractures of the septal cartilage and nasal bones are common in children; fractures of the facial bone are less frequent.[12] Soft tissue swelling after nasal fracture may make the diagnosis difficult, and roentgenograms often are not helpful. The nasal bones heal rapidly making the reduction difficult after 5 days. Early referral is helpful to assure timely examination under anesthesia and reduction of nasal fractures. If the nasal bones and septum heal in a poor position, subsequent growth may result in considerable deformity and airway obstruction. Late corrective procedure should be deferred until age 16 to 18 when growth should be complete. Fractures of the mandible are usually compound. Reduction and immobilization are required. Dislodged teeth should be saved and occasionally may be successfully reimplanted. Fractures of the zygoma and maxilla are rare in children. These fractures result from severe trauma such as automobile accidents. Open reduction is usually indicated.

Larynx. Laryngeal injuries should be suspected in children with head or chest trauma.[14] Symptoms may include hoarseness or stridor and subcutaneous emphysema. Tracheotomy may be required to establish an airway. Roentgenograms may help to establish a diagnosis. Further investigation by endoscopic examination and open surgical exploration should follow promptly. Mucosal lacerations are sutured, and cartilage fractures are reduced and stabilized with wire fixation. Internal stents may be required to assure an airway through the trachea and larynx. These measures are undertaken to avoid airway stenosis.

Cervical Esophagus. Corrosive esophagitis is destructive trauma to the esophagus that results in a loss of tissue in its walls.[8] All children with a history of ingestion of a potentially corrosive substance should be hospitalized. The presence or absence of oral or pharyngeal ulcerations is no sure indication of esophageal pathology. Treatment is undertaken to promote healing while preventing esophageal strictures. Since steroids are potent antifibroplastic and anti-inflammatory agents, steroid therapy should be instituted on admission. Antibiotics should be given to minimize infection in the ulcerated esophagus. A nasogastric tube is passed for feeding. Esophagoscopy should be delayed 2 to 5 days to allow the patient to stabilize. Also, esophageal ulcerations become more obvious after a short delay. The esophagoscope is advanced only to the first esophageal ulceration. If no esophageal ulcerations exist, treatment is suspended. The esophagus should heal from mild non-ulcerative esophagitis without stricturing. If ulcerative lesions are identified, treatment is continued, and interval esophagoscopy is performed to follow progress until healing is complete. If the esophageal lumen becomes obstructed by stricture, dilatation therapy is started.

REFERENCES

1. Beinfield, H. H.: Surgery for bilateral bony atresia of the posterior nares in the newborn. *Arch. Otolaryngol. 70*:1, 1959.
2. Bernstein, L.: Management of cleft lip and palate problems. *Otolaryngol. Clin. North Am. 3*:171, 1970.
3. Blumberg, J. B., J. K. Stevenson, R. J. Lemire and E. A. Boyden: Laryngotracheal cleft, the embryologic implications. Review of the literature. *Surgery 57*:559, 1965.
4. Bouhuys, A.: *Breathing.* Grune & Stratton, New York, p. 25, 1974.
5. Bremer, J. L.: *Congenital Anomalies of the Viscera.* Harvard University Press, Cambridge, Mass., p. 1, 1957.
6. Bunker, P. G.: Foreign body complications. *Laryngoscope 71*:903, 1961.
7. Calcaterra, T. C.: An evaluation of the treatment of subglottic hemangioma. *Laryngoscope 78*:1956, 1968.
8. Cardona, J. C., and J. F. Daly: Current management of corrosive esophagitis. *Ann. Otol. Rhinol. Laryngol. 80*:521, 1971.
9. Cramblett, H. G.: Croup—present day concept. *Pediatrics 25*:1071, 1960.
10. Crooks, J.: Non-inflammatory laryngeal stridor in infants. *Arch. Dis. Child. 29*:12, 1954.
11. Dennison, W. M.: The Pierre Robin Syndrome. *Pediatrics 36*:336, 1965.
12. Dingman, R. O. and P. Natvig: *Surgery of Facial Fractures.* W. B. Saunders Co., Philadelphia, p. 311, 1964.
13. Fearon, B. and R. Shortreed: Tracheobronchial compression by congenital cardiovascular anomalies in children: syndrome of apnea. *Ann. Otol. Rhinol. Laryngol. 72*:949, 1963.
14. Fitz-Hugh, G. S. and J. B. Powell: Acute traumatic injuries of the oropharynx, laryngopharynx and cervical trachea in children. *Otolaryngol. Clin. North Am. 3*:375, 1970.
15. Franceschetti, A. and D. Klein: The mandibulofacial dysostosis. A new hereditary syndrome. *Acta Ophthalmol. 27*:143, 1949.
16. Gardner, H. G., K. R. Powell, V. J. Roden and J. D. Cherry: The evaluation of racemic epinephrine in the treatment of infectious croup. *Pediatrics 52*:52, 1973.
17. Hamilton, W. J. and H. W. Mossman: *Human Embryology* (4th ed.). The Williams & Wilkins Co., Baltimore, p. 291, 1972.
18. Holder, T. M., D. T. Cloud, J. E. Lewis, Jr. and G. P. W. Pilling: Esophageal atresia and tracheoesophageal fistula. A survey of its members by the Surgical Section of the American Academy of Pediatrics. *Pediatrics 34*:542, 1964.
19. Holder, T. M., L. L. Leape and K. W. Asheraft: Congenital malformations of the trachea, bronchi and esophagus. In *Otolaryngology: Head and Neck,* Volume 3, M. M. Paparella and D. A. Shumbrick (Eds.). W. B. Saunders Co., Philadelphia, p. 685, 1973.
20. Holinger, P. H.: Foreign bodies in the air and food passages. *Trans. Am. Acad. Ophthalmol. Otolaryngol. 66*:193, 1962.
21. Jackson, C.: Foreign bodies in the air and food passages. In *Otolaryngology,* Volume 5, W. H. Ma-

loney (Ed.). Harper & Row Publishers, Hagerstown, Md., p. 1, 1974.
22. James, J. A.: Dexamethasone in croup. *Am. J. Dis. Child.* *117*:511, 1969.
23. Kartagener, M. and P. Stucki: Bronchiectasis with situs inversus. *Arch. Pediatr.* *79*:193, 1962.
24. Margolis, C. Z., D. L. Ingram and J. H. Meyer: Routine tracheotomy in Hemophilus influenzae Type B epiglottitis. *J. Pediatr.* *81*:1150, 1972.
25. Milko, D. A., G. Marshak and T. W. Striker: Nasotracheal intubation in the treatment of acute epiglottitis. *Pediatrics* *53*:674, 1974.
26. McGovern, F. H. and G. S. Fitz-Hugh: Surgical management of congenital choanal atresia. *Arch. Otolaryngol.* *73*:627, 1961.
27. Miller, R. D. and M. B. Divertie: Kartagener's syndrome. *Chest* *62*:130, 1972.
28. Newth, C. J. L., H. Levison and A. C. Bryan: The respiratory status of children with croup. *J. Pediatr.* *81*:1068, 1972.
29. Paradise, J. L.: Why T & A remains moot. *Pediatrics* *49*:648, 1972.
30. Pratt, L. W.: Tonsillectomy and adenoidectomy mortality and morbidity. *Trans. Am. Acad. Ophthalmol. Otolaryngol.* *74*:1146, 1970.
31. Proctor, B. and C. Proctor: Congenital lesions of the head and neck. *Otolaryngol. Clin. North Am.* *3*:221, 1970.
32. Proctor, D. F.: Physiology of the upper airway. In *Handbook of Physiology, Section 3, Respiration,* Volume 1, W. O. Fenn and H. Rahn (Eds.). American Physiological Society, Washington, D.C., p. 309, 1969.
33. Reid, J. M. and J. A. Donaldson: The indications for tonsillectomy and adenoidectomy. *Otolaryngol. Clin. North Am.* *3*:339, 1970.
34. Resouly, A.: Kartagener's syndrome. A case report and review of the literature. *J. Laryngol. Otol.* *86*:1237, 1972.
35. Ritter, F. N.: The diagnosis and treatment of suppurative sinus disease in children. *Otolaryngol. Clin. North Am.* *3*:290, 1970.
36. Silverman, W. A. and W. A. Blanc: The effect of Humidity on survival of newly born premature infants. *Pediatrics* *20*:477, 1957.
37. Singleton, G. T. and B. Hardcastle: Congenital choanal atresia. *Arch. Otolaryngol.* *87*:620, 1968.
38. Smith, J. L. and F. R. Stowe: The Pierre Robin syndrome (glossoptosis, micrognathia, cleft palate). *Pediatrics* *27*:128, 1961.
39. Snow, J. B.: The classification of respiratory viruses and their clinical manifestations. *Laryngoscope* *79*:1485, 1969.
40. Sprinkle, P. M.: Criteria for the diagnosis of adenotonsillitis. *Ann. Otol. Rhinol. Laryngol.* (*Suppl. 19*): *84*:25, 1975.
41. Sutow, W. W.: Cancer of the head and neck in children. *J.A.M.A.* *190*:414, 1964.

Bronchitis and Bronchiolitis

W. SHAIN SCHLEY AND ALFRED N. KRAUSS

9

Acquired Disease of the Bronchi

The bronchi distribute throughout the lungs. They range in size from the right main stem bronchus (12 to 16 mm in diameter in the adult) and the left main stem bronchus (10 to 14 mm in the adult) down to the bronchioles, airways generally 1 mm or less. In the human, bronchial branches arise by means of bifurcations. While every new branch is smaller than its parent, the total resulting cross-sectional area at every division is greater. The bronchi do not represent an abrupt transition in form at their origin from the trachea, and are similarly gradually transformed into the bronchioles at their end.[28] The main stem bronchi, where they arise at the tracheal bifurcation, are fibromuscular tubes supported by cartilage and lined with a mucosal epithelium. The segmental bronchi have irregular plates of cartilage, a muscular layer, and an abundance of mucous glands. The smaller bronchi have a prominent venous plexus and fewer glands than the preceding segmental bronchi. Bronchi and their surrounding tissues contain many nerve endings.

Bronchi play a prominent part in pulmonary reflexes, especially those that relate to pulmonary irritants. The muscular lining of these airways provides a means for active regulation of airway resistance mediated by these nerves. Pulmonary irritants, in addition to eliciting reflexes that may result in alterations of airway resistance, also may affect secretion of mucus at the bronchial level. Alterations of these mechanical and physical characteristics of the bronchi in disease provide a basis for understanding the pathogenesis of acquired disease of the bronchi.

ETIOLOGY

Congenital anomalies of the airways have been discussed in Chapter 8. Primarily, the diseases to be considered in this chapter are of infectious origin. In both children and adults, viruses are the major source of acute disease of the bronchi.[28,32] When bronchitis becomes chronic, or in bronchiectasis, bacteria assume a more important role. *H. influenzae* has been especially associated with bronchiectasis, although *S. aureus*, pneumococci, and *E. coli* have also been found in association with this disease.[4,19] Bronchiectasis has also occurred with tuberculosis and fungal infection.[44]

The bronchi are in the first line of defense against bacterial and viral infection. Various environmental, social, and hereditary factors have been associated with decreasing effectiveness of the bronchi in dealing with bacteria and other foreign material. Tobacco smoke has been shown to have a depressant effect on the ability of macrophages, taken from rabbit lungs, to inactivate *S. albus.*[22] The toxic element was found to be in the gaseous phase of the smoke. Gaseous pollutants, such as NO_2, have been associated with an increase in the incidence of bronchitis in school children.[35] These findings, from Tennessee, have been corroborated by more extensive epidemiologic studies from England and Wales.[5] The ability of the lungs to clear bacteria is reduced by cigarette smoke,[31] and this reduction is associated with an increase in the number and volume of mucous glands in their airways.[11] The mucus is of increased viscosity and interferes with bacterial clearance. Thus air pollutants arising from both industries and tobacco smoke act synergistically to promote infection in the lower respiratory tract of exposed individuals.[21]

Smoking, air pollution, and infection are all important factors in the development of lower airway disease in children and adults, but these aspects appear more frequently when a family has a history of cough and wheezing.[32] The relatives of allergic children have increased bronchial lability on exercise.[20] These studies suggest that, in addition to exposure to various airway irritants and pollutants, hereditary factors are important. Studies from England and Wales demonstrate an increased morbidity from bronchitis in children of semiskilled and unskilled workers.[5] The authors have suggested that this finding demonstrates the combined effects of poor environment, exposure to pollutants, and heredity.

BRONCHITIS

Bronchitis is a disease characterized by a cough with the production of sputum. As indicated in the previous section, chemical irritants, viruses, bacteria, fungi, and allergies may all result in inflammation of the bronchi. In children, this disease may occur in association with bronchiolitis, laryngotracheobronchitis (croup), and asthma.

It may occur at any time of the year, but bronchitis is most frequently associated with damp and cool seasons. Most commonly it is the result of viral infections, especially in children,[13,32] but may also be bacterial in origin. Staphylococci, pneumococci, and *H. influenzae* are the most frequently reported bacterial pathogens. Bronchitis also occurs in association with viral influenza, diphtheria, measles (rubeola), and smallpox. Dusts, especially those of heavy metals, may also result in bronchitis.

In its early stages, bronchitis is characterized pathologically by congestion and edema of the bronchial mucosa. Hypersecretion of the mucous cells follows. With progression of the illness, necrosis of the bronchial epithelium takes place, and desquamation of these cells into the bronchial lumen occurs. Following the acute illness, complete recovery may take place or scarring may occur.[13]

When a viral infection is the cause, the onset usually occurs over a 24-hour period. Like most viral infections, a low grade fever may be present accompanied by chills and prostration. After this initial syndrome, a "loose" cough begins, and the patient may begin to produce sputum. Rales and rhonchi, especially at the bases, are heard. In the adult, bronchitis usually lasts about 7 to 10 days.

Laboratory investigations are usually of little assistance. The radiologic findings are ordinarily nonspecific (Fig. 9-1) in the absence of pneumonia.[13,46] A chest roentgenogram should be performed, however, if pneumonia is suspected. Examination of the sputum and sputum cultures are helpful in identifying specific bacterial pathogens.

In the absence of specific bacterial pathogens, antibiotics are not indicated. Wheezing and coughing may be treated symptomatically with bronchodilators and expectorants. Postural drainage and humidification are important in maintaining the patency of the airways by their cleansing actions. Removal of any environmental factors, such as cigarette smoke, is also of great potential benefit.

BRONCHIECTASIS

This disorder is defined as dilation of the bronchi. It may be the result of bronchial injury early in childhood and, if not properly treated, may lead to severe disability and early death from pulmonary failure or cor pulmonale.

Most patients with bronchiectasis develop the disease before the age of 5 years.[1,15,16,19,47] Most authors are in agreement that about three-quarters of all patients become sick before their fifth birthday, and 30 to 40% of all patients develop their first symptoms before they are 12 months of age. Bronchiectasis is related to a preceding pneumonia in about one-third of all cases, and to pertussis in about one-sixth of all cases. Other com-

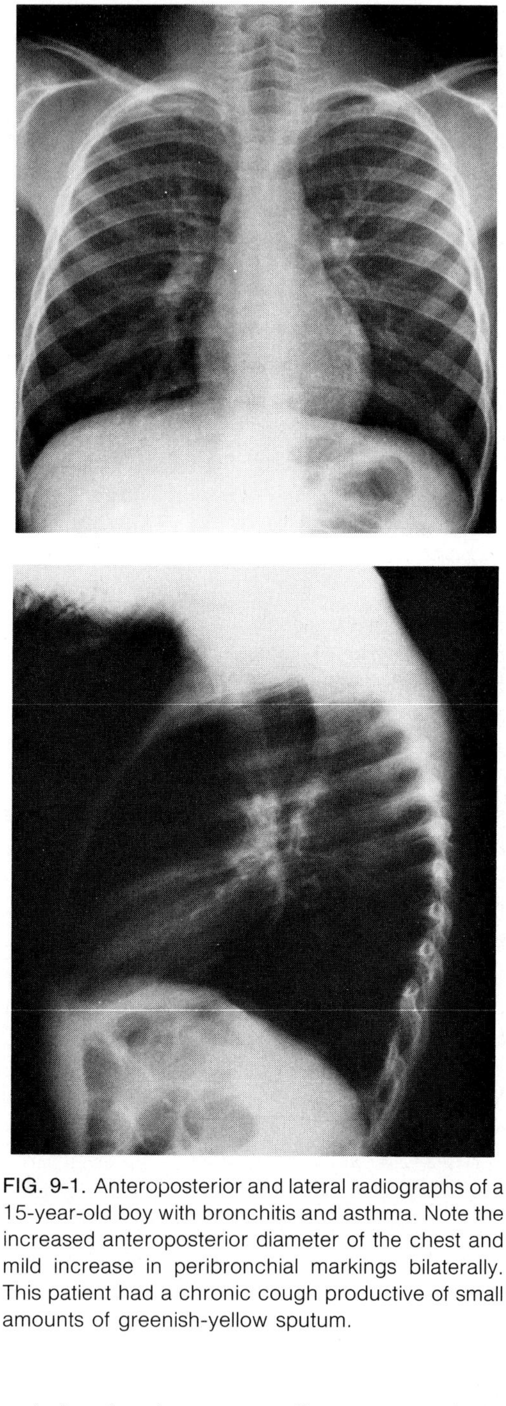

FIG. 9-1. Anteroposterior and lateral radiographs of a 15-year-old boy with bronchitis and asthma. Note the increased anteroposterior diameter of the chest and mild increase in peribronchial markings bilaterally. This patient had a chronic cough productive of small amounts of greenish-yellow sputum.

mon preceding events include tuberculosis, measles, and asthma. Bronchiectasis is also a sequel of cystic fibrosis and hypogammaglobulinemia. Congenital bronchiectasis may occur both as a result of congenital narrowing of airways with distal infection and as a result of Kartagener's syndrome (situs inversus, sinusitis, and bronchiectasis).

The patient with bronchiectasis usually complains of a chronic productive (or loose) cough. Depending on the presence of respiratory infection, the sputum produced may be white, yellow, or green, and may be foul-smelling.[6,19,47] Hemoptysis of varying severity is present in about 15% of patients. Other complaints include fever, sweats, and, in children, poor weight gain.[1,19,47] Although asthma is not a frequent initiating event in the patient with bronchiectasis, approximately 50% of bronchiectatic patients complain of asthma.[16,19,47] Sinusitis also occurs in a significant percentage of patients with bronchiectasis.[19]

Physical examination of the patient with bronchiectasis generally reveals localized crepitations and inspiratory rales.[6,19] In series of patients studied before antibiotic use became common, clubbing and cyanosis were relatively common. In more recent series, these findings are less common. Postural deformities are also frequent, especially in surgically treated patients, and height and weight are somewhat below normal.[16] Because bronchiectasis is associated with sinusitis, the sinuses should be carefully examined. In addition, the two other components of Kartagener's triad—sinusitis and situs inversus—should be sought.[23]

The early pathology of bronchiectasis is similar to that of bronchitis. In the case of bronchiectasis, however, progression of the disease with peribronchial fibrosis and dilation of the bronchi follows. The mucous glands may hypertrophy. Destruction of the bronchial cartilage in association with fibrosis is thought to be the cause of the bronchial dilation. In its early, reversible stages the dilation is tubular or cylindrical in appearance; in later, irreversible stages it is saccular.[1] Occasionally the inflammatory process may erode into vessels, causing hemoptysis. The lesions of tuberculosis, histoplasmosis, aspergillosis, hypogammaglobulinemia, Kartagener's syndrome, and cystic fibrosis may also be found if these conditions are present in association with bronchiectasis.

These pathologic changes are associated with a marked decrease in the clearance of particles from the airways. This clearance delay is greatly aggravated by smoking.[33] Patients with localized disease may not have significant alterations in their pulmonary function tests.[4] The presence of abnormalities in pulmonary function is not related to the type of bronchiectasis—cylindrical or saccular. In general, these patients demonstrate evidence of diffuse obstruction, with reductions in maximum breathing capacity (MBC), increased airway resistance, and increased residual volume/total lung capacity ratios (RV/TLC). An elevated dead space/tidal volume ratio and slow nitrogen washout are also present in some patients, although carbon monoxide diffusing capacity and arterial oxygen saturation are usually within normal limits. More sensitive tests of hypoxemia, such as the alveolar-arterial oxygen difference, may be mildly abnormal. Tests of pulmonary mechanics reveal reductions in dynamic compliance, frequency-dependent falls in compliance, and abnormal flow-volume loops in patients with bronchiectasis.[4,30]

Bronchiectasis may be localized or general in its distribution. It is bilateral in approximately one-third of cases. When unilateral, it occurs more frequently on the left. In general, the lower lobes are much more frequently affected than the upper lobes.[1,6,15,16,19,47] The distribution of bronchiectasis is important in determining therapy. In the absence of pneumonia, the plain film of the chest (Fig. 9-2) is usually not helpful in diagnosis.[6] Similarly, bronchoscopy is not helpful in this respect. Bronchos-

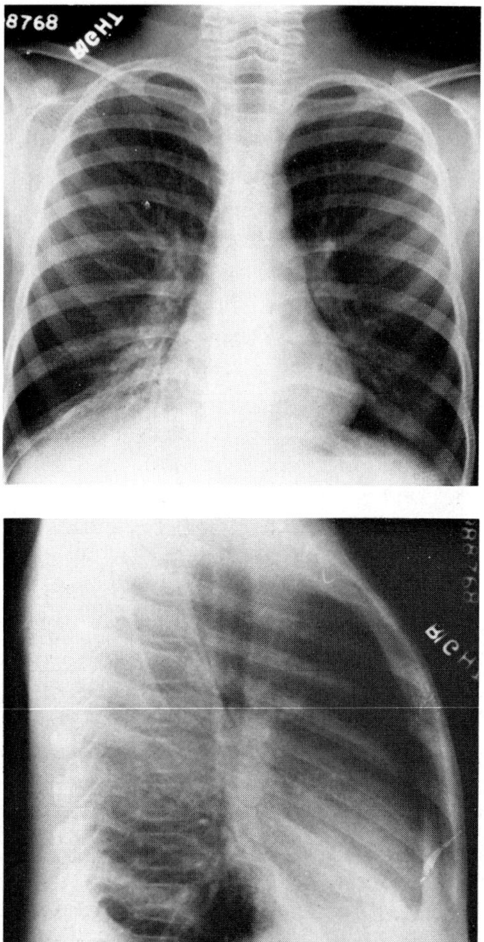

FIG. 9-2. Anteroposterior and lateral radiographs of an 8-year-old boy with surgically proven bronchiectasis of the right middle and lower lobes. Infiltrate is present on the right.

copy usually reveals inflammation of the mucosa and the presence of pus in the airways, but cannot be used to confirm the diagnosis or extent of bronchiectasis; for those aspects bronchography (Fig. 9-3) is necessary.[1,6,15,16,19,47]

Other laboratory aids should include skin tests for tuberculosis and fungi, sweat test for

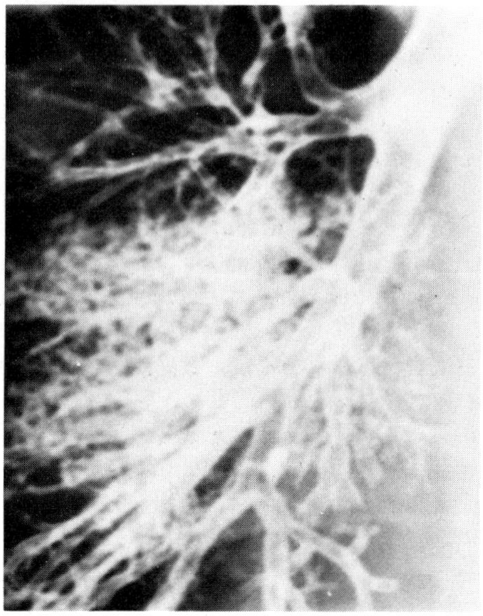

FIG. 9-3. Enlargement of a bronchogram of patient depicted in Figure 9-2. Note the dilation of bronchi and pooling of contrast material in affected bronchi at center and lower portions of the radiograph, and compare with delicate patterns of normal bronchi in the upper portion of the figure.

cystic fibrosis, sputum cultures for bacteria and fungi, and immunoelectrophoresis for detection of hypogammaglobulinemia.

With the advent of effective antibiotics, the therapy and prognosis of bronchiectasis have undergone a marked change. Intensive chemotherapy of the childhood respiratory illnesses recognized as precursors of bronchiectasis has resulted in a decreased incidence of this illness.[7,17] In addition, patients with established bronchiectasis also benefit from vigorous antibiotic therapy of bacterial infections. Postural drainage and expectorants are extremely valuable in maintaining clear and clean airways. Appropriate desensitization therapy should be offered asthmatic patients who will benefit from it. Asthma, however, has been associated with a poor prognosis in bronchiectasis.[16,47] In a long-term follow-up of bronchiectatic children into the antibiotic era, it was found that these children usually stabilized during the second and third decades of life.[16,17] Deaths occurred mainly in patients with severe bilateral disease, and were caused by either cor pulmonale or pulmonary failure.

Surgical procedure is indicated in patients with localized disease and mild to moderate symptoms.[7,16,17] Since operation is rarely an emergency in patients with bronchiectasis, a year of vigorous medical therapy is usually appropriate before surgical procedure is considered. The progress of the patient may be followed with bronchograms. Cylindrical bronchiectasis is frequently reversible. While a focal lesion causing bronchiectasis may not jeopardize the normal lung, cases of extension after removal of apparently localized disease have been encountered.[1] Bronchography correlates with the severity of the disease to a better degree than the physical examination, and therefore should be used as a guide to the use of surgical therapy.

Following successful surgical treatment in childhood, lung growth, measured by vital capacity, keeps pace with physical growth.[1] Successful therapy of bronchiectasis frequently results in disappearance of such physical signs as clubbing. However, dyspnea on exercise was found to persist, especially in patients who required operations.[16]

In summary, the bronchi serve an important function in the distribution of air throughout the lung. They also provide an important defense against bacterial, viral, and environmental pathogens. They may be injured by pollutants in such a way as to reduce their ability to perform these important functions. Since disease in childhood may lead to chronic disability and early death in adulthood, it is important for the pediatrician to recognize disease of the bronchi early in its course and to provide vigorous treatment. In addition, the pediatrician can perform an important role in preventive medicine by campaigning against smoking and air pollution, and thus prevent a lifetime of disease.

Bronchiolitis

Bronchiolitis is an acute infection of the lower respiratory tract, frequently occurring in children during the first year of life. Commonly preceded by an upper respiratory infection, its onset is rapid. The bronchioles and alveoli are the major areas affected by this illness, and the pathologic changes that take place in these areas account for the symptoms and signs of the patient with bronchiolitis. Investigation of this patient's medical history often provides the clinician with important clues as to the future course of respiratory illness in the child.

ANATOMY

Bronchioles are the first conducting airways that do not contain cartilage. In the human adult they are approximately 1 mm in diameter.[28] They are unsupported by cartilage, but have a very high proportion of smooth muscle in proportion to the diameter of their lumen. Krahl suggests that the term bronchiole be reserved for airways that are directly incorporated into the surrounding pulmonary parenchyma, that have few or no mucous-secreting structures, and that have a continuous epithelial lining of ciliated and nonciliated cells.[28] Fibroelastic elements within the walls of the bronchioles maintain the lumen of the airway and help regulate its diameter by exerting tension. Each bronchiole that arises from a bronchus gives rise to approximately 10 to 20 terminal bronchioles. The terminal bronchioles are not equipped with ciliated epithelial cells or goblet cells, but heavily granulated Clara cells, which secrete a clear liquid, make their appearance. Terminal bronchioles, in turn, branch into two respiratory bronchioles, which are so called because of the appearance of alveoli. The respiratory bronchioles may give rise to one or two more divisions. Further divisions are usually termed alveolar ducts. It can be seen that, because of the amount of smooth muscle bronchioles contain, and their position between the bronchi and the areas of pulmonary gas exchange, the bronchioles play a key role in the distribution of gas within the lung.

INCIDENCE AND ETIOLOGY

Bronchiolitis is commonly an illness of the young child. Holdaway, Romer, and Gardner reported that 77% of their cases were under the age of 6 months.[26] In 93% of cases of bronchiolitis another family member had a viral infection.[9] The pattern is, then, for a viral infection in an older individual to spread to an infant, who subsequently develops the clinical syndrome of bronchiolitis.

The virus most frequently associated with bronchiolitis is the respiratory syncytial virus (RSV). Depending on the method of sampling and the patient population, a viral cause is identified in 40 to 75% of all cases of bronchiolitis.[3,9,18,34,45] RSV accounts for 16 to 90% of virus isolations in bronchiolitis. Epidemics of bronchiolitis have been identified,[3,12,18,34,45] frequently in association with RSV, and these epidemics occur most frequently between December and May.[50] Sporadic cases also occur. Although these are most likely of viral origin, the relationship between sporadic bronchiolitis and asthma is an interesting one and is discussed in a later section, Course and Prognosis.

PATHOLOGY AND PATHOPHYSIOLOGY

Postmortem examination of patients dying after bronchiolitis reveals that the disease process is largely limited to the lungs.[10,27] Grossly, the lungs are markedly emphysematous. Mucous plugs may be found in the airways, and this condition may be associated with areas of atelectasis. The alveoli are more usually overdistended with air. Microscopically, the bronchioles are surrounded with lymphocytes, and a polymorphonuclear leukocytic infiltration is also seen in many cases. The alveolar cell walls may be edematous. Characteristic viral inclusion bodies are not seen with light microscopy in patients dying of bronchiolitis.

Air trapping occurs extensively in bronchiolitis because of the swelling and edema of the small airways. Inspiration is an active muscular process. The negative intrathoracic pressures generated during inspiration serve to dilate the airways and permit entry of air into the alveoli. Positive pressure generated during expiration tends to close the airways. Positive pressures must be generated because the normal process of relaxation does not generate enough pressure to allow complete expulsion of air during expiration when the bronchioles are obstructed, as in bronchiolitis. This process of air trapping results in the characteristic barrel chest of the infant with bronchiolitis. It also causes underventilation. Reynolds has shown that the hypoxemia resulting from the underventilation in bronchiolitis responds to low concentrations of supplemental oxygen.[39,42] This finding indicates that maldistribution of ventilation and not intrapulmonary venoarterial shunting is the cause of hypoxemia in bronchiolitis. The defect in oxygenation is usually repaired within 2 weeks.

Physiologic studies have documented that children with bronchiolitis have elevated respiratory frequencies when compared with normal children.[29,37,49] Minute volume is slightly higher and tidal volume slightly lower in these patients. Although Kreiger failed to demonstrate a significantly increased pulmonary resistance in her patients with bronchiolitis,[29] two later studies did show a significant rise in total and inspiratory and expiratory resistances.[37,49] The overall rise may be as great as 4.2 times normal, although the average is 2.7 times normal values. This change is associated with a doubling of the thoracic gas volume and a fall in pulmonary compliance to one-third of normal.[37] These changes are consistent with the findings of bronchiolar edema and emphysema at postmortem examination, and the thesis that bronchiolar obstruction accounts for the observed air trapping. Although the expected changes in mechanics are observed, they do not closely correlate with the observed changes in blood gas tensions,[37] suggesting that other mechanisms, such as small areas of atelectasis, may play a significant role in determining the precise clinical status of a particular patient.

SIGNS AND SYMPTOMS

Most patients with bronchiolitis are infants under the age of 6 months. The illness frequently begins as a mild cold, with inflammation of the nasal mucosa. Most patients have temperatures between 99° and 101° F by rectum. Only about 25% have rectal temperatures in excess of 102.5° F (39.1° C).[50] Signs of inflammation are generally limited to the nose, trachea, and bronchi. Conjunctivitis, purulent rhinitis, otitis, and laryngitis are not frequent in association with bronchiolitis. The onset of respiratory distress may be rapid. As indicated in the section on pathophysiology, the respirations become shallow and rapid, and rates of 40 to 80 breaths/min. are not unusual. As the illness progresses, pallor, cyanosis, limpness, and collapse may occur. Physical examination of the chest reveals an increased anteroposterior diameter.

Retractions are present in most patients, and wheezing occurs in about half.[9,45] Rales are also a frequent accompaniment of bronchiolitis. Breath sounds may diminish, and rhonchi may also be heard. In association with the increased diameter of the chest and the air trapping that takes place, the chest is usually hyperresonant to percussion. Any localized diminution in breath sounds or dullness should make the clinician recall the association between bronchiolitis and bronchopneumonia. In severe cases, where oral intake of fluids has been poor, the signs of dehydration may accompany bronchiolitis. The liver edge is often palpable 1 to 2 cm below the right costal margin because of overexpansion of the lungs. In the absence of congestive heart failure, the liver edge is sharp.

Radiographic examination of the chest reveals hyperlucency of the lungs (Fig. 9-4). The anteroposterior diameter of the chest is increased, and the diaphragm may be flattened. The increased diameter of the chest may make the heart appear small. Associated bronchopneumonia may be evident as increased peribronchial markings, and pulmonary linear streaking may also be evident.[46]

Differential diagnosis includes asthma, asthmatic bronchitis, and pneumonia. Although careful physical and radiologic examination should enable the clinician to differentiate bronchiolitis from pneumonia, the separation between bronchiolitis and asthma is more difficult. This distinction is particularly difficult when an infant is first seen with respiratory distress of rapid onset, low grade fever, and wheezing. Simon and Jordan have pointed out the great degree of similarity between respiratory syncytial-negative bronchiolitis and asthmatic bronchitis.[45] Patients with either RS-negative bronchiolitis or asthmatic bronchitis are more likely to have a higher total white cell count (14,000 to 15,000 WBC versus 12,000), a temperature over 102° F (45 versus 30%), and eosinophilia than the child with RS-positive bronchiolitis. RS-positive bronchiolitis is more likely to affect the infant under 6 months of age and to occur in epidemics. Systemic toxicity is not as great as bronchiolitis unassociated with RS virus. An allergic component is found less frequently in RS-positive patients than in RS-negative patients. None of these points, however, are absolute clinical indicators of a particular syndrome, and in general do not provide any assistance in prescribing therapy. The clinical response to bronchodilators is not a good differentiating point between asthma and bronchiolitis, since improvement in a bronchiolitic patient may be

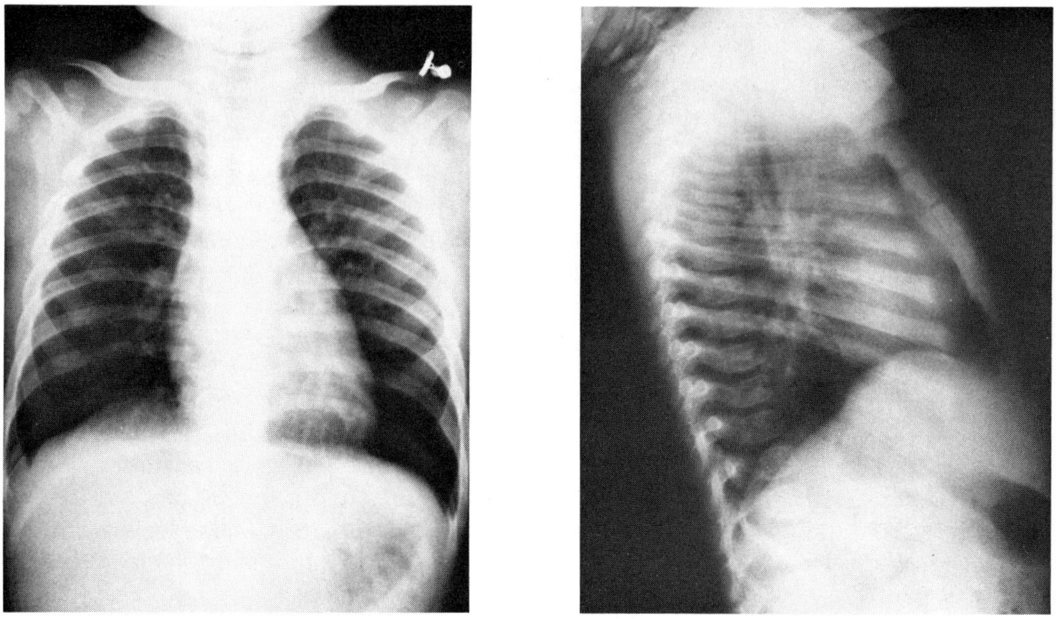

FIG. 9-4. Anteroposterior and lateral radiographs of $1\frac{1}{2}$-year-old infant with bronchiolitis. Note the increased amount of intrathoracic air and the lack of distinct pulmonary infiltrates. Diaphragm is flattened.

due to nonspecific effects on the airways. Aerosolized bronchodilators are of little value in bronchiolitis.[36]

THERAPY

The main principles of the treatment of bronchiolitis are to maintain an adequate level of arterial oxygenation and to prevent dehydration. To these purposes, oxygen should be provided in amounts sufficient to relieve cyanosis. Adequate amounts of fluids should be given either intravenously or by tube. There is no objective evidence of benefit from mist, expectorants, aerosols, or wetting agents.[27,36,42,50] Aminophylline and epinephrine may, in appropriate doses, be of value in the patient with a significant bronchospastic component. The routine use of these drugs is not to be advocated, however. Because of the increased volume of the lungs, the liver and spleen are often palpable. In association with the tachypnea and tachycardia that accompany bronchiolitis, the presence of a palpable liver has led many clinicians to diagnose congestive heart failure. The need for digitalis is rare.[42]

The liver of congestive heart failure has a rounded edge, in contrast to the normally sharp hepatic margin. A pulse rate of 160 to 180 beats per minute often occurs in bronchiolitis without heart failure. Extreme tachycardia, collapse, and hepatomegaly are all indications for the use of digitalis in bronchiolitis. It should be used to treat heart failure, not in the routine care of the patient with bronchiolitis. Sedatives are to be avoided. Anxiety in bronchiolitis is a sign of hypoxemia. Oxygen is the best sedative agent for the child with bronchiolitis. In the absence of bronchopneumonia, antibiotics are not indicated for viral bronchiolitis. *H. influenzae* has been associated with some outbreaks of bronchiolitis. In this instance, the use of antibiotics should be guided by cultures and sensitivities. Tracheotomy is of no value as the obstruction to airflow in bronchiolitis is intrapulmonary.

Controversy surrounds the use of steroids in bronchiolitis. Most studies evaluating the effects of steroid therapy have relied on clinical observations or duration of hospital stay, which may be affected by factors unrelated to the course of the illness or the efficacy of the medication. Dennis and colleagues found no objective evidence of benefits from the use of methylprednisolone in bronchiolitis, but nevertheless found it valuable for "desperate" situations.[9] High did not find steroids useful, however.[25] Dabbous and colleagues, using a modification of the Silverman retraction score, could demonstrate no significant differences in the course of patients receiving 5 mg/kg of prednisone on the first day of illness, and 2.5 mg/kg on the second day.[8] Reynolds and Cook suggest that steroids may be of value in extreme situations.[42] Objective trials using the techniques of pulmonary physiology to evaluate the progress of patients are needed to resolve the questions regarding the use of steroids in bronchiolitis.

Similar problems surround the use of aerosolized bronchodilators. Phelan and Williams were unable to demonstrate any effect of aerosolized orciprenaline or isoprenaline on infants with bronchiolitis.[36] In view of the problems associated with deposition of particles in small airways even in health, this finding is not surprising. It should be remembered when considering this route for administration of other drugs.

In summary, patients with bronchiolitis should receive adequate oxygen and fluids. When necessary, both should be regulated by means of arterial blood gases and determinations of serum chemistries. Sedatives are contraindicated in bronchiolitis. Anxiety should be treated with oxygen and good nursing care. Steroids and digitalis may be of value in the extremely ill patient, but are not to be used routinely. Bronchodilators, administered parenterally, may be of value in the patient with a significant bronchospastic component, but are not routinely indicated in bronchiolitis.

COURSE AND PROGNOSIS

Bronchiolitis is mainly a disease of ambulatory patients. Only one child in five is hospitalized.[27] With present-day therapy, the mortality of hospitalized patients is probably under 1%, although recent series have reported mortalities of up to 5%.[24] The clinical disease usually resolves within about 1 week. As indicated earlier, most physiologic abnormalities that accompany this illness have diminished or disappeared by this time.

The relationship between the occurrence of bronchiolitis in infancy and the later development of allergies has been studied by many groups of investigators. Wittig and Glaser found that 32 of 100 patients with bronchiolitis suffered from asthma, and 17 additional ones have nasal allergies, including hay fever.[48] A history of asthma or eczema was found in 44% of the families involved in this study. Eisen and Bacal, in a 4 to 14-year follow-up of 63 patients with one attack of bronchiolitis, found a 25% incidence of asthma and a 62% incidence of a family history of allergies.[14] Although Simon and Jordan felt that RSV-positive bronchiolitis did not have a major allergic component,[45] a recent study of 80 such patients, 66 of whom were less than 6 months of age at the time of illness, revealed that 56% had further wheezing and a family history of asthma.[43] Boesen's data[2] support those of Simon and Jordan. He found that, whereas only 10% of children ill before 1 year of age developed asthma in later childhood, 70% of those with bronchiolitis after 3 years of age did so. Polmar and colleagues found that patients with sporadic bronchiolitis had higher levels of IgE than patients with epidemic bronchiolitis.[38] IgE levels over the 95 percentile were found in 35% of their patients with sporadic bronchiolitis but only 6% of patients with epidemic bronchiolitis.

These studies suggest some overlap between two patient populations with bronchiolitis. One population consists largely of infants under 1 year of age who develop bronchiolitis in the setting of an epidemic of viral respiratory infection. A small percentage of these children may develop respiratory or other allergies later during childhood. The second group of children, composed mainly of older infants, develops bronchiolitis sporadically. Although a viral illness may initiate disease in these children, it is unaccompanied by an "epidemic" of respiratory illness. Attempts to recover viruses from these patients, especially RSV, frequently fail. This group has a high frequency of a positive family history for allergies. Many of these children (25 to 70%) will have recurrent wheezing or develop asthma.

REFERENCES

1. Avery, M. E., M. C. Riley and A. Weiss: The course of bronchiectasis in childhood. *Bull. Johns Hopkins Hosp. 109*:20, 1961.
2. Boesen, I.: Asthmatic bronchitis in children. *Acta Paediatr. Scand. 42*:87, 1953.
3. Chanock, R. M., H. W. Kim, A. J. Vagarsko, A. Deleva, K. M. Johnson, C. Cumming and R. H. Parrott: Respiratory syncytial virus. I. Virus recovery and other observations during the 1960 outbreak of bronchiolitis. *J.A.M.A. 176*:647, 1961.
4. Cherniack, N. S. and R. W. Carton: Factors associated with respiratory insufficiency in bronchiectasis. *Am. J. Med. 41*:562, 1966.
5. Colley, J. R. T. and D. D. Reid: Urban and social origins of childhood bronchitis in England and Wales. *Br. Med. J. 2*:213, 1970.
6. Crofton, J.: Diagnosis and treatment of bronchiectasis. I. Diagnosis. *Br. Med. J. 1*:721, 1966.
7. Crofton, J.: Diagnosis and treatment of bronchiectasis. II. Treatment and prevention. *Br. Med. J. 1*:783, 1966.
8. Dabbous, I. A., J. S. Tkachyk and S. J. Stamm: A double-blind study on the effects of corticosteroids in the treatment of bronchiolitis. *Pediatrics 37*:477, 1966.
9. Dennis, J. L., W. M. Palmer and R. W. Cleveland: Bronchiolitis in infants. *J.A.M.A. 172*:688, 1960.
10. Disney, M. E., B. R. Sandiford and J. Cragg: Epidemic bronchiolitis in infants. *Br. Med. J. 1*:1407, 1960.
11. Dunnill, M. S.: The contribution of morphology to the study of chronic obstructive lung disease. *Am. J. Med. 57*:506, 1974.
12. Editorial. Epidemic bronchiolitis. *Br. Med. J. 2*:1863, 1960.
13. Edwards, G.: Acute bronchitis—aetiology, diagnosis, management. *Br. Med. J. 1*:963, 1966.
14. Eisen, A. H. and H. L. Bacal: The relationship of acute bronchiolitis to bronchial asthma. *Pediatrics 31*:859, 1963.
15. Field, C. E.: Bronchiectasis in childhood. *Pediatrics 4*:21, 231, 355, 1949.
16. Field, C. E.: Bronchiectasis. *Arch. Dis. Child. 36*:587, 1961.
17. Field, C. E.: Bronchiectasis. *Arch. Dis. Child. 44*:551, 1969.
18. Freeman, G. L. and R. H. Todd: The role of allergy in viral respiratory tract infections. *Am. J. Dis. Child. 104*:330, 1962.
19. Glauser, E. M., C. D. Cook and G. B. Harris: Bronchiectasis: a review of 187 cases in children with follow-up pulmonary function studies in 58. *Acta Paediatr. Scand. Suppl. 165*:1, 1966.
20. Godfrey, S. and P. Konig: Exercise-induced bronchial lability in atopic children and their families. *Ann. Allergy 33*:199, 1974.
21. Green, G.: Cell dysfunction as a pathogenetic determinant in chronic bronchopulmonary disease. *Arch. Environ. Health 21*:481, 1970.
22. Green, G. G. and D. Carolin: The depressant effect of cigarette smoke on the in vitro antibacterial activity of alveolar macrophages. *N. Engl. J. Med. 276*:421, 1967.
23. Hartline, J. V. and P. S. Zelkowitz: Kartagener's syndrome in childhood. *Am. J. Dis. Child. 121*:349, 1971.
24. Heycock, J. D. and T. C. Noble: 1230 cases of acute bronchiolitis in infancy. *Br. Med. J. 2*:879, 1962.
25. High, R. H.: Bronchiolitis. *Pediatr. Clin. North Am. 4*:183, 1957.
26. Holdaway, D., A. C. Romer and P. S. Gardner: The diagnosis and management of bronchiolitis. *Pediatrics 39*:924, 1967.
27. Hubble, D. and G. R. Osborne: Acute bronchiolitis in children. *Br. Med. J. 1*:107, 1941.
28. Krahl, V. E.: Anatomy of the mammalian lung. In *Handbook of Physiology: Respiration,* Volume 1, W. O. Fenn and H. Rahn (Eds.). p. 213, 1964.
29. Krieger, I.: Mechanics of respiration in bronchiolitis. *Pediatrics 33*:45, 1964.
30. Landau, L. I., P. D. Phelan and H. E. Williams: Ventilatory mechanics in patients with bronchiectasis starting in childhood. *Thorax 29*:304, 1974.
31. Laurenzi, G. A., J. J. Guarneri, R. B. Endriga and J. P. Carey: Clearance of bacteria by the lower respiratory tract. *Science 142*:1572, 1963.

32. Leeder, S. R.: Role of infection in the cause and course of chronic bronchitis. *J. Infect. Dis. 131*:731, 1975.
33. Lourenco, R. V.: Distribution and clearance of aerosols. *Am. Rev. Respir. Dis. 101*:460, 1970.
34. Parrott, R. H., A. J. Vargosko, H. W. Kim and R. M. Chanock: Clinical syndromes among children. *Am. Rev. Respir. Dis. Suppl. 88*:73, 1963.
35. Pearlman, M. E., J. F. Finklea, J. P. Creason, C. M. Shy, M. M. Young and R. J. M. Horton: Nitrogen dioxide and lower respiratory illness. *Pediatrics 47*:391, 1971.
36. Phelan, P. D. and H. E. Williams: Sympathomimetic drugs in acute viral bronchiolitis. *Pediatrics 44*:493, 1969.
37. Phelan, P. D., H. E. Williams and M. Freeman: The disturbances of ventilation in acute viral bronchiolitis. *Aust. Paediatr. J. 4*:96, 1968.
38. Polmar, S. H., L. D. Robinson and A. B. Minnefor: Immunoglobulin E in bronchiolitis. *Pediatrics 50*:279, 1972.
39. Reynolds, E. O. R.: The effect of breathing 40% oxygen on the arterial blood gas tensions of babies with bronchiolitis. *J. Pediatr. 63*:1135, 1963.
40. Reynolds, E. O. R.: Recovery from bronchiolitis as judged by arterial blood gas tension measurements. *J. Pediatr. 63*:1182, 1963.
41. Reynolds, E. O. R.: Arterial blood gas tensions in acute disease of the lower respiratory tract in infancy. *Br. Med. J. 1*:1192, 1963.
42. Reynolds, E. O. R. and C. D. Cook: The treatment of bronchiolitis. *J. Pediatr. 63*:1205, 1963.
43. Rooney, J. C. and H. E. Williams: The relationship between proved viral bronchiolitis and subsequent wheezing. *J. Pediatr. 79*:744, 1971.
44. Rosenzweig, D. Y. and W. W. Stead: The role of tuberculosis and other forms of broncho-pulmonary necrosis in the pathogenesis of bronchiectasis. *Am. Rev. Respir. Dis. 93*:769, 1966.
45. Simon, G. and W. S. Jordan: Infectious and allergic aspects of bronchiolitis. *J. Pediatr. 70*:533, 1967.
46. Singleton, E. B. and M. L. Wagner: Radiologic atlas of pulmonary abnormalities in children. W. B. Saunders, Philadelphia, pp. 93, 153, 1971.
47. Strang, C.: Fate of children with bronchiectasis. *Ann. Intern. Med. 44*:630, 1956.
48. Wittig, H. J. and J. Glaser: The relationship between bronchiolitis and childhood asthma. *J. Allergy 30*:19, 1959.
49. Wohl, M. E. B., L. C. Stigol and J. Mead: Resistance of the total respiratory system in healthy infants and infants with bronchiolitis. *Pediatrics 43*:495, 1969.
50. Wright, F. H. and M. D. Breem: Diagnosis and treatment: management of acute viral bronchiolitis. *Pediatrics 35*:334, 1965.

Asthma

ELLIOT F. ELLIS

10

Asthma may be defined as a diffuse, obstructive pulmonary disease characterized by hyperreactivity of the airways to a variety of stimuli. The airway obstruction is intermittent, and reversibility may occur spontaneously or as a result of treatment. The reversible nature of the disease is an important physiologic and clinical feature of asthma that distinguishes it from emphysema (a condition rarely seen in childhood), in which the obstruction of the airways is, by and large, irreversible. The hyperreactivity or irritability of the airways in asthma manifests itself as bronchoconstriction following exposure of the asthmatic patient, in either a natural or a laboratory setting, to inhalation of cold air, strong odors, irritant fumes such as SO_2 and tobacco smoke,[99,105] acetylcholine (or its congener Mecholyl), and other pharmacologically active agents such as histamine released, for example, during an IgE-mediated allergic reaction.[73] The hyperreactivity of the airways is present to some degree in all asthmatics regardless of the principal provoking cause(s) of the acute episodes of airway obstruction. The essential elements of the definition of asthma are the increased responsiveness of the airways and the intermittency of the obstructive signs and symptoms.

Prevalence and Socioeconomic Considerations

While asthma occurs worldwide, it appears to be a disorder principally of urbanized populations. Many anecdotal references discuss homogenous population groups throughout the world, who are apparently free of asthma in their native setting but develop the disorder when they relocate in urban communities. The significance of these observations is not known, but the important influence of environmental factors in the pathogenesis of the disease is suggested. The incidence of asthma throughout the world is difficult to estimate from published material because of nonuniformity of diagnostic criteria and unreliability of questionnaires upon which much of the epidemiologic data is based. However, the information available indicates an incidence of 0.5 to 9% with a median of about 3.5%.[97] As a cause of chronic illness in childhood and morbidity leading to school absence, asthma is a disease of major importance on a global basis.[1,4,21,22]

Natural History

Asthma may have its onset at any period in life from infancy to old age. In some individuals, asthma bears a close association with atopic dermatitis (atopic eczema) and hay fever, and the asthmatic frequently suffers with either or both of the latter disorders.[68] In this group of individuals, one often finds a familial pattern in which the mother, father, or siblings of the propositus is afflicted with asthma, hay fever, or atopic eczema,[11,103] and some appear to have a predisposition to synthesize antibodies of the IgE species against common environmental antigens.[110] In other individuals with asthma, none of the above stigmata are noted. While few long-term studies of the natural history of asthma have been undertaken, those that exist indicate a good prognosis.[67,79] Most young asthmatic children have a remission of their disease with growth, and this improvement may be attributed in part to the age-related increase in cross-sectional diameter of the airways.[42,43] Another group of children with asthma may continue to have intermittent symptoms of airway obstruction throughout their lives, with little interference with their functioning or longevity. A minority of asthmatic children have a severe and progressively incapacitating form of the disease, which significantly interferes with their school attendance, participation in sports, and general day-to-day functioning.[107]

Etiology

Asthma is a complex disorder in which infectious, immunologic, autonomic nervous system, and psychologic factors may all be involved in an individual patient; these factors result in airway obstruction and the clinical signs and symptoms of asthma[82] (Fig. 10-1). Early in life, viral agents play a major role as precipitants of symptoms and, even in older children and adults, viral respiratory tract infection is frequently associated with exacerbations of coughing and wheezing.[9,36,37,46,54,65,70] Bacterial respiratory tract infection has not been shown to have an etiologic role in asthma,[10,31,37,65,70,89,92] nor does satisfactory evidence exist that "bacterial allergy" expresses itself as symptoms of airway obstruction.[53] Immunologic or allergic factors have long been considered to be of major importance in asthma, particularly by physicians in the United States. While it is abundantly clear that in some patients the principal cause of symptoms is IgE-mediated allergy to environmental factors such as danders, pollens, molds, house dust, and occasionally foods (so-called extrinsic asthma), in an equally large number of cases, particu-

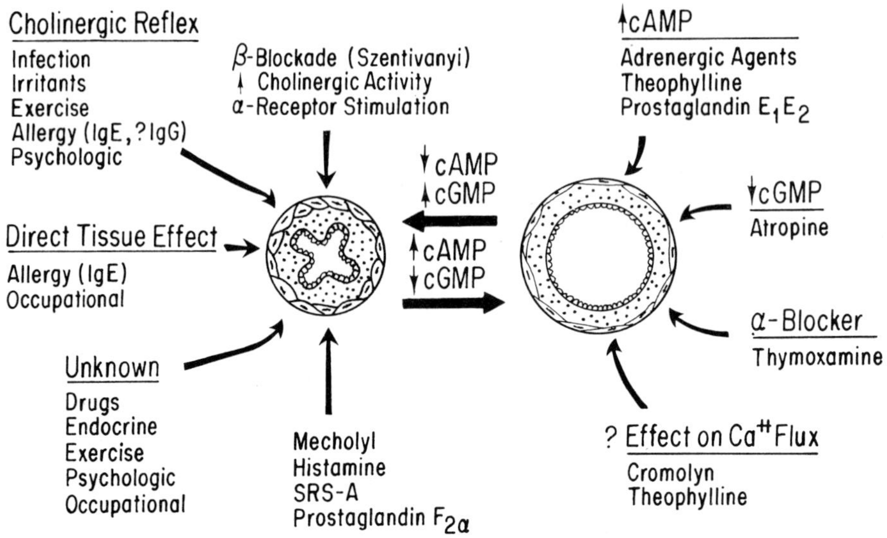

FIG. 10-1. The many precipitants of bronchoconstriction and their presumed mechanism of action. In the case of exercise, allergy, and occupational factors, several mechanisms leading to bronchoconstriction have been proposed. The intracellular concentration of the cyclic nucleotides, cAMP and cGMP, appears to be a principal determinant of smooth muscle tension, an important factor in airway diameter. Drugs used in asthma therapeutics and their effect on cAMP and cGMP metabolism and other factors are shown (see text).

larly during the first 2 years of life, allergic factors cannot be demonstrated (so-called intrinsic asthma).

Recent literature reflects a resurgence of interest in the role of the autonomic nervous system in the cause of asthma.[82,83] It is thought that airway caliber is regulated by cholinergic bronchoconstrictor influences transmitted via vagal pathways, opposed by bronchodilator influences mediated through a recently described nonadrenergic system[85a] and through the beta-adrenergic receptors in airway smooth muscle.[105,106] Cholinergic influence ordinarily predominates, and an airway "tone" can be abolished by atropine administration.[16] The cholinergic theory of asthma proposes that the disorder is due to overactivity of cholinergic bronchoconstrictor activity,[39,105] while the beta-blockade theory proposes that asthma is due to dysfunction of the beta-adrenergic receptor system, resulting in diminished sympathetic bronchodilator effect on the airways.[69,101] The observation that histamine released in an IgE-mediated allergic reaction causes an increase in bronchomotor tone, not only by a direct action on airway smooth muscle but also by reflex action consequent to stimulation of afferent vagal irritant airway receptors, indicates the interplay of the various mechanisms that influence airway caliber.[39]

The importance of psychologic factors in the pathogenesis of asthma has been emphasized by some behaviorists in the past, but current thinking, while not denying emotional factors as contributory, would not assign a primary etiologic role to psychologic influences.[58,66] The effects of a chronic illness such as asthma on a child and his family can be devastating, and many of the behavioral problems observed in chronic asthmatics may result from, rather than be causally related to the disease.

Pathophysiology

The fundamental pathophysiologic lesion in asthma is airway obstruction. The obstructive process is due to: (1) smooth muscle spasm, (2) mucous membrane edema, and (3) tenacious mucus.[24,104]

The contribution of each of these factors to the airway obstruction probably varies from patient to patient and during various stages of an attack. In rapid-onset asthma, in which symptoms appear in minutes, smooth muscle spasm is likely to be the predominant factor. In the prolonged episode, particularly during severe status asthmaticus, edema and tenacious mucoid secretions play major roles in the obstructive process. Both large airways, i.e., those greater than 2 mm in diameter, and small airways (less than 2 mm) are involved, and while large or small airway obstruction may be dominant in a given individual, airways of all dimensions are generally obstructed to varying degrees.[61,62] *Physiologic tests that are considered to measure predominantly large or small airway disease have been developed.* The airway obstruction leads to:

(1) Increased work of breathing and greatly increased oxygen consumption by muscles involved in respiration (intercostal, diaphragm, and accessory neck muscles).

(2) Uneven (nonuniform) ventilation of the lung with nonventilation of some areas, resulting in atelectasis distal to the obstructed airways and air trapping, and hyperinflation in other areas.[14,41,55,63]

(3) Relative increase in the elastic resistance of the lung due to atelectasis and trapped air. In adults a reversible decrease in pulmonary elastic recoil has been reported.[40,111]

(4) Abnormalities in blood gases.[64,81,84,95,102] In the initial stages of an asthmatic attack, arterial P_{CO_2} is usually decreased due to hyperventilation. As the obstruction worsens, alveolar hypoventilation supervenes, Pa_{CO_2} rises, and after blood buffer mechanisms are exhausted, pH falls. Arterial hypoxemia is almost always present in attacks of sufficient severity to require medical attention. The principal cause of the diminished Pa_{O_2} in asthma is continued perfusion of hypoventilated areas of the lung, i.e., areas with a low $\dot{V}_A/\dot{Q}$ (ventilation-perfusion) ratio.[81,102] Thus, a large A-a (alveolar-arterial) oxygen difference exists. In addition to the preceding abnormalities, some asthmatic adults[45] and children[19] have been reported to have a blunted ventilatory response to hypoxemia, suggesting an abnormality in the regulation of breathing. Pulmonary hypertension with ECG evidence of right heart strain has been observed in symptomatic asthmatics, particularly during severe attacks.[81]

Clinical Findings

The signs and symptoms of asthma—cough, wheezing, and dyspnea—in the typical case are generally sufficiently distinctive to permit diagnosis by physician and layman alike. The degree of wheezing varies, and since the latter is a manifestation of partial airway obstruction, relative absence of wheezing in the face of respiratory distress and poor air exchange on auscultation of the lungs is indicative of severe obstruction. During an attack, the affected child, depending upon severity of the episode, shows varying degrees of tachypnea, cyanosis, hyperinflation of the chest, use of diaphragm and accessory muscles of respiration, and dyspnea. In some children, cough, particularly persistent at night upon lying down and on exercise, and tachypnea and shortness of breath, also particularly notable following exercise, may be the predominant signs and symptoms of asthma. In many instances, wheezing, audible with the naked ear, is also present. The cough during an acute attack sounds "tight" and is generally nonproductive of mucus. As the attack subsides, tenacious mucoid sputum is produced, except in young children, who rarely expectorate. Children with asthma differ greatly in the frequency and degree of symptoms.[67] Some have only an occasional symptomatic episode, mild in degree and brief, precipitated perhaps by a known allergenic exposure, e.g., to cats or horses, and otherwise are entirely free of symptoms. Other asthmatics have a low-grade degree of coughing and wheezing much of the time, punctuated by severe exacerbations of symptoms following exposure to known allergens, viral infections, exercise, and nonspecific irritants. Thus, asthmatics are heterogenous not only in terms of cause(s) of their disease but also in terms of its clinical expression.

Status asthmaticus is a life-threatening form of asthma that, by common definition, is temporarily resistant to drugs that are usually effective in relieving an attack, i.e. epinephrine, isoproterenol, and aminophylline.[18,25] While status asthmaticus has no biochemical definition, most clinicians recognize it as a particularly severe episode of asthma that is treatment-resistant and cause for concern because of its possible progression to respiratory failure.

Diagnostic Tests

LABORATORY FINDINGS

Eosinophilia of the blood and the sputum is a regular finding in individuals with asthma regardless of whether allergic factors can be shown to have an etiologic role in the disease. Blood eosinophilia above 250 to 400 cells/mm^3 is the rule. A correlation has been made between the severity of asthma and the degree of the eosinophilia. Furthermore, the extent to which blood eosinophilia can be suppressed with corticosteroids has been used as an index of therapeutic efficacy of these agents.[26,44]

The sputum in uncomplicated asthma is highly distinctive.[30] Grossly it is tenacious, rubbery, and whitish. In the presence of infection, particularly in adults, the sputum may be yellowish. Microscopically, many eosinophils are found and are seen frequently arranged in sheets, but histiocytes and PMN's are also present in large numbers. Eosinophilic granules from disrupted cells may be seen throughout the sputum smear. Elongated dipyramidal crystals (Charcot-Leyden), originating from both eosinophils and basophils, or mast cells are commonly found. When infection is present and particularly in the face of a bronchitic element, polymorphonuclear leukocytes and bacteria predominate. The finding of sputum eosinophilia is highly suggestive of a diagnosis of asthma after a few less common pulmonary conditions have been excluded. In uncomplicated cases of asthma, sputum cultures rarely reveal pathogenic bacteria,[10] particularly when the specimen is obtained by the transcricoid approach (a difficult diagnostic procedure in children), which avoids contamination of the specimen with mouth and pharyngeal organisms.

Serum protein and immunoglobulin concentrations are generally normal in asthma, except for a finding of an elevated IgE concentration in some cases where reaginic allergy may have an etiologic role.

RADIOGRAPHIC STUDIES

Chest roentgenogram varies in appearance from normal to hyperinflated. Lung markings are commonly increased, particularly in chronic cases. Atelectasis, most often involving the right middle lobe, is common, particularly in young children, and may be a recurrent problem.[27,56,108] Small segmental areas of atelectasis are frequently observed during acute exacerbations of asthma and may be misinterpreted as pneumonitis. The rapidity with which they clear suggests that the densities do indeed represent atelectasis rather than pneumonitis.

An esophagogram should be considered as part of the evaluation of the infant or young child with suspected asthma in order to rule out congenital anomalies that might cause airway obstruction. An inspiratory and expiratory chest roentgenogram is extremely helpful in diagnosing foreign body aspiration as a cause of wheezing in childhood (Fig. 10-2).

Bronchoscopy is only rarely indicated in the study of a child with obstructive airway disease. In adults, the availability of the fiberoptic bronchoscope has provided a powerful new diagnostic tool. However, because of instrument size limitations, fiberoptic bronchoscopy is principally limited to the study of adolescents. Bronchoscopy can be a dangerous procedure in individuals with reactive airway disease, particularly when using non-fiberoptic instruments. Many complications have been encountered during the procedure, including severe bronchospasm and cardiac arrest. Bronchoscopy in an asthmatic should not be undertaken lightly, and it should never be undertaken because physicians, faced with a difficult and resistant case of asthma, are unable to think of anything else to do. For example, as noted previously, atelectasis, particularly involving the right middle lobe, may be a recurrent problem in poorly controlled asthma. Bronchoscopy in this circumstance rarely, if ever, results in either expansion of the atelectatic area or positive information that leads to improved management of the case.

Generally, bronchography in asthmatics is, except in carefully selected cases, a waste of time and money; rarely does it "provide new information necessary for specialized treatment."[86] Consideration must be given to the complications of contrast media and general anesthesia in regard to any anticipated yield from bronchography.[86]

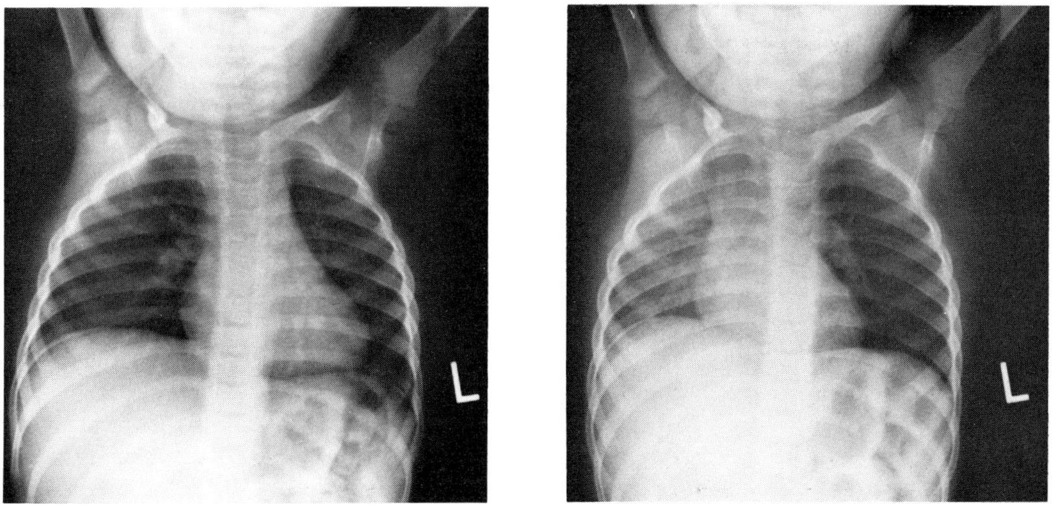

FIG. 10-2. An 18-month-old child had sudden onset of cough and wheezing. *A*, an inspiratory film with no abnormalities evident. However, on expiration, *B*, the left lung does not empty and the mediastinal structures shift to the right, suggesting obstruction of the left main stem bronchus, from which a nonopaque foreign body (piece of plastic) was subsequently removed during bronchoscopy.

LUNG SCANNING

Lung scanning with macroaggregates of albumin (MAA) labeled with ^{131}I is rarely indicated in children. It has been used primarily in diagnosis of thromboembolic disease, which occasionally enters into the differential diagnosis of asthma in adults. Radioactive xenon (^{133}Xe) is used in pulmonary function testing, particularly for the study of the ventilation-perfusion relationships.

OTHER DIAGNOSTIC TESTS

Allergy skin tests are useful in identifying environmental allergens that may play an etiologic role in the disease. Skin tests are customarily done to detect IgE antibody to inhalants (e.g., pollens, molds, epidermals, house dust) and other allergens suggested by the patient's history, e.g., foods. Specific IgE antibody to inhalants may also be detected by RAST (Radio-Allergosorbent Test) testing of the patient's serum,[48,49] but this procedure offers little advantage over properly done and interpreted skin tests and is more costly.

Inhalational bronchial challenge testing is done to establish the clinical significance of those allergens implicated by skin testing.[2,15,76,98] The importance attached to bronchial challenge testing as a diagnostic tool varies throughout the world. In certain Scandinavian countries, it is considered to be an indispensable part of the evaluation of the patient, particularly for selection of allergens for inclusion into a hyposensitization (immunotherapy) regimen,[3] while in the United States the procedure remains an investigative tool. The heightened sensitivity of asthmatics to inhalation of Mecholyl (methacholine) and histamine in terms of the amount required to cause bronchoconstriction is used for diagnostic purposes in cases in which the diagnosis of asthma is for some reason uncertain.[52,74,98] Children who are old enough to cooperate (generally at least 6 years of age) are tested with increasing concentrations of Mecholyl or histamine by inhalation while their airway response is monitored by pulmonary function testing. Asthmatics generally have a bronchoconstrictive response to minute amounts of these agents—amounts that would be insufficient to cause change in airway caliber in normal children or in children with pulmonary disorders other than asthma. Since the test procedure demands a considerable amount of caution and experience, it remains largely a tool limited to use in specialized centers.

The response of the asthmatic to exercise is quite characteristic and can be used as a diagnostic aid in cases in which the diagnosis is in question.[20,100] After a standardized workload is provided by having the child run on a treadmill, a decrease in lung function characteristic of asthma occurs about 5 minutes after completion of the exercise. Although its precise mechanism is unknown, the response seems to be quite specific for asthma.

Two drugs, aspirin and propranolol (the latter is rarely prescribed in children), may cause alarming attacks of asthma in some asthmatics.[32,57,88,112,113] The mechanism of aspirin-induced asthma, which usually occurs in a triad of nasal polyposis, asthma, and aspirin intolerance, is unknown.[57] In the case of suspected aspirin-induced asthma, great caution must be exercised if it is considered to be of sufficient importance to establish the diagnosis by test-dosing.

PULMONARY FUNCTION TESTING

Pulmonary function testing is valuable in the diagnostic evaluation of children with pulmonary disease in whom the diagnosis of asthma on clinical, laboratory, and radiographic grounds is uncertain. In those known to have asthma, pulmonary function tests are useful in assessing the degree of airway obstruction and disturbance in gas exchange, in measuring the airway response to inhaled allergens and chemicals such as histamine and methacholine (bronchial provocation testing), in quantifying the response to therapeutic agents, and in performing the long-term follow-up of the disease. Pulmonary function testing in asthma is most valuable when performed before and after aerosol bronchodilator administration, since the degree of reversibility of the airway obstruction at the time of the testing may be ascertained. Tests vary in their complexity, but a good deal may be learned from the application of relatively simple tests. Lack of cooperation usually prevents meaningful pulmonary function testing in children below 6 years of age.

Static Lung Volumes and Capacities. Various combinations of abnormalities may be seen with the important reservation that, in mild cases in remission, no abnormalities may be detected. From the tests most often used clinically, total lung capacity (TLC) is increased as are the functional residual capacity (FRC) and residual volume (RV).[13] The vital capacity may be normal or decreased and the tidal volume normal or increased.

Dynamic Lung Volumes and Capacities. Dynamic lung volumes, termed flow rates, provide an index of the degree of airway obstruction. Since expiratory flow is determined not only by the diameter of the airways but also by the elastic recoil forces of the lung, it is easy to see that flow at high lung volumes will exceed flow at low lung volumes. Tests that meaure flow at relatively large lung volumes, $FEV_{0.5}$ (forced expiratory volume in 0.5 second), PEFR (peak expiratory flow rate), MEFR (flow between 200 and 1200 cc), are to a considerable degree effort-dependent and are less satisfactory than tests that measure flow over a larger range of lung volume, FEV_1 (forced expiratory volume in one second), or tests that ignore the effort-dependent early portion of expiration and measure flow between 25 and 75% of the FVC (forced vital capacity), such as the MMF (maximum mid-expiratory flow), also known as the $FEF_{25\text{-}75\%}$ (forced mid-expiratory flow). The MMF is of particular value since it is considered to reflect obstruction of small airways.[62] Expiratory flow measurements at large lung volumes are insensitive to changes in peripheral airway resistance and reflect abnormalities principally in central airways.

Probably of greatest value is the expiratory flow-volume curve in which expired lung volume is plotted against flow rate. The flow-volume curve gives a clear graphic picture of flow at large and small lung volumes, and therefore presumably reveals abnormalities in both central and peripheral airways.[47]

All of the preceding tests of dynamic lung volumes show reduced capacity in children with asthma and return to normal values following administration of aerosolized bronchodilator. In mild asthmatics during asymptomatic periods, tests of dynamic lung function may give results within normal limits.

Functional residual capacity (FRC), which cannot be measured directly by spirometry, is determined with the nitrogen washout technique. Residual volume (RV) can be calculated once the FRC is known. Total lung capacity, FRC, and RV can also be determined with the body plethysmograph, which also may be used to measure airway resistance.[35]

Because of the airway obstruction in asthma, distribution of ventilation is frequently abnormal; i.e., various lung units fill and empty asynchronously. Maldistribution of ventilation may be determined by the single breath nitrogen test (SBN_2) and the 7-minute nitrogen washout test.

Another test of current interest for the detection of small airway disease is the measurement of "closing volume."[60] This volume is increased in some asthmatics and in chronic smokers. Unfortunately, the test is difficult to do in children. Studies in adult asthmatics have shown a loss of elastic recoil, which is reversible in many cases with remission of the disease.[40]

Diffusing capacity of the lung for carbon

monoxide (DL_{CO}) is generally normal in asthma,[7] whereas it is abnormal in emphysema (rarely seen in childhood), in which loss of functioning alveolar capillary bed accompanies increased lung volume, and also in many of the hypersensitivity pneumonidities, in which loss of functioning alveolar capillary bed accompanies decreased lung volume.[90]

Determination of arterial blood gas pressures and pH is essential in the adequate evaluation of the patient with asthma. During periods of remission Pa_{O_2}, Pa_{CO_2}, and pH may be normal. However, during symptomatic periods, low Pa_{O_2}, principally due to mismatching of ventilation and perfusion, is the rule.[102] A low Pa_{O_2} may persist for days to weeks after the acute episode is over.[61] Pa_{CO_2} is generally low during the early stages of an asthmatic attack owing to hyperventilation.[81] As the obstruction worsens Pa_{CO_2} rises and this sign is ominous. Blood pH remains normal until the buffering capacity of the blood is exhausted; then acidosis develops. Determination of alveolar-arterial O_2 gradient ($A\text{-}aO_2$) on room air and 100% O_2 breathing permits differentiation of hypoxemia due to ventilation-perfusion abnormality from that due to right-to-left shunts.

Differential Diagnosis

In infancy and early childhood the following must be considered in the differential diagnosis of asthma:

(1) *Congenital malformations.* Developmental anomalies of the respiratory, cardiovascular, or gastrointestinal systems may cause signs and symptoms of partial airway obstruction by intrinsic or extrinsic mechanisms. These causes of airway obstruction may be ruled out by a combination of history, x-ray contrast studies, and/or endoscopy.

(2) *Foreign bodies.* Opaque foreign bodies are readily visible by x-ray examination. Nonopaque foreign bodies are more of a problem, but generally a history of sudden onset of cough and wheezing in a previously well small child, combined with abnormal diaphragmatic movement on inspiratory and expiratory chest roentgenograms, establishes the diagnosis (see Fig. 10-2).

(3) *Infectious agents.* Viral infections of the upper respiratory tract that involve the glottis and the subglottis generally give rise to signs and symptoms of croup with inspiratory stridor, high pitched cough, and hoarseness, a clinical picture distinctive from the lower airway signs and symptoms of asthma. Primary bacterial infection of the lower airway in the absence of underlying disease, e.g., cystic fibrosis of the pancreas or immune deficiency disease, is rare in infants and children. On the other hand, viral agents, particularly RSV, can cause bronchiolitis, with a clinical picture virtually indistinguishable from asthma during the first 2 years of life. It is rare for an infant or young child to suffer more than one or two episodes of infectious bronchiolitis, so a history of recurrent episodes of obstructive airway disease should strongly suggest the diagnosis of asthma, *regardless of age.*

(4) *Underlying disorders.* Cystic fibrosis of the pancreas and immunologic deficiency disease should always be considered in a child with chronic lower respiratory tract symptoms and may be ruled out by a careful history, by sweat test, and by *in vivo* and *in vitro* evaluation of immunologic competence.

(5) *Chronic bronchitis* as a primary diagnosis is rare in childhood, at least in the United States, and children who carry this diagnosis are almost always found to have some underlying cause for their signs and symptoms of airway obstruction; appropriate studies show that many are suffering from asthma.

(6) *Hypersensitivity pneumonitis.* A group of recently elucidated pulmonary disorders, exemplified by farmers' lung in adults, has been shown to represent a hypersensitivity response to inhaled organic "dusts" such as the thermophilic actinomycetes. Patients

with hypersensitivity pneumonitis bear a superficial resemblance to asthmatics but generally have more in the way of constitutional symptoms after exposure to the offending substance and typically do not wheeze. Ventilatory studies are generally unremarkable but the diffusing capacity (DL_{CO}) is strikingly abnormal, in contrast to asthma in which DL_{CO} is not affected. While only rarely affecting children, hypersensitivity pneumonitis must always be included in the differential diagnosis of chronic pulmonary disease in children.[87]

(7) *Others.* A host of conditions that compromise the airway, including endobronchial tuberculosis, fungal diseases, bronchial adenoma, and foreign bodies, must be considered as possible causes of obstructive airway disease. The correct diagnosis can generally be established by careful history taking, pulmonary function tests, microbiologic studies including cultures and skin tests, and x-ray examination with contrast studies and occasionally lung scan. Other disorders that rarely occur in childhood may show the signs and symptoms of asthma, e.g., carcinoid, tropical eosinophilia, and other parasitic infestations that involve the lung during some phase of the disease. In each of these circumstances the history, which is usually atypical for asthma, may suggest the underlying disorder.

Complications of Asthma

During an acute attack of asthma, pneumothorax may occur as a sudden worsening of the patient's respiratory distress accompanied by sharp chest pains and a shift of the mediastinum on physical examination.[12,50] X-ray examination confirms the diagnosis. Mediastinal and subcutaneous emphysema due to alveolar rupture and dissection of air along vessels is occasionally observed during an asthmatic attack.[12] Atelectasis, usually involving the right middle lobe or even an entire lung, is more common.[80,108] Unless the collapse involves a substantial amount of lung tissue, the atelectasis is usually diagnosed only as a result of x-ray examination. Bronchiectasis apparently was a complication of asthma in the pre-antibiotic days, but only rarely does this occur today. While electrocardiographic evidence of acute cor pulmonale can occasionally be obtained during a severe episode of asthma, chronic cor pulmonale secondary to asthma rarely occurs in children. Contrary to popular opinion, asthma beginning in childhood does not lead to chronic obstructive emphysema if cigarette smoking is avoided.

Growth failure may be observed as a complication of asthma,[85] particularly in children with intractable disease. It may be difficult to separate the effects on growth due to chronic disease from the linear growth suppression produced by corticosteroids when these drugs are required in therapy. The problem is further complicated by constitutional factors; thus the height of the parents and siblings must be considered in assessing growth retardation in an asthmatic child. Chronic disability leading to loss of school and work and family disruption are significant complications of chronic intractable asthma. Obesity due to a combination of inactivity, overeating due to frustration, and steroid therapy is a particular problem in adolescent females with severe asthma.

Treatment

The three principal modalities of treatment of asthma are avoidance of known precipitants, hyposensitization, and drug therapy.

AVOIDANCE OF KNOWN PRECIPITANTS (IMMUNOLOGIC [ALLERGIC] AND NONIMMUNOLOGIC)

Identification and avoidance of known precipitants of asthma may result in amelioration of the disease. These precipitants include allergens, such as inhalants (e.g., danders, pollens, molds, and house dust) and foods (e.g., fish, eggs, and nuts) and irritants such as cold air, tobacco smoke, strong fumes, paint, disinfectants, and air pollutants (e.g., SO_2). Whereas air-cleaning devices of the electronic precipitator or high-efficiency particulate (HEPA) filter type are effective in removing particulate matter from the air in a confined space, their efficiency in homes under average living conditions is open to question. Furthermore, the devices are costly and should be rented, if possible, prior to purchase to determine their usefulness.

HYPOSENSITIZATION

No conclusive evidence exists that hyposensitization (immunotherapy) to known immunologic precipitants favorably influences the course of asthma. However, many allergists believe that a trial of hyposensitization is indicated when it has been established by history and allergy testing that the major precipitants of the asthma are inhalant allergens that cannot be completely avoided. Generally, such allergens are pollens, molds, and house dust but *not* danders of household or farm animals. This modality of therapy is best administered by a properly trained and qualified allergist. If no improvement is evident after 1 to 2 years of therapy, the injections should be discontinued. Far too many children continue to receive allergy extracts in the absence of good evidence that the injections have favorably influenced the course of their disease. This practice is a waste of the family's time and money.

PHARMACOLOGIC THERAPY

The principal modality of asthma management[17] is pharmacologic therapy. The effect of pharmacologic agents used in asthma therapeutics on intracellular cyclic 3′,5′ adenosine monophosphate (cyclic AMP) and cyclic 3′,5′ guanosine monophosphate (cyclic GMP) concentrations is seen in Figure 10-1. These nucleotides are thought to have an important role in the modulation of bronchoconstrictive mediator release[5] and tension of smooth muscle.[91] Drugs used in asthma therapeutics include both catecholamine (epinephrine, isoproterenol, and isoetharine) and related non-catecholamine adrenergics (metaproterenol, terbutaline, salbutamol, and ephedrine), theophylline (a methylxanthine), cromolyn sodium, corticosteroids, atropine and related anticholinergics, and a number of less widely used entities.

TREATMENT OF THE ACUTE ATTACK

An acute episode of asthma sufficient to cause respiratory distress is most effectively treated, with the least adverse side effects, by administration of an aerosol bronchodilator such as isoproterenol, isoetharine, metaproterenol, terbutaline, or salbutamol. These agents are available in freon-propelled canisters for self-administration and also in a solution that may be mixed with water or saline. For example, five drops of isoproterenol, 1:200, in 2 cc of saline solution, in a hand-held nebulizer aerosolized with compressed air (from an inexpensive compressor or even a bicycle pump) results in rapid relief of symptoms (Fig. 10-3). Patients and their parents must be cautioned about the adverse effects of the excessive use of aerosol adrenergic agents. The need for frequent (more often than every 3 to 4 hours) aerosol treatment, because of poor and short-lived bronchodilator response, is an indication that the attack is worsening and that the patient requires prompt medical attention. (Aerosol therapy is discussed further in Chapter 4.)

For the child who has particularly acute airway obstruction and is too "tight" to effectively inhale the aerosol, epinephrine HCl (adrenaline), 1:1000, given subcutaneously in a dose of 0.05 to 0.2 cc is an effective treatment. The side effects of epinephrine (pallor, tachycardia, jitteriness) are largely dose re-

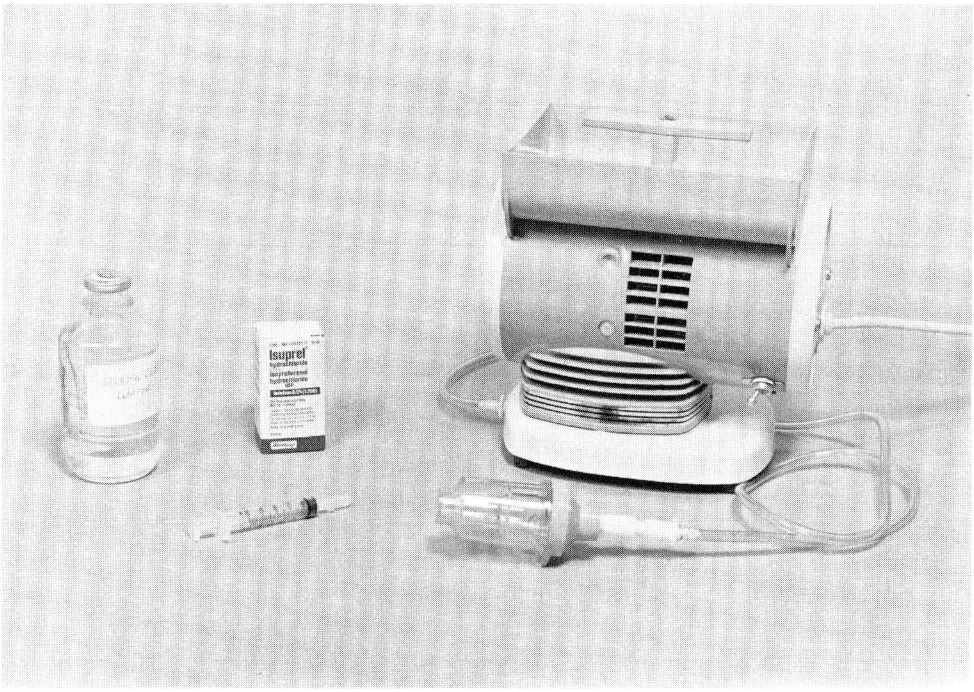

FIG. 10-3. The Maxi-myst unit is a convenient and inexpensive (about $80) source of compressed air for nebulization of adrenergic bronchodilator agents. Isoproterenol HCl (Isuprel) solution (5 drops in 2 cc of water or saline) or isoetharine (Bronkosol) (10 drops in 2 cc of water or saline solution) may be delivered to the airways at a rate controlled by the patient according to instructions provided. The unit is particularly useful for the child who awakens in the middle of the night with an acute attack of asthma. A Maxi-myst treatment permits effective management at home and obviates middle-of-the-night trips to the emergency room or doctor's office.

lated, and a relatively small dose, as recommended previously, injected at 20-minute intervals two or three times, frequently gives better response with fewer side effects than a large (0.3 to 0.4 cc) single dose.

If the child fails to respond satisfactorily to treatment with adrenergic drugs, aminophylline in a dose of 4 to 5 mg/kg body weight (25 mg/cc concentration, diluted 1:1 with saline solution or other intravenous fluid) is infused at a rate dictated by the degree of respiratory distress (but no more rapidly than 1 to 2 cc/min.).

Hypoxemia is invariably present in patients with asthma of sufficient degree to seek medical attention;[81] thus oxygen administration is indicated as part of the management of the acute episode. Furthermore, certain of the adrenergic aerosols (e.g., isoproterenol) and aminophylline can aggravate ventilation-perfusion imbalance and lead to a worsening of hypoxemia.[102] Lack of good response to the treatment with adrenergic agents and aminophylline indicates that a severe treatment-resistant state of asthma has developed (status asthmaticus), and the child should be hospitalized for intensive treatment.

STATUS ASTHMATICUS

A patient with a progressively severe attack of asthma, unresponsive to treatment with adrenergic drugs and theophylline, is by definition diagnosed as having status asthmaticus. Status asthmaticus should be viewed as a potentially life-threatening emergency because it can lead to respiratory failure. Infants and children suffering from status asthmaticus should be admitted to a hospital intensive care unit prepared to deal with all complications of this condition. Optimal treatment includes:

(1) Initial and serial determinations of arterial blood gas pressures and pH. These measurements are crucial since therapy will be guided by the arterial blood gas and pH status.

(2) Administration of humidified oxygen, preferably by nasal cannula (which causes less anxiety than a mask) at a concentration sufficient to maintain Pa_{O_2} between 70 and 90 mm Hg. In an infant or young child, a tent may be necessary to administer oxygen. Otherwise, mist tents should be avoided since mist may act as an airway irritant in some patients and actually aggravate the airway obstruction. Furthermore, little evidence is available that the water reaches the lower airways.[8] (See also discussion in Chapter 4.)

(3) Intravenous administration of a balanced electrolyte solution at 1–1½ times the maintenance requirements. Do not overhydrate the patient.

(4) Aminophylline, 25 mg/cc in a dose of 4 to 5 mg/kg of body weight diluted 1:1 with intravenous fluids and administered over 10 to 20 minutes every 6 hours. Alternatively, aminophylline may be given by a combination of a loading dose plus a constant infusion if equipment for constant infusion is available. A loading dose of 6.0 mg/kg of aminophylline is given over 20 minutes followed by a constant infusion dose of 1.1 mg/kg/hr.[77] If constant infusion equipment is not available, the calculated one hourly dose may be administered each hour over 10 minutes. Adjustment of the aminophylline dosage is greatly facilitated if plasma-theophylline concentrations can be measured periodically so that a theophylline-plasma concentration of 10 to 20 mcg/ml[71] of plasma is maintained.

(5) Methylprednisolone (Solu-Medrol) in a dose of 2 to 4 mg/kg body weight every 4 to 6 hours is administered intravenously. Methylprednisolone is preferred to hydrocortisone (Solu-Cortef) because of its negligible effect on electrolyte metabolism and its lesser cost for an equivalent amount of anti-inflammatory activity.

(6) Administration of aerosol bronchodilators, e.g., isoproterenol, 1:200, five drops in 2 cc water or saline solution, or Bronkosol, ten drops in 2 cc water or saline solution, every 2 to 3 hours or more often if necessary.

(7) Sodium bicarbonate in a dose of 1 to 3 mg/kg body weight or according to the formula $0.3 \times$ weight in kilograms $\times$ base deficit, administered over 20 minutes as required to maintain the pH above 7.2, particularly in the face of metabolic acidosis complicating respiratory acidosis.

(8) Chest roentgenogram to detect complications of status asthmaticus (pneumothorax, mediastinal emphysema, subcutaneous emphysema), atelectasis, and/or pneumonitis.

With therapy as just outlined, most patients improve within 18 to 30 hours, depending upon the severity of the episode. Respiratory failure as evidenced by the inability to maintain adequate Pa_{O_2}, progressive increase in Pa_{CO_2} particularly above 65 to 75 mm Hg, and decreasing pH indicate the need for nasotracheal intubation and ventilator-assisted respiration. A volume ventilator should be available since it is often impossible to adequately ventilate a patient with status asthmaticus with a pressure-cycled ventilator because of the high airway resistance that must be overcome.[23,109] The details of ventilator therapy are given in Chapter 3.

No evidence exists that bacterial infection precipitates status asthmaticus;[92] therefore antibiotics are not prescribed routinely in the absence of cultural, radiographic, and clinical evidence of bacterial infection. However, antibiotics may be considered when the patient is intubated and being ventilated with a respirator.

Bronchoscopy and administration of rectal ether have no place in the modern management of status asthmaticus.

A mild episode of asthma can often be managed by administration of oral bronchodilators. The adrenergic agents—metaproterenol, 5 to 10 mg; terbutaline, 2.5 to 5 mg; salbutamol, 2 to 4 mg; ephedrine, 6.25 to 12.5 mg (the latter is least desirable of the adrenergic agents)—as a single dose give relief in about 30 minutes.[6] Alternatively, theophylline in one of the many formulations available,[28] in a dose of 5 mg/kg body weight, is similarly effective when given orally. Administration of an adrenergic agent and theophylline simultaneously has a sound theoretic basis and may be useful in patients who get suboptimal bronchodilator response to either agent administered alone. Repetition of the preceding medication at 6-hour intervals for three to four doses generally suffices to relieve the mild exacerbation of asthma.

TREATMENT OF CHRONIC ASTHMA

Many asthmatic children are virtually free of symptoms except for the periodic exacerbations of coughing and wheezing associated with exposure to known allergens or other precipitants. Such patients may be treated with the short-term use of drugs as previously described. However, a significant number of asthmatics have, more or less, chronic low-grade symptoms of airway obstruction punctuated by acute exacerbations. They often benefit from regular around-the-clock administration of bronchodilator drugs, as attested to by decreased frequency of acute exacerbations, better school attendance, decreased sleep disturbance due to asthma, and improved exercise tolerance. Around-the-clock therapy may be initiated with some form of theophylline in a dose of 3 to 5 mg/kg body weight (anhydrous theophylline equivalent) given every 6 hours.[28] Theophylline has a relatively short half-life (2 to 3 hours in children, 4 to 5 hours in adults),[29] and thus should be given at least every 6 hours to maintain adequate plasma concentrations. Recent recognition of the substantial variability in the rate of theophylline metabolism[29] among individual patients stresses the need to monitor plasma or saliva theophylline concentrations (10 to 20 μg/ml of plasma appears to be optimal for bronchodilation).[71] This monitoring is especially important for patients who achieve inadequate therapeutic response or suffer adverse side effects on the usual dosing regimens.

If adequate bronchodilator control is not achieved with theophylline alone, oral adrenergic agents such as metaproterenol, terbutaline, salbutamol, or ephedrine may be administered on a 6-hourly basis with the theophylline. Fixed dose combinations of theophylline, ephedrine, and phenobarbital, though convenient, are often less satisfactory than the use of single entities. With the combination formulation, the physician is locked into a fixed ratio of theophylline to ephedrine, and a dose of either agent cannot be increased or decreased without affecting the dose of the other. Phenobarbital in the combination has not been proven to have any beneficial effect (it is presumably present as a sedative) and unnecessarily complicates treatment because it may produce adverse drug effects.

Those patients who continue to have an unacceptable degree of asthma despite regular administration of theophylline and adrenergic agents are candidates for trial on cromolyn sodium.[33] The drug is a lipid insoluble, relatively nontoxic white powder that is inactive by mouth and must be taken by inhalation from a capsule inserted into a specially designed, hand-held device called a Turbo-inhaler. Children under 5 to 6 years of age are generally unable to cooperate sufficiently to make effective use of the drug. Since patient compliance is essential, the age of the child must be considered before prescribing cromolyn. Cromolyn prevents both allergen-induced and nonallergen-induced release of the chemical mediators of bronchoconstriction. The drug is not a bronchodilator and should not be used in the treatment of an acute attack, but is administered prophylactically to prevent attacks. Cromolyn is effective when administered minutes before allergenic exposure and should be taken every 6 hours for optimal efficacy. It is useful not only in allergic (extrinsic) asthma but also in nonallergic (intrinsic) asthma, and is particularly effective in the prevention of exercise-induced asthma. Some patients have a remarkable response to cromolyn therapy within a week (if no improvement occurs after 3 to 4 weeks, the drug should be discontinued), while others with a comparable degree of asthma do not respond. The principal drawback to the drug is its cost, which amounts to $30 to $40 each month.

A small segment of the pediatric asthmatic population, despite optimal therapy in terms of environmental control measures, allergic management, and drug therapy as described previously, will suffer periodic episodes of severe asthma or will continue to have a degree of chronic asthma that interferes with normal day-to-day activity, such as school attendance, sports programs, and sleeping through the night. In those who suffer from periodic severe attacks, large doses of prednisone, 2 to 4 mg/kg body weight, given every 4 to 6 hours for 24 to 48 hours, with rapid withdrawal of the drug without a long weaning period once the child's condition improves, give good clinical results and minimal adverse effects.

In children with chronic, severe airway obstruction, the appropriate use of corticosteroids, given orally or topically in the form of one of the newly marketed aerosols, can be quite effective. Continuous low-dose oral steroid therapy, 2.5 mg/day or 20 to 30 mg every other day in alternate-day regimens, is associated with little or no measurable adverse effect.[72,85] It is abundantly clear that the many recorded adverse effects secondary to corticosteroid administration are principally dose and dosing-interval related. When steroids are given orally, only short-acting agents (principally prednisone, prednisolone, or methylprednisolone) should be used. The drug is administered as a single dose early in the morning (6 A.M. to 8 A.M.). Use of short-acting steroids in this way minimizes interference with hypothalamic-pituitary-adrenal (HPA) axis function. Whenever possible, alternate-day regimens of steroid administration are preferable to daily steroid administration. Generally, two to three times the estimated daily requirement is given as a single dose early in the morning every 48 hours. It should be emphasized that only short-acting steroids are suitable for alternate-day therapy, and drugs such as dexamethasone, triamcinolone, and betamethasone, because of their prolonged HPA axis-suppressive effects, should not be prescribed in alternate-day steroid regimens.

Initiation of continuous steroid therapy is accomplished by giving progressively smaller daily doses, for example, 40 mg, 30 mg, 20 mg, 10 mg, on successive days to bring the asthma under control. Alternate-day therapy is initiated by doubling the last daily dose and giving it every 48 hours as a single dose early in the morning. If the patient does well, the alternate-day dose is decreased at 10 to 14 day intervals by 5 mg initially, and then by 2.5 mg increments until the lowest dose compatible with acceptable control of symptoms is achieved. Conversion of a child already on a daily steroid regimen to alternate-day therapy is more difficult and requires gradual withdrawal of the drug on what is to become the "off" day while maintaining higher doses on the "on" day. Generally, it is advisable to continue theophylline medication on a regular basis since this treatment appears to reduce the steroid requirement.

Some asthmatic children with especially severe disease cannot be controlled with alternate-day steroid therapy and develop an unacceptable degree of symptomatology between 36 and 48 hours following the previous dose. These individuals must receive daily therapy, but even in this instance, if at all possible, the drug should be given in a single dose early in the morning.

The recent introduction of the surface-active topical steroids administered as an aerosol represents a major advance in corticosteroid management of asthma.[38] There is good clinical and laboratory evidence that the aerosol steroids act principally in the airways, with little systemic effect except in high doses. The dose of aerosol steroid (beclomethasone dipropionate or triamcinolone acetonide) varies from 400 to 1600 mg/day given in four divided doses according to the severity of the disease. Obviously the lowest dose possible compatible with acceptable control of symptoms should be used. During periods of exacerbation of asthma that may occur in the aerosol steroid-treated patient, oral steroid therapy should be reinstituted until the exacerbation is brought under control, for two reasons. First, the delivery of the aerosol steroid may be interfered with if airway obstruction increases. Second, the stress of the attack requires systemic glucocorticoid effect, particularly in severe asthmatics who have recently been converted to the aerosol drug. As with cromolyn, the aerosol steroids should be prescribed only for children who are old enough to properly inhale the drug. Recovery of Candida from the pharynx without evidence of clinical disease has been reported in adults treated with beclomethasone.[59]

OTHER THERAPEUTIC AGENTS

Because of the renewed interest in cholinergic regulation of airway caliber, atropine and related anticholinergics are being reevaluated in asthma therapeutics. As noted previously, airway irritability is the sine qua non of asthma, and the large airway bronchoconstrictor effects of many irritants on asthmatic airways can be blocked with atropine.[93] Until recently, the adverse effects of atropine in the doses required for therapeutic effects in the airways prevented its use clinically. A new aerosol drug known as SCH-1000 is under investigation in the United States and appears to have excellent anticholinergic activity in the airways, with minimal systemic side effects.[94] The long-term effects of the drug still require evaluation, but anticholinergic agents would appear to be of great value to the subpopulation of asthmatics who have particularly reactive airways and can become "frighteningly tight" over the course of minutes.

Alpha-adrenergic blocking agents (phentolamine and thymoxamine) have been used recently in the management of asthma.[75] The rationale for their use is based upon the presence of alpha-adrenergic receptors in tracheobronchial smooth muscle, which, when stimulated, cause bronchoconstriction.[78] Alpha-adrenergic antagonists block the stimulation of these receptors. At this time, it appears that alpha-adrenergic-induced bronchoconstriction plays a minor role in the pathogenesis of asthma in most patients.

Antihistamines have not been found to be useful in the treatment of asthma, particularly in therapy of the acute attack. In an occasional child, chronic administration of an antihistaminic drug seems to have a favorable effect.[51] Whether this effect is due to inhibition of histaminic activity on tracheobronchial smooth muscle or is due to the anticholinergic activity of some antihistamines is not known. Reluctance to use antihistamines in children with hay fever and asthma because of the possible "drying" effect of the histamine on bronchial secretions is unwarranted for the doses usually prescribed for the treatment of allergic rhinitis.

Iodides have long been used in the treatment of asthma for their alleged mucolytic effect. The latter has never been convincingly demonstrated, but an occasional patient appears to be improved while receiving iodide therapy. A therapeutic trial of 0.3 to 0.6 g of ssKI three times a day is sometimes attempted. Acneiform skin eruption in post-pubescent children and iodism are the principal adverse effects of iodide therapy, while an occasional goiter has been observed.[34] Glyceryl guaiacolate used as a mucolytic agent has little value. Similarly, acetylcysteine, because of its irritant effects on the airways, is contraindicated in asthma treatment.

Prostaglandins of the E series, which have bronchodilator activity,[96] and anti-SRS-A (slow-reacting substance of anaphylaxis) drugs are under investigation as possible therapeutic agents in asthma.

Sedatives or tranquilizers are best avoided in the treatment of asthma. When the disease is brought under control by the proper use of effective drugs, the need for sedatives and tranquilizers vanishes. The best sedative or tranquilizer for the anxious or "emotionally upset" asthmatic child is a sympathetic physician who knows how to treat the disease.

REFERENCES

1. Aas, K.: Allergic asthma in childhood. *Arch. Dis. Child. 44*:1, 1969.
2. Aas, K.: Bronchial provocation test in asthma. *Arch. Dis. Child. 45*:221, 1970.
3. Aas, K.: Diagnosis of immediate type respiratory allergy. *Pediatr. Clin. North Am. 22*:33, 1975.
4. Arbeiter, H. I.: How prevalent is allergy among United States school children? A survey of findings in the Munster (Indiana) school system. *Clin. Pediatr. 6*:140, 1967.
5. Austen, K. F.: A review of immunological, biochemical and pharmacological factors in the release of chemical mediators from the human lung. In *Asthma Physiology, Immunopharmacology, and Treatment,* K. F. Austen and L. M. Lichtenstein (Eds.) Academic Press, New York, p. 109, 1973.
6. Avner, S. E.: Beta adrenergic bronchodilators. *Pediatr. Clin. North Am. 22*:129, 1975.
7. Bates, D. V., B. T. Macklem and R. V. Christie: *Respiratory Function in Disease* (2nd ed.). W. B. Saunders Co., Philadelphia, p. 127, 1971.
8. Bau, S. K., N. Aspin, D. E. Wood and H. Levison: The measurement of fluid deposition in humans following mist tent therapy. *Pediatrics 48*:605, 1971.
9. Berkovich, S., S. J. Millian and R. D. Snyder: The association of viral and mycoplasma infections with recurrence of wheezing in the asthmatic child. *Ann. Allergy 28*:43, 1970.
10. Berman, S. Z., D. A. Mathison, D. D. Stevenson, E. M. Tan and J. H. Vaughan: Trans-tracheal aspiration studies in asthmatic patients in relapse with "infective" asthma and subjects without respiratory disease. *J. Allergy Clin. Immunol. 56*:206, 1975.
11. Bias, W. B.: The genetic basis of asthma. In *Asthma Physiology, Immunopharmacology and Treatment.* K. F. Austen and L. M. Lichtenstein (Eds.). Academic Press, New York, p. 39, 1973.
12. Bierman, C. W.: Pneumomediastinum and pneumothorax complicating asthma in children. *Am. J. Dis. Child. 114*:42, 1967.
13. Blackhall, M. I. and R. S. Jones: Lung volume and its subdivisions in normal and asthmatic males. *Thorax 28*:89, 1973.
14. Briscoe, W. A. and G. A. McLemore, Jr.: Ventilatory functions in bronchial asthma. *Thorax 7*:66, 1952.
15. Bronsky, E. A. and E. F. Ellis: Inhalation bronchial challenge testing in asthmatic children. *Pediatr. Clin. North Am. 16*:85, 1969.
16. Butler, J., C. G. Caro, R. Alcala and A. B. duBois: Physiological factors affecting airway resistance in normal subjects and in patients with obstructive respiratory disease. *J. Clin. Invest. 39*:584, 1960.
17. Chai, H. and R. W. Newcomb: Pharmacologic management of childhood asthma. *Am. J. Dis. Child. 125*:757, 1973.
18. Cotton, E. K. and W. Parry: Treatment of status asthmaticus and respiratory failure. *Pediatr. Clin. North Am. 22*:163, 1975.
19. Cropp, G. J. A.: Personal communication.
20. Cropp, G. J. A.: Exercise-induced asthma. *Pediatr. Clin. North Am. 22*:63, 1975.
21. Dawson, B., R. Illsley, G. Horobin and R. Mitchell: A survey of childhood asthma in Aberdeen. *Lancet 1*:827, 1969.
22. Derrick, E. H.: Childhood asthma in Brisbane. Epidemiologic observations. *Aust. Paediatr. J. 9*:135, 1973.
23. Downes, J. J., T. Fulgencio and R. C. Raphaely: Acute respiratory failure in infants and children. *Pediatr. Clin. North Am. 19*:423, 1972.
24. Dunnill, M. S.: The morphology of the airways in bronchial asthma. In *New Directions in Asthma,* M. Stein (Ed.). American College of Chest Physicians, Park Ridge, Ill., p. 213, 1975.
25. Editorial: Treatment of status asthmaticus. *Br. Med. J. 4*:563, 1972.
26. Editorial: The total eosinophil count in obstructive pulmonary disease. *N. Engl. J. Med. 292*:1182, 1975.

27. Eggleston, P. A. and B. H. Ward: Radiographic abnormalities in acute asthma in children. *Pediatrics 54*:442, 1974.
28. Ellis, E. F. and E. D. Eddy: Correspondence: anhydrous theophylline equivalence of commercial theophylline formulations. *J. Allergy Clin. Immunol. 53*:116, 1974.
29. Ellis, E. F., R. Koysooko and G. Levy: Pharmacokinetics of theophylline in children with asthma. *Pediatrics 58*:542, 1976.
30. Epstein, R. L.: Constituents of sputum. A simple method. *Ann. Intern. Med. 77*:259, 1972.
31. Evans, H. E., I. Mandl and L. Glass: Serum enzyme inhibitors, immunoglobulins and upper respiratory tract bacteria in asthma. *Am. Rev. Respir. Dis. 108*:672, 1973.
32. Falliers, C. J.: Aspirin and subtypes of asthma. Risk factor analysis. *J. Allergy Clin. Immunol. 52*:141, 1973.
33. Falliers, C. J.: Cromolyn sodium (disodium cromoglycate) prophylaxis. *Pediatr. Clin. North Am. 22*:141, 1975.
34. Falliers, C. J., H. Chai, W. P. McCann and E. F. Ellis: Controlled study of iodotherapy for childhood asthma. *J. Allergy 38*:183, 1966.
35. Ferris, B. G., Jr., J. Mead and L. H. Opie: Partitioning of respiratory flow resistance in man. *J. Appl. Physiol. 19*:653, 1964.
36. Freeman, G. L. and R. H. Todd: The role of allergy in viral respiratory tract infections. *Am. J. Dis. Child. 104*:330, 1962.
37. Gregg, I.: The role of viral infection in asthma and bronchitis. In *Symposium—Viral Diseases.* A. T. Proudfoot (Ed.). Held December 6 & 7, 1973, in the Hall of the Royal College of Physicians of Edinburgh. Royal College of Physicians, Edinburgh, p. 82, 1975.
38. Godfrey, S.: The place of a new aerosol steroid, beclomethasone dipropionate, in the management of childhood asthma. *Pediatr. Clin. North Am. 22*:147, 1975.
39. Gold, W. M.: Cholinergic pharmacology in asthma. In *Asthma Physiology, Immunopharmacology, and Treatment,* K. F. Austen and L. M. Lichtenstein (Eds.). Academic Press, New York, p. 169, 1973.
40. Gold, W. M., H. S. Kaufman, and J. A. Nadel: Elastic recoil of the lungs in chronic asthmatic patients before and after therapy. *J. Appl. Physiol. 23*:433, 1967.
41. Heckscher, T., H. Bass, A. Oriol, B. Rose, N. R. Anthonisen and D. V. Bates: Regional lung function in patients with bronchial asthma. *J. Clin. Invest. 47*:1063, 1968.
42. Hogg, J. C.: The effect of lung growth on the distribution of airways resistance. In *Identification of Asthma,* R. Porter and J. Birch (Eds.). Churchill Livingstone, London, p. 47, 1971.
43. Hogg, J. C., J. Williams, J. B. Richardson, P. T. Macklem, and W. M. Thurlbeck: Age as a factor in the distribution of lower-airway conductance and in the pathologic anatomy of obstructive lung disease. *N. Engl. J. Med. 282*:1283, 1970.
44. Horn, B. R., E. D. Robin, J. Theodore and A. Van Kessel: Total eosinophil counts in the management of bronchial asthma. *N. Engl. J. Med. 292*:1152, 1975.
45. Hudgel, D. W. and J. V. Weil: Asthma associated with decreased hypoxic ventilatory drive. A family study. *Ann. Intern. Med. 80*:622, 1974.
46. Huhti, E., T. Mokka, J. Nikoskelainen and P. Halonen: Association of viral and mycoplasma infections with exacerbations of asthma. *Ann. Allergy 33*:145, 1974.
47. Hyatt, R. E. and L. F. Black: The flow-volume curve: a current perspective. *Am. Rev. Respir. Dis. 107*:191, 1973.
48. Johansson, S. G. O., H. Bennich and T. Berg: In vitro diagnosis of atopic allergy. III. Quantitative estimation of circulating IgE antibodies by the radioallergosorbent test. *Int. Arch. Allergy Appl. Immunol. 41*:443, 1971.
49. Johansson, S. G. O., H. Bennich and T. Berg: The clinical significance of IgE. In *Progress in Clinical Immunology,* R. Schwartz (Ed.). Grune & Stratton, New York, p. 157, 1971.
50. Jorgensen, J. R., C. J. Falliers and S. C. Bukantz: Pneumothorax and mediastinal and subcutaneous emphysema in children with bronchial asthma. *Pediatrics 31*:824, 1963.
51. Karlin, J. M.: The use of antihistamines in asthma. *Ann. Allergy 30*:342, 1972.
52. Kiviloog, J.: Bronchial reactivity to exercise and methacholine in bronchial asthma. *Scand. J. Respir. Dis. 54*:347, 1973.
53. Koivikko, A.: Bacterial vaccine in childhood asthma. A double-blind study. *Acta Allergol. 28*:202, 1973.
54. Lambert, H. P. and H. Stern: Infective factors in exacerbations of bronchitis and asthma. *Br. Med. J. 3*:323, 1972.
55. Levine, G., E. Housely, P. MacLeod and P. T. Macklem: Gas exchange abnormalities in mild bronchitis and asymptomatic asthma. *N. Engl. J. Med. 282*:1277, 1970.
56. Lecks, H. I., T. Whitney, D. Wood and L. P. Kravis: Newer concepts in occurrence of segmental atelectasis in acute bronchial asthma and status asthmaticus in children. *J. Asthma Res. 4*:65, 1966.
57. Lockey, R. F. and D. L. Rucknagel: Familial oc-

currence of asthma, nasal polyps and aspirin intolerance. *Ann. Intern. Med. 78*:57, 1973.

58. Mattsson, Å.: Psychologic aspects of childhood asthma. *Pediatr. Clin. North Am. 22*:77, 1975.
59. McAllen, M. K., S. J. Kochanowski and K. M. Shaw: Steroid aerosols in asthma. An assessment of betamethasone valerate and a 12-month study of patients on maintenance treatment. *Br. Med. J. 1*:171, 1974.
60. McCarthy, D. S., R. Spencer, R. Greene and J. Milic-Emili: Measurement of "closing volume" as a simple and sensitive test for early detection of small airway disease. *Am. J. Med. 52*:747, 1972.
61. McFadden, E. R., Jr., R. Kiser and W. J. DeGroot: Acute bronchial asthma. Relations between clinical and physiologic manifestations. *N. Engl. J. Med. 288*:221, 1973.
62. McFadden, E. R., Jr. and D. A. Linden: A reduction in maximum mid-expiratory flow rate. A spirographic manifestation of small airway disease. *Am. J. Med. 52*:725, 1972.
63. McFadden, E. R., Jr. and H. A. Lyons: Airway resistance and uneven ventilation in bronchial asthma. *J. Appl. Physiol. 25*:365, 1968.
64. McFadden, E. R., Jr. and H. A. Lyons: Arterial blood gas tensions in asthma. *N. Engl. J. Med. 278*:1027, 1968.
65. McIntosh, K., E. F. Ellis, L. S. Hoffman, T. G. Lybass, J. J. Eller and V. A. Fulginiti: The association of viral and bacterial respiratory infections with exacerbations of wheezing in young asthmatic children. *J. Pediatr. 82*:578, 1973.
66. McLean, J. A. and A. Y. T. Ching: Follow-up study of relationships between family situation and bronchial asthma in children. *J. Am. Acad. Child Psychiatry 12*:142, 1973.
67. McNichol, K. N. and H. B. Williams: Spectrum of asthma in childhood I. Clinical and physiological components. *Br. Med. J. 4*:7, 1973.
68. McNichol, K. N. and H. E. Williams: Spectrum of asthma in children II. Allergic components. *Br. Med. J. 4*:12, 1973.
69. Middleton, E., Jr.: Autonomic imbalance in asthma with special reference to beta-adrenergic blockade. *Adv. Intern. Med. 18*:177, 1973.
70. Minor, T. E., E. C. Dick, A. N. DeMeo, J. J. Ouellette, M. Cohen and C. E. Reed: Viruses as precipitants of asthmatic attacks in children. *J.A.M.A. 227*:292, 1974.
71. Mitenko, P. A. and R. I. Ogilvie: Rational intravenous doses of theophylline. *N. Engl. J. Med. 289*:600, 1973.
72. Morris, H. G., I. Neuman and E. F. Ellis: Plasma steroid concentrations during alternate-day treatment with prednisone. *J. Allergy Clin. Immunol. 54*:350, 1974.
73. Nadel, J. A.: Neurophysiologic aspects of asthma. In *Asthma Physiology, Immunopharmacology, and Treatment.* K. F. Austen and L. M. Lichtenstein (Eds.). Academic Press, New York, p. 29, 1973.
74. Parker, C. D, R. E. Bilbo and C. E. Reed: Methacholine aerosol as test for bronchial asthma. *Arch. Intern. Med. 115*:452, 1965.
75. Patel, K. R. and J. W. Kerr: Effect of alpha receptor drug, thymoxamine, on allergen-induced bronchoconstriction in extrinsic asthma. *Clin. Allergy 5*:311, 1975.
76. Pepys, J. and B. J. Hutchcraft: Bronchial provocation tests in etiologic diagnosis and analysis of asthma. *Am. Rev. Respir. Dis. 112*:829, 1975.
77. Piafsky, K. M. and R. I. Ogilvie: Dosage of theophylline in bronchial asthma. *N. Engl. J. Med. 292*:1218, 1975.
78. Prime, F. J., S. Bianco, J. P. Griffin and P. L. Kamburoff: The effects on airways conductance of alpha-adrenergic stimulation and blocking. *Bull. Physiopathol. Respir. 8*:99, 1972.
79. Rackemann, F. and M. C. Edwards: Asthma in children. A follow-up study of 688 patients after an interval of 20 years. *N. Engl. J. Med. 246*:815, 1952.
80. Rakower, J., W. Pinkhas and H. Halberstadt: Massive asthmatic atelectasis. *Chest 27*:573, 1955.
81. Rebuck, A. S. and J. Read: Assessment and management of severe asthma. *Am. J. Med. 51*:788, 1971.
82. Reed, C. E.: The pathogenesis of asthma. *Med. Clin. North Am. 58*:55, 1974.
83. Reed, C. E.: Abnormal autonomic mechanisms in asthma. *J. Allergy Clin. Immunol. 53*:34, 1974.
84. Rees, H. A., J. S. Millar and K. W. Donald: A study of the clinical course and arterial blood gas tensions of patients in status asthmaticus. *Q. J. Med. 37*:541, 1968.
85. Reimer, L. G., H. G. Morris and E. F. Ellis: Growth of asthmatic children during treatment with alternate-day steroids. *J. Allergy Clin. Immunol. 55*:224, 1975.

85a. Richardson, J. and J. Béland: Nonadrenergic inhibitory nervous system in human airways. *J. Appl. Physiol. 41*:764, 1976.

86. Robinson, A. E. and J. B. Campbell: Bronchography in childhood asthma. *Am. J. Roentgenol. Radium Ther. Nucl. Med. 116*:559, 1972.
87. Salvin, R. G., T. S. Laird and J. D. Cherry: Allergic bronchopulmonary aspergillosis in a child. *J. Pediatr. 76*:416, 1970.
88. Samter, M. and R. F. Beers: Intolerance to aspirin. Clinical studies and considerations of its pathogenesis. *Ann. Intern. Med. 68*:975, 1968.
89. Sanders, S. and A. P. Norman: The bacterial flora of the upper respiratory tract in children with severe asthma. *J. Allergy 41*:319, 1968.

90. Schlueter, D. P.: Pulmonary hypersensitivity diseases. *Adv. Intern. Med. 18*:153, 1972.
91. Schultz, G., J. G. Hardman and E. W. Sutherland: Cyclic nucleotides and smooth muscle function. In *Asthma Physiology, Immunopharmacology, and Treatment,* K. F. Austen and L. M. Lichtenstein (Eds.). Academic Press, New York, p. 123, 1973.
92. Shapiro, G. G., P. A. Eggleston, W. E. Pierson, C. G. Ray and C. W. Bierman: Double-blind study of the effectiveness of a broad spectrum antibiotic in status asthmaticus. *Pediatrics 53*:867, 1974.
93. Simonsson, B. G., F. M. Jacobs and J. A. Nadel: Role of autonomic nervous system and the cough reflex in the increased responsiveness of airways in patients with obstructive airway disease. *J. Clin. Invest. 46*:1812, 1967.
94. Simonsson, B. G., B. Jonson and B. Ström: Bronchodilatory and circulatory effects of inhaling increasing doses of an anti-cholinergic drug, ipratropium bromide (SCH 1000). *Scand. J. Respir. Dis. 56*:138, 1975.
95. Simpson, H., J. O. Forfar and D. J. Grubb: Arterial blood gas tensions and pH in acute asthma in childhood. *Br. Med. J. 3*:460, 1968.
96. Smith, A. P.: Role of prostaglandins in the pathogenesis and treatment of asthma. In *Asthma Physiology, Immunopharmacology, and Treatment,* K. F. Austen and L. M. Lichtenstein (Eds.). Academic Press, New York, p. 267, 1973.
97. Smith, J. M.: Incidence of atopic disease. *Med. Clin. North Am. 58*:3, 1974.
98. Spector, S. L. and R. S. Farr: Bronchial inhalation procedures in asthmatics. *Med. Clin. North Am. 58*:71, 1974.
99. Sterling, G. M.: Mechanism of bronchoconstriction caused by cigarette smoking. *Br. Med. J. 2*:275, 1967.
100. Symposium on exercise and asthma. *Pediatrics* (*Suppl.*) *56*:843, 1975.
101. Szentivanyi, A.: The beta adrenergic theory of the atopic abnormality in bronchial asthma. *J. Allergy 42*:203, 1968.
102. Tai, E. and J. Read: Blood gas tensions in bronchial asthma. *Lancet 1*:644, 1967.
103. VanArsdel, P. P. and A. G. Motulsky: Frequency and hereditability of asthma and allergic rhinitis in college students. *Acta Genet. 9*:101, 1959.
104. Vaughan, J. H., E. M. Tan, D. A. Mathison, D. D. Stevenson, S. Z. Berman and A. I. Braude: Bronchial asthma: pathophysiology. In *Asthma Physiology, Immunopharmacology, and Treatment.* K. F. Austen and L. M. Lichtenstein (Eds.). Academic Press, New York, p. 1, 1973.
105. Widdicombe, J. G., D. C. Kent and J. A. Nadel: Mechanism of bronchoconstriction during inhalation of dust. *J. Appl. Physiol. 17*:613, 1962.
106. Widdicombe, J. G. and G. M. Sterling: The autonomic nervous system and breathing. *Arch. Intern. Med. 126*:311, 1970.
107. Williams, H. E. and K. N. McNichol: Prevalence, natural history and relationship of wheezy bronchitis and asthma in children. An epidemiological study. *Br. Med. J. 4*:321, 1969.
108. Wittig, H. J. and C. H. Chang: Right middle lobe atelectasis in childhood asthma. *J. Allergy Clin. Immunol. 39*:245, 1967.
109. Wood, D. W. and J. J. Downes: The management of respiratory failure in childhood status asthmaticus. Experience with 30 episodes and evolution of a technique. *J. Allergy Clin. Immunol. 42*:261, 1968.
110. Wood, C. B. and J. Oliver: Serum IgE in asthmatic children. Relation to age, sex, eczema and skin sensitivity tests. *Arch. Dis. Child. 47*:890, 1972.
111. Woolcock, A. J. and J. Read: Lung volumes in exacerbations of asthma. *Am. J. Med. 41*:259, 1966.
112. Yunginger, J. W., E. J. O'Connell and G. B. Logan: Aspirin-induced asthma in children. *J. Pediatr. 82*:218, 1973.
113. Zaid, G. and G. N. Beall: Bronchial response to beta-adrenergic blockade. *N. Engl. J. Med. 275*:580, 1966.

Cystic Fibrosis

MARTIN I. LORIN AND CAROLYN R. DENNING

11

It is surprising that a disease of such severity and with as many unusual features as cystic fibrosis could have gone unrecognized for so long. It was first described in 1936 by Fanconi.[52] Considered then a rapidly fatal disorder of infancy, it is today recognized as a major cause of chronic pulmonary disease in children and adolescents, responsible for more deaths in this age group than asthma and tuberculosis combined.[30] It is a genetically determined disease, affecting many organs both biochemically and clinically. Bronchopulmonary infection, gastrointestinal malabsorption, and elevated sweat sodium and chloride concentrations are the most characteristic manifestations and can be found in the majority of patients. Nasal polyps, chronic sinusitis, biliary cirrhosis, intestinal obstruction by inspissated fecal material, aspermia, and diabetes mellitus are additional clinical disturbances and complications not uncommon in cystic fibrosis.

The biochemical pathway by which the genetic abnormality of cystic fibrosis is translated into cellular dysfunction and the various clinical manifestations remain obscure. The primary derangement appears to be an aberration of exocrine secretion throughout the body, although it is not yet clear whether this deviant characteristic is due to an intrinsic abnormality of the exocrine cell itself, an abnormal serum factor, or an abnormality of autonomic innervation of the exocrine glands. Impaction of secretions in the ducts or ductules of various organs, with resultant obstruction, inflammation, and fibrosis, is the basic, gross, pathologic change. Farber, in 1945, postulated that this series of events was due to an abnormality of mucus production and introduced the term mucoviscidosis.[53] Although Farber's original concept remains valid, subsequent investigations have shown that the defect is not limited to mucus production, for nonmucous glands, such as the parotid and sweat glands, are functionally abnormal even though anatomically undisturbed.

Genetics

Cystic fibrosis is transmitted as an autosomal recessive trait. This conclusion was originally based on studies such as those of Danks[29] and Merritt,[132] who analyzed a great many family pedigrees, and was further supported by the report of Grand[70] that 11 out of 11 children born to women with cystic fibrosis were normal. The authors are aware of only one instance where a mother with cystic fibrosis gave birth to a child with cystic fibrosis.[152A] Still additional evidence confirming the autosomal recessive nature of cystic fibrosis has come recently from the in vitro demonstration of certain biochemical abnormalities in parents of children with this disease.[8,114] These biochemical disturbances, which are discussed later, are not associated with any clinical manifestations, are quantitatively less pronounced than in the patients themselves, and are present in both parents. Lobeck,[112] Danks,[29] and Merritt[132] believe that the available genetic data indicate that cystic fibrosis is probably determined by a single pair of alleles. Based on tissue culture study of skin fibroblasts, however, Danes has suggested that the disease can be caused by homozygosity of mutant genes at either of two distinct loci, each affected member of a kinship having involvement at the same locus.[28] The in vivo counterpart of this phenomenon, two distinct clinical syndromes or variants, has not been demonstrated.

Among Caucasians in different parts of the world, the reported incidence of cystic fibrosis varies from approximately one in 2000 to one in 3000 live births.[42] This incidence gives rise to an estimated gene frequency of 3 to 5%, which is surprisingly high for a potentially lethal gene, and has engendered speculation of a survival advantage for the heterozygotes. To date, such a survival advantage has not been demonstrated, although the results of some studies do suggest a reproductive advantage to the carrier state. Danks, for example, found that grandparents of children with cystic fibrosis averaged more live offspring than control families.[29]

The incidence of cystic fibrosis is lower among nonwhites than among whites. A survey of cystic fibrosis clinics in the eastern United States revealed that only 2% of the patients were Negro, although approximately 13% of the population in this area was black.[97] Kulczycki reported an incidence of 1 in 17,033 black newborns.[99A] Even this relatively low incidence of disease probably represents an admixture of white genes through intermating, as cystic fibrosis is almost unknown among African Negroes. Documented cases among Orientals are rare,[90] and the incidence has been estimated as only one in 90,000.[185]

Chromosomal abnormalities have not been reported in cystic fibrosis, and the finding of normal chromosomal patterns in seven patients is mentioned by di Sant'Agnese.[42]

Pathology and Pathophysiology (General)

Cystic fibrosis appears to involve the exocrine organs directly, while nonexocrine organs, such as the heart, islets of Langer-hans, and long bones, are involved only indirectly or secondarily. Physical and chemical changes have been described in various exocrine secretions, but these changes are not the same for the different organs involved, and to date, no single concept has been able to adequately explain the many and often dissimilar abnormalities found. Some exocrine secretions have not been fully investigated, even as regards such simple parameters as electrolyte composition, while for some others, reports of different workers have been conflicting and further studies are needed for clarification.

As some knowledge of the nonpulmonary aspects of cystic fibrosis is important for a full understanding of the respiratory pathophysiology, and essential to the proper diagnosis and treatment of patients afflicted with this disease, it is appropriate to examine, in some detail, the pathologic and pathophysiologic changes that occur in nonrespiratory organs, as well as the changes in the pulmonary system proper.

SWEAT GLANDS

The electrolyte composition of eccrine sweat from patients with cystic fibrosis is distinctly abnormal. Not only are the mean sodium and chloride concentrations significantly higher than normal, but also, almost no overlap exists between the values for patients with cystic fibrosis and for normal subjects, making the determination very useful diagnostically. This derangement of electrolyte composition of sweat is one of the most constant features of cystic fibrosis, being present in essentially all individuals with this disease.

Gibson reported the mean sweat chloride concentration in patients with cystic fibrosis to be 95 mEq/l, with a range of 80 to 122 mEq/l, as compared to a mean of only 21 mEq/l, and a range of 7 to 49 mEq/l for control subjects.[63] Di Sant'Agnese found a mean sweat sodium concentration of 103 mEq/l for cystic fibrosis patients and only 22 mEq/l for normal children.[41] Grand found that the concentration of sodium in the sweat of children with cystic fibrosis was reduced by the administration of aldosterone, although not to the same degree as in normal children.[69]

The mean sweat potassium in cystic fibrosis is also significantly elevated, but the ranges for disease and normal values overlap considerably.[41] Di Sant'Agnese reported the concentration of calcium in the sweat of patients with cystic fibrosis to be slightly elevated as compared to normal subjects.[36] Emrich found this to be true only at high rates of sweating.[50] Utilizing a rotational viscometer and pooled samples, Lorin noted the viscosity of sweat in this disease to be normal.[116] Emrich, however, measuring individual sweat samples with a miniature Ostwald viscometer, detected a slight increase in viscosity, which could be accounted for by the increased electrolyte concentration.[49]

The sweat glands appear normal both by light and by electron microscopy, except for the finding of fewer than normal secretory vacuoles in the mucoid cells.[136] The description by Munger[136] of virus-like particles in the gland could not be confirmed by Spicer.[161] Gibbs measured the concentration of various tissue enzymes in the sweat glands of normal subjects and in patients with cystic fibrosis and found no differences between the two groups.[62] The electrolyte abnormality appears to be due to a defective or blocked sodium reabsorption mechanism in the duct of the gland, as both the hydrostatic secretory pressure and the precursor fluid formed by the coiled portion have been shown to be normal.[157,160]

PANCREAS

Unlike the sweat glands, the pancreas in cystic fibrosis undergoes dramatic anatomic changes. At postmortem examination, dilatation of ducts and ductules, replacement of normal parenchyma by fibrous and adipose tissue, and the presence of cysts up to several millimeters in diameter are striking and give rise to the term, cystic fibrosis of the pancreas[15] (Fig. 11-1). On the basis of autopsy study of a series of patients dying at various ages, from a few days to a few years, Andersen reconstructed the sequence of events leading to these pathologic alterations.[1] Abnormal secretions precipitate in the acini and ducts with resultant obstruction and dilatation; intralobular ducts expand to form cysts.

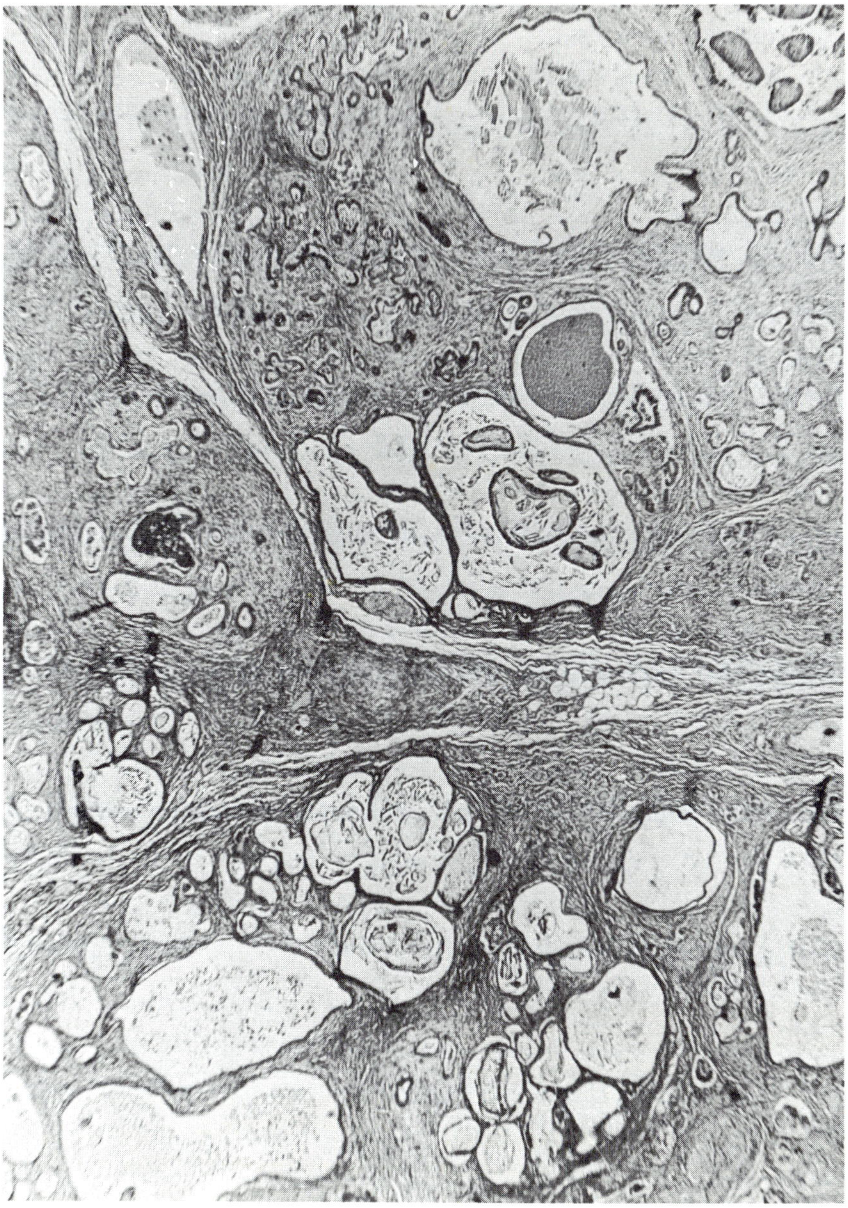

FIG. 11-1. Pancreas of a 9-year-old child with cystic fibrosis. Specimen shows multiple large cysts and widespread fibrosis. (From Andersen, D. H.: Pathology of cystic fibrosis. *Ann. N.Y. Acad. Sci. 93*:500, 1962.)

The acini become atrophic, and diffuse fibrosis develops within and between lobules (Fig. 11-1). Finally, the tissues are infiltrated by adipose cells. Antemortem, physiologic studies by Hadorn have led to the same conclusion.[74] Using a triple-lumen, double balloon duodenal tube to isolate and study pancreatic secretion, he concluded that the primary disturbance was a defect in water and bicarbonate secretion (ductal activity) and that the deficiency of enzyme secretion (acinar activity) was secondary to ductal obstruction and not a primary defect of the acinar cells.

The islet cells are relatively spared by the destructive and fibrotic changes, and Bodian noted that, although the number of islets decreased with advancing age, some normal islet tissue was present in all cases, including the oldest in his series, 13 years.[15] Kaiser concluded from the study of a relatively small group of patients that the diabetes of cystic fibrosis is generally a late complication due to progressive pancreatic changes.[94] Handwerger suggested that, since the characteristic complications and postmortem changes of diabetes were absent, and the decrease in number of beta cells was only moderate, the glucose intolerance (chemical diabetes) present in almost half of these patients was due to anatomic disorganization of the islets by pancreatic fibrosis, and an impaired release of insulin, rather than beta cell destruction per se.[76]

SALIVARY GLANDS

Anatomic changes in the various salivary glands are not as striking as those in some other exocrine organs, and Bodian noted that they were related to the proportion of mucus-secreting cells present.[15] Thus, the parotid gland appears essentially normal, while the submaxillary and, more so, the sublingual glands reveal accumulated secretion in the ducts and mild dilatation of ducts and acini, generally without atrophy or fibrosis.

The sodium content of mixed saliva from patients with cystic fibrosis is significantly greater than that of control subjects.[39] When the compositions of parotid and submaxillary saliva are studied separately, the abnormalities are, in general, found to be more pronounced for the submaxillary secretion. Thus, Mandel found a significant increase in the sodium concentration of submaxillary but not of parotid saliva.[118,119] Organic constituents, such as amylase and lysozymes, were also noted to be increased in submaxillary but not parotid secretion. Calcium levels in submaxillary saliva from patients with cystic fibrosis are almost double those of normal subjects.[21,119] Studies by Wiesmann, with a sodium sensitive electrode placed directly on the oral mucosa, led him to believe that the chief source of elevated salivary sodium is the small glands of the oral mucosa.[182]

In normal children both parotid and submaxillary saliva is clear, whereas in children with cystic fibrosis, submaxillary saliva is turbid,[21] an observation that has focused considerable attention on the glycoprotein composition of submaxillary secretion. Mandel noted a significant elevation of total protein concentration in submaxillary saliva from patients with cystic fibrosis, the protein bound carbohydrates, hexose and fucose, being increased proportionately.[119] Gugler reported several differences in the protein electrophoresis pattern of submaxillary saliva in patients with cystic fibrosis as compared to normal subjects.[73] However, these differences could be reversed by the addition of ethylenediaminetetraacetic acid (EDTA, which binds calcium) to the cystic fibrosis saliva, or by the addition of calcium to normal saliva. The differences, therefore, appear to be due to polymerization of normal glycoproteins by the excessive calcium present in the cystic fibrosis saliva, rather than to abnormal glycoproteins per se. To date, no immunologically unique glycoprotein has been demonstrated in cystic fibrosis saliva. The relationship of the high calcium content and glycoprotein polymerization to the precipitation of secretion in salivary glands and other exocrine organs is intriguing, but uncertain. The viscosity of submaxillary[116] or parotid saliva[100] in cystic fibrosis has not been shown to be significantly greater than normal.

LIVER

Although some hepatic changes are to be found in most autopsied cases of cystic fibrosis, the degree of involvement varies remarkably. The mildest cases show only distention of small bile ducts with eosinophilic concretions, ductal proliferation, and periductal fibrosis.[1] In the somewhat more advanced situation, focal biliary cirrhosis is present, while in the most severely affected patients the process is generalized, and a diffuse, multilobular, biliary cirrhosis develops.[15,37] Ultimately, the distortion, scarring, and regeneration lead to portal hypertension. It is believed that these changes are caused by the coagulation of abnormal secretions in the ductules and consequent obstruction, inflammation, and fibrosis. The results of examination of serial sections of the liver by Bodian are in agreement with this hypothesis.[15]

Fatty changes of the liver have been described, especially in untreated patients or in those who die after a protracted terminal phase with poor nutrition. Centrilobular congestion or necrosis is occasionally seen as a result of chronic hypoxia and cor pulmonale.[1] These disturbances are secondary rather than primary.

INTESTINES

The most characteristic intestinal changes are those described by Bodian as mucosis.[15] The intestinal glands are distended with secretions, the intestinal contents are thick and mucoid, and a layer of tenacious mucus covers the mucosa. Andersen noted inspissated secretions in the intestinal glands and hypersecretion of Brunner's glands.[1] Johansen reported that the mucus in the glands and goblet cells of the rectal mucosa appeared both more copious and more concentrated.[92]

Although the intestinal tract in this disease is commonly thought of in terms of diarrhea, steatorrhea, and malabsorption, it is evident that this organ is also subject to intraluminal obstruction by inspissated secretions and fecal material in a manner similar to the intraluminal obstruction of various other organs. The most well-known example of this phenomenon is meconium ileus, in which the small bowel, usually the terminal ileum, becomes impacted in utero with exceedingly thick meconium. The bowel proximal to the obstruction becomes distended, while the distal bowel is hypoplastic (microcolon). The intestinal obstruction appears more related to the degree of mucosis than to the extent of pancreatic insufficiency.[170] Elevated calcium levels in the meconium of infants with meconium ileus, as reported by Kopito, could be significant in view of the suggested role of calcium in binding and polymerizing glycoproteins into giant molecules that might well precipitate out of solution and cause the intestinal contents to become solid before they reach the large bowel.[96]

AUTONOMIC NERVOUS SYSTEM

Although anatomic abnormalities of the autonomic nervous system have not been described in cystic fibrosis, the fact that most of the exocrine glands and organs involved directly by the disease are innervated by this system has stimulated considerable interest in the possibility of a primary disturbance of autonomic function. Barbero has reviewed this aspect of cystic fibrosis, including the generally unsuccessful attempts to produce the disease in animals by chronic cholinergic stimulation or blockade.[6] Chernick demonstrated that parasympathomimetic stimulation of normal children produced changes in submaxillary saliva similar to those seen in cystic fibrosis.[21] It has also been shown that guanethidine, an adrenergic blocking agent, can clear the abnormal turbidity of submaxillary saliva in patients with cystic fibrosis, although other adrenergic blocking agents do not have this effect.[22]

Rubin demonstrated significant differences in pupillary reactivity between patients with cystic fibrosis and control subjects,[154] an observation of especial interest in that the pupil is a nonglandular, nonexocrine organ. Unfortunately, similar studies by Lowenfeld have failed to confirm these differences, and the area remains in need of further observations.[117]

SERUM FACTORS

Serum electrolytes are normal in cystic fibrosis, and electrophoretic examination of serum proteins, lipoproteins, and glycoproteins reveals only secondary, nonspecific changes.[26] The search for an abnormal or unique serum substance in this disease met with its first success in 1967, when Spock reported that serum from patients with cystic fibrosis added to explants of rabbit tracheal epithelium caused a disorganization of the ordinarily highly coordinated ciliary action.[163] It was further noted that the substance responsible for the ciliary dyskinesis resides in the euglobulin fraction of serum, and is present, although in lesser concentration, in the serum of heterozygotes. Bowman[16] and Lockhart[114] have demonstrated a similar effect on oyster cilia, although in their experiments the end point was the cessation of ciliary activity rather than dyskinesis. Again, the factor was also present in the serum of heterozygotes.

The nature and significance of this serum anticiliary factor is still unclear. Spock found it to be heat labile, nondialyzable, and present in two molecular fractions.[163] Chemically, it appears to be a cationic protein,[16A] found by Conover[24A] to be a small molecular weight polypeptide in the range of 1000 to 10,000 MW, by Bowman[16B] to be 6000 to 11,000 MW, and by Danes[28A] to be close to 5000 MW. Most investigators have found it associated with the immunoglobulin fraction in serum.[16C,156A,7A] Studies with fluorescein labeling, however, indicate that it does not behave like an antibody or bind to cilia.[78] Bowman has reported that the ciliary inhibitor can be dissociated from immunoglobulin.[18] The fact that the substance is present in the serum of heterozygotes, who have no disease, indicates that it is not the result of pulmonary damage or inflammation and suggests that it is a direct genetic effect. Yet, the same reasoning must cast doubt on its pathogenic role, since the heterozygotes are clinically completely well despite the presence of this substance. Wilson has reported serum protein differences between the patient with cystic fibrosis, the carrier, and the normal, based on isoelectric focusing in acrylamide gels.[183A] Ciliary beating of explants of respiratory epithelium from patients with cystic fibrosis was found by Spock to be normal.[162] In vivo observations in our laboratory have indicated that ciliary activity of the nasal mucosa is at least grossly normal in patients with cystic fibrosis. A finely powdered coloring agent was insufflated onto the ciliated portion of the nasal septum and its clearance to the posterior nasopharynx observed through a stereomicroscope. The pattern and direction of mucus flow, as indicated by the contrast material, were the same in patients with cystic fibrosis as in normal subjects. An excellent review of the current status of the factors related to cystic fibrosis has just been published.[120A]

SODIUM TRANSPORT

Since 1953, when di Sant'Agnese reported finding an increased sodium concentration in the sweat of patients with cystic fibrosis,[38] researchers have shown considerable interest in the mechanisms of sodium transport in this disease. Most investigations have indicated that renal handling of sodium is normal in cystic fibrosis,[38,41,69] although a study by

Robson raises the possibility of increased sodium reabsorption in the proximal renal tubules.[152] Intraerythrocyte sodium concentrations have been shown to be normal in this disorder, as has the efflux of sodium from these cells.[113] Balfe, however, has found a defect in the ovabain-sensitive sodium transport mechanism of erythrocytes from patients with cystic fibrosis as well as from their parents.[5]

Interesting observations by Mangos suggest that the derangement of sodium transport in cystic fibrosis is due to a blockage of the sodium pump rather than a defect per se.[120] Retrograde perfusion of the rat parotid gland with saliva or sweat from patients with cystic fibrosis renders the duct of the gland unable to reabsorb sodium. The sodium-transport inhibiting factor in sweat has also been shown to decrease the reabsorption of the sodium by the normal sweat gland in situ.[93] The relationship of the sodium-transport inhibiting factor to other organs such as the liver, pancreas, and lung remains to be determined.

Gibson has suggested that mucus, which normally functions to inhibit the flow of water and small ions, thereby protecting the cell membrane from osmotic, hydrostatic, and ionic gradients, is defective in cystic fibrosis, leading to an increased permeability across the membrane.[64] Presumably, under these conditions, the gradient necessary to produce a hypotonic secretion cannot be maintained and the secretion loses water.

For a more comprehensive discussion of the water and electrolyte abnormalities in the exocrine secretions of patients with cystic fibrosis, see *Cystic Fibrosis. Projections into the Future.*[120A]

Pathology and Pathophysiology (the Lung)

As the basic biochemical lesion in cystic fibrosis remains unknown, it is not surprising to find equal uncertainty and speculation about the mechanism by which this aberration leads to the chronic pulmonary obstruction and bronchopulmonary suppuration so characteristic of this disease. Reviewing the autopsy material of 36 cases, Zuelzer noted the earliest findings in the lungs to be plugging of bronchi and bronchioles by mucoid secretions, even before the appearance of inflammatory changes[189] (Figs. 11-2 and 11-3). He concluded that the essential change in the disease is the production of abnormally thick mucus by the bronchial glands and resultant obstruction of air passages. Andersen also noted occlusion of small airways by mucoid secretions to be an early pathologic finding, present even in the lungs of infants dying of meconium ileus and other nonrespiratory causes.[1] The finding of ductal obstruction by inspissated or precipitated secretion in other organs such as the pancreas, liver, gall bladder, and mucous salivary glands, in the absence of infection, seemed to warrant extrapolation to a similar mechanism in the lung, that is, the basic assumption that mucus retention is primary and, specifically, that it precedes bacterial infection.

MUCUS AND SPUTUM

Although the cause of the accumulation of secretion and debris in the bronchi and bronchioles is not known, it is commonly believed to be due to some physiochemical abnormality of mucus, as for example, an increased viscosity. One major obstacle to the resolution of this question has been the inaccessibility of uncontaminated tracheobronchial mucus for analysis and investigation. Expectorated sputum is invariably contaminated by saliva. Attempts to remove the saliva by decanting or absorbing onto gauze are inaccurate and arbitrary, as the serous and soluble portions of the sputum must be irrevocably mixed with the saliva. Even material obtained by bronchoscopic aspiration is, in these patients, contaminated by bacteria, cellular debris, and inflammatory products. Despite these limitations, however, studies of both

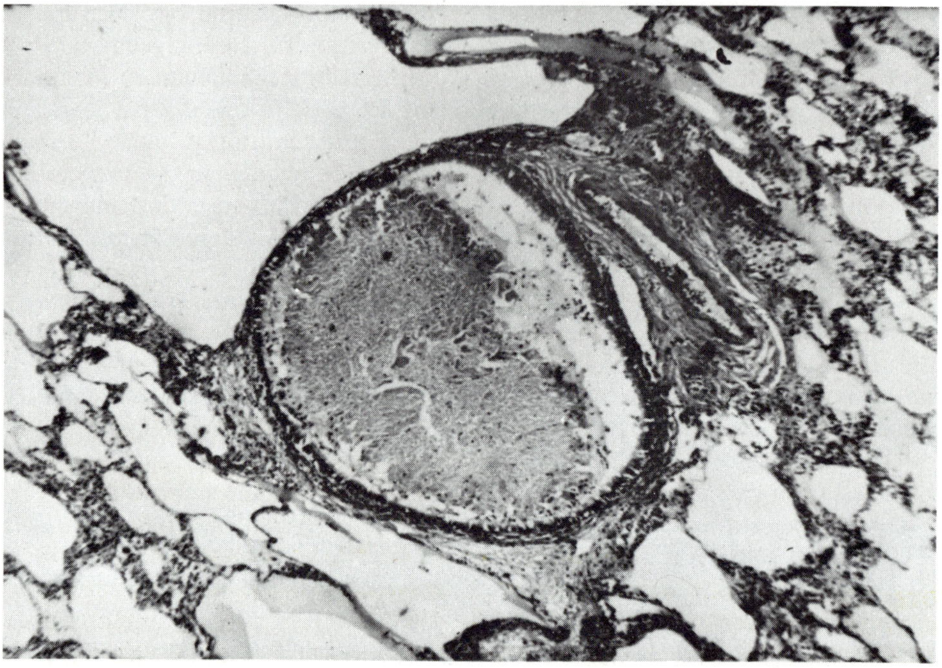

FIG. 11-2. Plugging of small airway by mucopurulent material. Lung section was taken from a 9-year-old child with cystic fibrosis, who, at the time of death from biliary cirrhosis, had only moderate pulmonary involvement. The bronchiole shown is almost completely occluded by the mass of mucus and cellular debris. Inflammatory reaction extends from the bronchiolar wall into the surrounding lung parenchyma. Involvement of the small airways occurs early in this disease.

expectorated and bronchoscopically obtained secretion have yielded interesting and clinically enlightening information, clarifying to some degree the secondary, if not the primary, changes within the lungs.

In 1960, Denton reported that the viscosity of sputum from children with cystic fibrosis was greater than that of tracheobronchial secretions obtained from normal children at the time of tonsillectomy.[34] He also found the viscosity of cystic fibrosis sputum to be greater than that of sputum from patients with acute or chronic bronchitis. It is now clear, however, that the sputum in cystic fibrosis owes its viscosity, at least in part, to its high content of DNA, a secondary phenomenon, reflecting the constant purulence of sputum in this disease. In 1969, Sturgess reported that the viscosity of cystic fibrosis sputum was comparable to, but not greater than that of purulent sputum from other chronic pulmonary diseases.[167] Feather claims that the viscosity of mucoid (nonpurulent) sputum from patients with cystic fibrosis is actually less than that of similar material from patients with asthma or chronic bronchitis.[54] His data, however, are open to question on several grounds. Purulence or nonpurulence of specimens was decided wholly on the basis of visual appearance. All of the mucoid cystic fibrosis sputum came from only two patients. Finally, it is doubtful that one ever obtains valid mucoid or nonpurulent sputum specimens from patients with cystic fibrosis. Data from our own laboratory (Fig. 11-4) indicate that such nonpurulent appearing specimens are chiefly saliva, presumably because patients with

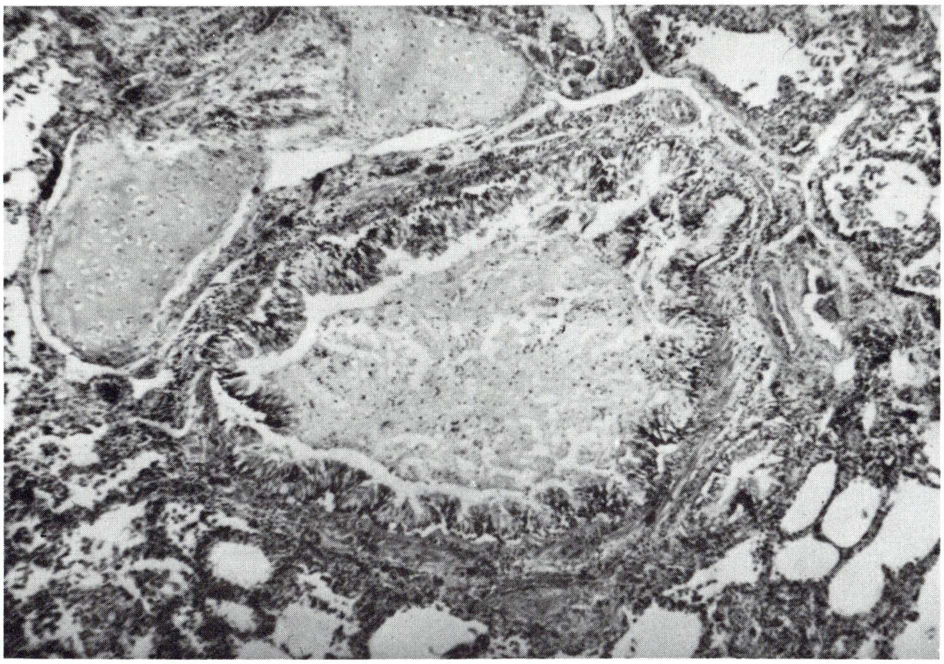

FIG. 11-3. Plugging of larger airway. Lung section taken from a 14-year-old child who died from severe pulmonary involvement of cystic fibrosis. The bronchus (note cartilage in wall) seen above is completely occluded by intraluminal secretion and debris. There is extensive inflammatory reaction in the bronchial wall and neighboring parenchyma. Involvement of large airways is a relatively late change in cystic fibrosis.

minimal bronchopulmonary infection raise such tiny amounts of sputum that relatively massive salivary contamination is inevitable. In view of the critical importance of the question of viscosity and other flow properties of sputum in this disorder, a great deal more investigation is called for, including measurements of such parameters as surface tension, spinnbarkeit, and viscoelasticity.

Much attention has been focused in this disease on the search for a biochemical derangement of sputum that could explain its presumed increased viscosity or tendency to accumulate in the airways. Since glycoproteins are a major component of mucus, an abnormality of glycoprotein synthesis has been postulated as the basic defect, but has never been convincingly demonstrated. Dische[43] and other workers[23] have noted an increased fucose to sialic acid ratio in duodenal fluid and submaxillary saliva from children with cystic fibrosis, and have suggested that this disturbance of the carbohydrate moiety of the glycoprotein could so alter the size or shape of the molecule as to increase its viscosity or decrease its solubility. Potter, however, found the ratio of fucose to sialic acid to be decreased rather than increased in sputum from patients with cystic fibrosis.[147] Studies by Chernick and Matthews revealed the DNA content of cystic fibrosis sputum to be very high, not only as compared to normal sputum (from patients with laryngectomy) but even as compared to sputum from patients with bronchiectasis.[24,124] The DNA itself, although increased in quantity, was found to be normal human DNA in regard to composition.[149]

The sodium concentration of tracheobronchial secretions or sputum from cystic fibrosis

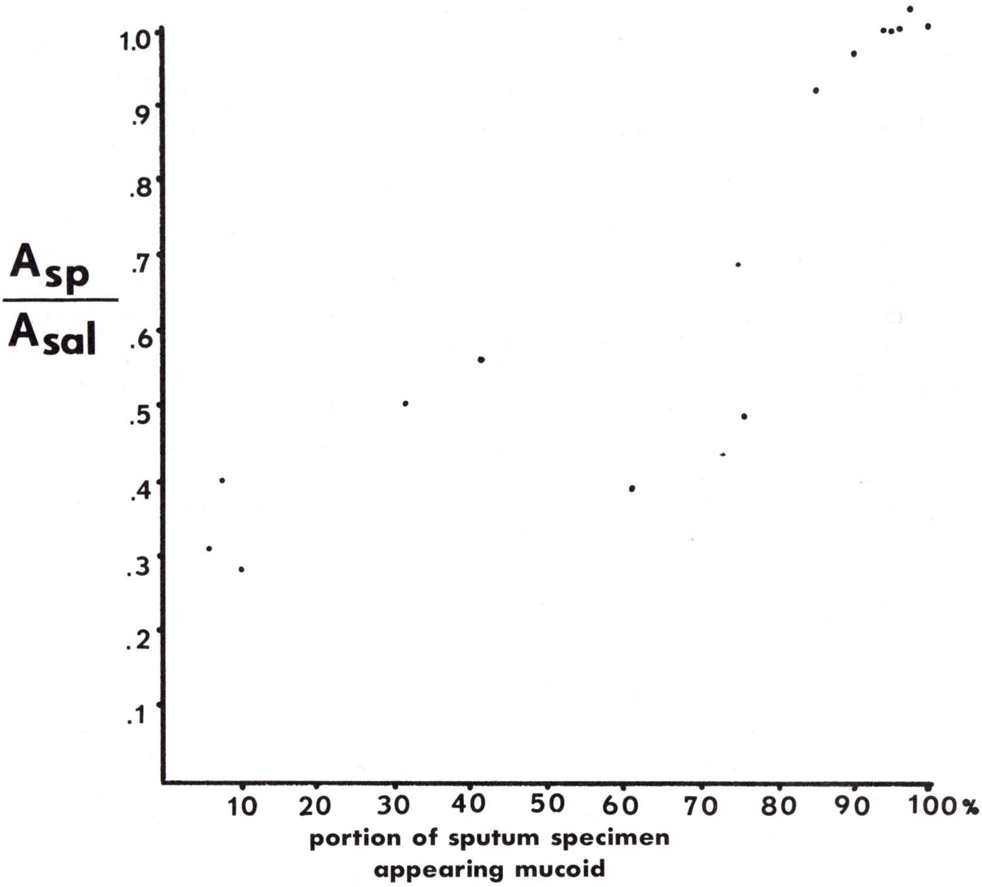

FIG. 11-4. Relation of mucoid appearance of sputum specimen to contamination with saliva. The concentration of amylase in the sputum specimen (A_{sp}) divided by the concentration of amylase in a simultaneously collected sample of mixed saliva (A_{sal}) gives a measure of the portion of the sputum specimen that is actually saliva. Each dot represents one sputum and one saliva specimen from a patient with cystic fibrosis. It should be noted that when the sputum specimen appears purely mucoid, the A_{sp}/A_{sal} ratio is around unity, indicating that the specimen is essentially saliva.

patients is less than that of comparable material from normal subjects or from patients with other chronic pulmonary conditions.[24,124] This phenomenon is secondary, as the increased content of nonelectrolyte solids (protein, amino acids, DNA, lipid) resulting from inflammation and exudation draws in water to reestablish osmotic equilibrium.[148] Working with secretions obtained by bronchoscopic aspiration, Chernick found the calcium concentration in cystic fibrosis to be double that in bronchiectasis. Since divalent cations, such as calcium, are believed to cross link mucoprotein molecules, he suggested that the elevated calcium content is the primary disturbance that increases the viscosity or otherwise alters the physical properties of the mucus. Chernick refers to studies in which the viscosity of snail mucus was increased by the addition of calcium chloride, and mentions his own similar results with tracheobronchial secretions.[24] In contrast however, Lieberman found that calcium chloride did not increase the viscosity of cystic fibrosis sputum, and that very high concentrations (0.5 m to 2.0 m) actually resulted in a decrease in viscosity.[105] Finally, it should be noted that, in less than complete agreement with the data of Chernick,[24] Matthews[124] found the calcium content of cystic fibrosis sputum to be only slightly greater than normal and less than that of bronchiectatic sputum.

Although no direct evidence is available to confirm that tracheobronchial secretions in cystic fibrosis are basically more viscid than normal, considerable indirect evidence exists to support such an hypothesis. This evidence is along two major lines. First are the data indicating that airway obstruction precedes infection of the tracheobronchial tree, and second are the observations that therapeutic measures that decrease sputum viscosity can reverse this obstruction, even in the absence of signs of infection.

Thus, Demuth noted airway obstruction, as manifested by impairment of intrapulmonary gas distribution, to be the earliest detectable sign of lung involvement in cystic fibrosis, preceding clinical or radiographic changes.[31] Kulczycki found evidence of air trapping on x-ray examination to be present before clinical signs of pulmonary disease.[99] Phelan reported increased thoracic gas volume and decreased airway conductance in a group of infants with cystic fibrosis, many of whom had the physiologic abnormalities in the absence of any clinical evidence of pulmonary infection.[143] Serum antistaphylococcal alpha-hemolysin titers were measured by Iacocca in normal subjects and in patients with cystic fibrosis.[88] Elevated antibody levels were present in cystic fibrosis, but only in those patients with clinically evident pulmonary involvement. In other words, serologic evidence of infection followed, rather than preceded, clinical signs of airway obstruction. Similarly, Huang noted that 25% of patients who had overaeration as the only roentgenographic change grew no pathogen from throat or bronchial aspirate cultures (these mild patients could not produce sputum).[86]

Aerosol and mist tent therapies have been shown by some workers to decrease airway resistance and improve pulmonary function in patients with cystic fibrosis. Matthews[122] and Doershuk[45] found that air trapping is lessened by the use of a night mist tent and, further, that the denser mist produced by ultrasonic nebulizers is more effective than that produced by the usual jet nebulizer. (This latter observation is in accord with the in vitro demonstration by Lifschitz that decrease in sputum viscosity is proportionate to the amount of water added[109].) In one study, only patients with mild involvement were included, as it was deemed unjustifiable to withhold mist therapy from those more seriously affected.[122] Even these patients (mean vital capacity (VC) 89% of predicted!) showed a decreased functional residual capacity (FRC) and residual volume (RV) after sleeping in a mist tent. In Phelan's series, improvement in thoracic gas volume and airway resistance followed a program of aerosol therapy in infants without signs of infection, as well as in those with such signs.[143]

These kinds of data support the concept that bronchial obstruction in cystic fibrosis is related to the accumulation of highly viscid material in the airways. A recent study of a small group of patients with cystic fibrosis disclosed a significant correlation between increasing sputum viscosity and decreasing forced expiratory volume $(FEV)_1$,[55] indicating either a more basic derangement of secretion viscosity in those patients with more severe pulmonary involvement or, perhaps more likely, an increase in sputum viscosity attendant on the greater degree of purulence in those patients with more advanced pulmonary damage. It is apparent that, even if viscosity changes are not the basic pulmonary disturbance in this disease, such changes are clinically important in the pathogenesis of the ultimately fatal pulmonary obstruction that occurs.

Mucus, too viscous to be properly cleared by the cilia, accumulates in the airways, where it acts both as an obstruction and as a culture media for bacteria. The obstruction is earliest and most severe in the periphery of the lung, where for aerodynamic reasons, cough is ineffective, and where, by virtue of the narrowness of the lumen, a small amount of mucus can produce significant or even total obstruction. Examination of pathologic material and physiologic data does indicate that the airway obstruction in cystic fibrosis occurs first in the bronchioles and only later in the large airways. Bodian, in his classic monograph on the pathologic changes of cystic fibrosis, emphasized the obstruction of bronchioles by mucus, pus or mucopus, and also noted that inflammatory changes occurred more regularly in the walls of the bronchioles than the bronchi.[15] Andersen similarly concluded, on the basis of examination of autopsy material, that obstruction and inflammation occurred first in the bronchioles and progressed from there to the bronchi.[1] Esterly's review of autopsy material from 84 cases of cystic fibrosis also revealed the most important obstructive changes to be in the bronchioles.[51] Mellins has reviewed the physiologic data indicating the progression of airway obstruction from smaller to larger airways in this disease.[130] He notes that early in the disease, the abnormal distribution of tidal volume and vital capacity, in the presence of normal airway resistance, maximum breathing capacity, and forced expiratory volume, indicates obstruction of small peripheral airways. Later, the finding of a reduced 1-second forced expiratory volume, while measured airway resistance is still normal, suggests the advent of dynamic expiratory compression of larger airways. In advanced cases, the development of increased airway resistance during quiet breathing finally suggests intraluminal obstruction of large airways.

LUNG DESTRUCTION

At first, obstruction is due only to retained mucus, but colonization by pathogenic bacteria, notably *S. aureus* and *P. aeruginosa*, occurs rapidly. These organisms then invade the mucosa and submucosal tissues, initiating a chronic infectious bronchiolitis and bronchitis. Eventually, the bronchial contents become predominantly inflammatory, with bacteria, desquamated epithelial cells, and necrotic leukocytes enmeshed in a coagulum of mucus and cellular debris. Inflammatory swelling and hyperemia of the mucosa add to the airway obstruction as does some degree of bronchospasm in most patients.

The combination of intraluminal debris, mucosal edema, and bronchospasm leads to considerable airway obstruction with a resultant increase in FRC and RV. Alveoli and alveolar ducts are overdistended, and in localized areas alveolar walls may rupture, with the formation of emphysematous blebs. However, true emphysema, as a diffuse process with thinning and atrophy of interalveolar septa, does not occur.[15,51] Small or large foci of atelectasis secondary to complete obstruction of bronchioles or subsegmental bronchi are common. Areas of pneumonia heal by organization so that regions of fibrosis appear, often intimately involved with the atelectatic tissues. Alveoli adjacent to the airways are especially prone to chronic pneumonitis and subsequent fibrosis. The pulmonary fibrosis seen in cystic fibrosis is clearly focal, chiefly peribronchial scar tissue and is not a diffuse interstitial fibrosis. Mucous gland hypertrophy and hyperplasia in the bronchi and bronchioles are prominent and often massive, but it is uncertain whether these conditions represent a response to the disease itself or to the secondary chronic infection. It is likely that both these factors are involved.

The ultimate destructive pulmonary change in cystic fibrosis is bronchiectasis (Figs. 11-5 and 11-6a). As early as 1952, when most patients with this disorder died in infancy or early childhood, Bodian described both tubular and saccular bronchiectasis, as well as bronchiolectasis, at autopsy.[15] Andersen also noted the frequency of bronchiectatic abscess cavities in the lungs of children dying

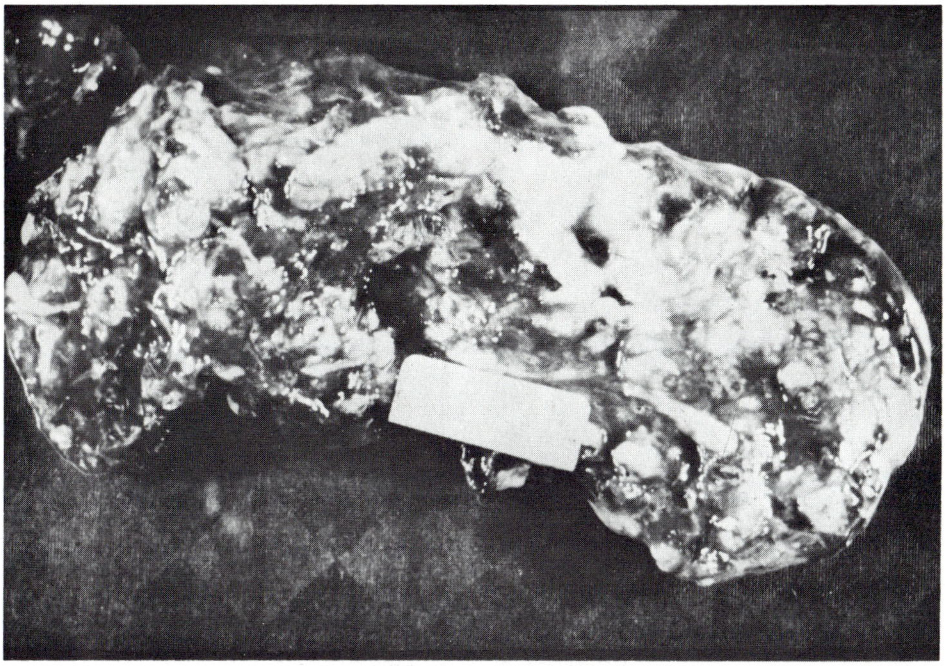

FIG. 11-5. Example of right upper lobe completely destroyed by bronchiectasis. This surgically resected specimen reveals total replacement of normal tissue by bronchiectatic abscess cavities and chronic pneumonitis.

of cystic fibrosis, and suggested that these cavities evolved from areas of chronic atelectasis and infection.[1] Esterly found bronchiectasis in 50% of infants dying before 6 months of age and in 100% of those dying after 6 months.[51]

Bronchiectasis in these patients results from a combination of factors. Increasing accumulation of mucopurulent material in the bronchial lumen provides a dilating pressure, while atelectasis of adjacent tissues removes the counterpressure of distended alveoli and facilitates outward bulging of the bronchial wall. Bacterial infection, inflammation, and destruction of the bronchial wall weaken its resistance to distortion and distention. The importance of mucoid impaction of the bronchi as a factor in the development of bronchiectasis in cystic fibrosis has been stressed by Waring.[175] Describing the radiologic appearance of the impaction as a finger-like or nodular density due to distention of the bronchi with mucopus, he noted evidence of the entity in one-third of his patients, and reported that its persistence for more than 1 month could be related to subsequent bronchiectasis in the same segment (Figs. 11-7 through 11-9a). These pus-filled, bronchiectatic cavities once formed are permanent and may act as reservoirs of bacteria, which subsequently infect other portions of the lung. They are the major source of the foul-smelling, purulent sputum as well as the anorexia, weight loss, anemia, and fever that often plague these patients in the advanced stage of the disease. Hypertrophied bronchial arteries in the walls of these bronchiectatic cavities are the origin of the gross and occasionally massive hemoptysis seen in cystic fibrosis patients. Lesser degrees of bleeding may come from capillaries and veins in the inflamed, hyperemic mucosa throughout the tracheobronchial tree.

Expiratory collapse of major airways in patients with cystic fibrosis has been demon-

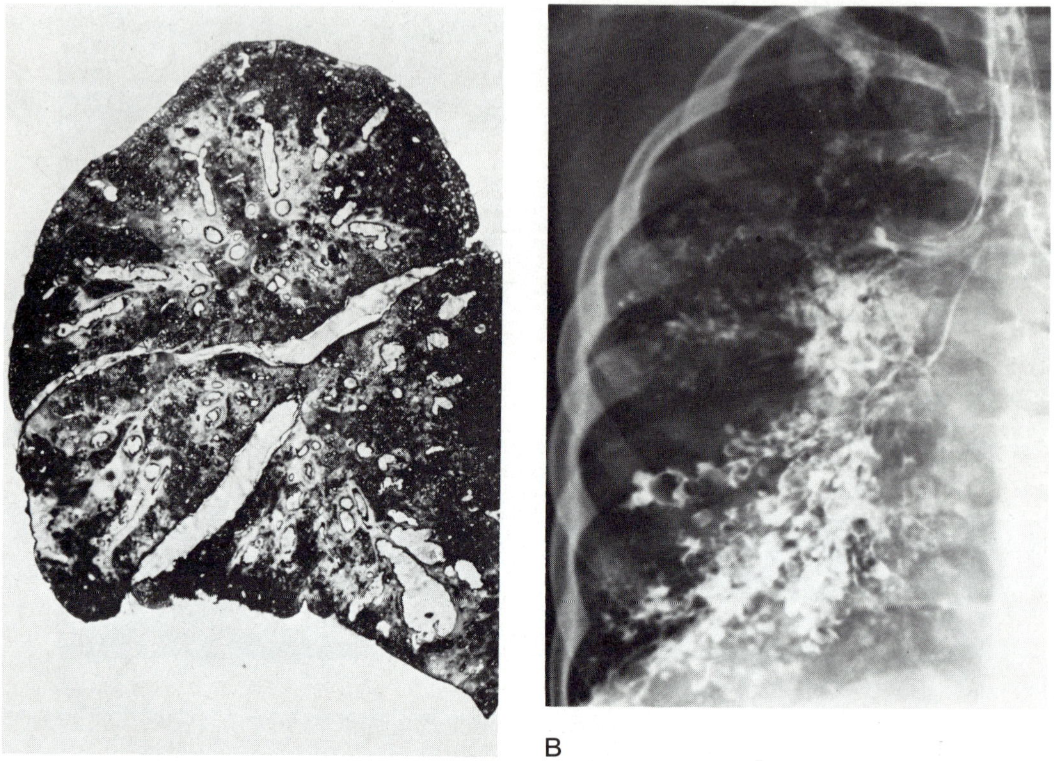

A B

FIG. 11-6. A, Whole lung preparation (Gough-Wentworth technique) from a 6-year-old child who died from pulmonary involvement of cystic fibrosis. Note marked dilatation of various size airways filled with mucopus. There is also peribronchial fibrosis, extensive bronchopneumonia, and patchy atelectasis. (From Goldring, R. M., et al.: Pulmonary hypertension and cor pulmonale in cystic fibrosis. *J. Pediatr.* *65*:501, 1964.); B, Widespread, grape-like bronchiectasis in the right middle and lower lobe is demonstrated by bronchography in the case of this young girl with cystic fibrosis. Today, bronchography is seldom indicated or necessary in the management of patients with this disease.

strated by cinebronchography, and contributes not only to air trapping but also to tussive insufficiency.[131] The larger bronchi, their walls weakened by years of chronic purulent bronchitis, cannot withstand the exceedingly high transmural pressures generated during cough in the presence of severe peripheral airway obstruction. The intraluminal pressure drop across the obstructed peripheral airways during expiratory flow is so great that pressure within the larger bronchi is very low even when the driving intrapleural pressure is enormous. This drop results in an increased transmural pressure that is sufficient to collapse the airway, trapping secretions as well as air. Rather than being expelled with a single bechic blast, as a cork from a popgun, the secretions must be milked along slowly and squeezed out of the collapsing airway as toothpaste out of a tube.

Airway obstruction is the major cause of progressive ventilatory insufficiency and death by asphyxiation in cystic fibrosis. Destruction of lung parenchyma by peribronchial fibrosis, bronchiectasis, chronic pneumonitis, atelectasis, alveolar rupture, and cyst formation all contribute to the ventilatory impairment and ultimate respiratory failure.

Although some autoantibodies have been detected in serum and sputum of patients

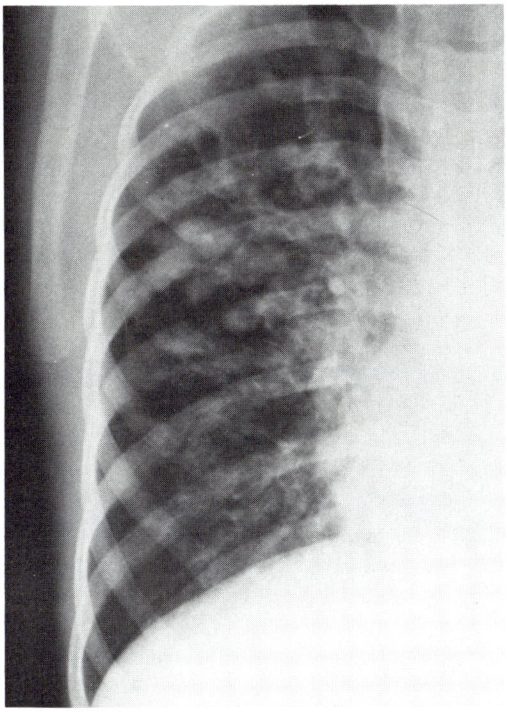

FIG. 11-7. Mucoid impaction. Branching, finger-like radiodensities are noted in the right upper lobe on the conventional chest roentgenogram.

with cystic fibrosis, there is little evidence to suggest that they are a primary factor in the pathogenesis of this disease. They are probably secondary to inflammation and tissue destruction. Serum antibodies to pancreatic extract were found in one study,[137] but not in another.[165] Blanc reported autoantibodies to the pancreas and submaxillary gland in 3 of 17 patients with cystic fibrosis.[12] Stein found, in sputum from patients with this disease, antibodies to extracts of cystic fibrosis lung and pancreas, but not to normal lung or pancreas.[165]

INFECTION

The frequency with which *S. aureus* and *P. aeruginosa* are recovered from the sputum of patients with cystic fibrosis has focused attention on these organisms as being, perhaps, uniquely related to the pathogenesis of the pulmonary lesions. That the lungs in this disease are destroyed by chronic bacterial infection cannot be disputed. These patients are born with anatomically normal lungs, which by the time of death are diffusely inflamed, pus filled, bronchiectatic, and scarred. Are the Staphylococcus and Pseudomonas simply the most available opportunists, or does some abnormality of tracheobronchial mucus in this disease favor their growth in particular? It is clear that their presence is pathogenic and not saprophytic. Iacocca recovered one or both of these organisms from all levels of the tracheobronchial tree at autopsy.[89] Pathologic evidence of chronic bacterial infection in these patients includes: bronchopneumonia, suppurative bronchiolitis, peribronchiolitis, and abscess forma-

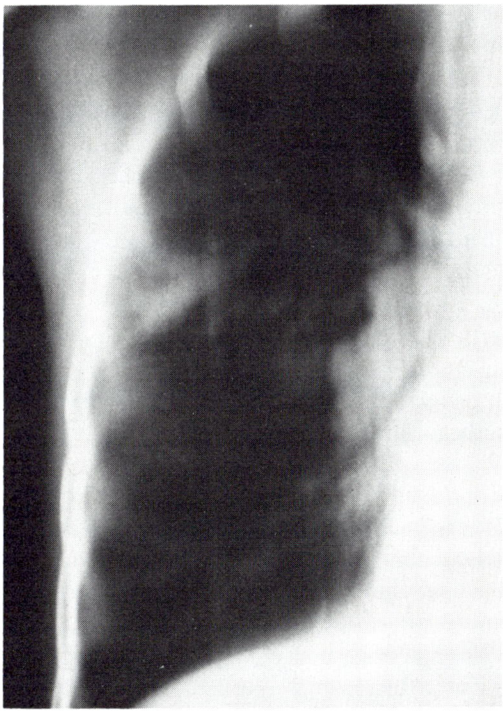

FIG. 11-8. Mucoid impaction. Often, the mucoid impactions are more clearly discernible on tomographic examination. Here, the impaction is clearly visible in the anterior segment of the right upper lobe.

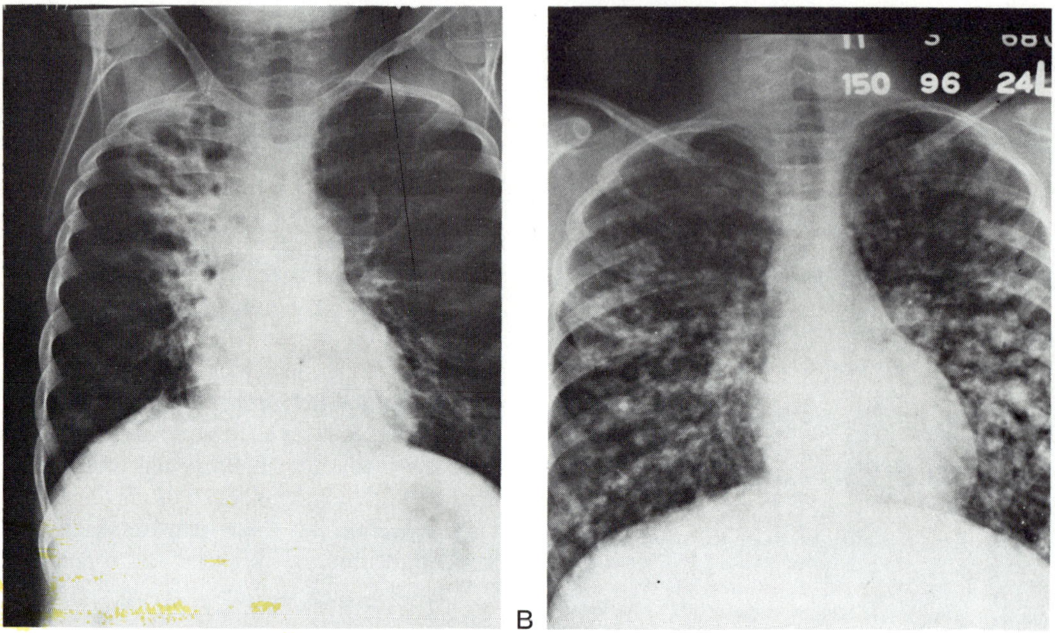

A B

FIG. 11-9. A, Bronchiectasis. A chronically atelectatic and bronchiectatic right upper lobe is readily evident in this roentgenogram of the chest of an 8-year-old boy with cystic fibrosis; B, Widespread mucoid impactions and peribronchial abscesses. Roentgenogram taken several weeks before death.

tion.[1,15] Expectorated sputum is heavily laden with sloughed bronchial mucosal cells, polymorphonuclear leukocytes, and collagen fibers. Its rich content of DNA, lipids, amino acids, and potassium reflects active tissue destruction and cellular death.[24,124] High serum levels of antibodies against Staphylococcus and Pseudomonas are regularly found in patients with cystic fibrosis, whereas antibodies against common saprophytes such as *Neisseria catarrhalis* are not to be found.[18,75,88] Pulmonary infection in this disease is not limited to *S. aureus* or *P. aeruginosa,* almost every known pathogen having been recovered at one or another time from some patient. Serum antibodies against *K. pneumoniae* and *H. influenzae* have also been detected in patients with cystic fibrosis.[18,75]

Routine tests of immunologic competence have revealed no abnormalities in cystic fibrosis, and infection outside the respiratory system is rare.[75] Serum levels of IgG and IgA are elevated in response to chronic pulmonary infection, as would be expected. Secretory IgA is present in saliva and tracheobronchial secretions. The only report so far of a possible immunologic defect in this disease has been that of Boxerbaum, who stated that serum from patients with cystic fibrosis inhibited the phagocytosis of *P. aeruginosa* by rabbit alveolar macrophages in an in vitro system.[17] The same serum had no effect on the phagocytosis of *S. aureus* or *S. marcescens.* If confirmed, this exciting development could open many new lines of research in cystic fibrosis.

In 1966, Doggett reported the frequent occurrence of mucoid strains of Pseudomonas in the sputum of patients with cystic fibrosis and hypothesized that this variant of the organism was unique to this condition, perhaps induced by some factor in the host himself.[46] Doggett also suggested that the capsular slime produced by this organism was a primary factor in the viscosity and insolubility of sputum in this disease. It was subsequently shown, however, that the mucoid strain is phage induced and is also found in patients with other types of chronic lung disease.[19] Mucoid strains do, in general, seem to be most common in patients with advanced cystic fibrosis, but this rule is far from universal, and whether it is cause or effect has yet to be determined.

The search for a factor other than the physical retention of secretions, which could explain the ease with which bacteria invade and colonize the tracheobronchial tree in cystic fibrosis, has met with only limited success. May reported that a sterilized filtrate of sputum from patients with cystic fibrosis appeared to support the growth of *S. aureus* somewhat better than did comparable material from patients with bronchiectasis.[125] He found an increased content of p-hydroxyphenylacetic acid (p-HPAA) in the urine of patients with cystic fibrosis and showed that under certain circumstances, p-HPPA can enhance the growth of *S. aureus.* He suggested, but did not actually demonstrate, that an elevated content of p-HPAA existed in cystic fibrosis sputum.

COR PULMONALE

Cor pulmonale (Fig. 11-10) is such a common accompaniment of severe, long-standing pulmonary involvement in cystic fibrosis that its pathophysiology must be considered along with the pathophysiology of the pulmonary disorder itself. The primary determinant of cor pulmonale is chronic hypoxemia and pulmonary arteriolar constriction. Focal areas of destruction of the pulmonary capillary bed by scarring and fibrosis contribute to the increased pulmonary resistance, but do not by themselves cause pulmonary hypertension.

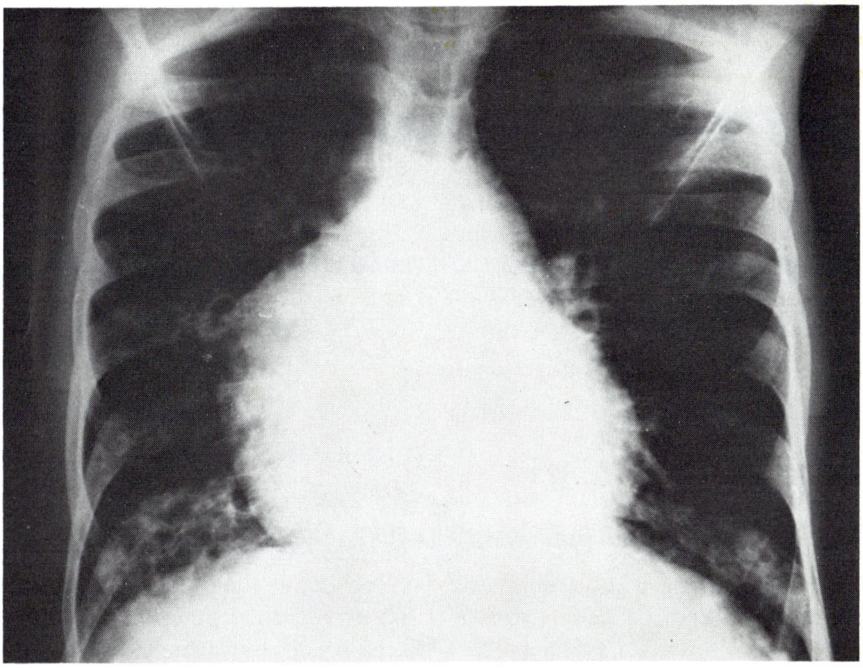

FIG. 11-10. Cor pulmonale. Chest roentgenogram of a 14-year-old boy with severe pulmonary cystic fibrosis and secondary cor pulmonale. Note the massive right ventricular enlargement evident in this case.

The role of hypoxia in the genesis of pulmonary hypertension and cor pulmonale in this disease was first emphasized by Goldring, who showed during cardiac catheterization that the elevated pulmonary artery pressure could be reduced by the administration of 100% oxygen.[65] Moss also found a reduction of pulmonary artery pressure following correction of hypoxemia, but noted that this reduction was neither invariable nor complete and suggested that additional factors were involved.[135] Symchych reported the finding of medial hypertrophy of pulmonary arterioles at autopsy.[169] Although this hypertrophy is presumably a reaction to chronic hypoxemia, it would not be immediately reversible by oxygen. Alveolar overdistention, characteristic of this disease, may compress alveolar capillaries and contribute to the increased vascular resistance. Dilated bronchial arteries and bronchopulmonary anastomoses have also been suggested as factors augmenting the pulmonary hypertension in these patients.

Moss reported that cor pulmonale, defined as an increased pulmonary vascular resistance, was generally present if the vital capacity was reduced below 60% of predicted.[134] It should be emphasized that pulmonary hypertension is much more common than clinical signs of right ventricular failure, and elevation of right ventricular pressure may precede clinical signs of cor pulmonale by many years. Patients with cystic fibrosis may die of ventilatory failure without clinically evident right heart failure, but the reverse is rarely true.

Clinical Manifestations (Pulmonary)

The earliest pulmonary manifestations of cystic fibrosis are characteristically those of chronic bronchitis—cough and airway obstruction. At this stage the lungs are clear to auscultation, and cough may or may not be productive of sputum. As the disease progresses, the major expressions become those of bronchiectasis—purulent sputum, pulmonary rales, and peribronchial infiltrative changes on the roentgenogram. Systemic signs such as fatigue, weight loss, and elevated erythrocyte sedimentation rate may make their appearance at this time. The final stage of the disease is dominated by progressive ventilatory insufficiency and cor pulmonale. As is the case with other organ systems in this disease, the spectrum of severity of pulmonary involvement is wide, so that occasionally "late" changes may be seen in infancy, while some adolescents or adults may show only "early" or mild lung involvement.

With the notable exception of infants born with meconium ileus, who are at risk of developing pneumonia and atelectasis postoperatively, pulmonary symptoms are not usually evident in the *immediate* neonatal period.[80] Beyond the first week or two of life, however, respiratory symptoms become increasingly common and are eventually present in most infants with this disease. Symptoms may begin insidiously, with frequent cough, fussiness, and decreased appetite, or suddenly, with fever, rales, and respiratory distress. Failure to respond to conventional antibiotic therapy, or relapse soon after these drugs are discontinued, may be the first clue to the underlying chronic problem. The presence of wheezing, not uncommon among infants with cystic fibrosis, may lead to an initial erroneous diagnosis of asthma or bronchiolitis. In contradistinction to the presenting symptoms during infancy or early childhood, other patients may have mild symptoms for many years before the true cause is recognized. Such patients may be mislabeled as "allergic" or "bronchitic," and considerable lung damage may have already occurred by the time the correct diagnosis is established. Shwachman reported a series of patients surviving to 17 years or beyond, and therefore, presumably, with basically mild disease.[159] He noted that almost half of these patients were not diagnosed until they were more than 10 years old.

COUGH AND SPUTUM

When pulmonary involvement is mild, cough is apt to be dry and nonproductive. It is also episodic, disappearing for months, only to return with the next cold or minor respiratory infection. The cough is not pathognomonic at this time, and only its persistence might lead one to suspect cystic fibrosis. Eventually, however, the cough becomes wetter and more rattly in sound, and is productive of sputum. Even if the child does not expectorate, one may detect the gurgling sound as the secretions are brought to the oropharynx and the sudden disappearance of the sound as they are swallowed. Once sputum is regularly produced, infection of the tracheobronchial tree is invariably established, and the sputum rarely fails to yield a pathogenic organism on culture. Feigelson was able to recover *S. aureus* and/or *P. aeruginosa* from all his patients who produced sputum.[58] Huang recovered one or both of the same organisms from 95% of her patients with moderate or severe disease.[86] Initially, the sputum consists of small yellow or light green plugs suspended in a mucoid, translucent fluid, which is probably chiefly saliva. Later, the specimen becomes more viscous, more copious, and more foul smelling.

The pitiful sight of the child with advanced cystic fibrosis coughing fitfully again and again, with eyes bulging, lips cyanotic, and neck veins distended, as he slowly and agonizingly raises a thimbleful of thick, tenacious sputum, is only too familiar to both parent and physician. Difficulty in expectoration at this stage is related to expiratory collapse of major airways as well as to the increased viscoelasticity of the secretions themselves. The appearance and odor of the sputum and the specter of the cough are often disturbing to those about him and add to the patient's difficulties with social adjustments.

PHYSICAL EXAMINATION

Digital clubbing is a regular and relatively early finding in cystic fibrosis, often present before more definitive evidence of bronchiectasis, such as persistent rales, purulent sputum, or chronic infiltrative changes on chest roentgenogram. Why clubbing should be so common in this disease, while it is so unusual in asthma, the other major airway obstructive disease of childhood, is unclear but is a useful diagnostic feature. The related phenomenon of hypertrophic pulmonary osteoarthropathy (HPO) is also seen in patients with cystic fibrosis, although generally only in those with advanced lung disease. Grossman reported radiologic changes of HPO in 3 of 18 patients with moderate to severe pulmonary involvement.[72] The most commonly affected sites were the distal tibia and fibula, with periosteal new bone formation as the major radiographic finding. Clinical manifestations include pain and tenderness over the involved area and swelling of the joint or extremity, all of which tend to worsen with exacerbations of the pulmonary disease, and may improve as lung infection remits. Pain and swelling may precede the radiologic changes by months. Joint swelling may be hard to differentiate from early cor pulmonale.

The chest appears round and hyperinflated (Fig. 11-11), and the percussion note is hyperresonant. In advanced disease, frank barrel chest deformity and dorsal kyphosis occur. Stamm reported an increased chest circumference relative to body surface area to be a fairly consistent finding in children with cystic fibrosis, regardless of the severity of pulmonary involvement.[164] Waring, on the other hand, found that an increased thoracic index (thoracic depth divided by width) was

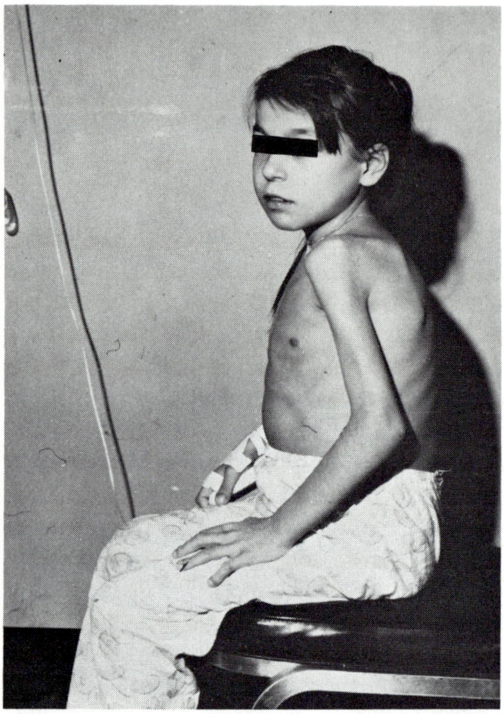

FIG. 11-11. 12-year-old girl with severe cystic fibrosis. Note the poor nutritional status and the full, rounded chest.

present only in patients with significant lung involvement.[177] Another common sign of pulmonary overinflation is the lack of lateral expansion of the lower rib cage during inspiration, indicating a flat, relatively fixed diaphragm.

Pulmonary rales are not an early finding in this disorder and indicate serious pulmonary involvement, either acute or chronic. Rales that persist despite proper therapy are presumptive evidence of bronchiectasis. Although significant radiographic changes often occur in the absence of auscultatory findings, the reverse is rarely true, and the child with rales almost always has some discernible abnormality on chest roentgenogram, although not always in the exact area of the rales. If routine auscultation fails to reveal rales, they can occasionally be elicited by having the patient exhale completely down to residual lung volume and then listening over the area in question as he breathes in. The expiratory maneuver down to residual volume closes the narrowed and compliant airways so that their mucus-coated surfaces oppose. On the following inspiration these surfaces pop apart producing the characteristic medium rales. One may also hear coarser rales through both inspiration and expiration in patients with cystic fibrosis. These rales are generated by the flow of air bubbling through mucus or mucopus in the bronchi. The very fine crackling rales of alveolar fluid are rarely heard.

SYSTEMIC SIGNS

These signs of pulmonary infection are modified by the chronic nature of the infection and the adequate immunologic response. Despite the constant presence of pus within the lungs, empyema and metastatic infection outside the thorax are remarkably rare. Fever and leukocytosis may be absent even in the presence of bronchiectasis and frank abscess cavities. With severe bronchiectasis the serum gamma globulin level is elevated, often exceeding 2 g%. Appetite and weight are sensitive indicators of pulmonary infection. Untreated children with cystic fibrosis usually have ravenous appetites because of the pancreatic achylia and intestinal malabsorption. Dietary management and pancreatic replacement therapy return the appetite to normal, but pulmonary infection depresses it remarkably. With severe pulmonary disease cachexia may be extreme, due to several factors: the anorexia, general toxicity, and weight loss of chronic infection; flattened diaphragms, which compress the abdominal viscera causing a feeling of satiation; and the increased work of breathing, which may be three times normal.[25]

Polycythemia is not seen as frequently in these patients as might be anticipated, probably because of a superimposed chronic anemia of infection. Decreased intestinal absorption of iron secondary to exogenous pancreatic replacement therapy has also been described and may contribute to the failure of red cell response.

DIAGNOSIS

Most patients appear at the clinic with respiratory or gastrointestinal symptoms or both. However, it is understandable that, if these major organ systems are relatively spared, the patient may seek medical attention because of symptoms in other organs. Nasal polyps, hyponatremic dehydration, and biliary cirrhosis have all, on occasion, been the presenting complaint of cystic fibrosis. The diagnosis is almost always established by the clinical picture of pulmonary and/or gastrointestinal involvement and a positive sweat test. Fortunately, elevated sweat electrolytes have few other causes (adrenal insufficiency, glucose-6-phosphatase deficiency glycogen storage disease, ectodermal dysplasia). The sweat abnormality is one of the most consistent derangements in cystic fibrosis, and documented cases with normal values for sweat electrolytes are exceedingly rare.

The test should be performed by pilocarpine iontophoresis only. Older methods in which the arm or the entire patient is enclosed in a plastic bag are totally unsatisfactory. In the hands of a well-trained, experienced technician the pilocarpine iontophoresis sweat test is extremely accurate and reliable, but in the laboratory that performs only two or three of these tests a year, spurious results are not uncommon. The most reliable and accurate test is a quantitative measure of sodium and chloride from sweat collected onto gauze pads or filter paper and the NaCl eluted. Several current screening tests use pilocarpine iontophoresis as the stimulus to sweating and then directly measure skin conductivity. Though appealing for ease in operation and measurement, they do not yet afford the user the high degree of accuracy essential to this test. The direct reading chloride electrode, placed on the skin, has not, in our experience, given consistent or reliable results. The Cystic Fibrosis Foundation is currently initiating a collaborative study on sweat test methodologies, to determine the most effective, reliable method in use today.

The importance of referral to a large medical center or a cystic fibrosis clinic for confirmation of the diagnosis cannot be overemphasized. In the unusual case where the results of the sweat test are inconstant or of borderline value (40 to 60 mEq/l of chloride), duodenal aspiration for assay of pancreatic trypsin is often useful (provided the patient has pancreatic insufficiency). Tests of malabsorption, such as stool fat or serum carotene, are not sufficiently specific to confirm the diagnosis of cystic fibrosis, although they may be helpful in evaluating the degree of gastrointestinal involvement.

RADIOLOGY

Chest roentgenographic changes become more characteristic as the disease progresses, and the roentgenographic picture of advanced cystic fibrosis can hardly be confused with any other pediatric entity. Early in the illness overaeration, flattened diaphragms, and a full anteroposterior diameter of the thorax may be the only changes noted (Fig. 11-12). Pneumonia and atelectasis around the segmental and subsegmental bronchi, whenever they appear, give rise to the familiar peribronchial densities seen in this disorder. Bronchial shadows become more prominent as edema and infiltration of the bronchial wall and surrounding parenchyma make these regions radiodense. If the axis of the bronchus is perpendicular to the x-ray beam, these shadows appear as parallel "tram lines." If the bronchus is parallel to the x-ray beam, it appears in cross section as "peribronchial cuffing" (Fig. 11-13).

It should be noted that, although the disease pathologically begins in the bronchioles and smaller airways, radiologically it is first

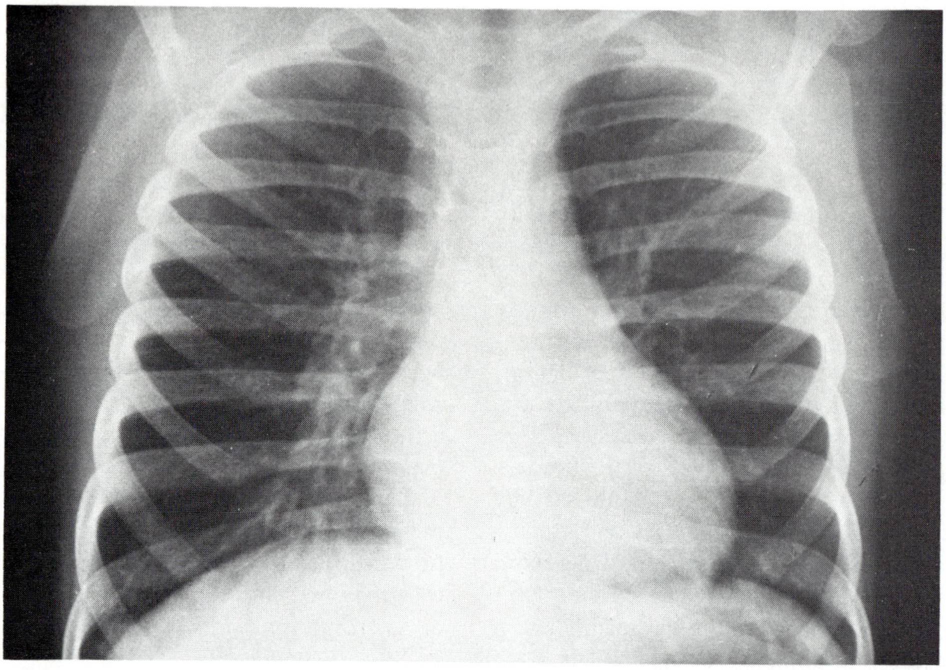

FIG. 11-12. Chest roentgenogram of a 7-year-old girl with mild (early) pulmonary involvement. Air trapping, as manifested by low, flat diaphragms, is only modest. There are abnormal peribronchial markings especially in the right lower lobe, and the right hilar region is full.

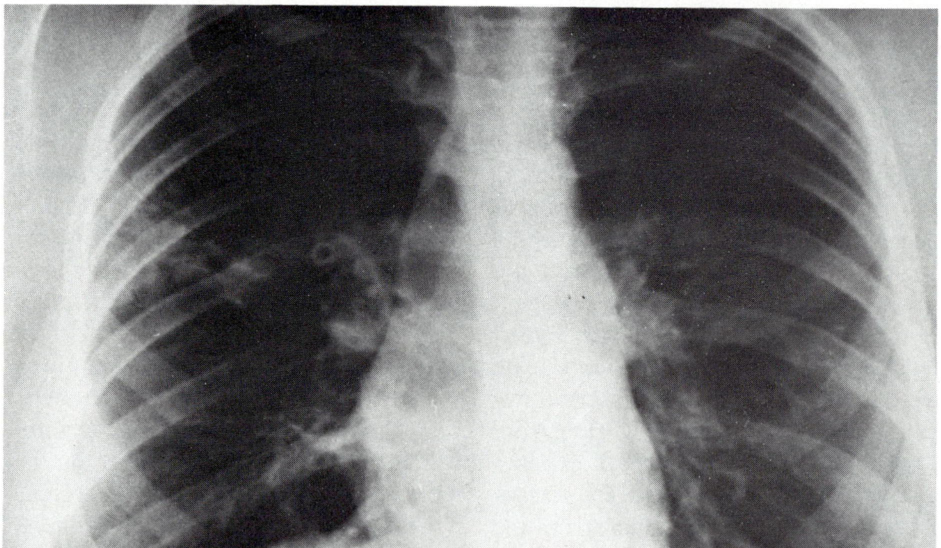

FIG. 11-13. Peribronchial cuffing. The characteristic bronchial thickening and peribronchial densities in cystic fibrosis, when seen "end-on" roentgenographically, appear as radiodense cuffs.

noted in and around the larger airways simply because the bronchiolar changes are too small to be visible on the roentgenographic film. As the areas of chronic pneumonitis and atelectasis increase, so do the abnormal densities on chest film, especially in the central regions. Hilar adenopathy is common, often enmeshed in gross, peribronchial inflammatory changes (Figs. 11-14 and 11-15). The periphery of the lung appears spared, but in reality is overinflated and hyperlucent with a paucity of lung markings. Dilated, thick-walled bronchi may be visible on plane film, but are best appreciated on tomograms. Large subpleural blebs may be visible, especially in the upper lobes (Fig. 11-16). Mucoid impactions of segmental and subsegmental bronchi appear as soft, branching densities following the paths of the bronchi, or as soft nodules when seen end-on (Figs. 11-7 and 11-8).

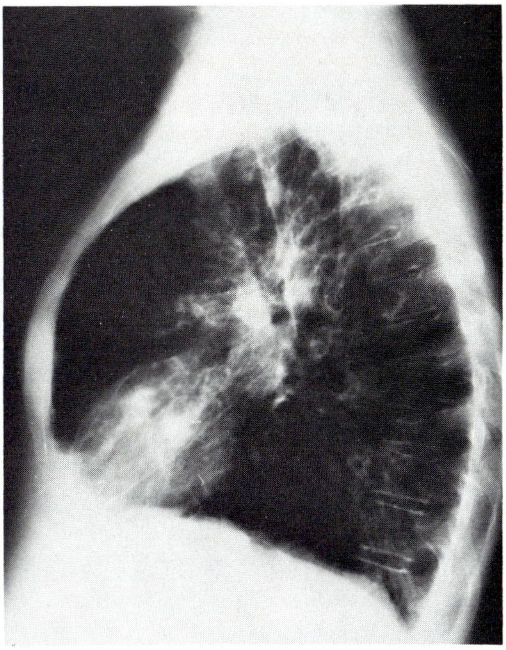

FIG. 11-15. Lateral view of patient in Figure 11-14. Note the markedly increased anteroposterior diameter of the thorax and the bowing of the sternum and the thoracic vertebral column. The diaphragm is severely flattened. The peribronchial changes are also noted, as on the posteroanterior view.

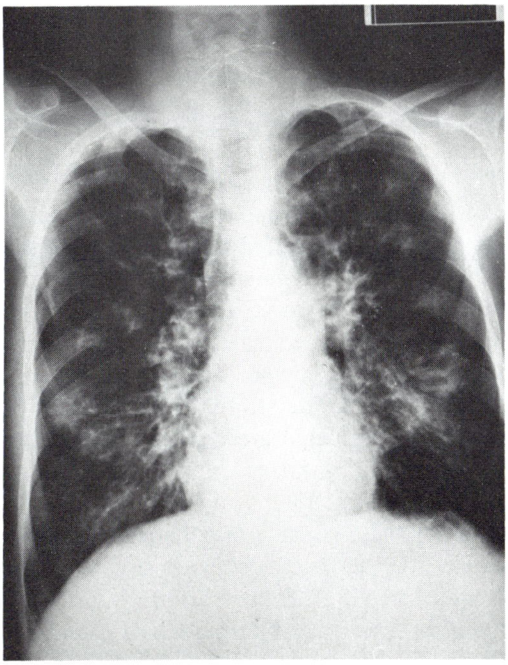

FIG. 11-14. Posteroanterior chest roentgenogram of a 17-year-old boy with severe pulmonary involvement by cystic fibrosis. Bilateral peribronchial and parenchymal changes are extensive and severe. An abscess cavity with fluid level is evident in the left upper lobe. Diaphragms are very low.

Unlike most other diseases resulting in bronchiectasis, cystic fibrosis has no tendency to spare the upper lobes, even in the early stages. Radiographic evidence of lung destruction is distributed among all lobes and bronchopulmonary segments.

PULMONARY FUNCTION

In general, the degree of abnormality of pulmonary function tests parallels the clinical severity of the illness, although exceptions are occasionally seen.[25,129,188] Measurements of airway obstruction are the most useful clinical tests, and many workers have found the maximum midexpiratory flow rate (MMEF)

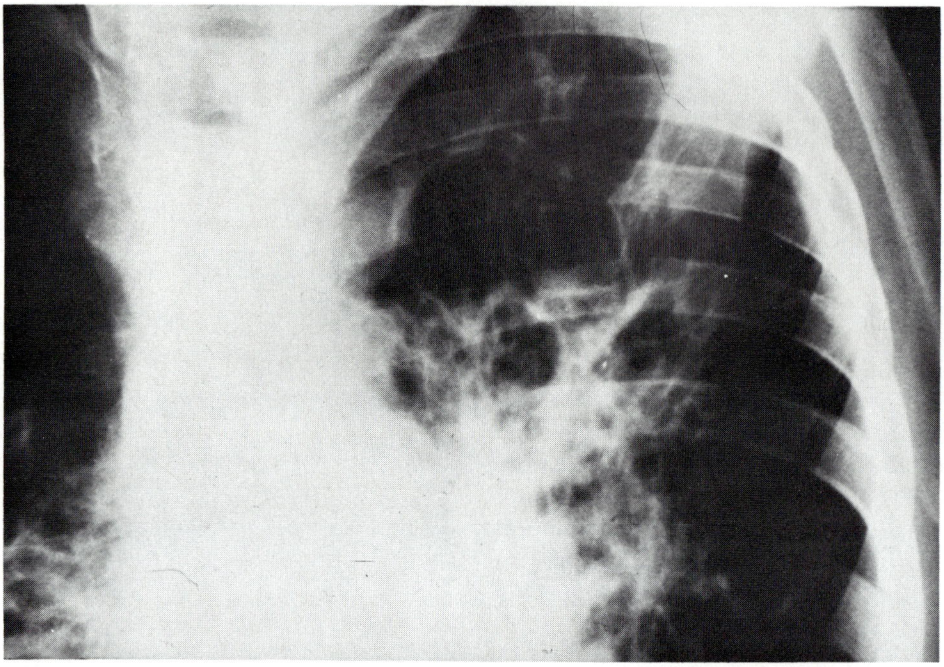

FIG. 11-16. Cystic changes in the left upper lobe of an 18-year-old boy with cystic fibrosis. Such changes are common in older children with this disease.

to be the most sensitive test in this regard.[56,188] Most sensitive is not necessarily synonymous with most useful, and there has been considerable discussion as to the best pulmonary function test to monitor this disease. In reality no one best test exists. Rather, the physician in charge must avail himself of whatever pulmonary function data are available and interpret them in conjunction with the entire clinical picture.

Early in the disease, when pulmonary involvement is minimal, the MMEF may well be the most discerning of the routinely available tests, detecting pulmonary abnormalities before the physical or x-ray examination. When lung disease is clinically evident, however, other tests of pulmonary function are more likely to be of help in following the course of the respiratory involvement. Both the VC and the FEV_1 have less day-to-day variability than the MMEF in patients with cystic fibrosis, and should therefore better reflect the overall progress of the patient.[103] The VC and FEV_1 decrease, while the FRC and RV increase as lung disease worsens. It is not uncommonly noted that in the most severely affected patients the RV as determined by helium dilution is not as increased as might be anticipated and that the TLC is less than 100% of predicted. This finding appears to be artifactual, due to the fact that some of the most obstructed areas cannot equilibrate with the helium during the allotted time period of the test. Plethysmographic measurement of TLC in a group of patients with cystic fibrosis failed to reveal any with decreased TLC.[9] Of the various pulmonary function tests available, the RV/TLC[25] and (RV/TGV)p[9] correlate best with the clinical status of the patient. Other tests, such as VC, FEV_1, MMEF, airway resistance, and single breath nitrogen test, also have been shown to correlate with the clinical condition of the patient, although not quite as well as the

RV/TLC or (RV/TGV)p.[9,25] The diffusing capacity of the lung is normal or only slightly reduced.[146]

When pulmonary involvement is severe, monitoring of arterial blood gases becomes critical. As with other obstructive airway diseases, decreased Po_2 precedes an elevation of Pco_2. The former reflects uneven distribution of tidal air and altered ventilation-perfusion ratios, while the latter indicates inadequate alveolar ventilation and hence respiratory failure.

COMPLICATIONS OF PULMONARY DISEASE

Cor Pulmonale. Defined as an elevated pulmonary vascular resistance, cor pulmonale occurs so regularly in severe cystic fibrosis that it could almost be viewed as the natural end point of pulmonary involvement rather than as a complication.[134] Clinically evident cor pulmonale, however, is seen less regularly, and it is not uncommon for patients to die of ventilatory insufficiency with no discernible evidence of right heart failure. Clinical signs of right-sided cardiac failure are considerably obscured by manifestations of the lung disease itself.[156B] Tachypnea, tachycardia, and dyspnea are signs of airway obstruction as well as cardiac failure. Cyanosis may reflect pulmonary rather than cardiac insufficiency. A palpable liver may be due to low, flattened diaphragms and not to hepatomegaly. The swelling of hypertrophic pulmonary osteoarthropathy may be confused with the edema of cardiac failure. Pulmonary hyperaeration makes the heart appear small on radiologic examination and displaces the QRS loop of the ECG posteriorly.

Strober[166] and Pittman[145] found, in older patients with advanced pulmonary cystic fibrosis, that hypoalbuminemia was dilutional and not nutritional. The expanded plasma volume, they suggested, was an early sign of cor pulmonale. It is common in such patients to see the serum albumin concentration return to normal following adequate diuretic therapy. Other clinical clues to the development of cor pulmonale are weight gain in a patient who is otherwise doing poorly, puffy face, fatigue or weakness out of proportion to the pulmonary disease or to the dyspnea, orthopnea, venous distention, and difficulty raising sputum. As hypoxemia is probably the major determinant of cor pulmonale, patients who are significantly or progressively hypoxic should be observed closely for signs of impending right heart failure.

Pneumothorax. As more and more patients with cystic fibrosis are surviving to adolescence and adulthood, this complication has become increasingly frequent, occurring in between 2 and 3% of patients (Fig. 11-17). Several authors have reported large series of patients with this complication,[14,107] and it is evident that pneumothorax is most common in older patients, being infrequent before the age of 10 years. Shortness of breath and the abrupt onset of chest pain are the most common complaints, and decreased breath sounds over the involved hemithorax the most common physical finding. Severe respiratory distress and even death may result from tension phenomena or from further pulmonary embarrassment in a patient who has already sustained severe respiratory damage.

Most cases of pneumothorax in this disease result from the rupture of a subpleural bleb or pulmonary cyst directly into the pleural space. Such cysts may be visible on plane roentgenographic film of the chest (Fig. 11-16) and are most common in the upper lobes. Palpable subcutaneous emphysema was present at the time of admission in only two of 36 episodes of pneumothorax reported by Lifschitz.[107]

Hemoptysis. Blood-tinged sputum is seen commonly; gross hemoptysis, fortunately, is less frequent. The former is most likely the result of venous bleeding or capillary oozing from an inflamed bronchial mucosa, while the latter indicates rupture of a dilated bronchial artery in an area of atelectasis. The course of

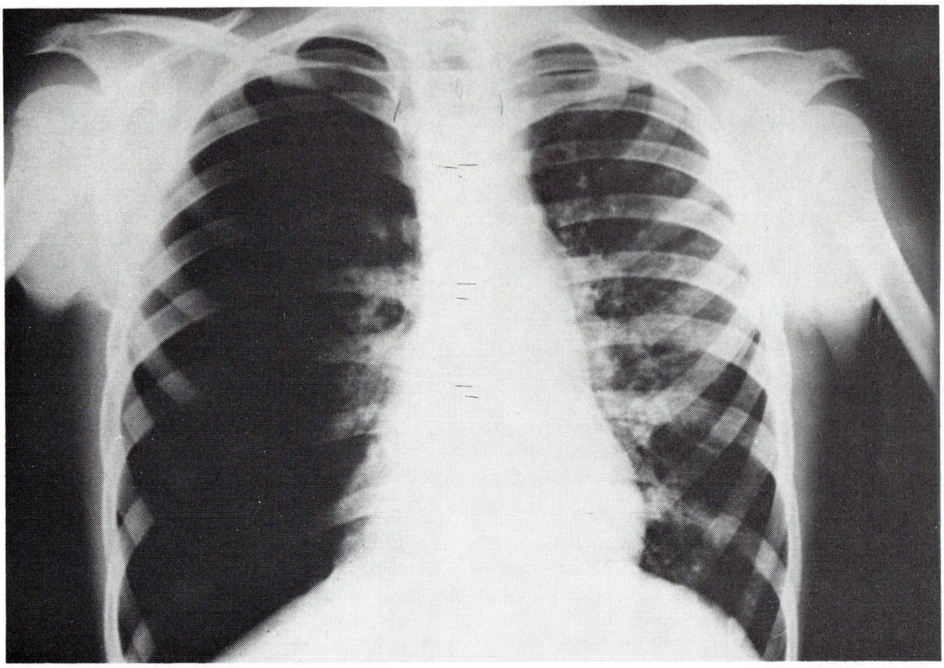

FIG. 11-17. Right pneumothorax with total pulmonary collapse. Patient was a 17-year-old boy with cystic fibrosis.

massive hemoptysis is variable; although it may remit for long periods of time, it clearly tends to recur. Holsclaw reported that 13 of 19 patients with massive hemoptysis were dead within 6 months of the initial episode. Some of the deaths were directly related to the hemoptysis while others reflected the severity of the underlying disease.[81]

Atelectasis. Subsegmental atelectasis is so common as to be considered a feature of the disease rather than a complication. Lobar atelectasis, however, is seen less regularly although it is by no means uncommon. Occasionally, collapse of a lobe may be acute because of a mucous plug. Such a situation may be rapidly reversible by appropriate therapy (Fig. 11-16). More often, however, obstruction and atelectasis are associated with considerable bronchopulmonary infection. The bronchial mucosa is inflamed and edematous, the lung parenchyma itself infected. Enlarged peribronchial and hilar lymph nodes may also contribute to bronchial obstruction. Under these conditions reexpansion is difficult to achieve, and bronchiectasis, if not already present, develops quickly in the obstructed, collapsed lobe, which is soon completely destroyed by infection.

Other Complications. Pneumonia and bronchiectasis are both too integral a part of the pulmonary disease to be considered as complications and have already been discussed in some detail. It cannot be emphasized too strongly that the pneumonia seen in this disease is rarely an acute infection by a new microorganism associated with fever, toxicity, and roentgenographic change, but rather is an exacerbation of existing chronic infection, a shift of the balance between host and parasite, and an extension of infection to new regions of the lung. Radiographic evidence of such change may be obscured by the chronic changes.

Empyema is rare. Pulmonary botryomycosis, a purulent-granulomatous pneumonia due most often to *S. aureus* or a fungus, has been reported, but also is rare.[95] Allergic bronchopulmonary aspergillosis is a rare complication of cystic fibrosis but has been reported.[141A]

Clinical Manifestations (Extrapulmonary)

The nonpulmonary clinical manifestations of cystic fibrosis are varied and can, in their own right, be disabling or fatal. If pulmonary involvement is mild, it is not uncommon for a patient with cystic fibrosis to have symptoms that involve another organ or system. In infancy, gastrointestinal problems may commonly outweigh respiratory problems. In childhood and occasionally even adolescence, we see patients in whom the clinical symptomatology is almost entirely nonpulmonary. Finally, it should be noted that even in infants and children who come to the clinic because of pulmonary signs or symptoms, it may be the nonpulmonary manifestations, such as nasal polyps or chronic steatorrhea, that first arouse a suspicion of cystic fibrosis.

GASTROINTESTINAL SYSTEM

The gastrointestinal expression of cystic fibrosis is often characterized by pancreatic insufficiency, malabsorption, steatorrhea, and growth retardation. This gastrointestinal disorder is usually accompanied by a voracious appetite unless pulmonary infection occurs, in which situation various degrees of anorexia are the rule. The typical stool is not watery, but rather is large, loose, greasy, and characteristically foul smelling. Undernutrition and failure to thrive are commonly seen in infants with this disease. Nutritional hypoproteinemia may develop in infants receiving a low protein formula such as breast milk or in those receiving soybean preparations. Fecal loss of fat soluble vitamins is excessive, and clinical deficiency of vitamins A and K has been reported. Interestingly, rickets has not been noted as a complication of cystic fibrosis.[40] Clinical evidence of vitamin E deficiency is not apparent, although blood levels are low[173] and ceroid-pigment in smooth muscle fibers has been described at autopsy.[13] At least 10% of patients with cystic fibrosis have normal pancreatic function, and this group is usually spared from the gastrointestinal complications described in this section.

Duodenal ulcers are surprisingly rare in cystic fibrosis, considering the regularity with which such lesions can be produced experimentally by diversion of the pancreatic secretion.[4] Rectal prolapse is common, especially in untreated infants and toddlers, and should always arouse the suspicion of cystic fibrosis.

These patients are also subject to partial or complete intestinal obstruction by solidification of intestinal contents in the small bowel and by impaction of the hard stool in the dilated, redundant colon. The classic example of this phenomenon is meconium ileus of the newborn, in which condition some segment of the intestines, usually the terminal ileum, becomes impacted and obstructed in utero (Fig. 11-18). Abdominal distention usually develops within a few hours of birth, followed by vomiting of bile-stained material and the failure to pass meconium. The most constant roentgenographic finding in the uncomplicated case is uneven distention of intestinal loops.[104] The most common complication is intrauterine rupture of the bowel and meconium peritonitis.[47] If this condition occurs sufficiently before birth, peritoneal calcifications may be present on x-ray examination of the abdomen at birth.

A somewhat similar picture can occur at any age and is referred to as meconium ileus equivalent.[87,91] The obstruction may be complete and acute, or incomplete and chronic. Some patients have had recurrent bouts of obstipation and intestinal obstruction. Some have been originally misdiagnosed as having Hirschsprung's disease. The characteristic roentgenographic picture in these patients is massive accumulation of bubbly stool in the large and small bowel. Intussusception is a rare complication of the same mechanism, the hard stool in the small bowel presumably acting as a lead point.[59]

PANCREAS

Acute pancreatitis appears to be uncommon although no data exist as to its actual frequency. Di Sant'Agnese[40] mentions it as a cause of abdominal pain in these patients, and Shwachman has reported recurrent pancreatitis in 10 older patients with cystic fibrosis.[159A] Pancreatic calcifications have been noted rarely on x-ray examination of the abdomen. Clinically evident diabetes mellitus is a not too unusual complication of cystic fibrosis, especially after the age of 10 to 12 years. It differs from ordinary juvenile diabetes in that ketoacidosis is exceedingly rare.

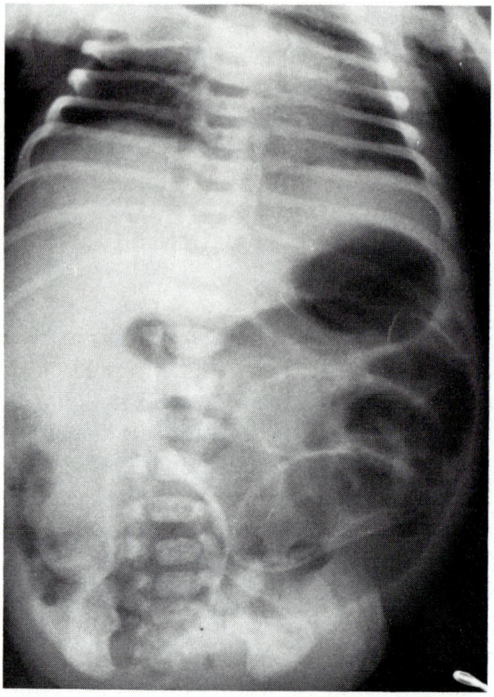

FIG. 11-18. Meconium ileus. Note the markedly distended loops of small bowel. Patient was a 24-hour-old male infant with abdominal distension and failure to pass meconium. Meconium ileus was confirmed at operation.

LIVER

Although evidence of biliary cirrhosis can be found in over 20% of cases at necropsy, only a much smaller percentage develop signs or symptoms of hepatic involvement during life. The typical clinical picture as described by di Sant'Agnese includes hepatosplenomegaly, portal hypertension, hypersplenism, and ascites.[37] Bleeding from esophageal varices is the usual mode of death in these patients. Disturbances of prothrombin time are frequent. Jaundice is uncommon. Surprisingly, clinical signs of gall bladder disease are rarely noted.

EAR, NOSE AND THROAT

Nasal polyps are rather common in cystic fibrosis, and since they are otherwise unusual in children, their presence should always suggest the possibility of this disease. Clinical evidence of chronic sinusitis is infrequent, while roentgenographic evidence of sinus involvement, especially the maxillary sinuses, is seen quite regularly. The dental staining so characteristic of this disease is related primarily to the use of tetracycline-like drugs in infancy and early childhood, although the disease itself can cause some darkening of the teeth. Dental caries are not especially frequent. Chronic enlargement of the submaxillary glands has been noted. Recurrent otitis media is not seen as frequently as one might expect, perhaps because these children usually receive antibiotics with each respiratory infection. Recently, however, audiometric surveys have suggested that a considerable percentage of these children have a middle ear hearing loss.[98]

SWEAT

The physiologic disturbance of the sweat gland is manifested clinically by the excessive loss of salt in the sweat and a tendency to hyponatremic dehydration in hot weather, especially when the patient has diarrhea, vomiting, or prolonged high fever. Interestingly, some parents have noted a salty taste when kissing the infant. The same diagnostic maneuver has been applied on occasion by the astute physician.

HEART

Cor pulmonale has been discussed previously. Myocardial fibrosis has been described in patients with cystic fibrosis.[7,60] In older patients, in association with advanced pulmonary disease, such fibrosis might be secondary to chronic cor pulmonale and myocardial hypoxia. However, a report does exist of three children below 25 months of age with only mild respiratory disease who died from cardiac failure and on autopsy were found to have myocardial fibrosis and regions of myocardial necrosis centered around normal, permeable blood vessels.[77] The cause of such changes is unknown.

EMOTIONAL

Intellect is one of the few functions undisturbed by cystic fibrosis. Emotional and behavioral problems arising from the stresses and strains of living with such a devastating disease, on the other hand, are common. Andersen has emphasized the stress that this disease places upon the entire family unit.[2] McCollum reviewed the economic impact of cystic fibrosis upon the family and found it catastrophic for most families of moderate income.[126] This economic drain places further emotional stress upon the parents.

Parental adaptation to the child with cystic fibrosis can be divided into four phases: prediagnostic (typically a period of parental anxiety), confrontational, long-term adaptive, and terminal.[127] Denial, a useful defense mechanism in the long-term adaptive stage, is seriously impeded by the intrusive characteristics of the disease and its treatment.

Tropauer noted that the anxieties and conflicts related to this disease vary according to the patient's age. As might be anticipated, adolescence is a particularly trying time since "the relative invalidism and necessity of daily care prolong the dependent relationship between the sick child and his parents. This is intensified when physical limitations and recurrent, acute illnesses interrupt the natural association with his friends that helps the teenager emancipate himself from the family and gain independence."[171] Denning has comprehensively described the psychologic and social aspects of cystic fibrosis.[31A]

GENITOURINARY

No primary, clinical involvement of the kidneys occurs in cystic fibrosis, although severe hypoxia, cor pulmonale, and renotoxic antibiotics may all result in some secondary disturbances of renal function.

Conception, gestation, and delivery may all be accomplished by women with cystic fibrosis, although not without risk of severe or even fatal exacerbation of pulmonary disease.[70]

The majority of males with cystic fibrosis are azoospermic and infertile.[32] It is clear that the azoospermia is due to an obliterated, atrophic vas, but whether the condition of the vas is itself due to maldevelopment or to obstruction and fibrosis is still uncertain.[102,128,140,141]

Treatment

Although no cure exists for cystic fibrosis, proper treatment can have a profound effect on the patients' well-being and length of survival. The introduction of the sweat test in

1953 and subsequent refinements in diagnostic acumen have undoubtedly contributed to the apparent improvement in survival by permitting recognition of individuals with milder or atypical disease who were missed in former years.[38] Nevertheless, the improved outlook is basically real and presumably related to therapy. At Babies Hospital in New York City, for example, the number of deaths due to cystic fibrosis in children below 5 years of age declined from seven in 1961 to only one in 1971 despite an increase in the number of such patients seen yearly. Life table studies of Warwick indicate an increased survival with the use of antibiotics and dietary management, and a still greater increase with the introduction of mist tents, aerosol treatments, and postural drainage.[179,180,180A] Similar studies of Huang have led to essentially the same conclusions.[84] In 1964, Doershuk reported the results of a comprehensive therapeutic program for patients with cystic fibrosis.[44] Of 96 patients followed for an average of 37 months, only 3% died and only 4% showed progression of lung disease. The superior results obtained were thought to indicate the benefits of early, aggressive, and comprehensive therapy in dealing with this disease.

PULMONARY THERAPY

Since most of the morbidity and almost all of the mortality in cistic fibrosis is the result of pulmonary involvement, treatment of the pulmonary lesion is a critical aspect of any therapeutic program. Prophylactic pulmonary therapy is based upon attempts to restore the tracheobronchial cleansing mechanism. The goal is to prevent or forestall bronchopulmonary infection and bronchiectasis, which herald the inexorable progression to pulmonary suppuration and lung destruction.

Mist Tents. For many workers in the field of cystic fibrosis, pulmonary therapy begins with the use of the night mist tent as a means of delivering water to the patient's airways so as to thin the secretions therein. The equipment used must produce a high density mist of appropriate droplet size. Keeping in mind that one wishes to deposit the water in the airways and not in the alveoli, a range of droplet size between 1 and 5 μ would appear satisfactory.[142,183] Most ultrasonic nebulizers, as well as some of the newer jet-type nebulizers, produce droplets in this range. The ultrasonic units, however, are able to generate a denser mist, for the rate of nebulization is greater and is independent of the rate of air flow. A 10% solution of propylene glycol may be used instead of plain water to stabilize droplet size and increase mist density, especially with jet-type units (Fig. 11-19).

The mist tent was originally suggested by Denton in 1955,[35] but the Cleveland group under the direction of Matthews and Doershuk has probably been the most aggressive in its use. These workers observed a large group of patients for several months, during which time they continued to receive full treatment with the exception of the mist tent. No significant change in pulmonary function occurred during this control period. The mist tent was then added to the treatment program, and repeat measurements after 1 month showed statistically significant improvement of essentially all parameters of airway obstruction. When the tents were discontinued, pulmonary function deteriorated to its prior level.[45,122] Norman[139] and Zapletal,[186] in similar studies, were unable to confirm the findings of Matthews and Doershuk. Other investigators including Waring,[176] Motoyama,[135B] Chang,[20A] and Rosenbluth[153] have found no evidence of improvement in pulmonary mechanics during the period of mist tent use.

Wolfsdorf and co-workers have argued that most of the aerosolized water is deposited in the nose and mouth and that little reaches beyond the carina.[184] Their studies with technetium 99^{m} labeled aerosols in normal subjects did indicate that only a small amount of radioactivity could be detected distal to the carina. However, their scanning procedure to determine the amount of radioactivity deposited in the lungs required about $1\frac{1}{2}$ hours, during which time the mucociliary apparatus would be carrying the deposited material cephalad at a rate of about 1 cm/min.[27,150] Morrow found that approximately 50% of deposited 5 μ particles were cleared from the tracheobronchial tree in 1 hour.[133] This ongoing process would have minimized the peripheral radioactivity detected by Wolfsdorf and associates.[121] These authors calculated that an adult patient sleeping 8 hours in an ultrasonic mist tent would deposit 16 cc of water in his lower respiratory tract and considered this amount insignificant.[184]

Lifschitz, however, showed by in vitro dilution studies that 16 cc of plain water was able to reduce by 50% the viscosity of 50 cc of cystic fibrosis sputum.[109] He considered this reduction to be a significant mucolytic effect on a significant volume of sputum, and concluded that even 16 cc of water deposited in the airways would be clinically important. In the early stages of cystic fibrosis the distal airways, and in the later stages even the larger airways contain mucopurulent material and should benefit from the deposition of water droplets therein. Yet, Rosenbluth could demonstrate no consistent effect of mist tent therapy on the water content or viscosity of sputum in these patients.[153] The routine prescription of mist tents for patients who perceive no subjective benefit from their use is an unresolved problem.

Occasional patients are unable to tolerate the mist tent. Children with asthma in addition to cystic fibrosis may develop bronchospasm, dyspnea, and severe subjective distress when exposed to dense ultrasonic mist. Relief by bronchodilators is only temporary, and such patients are unable to sleep in the tent. Patients with severe pulmonary disease and

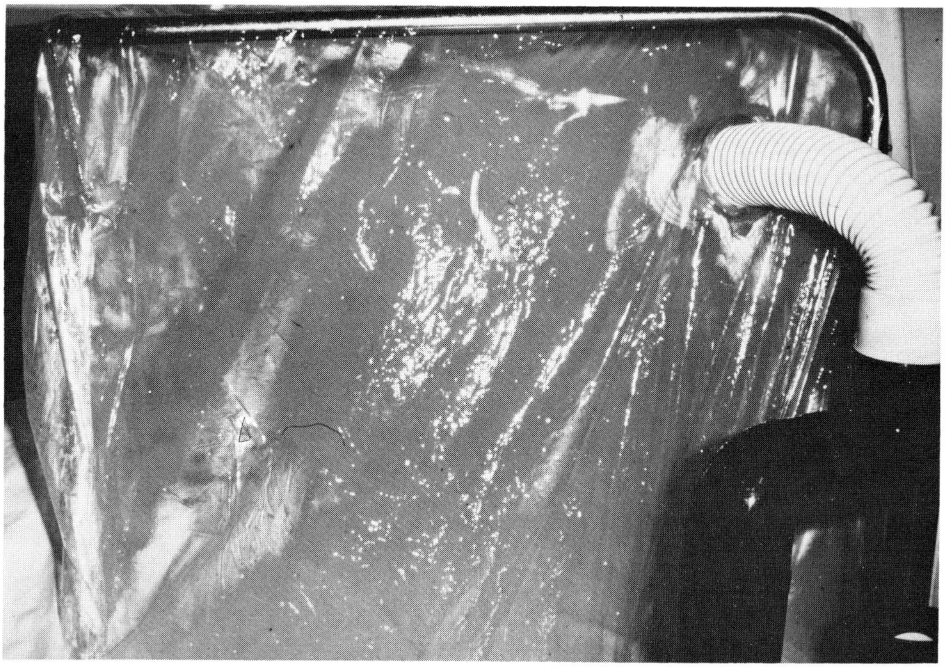

FIG. 11-19. Properly functioning high density mist tent. Note that the mist is dense enough to obscure the patient within the tent.

ventilatory failure may also become intolerably uncomfortable and dyspneic in a mist tent. Whether the changes occur because of bronchial irritation and bronchospasm, deposition of water droplets in the already critically narrowed airways, or emotional reaction precipitated by fear of isolation, separation, and death is not known.

Aerosol Therapy. Whereas the mist tent can provide a large volume of water over many hours, intermittent aerosol therapy (with or without IPPB) can provide only a small volume over a brief period of time. Since only a fraction of the nebulized material deposits in the target area due to airway obstruction by abnormal secretions, it is almost mandatory that a pharmacologically active substance be used for this type of therapy. Water or saline solution alone, in these relatively small amounts, would be unlikely to accomplish anything other than perhaps stimulating cough. It has been shown that patients with minimal airway disease have even distribution of aerosol particles throughout the lung.[1A]

If reduction of sputum viscosity (mucolysis) is the goal, one should select agents that perform this task as a chemical process rather than simply by dilution. The most commonly employed drugs of this type are acetylcysteine and deoxyribonuclease, both of which have demonstrated in vitro a profound mucolytic effect on sputum from patients with cystic fibrosis.[105,158] Acetylcysteine has the advantages of being less expensive, more stable, more convenient, and less allergenic. Hypertonic saline solution (3 or 5%) has also been employed as a mucolytic agent, but is less effective in vitro than either of the two agents just discussed, while seeming to be more irritating in vivo, often producing bloody sputum.

The in vitro mucolytic effect of these agents is incontrovertible, but their in vivo clinical efficacy has not been conclusively demonstrated. Certainly, many patients feel that these drugs help them raise secretions and make coughing easier, but objective evidence of improvement in airway resistance or other parameters of pulmonary function is scarce and unconvincing.[83,151] Whether the use of such agents is worth the time, expense, and possible side effects involved would appear, at present, to be decided chiefly on subjective grounds.

A second class of drugs administered by the aerosol route is designed to widen the airways by relieving bronchospasm and/or mucosal edema. Early, poorly controlled studies on small numbers of patients failed to show any benefit from bronchodilators in patients with cystic fibrosis.[25,181] More recent studies on larger numbers of patients, with proper controls and statistical analysis, have demonstrated a significant response to nebulized bronchodilator agents.[57,61,108] Lifschitz found that aerosols of either isoproterenol or racemic epinephrine increased FEV and FEV_1 in patients with cystic fibrosis, including those who had no history of wheezing.[108] Edema of the bronchial mucosa is also present in these patients and is frequently noted during bronchoscopy. Matthews has suggested the use of a vasoconstrictor such as phenylephrine to decongest the inflamed bronchial mucosa.[123]

The administration of antimicrobial agents by aerosolization has been widely recommended in the treatment of cystic fibrosis and other diseases associated with pulmonary suppuration, although the evidence to document the clinical value of this mode of therapy is less than conclusive.[10,79,123] Huang has reported that, while the sputum level of most antibiotics is very low after even large systemic doses, aerosol administration of the same antibiotics achieved therapeutic concentrations in the sputum.[85] The aerosol route also permits convenient home use of antibiotic agents that are not absorbed orally and would otherwise require parenteral administration. Systemic absorption of kanamycin, for example, has been found to be very low after aerosol administration, and long-term therapy is usually well tolerated and free of serious side effects.[110]

Aerosol medications may be administered with or without IPPB. The simplest equipment is a small, jet nebulizer driven by an oil-free, electrical air compressor (Fig. 11-20). The nebulized solution is delivered via a plastic mask held over the infant's or child's face, exhalation ports permitting the escape of air during expiration. Older children use a mouthpiece instead of the mask. Although this method is wasteful of medication, since nebulization continues during expiration, it has the important advantages of being simple, safe, and relatively inexpensive. Upkeep is modest and sterilization simple. Patient cooperation is not critical, and there is no danger of delivering excessive pressure to the lung. If desired, the medications may be administered by IPPB, especially for the patient who is severely ill with small vital capacity, small tidal volume, and elevated arterial P_{CO_2}. The theoretic dangers of increasing air trapping or producing a pneumothorax by the use of IPPB must be kept in mind when prescribing this type of therapy.[123] No data are available to warrant the routine use of IPPB rather than simple aerosol in the majority of patients with cystic fibrosis.

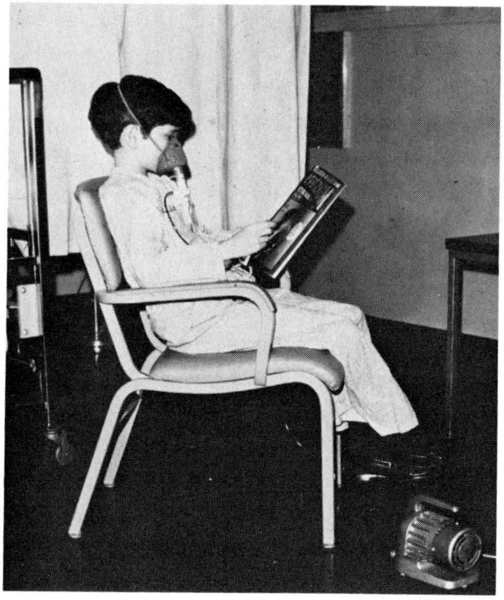

FIG. 11-20. Youngster receiving aerosol therapy by small compressor and jet nebulizer. In this age group the use of a mouthpiece is actually preferable to the mask shown.

All equipment, both for the mist tent and for intermittent aerosol, must be kept scrupulously clean. Each piece should be cleansed and carefully dried after each use and "sterilized" periodically. A convenient means of home sterilization is hot soapy water followed by a 1-hour soak in dilute white vinegar (8 parts vinegar to 18 parts water). A final double rinse in alcohol favors evaporation from inner parts and thorough drying.

Bronchial Drainage. Having thinned the secretions and dilated the airways, it now remains to move the secretions from the smaller and more peripheral airways where cough is ineffective to the larger, central bronchi where the material can be evacuated by cough. To this end, gravity, percussion, and vibration are utilized in the technique of bronchial drainage (also referred to as postural drainage).

The patient is positioned specifically for each pulmonary segment, so that the segmental bronchi are as nearly vertical as is commensurate with the patient's comfort (Fig. 11-21). The parent or therapist then claps vigorously with cupped hand(s) for approximately 2 minutes over the area of the chest corresponding to the segment or segments being drained in an attempt to dislodge the secretions impacted in the peripheral airways. Following percussion, vibration is performed over the segment being treated by gently compressing the chest and vigorously vibrating the area while the patient is exhaling as long as possible through pursed lips. This procedure is repeated five times. The final component of bronchial drainage is to encourage the patient to cough and expectorate as much mucus as possible per segment.

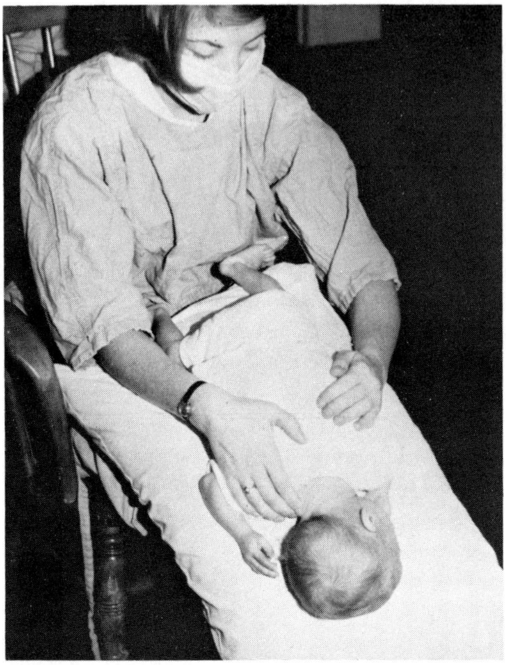

FIG. 11-21. Physical therapist administering postural drainage to an infant. The posterior segment of the left lower lobe is being clapped as the infant is held comfortably on the lap.

The classic analogy is smacking the bottom of an inverted ketchup bottle to initiate flow of thick ketchup. Since cystic fibrosis is a generalized disease with no tendency to spare the upper lobes, all areas of the lung, including the upper lobes, should be treated routinely and prophylactically.

For patients with significant pulmonary involvement, bronchial drainage is a critical part of the treatment program. The increased volume of sputum expectorated is obvious to both patient and physician. Subjective improvement is usually gratifying and many patients are almost free of cough for several hours following such a session. The importance of drainage as part of the overall treatment program has been emphasized by Matthews, who noted signs of increased airway obstruction when drainage was omitted from the treatment schedule.[123] Denton reported increased expectoration of sputum following bronchial drainage with a mechanical percussor as compared to a control period with positioning and a placebo percussor (noise but no vibrations).[33] Lorin found that the volume of sputum produced by bronchial drainage in a group of cystic fibrosis patients was double that produced by an equal period of cough alone. He further noted that the mean volume of sputum per cough was also significantly increased by drainage, indicating that the process accomplishes more than simply stimulating cough[115] (Table 11-1). It is an effective means of dislodging secretions from small, peripheral airways and propelling them to the larger, central airways from which they can be coughed up.

Aerosol treatments followed by bronchial drainage are generally prescribed two or three times a day at home and four times a day in the hospital. Treatments are best not per-

TABLE 11-1. Effect of Postural Drainage on Sputum Expectoration in Patients with Cystic Fibrosis*

	Control Period	Postural Drainage	P
Total volume of sputum expectorated	1.6 cc	3.4	<0.0001
Consistency of sputum specimen	28	32	Not statistically significant
Volume of sputum expectorated per cough	0.33 cc	0.56	<0.001

* Data from controlled study of Lorin and Denning, *Amer. J. Physiol. Med. 50:*215, 1971, showing significant augmentation of sputum volume by postural drainage in patients with cystic fibrosis. The higher "consistency" (a measurement akin to viscosity) of the sputum produced by drainage, although not statistically significant, rules out the possibility that the increased volume resulted from increased contamination with saliva.

formed for at least an hour following a meal to avoid discomfort or vomiting. As such treatments need to be continued indefinitely, efforts should be made to keep the sessions pleasant and free of emotional conflicts. Understanding, compromise, and love are indispensable ingredients of a successful program of pulmonary therapy.

Antimicrobial Agents. Prior to the development of effective antimicrobial drugs, children with cystic fibrosis generally died of pneumonia during the early years of life. First the discovery of penicillin, then the development of broad spectrum antibiotics, the evolution of penicillinase-resistant penicillins and other reliable antistaphylococcal drugs, and finally the production of effective antipseudomonal agents have all been landmark achievements in the battle against cystic fibrosis. The availability of these agents as well as an increased therapeutic aggressiveness have both contributed to the improved survival of these patients.[129A] The phenomenon of changing bacterial flora and the development of resistance to these drugs have limited their ultimate success, however, and have led many students of this disease to abandon the routine, prophylactic use of antimicrobial drugs in favor of a more individualized program, prescribing the drugs for specific clinical indications. The use of antibiotics varies from clinic to clinic, and the following discussion is intended only as a critique of the rationale of such therapy in patients with cystic fibrosis.

The recovery of *S. aureus, P. aeruginosa,* or other potential pathogens from sputum culture should not be considered a priori indication for antimicrobial therapy. Indeed, most patients with cystic fibrosis are at least colonized, if not infected, with one or more of these bacteria, and they generally persist even after antibiotic treatment. Only in the very earliest stage of the disease is one justified in conceptualizing the infectious process in the conventional sense of the patient being free of infection at one point in time, becoming infected at another point, and again being free of infection at a final point after therapy. Beyond this early and generally brief period, the critical concept for rational antibiotic therapy is that the cystic fibrosis patients and their pathogenic bacteria exist together in a dynamic, host-parasite relationship. Whenever this relationship can be held stable (no progression of lung damage or increase in symptomatology), without antibiotics, these agents are withheld. Whenever the balance is tipped in favor of the parasite, antimicrobial therapy is introduced in an attempt to intervene and restore the previous balance, thereby preventing pulmonary damage.

At different stages of the disease the need for antimicrobial agents may vary widely. Consider, for example, the child with mild pulmonary involvement. He coughs only when he runs or laughs hard or has postural drainage. He produces practically no sputum. This description is his baseline. Suddenly, with or without signs of an upper respiratory infection, his cough increases and becomes more productive. He has no fever but may feel less "full of pep" than usual, and his appetite may drop off a bit. Roentgenogram of the chest is unchanged, and repeat sputum culture reveals no new bacterial pathogen. Appropriate oral antibiotic therapy is begun and continued until after he has returned to his previous clinical baseline.

Now consider the patient with more advanced pulmonary disease. Cough is severe and productive. Chest roentgenogram reveals peribronchial fibrosis, chronic peribronchial infiltrations, and atelectasis; the diaphragms are flat and the anteroposterior diameter of the thorax is markedly increased. It is evident that pulmonary disease is not only severe but also progressing, and more vigorous and more prolonged antibiotic therapy is initiated in the hope of slowing the rate of pulmonary destruction. As the courses of antibiotic treatment become longer and the periods between become shorter, bacterial resistance to these drugs increases and clinical response becomes less evident and less certain. Reliance on aerosol antibiotics increases. Admission to the hospital for parenterally administered antibiotic therapy becomes necessary and increasingly frequent. In the final stage of the disease, when the patient has advanced bronchiectasis, severe airway obstruction, copious sputum, markedly diminished pulmonary function, and impending ventilatory failure, the physician often searches desperately for some combination of antibiotics that will control symptoms and permit the patient to continue to function.

It is often difficult or impossible to ascertain what has shifted the precarious balance between patient and bacteria. Certain exogenous viral infections such as measles or influenza are well recognized as being capable of upsetting the status quo in such patients but can account for only a small percentage of the exacerbations seen. In the younger and milder patients, acute worsening of pulmonary symptoms often appears related to minor upper respiratory infections; with older and sicker patients, exacerbations more often occur without an obvious precipitating cause. Such exacerbations in cystic fibrosis do not ordinarily signify pneumonia in the conventional sense. Certainly, it is not a case of normal lung tissue being invaded by a foreign microorganism. Rather, bacteria with which the patient has lived for many years and against which he has developed adequate serum antibodies have now, for some reason, increased their activity or spread to previously spared portions of the lungs or bronchial tree.

Patients with cystic fibrosis may reach extraordinary degrees of lung damage without ever having had an acute episode of pneumonia in the usual sense. Radiographic change may also be gradual and subtle. Increased cough (especially a night cough) or a significant change in the quantity or nature of the sputum are generally the most reliable signs of increased infection in the patient with mild or moderate lung disease. Increased dyspnea, fatigue, anorexia, and weight loss are the corresponding, most useful signs in the patient with advanced pulmonary involvement.

Frequent sputum cultures and the determination of in vitro antibiotic sensitivity of recovered pathogens are helpful in the rational selection of antimicrobial agents. In younger children who do not expectorate, suctioning of the posterior pharynx generally induces cough and sputum. Iacocca has reported reasonably good correlation between the results of throat culture and the results of culturing the sputum or bronchoscopically obtained secretions in patients with cystic fibrosis.[89] It is neither necessary nor wise to await the results of a culture taken at the time of an acute exacerbation before starting therapy. The choice of agent should be determined by the most recent prior culture and past responsiveness, and changed later if necessary.

When the patient is in the hospital, either because of a severe, acute exacerbation or because of a progressive downhill trend, all aspects of therapy are intensified and antibiotics are administered parenterally, preferably by the intravenous route. Eradication of the offending microorganism is an unrealistic goal in most cases. The objectives of therapy are to lessen airway obstruction by decreasing the degree of purulent bronchitis and bronchiolitis, to reverse recent parenchymal extension of infection, and to alleviate the systemic signs of infection, even though the infection itself cannot be eliminated, and the abscess cavities cannot be sterilized. In the presence of significant pulmonary involvement, elimination of all pathogens from the sputum is impossible. Although it is not uncommon to see the disappearance of Hemophilus, Klebsiella, or Staphylococcus species after appropriate antibiotic therapy, these organisms are usually superseded by Pseudomonas or occasionally Enterobacter or Proteus species.

Bronchopulmonary Lavage. Although not a routine procedure in the treatment of this disease, lavage has been employed by a number of cystic fibrosis centers. As part of a planned, comprehensive, therapeutic approach it appears to offer some promise of symptomatic benefit as well as improvement in pulmonary function.[20,101,1B] It is too early to assess the possible effect of bronchopulmonary lavage on life expectancy or ultimate outcome, although one would not anticipate a dramatic effect. Better antibiotic coverage, improved post-lavage care, and the more judicious selection of patients have combined to decrease the originally high mortality for the procedure itself.

Anabolic Steroids. These agents appear to have a limited but definite role in the management of this disease. The therapeutic effect may not necessarily be related to the anabolic effect per se, although the increased appetite, weight gain, and improvement in strength and exercise tolerance are certainly gratifying end results in themselves. It has been recognized for some time that, whereas prior to puberty the survival of males and females with cystic fibrosis was the same, after the onset of puberty the death rate for females increases far more rapidly than does the rate for males. Empirical trials of androgenic hormones suggested clinical benefit,[66] and subsequent controlled studies demonstrated improvement of pulmonary function, at least for females treated with these agents.[48]

Therapy of the End Stage Pulmonary Lesion. The final phase of cystic fibrosis is usually characterized by ventilatory failure and cor pulmonale, and treatment must be directed at the cardiopulmonary system as a unit. All available modalities are employed to relieve airway obstruction and to control pulmonary infection. Hypoxia is usually more severe than hypercapnia because of the uneven distribution of inspired air and resultant abnormal ventilation-perfusion ratios throughout the lung. Hypoxemia should be corrected by the cautious and controlled administration of oxygen, as by nasal catheter or by concentration-controlling masks. Concentration of oxygen in a tent is difficult to control or keep constant. Attempts to raise the arterial oxygen saturation much over 75% may result in an excessive rise in arterial Pco_2. Blood gases must be monitored closely and the ambient oxygen concentration or the flow rate of nasal oxygen adjusted to the optimal value short of an unacceptable increase in arterial Pco_2.

Correction of hypoxemia to relieve pulmonary arteriolar vasoconstriction is a major part of the treatment of cor pulmonale. Diuretics and digitalis are indicated in the presence of cardiomegaly, hepatomegaly, venous distention, or edema.[181A] Moss has indicated the difficulty of diagnosing cor pulmonale in patients with cystic fibrosis.[134] Tachypnea and tachycardia occur secondary to the lung disease. The liver may be palpable because of a depressed and flattened diaphragm. Pulmonary air trapping and voluminous lungs make the heart appear small on roentgenogram. Both the ECG and the vectorcardiogram are influenced by changes in heart position secondary to hyperaeration and correlate poorly with the presence of cor pulmonale.[106] Low serum albumin may be a useful indicator of hypervolemia in these patients.[166] Moss has suggested digitalization before the advent of obvious clinical signs of cor pulmonale, since some experimental evidence in animals suggests that the prophylactic use of digitalis is of value.[134] However, firm evidence of such prophylactic value is lacking. Recent studies indicate that digoxin, a lipid soluble drug, is adequately absorbed by patients with cystic fibrosis.[135A] The use of drugs such as tolazoline hydrochloride specifically to reduce pulmonary arteriolar resistance has been reported as showing encouraging results, and further studies are being conducted.

Artificial ventilation via tracheostomy or endotracheal intubation is not routinely indicated for ventilatory failure in these patients because of the terminal nature of the illness and the extent of irreversible pulmonary damage present. Negative pressure, Drinker-type respirators avoid the trauma of tracheostomy or intubation, but are less efficient and interfere with cough and postural drainage. The decision to use any mechanical ventilator in a patient with cystic fibrosis must be highly individualized. Certainly today with the more potent diuretic and antimicrobial agents available, it is no longer rare for patients to recover from even severe ventilatory failure with or without cor pulmonale. Such recovery may be relatively complete or only partial, and for these patients the final phase of the disease may last years rather than days or weeks. For those unfortunate patients who must live out their final months or years as respiratory invalids, psychologic and economic support often becomes the critical issue.

Pulmonary Complications. Tension pneumothorax is treated primarily by closed thoracotomy and underwater tube drainage. Lesser degrees of pneumothorax may or may not require mechanical intervention, depending upon the extent of pulmonary collapse and the presence or absence of respiratory distress. Postural drainage must be modified and abbreviated while the chest tube is in place, but need not necessarily be discontinued. Appropriate and adequate antibiotic therapy should be instituted to prevent both empyema and the spread of intrapulmonary infection during the period of relative chest immobilization. Antibiotics may also lessen the degree of purulent bronchitis and thereby decrease airway obstruction, favoring closure of the air leak.

With such therapy most air leaks cease in a few days, although recurrences are not uncommon.[14,107] Refractory cases require open thoracotomy, excision, and/or oversewing of subpleural blebs, and some form of pleuroparietopexy.[107] The value of injection of sclerosing agents into the pleural space is uncertain. All of these therapeutic modalities need to be studied in a systematic, controlled fashion.[165A]

Hemoptysis is a common complication of cystic fibrosis. Blood-tinged sputum usually indicates oozing from infected and inflamed bronchial mucosa, and more often than not, it responds satisfactorily to vigorous antibiotic therapy. Potentially irritating aerosols (hypertonic saline, acetylcysteine, deoxyribonuclease) should be temporarily discontinued. Isoproterenol should be avoided because of its vasodilatory effect; racemic epinephrine is a vasoconstrictor and may be substituted. Frank hemoptysis is less common, but more serious, indicating rupture of a dilated bronchial artery.

When massive hemoptysis occurs, the patient should be kept relatively quiet and placed on modified bed rest. In such cases, one is caught in a therapeutic dilemma between the desire to suppress cough and therefore avoid dislodging the blood clot, and the fear that cough suppression will lead to accumulation of secretions and aggravate the pulmonary infection. Bronchial drainage may have to be temporarily stopped or modified. Mild sedatives or tranquilizers are useful to allay anxiety and decrease physical activity, but codeine and other cough suppressants are best avoided or used cautiously. Antibiotics are indicated, not only to prevent spread of infection during the period of restrained cough, but also to permit healing and epithelialization of the mucosa overlying the eroded blood vessel in the bronchiectatic cavity. The prothrombin time should be checked because of the impaired absorption of the fat soluble vitamin K and the frequency of biliary cirrhosis in these patients. Vitamin K may be administered parenterally if indicated. Blood loss is replaced by the transfusion of whole blood as required. Death, if it occurs, is usually by asphyxiation rather than by exsanguination. Although pneumonectomy for life-threatening hemoptysis in this disease has been successful,[81] it should be undertaken only as a desperate measure. Aside from the question of pulmonary reserve is the distinct possibility of significant bleeding from the remaining lung in the near future.

Acute lobar atelectasis is treated by a general increase in all aspects of pulmonary therapy, especially bronchial drainage. If this therapy fails to reexpand the lobe, bronchoscopy should be undertaken promptly. This procedure affords an opportunity to suction or wash out the impacted bronchus and also provides material for culture to identify the microorganisms present. Chronically atelectatic lobes are, in these patients, invariably destroyed by bronchiectasis. If fever or other systemic signs persist, lobectomy may be considered, but careful evaluation of the patient's overall pulmonary status as well as his overall general condition is mandatory. Lobectomy should be undertaken only if it is believed that the symptomatic benefit to be obtained outweighs the risks and discomforts of a surgical procedure.

TREATMENT OF NONPULMONARY LESIONS

Malabsorption. Since the majority of patients with cystic fibrosis have pancreatic insufficiency,[42,68] it is important to treat this aspect of the disease adequately so as to maintain normal or near normal growth and development as well as to prevent complications such as rectal prolapse or specific vitamin deficiency. For infants and young children the caloric intake should be increased to at least twice normal, while the protein intake may need to be as high as 4 to 5 g/kg/day. A high protein, low fat formula, such as Probana, is given for the first year of life; double-strength skim milk is given thereafter. Strained meats should be started as early as 2 months of age and the infant given three solid feedings daily of meat, vegetable, and fruit. Cereal is best avoided during the first 12 months in order to allow room for higher protein foods in an infant whose gastric capacity is limited. The degree of restriction of dietary fat is individualized in that the physician can allow as much fat as is tolerated. An excellent review of the dietary management of cystic fibrosis has been reported by Mike.[132A]

Further treatment of pancreatic insufficiency is accomplished by the oral administration of a pancreatic enzyme preparation such as Pancreatin, Panteric, Viokase, or Cotazym. The choice of preparation and the dosage must be individualized to attain maximal growth and weight gain as well as freedom from symptoms of pancreatic insufficiency. The therapeutic effects of pancreatic replacement therapy are decrease in abdominal distention and discomfort; decrease in the frequency of stools, which also become smaller, more solid, and less foul smelling; and adequate weight gain. The appetite should return to normal.

A water-miscible, multivitamin preparation should be given in sufficient amounts to assure the intake of 10,000 units of vitamin A daily. Additional supplementation with vitamin B complex and vitamin E is also recommended.[3,178] Vitamin K is administered only in times of special need, such as in infants with hypoprothrombinemia and in older patients with bleeding thought to be due to a prolonged prothrombin time. A liberal salt intake is necessary, especially during hot weather or febrile episodes, because of the excessive sodium loss in the sweat. Young children are encouraged to salt their food liberally; older patients can take enteric-coated salt tablets.

Rectal Prolapse. This condition is, in general, best treated by control of malabsorption as outlined previously. When acute, the prolapse is manually reduced by the patient, the parent, or the physician. In infants with recurrent prolapse, it is sometimes useful to tape the buttocks together between bowel movements, while attempting to control the malabsorption. Surgical procedures to prevent recurrence are almost never indicated or necessary.

Meconium Ileus. When unaccompanied by complications such as volvulus, perforation, atresia, or peritonitis, many infants with meconium ileus can be successfully treated in a nonsurgical fashion by the use of Gastrografin enemas.[138,174] One must not assume, however, that the nonoperative approach is applicable to all cases of meconium ileus. Certainly, those patients with the aforementioned complications require immediate surgical procedure. The action of the Gastrografin is believed to be due to its high osmolarity, drawing water into the bowel lumen, softening the viscid meconium, and loosening it from the bowel wall. Generally, 60 to 90 cc of the undiluted, radiopaque material is instilled into the colon via a No. 8 French catheter, under fluoroscopic control. It is imperative that an intravenous infusion be in place during the procedure to maintain fluid balance as the hypertonic material is administered.

Several different surgical procedures have been recommended for those infants who require an operation. These procedures include the Mikulicz resection of the ileum,[71] a primary end-to-end anastomosis,[168] and resection with a Roux-en-Y anastomosis with distal ileostomy.[11] The preferred surgical procedure at the Babies Hospital in New York City is resection and proximal "chimney" anastomosis.[155,156] This procedure consists of resection of the most dilated segment of ileum and a side-to-end anastomosis joining the side of the proximal limb to the end of the distal limb. A soft polyethylene catheter is inserted into the proximal limb, guided through the anastomosis, and threaded into the distal bowel. The end of the proximal limb (with the catheter) is brought out through a stab wound in the abdominal wall. The end enterostomy permits immediate and adequate decompression.

In the postoperative period, solutions of pancreatic enzymes or acetylcysteine are instilled into the distal bowel via the catheter, helping clear the bowel of its meconium. Once the solutions have been instilled, the proximal limb is clamped intermittently until adequate decompression has taken place and peristalsis has resumed. When the edema of the anastomosis has subsided and the distal bowel enlarged sufficiently from feedings via the catheter so that some of the contents of the proximal bowel pass through the anastomosis, the catheter is removed and the stoma of the proximal bowel is completely occluded. After normal intestinal function is fully established, the enterostomy is excised below the skin level. Most of these openings then close spontaneously.

For those patients requiring surgical intervention, careful adherence to the maintenance of optimal fluid and electrolyte balance, caloric needs, and control of pulmonary infection is essential. On occasion, intravenous hyperalimentation has been lifesaving in these patients.

Meconium Ileus Equivalent. Abdominal pain is a common complaint in patients with cystic fibrosis, and palpable fecal masses in both lower quadrants are frequently noted in the course of a routine physical examination. These masses are usually mobile and nontender. In an otherwise asymptomatic patient, observation and conservative management are all that is generally needed, for the masses usually pass spontaneously within days to weeks. It is sometimes helpful to liberalize the dietary fat intake, adjust the dosage of pancreatic enzymes, and administer stool-softening agents (e.g., dioctyl sodium sulfosuccinate). It is postulated that these fecal masses, adherent to the wall of the cecum and colon, stimulate intestinal peristalsis with resultant abdominal pain. Less frequently, the pain may become severe, and signs of acute intestinal obstruction such as vomiting and abdominal distention develop, necessitating hospitalization.

The obstruction usually responds to conservative treatment consisting of enemas and, on occasion, decompression of the small intestine by a Miller-Abbott tube. Pancreatic enzymes and acetylcysteine may be given orally or instilled through the tube. Enemas of many different types have been tried including those containing detergents, acetylcysteine, and Gastrografin. The most effective of these seems to be Gastrografin, as described previously. The same precautions for its use must be followed and the volume of the enema adjusted to the size and age of the patient. Rarely, a patient may not respond to the conservative medical program just outlined, and requires surgical procedure to relieve the intestinal obstruction. One must also be alert to the possibility of an intussusception or volvulus complicating the meconium ileus.[82]

Adolescent and young adult patients with cystic fibrosis are frequently bothered by severe, recurrent abdominal pain. These patients seem to have an incomplete obstruction of the large bowel and may be helped by the oral administration of acetylcysteine on a regular daily basis.[67,111]

Biliary Cirrhosis. The majority of patients with cystic fibrosis who are found to have biliary cirrhosis at autopsy have had few, if any, symptoms referable to the liver during life and required no special treatment in this regard. However, about 2% of patients with this disease seem to have more severe or progressive liver disease, resulting in the syndrome of portal hypertension. Edema and ascites are treated conservatively and symptomatically with diuretic agents and cautious salt restriction. Bleeding from ruptured esophageal varices poses the most immediate threat to life, and various portosystemic shunting procedures have been tried with varying degrees of success. It is wise to administer extra vitamin K at such times. There has been only limited experience with elective shunts in patients who have demonstrable varices but have never bled. Most workers in this area do not consider performing a shunt until the patient has had at least one bleeding episode.[172] There are two reasons. First many such patients go for years without bleeding, and many die from their pulmonary disease before bleeding develops. Second, hepatic failure may develop after a shunt in patients with marginally functional livers.

Nasal Polyps. These polyps, seen commonly in patients with cystic fibrosis, seem to present the problem of chronic recurrence in some patients more than in others. Those patients who have mild to moderate nasal obstructive symptoms may be satisfactorily managed by daily use of a steroid-containing cream (Neomedrol in Veriderm Cream 0.25%). This cream, which is applied into the nose and snuffed (much like tobacco snuff), seems to shrink the polyp, allowing a better airway. Those patients who are more severely obstructed by the polyps and who are uncomfortable benefit by the surgical removal of their polyps, followed by daily use of the steroid cream. Some patients may require repeated polypectomies.

Emotional. Some of the relatively common emotional problems (such as depression and anxiety) experienced by patients with cystic fibrosis are improved by antidepressant medications and tranquilizers. It is not just the patient but his entire family who need comprehensive, early counseling and guidance in order to minimize the emotional ravages of this disease. A psychiatrist or psychologist should be an integral member of the treatment team as well as a medical social worker, nurse, physical therapist, geneticist, nutritionist, clinic coordinator, and physicians who have a special feeling for handling problems of the chronically ill. At many cystic fibrosis centers, group psychotherapeutic sessions have been started for adolescent patients with cystic fibrosis as well as for their parents. These sessions have generally met with the enthusiastic approval of the participants, although it would be premature to predict their impact on a long-term basis.

REFERENCES

1A. Alderson, P. O., R. H. Secker-Walker, D. B. Strominger, J. Markham and R. L. Hill: Pulmonary deposition of aerosols in children with cystic fibrosis. *J. Pediatr. 84*:479, 1974.

1B. Altman, R. P., L. L. Kulczycki, J. G. Randolph and J. E. McClenathan: Bronchoscopy and bronchial lavage in children with cystic fibrosis. *J. Pediatr. Surg., 8*:809, 1973.

1. Andersen, D. H.: Pathology of cystic fibrosis. *Ann. N.Y. Acad. Sci. 93*:500, 1962.
2. Andersen, D. H.: Cystic fibrosis and family stress. *Children 7*:1, 1960.
3. Andersen, D. H.: Celiac syndrome. III. Dietary therapy for congenital pancreatic deficiency. *Am. J. Dis. Child. 70*:100, 1945.
4. Alterman, K.: Duodenal ulceration and fibrocystic pancreas disease. *Am. J. Dis. Child. 101*:210, 1961.
5. Balfe, J. W., C. Cole and L. G. Welt: Red-cell transport defect in patients with cystic fibrosis and in their parents. *Science 162*:689, 1968.
6. Barbero, G. J. and W. S. Chernick: Role of the autonomic nervous system in cystic fibrosis. In *Third International Conference on Research and Pathogenesis of Cystic Fibrosis of the Pancreas.* Wickersham Printing Co., Lancaster, Pa., p. 208, 1964.
7. Barnes, G. L., J. F. Gwynne and J. M. Watt: Myocardial fibrosis in cystic fibrosis of the pancreas. *Aust. Paediatr. J. 6*:81, 1970.
7A. Barnett, D. R., M. S. Shanfield, M. I. McCombs and B. H. Bowman: Isoelectric focusing and IgG allotyping of the serum fraction containing the cystic fibrosis ciliary inhibitor. *Tex. Rep. Biol. Med. 31*:709, 1973.
8. Bearn, A. G. and B. S. Danes: A genetic study of cystic fibrosis of the pancreas in cell culture. *Trans. Assoc. Am. Physicians 82*:248, 1969.
9. Beier, F. R., A. D. Renzetti, M. Mitchell and S. Watanabe: Pulmonary pathophysiology in cystic fibrosis. *Am. Rev. Respir. Dis. 94*:430, 1966.
10. Bilodeau, M. and J. Roy: Aerosoltherapie à la kanamycine dans 200 cas de suppuretions broncho-pulmonaires. *Can. Med. Assoc. J. 89*:537, 1963.
11. Bishop, H. C. and C. E. Koop: Management of meconium ileus. *Ann. Surg. 145*:410, 1957.
12. Blanc, W. A.: Immunocytological techniques in cystic fibrosis of the pancreas. In *Third International Conference on Research and Pathogenesis of Cystic Fibrosis,* P. A. di Sant'Agnese (Ed.).: Wickersham Printing Co., Lancaster Pa., p. 327, 1964.
13. Blanc, W. A., J. D. Reid and D. H. Andersen: Avitaminosis E in cystic fibrosis of the pancreas. *Pediatrics 22*:494, 1958.
14. Boat, T. F., P. A. di Sant'Agnese, W. J. Warwick and S. A. Handwerger: Pneumothorax in cystic fibrosis. *J.A.M.A. 209*:1498, 1969.
15. Bodian, M.: *Fibrocystic Disease of the Pancreas.* Heinemann Ltd., London, p. 86, 1952.
16. Bowman, B. H., L. H. Lockhart and M. L. McCombs: Oyster ciliary inhibition by cystic fibrosis factor. *Science 164*:325, 1969.
16A. Bowman, B. H., D. R. Barnett, R. Matalon, B. S. Danes and A. G. Bearn: Cystic fibrosis fractionation of fibroblast media demonstrating ciliary inhibition. *Proc. Natl. Acad. Sci. 70*:548, 1973.
16B. Bowman, B. H., B. J. Lankford, G. M. Fuller, S. D. Carson, A. Kurosky and D. R. Barnett: Cystic fibrosis: The ciliary inhibitor is a small polypeptide associated with immunoglobulin G. *Biochem. Biophys. Res. Commun. 64*:1310, 1975.
16C. Bowman, B. H., M. L. McCombs and L. H. Lockhart: Cystic fibrosis: characterization of the inhibitor to ciliary action in oyster gills. *Science 167*:871, 1970.
17. Boxerbaum, B., M. Kagumba and L. W. Matthews: Selective inhibition of fibrosis serum. *Am. Rev. Respir. Dis. 108*:777, 1973.
18. Burns, M. W.: The significance of various bacteria in chronic bronchial disorders as determined by bacterial antibody detection. *Aust. Ann. Med. 17*:289, 1968.
19. Carlson, D. M. and L. W. Matthews: Polyuronic acids produced by Pseudomonas aeruginosa. *Biochemistry 5*:2817, 1966.
20. Cezeaux, G., J. Telford, G. Harrison and A. S. Keats: Bronchial lavage in cystic fibrosis. *J.A.M.A. 199*:15, 1967.
20A. Chang, N., H. Levison, K. Cunningham, D. N. Crozier and O. Grosett: An evaluation of nightly mist tent therapy for patients with cystic fibrosis. *Am. Rev. Respir. Dis. 107*:672, 1973.
21. Chernick, W. S., G. J. Barbero, and F. M. Parkins: Studies on submaxillary saliva in cystic fibrosis. *J. Pediatr. 59*:890, 1961.
22. Chernick, W. S. and G. J. Barbero: Reversal of submaxillary salivary alterations in cystic fibrosis by guanethidine. *Bibl. Paediatr. 86*:125, 1967.
23. Chernick, W. S. and G. J. Barbero: Studies on human tracheobronchial and submaxillary secretions in normal and pathophysiological conditions. *Ann. N.Y. Acad. Sci. 106*:698, 1963.
24. Chernick, W. S. and G. J. Barbero: Composition of tracheobronchial secretions in cystic fibrosis of the pancreas and bronchiectasis. *Pediatrics 24*:739, 1959.
24A. Conover, J. H., E. J. Conod and K. Hirschhorn: Studies on ciliary dyskinesia factor in cystic fibrosis. *Life Sci. 14*:253, 1974.
25. Cook, C. D., P. J. Helliesen, L. Kulczycki, H. Barrie, L. Friedlander, S. Agathon, G. B. C. Harris and H. Shwachman: Studies of respiratory physiology in children. II. Lung volumes and mechanics of respiration in 64 patients with cystic fibrosis of the pancreas. *Pediatrics 24*:181, 1959.
26. Crosato, M. and G. C. Mussa: Cellulose acetate electrophoretic determination of serum proteins, lipoproteins, and glycoproteins in infantile mucoviscidosis. *Minerva Pediatr. 20*:2326, 1968.
27. Dalhamn, T.: Mucous flow and ciliary activity in the trachea of healthy rats and rats exposed to respiratory irritant gases. *Acta Physiol. Scand. 36 (Suppl. 123)*:1, 1956.

28. Danes, B. S. and A. G. Bearn: Cystic fibrosis of the pancreas: a study in cell culture. *J. Exp. Med. 129*:775, 1969.

28A. Danes, B. S., S. D. Litwin, T. H. Hutteroth, H. Cleve and A. G. Bearn: Characterization of cystic fibrosis factor and its interaction with human immunoglobulin. *J. Exp. Med. 137*:1538, 1973.

29. Danks, D. M., J. Allan and C. M. Anderson: Genetic study of fibrocystic disease of pancreas. *Ann. Hum. Genet. 28*:323, 1965.

30. Dees, S. C.: Asthma. In *Disorders of the Respiratory Tract in Children,* E. L. Kendig (Ed.). W. B. Saunders Co., Philadelphia, p. 449, 1967.

31. Demuth, G. R., W. F. Howatt and N. S. Talner: Intrapulmonary gas distribution in cystic fibrosis. *Am. J. Dis. Child. 103*:129, 1962.

31A. Denning, C. R., M. M. Gluckson and I. Mohr: Psychological and social aspects of cystic fibrosis. In *Cystic Fibrosis: Projections into the Future.* Symposia Specialists, Miami, p. 127, 1976.

32. Denning, C. R., S. C. Sommers, and H. J. Quigley: Infertility in male patients with cystic fibrosis. *Pediatrics 41*:7, 1968.

33. Denton, R.: Bronchial secretions in cystic fibrosis: effects of treatment with mechanical percussion vibration. *Am. Rev. Respir. Dis. 86*:41, 1962.

34. Denton, R.: Bronchial obstruction in cystic fibrosis: rheological factors. *Pediatrics 25*:611, 1960.

35. Denton, R.: The clinical use of continuous nebulization in bronchopulmonary disease. *Dis. Chest 28*:123, 1955.

36. di Sant'Agnese, P. A. in discussion with C. C. Lobeck and N. R. McSherry: Ionic composition of pilocarpine induced sweat in relation to gland output during aging and in cystic fibrosis. *Bibl. Paediatr. 86*:41, 1967.

37. di Sant'Agnese, P. A. and W. A. Blanc: A distinctive type of biliary cirrhosis of the liver associated with cystic fibrosis of the pancreas. *Pediatrics 18*:387, 1956.

38. di Sant'Agnese, P. A., R. C. Darling, G. A. Perera and E. Shea: Abnormal electrolyte composition of sweat in cystic fibrosis. *Pediatrics 12*:549, 1953.

39. di Sant'Agnese, P. A., H. Grossman, R. C. Darling and C. R. Denning: Saliva, tears, and duodenal contents in cystic fibrosis of the pancreas. *Pediatrics 22*:507, 1958.

40. di Sant'Agnese, P. A. and M. J. Lepore: Involvement of abdominal organs in cystic fibrosis of the pancreas. *Gastroenterology 40*:64, 1961.

41. di Sant'Agnese, P. A. and G. F. Powell: The eccrine sweat defect in cystic fibrosis of the pancreas. *Ann. N.Y. Acad. Sci. 93*:555, 1962.

42. di Sant'Agnese, P. A. and R. C. Talamo: Pathogenesis and physiopathology of cystic fibrosis of the pancreas. *N. Engl. J. Med. 277*:1287, 1343, 1399, 1967.

43. Dische, Z., P. A. di Sant'Agnese, C. Pallavicini and J. Youlos: Composition of mucoprotein fractions from duodenal fluid of patients with cystic fibrosis and from controls. *Pediatrics 24*:74, 1959.

44. Doershuk, C. F., L. W. Matthews, A. S. Tucker, H. Nudelman, G. Eddy, M. Wise and S. Spector: A 5 year clinical evaluation of a therapeutic program for patients with cystic fibrosis. *J. Pediatr. 65*:677, 1964.

45. Doershuk, C. F., L. W. Matthews, C. T. Gillespie, M. D. Lough and S. Spector: Evaluation of jet-type and ultrasonic nebulizers in mist tent therapy for cystic fibrosis. *Pediatrics 41*:723, 1968.

46. Doggett, R. G., G. M. Harrison, R. N. Stillwell and E. S. Wallis: Atypical Pseudomonas aeruginosa associated with cystic fibrosis of the pancreas. *J. Pediatr. 68*:215, 1966.

47. Donnison, A. B., H. Shwachman and R. E. Gross: Review of 164 children with meconium ileus. *Pediatrics 37*:833, 1966.

48. Dooley, R. R.: Pulmonary function change in cystic fibrosis patients treated with norethandrolone. *Am. Rev. Respir. Dis. 99*:990. 1969.

49. Emrich, H. M., E. Stoll, B. Friolet, J. P. Colombo, E. Rossi and R. Richterich: Excretion of different substances in the sweat of children with cystic fibrosis and controls. *Bibl. Paediatr. 86*:58, 1967.

50. Emrich, H. M., E. Stoll, B. Friolet, J. P. Colombo, R. Richterich and E. Rossi: Sweat composition in relation to rate of sweating in patients with cystic fibrosis of the pancreas. *Pediatr. Res. 2*:464, 1968.

51. Esterly, J. R. and E. H. Oppenheimer: Cystic fibrosis of the pancreas: structural changes in peripheral airways. *Thorax 23*:670, 1968.

52. Fanconi, G., E. Vehlinger and C. Knauer: Des Coeliakiesyndrom bei angeborener zystischer Pankreasfibromatose und Bronchiektasien. Wien. Med. *Wochenschr. 86*:753, 1936.

53. Farber, S.: Some organic digestive disturbances in early life. *J. Michigan Med. Soc. 44*:587, 1945.

54. Feather, E. A. and G. Russell: Sputum viscosity in cystic fibrosis of the pancreas and other pulmonary diseases. *Br. J. Dis. Chest 64*:192, 1970.

55. Feather, E. A. and G. Russell: Sputum viscosity and pulmonary function in cystic fibrosis. *Arch. Dis. Child. 45*:807, 1970.

56. Featherby, E. A., T. R. Weng, D. N. Crozier, A. Duic, B. J. Reilly and H. Levison: Dynamic and static lung volumes, blood gas tensions, and diffusing capacity in patients with cystic fibrosis. *Am. Rev. Respir. Dis. 102*:737, 1970.

57. Featherby, E. A., T. R. Weng, and H. Levison: The effect of isoproterenol on airway obstruction in cystic fibrosis. *Can. Med. Assoc. J. 102*:835, 1970.

58. Feigelson, J. and Y. Pecau: Bacteriological studies of bronchial secretions in 19 cases of cystic fibrosis. *Bibl. Paediatr. 86*:214, 1967.

59. Flux, M.: Intussusception in a patient with cystic fibrosis. *South. Med. J. 60*:1184, 1967.
60. Fridman-Manduzio, A. and J. Haot: Myocardial lesions in mucoviscidosis. *Brux. Med. 50*:458, 1970.
61. Gandevia, B. and C. Anderson: Effect of a bronchodilator aerosol on ventilatory capacity in fibrocystic disease of the pancreas. *Arch. Dis. Child. 34*:511, 1959.
62. Gibbs, G. E.: Quantitative microdetermination of enzymes in sweat glands in cystic fibrosis. *Bibl. Paediatr. 86*:95, 1967.
63. Gibson, L. E. and R. E. Cooke: A test for concentration of electrolytes in sweat in cystic fibrosis of the pancreas, utilizing pilocarpine by iontophoresis. *Pediatrics 23*:545, 1959.
64. Gibson, L. E., W. J. Matthews, P. T. Minihan and J. A. Patti: Relating mucus, calcium, and sweat in a new concept of cystic fibrosis. *Pediatrics 48*:695, 1971.
65. Goldring, R. M., A. P. Fishman, G. M. Turino, H. I. Cohen, C. R. Denning and D. H. Andersen: Pulmonary hypertension and cor pulmonale in cystic fibrosis of the pancreas. *J. Pediatr. 65*:502, 1964.
66. Good, T. A. and S. P. Bessman: Anabolic steroids in cystic fibrosis. *Am. J. Dis. Child. 111*:272, 1966.
67. Gracey, M. V. Burke and C. M. Anderson: Treatment of abdominal pain in cystic fibrosis by oral administration of n-acetylcysteine. *Arch. Dis. Child. 44*:404, 1969.
68. Grand, R. J.: Changing patterns of gastrointestinal manifestations of cystic fibrosis. *Clin. Pediatr. 9*:588, 1970.
69. Grand, R. J., P. A. di Sant'Agnese, R. C. Talamo and J. C. Pallavicini: Effects of exogenous aldosterone on sweat electrolytes. *J. Pediatr. 70*:357, 1967.
70. Grand, R. J., R. C. Talamo, P. A. di Sant'Agnese and R. H. Schwartz: Pregnancy in cystic fibrosis of the pancreas. *J.A.M.A. 195*:993, 1966.
71. Gross, R. E.: *Surgery of Infancy and Childhood.* W. B. Saunders Co., Philadelphia, p. 183, 1953.
72. Grossman, H., C. R. Denning and D. H. Baker: Hypertrophic osteoarthropathy in cystic fibrosis. *Am. J. Dis. Child. 107*:1, 1964.
73. Gugler, E., C. J. Pallavicini, H. Swerdlow and P. A. di Sant'Agnese: Role of calcium in submaxillary saliva of patients with cystic fibrosis. *J. Pediatr. 71*:585, 1967.
74. Hadorn, B., G. Zappi, D. H. Shmerling, A. Prader, I. McIntyre and C. M. Anderson: Quantitative assessment of exocrine pancreatic function in infants and children. *J. Pediatr. 73*39, 1968.
75. Halbert, S. P.: Immunological aspects of cystic fibrosis. *Bibl. Paediatr. 86*:144, 1967.
76. Handwerger, S., J. Roth, P. Gordon, P. di Sant'Agnese, D. Carpenter and G. Peter: Glucose intolerance in cystic fibrosis. *N. Engl. J. Med. 281*:451, 1969.
77. Hermier, M., R. Gilly, J. Gilly, J. Raveau and M. Bovier-Lapierre: Myocardial necrosis and sudden death in childhood mucoviscidosis. *Pediatrie 22*:931, 1967.
78. Herzberg, V., L. Calvert and B. H. Bowman: Evidence that the ciliary inhibitor or cystic fibrosis is not an antibody. *J. Clin. Invest. 52*:2732, 1973.
79. High, R. H., A. Sarria and N. N. Huang: Kanamycin in the treatment of infections in infants and children. *Ann. N.Y. Acad. Sci. 76*:289, 1958–59.
80. Holsclaw, D. S., H. B. Eckstein and H. H. Nixon: Meconium ileus, *Am. J. Dis. Child. 109*:101, 1965.
81. Holsclaw, D. S., R. J. Grand and H. Shwachman: Massive hemoptysis in cystic fibrosis. *J. Pediatr. 76*:829, 1970.
82. Holsclaw, D. S., C. Rocmans and H. Shwachman: Intussusception in patients with cystic fibrosis. *Pediatrics 48*:51, 1971.
83. Howatt, W. F. and G. R. DeMuth: Double blind study of the use of acetylcysteine in patients with cystic fibrosis. *Univ. Mich. Med. Ctr. J. 32*:82, 1966.
84. Huang, N. N., C. N. Marci, J. Girone and A. Sproul: Survival of patients with cystic fibrosis. *Am. J. Dis. Child. 120*:289, 1970.
85. Huang, N. N., A. Sarria and R. H. High: A limited study on the use of Kanamycin in patients with fibrocystic disease of pancreas. In *Antibiotics Annual,* H. Welch and F. Marti-Ibanez (Eds.). Medical Encyclopedia, New York, p. 687, 1958–1959.
86. Huang, N. N., E. L. Vanloon and K. T. Sheng: Flora of the respiratory tract of patients with cystic fibrosis of the pancreas. *J. Pediatr. 59*:512, 1961.
87. Hunton, D. B., W. K. Long and H. Y. Tsumagari: Meconium ileus equivalent: an adult complication of fibrocystic disease, *Gastroenterology 50*:99, 1966.
88. Iacocca, V. F. and J. Barbero: Serum antistaphylococcal alpha-haemolysin titres in cystic fibrosis. *Arch. Dis. Child. 43*:220, 1968.
89. Iacocca, V. F., M. S. Sibinga and G. J. Barbero: Respiratory tract bacteriology in cystic fibrosis. *Am. J. Dis. Child. 106*:315, 1963.
90. Ikai, K.: Cystic fibrosis cases found by re-examination of histology of pancreas and postmortem protocol in Japanese children and sweat tests on siblings. *Acta Paediatr. Jpn. 7*:23, 1965.
91. Jaffe, B. F., W. P. Graham III and L. Goldman: Postinfancy intestinal obstruction in children with cystic fibrosis. *Arch. Surg. 92*:337, 1966.
92. Johansen, P. G. and R. Kay: Histochemistry of rectal mucus in cystic fibrosis of the pancreas. *J. Pathol. 99*:299, 1969.
93. Kaiser, D., E. Drack and E. Rossi: Effect of cystic

fibrosis sweat on sodium reabsorption by the normal sweat gland. *Lancet 1*:1003, 1970.
94. Kaiser, G., K. Zuppinger and E. Joss: Mucoviscidosis and diabetes mellitus. *Helv. Paediatr. Acta 25*:135, 1970.
95. Katznelsen, D., G. F. Vawter, G. E. Foley and H. Shwachman: Botryomycosis, a complication in cystic fibrosis. *J. Pediatr. 65*:525, 1964.
96. Kopito, L. and H. Shwachman: Mineral composition of meconium. *J. Pediatr. 68*:313, 1966.
97. Kramm, E. R., cited in P. A. di Sant'Agnese and R. C. Talamo: Pathogenesis and physiopathology of cystic fibrosis of the pancreas. *N. Engl. J. Med. 277*:1287, 1967.
98. Kulczycki, L. L., J. S. Butler, D. McCord-Dickman and G. R. Herer: The hearing of patients with cystic fibrosis. *Arch. Otolaryngol. 92*:54, 1970.
99. Kulczycki, L. L. and J. M. LoPresti: Mucus retention and overinflation as basic pulmonary complications in cystic fibrosis. *Bibl. Paediatr. 86*:207, 1967.
99A. Kulczycki, L. L. and V. Schauf: Cystic fibrosis in blacks in Washington, D.C. *Am. J. Dis. Child. 127*:64, 1974.
100. Kutcher, A.: Personal communication.
101. Kylstra, J. A., D. C. Rausch, K. D. Hall and A. Spock: Volume controlled lung lavage in the treatment of asthma, bronchiectasis and mucoviscidosis. *Am. Rev. Respir. Dis. 103*:651, 1971.
102. Landing, B. H., T. R. Wells and C. I. Wang: Abnormality of the epididymis and vas deferens in cystic fibrosis. *Arch. Pathol. 88*:569, 1969.
103. Laraya-Cuasay, L., S. D. Braverman, M. A. Capitano and N. N. Huang: Day to day variability of pulmonary function tests in patients with cystic fibrosis. Presented at The Cystic Fibrosis Club, Twelfth Annual Meeting, Atlantic City, N.J., April, 1971.
104. Leonidas, J. C., W. E. Berdon, D. H. Baker and T. V. Santulli: Meconium ileus and its complications. *Am. J. Roentgenol. Radium Ther. Nucl. Med. 108*:598, 1970.
105. Lieberman, J.: Measurement of sputum viscosity in a cone plate viscometer. Evaluation of mucolytic agents in vitro. *Am. Rev. Respir. Dis., 97*:662. 1968.
106. Lieberman, J., C. F. Doershuk, C. Rapp and L. Matthews: Vectorcardiogram in cystic fibrosis. *Circulation 35*:552, 1967.
107. Lifschitz, M. I., F. O. Bowman, C. R. Denning and R. H. Wylie: Pneumothorax as a complication of cystic fibrosis. *Am. J. Dis. Child. 116*:633, 1968.
108. Lifschitz, M. I. and C. R. Denning: Assessment of bronchospasm in patients with cystic fibrosis. *Am. Rev. Respir. Dis. 99*:399, 1969.
109. Lifschitz, M. I. and C. R. Denning: Quantitative interaction of water and cystic fibrosis sputum. *Am. Rev. Respir. Dis. 102*:456, 1970.
110. Lifschitz, M. I. and C. R. Denning: Safety of Kanamycin aerosol. *Clin. Pharmacol. Ther. 12*:91, 1971.
111. Lillibridge, C. R., J. M. Docter and S. Eidelman: Oral administration of n-acetylcysteine in the prophylaxis of meconium ileus equivalent. *J. Pediatr. 71*:887, 1967.
112. Lobeck, C. C.: Cystic fibrosis. In *The Metabolic Basis of Inherited Disease,* 3rd edition, J. B. Stanbury, J. B. Wyngaarden and D. S. Fredrickson (Eds.). McGraw-Hill, New York, p. 1605, 1972.
113. Lobeck, C. C. in discussion with G. Giebisch: Use of micropuncture techniques in the study of electrolyte gradients in single nephrons. In *Third International Conference on Research and Pathogenesis of Cystic Fibrosis of the Pancreas.* Wickersham Printing Co., Lancaster, Pa., p. 107, 1964.
114. Lockhart, L. H., B. H. Bowman and D. Peters: Effect of cystic fibrosis serum upon oyster cilia. *South. Med. J. 61*:1356, 1968.
115. Lorin, M. I. and C. R. Denning: Evaluation of postural drainage by measurement of sputum volume and consistency. *Am. J. Phys. Med. 50*:215, 1971.
116. Lorin, M. I., C. R. Denning and I. D. Mandel: Viscosity of exocrine secretions in cystic fibrosis: sweat, duodenal fluid and submaxillary saliva. *Biorheology 9*:27, 1972.
117. Lowenfeld, I.: Personal communication.
118. Mandel, I. D., R. H. Thompson, S. Wotman, M. Taubman, A. H. Kutscher, E. V. Zegarelli, C. R. Denning, J. T. Botwick and B. S. Fahn: Parotid saliva in cystic fibrosis. *Am. J. Dis. Child. 110*:646, 1965.
119. Mandel, I. D., A. Kutscher, C. R. Denning, R. H. Thompson and E. V. Zegarelli: Salivary studies in cystic fibrosis. *Am. J. Dis. Child. 113*:431, 1967.
120. Mangos, J. A., N. R. McSherry and P. J. Benk: Sodium transport inhibitory factor in saliva of patients with cystic fibrosis. *Pediatr. Res. 1*:436, 1967.
120A. Mangos, J. A. and R. C. Talamo (Eds.): *Cystic Fibrosis, Projections into the Future.* Stratton Intercontinental Medical Book Corp., New York, 1976.
121. Matthews, L. W. and C. F. Doershuk: Mist therapy reconsidered twice more. *Pediatrics 43*:902, 1969.
122. Matthews, L. W., C. F. Doershuk and S. Spector: Mist tent therapy in treatment of the obstructive pulmonary lesion of cystic fibrosis. *Pediatrics 39*:176, 1967.
123. Matthews, L. W., C. F. Doershuk, M. Wise, G. Eddy, H. Nudelman and S. Spector: A therapeutic regimen for patients with cystic fibrosis. *J. Pediatr. 65*:558, 1964.
124. Matthews, L. W., S. Spector, J. Lemm and J. L.

Potter: Studies on pulmonary secretions: over-all chemical composition of pulmonary secretions from patients with cystic fibrosis, bronchiectasis, and laryngectomy. *Am. Rev. Respir. Dis. 88*:199, 1963.

125. May, R. J.: Non-mucoid factors affecting bacterial growth. In *Proceedings of the Fifth International Cystic Fibrosis Conference,* D. Lawson (Ed.). Cystic Fibrosis Research Trust, London, p. 169, 1969.
126. McCollum, A. T.: Cystic fibrosis: economic impact upon the family. *Am. J. Public Health 61*:1335, 1971.
127. McCollum, A. T. and L. E. Gibson: Family adaptation to the child with cystic fibrosis. *J. Pediatr. 77*:571, 1970.
128. McIntosh, R.: Cystic fibrosis of the pancreas in patients of over ten years of age. *Acta Paediatr. 43* (*Suppl. 100*):469, 1954.
129. Mearns, M. B.: Simple tests of ventilatory capacity in children with cystic fibrosis. *Arch. Dis. Child. 43*:528, 1968.

129A. Mearns, M. B.: Treatment and prevention of pulmonary complications of cystic fibrosis in infancy and childhood. *Arch. Dis. Child. 47*:5, 1972.

130. Mellins, R. B.: The site of airway obstruction in cystic fibrosis. *Pediatrics 44*:315, 1969.
131. Mellins, R. B., O. R. Levine, R. H. Ingram and A. P. Fishman: Obstructive disease of the airways in cystic fibrosis. *Pediatrics 41*:560, 1968.
132. Merritt, A. D., B. L. Hana, C. W. Todd Jr. and T. L. Myers: Incidence and mode of cystic fibrosis. *J. Lab. Clin. Med. 60*:998, 1962.

132A. Mike, E. M.: Practical dietary management of patients with the celiac syndrome. *Am. J. Clin. Nutr. 7*:463, 1959.

133. Morrow, P. E.: Experimental studies of inhaled materials. *Arch. Intern. Med. 126*:466, 1970.
134. Moss, A. J.: Cor pulmonale in cystic fibrosis. *Bibl. Paediatr. 86*:187, 1967.
135. Moss, A. J., W. H. Harper, R. R. Dooley, J. F. Murray and J. F. Mack: Cor pulmonale in cystic fibrosis of the pancreas. *J. Pediatr. 67*:797, 1965.

135A. Moss, A. J., S. Finkelstein, B. S. Crudup, G. A. Young, R. R. Dooley and A. B. Osher: Absorption of digoxin in cystic fibrosis. *J. Pediatr. 86*:295, 1975.

135B. Motoyama, E. K., L. E. Gibson and C. J. Zigas: Evaluation of mist tent therapy in cystic fibrosis using maximum expiratory flow volume curve. *Pediatrics 50*:299, 1972.

136. Munger, B. L., S. W. Brusilow and R. E. Cook: Electron microscopic study of eccrine sweat glands in patients with cystic fibrosis of the pancreas. *J. Pediatr. 59*: 497, 1961.
137. Murray, M. J. and A. P. Thal: The clinical significance of circulating pancreatic antibodies. *Ann. Intern. Med. 53*:548, 1960.
138. Noblett, H. R.: Treatment of uncomplicated meconium ileus by Gastrografin enema. *J. Pediatr. Surg. 4*:190, 1969.
139. Norman, A. P. and M. Hall: Nocturnal mist therapy in cystic fibrosis. *Practitioner 206*:786, 1971.
140. Olson, J. R. and D. K. Weaver: Congenital mesonephric defects in male infants with mucoviscidosis. *J. Clin. Pathol. 22*:725, 1969.
141. Oppenheimer, E. H. and J. R. Esterly: Observations on cystic fibrosis of the pancreas. *J. Pediatr. 75*:806, 1969.

141A. Ores, C. N., H. C. Neu and C. R. Denning: Allergic bronchopulmonary aspergillosis. Cystic Fibrosis Club Abstracts, 16th Annual Meetings, Denver, Colo., April 15, 1975.

142. Patterson, C. D. and G. H. Kamp: Retention of liquid aerosols in the lung. *Am. Rev. Respir. Dis. 95*:443, 1967.
143. Phelan, P. D., M. Gracey, H. E. Williams and M. Anderson: Ventilatory function in infants with cystic fibrosis. Physiological assessment of inhalation therapy. *Arch. Dis. Child. 44*:393, 1969.
145. Pittman, F. E., C. R. Denning and H. G. Barker: Albumin metabolism in cystic fibrosis. *Am. J. Dis. Child. 108*:360, 1964.
146. Polgar, G. and V. Promadhat: *Pulmonary Function Testing in Children.* W. B. Saunders Co., Philadelphia, p. 218, 1971.
147. Potter, J. L., L. W. Matthews, J. Lemm and S. Spector: Human pulmonary secretions in health and disease. *Ann. N.Y. Acad. Sci., 106*:692, 1963.
148. Potter, J. L., L. W. Matthews, S. Spector and J. Lemm: Studies on pulmonary secretions from patients with cystic fibrosis, bronchiectasis, and laryngectomy. *Am. Rev. Respir. Dis. 96*:83, 1967.
149. Potter, J. L., S. Spector, L. W. Matthews and J. Lemm: Studies on pulmonary secretions: nucleic acids in whole pulmonary secretions from patients with cystic fibrosis, bronchiectasis, and laryngectomy. *Am. Rev. Respir. Dis. 99*:909, 1969.
150. Quinlan, M. F., S. D. Salman, D. L. Swift, H. N. Wagner and D. F. Proctor: Measurement of mucociliary function in man. *Am. Rev. Respir. Dis. 99*:13, 1969.
151. Reas, H. W.: Use of n-acetylcysteine in the treatment of cystic fibrosis. *South. Med. J. 56*:1271, 1963.
152. Robson, A. M., S. Tateishi, J. R. Ingelfinger, D. B. Strominger and S. Klahr: Renal function in patients with cystic fibrosis. *J. Pediatr. 79*:42, 1971.

152A. Rodnan, J.: Personal communication.

153. Rosenbluth, M. and V. Chernick: Influence of mist tent therapy on sputum viscosity and water content in cystic fibrosis. *Arch. Dis. Child. 49*:606, 1974.
154. Rubin, L. S., G. J. Barbero, W. S. Chernick and M. S. Sibinga: Pupillary reactivity as a measure of

autonomic balance in cystic fibrosis. *J. Pediatr. 63*:1120, 1963.

155. Santulli, T. V.: Meconium ileus. In *Pediatric Surgery*, W. T. Mustard et al. (Eds.). Year Book Medical Publishers, Chicago, p. 851, 1969.
156. Santulli, T. V. and R. A. Amoury: Congenital anomalies of the gastrointestinal tract. *Pediatr. Clin. North Am. 14*:21, 1967.

156A. Schmoyer, I. R., S. P. Brooks and J. F. Fischer: Isolation and characterization of ciliary dyskinetic factor from cystic fibrosis serum. *Life Sci. 2*:1037, 1972.

156B. Siassi, B., A. J. Moss and R. R. Dooley: Clinical recognition of cor pulmonale in cystic fibrosis. *J. Pediatr. 78*:794, 1971.

157. Schulz, I. J. and G. Peter: Micropuncture studies of abnormality in sweat formation in cystic fibrosis. *Fed. Proc. 26*:287, 1967.
158. Sheffner, A. L., E. M. Medler, L. W. Jacobs and H. P. Sarett: In vitro reduction in viscosity of human tracheobronchial secretions by acetylcysteine. *Am. Rev. Respir. Dis., 90*:721, 1964.
159. Shwachman, H., L. L. Kulczycki and K. T. Khaw: Studies in cystic fibrosis. *Pediatrics 36*:689, 1965.

159A. Shwachman, H., E. Lebenthal and K. T. Khow: Recurrent acute pancreatitis in patients with cystic fibrosis with normal pancreatic enzymes. *Pediatrics 55*:86, 1975.

160. Slegers, J. F. G.: Cryoscopy of sweat glands in normal subjects and patients with cystic fibrosis. In *Third International Conference on Research and Pathogenesis of Cystic Fibrosis of the Pancreas.* Wickersham Printing Co., Lancaster, Pa., p. 119, 1964.
161. Spicer, S. S. cited by P. A. di Sant'Agnese and R. C. Talamo: Pathogenesis and physiopathology of cystic fibrosis of the pancreas. *N. Engl. J. Med. 277*:1287, 1967.
162. Spock, A.: Personal communication.
163. Spock, A., H. M. C. Heick, H. Cress and W. S. Logan: Abnormal serum factor in patients with cystic fibrosis of the pancreas. *Pediatr. Res. 1*:173, 1967.
164. Stamm, S. J. and J. Docter: Chest measurements as an aid in the diagnosis of cystic fibrosis. *Dis. Chest 47*:98, 1965.
165. Stein, A. A., F. C. Manlapas, K. F. Soike and P. R. Patterson: Specific isoantibodies in cystic fibrosis. *J. Pediatr. 65*:495, 1964.

165A. Stowe, S. M., T. F. Boat, H. Mendelsohn, R. C. Stern, A. S. Tucker, C. F. Doershuk and L. W. Matthews: Open thoracotomy for pneumothorax in cystic fibrosis. *Am. Rev. Respir. Dis. 111*:611, 1975.

166. Strober, W., G. Peter and R. H. Schwartz: Albumin metabolism in cystic fibrosis. *Pediatrics 43*:416, 1969.
167. Sturgess, J. and L. Reid: New pattern of sputum viscosity. In *Proceedings of the Fifth International Cystic Fibrosis Conference,* D. Lawson (Ed.). London, Cystic Fibrosis Research Trust, p. 368, 1969.
168. Swenson, O.: *Pediatric Surgery* (3rd ed.). Appleton-Century-Crofts, New York, p. 679, 1969.
169. Symchych, P. S.: Pulmonary hypertension in cystic fibrosis: descriptive and morphometric analysis of the pulmonary vasculature. *Arch. Pathol. 92*:409, 1971.
170. Thomaidis, T. S. and J. B. Arey: Intestinal lesions in cystic fibrosis of the pancreas. *J. Pediatr. 63*:444, 1963.
171. Tropauer, A., M. N. Franz and V. W. Dilgard: Psychological aspects of the care of children with cystic fibrosis. *Am. J. Dis. Child. 119*:424, 1970.
172. Tyson, K. R. T., S. R. Schuster and H. Shwachman: Portal hypertension in cystic fibrosis. *J. Pediatr. Surg. 3*:271, 1968.
173. Underwood, B. A. and C. R. Denning: Blood and liver concentrations of vitamins A & E in children with cystic fibrosis of the pancreas. *Pediatr. Res. 6*:26, 1972.
174. Wagget, J., D. G. Johnson, P. Berne and H. C. Bishop: The nonoperative treatment of meconium ileus by Gastrografin enema. *J. Pediatr. 77*:407, 1970.
175. Waring, W. W., C. H. Brunt and B. C. Hilman: Mucoid impaction of the bronchi in cystic fibrosis. *Pediatrics 39*:166, 1967.
176. Waring, W. W. and F. L. Seleny: Mist tent effects on ventilatory mechanics and other factors in cystic fibrosis (Abstract). *Pediatr. Res. 6*:431, 1972.
177. Waring, W. W., E. S. Golladay, S. E. Acker and B. C. Hilman: Shape and size of the thorax in children with chronic lung disease. *South. Med. J. 58*:1582, 1965.
178. Warwick, W.: Vitamin administration. In *Guide to Drug Therapy in Patients with Cystic Fibrosis,* N. N. Huang (Ed.). National Cystic Fibrosis Research Foundation, Atlanta, Ga., p. 48, 1972.
179. Warwick, W. J. and S. Monson: Life table studies of mortality. *Bibl. Pediatr. 86*:353, 1967.
180. Warwick, W. J. and R. E. Pogue: Computer studies in cystic fibrosis. In *Proceedings of the Fifth International Cystic Fibrosis Conference,* D. Lawson (Ed.). Cystic Fibrosis Research Trust, London, p. 320, 1969.

180A. Warwick, W. J., R. E. Pogue, H. U. Gerber and C. J. Nesbitt: Survival patterns in cystic fibrosis. *J. Chronic Dis. 28*:609, 1975.

181. West, J. R., S. M. Levin and P. A. di Sant'Agnese: Pulmonary function in cystic fibrosis of the pancreas. *Pediatrics 13*:155, 1954.

181A. Whitman, V., R. C. Stern, P. Bellet, C. F.

Dorshuk, J. Liebman, T. F. Boat, G. Borkat and L. W. Matthews: Studies on cor pulmonale in cystic fibrosis: I. Effects of diuresis. *Pediatrics 55*:83, 1975.

182. Wiesmann, V. N., T. F. Boat and P. A. di Sant'Agnese: Sodium concentration in unstimulated parotid saliva and on oral mucosa in normal subjects and in patients with cystic fibrosis. *J. Pediatr. 76*:444, 1970.

183. Williams, T. J.: Localization of material aerosolized by ultrasonic nebulizer as determined by a colorimetric method. *Proceedings of First Conference on Clinical Applications of the Ultrasonic Nebulizer 25*:25, 1966.

183A. Wilson, G. B., T. L. John and J. R. Fonseca: Demonstration of serum protein differences in cystic fibrosis by isoelectric focusing in thin-layer acrylamide gels. *Clin. Chim. Acta 49*:79, 1973.

184. Wolfsdorf, J., D. L. Swift and M. E. Avery: Mist therapy reconsidered; an evaluation of the respiratory deposition of labelled water aerosols produced by jet and ultrasonic nebulizers. *Pediatrics 43*:799, 1969.

185. Wright, S. W. and N. E. Morton: Genetic studies on cystic fibrosis in Hawaii. *Am. J. Hum. Genet. 20*:157, 1968.

186. Zapletal, A., E. K. Motoyama, L. E. Gibson and A. Bouhuys: Pulmonary mechanics in asthma and cystic fibrosis. *Pediatrics 48*:64, 1971.

188. Zelkowitz, P. S. and S. T. Giammona: Cystic fibrosis: pulmonary studies in children, adolescents, and young adults. *Am. J. Dis. Child. 117*:543, 1969.

189. Zuelzer, W. W. and W. A. Newton: Pathogenesis of fibrocystic disease of the pancreas. *Pediatrics 4*:53, 1949.

Pneumonia Caused by Bacteria, Mycoplasmata, Viruses, and Pneumocystis

JOHN C. RIBBLE AND STANLEY E. READE

12

Pneumonia, for the purposes of this discussion, is defined as a microbial disease of the lung, involving the alveoli and/or the interstitial supporting pulmonary tissue. Pneumonias caused by bacteria, mycoplasmata, viruses, and pneumocystis are discussed in this chapter. Mycobacterial infections are presented in Chapter 13, and upper airway diseases are detailed in Chapters 8 and 9.

Incidence

The nationwide incidence of pneumonia is difficult to assess inasmuch as it is not a reportable disease in the United States. Information derived from two family studies in Cleveland[9] and in New York,[13] and from a study of children 2 to 10 years old in Seattle,[15] place the incidence of pneumonia as 0.1 to 0.3 cases per person per year. From 1955 to 1959, pneumonia was diagnosed at a rate of 823 cases per 100,000 patient visits per year to the Pediatrics Outpatient Department of a large urban hospital.[32]

Mortality figures (1966) indicate that fatal "influenza and pneumonia" accounted for 10.9 deaths per 100,000 population of children 1 to 4 years of age and 2 per 100,000 of those 5 to 14 years of age.[40]

Etiology

Pneumonia can be caused by viruses, rickettsiae, mycoplasmata, bacteria, fungi, and parasites. Identification of the microbes responsible for pneumonia in an individual patient can be difficult, and the results of diagnostic tests may be equivocal. The only sure way to establish the cause of pneumonia is to examine the fluid or tissue removed directly from the infected lung. In the past several years, interest has been revived in the use of lung puncture and aspiration to diagnose pneumonia.[22] This technique may be attended by serious complications, fortunately rare, such as pneumothorax, thoracic hemorrhage, and introduction or spread of infection. Therefore, it should be used only when serious pneumonia is present and its cause is uncertain, and when treatment is having no effect on the disease. These circumstances arise most often in the child with immunodeficiency or immunosuppression. The technique consists of introduction of a needle into the parenchyma of the lung, aspiration of fluid, maintenance of suction, and withdrawal of the needle.

Indirect measures for diagnosis include cultures of secretions of the nose and throat and of sputum. The usual culture of the nose and throat is not a useful diagnostic method inasmuch as bacteria capable of causing pneumonia are found in the upper airway secretions of a large percentage of healthy children. Examination of expectorated sputum is of more diagnostic value but frequently it is contaminated with saliva, making it difficult or nearly impossible to obtain adequate specimens from infants and young children.

Transtracheal intubation has been suggested for the recovery of sputum from the depths of the trachea where it is unlikely to be contaminated with pharyngeal secretions.[34] With precautions to maintain sterility, the needle is inserted through the cricothyroid membrane into the tracheal lumen. A catheter is passed through the needle, the needle removed, and the catheter passed down into the trachea. A small amount of saline solution is injected and then aspirated. This procedure offers a greater likelihood of obtaining a pathogen and less chance of contamination with microbes unrelated to the pneumonia. In one series, a single organism was obtained from material removed by transtracheal aspiration in 75% of the specimens—a sharp contrast to the many organisms that are routinely identified in expectorated sputum.

Realizing the difficulties in making a precise etiologic diagnosis, it is reasonable to examine the evidence that certain agents are responsible for pneumonia. The evidence that certain viruses can cause pneumonia comes mainly from studies that compare the frequency of virus isolation from respiratory secretions of children with pneumonia to the frequency of virus isolation from age-matched subjects with no respiratory illness. Table 12-1 summarizes three studies and indicates that "respiratory viruses" could be isolated from the secretions of about 30% of infants and children with pneumonia, but from only 4 to 7% of control subjects, indicating that these viruses were causing the disease. [23,24] The specific viruses recovered from patients with pneumonia are summarized in Table 12-2, which includes data from four separate studies.[6,23,24] Respiratory syncytial viruses, isolated most frequently from infants under 1 year of age, were found in 10 to 15% of patients with pneumonia, and parainfluenza viruses from 5 to 7%. In more than 50% of children with pneumonia, no viral agents were isolated nor was there serologic evidence of infection with any of the viruses usually associated with respiratory tract infection.

Mycoplasma organisms have been shown to be the cause of pneumonia by similar types of studies. *M. pneumoniae* strains were iso-

TABLE 12-1. Isolation from Upper Airway of Respiratory Viruses (Respiratory Syncytial, Parainfluenza, Influenza, Adenoviruses, and Rhinoviruses) and Bacteria from Children with Pneumonia Compared to Isolations from Control Children with No Respiratory Illness

Study	Respiratory Viruses		Pneumococci		H. influenzae		Mycoplasma	
	Pn*	C†	Pn	C	Pn	C	Pn	C
1[8]	20.6‡	3.9	39.6	27.5	8.2	7.8	12.6	2.0
2[8]	31.1	5.5	65.3	39.6	25.0	4.4	5.1	0
3[9]	33.3	6.9	53.4	40.0	3.4	1.7	—	—

* Children with pneumonia
† Controls
‡ Percent of children yielding agent

lated from 5 to 15% of children with pneumonia (most frequently from those 5 to 9 years of age) and could be recovered in only 2% or less of control subjects.

What is the evidence that certain bacteria may cause pneumonia? Cultures of blood and empyema fluid, of material aspirated from involved lung, and of pulmonary tissue obtained at autopsy have clearly identified pneumococci, staphylococci, *H. influenzae,* streptococci, and Klebsiella species as important causes of pneumonia. Population studies (Table 12-1) have not shown striking differences in the recovery of these organisms from respiratory secretions of patients with pneumonia as compared to healthy children.

Host Defenses and General Pathology

Except for the first few hours of life, infectious microbes are always present in the upper respiratory tract. Protection from infection with these agents is afforded by several processes. Most of them have been identified in adults and older children, and the investigation of defense mechanisms in infants is not complete.

The properly functioning epiglottis serves as a mechanical barrier to inhalation of particulate and liquid material. A forceful expulsion or coughing up of extraneous substances occurs if they gain access to the respiratory

TABLE 12-2. Recovery of "Respiratory" Viruses from Children with Pneumonia Compared to Recovery from Control Children with No Illness

Study	RSV		Parainfluenza		Influenza		Adenovirus		Rhinovirus	
	Pn*	C†	Pn	C	Pn	C	Pn	C	Pn	C
1[10]	9.5‡	0	2.4	0	0	0	5.5	3.9	4.4	1.7
2[8]	9.9	3.9	6.5	0	—	—	3.8	0	—	—
3[8]	14.9	1.1	5.2	0	—	—	6.3	4.4	—	—
4[9]	13.3	0	6.7	1.5	5.5	0.8	4.4	1.5	2.2	3.1

* Children with pneumonia
† Controls
‡ Percent of children yielding agent

tract. Intubation and assisted ventilation can force infected particles past the usual protective barriers, and weakness or sedation can diminish the effectiveness of the cough.

Small particles or droplets, some containing infectious agents, can descend freely past the epiglottis along with the inspired air, and unless they are irritating, they do not trigger the expulsion reflex. Nevertheless, these tiny particles can be removed from the respiratory system by the cilia-mucus system. The small hairlike appendages induce the mucus lining the airways to flow in one direction—toward the mouth. The particles in the escalating stream of mucus are carried to the upper tract where they are expelled, expectorated, or swallowed. Cilia can be detected in human fetuses between the thirteenth and twentieth weeks of gestation, but their functional capacity during early life is not known. The ciliated cells may be destroyed or their function impaired during the course of viral respiratory infections, thus predisposing to bacterial superinfection of the lower tract.

If foreign material reaches the alveoli of the lung, it may be engulfed by the macrophages lining the alveoli. Furthermore, extraneous matter in the alveoli calls forth granulocytes from the circulating blood, and under optimal circumstances these cells ingest and destroy foreign invaders. Phagocytosis and killing of bacteria result from the interaction of microorganisms, serum opsonins, complement, and granulocytes. The opsonins for many gram-positive bacteria, among them pneumococci, staphylococci, and streptococci, are mainly IgG whereas the opsonins for *E. coli* and several other gram-negative bacteria are, for the most part, IgM. Phagocytosis and killing of many gram-positive bacteria can be demonstrated in vitro when blood from full-term infants is tested. The full-term infants' blood has an adequate number of active granulocytes and a sufficient concentration of IgG opsonins obtained from the mother by transfer across the placenta. Destruction of gram-negative bacteria by the blood of full-term infants is not optimal, not because of any abnormality of their granulocytes but because the necessary IgM opsonins are not usually transferred to the infant. Premature babies may have impaired phagocytosis of both gram-positive and gram-negative bacteria because of deficiencies in both IgG and IgM. The IgG deficiency in prematures can be explained by noting that the major portion of these globulins cross the placenta late in gestation. Fetuses of less than 20 weeks have less than 100 mg/ml IgG; at 30 weeks the level is about 400. The IgG levels increase from 600 to 700 at the thirty-fifth week of gestation to the normal adult level of 1200 mg/ml at the time of birth.

Inflammatory reactions may occur in three areas of the lung: the alveoli, the walls of the airways, and the interstitial and perivascular spaces of the parenchyma. Involvement of each of these sites results in a distinctive roentgenographic pattern in older children and adults. (In infants it is rare to see inflammation confined to only one of these areas.)

Pneumococci, for example, incite an alveolar inflammatory exudate that fills the air spaces without resulting in any loss of their volume. The fluid in the alveoli has the roentgenographic density of water and thus highlights the air in the bronchi and bronchioles, producing an "air bronchogram." The exudate can extend centripetally to adjacent alveoli through the canals of Lambert and pores of Cohn and may, in this way, cross over the boundaries of the anatomic segments of the lung—indeed, whole lobes may be involved by the inflammatory process.

Staphylococci usually infect the bronchial walls and the tissue surrounding them. This infection leads to densities of some individual lobular segments interspersed among uninvolved ones and results in the patchy roentgenographic picture known as bronchopneumonia.

Viruses usually affect the interstitial spaces of the lung parenchyma resulting in a "reticulonodular" pattern representing the swollen supporting structures of the lung. The inflammation usually spreads to some of the alveoli, producing a stippling of densities in addition to the reticular pattern. Involvement of the perivascular spaces leads to blurring of the usual sharp margins of the blood vessels that can be seen in the roentgenogram radiating from the hilum, and to thickening of the septa between the lobules.

Bacterial Pneumonias

PNEUMOCOCCUS (Fig. 12-1)

S. pneumoniae (pneumococci) are gram-positive diplococci that grow well on blood agar with characteristic green hemolysis. Pneumococci can be typed by using antiserum prepared against specific capsular polysaccharides in the quellung or capsular-swelling reaction. Typing can be useful for rapid identification of pneumococci in sputum or empyema fluid and for epidemiologic purposes. In addition, some clinical presentations are related to the serologic types of the infecting pneumococcal organisms. For instance, type 3 causes the most serious illnesses, including lung abscesses that are not consequences of infection with other serotypes. Type 14 infections may result in hemolytic anemias as a result of antibody produced against the type 14 polysaccharide, which cross-reacts with the blood group A antigen.

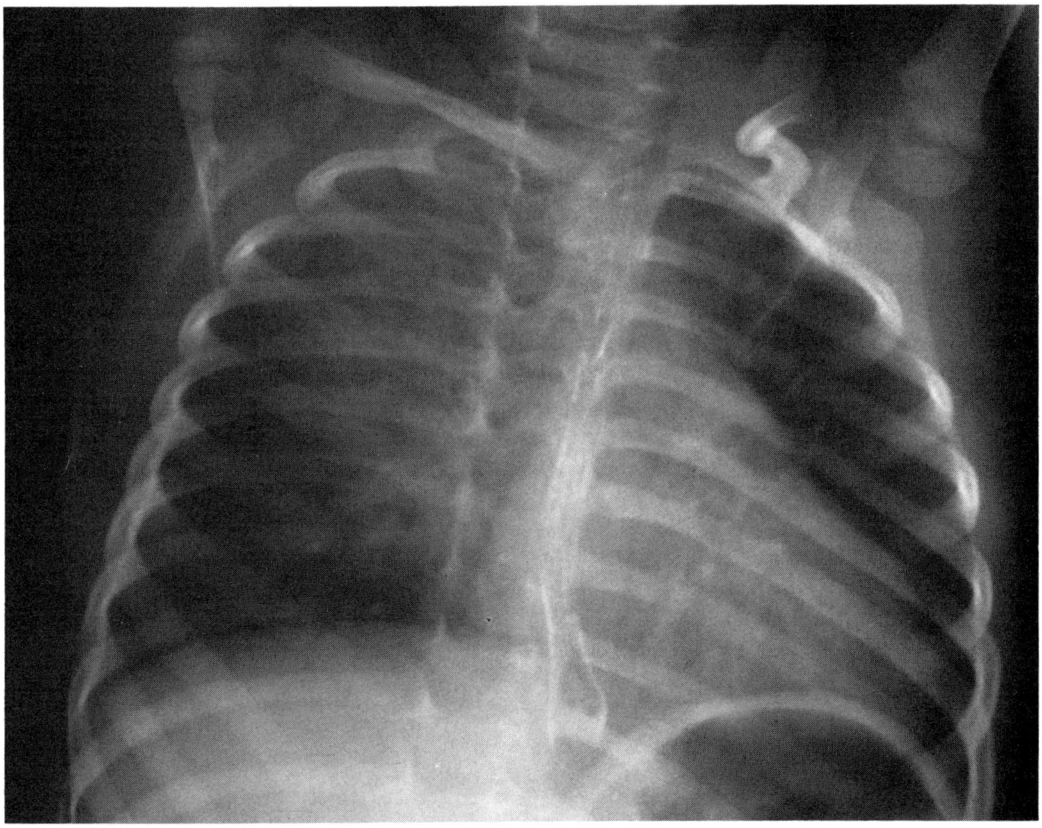

FIG. 12-1. Pneumococcal pneumonia showing consolidation of right upper lobe.

Wood and his associates have studied pneumococcal pneumonia in experimental animals and have examined the progress of the disease from its inception to resolution.[42] They demonstrated that, when infection begins in a bronchial segment, the lesion spreads centrifugally carrying pneumococci in edema fluid. Then, red cells and white cells enter and fill the alveoli leading to consolidation, followed by the appearance of macrophages, which characterize the stage of resolution and subsiding inflammation. Pneumococci may be killed by granulocytes in the process of phagocytosis. Those bacteria that are not destroyed in the lungs are carried to the regional lymph nodes via lymphatics where further removal takes place. If these defenses are not completely successful, bacteria can then enter the blood via the thoracic duct, leading to possible dissemination of pneumococci to extrapulmonary sites.

Pneumococcal pneumonia frequently follows a mild upper respiratory tract infection. After a day or two of minor symptoms such as a stuffy nose and low-grade fever, the child develops a temperature greater than 38.5° C, fast breathing with retractions, cough, and occasionally pleuritic chest pain. Vomiting, abdominal pain, distention, and ileus may occur and can mimic an acute abdomen. A single chill may introduce the severe stage of the illness and is thought to result from the entrance of bacteria into the blood. The physical signs depend upon the distribution and the stage of development of the pneumonia. Typical findings of consolidation may be present as well as signs of pleural fluid. In patients with patchy involvement, the signs of consolidation are absent and there may be widely scattered rales. Physical signs are hard to elicit in infants and they should always be confirmed by radiography.

In the untreated disease, fever and signs of serious illness persist for 4 to 7 days. Patients who receive appropriate antibacterial therapy usually become afebrile within 12 to 24 hours, and persistence of fever for longer periods strongly suggests the presence of a complication of pneumococcal pneumonia such as an undrained empyema.

The difficulties in establishing a precise diagnosis of pneumococcal pneumonia are outlined in the section on Etiology. Positive blood cultures or isolation of pneumococci from pleural fluid or from directly aspirated lung fluid are the only certain ways of establishing the diagnosis.

Uncomplicated pneumococcal pneumonia can be successfully treated by the administration of procaine penicillin—300,000 units twice a day intramuscularly. Oral penicillin should not be relied upon for the treatment of pneumonia in a seriously ill child. Ampicillin is effective against pneumococci as well as *H. influenzae,* and it is commonly used to treat children with presumed bacterial pneumonia when the cause is uncertain. Penicillinase-resistant penicillins are also active against pneumococci, and if they are being used to treat suspected staphylococcal infection, it is not necessary to add another agent to treat possible pneumococcal disease. Cephalosporin derivatives or erythromycin can be used in patients with a history of penicillin allergy. Antibiotic therapy should be continued for 5 to 10 days in patients with uncomplicated pneumococcal pneumonia. If complications are present, larger doses of penicillin are recommended; 200,000 units/kg/day intravenously is adequate to treat pneumococcal meningitis and persistent infection in the pleural space, joints, or other organs. Antibiotic therapy alone is not adequate to cure empyemas, which must be drained through either a needle or small chest tube. More extensive or prolonged drainage is rarely necessary.

Example

A 5-month-old girl with Down's syndrome was admitted because of tachypnea and dyspnea. Two days before admission she had a slight cough, runny nose, and decreased appetite, but no fever. On the day before admission, she looked blue and had wheezing respirations. At the time of admission, her temperature was 37.2° C and the examination of her lungs was normal. A chest roentgenogram showed an enlarged heart, a prominent pulmonary artery, and overcirculated but not infiltrated lung fields. She was not treated with antibiotics. Over the next 2 days she developed rhonchi and rales in the right lung field and had mild intercostal retraction. On the third hospital day she developed fever as high as 39° C, a white count of 34,000, and a perihilar infiltrate, which increased over the next 24 hours. Blood, nose, and throat cultures grew *S. pneumoniae* type 4.

She was treated with intramuscular penicillin (50,000 units/kg/day), and she became afebrile and the infiltrates resolved. The patient's cardiac lesion was identified as a complete atrioventricular canal with a large left-to-right shunt. This case illustrates the evolution of pneumococcal pneumonia from the preceding upper respiratory infection, which lasted for about 5 days, followed by the development of fever, pulmonary infiltrate leukocytosis, and blood cultures positive for pneumococci. Prompt clinical improvement ensued after the beginning of penicillin treatment.

PRIMARY STAPHYLOCOCCUS (Fig. 12-2)

Primary staphylococcal pneumonia is related to aspiration of infected material and the formation of one or a few localized areas of pulmonary disease. Secondary staphylococcal pneumonia is a complication of bacteremia and is characterized by many small lesions scattered throughout both lungs.

Staphylococci are gram-positive cocci that grow readily in most laboratory culture media. Two species are responsible for human disease. *S. aureus,* identified by its production of coagulase and its ability to ferment certain sugars, is the more important pathogen. *S. epidermidis* is coagulase-negative and is less frequently implicated in disease. This strain may cause infection of foreign bodies inserted into the head for the relief of hydrocephalus or appliances such as prosthetic heart valves. *S. aureus* strains can be grouped and typed serologically, but usually bacteriophage typing is used to categorize these bacteria. Most of the nursery epidemics of the late 1950's and early 1960's were due to staphylococci lysed by phages 80 and 81 or by the group 1 phages 29, 52, and 52A. During epidemic periods most cases of staphylo-

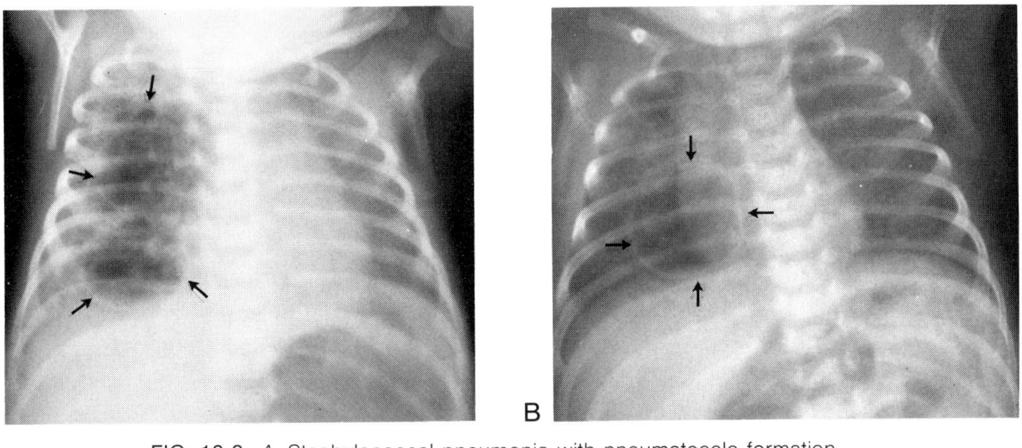

A B

FIG. 12-2. *A*, Staphylococcal pneumonia with pneumatocele formation. *B*, Coalescence of cysts with reduction in size during 10-day interval.

coccal pneumonia are due to the prevalent epidemic strains; however, staphylococci of any phage type or "non-typable" strains may cause pneumonia. *S. epidermidis* rarely, if ever, causes pulmonary disease.

S. aureus strains produce a number of toxins and enzymes that induce death of experimental animals, tissue necrosis, lysis of red cells, inactivation of white blood cells, destruction of penicillin, and activation of fibrinolytic systems. There is, however, no direct correlation between the production of these substances and the pathogenicity of a given strain of *S. aureus.*

Primary staphylococcal pneumonia is seen most frequently in infants under the age of 6 months and is due to infection acquired during residence in the newborn nursery, even though the disease does not appear until the infant is several weeks old. Staphylococcal infection in the nursery is spread from carriers and from infected babies to susceptible infants by direct contact and possibly via the air. Only a few staphylococci (around 10 bacteria) are capable of inducing colonization of a newborn infant. Because of the low infectious dose, it is very difficult to prevent the spread of staphylococci by altering the environment.

Staphylococcal pneumonia in infants and children has decreased in frequency since the period when epidemics were common. At the Hospital for Sick Children in Toronto, the average number of cases from 1959 to 1963 was 35 a year, but in 1969 only 3 patients with staphylococcal pneumonia were seen.[39] The reasons for the decline in incidence are not known. The reduction is perhaps related to the cyclic nature of epidemics of staphylococcal disease and to the use of penicillinase-resistant penicillins for treatment of early staphylococcal infections, thus preventing more serious diseases like pneumonia.

Staphylococci are aspirated and infect the bronchi with the production of pus and changes in the mucosa. The pulmonary involvement follows the distribution of affected bronchi and involves lobules or segments. The infected alveoli contain myriads of bacteria, edema fluid, and pus cells. As the infection progresses, it destroys the walls of the alveoli with the formation of air-filled cavities, pneumatoceles, which may be under pressure and occasionally may rupture with the production of pyopneumothorax. The accumulation of air in the pneumatocele results from a valve-type bronchial obstruction that allows entry of air into the cavity but impedes its egress. In infants and small children, primary staphylococcal pneumonia is frequently accompanied by infection of the pleural space and a significant collection of empyema fluid.

The onset may be insidious or fulminant. Widespread involvement of the lungs may be discovered by physical examination or by roentgenogram after a few days of what has been regarded as a mild upper respiratory tract infection. High temperature, tachypnea, labored and grunting respirations, abdominal distention, and vomiting may supervene and call attention to the severity of the disease. Physical examination may not be of great value in making the diagnosis, but in older children the signs of pleural fluid may be detected. The white blood cell count is usually elevated with young cell forms, but the count may be below normal in patients with overwhelming disease. Most patients with staphylococcal pneumonia have *S. aureus* in their anterior nares or throats and blood cultures are positive in 30 to 40%. Empyema fluid contains white blood cells and easily visible staphylococci if prolonged antibiotic therapy has not preceded the removal of the fluid.

The clinical picture and the radiographic findings are characteristic, and the diagnosis is seldom in doubt. Streptococcal pneumonia with empyema may resemble staphylococcal pneumonia including even the production of pneumatoceles. The diagnosis can be established by culture. Aspiration pneumonia with lung abscesses may occasionally mimic staphylococcal pneumonia, but the clinical setting and the culture findings should distinguish the two conditions. Pneumococcal pneumonia may be accompanied by pleural fluid but lung destruction is uncommon.

Before the availability of penicillinase-resistant penicillin, the therapy for staphylococcal pneumonia consisted of administration of a variety of antibiotics and removal of empyema fluid by continuous chest tube drainage or by rib resection with open drainage. Hospitalization was frequently prolonged for weeks or months, and the mortality rate was between 12 and 50%. Since the availability of better antistaphylococcal antibiotics, the duration of the course of treatment for staphylococcal pneumonia has been shortened and the need for extensive surgical drainage of empyemas has diminished. Stiles et al. recommend that drainage be carried out by needle aspiration or occasionally by chest tube left in place for no more than 24 hours.[37] They feel that open drainage is almost never indicated. Antibiotic treatment should consist of methicillin (150 to 200 mg/kg/day intravenously or intramuscularly), and it should be administered every 4 hours. Other penicillinase-resistant penicillins or cephalosporin derivatives may also be used. The duration of therapy depends upon the response to therapy. The treatment should continue until the patient is afebrile and pulmonary infiltrates have resolved. It is not necessary to continue treatment just because pneumatoceles persist inasmuch as they may remain for several weeks or months with no symptoms and resolve without additional antibacterial therapy.

Example

A 4-month-old boy entered the hospital because of fever for 5 days and labored respirations for 1 day. Three weeks before admission he had a small post-auricular abscess due to *S. aureus,* which was incised and drained, but no antibiotic therapy had been given.

The baby had a temperature of 39.8° C and grunting respirations of 60 per minute. At the left base of the lung posteriorly there were decreased breath sounds and dullness to percussion. The radiograph of the chest indicated pleural effusion and pneumatoceles. The pleural fluid was purulent and contained many staphylococci. The white blood count was 36,000 per cubic millimeter. The patient was treated with methicillin (150 mg/kg/day) for 3 weeks; in addition, a small chest tube was inserted and remained in place for 1 week. The patient became afebrile within 3 days, and the lungs showed continued improvement even though the pneumatoceles persisted for several months.

HEMOPHILUS INFLUENZAE

H. influenzae is a pleomorphic gram-negative coccobacillus that grows best on chocolate agar in environments with high CO_2 concentration. The organisms can be categorized by the antigenicity of their polysaccharide capsules as types a, b, c, d, e, or f. Nearly all serious infections with Hemophilus species are due to type b strains.

Serious *H. influenzae* infections are seen primarily in children under the age of 5, but serious infections have occurred in older children and adults; these infections include meningitis, arthritis, bacteremia, and pneumonia. Proven *H. influenzae* pneumonia is a rarity. A review of 991 cases of pneumonia and empyema cited that none was due to Hemophilus. In other large series, single examples of pneumonia and empyema have been due to this organism.[37]

It is probable that most cases of *H. influenzae* pneumonia are the result of descending infection from the upper airways. Inflammatory response is provoked, with various degrees of pulmonary involvement. It is frequently suggested that Hemophilus causes patchy widespread bronchopneumonia, but the best documented cases have demonstrated lobar consolidation.[28]

Patients with lobar pneumonia due to Hemophilus are seriously ill. The disease is frequently preceded by an upper respiratory infection, and then 1 to 7 days later the onset of high fever, labored respirations, and vomiting. The physical examination indicates consolidation and occasionally the presence of pleural fluid. Usually leukocytosis is greater than 25,000. Hemophilus can be cultured from the blood and is usually present in empyema fluid before antimicrobial therapy is begun. If the organisms are abundant in pleural fluid, a direct quellung reaction with type b antiserum can lead to prompt diagnosis.

Therapy consists of general care of the patient and administration of appropriate antibiotics and needle drainage of empyema, if present. Ampicillin (200 mg/kg/day intravenously) given every 4 hours constitutes proper antimicrobial therapy. Chloramphenicol can be used if the patient has an allergy to ampicillin or if the strain is resistant to ampicillin. The course of the pneumonia is usually ameliorated by appropriate therapy and defervescence is prompt. Pulmonary changes may resolve more slowly; they may be present for 2 weeks or longer.

PNEUMONIA OF THE NEWBORN

This condition may be acquired during intrauterine life, during the course of or just before delivery, or shortly after birth. Pneumonia acquired in utero several days or more prior to delivery is recognized mainly in stillborn infants, inasmuch as the disease is frequently lethal to the fetus. Obstetric complications, prolonged rupture of the membranes, and intrauterine asphyxia predispose to this condition, which may result from aspiration of infected amniotic fluid or be caused by seeding of microorganisms from an infected placenta or from the blood of a mother with bacteremia. Contamination of the respiratory tract just before, or at the time of, delivery is usually due to aspiration of infected material.

The organisms identified in newborn infants with pneumonia acquired shortly before, or at the time of, delivery are: streptococci (not group A), *E. coli,* and other gram-negative bacteria. It is frequently difficult to be certain that the inflammation in the lungs results from the action of the microorganisms rather than from the irritation caused by meconium or other aspirated debris. Pneumonia acquired several days after delivery most often results from acquisition of organisms from other infants or attendants in the nursery environment.

Recent studies have elucidated the picture of pneumonia in newborn infants infected with group B streptococci,[1] and this specific illness is discussed more fully. Group B streptococci can be identified by their ability to grow in media containing sodium hippurate and more definitively by the detection of the group B antigen in the streptococcal cell walls by a precipitin test. They can be further subdivided into types I (and subtypes), II, and III. These organisms are found in the birth canal of more than 10% of parturient women and have become increasingly recognized as the cause of perinatal disease in both infants and mothers. Several forms of illness in the neonate result from infections with these bacteria, but among the most severe is the pneumonia and bacteremic disease that occurs in newborn infants in the first few hours of life.

This form of pneumonia in the young neonate is predominantly a disease of premature infants and commonly follows prolonged rupture of the membranes. The clinical picture is similar to that of the respiratory distress syndrome (RDS), with grunting and retraction evident before 3 hours of life. Significant apnea requiring stimulation and resuscitation is frequently present. Greyness, hypotension, and other signs of shock appear early in the course. The infants with group B streptococcal pneumonia require respiratory assistance although Ablow et al. indicate that the compliance of the lung is greater than in infants suffering from RDS.[1] The outstanding feature of the clinical illness is its rapidly lethal course, with death occurring in most instances within 24 to 36 hours.

The radiographs of the chest may show segmental or lobar involvement, or they may resemble those seen in RDS—diffuse granular infiltrates and the presence of air bronchograms. Lungs examined post mortem show some degree of atelectasis, interstitial hemorrhage, and hyaline membranes containing streptococci. This form of pneumonia is frequently lethal even if penicillin (to which group B streptococci are quite sensitive) is administered in the first few hours of life. The failure of therapy has stimulated interest in means of prevention of the illness, such as treatment of mothers carrying group B streptococci shortly before delivery. The best time for and form of prophylaxis remain to be determined.

GROUP A STREPTOCOCCUS

Pneumonia caused by group A streptococci occurred in infants, children, and adults in the pre-antibiotic era, usually as a complication of influenza or measles, as a double infection with pneumococci, or superimposed on acute viral upper respiratory infections. It also occurred in patients with chronic lung disorders such as asthma, bronchiectasis, abscess, tuberculosis, or cystic disease. Occasionally, streptococcal pneumonia was not preceded by any illness. For instance, 10 of 55 patients reported in 1941 had streptococcal pneumonia that was considered "primary."[20]

Since the introduction of antimicrobial drugs, streptococcal pneumonia has been a rare disease, and it is difficult to generalize about its present clinical forms. In an epidemic in New England in 1958, six of 174 patients with proven group A streptococcal infections had pneumonia.[3] In two patients, pneumonia followed insertion of a tracheostomy, and in two others it was preceded by streptococcal pharyngitis. The patients had a variety of roentgenographic changes ranging from accentuation of bronchial markings to extensive bronchopneumonia, segmental or lobar consolidation, and pneumatoceles. One patient had findings suggestive of multiple pulmonary infarctions.

The onset of streptococcal pneumonia is abrupt. The diagnosis is made by identifying group A streptococci in sputum, blood, or empyema fluid. Streptococcal pneumonia should be treated with penicillin (200,000 units/kg/day) given parenterally. Empyemas may require surgical drainage.

KLEBSIELLA

K. pneumoniae is primarily a disease of adults, notably old alcoholics, but it has been well documented in infants and children.[11,25,38] Klebsiella is classified in the Klebsiella-Aerobacter-Serratia group of organisms and belongs to the family Enterobacteriaceae. The organisms are gram-negative, nonmotile rods with capsules. More than 70 different types have been identified on the basis of the polysaccharide capsular antigens. Infection of the lung with Klebsiella organisms results in alveolar exudate, in congestion of alveolar walls, and eventually in necrosis of lung tissue with abscess and pneumatocele formation.

The clinical picture of Klebsiella infection in infants is hard to characterize. In one well-documented case of a 7-week-old premature infant, coryza, anorexia, somnolence, and dyspnea began 2 days before admission to the hospital.[29] The baby, when seen at the hospital, was grey and grunting with rales; the roentgenographic picture showed "bronchopneumonia with air bronchograms." Tracheal secretions contained many gram-negative rods, later identified as Klebsiella. The baby died 41 hours after admission, and the lungs showed bronchopneumonia with necrosis of alveolar septae. Although the lungs grew Klebsiella in pure culture, bacteria were not seen in microscopic sections. Others have reported pneumatoceles in infants in association with well-documented *K. pneumoniae.*

As in other forms of pneumonia, it is imperative to base the diagnosis of Klebsiella infection upon the detection of causative organisms in blood or secretions removed directly from the lung. Klebsiella organisms are not part of the normal flora of the upper respiratory tract in the general population, but they grow there in abundance in many patients who have been treated with antimicrobial drugs.

In vitro studies indicate that most strains of Klebsiella are susceptible to cephalothin, cefazolin, chloramphenicol, colistin, gentamicin, kanamycin, polymyxin b, and tobramycin, although this susceptibility may vary depending upon time and geographic location. Appropriate therapy includes cephalothin and gentamicin pending results of sensitivity testing.

Mycoplasma Pneumonia

The condition known for several years as primary atypical pneumonia, then Eaton's agent pneumonia, has now been named on the basis of the causative organism.

In 1962, Chanock, Hayflick, and Barile were able to cultivate the organism in artificial media, and they found that it was a Mycoplasma, subsequently termed *Mycoplasma pneumoniae.*[5] The agent is a small bacterium without a rigid cell wall, and it can be grown on artificial media if appropriate nutritional enrichment and proper osmolarity are supplied. *M. pneumoniae* lyses mammalian erythrocytes as a result of their production of hydrogen peroxide. The extent of hemolysis distinguishes *M. pneumoniae* from most other strains of Mycoplasmata encountered in humans.

A study done in the Seattle Group Health Cooperative from 1963 to 1968 demonstrated that about 20% of all pneumonia encountered there was associated with *M. pneumoniae* infections and that children 5 to 9 years of age had the highest attack rates.[15] *M. pneumoniae* was endemic in the study population at a rate of 2 to 3 cases per month, but occasionally clusters of patients increased the rate by 3 or 4 times. The disease was most common in large families, probably introduced there by school-age children. Males were more commonly infected and had more serious disease.

M. pneumoniae organisms are inhaled and then adhere tightly to the surface of respiratory epithelium. Infected cultures of respiratory epithelial cells show diminished ciliary activity and eventually cytopathic effects. *M. pneumoniae* may enter cells but no evidence exists that it produces toxic substances to account for injury of cells.

Since this form of pneumonia is not usually fatal, the tissue changes have not been extensively studied. The lungs are heavy and edematous with thickened bronchial walls. Many of the alveoli are filled with edema fluid, red cells, and macrophages; sometimes hyaline membranes are present. The alveoli and alveolar ducts contain focal areas of chronic inflammatory disease. The bronchioles are infiltrated with lymphocytes and the epithelium proliferates. After recovery, the lungs display pleural adhesions over the most severely affected parts.

The incubation period of the disease is not definitely established and may be as short as 5 days or as long as 3 weeks. In disease transmitted to volunteers, the incubation period is 9 to 12 days.

The illness usually begins with upper respiratory symptoms and fever followed by lower tract involvement. Cough occurs in 99%, and chills, headache, sore throat, and malaise are present in more than half of the patients. Less frequently, bullous myringitis or a mild skin rash occurs.

There are discrepancies between the physical findings in the chest and the appearance of the chest roentgenogram. Frequently, the physical findings are minimal or absent although the radiograph shows definite areas of infiltration, usually in the lower lobes. There may be harsh breath sounds, rhonchi, and occasionally rales. Pleuritic pain is not common nor is pleural fluid.

In untreated cases, fever and other symptoms can persist for 1 to 2 weeks, and roentgenographic changes may remain for longer periods. If appropriate treatment is begun early in the course of the disease, the fever and other symptoms are ameliorated within 3 or 4 days and the roentgenographic changes last no longer than 10 days.

Shulman et al. have reported unusually severe mycoplasmal pneumonia in several children with sickle-cell disease.[35] Clinical features included pneumonia involving more than one lobe, white cell counts over 25,000, prolonged fever, pleuritic pain, and pleural effusion. Moderate leukocytosis occurs in about one-fourth of the patients and white cell counts greater than 15,000 per cubic millimeter in about 5%.

The precise etiologic diagnosis can be made by the isolation of *M. pneumoniae* from the upper airway secretions or from sputum, and by demonstration of a rise in specific complement-fixing antibodies. Cold agglutinins are present in about one-half of the patients with serologic proof of *M. pneumoniae* pneumonia but are not specific inasmuch as they may occur in other types of nonbacterial pneumonia.

In a controlled study carried out among military recruits with serologically proven *M. pneumoniae* pneumonia, the administration of 0.9 g/day of demeclocycline for 6 days significantly reduced the duration of fever (from 10 to 3 days), rales, cough, and fatigue. Treatment stopped the progression and accelerated the clearing of the pulmonary process.[21] *M. pneumoniae* is inhibited in vitro by erythromycin. Treatment with this agent is as effective as treatment with tetracycline and should be used in children because of the deposition of tetracycline in the calcifying dental enamel and staining of the teeth.[31] The dose of erythromycin is 30 to 50 mg/kg/day in four or five divided doses.

Even though tetracycline and erythromycin are useful in treatment of the pneumonia, neither of these antibiotics routinely eradicates *M. pneumoniae* from the upper airway, and about one-half of treated individuals still harbor the organisms 10 to 20 days after treatment. These asymptomatic carriers can disseminate the organisms and be responsible for new cases of the disease.[36]

Viral Pneumonias

RESPIRATORY SYNCYTIAL VIRUS

Respiratory syncytial virus (RSV) is the single most important nonbacterial pathogen of the respiratory tract during early life.[6] It is the major cause of bronchiolitis, having been detected in 40% of patients by virus isolation or serologic study. RSV is a significant cause of pneumonia in infants and can be detected in about one-fourth of hospitalized patients with pneumonia.

The RSV is a paramyxovirus containing single-stranded RNA and surrounded by an envelope. It is susceptible to inactivation by many chemical and physical processes and must be handled carefully in the laboratory in order to preserve its ability to replicate in cell cultures.

RSV infection produces yearly epidemics that may occur in fall, winter, or spring, but each year the peak of serious respiratory disease in children coincides with the time of the RSV epidemic. Infants admitted to hospital with RSV infection of the respiratory tract were shown to shed large amounts of virus steadily for at least 5 days of illness.[16] These conditions obviously facilitate person-to-person transmission and explain the highly contagious nature of the disease.

Essentially all adults possess RSV neutralizing antibodies that can be passed transplacentally. It is surprising, therefore, to find that approximately 20% of moderate to severe respiratory tract disease in the first 6 months of life is caused by RSV, even though one-half of these infants already have neutralizing antibodies at the beginning of their illness. This finding indicates that specific neutralizing antibodies must be less effective in inhibiting RSV than many other viruses.

The development of lower respiratory disease is greatest during the initial infection with RSV. Small infants are most likely to develop bronchiolitis. In this disease, interaction of the virus with antibody from the mother may produce an immunologic reaction that plays a role in the syndrome of bronchiolitis.[14] RSV pneumonia as an isolated process occurs in somewhat older infants, after their maternally transmitted antibody has disappeared, and the lesions result from cytotoxic effects of the virus on lung tissue.

Patients with bronchiolitis may develop pneumonia. In fact, in about two-thirds of instances of pneumonia due to RSV, the patients display some of the features of bronchiolitis. Nasal discharge and sneezing are the first symptoms of bronchiolitis with the gradual development over a day or two of respiratory distress with cough, dyspnea, and irritability. This condition is frequently accompanied by temperatures of 38° C to 38.5° C, but fever may be absent. The infants are almost always tachypneic and may be in extreme distress with cyanosis. Rales are commonly heard at the end of inspiration; expiration is prolonged, and wheezes are prominent. Pneumonia caused by RSV in the absence of bronchiolitis resembles other viral pneumonias. It frequently begins as an upper respiratory infection, but the child does not improve and starts to cough and have grunting, rapid respirations. The diagnosis in both groups of patients is made by the roentgenogram, with interstitial pneumonia in most, or all, of the lobes the most constant finding. In addition, lobar or segmental consolidation may be especially prevalent in the right upper lobe, but pneumatoceles are not reported. Pleural fluid in very small amounts may be seen. The interstitial infiltrate clears within 7 to 10 days, but the area of consolidation may disappear more slowly.[33]

The specific diagnosis of RSV infection depends upon the isolation of the virus from nasopharyngeal secretions or the demonstration of a rising antibody titer using complement fixation. The white cell count is usually normal, not depressed as in many viral illnesses. Bacterial superinfection is not commonly a cause of pneumonia in children with RSV infection, and bacterial cultures from the nasopharynx ordinarily reveal normal flora.

Infants with bronchiolitis should be placed in cold vapor with oxygen, if necessary, and intravenous fluids should be used to maintain hydration. Antibacterial agents should not be used unless bacterial infection is likely.

ADENOVIRUS

Adenoviruses are the cause of at least 8 to 9% of respiratory diseases in hospitalized children, especially those 6 months to 4 years of age.[7,30] These viruses cause acute nonspecific upper respiratory infection, pharyngitis, pharyngoconjunctival fever, as well as pneumonia, which may appear as an added feature to the other clinical syndromes. Types 3, 4, 7, 21, and occasionally types 1 and 2, have been especially associated with pneumonia.

Each adenovirus is an icosahedron composed of 252 capsomeres surrounding a double-stranded core of DNA. These viruses multiply in the nuclei of cells with the formation of inclusions, and, in cell cultures, they induce rounding and clumping of cells with features that vary depending on which of the more than 30 types of adenovirus is present. These agents are recovered with the greatest frequency when primary human embryonic kidney cells are used for isolation, although they multiply in continuous lines of other human cells.

Adenoviruses can produce latent infection in tonsils, adenoids, and other human lymphoid organs, making it difficult to identify with certainty whether illnesses are the result of acquired infection with adenoviruses or are coincidental occurrences associated with the carrier state.

Several patients, mostly young children with pneumonia due to adenovirus infection, have died, and the lungs in this severest form of the disease have been markedly involved, showing injury to bronchial, bronchiolar, and alveolar epithelium and necrosis of bronchial and tracheal walls. Areas of inflammation display cells with intranuclear inclusions and enlarged epithelial cells with loss of nuclear membranes and dispersal of nuclear material into the cytoplasm.

The usual onset of adenovirus pneumonia is sudden, showing features of upper respiratory symptoms with fever, rhinorrhea, and cough. Nearly all patients have a red throat, and they may have conjunctivitis and morbilliform skin eruption. The cough becomes severe and paroxysmal, and rales and rhonchi can be heard. The radiograph reveals predominantly peribronchial interstitial disease but in serious cases may show areas of consolidation and necrosis of the parenchyma. Vomiting, diarrhea, meningismus, hepatomegaly, petechiae, or other signs of bleeding may complicate pneumonia. Fever, 38 to 39° C, may last for 4 to 5 days, but roentgenographic findings remain after the general symptoms have diminished.

The specific diagnosis is made by isolation of the virus (complicated by the carrier state) or by serologic methods. The simplest test for identifying adenovirus infection is complement fixation, which can be supplemented by neutralization or hemagglutination tests, which allow identification of type-specific antibody.

VARICELLA (Fig. 12-3)

Varicella pneumonia occurs in as many as 50% of adult patients with chicken pox but is distinctively uncommon in normal children with the disease (less than 1%). However, pneumonia is more frequent and unusually severe in children with immunodeficiencies or malignancies, and in those who are receiving immunosuppressive therapy. In one group of patients treated for cancer, 15 of 60 children with varicella developed pneumonia.[12]

The varicella-zoster virus is one of the agents of the herpesvirus group. It is icosahedral, has a DNA core, and is surrounded by a lipid envelope. During the first exposure, the virus infects the respiratory tract where it multiplies locally, then spreads via the blood to skin and visceral organs. The virus may remain dormant for years, then reappear causing lesions distributed along dermatomes (shingles) or, in patients with immunodeficiencies, it may involve other areas of the skin or viscera.

When the varicella-zoster virus affects the lungs, it results in inflammation with infiltration of the alveolar septa by mononuclear cells. The alveoli contain fluid and multinucleated giant cells with intranuclear inclusions.

Pneumonia begins 1 to 6 days after the appearance of the varicella rash. The first evidence of the disease is chest pain in about one-half of the patients. Hemoptysis occurs in about one-third. Dyspnea is frequently striking, and cyanosis may supervene. Physical findings are minimal or absent, but the chest roentgenogram indicates widespread involvement of the lungs as well as a typical nodular appearance.[27] Varicella pneumonia may be complicated by bacterial superinfection with *S. pneumoniae* or *S. aureus*.

If an immunosuppressed patient with no prior history of the disease is exposed to varicella, the suppressive therapy should be stopped or decreased to the lowest possible doses during the incubation period of the disease. This change in suppressive therapy probably reduces the risk of developing overwhelming disease with pneumonia and other visceral lesions. Zoster immune globulin, if given within 3 days of exposure, de-

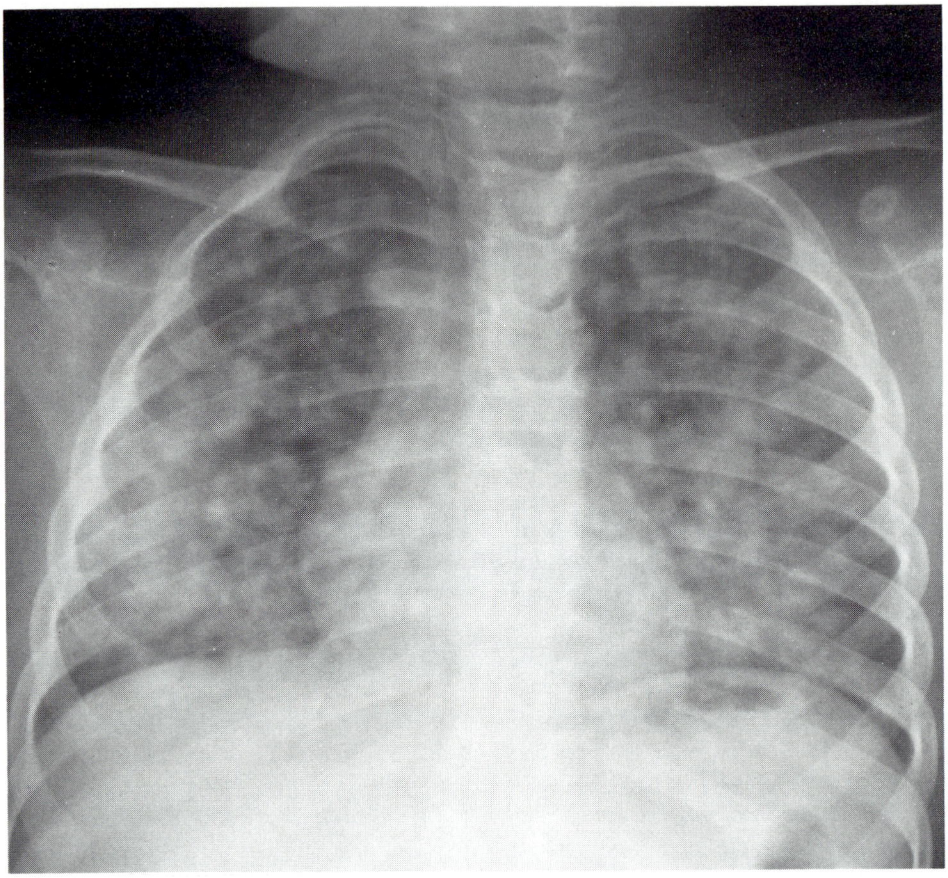

FIG. 12-3. Chicken pox pneumonia exhibiting relatively discrete central and mid-zonal alveolar densities, sparing the lung periphery.

creases the severity of the disease and the likelihood of pneumonia.[4] Commercially available gamma globulin in large doses (0.2 to 0.4 ml/lb) may exert a slight attenuating effect. Chemotherapy of varicella-zoster infections is experimental, and no clear recommendations can be made. 5-iodo-2′-deoxyuridine may decrease mortality. Cytosine arabinoside, though claimed to be of value, is probably without beneficial effect.

MEASLES

Measles pneumonia or giant-cell pneumonia may occur as a complication of measles in children with neoplastic disease,[26] as an isolated manifestation of measles in chronically ill or immunosuppressed children, [10] or as a part of the altered form of measles that occurs in those made partially immune by immunization with inactivated measles vaccine.[43]

Measles virus belongs to the paramyxovirus group and contains single-stranded RNA. The virus infects the patient via the respiratory tract, multiplies locally there, and then spreads via the blood to the skin and other organs. When the virus infects the lung, peribronchiolitis and alveolitis are present with macrophages and inclusion-bearing giant cells in the alveoli.[2]

When pneumonia complicates measles in children with diminished immunocompetence or neoplasia, it may appear at the time of, before, or several days after the onset of the rash. Marked and widespread interstitial change and hilar adenopathy are visible in the radiograph, but physical findings are variable in their intensity.

Patients who have measles pneumonia with no rash have interstitial pneumonia similar to that seen in patients with typical skin manifestations. The diagnosis can be proved only by demonstration of giant cells in the lungs and by identification of the measles virus.

Atypical measles occurring in persons previously vaccinated with inactivated virus can be a severe disease with high fever, abdominal pain, and a rash that is frequently hemorrhagic or vesicular and present on the extremities including the palms and soles. Pneumonia occurs frequently in these patients, with roentgenographic changes indicative of lobular or segmental infiltration, hilar lymphadenopathy, and pleural effusion. Nodular lesions in the lungs may persist for several months after the patient has apparently recovered from the rest of the disease.[43]

CYTOMEGALOVIRUS

Cytomegalovirus (CMV) infection is common in the population, but disease is rare. Many healthy children are carriers and excrete CMV in their urine and saliva during the first year of life. Complement-fixing antibodies are present in about 50% of the population aged 18 to 25 years and in 80% of those over 35 years.[41] When disease occurs in newborns or infants under 4 months of age, it usually is severe and progressive.

CMV is one of the herpesvirus group. It is icosahedral, contains double-stranded DNA, and has a lipid envelope. The virus is transmitted to the fetus via the placenta from an infected mother. It may also be spread by blood transfusions or by infected urine or respiratory secretions. CMV infects cells of the salivary glands, brain, kidneys, liver, and lungs. Infected cells contain intranuclear and intracytoplasmic inclusions. Pneumonia is characterized by protein-rich fluid and mononuclear cells in both the interstitium and the alveoli.

Disseminated CMV disease has been studied most thoroughly in newborns and infants, but it is also recognized in older immunosuppressed patients, especially recipients of renal transplants. In the transplanted patients, the lungs are the primary site of overt disease due to CMV. This appearance may represent either activation of latent infection or acquisition from an exogenous source. The clinical picture is varied and resembles that described for other nonbacterial pneumonias, with dyspnea and fewer physical findings than would be expected from the appearance of the chest roentgenogram. The radiographic findings include diffuse, panlobular involvement of the interstitial areas of the lung.[8]

CMV can be cultured in human fibroblasts from respiratory secretions, from lung tissue, or from urine, and giant cells bearing inclusions may be identified in urine. Immunofluorescence, indirect hemagglutination, and complement fixation may be used to detect rising antibody titers to CMV.

Pneumocystis Pneumonia (Fig. 12-4)

Pneumonia due to Pneumocystis was first associated with epidemic disease in premature and very young infants in Europe after World War II. In the United States, pneumonia due to this organism now occurs mainly in immunodeficient or immunosuppressed patients, particularly those with altered cell-mediated immunity. It is especially common in patients receiving corticosteroids as a part of an immunosuppressive regimen.[18]

Pneumocystis parasites are thought to be protozoa with both trophozoite and cyst

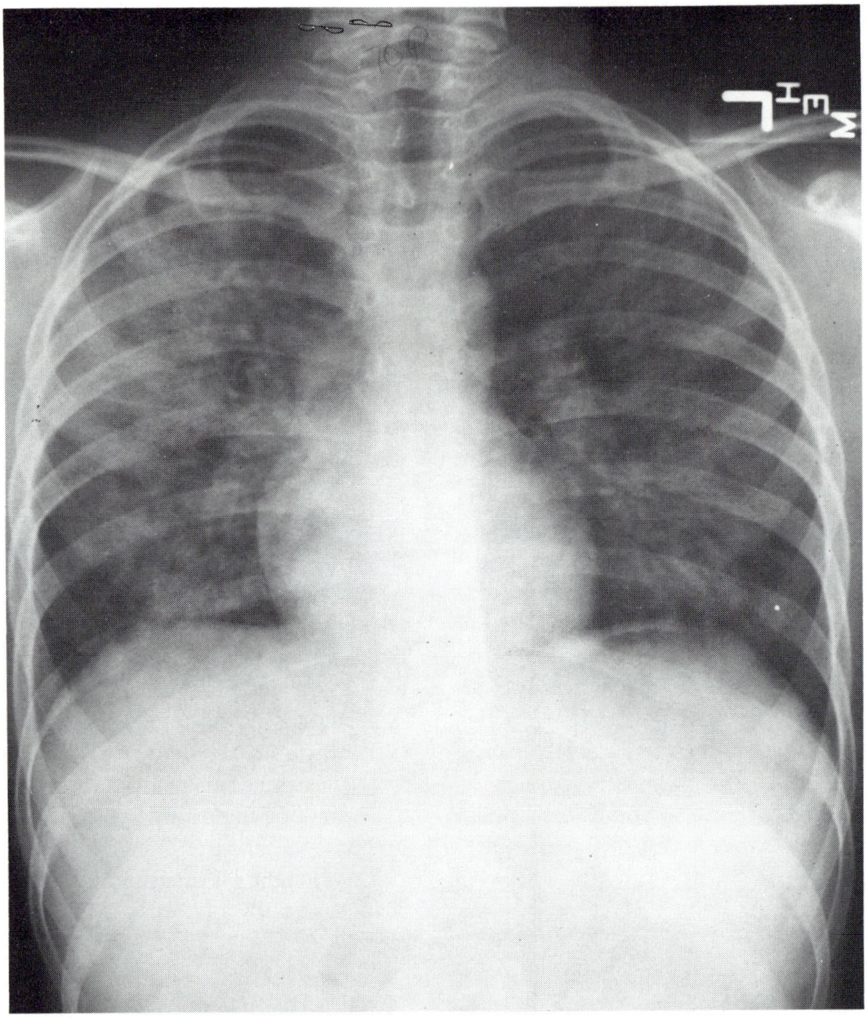

FIG. 12-4. *Pneumocystis* pneumonia with predominantly mid-zonal pulmonary densities bilaterally.

forms. The trophozoite is 1.5 μ, and the cyst is up to 7 μ in diameter with few intracellular organelles. *P. carinii* is the species name for the organism found in the lungs of rodents. It is believed that Pneumocystis species found in humans can infect only other humans and is, therefore, not *P. carinii.* The parasite causing human disease is, more appropriately, called just Pneumocystis, without further modification until more precise knowledge is available.[19]

Epidemics of Pneumocystis pneumonia in European nurseries represent baby-to-baby spread, and isolation of affected infants can prevent spread of the disease. Older susceptible individuals can acquire the organism from a patient with Pneumocystis pneumonia. It is also possible that Pneumocystis may exist in a latent form in previously infected persons, and that it becomes activated when the individual is immunosuppressed.

When the disease is produced in experimental animals, the cysts of Pneumocystis are first observed within the cytoplasm of alveolar septal cells, and little inflammatory response appears. Trophozoite forms then proliferate and mature inside the cysts and escape into the alveoli through breaks in the cyst wall. Eventually, intact as well as empty collapsed cysts and free trophozoites can be found in a proteinaceous, lipid-rich coagulum in the alveoli. Only in later states does evidence of host response appear, as alveolar-cell hypertrophy and interstitial infiltration with lymphocytes and plasma cells.

In the epidemic form of the disease among infants, the onset is insidious. The first signs are restlessness, followed by tachypnea and slight cyanosis. One or two weeks are required for the development of the full clinical picture of severe respiratory distress with marked retractions, cyanosis, and cough. Fever is minimal or absent. At times, air can be identified radiologically in the interstitium of the lungs, and it may spread to the mediastinum or other adjacent tissues.

The first symptoms in children or adults with cancer or immunodeficiency are unexplained fever, vomiting, diarrhea, a nonproductive cough, and anterior chest pain. The patients appear ill and display tachypnea, dyspnea, and cyanosis. However, rales and rhonchi may be absent. The extent of the disease is often indicated only by the chest roentgenogram. Leukemia lymphomas, neuroblastoma, reticulum cell sarcoma, and other solid tumors are the neoplasms associated with Pneumocystis infection. Paradoxically, Pneumocystis pneumonia commonly occurs during remission of the underlying disease. The radiograph displays a fine granular pattern, which is first evident in the hilar areas and then spreads to the periphery. These changes frequently involve the whole lung field and are indicative of both alveolar and interstitial involvement. Interstitial emphysema, pneumothorax, or pneumomediastinum may occur but usually without pleural reaction and without hilar lymphadenopathy.

DIAGNOSIS

The identification of the parasite is necessary for the diagnosis. The Pneumocystis may occasionally be found in the sputum, but when it cannot be found there or when no sputum is produced (a particular problem in young children), one must resort to other methods. Bronchial brushing is probably the safest procedure and is reported to yield a positive identification in 60% of cases of Pneumocystis pneumonia. Pulmonary hemorrhage is a possible complication particularly in patients with altered bleeding or clotting mechanisms. Needle or open-lung biopsies are associated with higher complication rates, and the diagnostic yield ranges from 50 to 64%.

Sputum or other material for examination should be preserved in a fixative as used for Papanicolaou procedures, and stained with Gomori's methenamine silver or Gram-Weigert. Pneumocystis can also be identified in frozen sections of biopsy material.

Specific therapy with pentamidine has proved effective in at least 50% of cases. In these patients the symptoms have disappeared, and the chest roentgenogram has reverted to normal or to the pre-pneumonitis state. This drug is available from the Parasitic Drug Service of the Center for Disease Control, Atlanta, Georgia, and is released for therapy if a clinical picture of Pneumocystis pneumonia exists, and the organism has been identified or appropriate studies are pending. The usual dosage is 4 mg/kg/day intramuscularly.

Adverse effects from pentamidine are relatively uncommon. They include reversible renal damage, local reactions at the injection sites, and hepatotoxicity. Immediate reactions such as hypotension and hypoglycemia may occur following intravenous administration.

Recently, trimethoprim-sulfamethoxazole (TMP-SMX) has been used in clinical trials.[17] Patients chosen for the studies have had less severe cases of Pneumocystis, but using 20 mg TMP-100 mg SMX/kg/day, 12 of 14 patients recovered. Adverse reactions from this combination are very unusual (0.01%) and are usually in the form of cutaneous sensitivity or gastrointestinal reactions.

REFERENCES

1. Ablow, R. C., S. G. Driscoll, E. L. Effmann, I. Gross, C. J. Jolles, R. Uauy and J. B. Warshaw: A comparison of early-onset group B streptococcal neonatal infection and the respiratory distress syndrome of the newborn. *N. Engl. J. Med. 294*:65, 1976.
2. Archibald, R. W. R., R. O. Weller and S. R. Meadow: Measles pneumonia and the nature of the inclusion-bearing giant cells: a light and electron-microscope study. *J. Pathol. 103*:27, 1971.
3. Black, P. H., M. N. Swartz, J. T. Sharp, L. J. Kunz, J. Stokes and R. B. McFarland: Severe streptococcal disease: observations during an epidemic occurring in southern New England, 1958–59. *N. Engl. J. Med. 264*:898, 1961.
4. Brunell, P. A., A. A. Gershon, W. T. Hughes, H. D. Riley and J. Smith: Prevention of varicella in high-risk children: a collaborative study. *Pediatrics 50*:718, 1972.
5. Chanock, R. M., L. Hayflick and M. F. Barile: Growth on artificial medium of an agent associated with atypical pneumonia and its identification as a PPLO. *Proc. Natl. Acad. Sci. U.S.A. 48*:41, 1962.
6. Chanock, R. M. and R. H. Parrott: Acute respiratory disease in infancy and childhood: present understanding and prospects for prevention. *Pediatrics 36*:21, 1965.
7. Chany, C., P. Lepine, M. Lelong, Le-Tan-Vinh, P. Satge and J. Virat: Severe and fatal pneumonia in infants and young children associated with adenovirus infections. *Am. J. Hyg. 67*:367, 1958.
8. Craighead, J. E.: Pulmonary cytomegalovirus infection in the adult. *Am. J. Pathol. 63*:487, 1971.
9. Dingle, J. H., G. F. Badger and W. S. Jordan: *Illness in the Home. A Study of 25,000 Illnesses in a Group of Cleveland Families.* Press of Western Reserve University, Cleveland, 1964.
10. Enders, J. F., K. McCarthy, A. Mitus and W. J. Cheatham: Isolation of measles virus at autopsy in cases of giant-cell pneumonia without rash. *N. Engl. J. Med. 261*:875, 1959.
11. Epstein, B. A., J. J. O'Brien, S. Rosenthal and P. B. Welty: Klebsiella pneumonia following an apparent staphylococcal pneumonia in a four-year-old child. *Clin. Pediatr. 14*:673, 1975.
12. Feldman, S., W. T. Hughs and C. B. Daniel: Varicella in children with cancer: seventy-seven cases. *Pediatrics 56*:388, 1975.
13. Fox, J. P., L. R. Elveback, T. Spigland, T. E. Frothingham, D. A. Stevens and M. Huger: The virus watch program: a continuing surveillance of viral infections in metropolitan New York families. *Am. J. Epidemiol. 83*:389, 1966.
14. Gardner, P. S., J. McQuillin and S. D. M. Court: Speculation on pathogenesis in death from respiratory syncytial virus infection. *Brit. Med. J. 1*:327, 1970.
15. Grayston, J. T., H. M. Foy and G. E. Kenny: Mycoplasmas (PPLO) in human disease. *D.M.* Dec., 1967.
16. Hall, C. B., R. G. Douglas and J. M. Geiman: Quantitative shedding patterns of respiratory syncytial virus in infants. *J. Infect. Dis. 132*:151, 1975.
17. Hughes, W. T., S. Feldman and S. K. Sanyal: Treatment of Pneumocystis carinii pneumonitis with trimethaprimsulfamethazole. *Can. Med. Assoc. J. 112*:475, 1975.
18. Hughes, W. T., R. A. Price, H-K. Kim, T. P. Coburn, D. Grigsby and S. Feldman: Pneumocystis carinii pneumonia in children with malignancies. *J. Pediatr. 82*:404, 1973.
19. Jones, T. A.: Letter to the editor: pneumocystis. *N. Engl. J. Med. 293*:404, 1975.
20. Keefer, C. S., L. A. Rantz and C. H. Rammelkamp: Hemolytic streptococcal pneumonia and empyema; a study of 55 cases with special reference to treatment. *Ann. Intern. Med. 14*:1533, 1941.
21. Kingston, J. R., R. M. Chanock, M. A. Mufson, L. P. Hellman, W. D. James, H. H. Fox, M. A. Manko and J. Boyers: Eaton-agent pneumonia. *J.A.M.A. 176*:118, 1961.
22. Klein, J. O.: Diagnostic lung puncture in the pneumonias of infants and children. *Pediatrics 44*:486, 1969.
23. Loda, F. A., W. A. Clyde, W. P. Glezen, R. J. Senior, C. I. Sheaffer and F. W. Denny: Studies on the role of viruses, bacteria, and M. pneumoniae as causes of lower respiratory tract infections in children. *J. Pediatr. 72*:161, 1968.
24. Mascaset, F. F., P. A. Kidd, C. R. Boland and H. A. Wenner: The etiology of acute respiratory infections. *J. Pediatr. 72*:829, 1968.
25. Miller, B. W., H. W. Orris and H. H. Taus: Friedländer's pneumonia in infancy. *J. Pediatr. 31*:521, 1947.
26. Mitus, A., J. F. Enders, J. M. Craig and A. Holloway: Persistence of measles virus and depression of antibody formation in patients with giant-cell pneumonia after measles. *N. Engl. J. Med. 261*:882, 1959.
27. Nisenbaum, C., K. Wallis and E. Herczeg: Varicella pneumonia in children. *Helv. Paediatr. Acta 24*:212, 1969.
28. Nyhan, W. L., D. R. Rectanus and M. D. Fonsek: Hemophilus influenzae type b pneumonia. *Pediatrics 16*:31, 1955.
29. Papageorgiou, A., C. R. Bauer, B. D. Fletcher and L. Stern: Klebsiella pneumonia with pneumatocele formation in a newborn infant. *Can. Med. Assoc. J. 109*:1217, 1973.

30. Pinkerton, H. and S. Carroll: Fatal adenovirus pneumonia in infants. *Am. J. Pathol. 65*:543, 1971.
31. Rasch, J. R. and W. J. Mogabgab: Therapeutic effects of erythromycin on Mycoplasma pneumoniae. *Antimicrob. Agents Chemother. 5*:693, 1965.
32. Ravitch, M. M. and R. Fein: The changing picture of pneumonia and empyema in infants and children. *J.A.M.A. 175*:1038, 1961.
33. Rice, R. P. and F. Loda: A roentgenographic analysis of respiratory syncytial virus pneumonia in infants. *Radiology 87*:1021, 1966.
34. Schreiner, A., A. Digranes and O. Myking: Transtracheal aspiration in the diagnosis of lower respiratory tract infections. *Scand. J. Infect Dis. 4*:49, 1972.
35. Shulman, S. T., J. Bartlett, W. A. Clyde and E. M. Ayoub: The unusual severity of mycoplasmal pneumonia in children with sickle-cell disease. *N. Engl. J. Med. 287*:164, 1972.
36. Smith, C. B., W. T. Friedewald and R. M. Chanock: Shedding of M. pneumoniae. *N. Engl. J. Med. 276*:1172, 1967.
37. Stiles, Q. R., G. G. Lindesmith, B. L. Tucker, B. W. Meyer and J. C. Jones: Pleural empyema in children. *Ann. Thorac. Surg. 10*:377, 1970.
38. Thaler, M. M.: Klebsiella-aerobacter pneumonia in infants. A review of the literature and report of a case. *Pediatrics 30*:206, 1962.
39. Turner, G. A. P.: Staphylococcal pneumonia. A contemporary rarity. *Clin. Pediatr. 11*:69, 1972.
40. Vital statistics of the United States, Volume II. National Center for Health Statistics, U.S. Dept. Health, Education, and Welfare, 1966.
41. Weller, T. H. and J. B. Hanshaw: Virologic and clinical observations on cytomegalic inclusion disease. *N. Engl. J. Med. 266*:1233, 1962.
42. Wood, W. B. and M. R. Smith: Host-parasite relationships in experimental pneumonia due to pneumococcus type III. *J. Exp. Med. 92*:85, 1960.
43. Young, L. W., D. I. Smith and L. A. Glasgow: Pneumonia of atypical measles. *Am. J. Roentgenol. 110*:439, 1970.

Pulmonary Tuberculosis in Children

STANLEY READ

13

Although the number of new cases of tuberculosis has declined markedly over the last 20 to 30 years, tuberculosis still remains a clinically important disease entity. New reported cases in 1975 showed an incidence of 15.74/100,000 population as compared with 24.38/100,000 in 1966. With respect to the various age groups, in 1974, there were 7.5/100,000 in the 0 to 4 year group, 2.6 in the 5 to 14 year group, and 6.3 in the 15 to 24 year group. The highest incidence was in the group over 65 years of age with a rate of 32.5/100,000.[5]

The majority of cases of tuberculosis occurring before puberty are of the primary pulmonary type, which represents the initial infection with *Mycobacterium tuberculosis.* Sensitization of the delayed type occurs, and the sensitized immune system, reacting with the initial focus of infection, gives rise to the primary complex. The primary complex consists of the pulmonary focus plus enlargement of lymph nodes draining the area. Ninety-five percent of primary foci occur in the lungs, and these lesions are usually benign and heal completely. Most of the complications of primary tuberculosis occur within a year of the onset of the disease. As long as primary tuberculosis is diagnosed and treated early, the risks of early and, probably, of late complications can be greatly reduced.[4]

Pathogenesis

Mycobacteria reach the lungs via the respiratory tract, most often by droplet infection from an individual with active pulmonary disease. The majority of disease is caused by *M. tuberculosis,* but on occasion may be due to *M. bovis, M. avium,* or atypical mycobacteria. All mycobacteria are typically resistant to decolorization with an acid-alcohol solution (acid-fast) and are slightly bent or curved slender rods. They are differentiated by their in vitro growth characteristics. Human disease due to *M. bovis* has become rare in areas where tuberculosis in cattle has been controlled. Disease due to *M. avium* and atypical mycobacteria is also uncommon. All the mycobacteria have some antigens in common, and infection with a strain other than *M. tuberculosis* will likely result in a weakly positive skin reaction to tuberculin prepared from *M. tuberculosis.*

In the primary tuberculous infection the bacilli multiply in a focus in the lung and create a small focal area of inflammatory exudate. In the early stages, this infection is not usually visible on roentgenogram. Very early in the course of the infection, lymphatic spread to the regional lymph nodes occurs, and an early transient bacteremia develops. Primary pulmonary foci are usually single, but occasionally two or more characteristic lesions are present.

Within 2 to 6 weeks after initiation of infection, delayed type hypersensitivity becomes apparent. At this time, perifocal cellular infiltration in the area of the infective focus in the lung increases rapidly and the regional nodes (usually hilar) enlarge. Usually it is during this period that the typical radiographic picture of the primary complex becomes evident. Also, at this time the tuberculin skin test first becomes positive.

Clinical Findings

In most cases, the onset of primary tuberculosis is insidious. Initially the child appears well. After an early, mildly febrile period, the temperature may return to normal, and the only sign may be increased fatigability. In a few weeks, low grade fever with two or three spikes per week to 38° or 38.5° C may develop. Usually no signs are apparent on physical examination during the early stages of primary tuberculosis.

Rarely, a child may be born with congenital tuberculosis.[6] This type occurs only when the mother has active miliary tuberculosis during the pregnancy. The newborn has evidence of disseminated disease with hepatosplenomegaly and, at autopsy, involvement of the major organ systems.

Occasionally, the onset of primary tuberculosis is dramatic, resembling lobar pneumonia. It begins with high fever, clinical and roentgenographic evidence of lobar consolidation, and leukocytosis. Although the fever and leukocytosis subside in a few days, the chest roentgenogram remains unchanged. The tuberculin test is positive at the beginning of the pneumonic onset. The reason for this initial reaction is not understood.

Hematogenous dissemination of tubercle bacilli probably occurs during the initial stages of all primary infections. However, the consequences of this spread apparently depend upon a number of factors, including the number of bacilli and specific and nonspecific host resistance factors. Foci can form in kidneys, adrenals, brain, meninges, bone, and other tissues. The organisms in these foci may, in some cases, survive and produce active disease at a later time.

Roentgenographic Findings

The primary complex (Fig. 13-1), lung parenchymal lesion and enlarged hilar lymph nodes, appears early in the disease and persists unchanged for at least 3 months before gradually decreasing in size. It often remains visible for 6 to 8 months and may persist for up to 2 years. Apparently, the appearance and course of the primary complex are affected little by therapy.

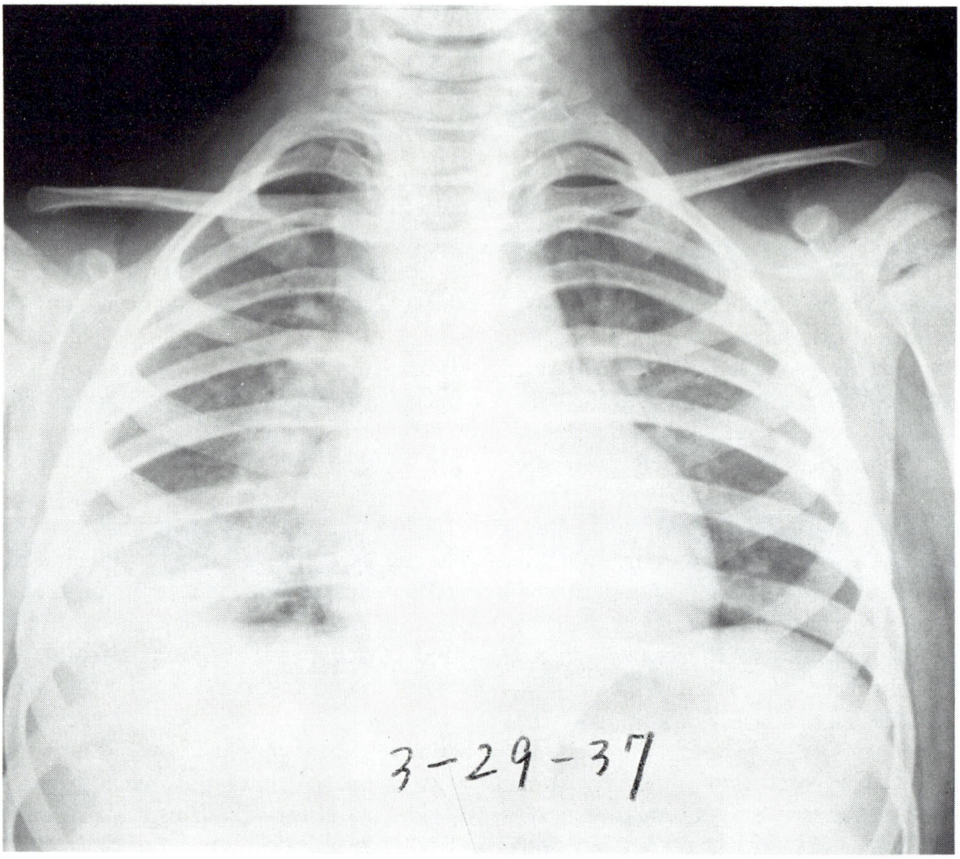

A

FIG. 13-1. *A*, Chest roentgenogram of a 6-year-old boy with pulmonary tuberculosis showing the primary complex. The primary focus is seen in the right lower lobe, and there is right hilar lymphadenopathy.
B, Roentgenogram of the same patient 5 years later shows residual calcification at the site of the primary focus and in the hilar lymph node area.

The primary focus can occur anywhere in the lung but is rarely seen in the apices. It occurs more often in the right lung than in the left. Segmental obstruction due to endobronchitis is probably a significant contributory factor to the initial density. Before chemotherapy was available, more than 90% of the primary lesions eventually developed calcifications. With improved chemotherapy, less calcification is seen, and now many treated children eventually have a normal roentgenogram.

Diagnosis

The tuberculin skin test is the standard method of testing for infection with *M. tuberculosis*. This test is the prototype of the delayed-type hypersensitivity reaction, and a positive reaction signifies not only the possibility of currently active tuberculosis, but also any infection in the past. The tuberculin skin test is performed by intradermal injection of 0.1 ml of a purified protein derivative (PPD) of *M. tuberculosis*. The reac-

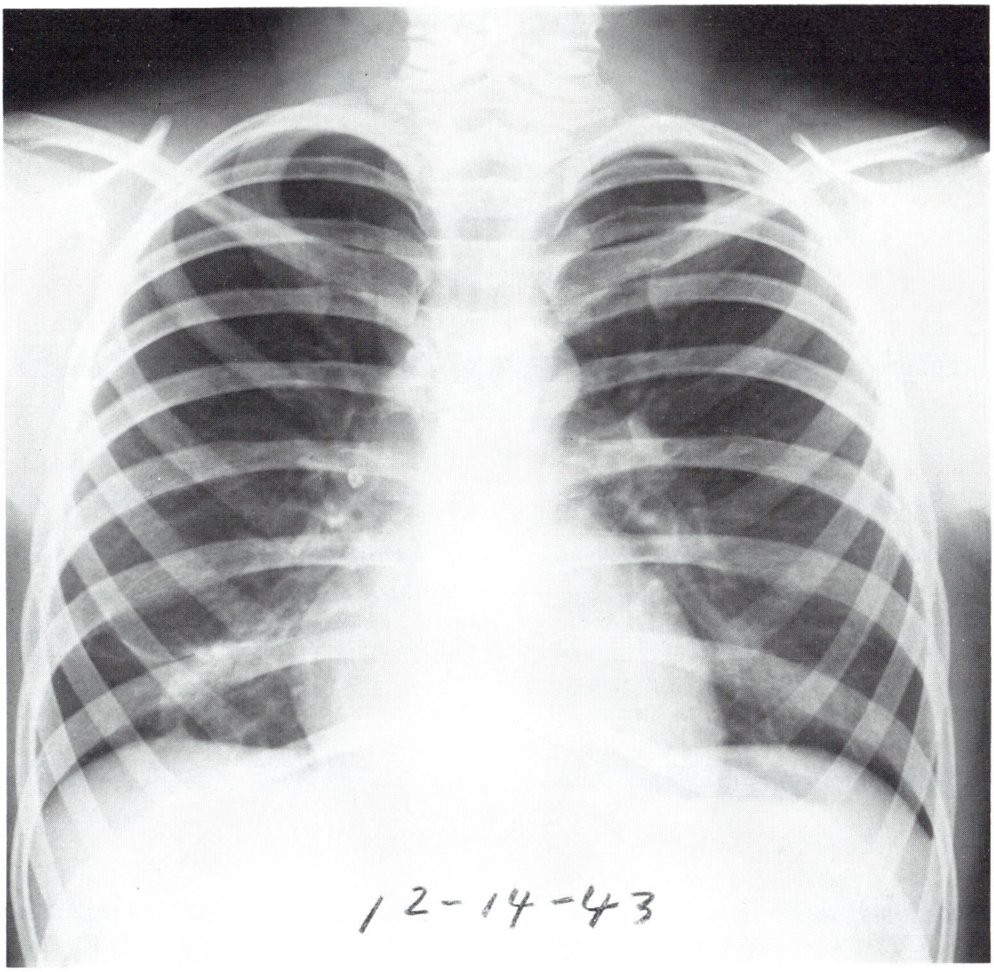

B

FIG. 13-1. Continued.

tion is examined in 48 hours and the diameter of the area of induration measured. A diameter of greater than 10 mm is considered positive. In general, PPD at a strength of 5 tuberculin units (TU) is used. Reactions from strengths greater than 50 TU must be interpreted with care, as a high incidence of nonspecific reactivity occurs.

A modification of the standard tuberculin test procedure, the tine test, is in widespread use because of the ease of administration and high degree of correlation with the intradermal injections. A test is considered positive if one or more papules result with more than 2 mm of induration. If the results of the tine test are at all questionable, an intradermal test should be performed.

Since most tuberculosis infections occur via the respiratory tract, chest roentgenogram is of diagnostic help. In recent converters, roentgenogram is only of value in determining the location and extent of involvement. The typical findings have been discussed previously.

The ultimate proof of a tuberculosis infection is the demonstration of bacteria. This bacterial proof is particularly difficult in children because of problems in obtaining a sputum specimen. Also, the number of organisms in primary tuberculosis is small. If sputum is obtained, a direct smear stained by the Ziehl-Neelsen technique should be examined, and material cultured on Löwenstein-Jensen medium. If sputum cannot be obtained, gastric aspirate should be performed on 3 successive days, early in the morning after an overnight fast. In some series, as many as 50 to 90% of children with radiologic evidence of primary pulmonary tuberculosis had positive cultures from gastric lavage material.

Course

In most cases of primary pulmonary tuberculosis, even without antimicrobial therapy, the initial lesion remains benign with no symptoms or signs. Treatment with isoniazid results in reversion of the tuberculin test to negative in 87% of those treated within 6 months of conversion. Occasionally the primary complex progresses locally, and before antibiotics, two out of three such children died.

Most chronic pulmonary tuberculosis develops in children whose first infection occurs after 7 years of age. The risk is greater for girls than boys and is higher in the adolescent period.

CHRONIC PULMONARY TUBERCULOSIS

Chronic pulmonary tuberculosis is rare in children. In a group of 2500 children followed at Bellevue Hospital in Manhattan, only 150 patients below 15 years of age developed this form of tuberculosis. The disease may be the result of an exogenous reinfection, although most cases are thought to be from endogenous foci.

Because of the hypersensitivity to the organisms in these cases, the bacilli are localized, forming initially an area of bronchopneumonia. The lesion increases in size with multiplication of organisms, accumulation of mononuclear cells, and macrophages. Eventually the lesion ulcerates, liquefaction occurs, and this material, containing tubercule bacilli, is disseminated through the bronchi. The initial lesions occur most commonly in the apical or subapical areas. Usually by the time that radiologic studies show spread from the initial lesion, a highlight, representing a cavity, can be seen in this initial lesion (Fig. 13-2). Healing is by resolution, encapsulation, fibrosis, and calcification.

BCG

The BCG vaccine was developed by Calmette and Guérin from a bovine strain of Mycobacterium and introduced as a live vaccine in 1922. Most studies have shown that BCG vaccination is effective in prevention of tuberculosis although a few studies have failed to show any effect.[2,3] It is generally conceded to be a safe vaccine with only occasional complications, which include disseminated disease, cold abscesses of local lymph glands, erythema nodosum, and secondary infection and ulceration at the site of the injection.

It is generally recommended that BCG be used in areas of the world where the risk of infection is high. It is given only to tuberculin negative individuals. In the United States, since the tuberculosis infection rate is low, the risk of infection is also low; hence widespread use of BCG would prevent little tuberculosis. It is only considered appropriate for individuals living or working in high-risk areas, e.g., health care personnel. It should not be given to individuals who are immunosuppressed or immunodeficient because they are unlikely to respond and the risk of complications is increased.

PREVENTION OF SEQUELAE OF PRIMARY INFECTION

Since it is believed that 90% of new cases of tuberculosis in the United States arise

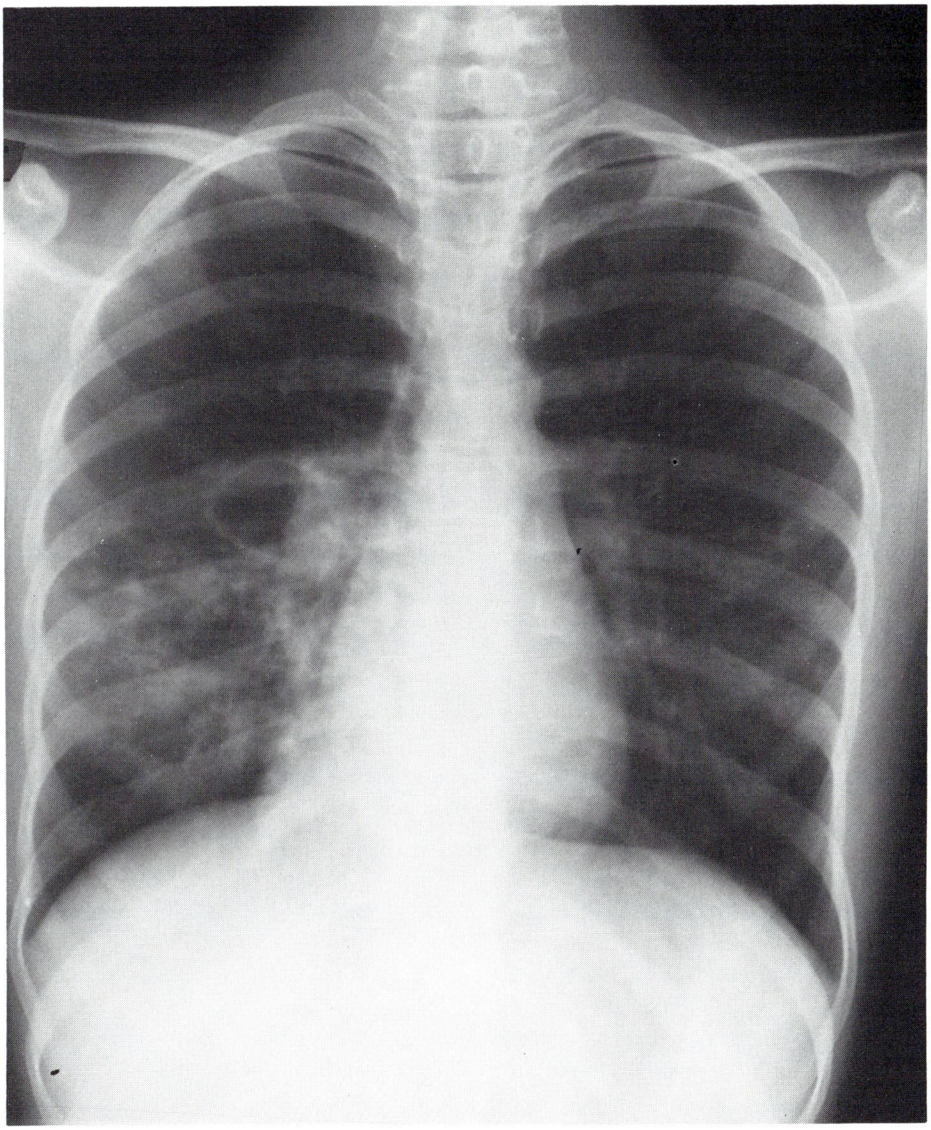

FIG. 13-2. 14-year-old girl with a cavitary lesion in her right lung. Acid-fast bacilli were seen on sputum smear.

endogenously from previous foci of infection,[4] treatment of the initial infection should markedly decrease the number of new cases. The objective is to eliminate organisms that may persist in the lung and other areas of the body as the result of the early hematogenous spread. It has been shown that in some individuals such foci of viable organisms can persist for many years without any clinical manifestations, until such time as the defense mechanisms are compromised. At that time, the mycobacteria begin replicating and cause disease.

Several high risk groups have been identified for treatment:

(1) Recent converters: These individuals

have a 1:30 chance of developing active tuberculosis in the first year after infection.

(2) Household contacts of newly developed, active cases.

(3) Tuberculin positive adolescents even if chest roentgenogram is normal. Adolescence is a particularly high risk period for the development of active pulmonary tuberculosis.

The recommended therapy for individuals in these groups is isoniazid (INH), 10 mg/kg/day up to a maximum daily dose of 300 mg/day, for 1 year.[1]

Treatment and Prognosis

Antibiotics are the treatment of choice for tuberculosis. The management of primary tuberculosis with INH has been discussed. Progressive primary tuberculosis and chronic pulmonary tuberculosis should be treated using a two-drug regimen. This approach has two major objectives: (1) prevention of emergence of resistant strains and (2) adequate antibiotic coverage in the event that the strain of *M. tuberculosis* is resistant to one of the drugs. It has been reported that in the United States as many as 8% of strains of *M. tuberculosis* are resistant to INH.[3] Duration of treatment should be for 18 to 24 months. Several possible regimens are acceptable. INH (10 mg/kg) and ethambutol (15 mg/kg) can be given for the duration of the treatment. Although ethambutol is a relatively poor antituberculosis drug, when used in combination with INH, it appears to prevent the emergence of INH-resistant strains. INH may also be combined with rifampin,[3] which is a much more active antituberculous drug. Other possible drugs for use in combination with INH include streptomycin, which has as one of its disadvantages that it must be given intramuscularly, or para-aminosalicylic acid, which must be given in large volumes by mouth and is very irritating to the gastrointestinal tract.

Side effects of INH include primarily hepatotoxicity, which is less common in children than in older patients. Consequently, liver enzymes must be followed on a regular basis and the drug stopped if hepatitis develops. Rifampin also causes hepatotoxicity, and it has been reported to have immunosuppressive properties. Ethambutol in high doses has been reported to cause retrobulbar neuritis. However, in doses of 15 mg/kg no more visual toxicity appears than when regimens not including ethambutol are used.

Intermittent therapy has recently been recommended in certain adult patients after a successful initial phase of daily treatment has been completed.[7] The success of the initial treatment is judged by negative cultures, usually during a period of 1 to 4 months. Intermittent treatment consists of twice weekly administration of either INH (15 mg/kg, PO) and streptomycin (25 to 30 mg/kg, IM), or INH (15 mg/kg, PO) and ethambutol (50 mg/kg, PO).

REFERENCES

1. Barlow, P. B., M. Black, D. L. Brummer, G. W. Comstock, I. N. Dubin, P. Enterline, M. L. Gibson, G. E. Hardy, Jr., J. A. Harrel, R. F. Johnston, D. C. Kent, B. A. Marvin, N. C. McCaig, J. R. Mitchell, and J. W. Mosley: Preventive therapy of tuberculous infection. *Am. Rev. Respir. Dis: 110*:371, 1974.
2. Chamberlayne, Earl C. (Ed.): Immunization in tuberculosis. DHEW Publication No. (NIH) 72-68, 1971.
3. Johnston, R. F., and K. H. Wildrick: The impact of chemotherapy on the care of patients with tuberculosis. *Am. Rev. Respir. Dis. 109*:636, 1974.
4. Lincoln, E. M. and E. M. Sewell: *Tuberculosis in Children.* McGraw-Hill, New York, 1963.
5. Morbidity and Mortality Weekly Report, Annual Supplement Summary, Vol. 24, No. 54, August, 1976.
6. Pai, P. M., and P. R. Parikh: Congenital miliary tuberculosis. A case report. *Clin. Pediatr. 15*:376, 1976.
7. Sbarbaro, J. A., P. B. Barlow, M. W. Craig, R. F. Johnston, W. P. Reagan, and L. B. Reichman: Intermittent chemotherapy for adults with tuberculosis. *Am. Rev. Respir. Dis. 110*:374, 1974.

Principles and Techniques of Neonatal Intensive Care

WILLIAM W. FRAYER AND PETER A. M. AULD

14

Successful management of problems of the newborn infant with respiratory distress relies on a thorough understanding of the underlying pathophysiology, rapid recognition of abnormal conditions, and prompt institution of definitive therapy. The problems are relatively few, whereas the number of therapeutic modalities has mushroomed in the last decade as etiological factors have become better understood. The increased emphasis on therapeutic manipulation has frequently resulted in a fragmented approach to the ill infant. Often detailed manipulations are carried out with exquisite precision, but fundamental metabolic and thermal needs may be overlooked. In addition, it must be recognized that specific therapy against the primary disease may itself produce serious side effects and complications that can be equally damaging to the patient.

From a problem-oriented viewpoint, two categories must be recognized: (1) ongoing needs, which change continuously, and (2) acute needs, which require prompt intervention. Ongoing needs include thermoregulation, nutrition, fluid and electrolyte balance, and surveillance. Acute needs include such problems as hypoxia, shock, metabolic and respiratory acidosis, hyperbilirubinemia, and coagulopathy.

Until an infant is sufficiently recovered to permit homeostatic mechanisms and routine infant care to meet his fundamental requirements on an indefinite basis, the four ongoing problems should be reviewed at least daily.

This chapter discusses the background and practical aspects of care associated with all of the ongoing needs of the ill newborn as well as specific diagnostic and therapeutic procedures that apply to acute respiratory and cardiovascular problems.

Ongoing Problem I—Thermal Regulation

The importance of providing an optimal thermal environment at minimal metabolic cost cannot be overemphasized. The zone of safety is very narrow and difficulty ensues when environmental temperature is either too low or too high.

FACTORS INFLUENCING THERMAL REGULATION

Prior to delivery, the fetal temperature is slightly higher than the mother's (0.5° C), and thermoregulation occurs by dissipation of heat through the placenta.[1,66] At delivery, the environment is at least 10° C colder than in utero, and the requirement for endogenous heat production becomes an immediate ongoing problem. The high surface area : body weight ratio places the infant at a disadvantage in which heat loss is favored. In addition, the low weight of the smaller infants results in diminished heat production. Surface area : body weight ratio is about three times that of an adult. Additional disadvantages in terms of thermal regulation accrue because of poor vasomotor control, absence of fat insulation,[49] and increased thermal conductance.

MAINTENANCE OF BODY TEMPERATURE

All infants strive to maintain a constant core body temperature.[1] Normal core temperatures are not the same for all infants. The normal temperatures of premature or small for gestational age infants are consistently below the temperature range of term infants.[9,23,67,84]

The environmental temperature that permits minimum oxygen consumption is called the neutral thermal temperature zone.[50] The smaller the infant, the higher the neutral thermal temperature and the narrower its range (Fig. 14-1). When an infant is exposed to temperatures below the neutral thermal zone, a two- or threefold rise in oxygen consumption occurs, Pa_{O_2} decreases, and metabolic acidosis results (Fig. 14-2). In very small infants, hypoglycemia may occur as well.[64,65] Infants nursed in a cool environment have an increased mortality rate,[10,23,83] and the caloric cost to these infants results in decreased growth.[41] In the case of an infant born with birth asphyxia, the metabolic expenditure with cold stress may be much increased.[8] Excessive heating of infants above the neutral thermal zone can also increase oxygen consumption. Rapid elevation of environmental temperature causes a decrease in minute ventilation or apnea.[76]

Maintenance of body temperature involves establishment of a balance between endogenous heat production and heat loss. A cold stress is a stimulus to non-shivering thermogenesis. Newborn infants are unable to produce heat by shivering, although increased muscular activity may accomplish the same metabolic result. The principal source of heat is chemical thermogenesis occurring in deposits of brown fat.[22] This tissue is located in the nape of the neck, para-aortic, suprarenal, and supra-adrenal areas (Fig. 14-3). Brown fat is rich in mitochondria possessing multiple fat vacuoles, an abundant blood supply, and a highly developed sympathetic innervation. The temperature gradient between skin and the environment is the most sensitive regulating factor, with the face and nose being particularly important temperature sensitive areas.[68] Norepinephrine released during cold stress activates cyclic AMP in brown fat,

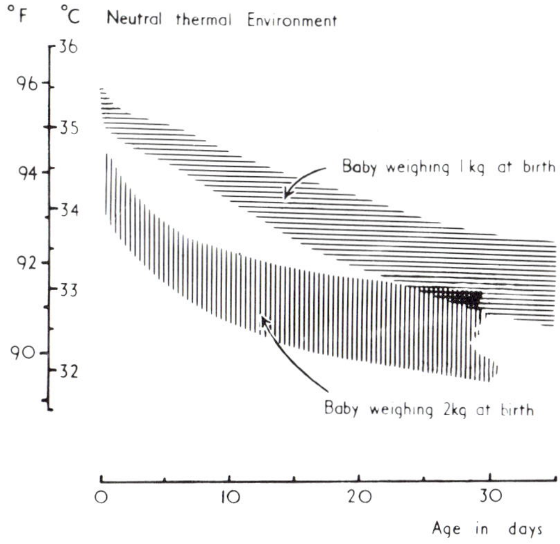

FIG. 14-1. Neutral thermal temperature as a function of age for 1- and 2-kg infants in an incubator environment at 50% relative humidity. (From Hey, E. N. and G. Katz.[49])

which in turn activates enzymes for hydrolysis of triglycerides. Triglycerides are broken down to glycerol and non-esterified fatty acids, which are oxidized to produce heat. Small infants are deficient in norepinephrine and thus are even more vulnerable to cold stress. As free fatty acids compete with albumin for bilirubin binding, prolonged cold stress could increase the risk of kernicterus at relatively low bilirubin concentrations.

Infants lose heat by conduction, convection, evaporation, and radiation, each mechanism being of importance in relation to therapeutic modalities. Conductive losses occur by direct transfer of heat from the body to cooler surfaces, e.g., cool bed linen. Heat loss by convection requires a cool current of air blowing on the skin, as may occur in open infrared heaters. Evaporative losses occur due

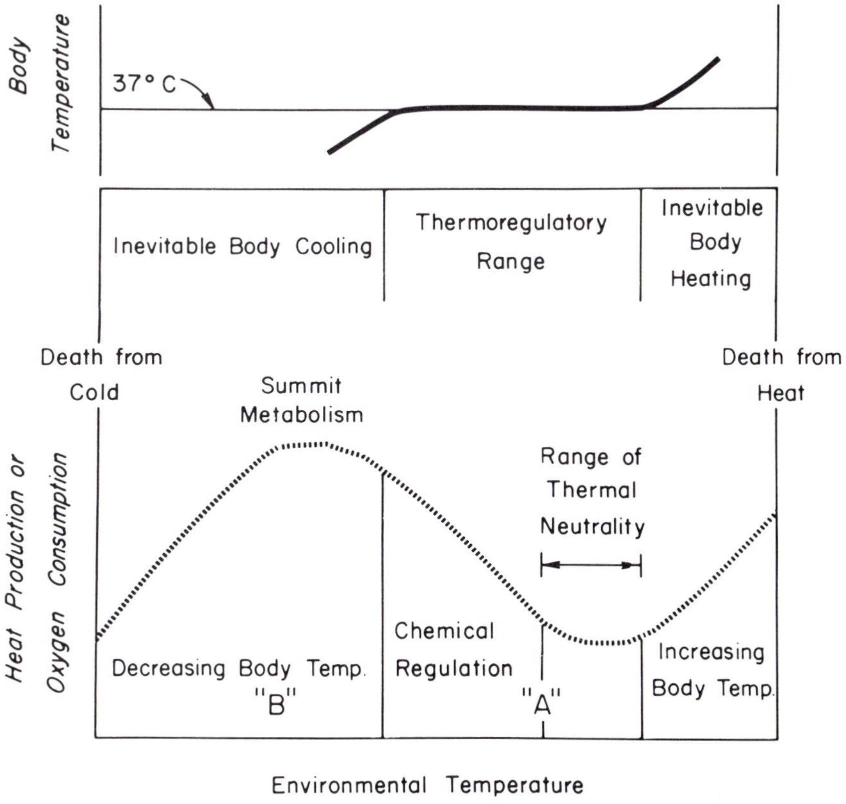

FIG. 14-2. The relationship of body temperature and oxygen consumption. (From Merenstein, G. and L. Blackmon: *Care of the High Risk Newborn.* Children's Hospital, San Francisco, 1971.)

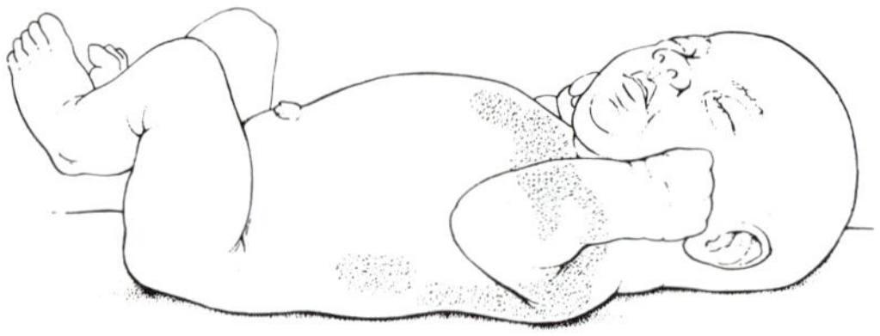

FIG. 14-3. The principal locations of brown fat in newborn infants. (Modified from Dawkins, M. R. and D. Hull: The production of heat by fat. *Sci. Am.* *213*:62, 1965.)

to evaporation of water from the skin and from the respiratory tract. This type of loss may account for as much as 25% of total heat loss. Premature infants may experience greater heat loss as a result of increased insensible water loss.[37] Infants lose significant quantities of heat by way of radiation, for example, from the infant to the cooler plastic of the incubator.

CLINICAL CONSIDERATIONS

Thermal stress at the time of birth is virtually unavoidable. Dahm and James have demonstrated the important role of evaporative heat loss in lowering body temperature in the delivery room.[19] Figure 14-4, which was

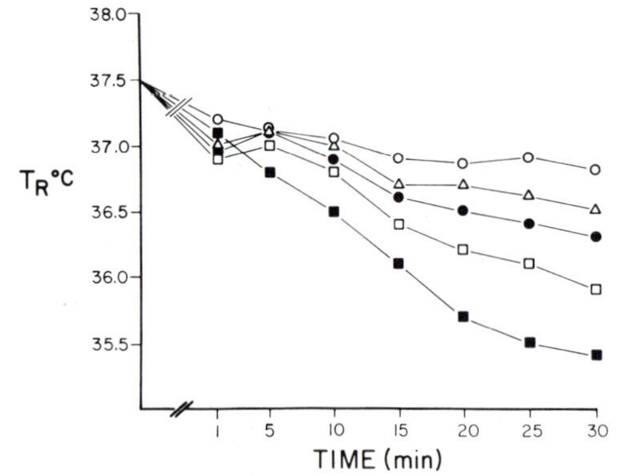

FIG. 14-4. Mean deep body temperature during the first 30 minutes of life for five groups of infants: ■ wet infants in room air; □ dry infants in room air, ● wet infants under a radiant heater, △ dry infants wrapped in a blanket, ○ dry infants under the radiant heater. (From Dahm.[19])

taken from their study, illustrates comparative cooling curves in various environments with and without drying. The most desirable environment for the newborn from this standpoint is dry, with the infant under a radiant warmer. Both premature and small for gestational age infants cool more rapidly than the term infant since their subcutaneous fat layer is much thinner.[49]

The increased oxygen requirement of thermal stress presents a problem for the infant who is asphyxiated at birth. Although attention in the delivery room may be directed at cardiopulmonary factors, response and outcome also depend on prompt drying and warming.

Radiant warming devices are essential equipment in all delivery rooms and should be used routinely. Transfer from the delivery room to the nursery should utilize prewarmed transport incubators.

Nursery Care. A neutral thermal environment is required for all infants. The requirements for establishing thermoneutrality depend on the age and size of the baby, as well as whether he is clothed or naked. The graphs in Figure 14-5 compare the temperatures required to maintain thermoneutrality for both naked and clothed (diaper, shirt, and blanket) infants weighing 1, 2, and 3 kg. The naked infant tolerates a much narrower range of environmental temperatures than the clothed infant.

Intensive Care. In an intensive care environment, the infant should be naked so that he may be observed properly. The high skin temperature required for thermoneutrality necessitates use of an extra source of heat. Since the turn of the century, incubators have been used with success. Presently both incubators and open radiant warmers are used for infant care.

Radiant warmers are indicated whenever special procedures are to be performed or when routine care requires frequent access to the patient. An incubator environment is unsuitable in these situations because of the

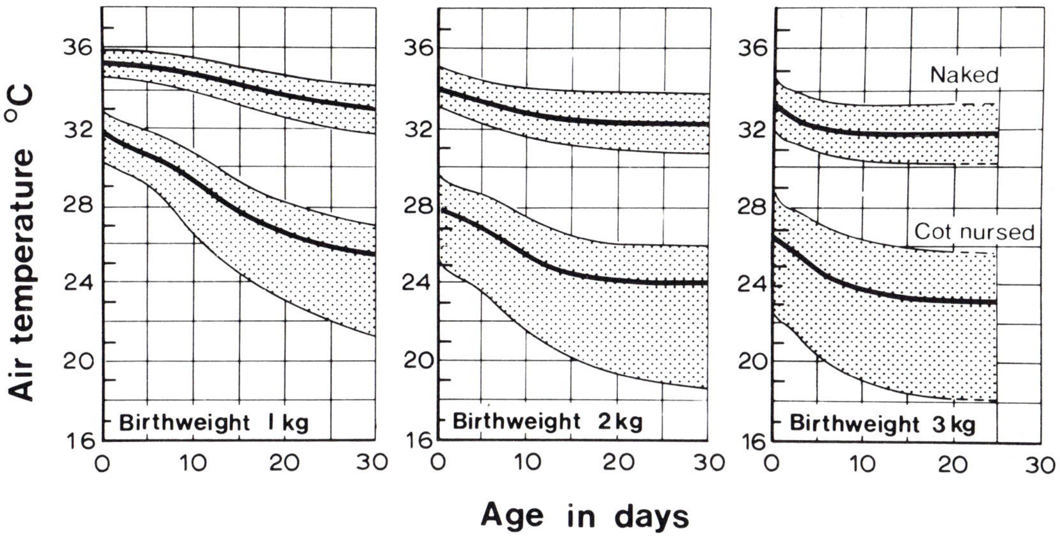

FIG. 14-5. Changes in optimal temperature over the first month of life for 1-, 2-, and 3-kg infants. The shaded area indicates the range and the solid line the optimum temperature of an environment in which an infant can maintain a normal core temperature without increasing either heat production or evaporative water loss by more than 25%. (From Avery, G. B.: *Neonatology—Pathophysiology and Management of the Newborn.* J. B. Lippincott Co., Philadelphia, 1975. Redrawn from Hey, E. N. *In* Recent Advances in Paediatrics (D. Gairdner and D. Hull (Eds.). London, Churchill, 1971.)

increased thermal stress imposed by frequent opening of the portholes or door. Although radiant heaters may be used both with and without servo control, the danger of severe burns makes continuous or unattended operation highly undesirable. Precautions required with servo control center on secure and proper placement of the thermistor temperature probe. If it is placed in a skin fold or beneath the infant, it will be effectively insulated, and skin and core temperature may fall considerably before this change is sensed by the warmer.

Infants who are being cared for in radiant warmers or are receiving phototherapy should be closely monitored for fluid balance. Insensible loss may double as a result of evaporation from the skin.[73,103,107] Cold gas coming from respirators, tanks, or wall outlets may also unnecessarily increase heat production.

Occasionally it is not possible to maintain acceptable core temperatures in infants who are in shock or have poor skin perfusion. Radiant warming depends on blood flowing through the skin to carry heat to the viscera. When this flow is decreased, skin temperatures may remain normal, but insufficient heat transfer to other organs may result in a lowering of core temperature. When radiant warmers are in use, rectal temperatures should be taken hourly. Infants whose temperatures are unstable under radiant heat should be placed in isolettes and may require heating blankets in order to stabilize body temperatures.

Incubators should be used as the routine treatment environment for infants requiring intensive care. They are specifically indicated for patients who are infected (in order to minimize the danger of cross infection) and for infants who cannot maintain their temperature under a radiant warmer. Incubators may also be operated with or without servo control. The effectiveness of servo control in incubators is not as great as that of a radiant warmer in maintaining constant skin temperature. The same precautions regarding temperature probe placement apply to both radiant warmers and incubators. When operated with constant heat output, the rate of heating is adjusted to maintain the environmental temperature appropriate for the baby's weight, as indicated in Table 14-1. Difficulty may be encountered in maintaining this temperature if treatment requires frequent access or repeated opening of the door. In these situations servo operation should be selected or the infant should be moved to a radiant warmer. In small infants excessive insensible water loss may be noted by decreased urine volume and a higher than usual urine specific gravity. This water loss may be minimized by the use of a heat shield (Fig. 14-6),[37] which may also reduce incidental thermal stress. Axillary temperatures are acceptable for infants in incubators.

Infants who are no longer acutely ill and weigh more than 1500 g generally do not require added heat. Appropriate clothing for an infant ordinarily includes a long-sleeve shirt, diaper, and a blanket with sheet. In this setting, minimal oxygen consumption occurs when the ambient temperature is 25° C.[48] Axillary temperatures should be taken at least every 4 hours to identify the infant with unstable temperature and to detect overheating.

TABLE 14-1. Optimal Incubator Temperatures for Infants of Various Weights (Assuming Infants Unclothed and 50% Humidity)

Weight (g)	C°	F°
Less than 1000	35–36	95–96
1000–1500	34–35	93–95
1500–2000	33–34	91–93
2000–2500	32–33	89–91
2500–3500	32	88–89
Over 3500	31	87–88

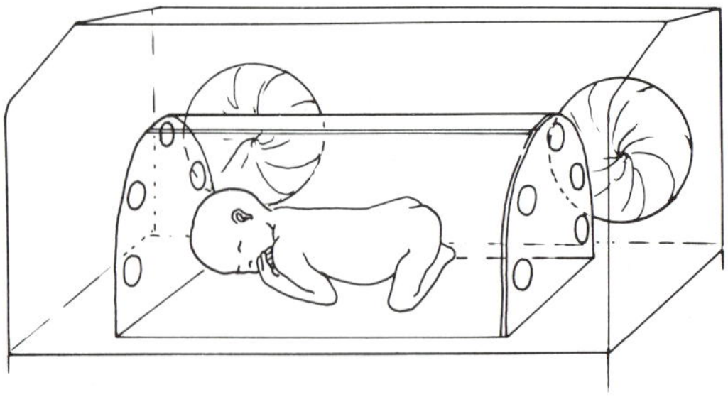

FIG. 14-6. An infant inside a heat shield intended for use inside an incubator.
(From Fanaroff[37] and From Klaus, M. H. and A. A. Fanaroff: *Care of the High Risk Neonate*. W. B. Saunders Co., Philadelphia, 1973.)

Ongoing Problem II—Surveillance

Surveillance is the essence of intensive care. It consists primarily of continuous evaluation by a skilled observer who, in addition to recording the details concerning intake, output, and vital signs, is also able to discern the subtle signs that suggest impending difficulty. Because of the overwhelming importance of oxygenation and tissue perfusion, proper surveillance also includes continuous electronic monitoring of vital signs and repeated assessment of blood gas and acid-base status.

A detailed discussion of nursing responsibilities is not possible here. However, a simple tabulation of observations or measurements performed underscores the overwhelming importance of skilled observation by an intensive care nurse.

Vital Signs
- Record of temperature, pulse, respirations, and blood pressure
- Record of apneic or bradycardic episodes

Intake/Output
- Formula: caloric content, route of feeding, volume taken
- Emesis: volume and guaiac testing

Drainage: volume measurement with guaiac testing
Urine: volume measurement, specific gravity measurement, dipstick testing for pH, glucose, protein, bilirubin, and blood
Stool: appearance, consistency, size

Ventilation
Measurement of FI_{O_2}
Observations of signs of respiratory distress: grunting, flaring, cyanosis, or retractions
Documentation of parameters of assisted ventilation: amount of distending airway pressure, ventilatory rate, I : E ratio, peak airway pressure

Physical Dimensions
Weight, girth, and head circumference

Environment
Bassinette, incubator, or infrared warmer
Use of phototherapy
Environmental temperature
Qualitative observations (e.g., sweating)

This information may give advance warning of problems such as sepsis, shock, or renal failure and is obviously essential in assessing the progress of a patient's illness. When unanticipated problems occur, these data are required as a basis for immediate therapy. Neonatal intensive care units should maintain a written record that includes all of the items on the preceding list.

MONITORING

Effective continuous surveillance has become possible only with the advent of electronic monitoring. Isolated determinations of pulse, respirations, or even blood pressure are not sufficient for many ill infants. Reliable detection of apnea or bradycardia is only possible with electronic monitoring.

Goals. Hypoxemia or tissue hypoxia either from poor oxygenation or poor perfusion can be tolerated only briefly without irreversible damage. It is therefore essential in unstable infants to provide some type of continuous rather than intermittent observation, which includes evaluation of hypoxia or hypoxemia.

Cardiac rate has been the function of choice, largely because appropriate monitors were the first to be of practical clinical value. It has remained most important because cardiac rate is extremely sensitive to the state of oxygenation and responds promptly to apnea.

Although the concept of alarms is inseparably connected with the idea of monitoring, the simple detection of high or low heart rate, respiratory rate, blood pressure, or temperature is no longer sufficient. It is reasonable to expect that the device which detects these abnormalities will also be able to provide accurate instantaneous and average measurements of the particular function, thereby obviating the need for repeated manual measurement. It is also reasonable to expect that the device will indicate whether its transducer or electrode is in satisfactory operating condition. The goal of continuous electronic surveillance, then, is to provide ongoing accurate measurement of particular vital signs, with activation of an alarm if the measurement exceeds a preset limit or if the reliability of the measurement is for any reason in question. Thus, alarms will go off more often than when real abnormalities exist. However, this practice is the only insurance that the reverse—alarms not going off when a problem does exist—is unlikely to occur.

Heart Rate Monitoring. Heart rate monitoring is accomplished by measuring the R-R interval in the patient's ECG. The electrodes used most often are adhesive electrodes applied at three positions on the thorax. Electrode "blankets" that require no cream on the conductive surfaces are also available. Because electrode placement is often variable and the sensitivity required for successful monitor operation is not standard, the tracing obtained is generally not useful as a diagnostic cardiogram.

Several sources of error may be encountered during heart rate monitoring in infants. Inaccurate rate determination may occur in machines designed for adults. Many of these monitors contain special electronic circuitry which avoids interference from electronic pacers. Because the infant's QRS complexes have a very steep slope in the R wave, they may be rejected as "pacer spikes" and thus give erroneously low counts and more frequent activation of the alarm. Thus care should be taken to ensure that this problem cannot occur in equipment planned for use on newborns. Special monitors presently available will count accurately even very rapid infant heart rates.

A second type of error is double rate counting. This problem occurs when the monitor mistakes a T wave for a QRS complex and includes it in the rate measurement. Double counting represents a particular hazard to the infant since the rate measured is erroneously high and bradycardia alarms will not be activated properly. This problem may also be avoided by selecting monitors with special circuits that distinguish between QRS and T waves regardless of lead placement or gain setting. In some instruments careful electrode placement and/or appropriate adjustments of the gain controls may be effective remedies.

Respiratory Rate Monitoring. Several basic types of apnea (respiratory rate) monitors are available. However, only one type has general usefulness as a respiratory rate monitor. Various types of mattresses and blankets are used as apnea monitors, but do not provide reliable respiratory rate information. Impedance pneumography, however, has gained widespread acceptance as a valid technique for measuring respiratory rate. The method relies on changes in electrical impedance measured across the chest as a result of changing volumes of air within. Ordinarily these monitors use the same electrodes placed for ECG monitoring—an obvious advantage.

In general this method is not as accurate as heart rate monitoring. Motion artifact sometimes occurs. Also, when the depth of inspiration varies significantly from breath to breath, some breaths may escape counting. Perhaps the most serious drawback is with instruments that require the adjustment of a sensitivity control. When these monitors are set for maximal sensitivity, the small changes in transthoracic impedance that occur as blood flows through the lungs with each heartbeat may be counted as breaths. Thus, in an apneic patient, the reading would be the same as heart rate and true apnea would be missed. Some devices can avoid this especially dangerous pitfall by constantly comparing the heart and respiratory rates and readjusting the sensitivity automatically. These monitors give an alarm promptly if the only detectable signal is at heart rate frequency.

Blood Pressure Monitoring. Blood pressure measurements may be made in infants either by a cuff with ultrasonic pickup for detecting blood flow changes or directly from an intravascular catheter and pressure transducer. While the first is the most widely used, it is only valuable for intermittent measurements. The only method for continuous monitoring of blood pressure is the use of a calibrated transducer on an intra-arterial catheter. Although numerous potential hazards are associated with this procedure, many clinical situations warrant the risk. Virtually all complications may be attributed to the presence of the intra-arterial catheter, most commonly umbilical artery catheters. Complications are the result of either infection or thromboembolic phenomena. Once the decision to place a catheter for monitoring has been made, consideration should be given to aspects that may affect the quality and accuracy of blood pressure monitoring. One of the most important of these considerations is catheter size. In plastic catheters smaller than No. 5 Fr., the tracing is often overdamped because of the narrow lumen. This damping produces an artificial decrease of the systolic and elevation of the diastolic pressures.

The most acceptable approach to catheter

maintenance requires the use of an additional coupling device that permits continuous infusion of fluid by a peristaltic pump. This device contains a pressure limiting valve that prevents the added fluid from affecting the pressure measurement. Together with this device, a miniature solid state pressure transducer is used. All equipment is gas sterilized so that bedside sterilization is not necessary. When the assembly is complete (Fig. 14-7), it lies on the mattress beside the infant. The error in this system is an acceptable 1 to 2 mm Hg. Calibration is routinely checked against a mercury pressure manometer before sterilization so that when the transducer is assembled at the bedside, the only calibration necessary is zero adjustment and electronic calibration using the internal standard of the monitor. At the time of assembly, particular attention should be paid to eliminating even the smallest bubbles of air from the line, stopcocks, continuous flow adapter, and the transducer itself.

When blood pressure monitoring equipment is in use, it is essential to have a continuous display of the pressure waveform. Because catheter sludging or clotting may occur unpredictably and also because air can enter the system either from the flushing solution source or by inadvertent injection when medications are added or blood is drawn, the shape of the pressure wave should be periodically observed as a matter of routine. The waveform normally has sharp features particularly at the top of the systolic upstroke. It should also be possible to identify the dicrotic notch that occurs with aortic valve closure. If these features are not present, it is likely that the measurement is inaccurate. In this case the patency of the catheter should be carefully investigated by drawing back—never by flushing. An attempt should also be made to free the line of any tiny air bubbles both by forward flushing if no clots are present in the line and by flushing toward the transducer. The importance of technique cannot be overemphasized. The monitor measures pressure based solely on the waveform presented to it.

When selecting equipment for use with newborn infants, it is desirable to choose a

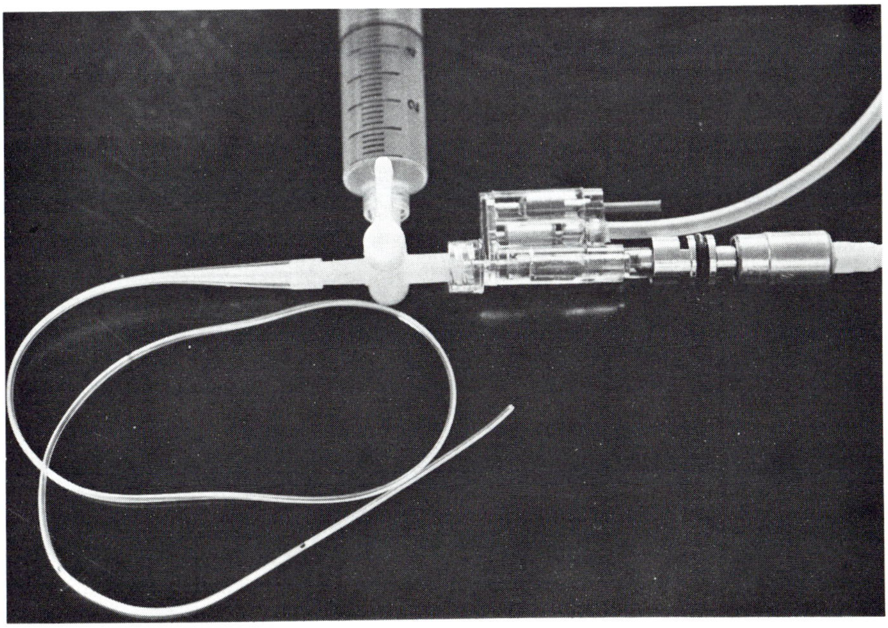

FIG. 14-7. An assembly for blood pressure monitoring with continuous infusion of fluid through the catheter.

monitor that offers a pressure scale compatible with the normal range of pressures in infants. Most adult monitors offer a full scale deflection of 0 to 300 mm Hg. Since the normal pressure in an infant is 50 to 70/30 to 40, an instrument with a full scale reading of 100 mm Hg would be useful. This type ordinarily makes it possible to maintain the oscilloscope display calibration while enjoying a trace that is large enough to interpret.

Once a monitor has been calibrated, it is possible for calibration drift to occur with time. This drift may be caused by a change in temperature of the transducer as it warms up. Another cause is damage to the transducer. Monitors that use vacuum tube circuitry are particularly susceptible to drift. Most new transistorized or solid state monitoring equipment is quite stable. Because drift can occur, it is necessary to recheck the calibration periodically. After the initial connection, recalibration should be done hourly for the first 3 hours. Afterwards, one check every 8 hours is sufficient. This rechecking procedure should consist of checking the zero reading by exposing the transducer to atmospheric pressure. (The zero reading is the one most likely to drift.) Calibration should be carried out according to the manufacturer's recommendation. If the height of the patient relative to the transducer is altered, zero and calibration must be readjusted.

Central venous pressure may be monitored with the same equipment. The venous catheter is positioned so that the tip is just above the right atrium. The monitoring equipment is usually set to indicate an average value. On some equipment, a special setting for CVP monitoring provides extra precision in calculating the pressure measurement.

Temperature Monitoring. The critical importance of temperature regulation in the premature and newborn infant has been discussed. The use of temperature monitors may be helpful in the management of particularly small infants in whom thermal instability may be a serious problem. Temperature monitoring is one of the most accurate processes available and requires only the fixation of a thermistor probe in order to measure axillary, skin, or rectal temperature. One must be certain that the probe is not directly exposed to the infant's source of heat. Small foam insulation discs are available for skin probes for infants under infrared warmers. Accidental dislodgement of the probe results in prompt cooling, and alarms will sound if set to appropriate physiologic limits. Most monitoring equipment is more accurate than the ordinary glass hospital thermometer.

UMBILICAL CATHETERS

Umbilical vessel cannulization is recommended for many infants requiring intensive care, as a means of providing a secure line for fluid and medication administration, obtaining arterial blood gas specimens, and monitoring arterial blood pressure. As mentioned, umbilical catheterization increases risk of infection and thromboembolic phenomena, as well as numerous other complications. Thus it merits careful consideration.

Umbilical Venous Catheters. Umbilical venous catheters are easily placed, have a low incidence of complication, and are often used for fluid administration or transfusion. If placed high in the inferior vena cava, they may also be used for central venous pressure determinations.

Indications. Infants requiring intensive care who will have parenteral fluid or transfusion requirements for more than 48 hours should be considered for umbilical venous catheters. The catheter should be a No. 5 Fr. polyvinylchloride, radiopaque, end-hole catheter. It should be placed with strict adherence to aseptic technique and special attention to the preparation and maintenance of a sterile field. Sepsis is the most serious and common complication. Catheter position may be estimated as indicated in Figure 14-8, and following placement, it should be checked routinely by roentgenogram. Position is ac-

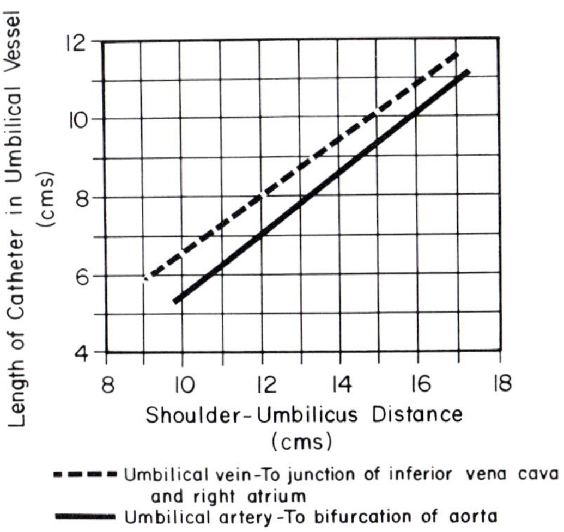

A

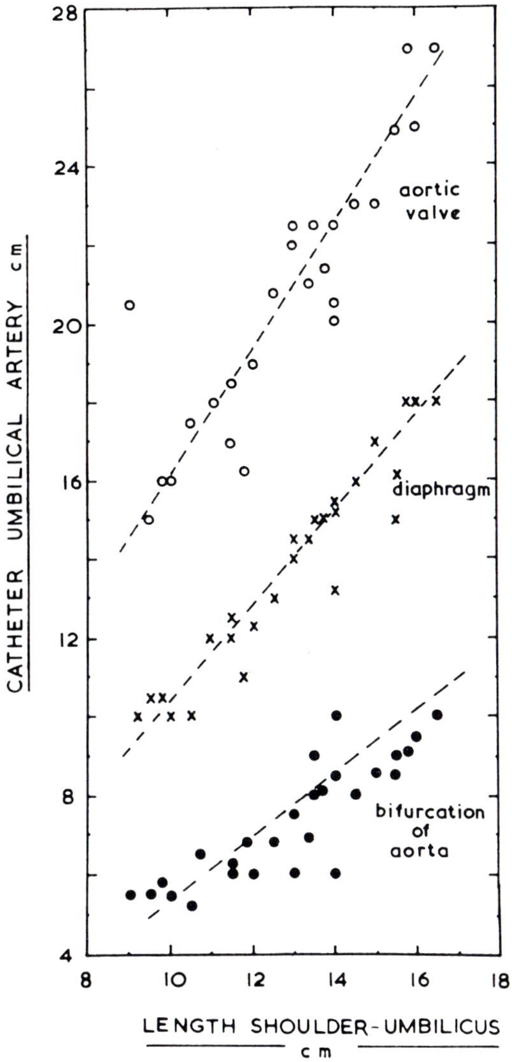

B

FIG. 14-8. Relationship between the shoulder-to-umbilicus measurement and the length of umbilical vessel catheter required to reach important anatomic landmarks.

A: (From Klaus, M. H. and Fanaroff, A. A.: *Care of the High Risk Neonate.* W. B. Saunders Co., Philadelphia, 1973.)

B: (From Avery, G. B.: *Neonatology—Pathophysiology and Management of the Newborn.* J. B. Lippincott Co., Philadelphia, 1975.)

ceptable if the catheter tip is in the inferior vena cava or umbilical vein. A catheter that is resting in a hepatic vessel should be withdrawn until the tip is in the umbilical vein. Attempts at repositioning in the inferior vena cava are usually fruitless. To minimize the risk of accidental decannulation, all catheters should be securely sutured in place and infusion controlled by a pump to avoid clotting. A stopcock should be provided as shown in Figure 14-7 to permit administration of medication or blood sampling.

Venous catheters may be safely maintained for periods of several weeks with proper care. However, leaking, gas in the portal system on roentgenogram, necrotizing enterocolitis or omphalitis are all indications for prompt, permanent removal of the catheter.

Infants whose catheters are placed after 24 hours of life are given broad spectrum antibiotic coverage because of the more than 85% incidence of colonization of the umbilical cord by this time. The only other indication for antibiotic coverage would be suspected contamination at the time of placement.

Umbilical Artery Catheters. The risk of much more serious complication from thromboembolism and vasospasm distinguishes umbilical arterial catheterization from the relatively routine catheterization of the umbilical vein. Umbilical arterial catheters should be placed only when the risk: benefit ratio is favorable and, while in place, should be maintained with scrupulous care and attention to early signs of complications so that the catheter may be removed promptly.

Indications. Any premature infant with moderate or severe respiratory distress should have an umbilical artery catheter for blood gas monitoring. Major surgery is also an indication for umbilical arterial blood pressure monitoring during the procedure.

Infants weighing less than 1200 g without respiratory distress have an increased likelihood of developing hypoxemia. Should respiratory distress develop in these infants, an umbilical artery catheter would be appropriate for both blood gas and blood pressure surveillance. It is ordinarily technically possible to place umbilical artery catheters in the majority of infants up to 5 days after birth. If an umbilical venous catheter is placed on admission, the possible future need for an arterial catheter should be anticipated and a short umbilical stump left.

Procedure. As with umbilical venous catheters, strict asepsis is essential. Catheterization is easiest if the artery is exposed by clean excision of the top of the umbilical stump. The artery may then be located easily as it protrudes slightly above the cut surface. Any clotted blood may be gently removed with fine forceps. Dilatation of the vessel is usually necessary and may be done by carefully introducing closed fine forceps and allowing them to open slightly several times. Probing is often damaging as false lumens are created and the risk of bleeding is increased. The catheter may be introduced after dilatation and inserted to a predetermined length. The catheter is safely positioned if the tip is between T-4 and the diaphragm or below L-2, as shown in Figure 14-9. The length of the catheter (in cm) required to reach T-7 or T-8 may be estimated by dividing the infant's length (in cm) by three and adding 1 cm (see Fig. 14-8).

Because of the risk of thrombosis and embolization, no infant should have an umbilical arterial catheter for more than 4 days. As with umbilical venous catheters, leaking, necrotizing enterocolitis, or omphalitis require permanent removal. If vasospasm causes toes to turn blue, catheters positioned above the diaphragm may be withdrawn to below L-2 or removed and replaced in the opposite umbilical artery. Both for ease of placement and for accurate blood pressure monitoring, a No. 5 Fr. end-hole, radiopaque polyvinylchloride catheter should be used and its position checked routinely by roentgenogram after placement or position adjustment. Heparin is not necessary and the continuous infusion technique described under blood pressure monitoring is recommended.

Complications. Although sepsis and thromboembolism are the most frequent complications observed with umbilical catheters, others also occur (Table 14-2). All are serious, and for this reason signs or symptoms suggestive of any of these warrant removal of the catheter and subsequent reliance on peripheral intravenous infusions or cutdowns as necessary. Blood specimens for gas tension and pH analysis may be obtained successfully in almost all infants from the radial, temporal, or brachial arteries. Femoral

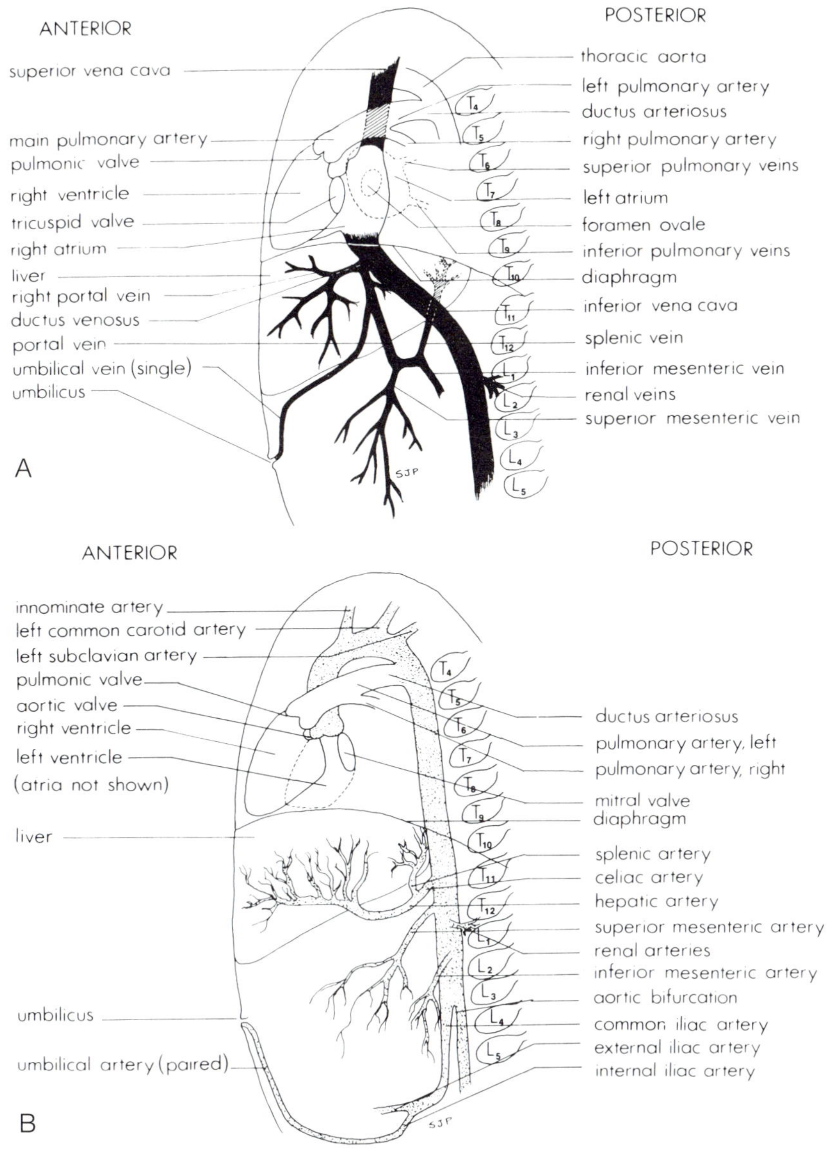

FIG. 14-9. The relationship between vertebral bodies as radiographic landmarks and the overlying vascular structures. (From Wesenberg, R. L.: *The Newborn Chest.* Harper & Row Publishers, Hagerstown, MD., 1973.)

sticks should be avoided, except in the most serious emergencies, because of the risk of septic hip necrosis.

OXYGEN MONITORING

Assessment of oxygenation in infants with cardiorespiratory problems is extremely important. It is usually determined from arterial blood specimens. Recently, continuous monitoring devices that measure Po_2 from a catheter in the aorta or transcutaneously have been introduced to supplement arterial blood gas (ABG) determinations.[51-54,90]

Arterial blood gas determinations should be performed on specimens drawn from ei-

TABLE 14-2. Complications of Umbilical Vessel Catheterization[36,45,63,97]

Septicemia
Perforation of the Peritoneum
Hemorrhage
Thrombosis
Arteritis
Necrosis of Toes
Extravasation of Fluid
Catheter Plugging
Improper Placement
Catheter Dislodgement

ther the right radial or temporal arteries since these specimens are not affected by ductal shunting. However, after many specimens it may be necessary to use the left arm or brachial arteries. When the need for frequent assessment exists, an umbilical arterial catheter should be placed (p. 394).

Continuous monitoring techniques have not replaced absolute measurements from arterial blood samples, but they may indicate trends or relative changes in gas tensions. Two types of device are in use—one of which is still developmental. Umbilical artery catheters are available with a built-in polarographic oxygen electrode. A small bedside meter provides a continuous indication of the measured Po_2. These instruments may drift and require frequent recalibration. Consequently, arterial blood gas determinations are still necessary.

The second technique for continuous oxygen monitoring, developed by Hüch and Hüch, utilizes a heated Clark electrode fixed on the patient's skin. The instrument maintains a local skin temperature high enough to "arterialize" the regional capillary blood flow. Oxygen diffusing through the infant's skin is measured by the electrode and indicated on either a meter or paper tape recording. When skin perfusion is good, these transcutaneous measurements have correlated well with simultaneous ABGs. Poor perfusion may result in unreliable determinations.[51-54]

Ongoing Problem III—Nutrition, Fluids, and Electrolytes

Nutritional, fluid, and electrolyte balance becomes a continuing problem for the clinician treating infants whenever oral feeding is impossible or inadequate due to immaturity, gastrointestinal obstruction or malformation, or respiratory distress.

It is only during the last weeks of gestation that an infant acquires any significant nutritional reserves. The differences in total body content of water, carbohydrate, protein, and fat between infants at various birth weights is shown in Figure 14-10. Thus the consequences of malnutrition depend upon the weight and maturity of the infant. Heird's theoretical calculation of survival time for these infants, shown in Table 14-3, further dramatizes this major limitation in smaller infants.

Calories alone are not sufficient to maintain a premature or starving infant. Protein catabolism cannot usually be stopped by the administration of solutions containing only dextrose. Dextrose infusion rates of 10 g/kg/day are effective in reducing protein catabolism, but in most infants negative nitrogen balance persists at 48 hours.[4] Respiratory distress may raise protein catabolism to 497 mg/kg over the same period.[72] In the face of inadequate nutritional intake, infants also sacrifice body stores of glycogen, fat, and trace elements.[86,102] Perhaps the most dangerous consequence of malnutrition in the newborn is the demonstrated irreversible reduction of brain size and cell number.[105] Although all tissues are growing rapidly at the time of birth, the late development of the central nervous system and its particularly rapid rate of growth in the last weeks of gestation appear to make it particularly vulnerable.[20,25-28,99,100,106]

The goal of nutritional therapy is to provide appropriate substrates and environment

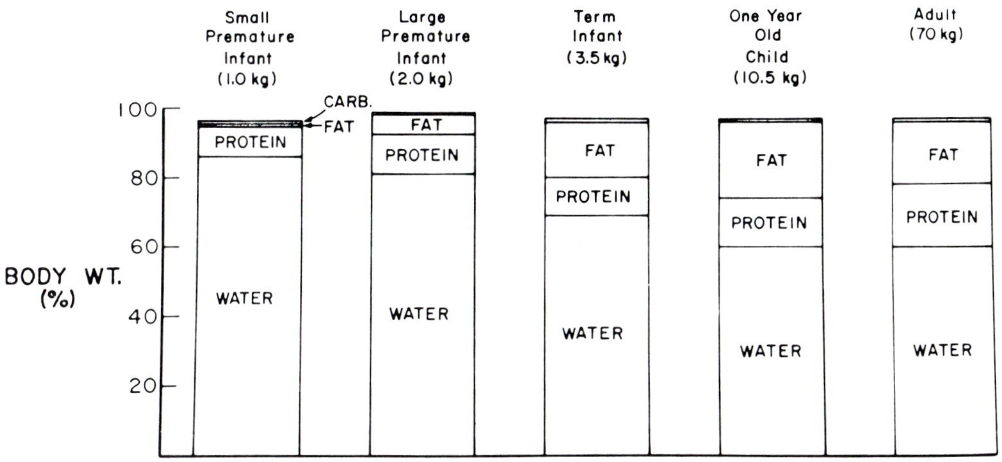

FIG. 14-10. Body composition of premature and full term infants, children and adults. (From Heird, W. C.[46])

to permit the continuation of growth that would have occurred in utero. Although it is not possible to duplicate the uterine environment, an understanding of intrauterine growth and its requirements is essential to the formulation of any nutritional plan for a sick infant. It is debatable whether the goal is also to duplicate the intrauterine growth rate. Because nutritional therapy plays such an important part in the management of the infant with respiratory distress, the rationale for therapy is presented in detail.

GROWTH

Data from Lubchenko and Kloosterman indicate that weight increases exponentially during most of the last trimester of pregnancy (Fig. 14-11); i.e., the rate of weight gain is proportional to the size of the fetus. This relationship is true until about the thirty-sixth week of gestation when the rapid rate subsides. It is also known that many substances accumulate at exponential rates in the body of the fetus. Table 14-4 compares the rates of accumulation of various minerals, nitrogen, fat, and water during the last trimester. These values corrected for body weight are expressed as amount/kg/day in Table 14-5. From this information it is evident that, although nitrogen and many minerals are accumulated at fairly uniform rates, the growth requirements of the fetus are changing. With increased mineralization of the skeleton near term, rates of accumulation of calcium and phosphorus increase significantly. The accretion rate for fat also rises. This information must be taken into account in formulating any plan for oral or parenteral nutrition.

TABLE 14-3. Calculated Survival Time in Days in Starvation and Semistarvation.*

	Water only	10% Dextrose†
Small premature infant	4	11
Large premature infant	12	30
Full-term infant	33	80
Adult	90	350

*From Heird, W. C. et al.: Intravenous alimentation in pediatric patients. *J. Pediatr. 80*:351, 1972.

†75 ml/kg/day for infant; 3 l/day for adult.

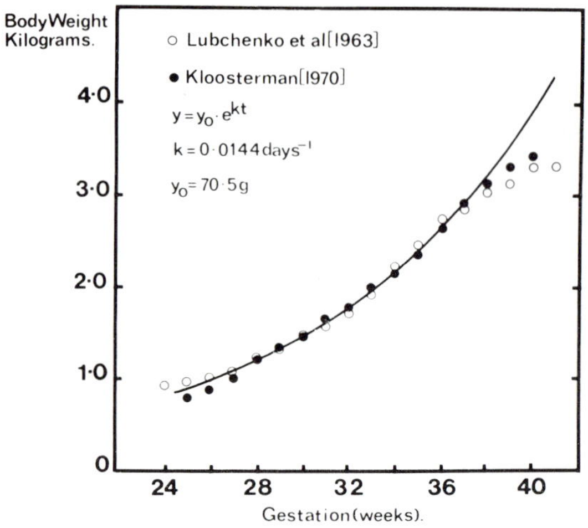

FIG. 14-11. Comparison of the means of two intrauterine growth curves showing that growth is exponential during the last trimester of pregnancy. (From Shaw, J. C. L.[81])

CALORIC AND FLUID REQUIREMENTS

An infant's caloric requirements are influenced by weight, gestational age, chronologic age, the existence of fetal malnutrition, and presence of disease. An infant typically utilizes about 120 calories/kg/day while growing. The specific factors that contribute to this requirement are shown in Table 14-6. On the first day of life, a full-term infant's basal caloric requirement is 35 cal/kg/day. By the second day this figure has risen to 45 cal/kg/day. Although small premature infants may have similar requirements at birth, by 3 weeks of age this number may reach 60 cal/kg/day in comparison to the 50 cal/kg/day requirement of the term infant.[86]

Infants who are small for gestational age

TABLE 14-4. Calculated Daily Rates of Accumulation of Various Substances by the Human Fetus at Different Periods of Gestation*

Substance	Weeks of gestation						
	24	26	28	30	32	34	36
Nitrogen, mg/day	159	207	269	349	452	587	761
Sodium, mg/day	15	18	23	28	33	43	53
Potassium, mg/day	15	19	24	31	39	50	64
Calcium, mg/day	59	79	105	140	186	248	330
Phosphorus, mg/day	36	47	62	82	108	142	188
Magnesium, mg/day	1.9	2.4	3.1	3.9	5.0	6.4	8.1
Iron, mg/day	0.8	1.1	1.4	1.9	2.5	3.3	4.3
Copper, μg/day	39	52	67	88	116	151	199
Zinc, μg/day	169	208	256	316	389	480	591
Fat, g/day	0.25	0.43	0.75	1.32	2.31	4.0	7.1
Water, g/day	7.6	9.7	12.3	15.7	20.0	25.6	32.6

*From Shaw, J. C. L.[81]

TABLE 14-5. Rates of Accumulation of Various Substances by the Human Fetus at Different Periods of Gestation (Expressed per kg of Body Weight per Day)*

Substance	Weeks of gestation 24	26	28	30	32	34	36
Nitrogen, mg	319	324	330	334	341	345	350
Sodium, mg	28	28	27	27	24	25	24
Potassium, mg	30	30	30	30	29	29	30
Calcium, mg	118	124	129	133	140	145	151
Phosphorus, mg	70	73	76	78	80	84	86
Magnesium, mg	3.8	3.7	3.8	3.8	3.8	3.7	3.7
Iron, mg	1.6	1.7	1.7	1.8	1.9	1.9	2.0
Copper, μg	78	80	83	85	87	89	92
Zinc, μg	337	326	315	302	293	282	272
Fat, g	0.5	0.6	0.9	1.3	1.7	2.4	3.2
Water, g	15.2	15.1	15.1	15.0	15.0	15.1	14.7

*From Shaw, J. C. L.[81]

have been shown to have a higher metabolic rate than prematures of the same weight. It has been suggested that this higher rate is a result of the disproportionate size of the brain (which has a high metabolic rate) in relation to body weight.[61,96] For these patients, caloric intake may have to be increased above standard allowances in order to obtain satisfactory growth. Infants with respiratory distress can be expected to have an increased requirement for calories because of the increased work of breathing. In this regard, it is relevant to note that the oxygen cost of breathing in the premature infant is greater than that in the adult.[94]

TABLE 14-6. Estimate of Caloric Expenditure During the Neonatal Period*

Activity	Caloric expenditure (kg/24 hr)
Minimal (nongrowing) expenditure	
Resting	50
Intermittent activity	0–15
Occasional cold stress	0–10
Total	50–75
Additional expenditure with growth	
Specific dynamic action	10
Fecal losses	10
Added requirement for growth	25
Total	45
Total caloric expenditure	95–120

*From Driscoll, J. M., Jr.[29]

Protein. Insufficient protein intake in either oral or parenteral regimens may result in hypoproteinemia and growth failure. If a nitrogen accretion rate of 350 mg/kg/day is assumed, the amount of protein that must be retained in order to meet this need is 2.1 g/kg. Normal growing infants who are breast-fed provide another index of protein requirement. Most breast milk contains 1.6 g of protein/100 cal. This figure considered in light of caloric requirements agrees quite closely with the number derived from accretion. Studies on infants who have received protein preparations parenterally have demonstrated growth with 1.7 g/kg/day.[87-89] Although oral intake as high as 9 g/kg/day has been correlated with improved growth,[88] doses for parenteral infusion should be limited to 2.5 mg/kg/day. Doses in excess of 3.5 g/kg/day are associated with hyperammonemia, aminoacidemia, and acidosis in infants weighing less than 1500 g.[30] This problem may be due in part to the immaturity of enzyme systems involved in the metabolism of certain amino acids, notably cystathionine synthetase in the conversion of methionine to cystine. Some evidence also suggests that amounts of parenteral protein in excess of 4 g/kg/day may be associated with impaired central nervous system function later in life in selected groups of patients.[43]

The goal of protein administration is to provide a source of nitrogen that can be utilized for anabolism without azotemia, hyperammonemia, or hyperaminoacidemia. When parenteral administration is required, protein may be administered either as hydrolysates of fibrin and casein or as mixtures of crystalline, synthetic L-amino acids. The synthetic amino acid mixture is preferable to the hydrolysate preparation in many ways. Its composition can be controlled more precisely, resulting in less variability from batch to batch. All protein is present in the form of amino acids so that the uncertain metabolism of small peptides is not a factor in nitrogen availability. They also have a lower titratable acid content and lower ammonium content. Problems that have been associated with the synthetic preparation include acidosis resulting from the net cation gap at physiologic pH and abnormal elevations of plasma concentrations of glycine and arginine, which suggests that the optimal concentration of component amino acids has not yet been determined.[46]

Fat. Fat normally accounts for between 35 and 45% of an infant's total caloric intake. It is a desirable food component because it provides 9 cal/g and consequently contributes much to the infant's energy requirements. Polyunsaturated fatty acids (linoleic and arachidonic) cannot be synthesized by humans and consequently must be provided exogenously. If less than 0.5% of all calories are provided as linoleic acid, skin changes and effects on megakaryocytes are observable. This effect does not occur if the level of linoleic acid is raised to 1 or 2%.[40] Consequently, it is generally felt that the requirement for fat is met if 2% of an infant's total caloric requirement is present as linoleic acid.

Formulas for oral feedings are not considered palatable unless the fat content is between 20 and 50%. Most commercial preparations that are designed to simulate breast milk contain about 35% fat. Safflower, oleo, corn or coconut oils are the most common sources of fat. These oils have been found to be the most readily absorbed and digested by both term and premature infants.

Parenteral preparations containing fat have been available for a number of years in Europe and Canada, where an extensive literature has accumulated.[3,7,15,82] Only one product has been licensed for use in the United States (Intralipid), and clinical experience here has been confined to research trials. Its application to the critically ill neonate requires further evaluation. It is supplied as a 10% emulsion with a milky white appearance. The major components are soybean oil (10%), egg yolk phospholipids (1.2%), glycerine (2.25%), and water for injection. The major fatty acids are linoleic (54%), oleic (26%), palmitic (9%), and linolenic (8%). The fat particles have the same physical characteristics as natural chylomicrons and are metabolized through the same pathways. Heparin has been shown to facilitate the clearance of lipid, but is not employed in the neonate because of its anticoagulant properties.[15] Most of the existing regimens for lipid administration supply 40 to 50% of the total caloric requirement as fat with a maximum dose of 3 to 4 g/kg/day. This dose represents 30 to 40 cc/kg/day of the 10% Intralipid preparation. These figures are based empirically on the average oral diet.[3,7,82]

Documented adverse reactions to Intralipid are rare, but include dyspnea, cyanosis, allergic reactions, hyperlipemia, hypercoagulability, emesis, hyperpyrexia, thrombocytopenia, hepatomegaly, splenomegaly, and transient abnormalities in liver function tests. The administration of any fat emulsion preparation should be accompanied by careful surveillance of serum chemistry values as well as inspection of plasma routinely to assure that the dose administered is being completely cleared by the infant. Depending on gestational age, the activity of lipoprotein lipase may be as low as one-third normal.

Carbohydrate. Carbohydrates are the principal source of calories for infants receiving either oral or parenteral nutrition. No specific requirement exists for carbohydrate intake, but clinical conditions such as hypoglycemia or severe negative nitrogen balance may be alleviated by the administration of dextrose solutions. One of the most common fluid regimens for full-term and premature newborn infants provides 10% dextrose and water at an infusion rate of 100 cc/kg/day.[33] This regimen provides 10 g/kg/day of dextrose with 30 to 40 cal/kg/day. This amount does not meet the basal requirements of a newborn. In premature newborn infants, glucose utilization or disappearance rates are particularly low at birth, rising after 48 hours.[34,80] This change in rate permits progression of glucose infusion over the first week to doses as high as 20 g/kg/day, thereby effectively doubling its usefulness. Not all infants routinely tolerate this high dose schedule without developing hyperglycemia and glycosuria. Because of the danger of hyperosmolarity, frequent checking of serum glucose concentrations is essential whenever higher doses are being administered. It is also important to note that, as dextrose concentrations are raised, small variations in infusion rate may provoke large transient elevations of serum glucose as a result of the infant's decreased ability to regulate insulin secretion rapidly. These transient elevations may also produce temporary glycosuria.

Sodium and Potassium. The requirement for sodium in either diet or parenteral regimen is variable during the newborn period, ranging from 1 to 3 mEq/kg/day.[29] While part of this total is incorporated in incremental tissue growth, most of this allowance replaces sodium that is lost in urinary output as a result of immature tubular function. Overheating may also initiate sweating, which further increases loss. Because of the variability of this requirement, parenteral administration should be adjusted in accordance with serum values.

The requirement for potassium is approximately the same as that for sodium at 1 to 2 mEq/kg/day.[29] This need may be decreased by any process that releases intracellular potassium, such as catabolism or hemolysis. For infants who are not being fed orally, it is usually appropriate to include potassium in intravenous fluids on the second day of life if urinary output is established. As with sodium, fluctuation of serum values may require adjustment of the concentration of potassium in infusates.

In addition to maintenance requirements, sodium, potassium, and water lost in nasogastric or other drainage may require replacement. Drainage fluid should be sent for laboratory determination of electrolyte concentrations and both volume and electrolyte losses replaced.

Calcium and Phosphorus. Both term and premature infants have a high requirement for calcium and phosphorus. The accretion rate at 36 weeks' gestation is 151 mg/kg/day for calcium and 86 mg/kg/day for phosphorus.[57,101] Most of this amount is incorporated in skeletal mineralization. In order to provide enough elemental calcium to allow intrauterine accretion rates to continue, 1.7 g/kg/day of calcium gluconate would be required parenterally. This dose far exceeds the usual maximum. In addition to the problems of infusion of calcium salts, calcium incorporation in bone produces hydrogen ion that must be excreted. If allowed to proceed at intrauterine rates, mineralization would produce 2 to 3 mEq/kg of hydrogen ion daily.[81]

Calcium salts may be administered either orally or parenterally. In a term infant, approximately 45% will be absorbed from the gastrointestinal tract.[40] Calcium gluconate may be given orally four or five times daily at a dose of 0.5 to 1.0 g/kg/dose. This dose should be diluted with formula or juice to a 5% solution. It provides up to 360 mg of elemental calcium daily. Parenteral dosage is restricted because of the possibility of bradycardia during or following administration. If added to a solution for infusion, the concentration should be adjusted so that the infant receives no more than 500 mg/kg/24 hours (45 mg elemental calcium).

Complications of calcium therapy may include hypocalcemia, hypercalcemia, and occasionally osteoporosis if parenteral therapy is prolonged. Hypocalcemia may be corrected by adjusting the concentration of the infusate and making certain that the volume administered provides the anticipated dose. Hypercalcemia may occur if insufficient quantities of phosphorus are present to permit mineralization. Readjustment of the calcium : phosphorus ratio will correct this problem.

Phosphorus is important in bone mineralization, urine buffering, and normal cellular enzyme function especially in red blood cells.[95] It is readily available in adequate quantities from most infant formulas or breast milk. Given parenterally, its concentration should be approximately equal to the concentration of calcium. A dose of 0.5 to 1.0 mEq/kg/day is appropriate. Deficiency of phosphorus may result in hypercalcemia, hypophosphatemia, and increased affinity of red blood cells for oxygen. All of these effects may be reversed by the adjustment of the phosphorus content of either the oral intake if the formula has a low phosphorus content or the parenteral infusate.

Trace Elements. In addition to requiring the major electrolytes, the infant needs magnesium, copper, zinc, iron, and iodine. Magnesium is usually added to infusates as $MgSO_4$ at a dose of 0.5 mEq/kg/day. Although copper deficiency has been described, zinc, iron, iodine, and copper are not provided in any conventional parenteral preparation. Although they may be present as contaminants in solution, it is desirable to provide for their regular administration as elements of normal plasma. If transfusion is occurring at least weekly because of anemia, needs for trace elements are probably being met. If not, transfusion with plasma for nutritional needs should be considered weekly.

Fluids. Fluid requirements are established by the amount of fluid lost. Infants lose water by urination, defecation, and evaporation from lungs and skin. Table 14-7 summarizes these losses.

Urinary output in infants is determined to a large degree by the amount of solute excreted. The concentrating capacity of the newborn kidney is about half that of an older child or adult at 700 mOsm/l.[29] The result is a greater loss of fluid with a given quantity of solute. This solute may be either electrolytes administered parenterally or metabolic byproducts produced endogenously. Normally functioning kidneys may excrete from 20 to 60 cc/kg/day. By several days of age 50 cc/kg/day is typical.[29]

Stool losses are usually small and account for about 5 to 10 cc/kg/day. Additional losses may result from nasogastric or ostomy drainage as well as from surgical drains. This volume should be replaced and electrolyte content measured for replacement also.

Evaporative losses from skin and respiratory tract (insensible loss) may account for up to 40 cc/kg/day depending on the relative

TABLE 14-7. Water Losses in Premature and Full-Term Newborn Infants

Source	Quantity (ml/kg/day)
Evaporative	
Skin and respiratory tract	21–30
Infants weighing < 1250 g	60–120
Urinary Output	25–62
Stool	2
Total	48–184

humidity of the infant's environment. Approximately half of this loss may be attributed to respiratory evaporation. This factor is important particularly for patients receiving air-oxygen mixtures that have been humidified to nearly 100%. The fluid requirement may be as much as 20 cc/kg/day lower in these cases. It has been demonstrated that respiratory humidifiers may, beyond decreasing fluid losses, serve as sources of additional fluid in a small number of instances.

Insensible loss from the skin is influenced both by environmental humidity (lower in the humidified isolette) and by the presence of nonionizing radiation. This type of radiant energy could come either from infrared warmers or from conventional phototherapy units. Each source has about the same effect and together may triple an infant's insensible loss.[73,103,107]

Dehydration in infants may result in weight loss, decreased urinary output, loss of skin turgor, dryness of mucous membranes, increased urinary specific gravity (normally less than 1.010), or evidence of hemoconcentration. Weight loss may not be measurable until dehydration is severe and then must be distinguished from primary malnutrition. Decreased urinary output is a sensitive early finding, but must be differentiated from primary renal disease. In urine free of protein and blood, elevated specific gravity should be considered an indication of dehydration. Since all newborns are not able to concentrate their urine, the absence of urine specific gravity elevation should not be taken as a sign of normal hydration. Values above 1.010 should be considered abnormal. Changes in skin turgor and mucus production are both associated with moderately severe dehydration and require prompt treatment.

Complications associated with fluid therapy are almost invariably related to the rate at which fluid is administered. Infants have a limited capacity to excrete a free water load even when well. Overhydration may produce peripheral edema, heart failure, or pulmonary edema if severe. Special care should be taken in the treatment of dehydrated infants to avoid rapid rehydration. Isotonic dehydration should be treated over a period of 24 hours. Hypertonic dehydration, however, requires slower rehydration (48 to 72 hours) to minimize the effects of intracranial fluid re-equilibration.

Vitamins. Vitamin deficiency syndromes occur when infants receive parenteral alimentation unless a vitamin supplement is added. Oral feeding with conventional formulas usually provides sufficient quantities of vitamins. In infants who cannot be fed sufficient quantities of formula, supplementation with a multivitamin preparation may be necessary. All premature infants receiving either breast milk or cows' milk based formulas should receive supplemental doses of vitamins C and D. Vitamins for parenteral administration are usually combined in fixed ratios. The contents of one such solution are shown in Table 14-8.

ORAL FEEDING

Breast milk and formulas that simulate it produce nearly equivalent growth rates.[40] Provided sufficient quantities can be ingested to meet caloric needs, the only concern for the physician is vitamin supplementation and

TABLE 14-8. Contents of a Standard Parenteral Vitamin Solution

Each 10 ml contains	
Ingredient	Quantity
Vitamin A	10,000 U
Ergocalciferol	1,000 U
Vitamin E	5 IU
Thiamine hydrochloride	50.0 mg
Riboflavin	10.0 mg
Pyridoxine hydrochloride	15.0 mg
Niacinamide	100.0 mg
Dexpanthenol	25.0 mg
Ascorbic acid	500.0 mg

iron intake. Both breast and cows' milk contains little iron and low concentrations of vitamins A, C, and D. Iron is ordinarily provided by infant cereals that are supplemented. Premature infants, because of decreased total body iron stores, should receive supplemental ferrous sulphate (8 to 15 mg Fe^{++}/day orally, divided b.i.d.) after the twelfth week of life. Commercial preparations are available which contain vitamins A, C, and D in appropriate proportions. Daily requirements are shown in Table 14-9.

NASOGASTRIC AND NASOJEJUNAL FEEDINGS

Adequate nipple feeding may be impossible due to immaturity or unwise in the presence of respiratory distress. Gavage or nasojejunal feeding may alleviate nutritional problems in these circumstances.

Infants weighing less than 1500 g seldom take adequate quantities of formula spontaneously. Although softer premature nipples may improve intake in these small infants, it is usually necessary to provide additional fluids and calories. In the absence of respiratory distress, this supplement can be given by slow gravity feeding through an indwelling nasogastric tube. Depending on the size of the infant, a feeding tube of size No. 5 or 7 Fr. may be readily passed through one nostril and advanced to the stomach. This distance may be estimated by the distance between the tips of the ear and the xyphoid process. The tube should be secured with tape with special care to avoid pressure on the nares. Many available tubes are made of polyvinylchloride and should therefore be changed every 24 to 48 hours to avoid hardening and gastric irritation.

Tube feeding should begin with small volumes and be incremented as tolerated. Vomiting or abdominal distention are indicators of too rapid progression. Failure of gastric emptying as demonstrated by aspiration of significant quantities of formula before the next feeding may indicate too frequent feedings or overfeeding. In this circumstance the feeding interval should be prolonged before limiting intake. These infants may tolerate fewer, larger feedings better than smaller, frequent ones.

Other complications of gavage feeding concern the feeding tube. Pressure caused by the tube may damage nasal soft tissue structures. Traumatic placement or prolonged use of a single catheter may produce mucosal erosion or occasionally gastric perforation.

Direct feeding into the stomach is contraindicated whenever the risk of regurgitation is increased. The risk is especially high if the infant has tachypnea or is receiving any type of respiratory therapy. Nasojejunal feeding bypasses this problem. It requires placement of a nasogastric catheter that is pliable and long enough to be moved by peristalsis through the pylorus. The tube may then be advanced in small increments until the tip is in the jejunum. Catheters for this purpose should be made of silastic so that frequent replacement is not necessary. Tubes made from polyvinylchloride are hazardous because they harden on exposure to intestinal secretions. A plastic stylette may be necessary to pass the tube into the stomach. As the tube

TABLE 14-9. Vitamin Supplementation Requirements for Infants Receiving TPN*

Vitamin	Requirement (24 hrs)
Vitamin A	70–200 IU
Thiamine	0.2 mg/1000 cal
Riboflavin	0.3 mg/1000 cal
Pyridoxine	9 mcg/g protein
Ascorbic acid	10 mg
Vitamin D	100–200 IU
Vitamin E	0.34–0.45 IU
Niacin	4.4 mg/1000 cal
Folic acid	5–50 mcg
Vitamin K	5 mcg
Vitamin B_{12}	Less than 1 mcg

* Modified from Shaw, J. C. L.[81] and W. C. Heird.[46]

tip passes the pylorus, the pH of secretions aspirated changes from acid to alkaline. Feedings may be either by gravity or by continuous infusion with a peristaltic pump. Complications, except for regurgitation, are the same as for gavage feeding.

PARENTERAL NUTRITION

For therapeutic purposes, parenteral alimentation should be defined as any form of intravascular administration of nutrient substances. This concept embraces both the routine infusion of dextrose and the administration of more complex regimens including carbohydrates, protein, fats, minerals, vitamins, and trace elements through deep vein catheters. It also encourages a unified approach to the ubiquitous nutritional problems encountered in neonatal intensive care.

Indications. Infants who are premature or small for gestational age have low energy reserves and cannot tolerate starvation for even a few hours. Some form of parenteral alimentation is indicated for any infant unable to take adequate, regular feedings. If an infant will not be able to take feedings for 48 hours, a progressive regimen of protein and fat as well as dextrose should be begun. Since sufficient calories for growth will not be available for nearly a week, an early start is important. Should an infant's clinical condition improve unexpectedly, alimentation may be modified or discontinued.

Administration. Parenteral alimentation may be administered through peripheral or central intravenous lines. If peripheral intravenous catheters are used, the dextrose concentration must be limited to 10% to avoid sclerosing the vessel. Lines placed in central veins with high flow permit solutions with higher dextrose concentrations, but if concentrations of dextrose above 10% are used, the risk of infection is increased and special precautions must be observed in both the insertion and daily maintenance of these catheters.[42,69] When dextrose concentration is limited, the only way of increasing the number of calories administered is by increasing the fluid administration rate. This procedure has obvious limitations, and often it is necessary to infuse higher concentration dextrose solutions.

Central Vein Catheters. Central vein catheters must be placed under sterile conditions in an operating room. The desired position is the superior vena cava just above the heart. Although this placement may be achieved by umbilical vein catheterization, cutdown or percutaneous catheterization of either the external or internal jugular vein is preferable. The method described by Dudrick and Wilmore in 1968,[104] illustrated in Figure 14-12, is frequently used because it avoids exposure of the point at which the catheter enters the vessel. After inserting a catheter in

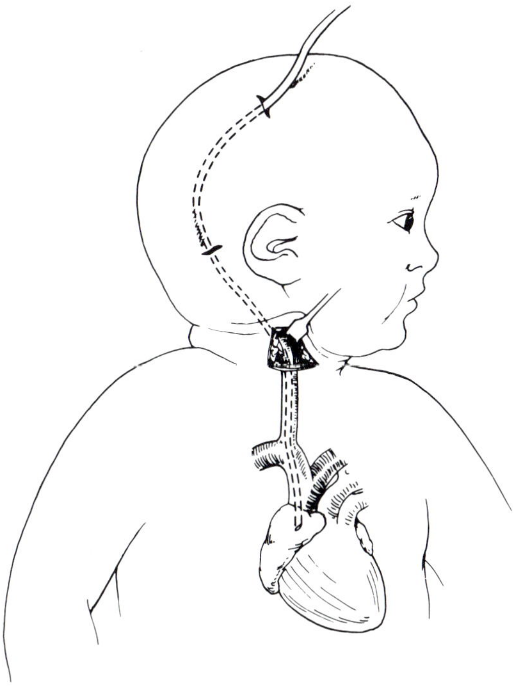

FIG. 14-12. Placement of a catheter for parenteral alimentation in the internal jugular vein according to the method of Dudrick and Wilmore. (From Avery, G. B.: *Neonatology—Pathophysiology and Management of the Newborn,* J. B. Lippincott Co., Philadelphia, 1975.)

the superior vena cava through a neck incision over either jugular vein, the proximal end of the catheter is tunnelled to a stab wound in the scalp where it exits, permitting closure and healing of the neck incision. Alternatively, some surgeons may permit the catheter to exit directly from the neck wound. Here it becomes particularly important to maintain an occlusive dressing with antibiotic ointment over the wound site around the catheter. With either technique, special attention should be given to a method of anchoring the catheter that protects it from accidental withdrawal if tension is accidentally applied. One such method is shown in Figure 14-13.

Because of the increased risk of infection, all catheter connections are routinely made observing careful sterile technique. Once connected, the line should not be opened or entered for drawing blood or giving medications. The administration setup should contain a volumetric administration set, appropriate tubing for a peristaltic pump, and a 0.22-μ filter to remove any particulate matter, bacteria, or fungi. If a lipid emulsion is to be infused, preparation should be made at the time connections are made. Figure 14-14 shows an appropriate setup. Once the lipid infusion is complete, the stopcock may be turned off, but all connections should remain intact until the entire administration set is changed.

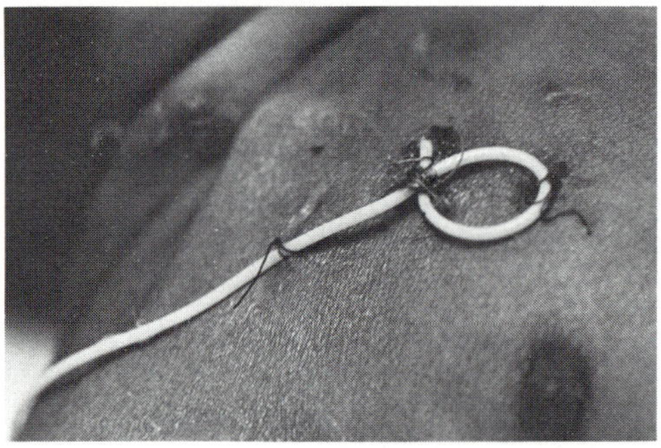

FIG. 14-13. An alternative method of catheter placement and fixation for parenteral alimentation.

Solutions for parenteral alimentation are ordered individually for each patient to permit the continuous adjustment of dextrose, protein, and electrolyte concentrations. This adjustment is necessary because the infant's inability to regulate insulin secretion requires gradual increase in dextrose concentration until appropriate levels can be reached. Infants also differ in tolerance for protein solutions and electrolyte requirements. If a stock solution cannot be used, solutions for parenteral alimentation should be prepared under the supervision of a trained pharmacist working at a laminar flow hood.

Knowledge of intrauterine growth and its requirements provides a theoretic basis for parenteral nutrition. Although electrolytes may be administered under the previously described guidelines, some special considerations pertain to regimens for carbohydrate, protein, and fat.

Carbohydrate Administration. Most infants will tolerate dextrose administration at 10 g/kg/day provided the administration is uniform. This dose may be increased at a rate of 1 g/kg/day until a maximum dose of 20 g/kg/day is reached.[2] The concentration of dextrose depends on the infant's fluid requirements or ability to tolerate fluid loading. In patients with good renal function, caloric intake can be increased at fixed dextrose concentrations by increasing the administration rate. Another factor that may limit the concentration of dextrose is the available route of administration. Concentrations higher than 10% can be given only into central veins, and special precautions against infection must be observed. Complications of dextrose administration, including hyperglycemia and glucosuria with diuresis, may also limit dextrose infusion.

Protein Administration. Synthetic L-amino acids may be combined with dextrose on the second day of parenteral supplementation or alimentation. A starting dose of 1 g/kg/day is appropriate, and over an 8-day period this dose may be increased to 2.5 g/kg/day as

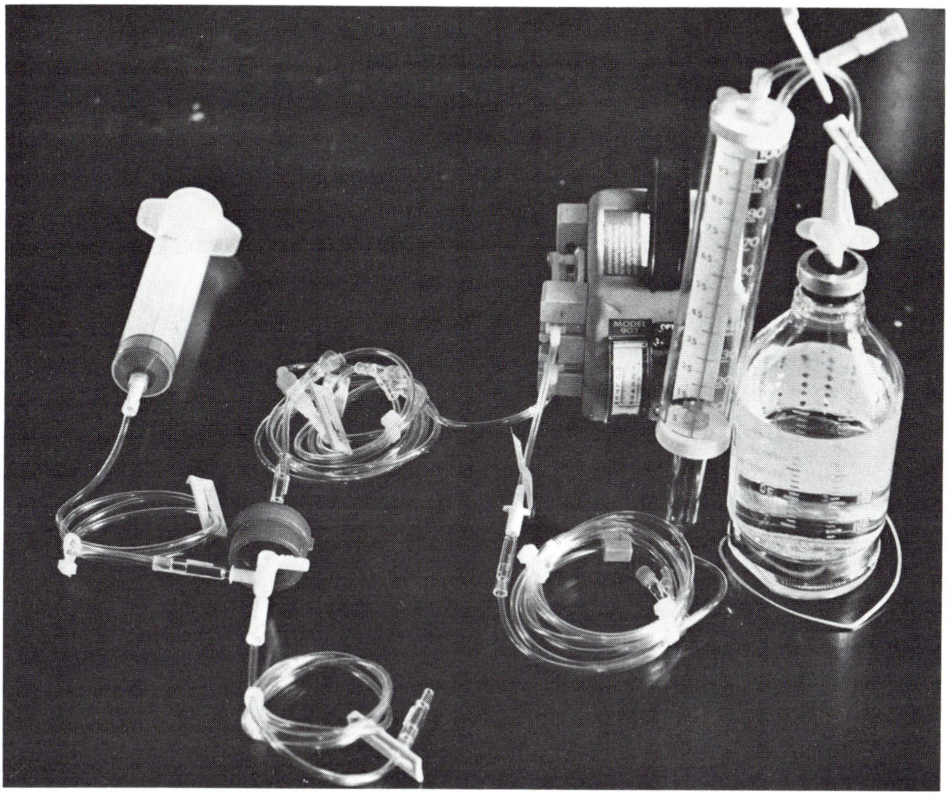

FIG. 14-14. A completely closed system for the administration of all parenteral nutrients. Dextrose, protein, electrolytes and water are pumped from the volumetric administration set through a Millipore filter to a stopcock, which permits the simultaneous infusion of Intralipid by syringe pump.

nonprotein calories supplied increase. The dose of protein is limited by the number of nonprotein calories available. The recommended proportion is 150 nonprotein calories to 1 g of nitrogen or for Freamine II, 6:1 nonprotein:protein calories.[70]

Fat Administration. Although highly desirable as a source of calories, the rate of parenteral administration of lipid may be limited by an infant's inability to clear it from plasma. Hyperbilirubinemia is an absolute contraindication to parenteral fat administration. Free fatty acids generated by metabolism of Intralipid compete with bilirubin for albumin binding and thereby decrease the reserve binding capacity. This reduction may increase the risk of kernicterus at much lower levels of jaundice.[16] Parenteral fat administration should be begun with a test dose of 1 g/kg/day on the second day of a parenteral alimentation regimen. Plasma should be inspected in a hematocrit tube following completion of the dose to be certain that fat metabolism is adequate. This dose may be increased daily over a period of 8 days until the dose reaches 4 g/kg/day. General routine guidelines for solution preparation are shown in Table 14-10. The progressive regimen recommended and the relative caloric contributions of the principal nutrients are outlined in Table 14-11.

Complications of Parenteral Alimentation. The most important complication of parenteral alimentation is infection. Fastidiousness

TABLE 14-10. Guidelines for Preparation of Solutions for Parenteral Alimentation

Solution	Quantity
Daily Requirements	
Dextrose	Up to 20 g/kg/day as tolerated
Protein	Up to 2.5 g/kg/day
Na	1–3 mEq/kg
K	1–3 mEq/kg
Ca	0.5–2 mEq/kg
P	0.25–0.50 mM per kilogram per day
Mg	0.5–1 mEq/day
Multivitamins	2 cc/kg
Intralipid	Up to 40 cc/kg IV given daily
Intermittent Requirements	
Vitamin K	1 mg IM or IV given weekly
B_{12}	1 μg/day IM or IV given weekly
Folic acid	50 μg/day IV given daily or weekly
Trace minerals	Weekly transfusions of whole blood or fresh plasma—10 cc/kg

at the time of insertion of the catheter and meticulous daily care minimize the incidence. However, infections with candida, staphylococci, and enteric organisms are not rare. Infants with parenteral alimentation catheters should be observed with special care for early signs of sepsis and worked up promptly. If sepsis is documented, the catheter must be removed. Other complications of intravascular catheters as well as the metabolic complications of parenteral alimentation are shown in Table 14-12. It is important to note that the majority of serious complications of alimentation with central catheters may be eliminated if the infant will tolerate larger volumes of fluid at lower solute concentrations given through a peripheral intravenous catheter. It is frequently possible to obtain the same caloric intake associated with central venous catheters.

Surveillance. The numerous potential metabolic complications make a surveillance routine mandatory for any patient receiving parenteral alimentation of any form. Most abnormalities are likely to appear during the first week of treatment; consequently this period of changing therapy merits special attention. An appropriate schedule for biochemical surveillance, which should be closely followed for any patient at risk, is shown in Table 14-13.

The remainder of this chapter discusses

TABLE 14-11. A Progressive Regimen for Total Parenteral Alimentation

	Nutrient (g/kg)			
Day	Carbohydrate	Protein	Fat	Total calories
1	10	—	—	34
2	11	1.0	1	52
3	12	1.0	2	67
4	13	1.5	2	72
5	14	1.5	3	87
6	15	2.0	3	92
7	16	2.0	4	107
8	17	2.5	4	112

TABLE 14-12. Complications Experienced with Total Parenteral Alimentation

Catheter	Metabolic
Sepsis	Persistent glycosuria
Extravasation of fluid	Acidosis
Local skin infections	Radiographic bone changes
Plugging or dislodgement	Hyperammonemia
Thrombosis of major vessel	Dehydration
Improper placement	Hepatic damage
	Postinfusion hypoglycemia
	Hypocalcemia
	Hypophosphatemia
	Hypokalemia
	Skin rash
	Essential fatty acid deficiency
	Copper deficiency

*From Avery, G. B.: *Neonatology—Pathophysiology and Management of the Newborn.* J. B. Lippincott Co., Philadelphia, 1975.

TABLE 14-13. A Surveillance Schedule for Infants Receiving Parenteral Alimentation

Variable	Frequency
Measurements	
Weight	Daily
Head circumference and length	Baseline and weekly
Blood Chemistries	
Electrolytes	Daily until stable,
Ca, glucose, BUN	then 2x weekly
P, Mg, SGPT, Pro-time	
Fractionated bilirubin	
Bile acids, protein	Baseline and weekly
Plasma aminogram	
Ammonia, triglycerides	Baseline
Fluid Balance	Daily
Intake volume	
Output volume	
Urinary specific gravity	
Urinary glucose (Dipstick)	

management of the acute, life-threatening problems of the infant with respiratory distress, including hypoxia, acidosis, and shock. Since similar modes of therapy are often used for more than one problem (e.g., assisted ventilation may be indicated for both hypoxia and respiratory acidosis), some duplication is unavoidable in this problem-oriented approach.

Acute Problem I—Hypoxia

PHYSIOLOGY AND ETIOLOGY—FACTORS AFFECTING TISSUE OXYGENATION

A decreased Pa_{O_2} is present in virtually every infant with respiratory distress, whether the cause is hyaline membrane disease (HMD), congenital heart disease, or congenital malformations such as diaphragmatic hernia. Significant hypoxemia is that level of Pa_{O_2} that results in tissue hypoxia. Thus in planning therapy, consideration must be given to factors that influence oxygen delivery to the tissues, such as cardiac output, distribution of peripheral blood flow, hemoglobin level, 2,3-diphosphoglycerate (DPG) activity, and pulmonary factors. The term, critical Po_2, has been used to define the level of oxygen pressure below which diffusion into the cell is impaired and organ function disturbed. A critical range of Po_2 between 20 and 30 mm Hg has been suggested for the adult.[74] An accumulation of lactic acid and resultant metabolic acidosis could be regarded as an indication that a critical Po_2 has been reached, although it may not be possible to determine the particular organ or tissues involved.

Premature infants are known to be deficient in 2,3-DPG,[75] and in contrast to the full-term infant, they do not increase its production in response to hypoxia.[75] Normally the deficiency of this enzyme in fetal life is looked on as an advantage since it favors oxygen uptake and retention by fetal red cells.[31,32] Their oxygen-hemoglobin dissociation curve is shifted to the right (Fig. 14-15). For the premature or other infant with respiratory distress, this deficiency or any other condition such as acidosis that causes such a shift in dissociation can be a serious disadvantage since oxygen availability to tissues is limited. For this reason and because of the limited capacity of fetal red cells for production, some investigators have suggested restoration of normal 2,3-DPG activity and content by exchange transfusion of infants at risk with whole blood from adults.[24] At present insufficient information exists to document the efficacy of this procedure and it is therefore not recommended.

Very little is known about the infant's ability to change cardiac output and control the distribution of peripheral blood flow. It is unlikely that the newborn can appreciably increase cardiac output in response to tissue demand for oxygen. If one can extrapolate from studies on lower animals such as the

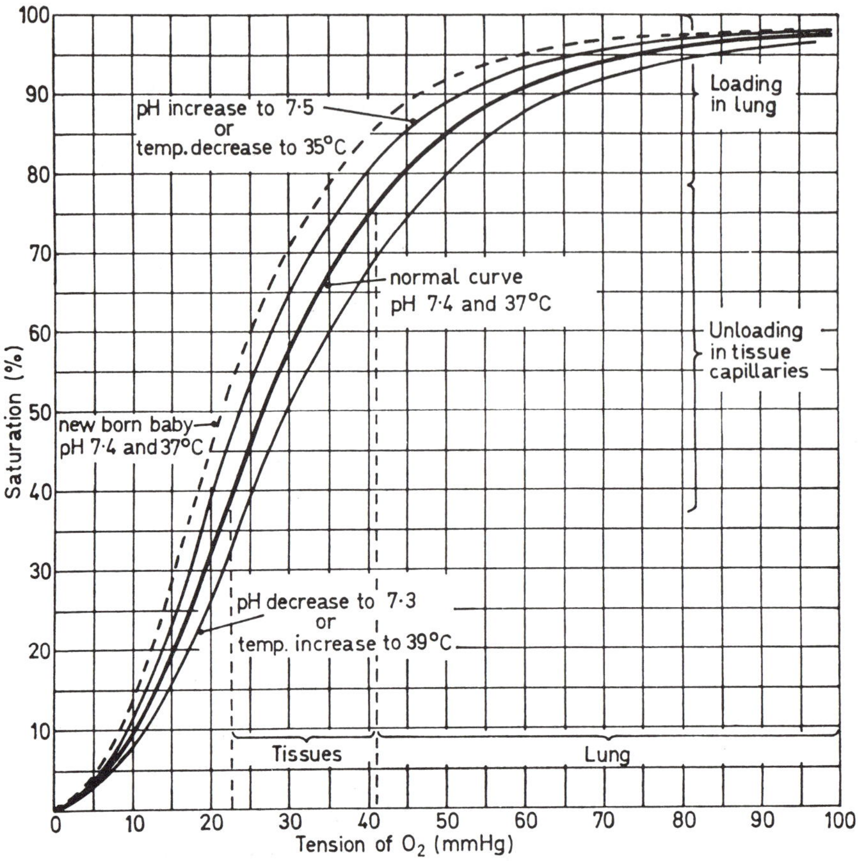

FIG. 14-15. Dissociation curve for oxyhemoglobin, showing effects of various influences on its position. (Data compiled by Severinghaus. From Cotes, J. E.: *Lung Function.* Blackwell Scientific Publications Ltd., Oxford, 1968.)

sheep, the fetal and newborn hearts have a low compliance, which limits increases in stroke volume. It is also unlikely that large increases in cardiac output can be achieved by increasing heart rate.[77] Indeed, in most distressed infants a fixed heart rate is the rule. Again, little is known as to whether the premature infant, particularly one in distress, can redistribute cardiac output by changes in peripheral circulation in response to hypoxia. The fetal sheep can redistribute blood flow from the periphery to vital central areas in response to hypoxia in utero.[78] Krauss and co-workers have been able to demonstrate a similar response in normal infants, but it is absent in some distressed infants. Here limb blood flow was measured in response to airway occlusion (dive reflex) and upward tilting (baroreceptor response). The absence of the self-protective reflex in these two test situations raises many further questions—all unanswered—regarding sympathetic regulatory functions in distressed infants.[58]

Oxygen consumption in the first day of life is approximately 4.5 ml/kg/min. rising to over 6 ml/kg/min. by the end of the first week. The newborn infant, especially when premature, has little reserve in meeting his oxygen needs. Stresses such as hypothermia may raise oxygen consumption to 15 ml/

kg/min. The following calculation indicates how marginal the reduction can be in providing oxygen to tissues; e.g. a 1-kg infant with hemoglobin 17 g/100 ml, blood volume 100 ml, and cardiac output 150 ml/kg/min. will transport 30 ml/kg/min. of oxygen at 100% saturation of hemoglobin. In disease situations where oxygen saturation is lowered, the oxygen delivery will be grossly inadequate. In view of all these considerations and because of limitations in response available to the infant, every effort must be made to minimize oxygen consumption in respiratory distress.

In pulmonary disease of the newborn almost all hypoxia is due to right-to-left shunts. In HMD right-to-left shunts occur in the lungs[71] and through the foramen ovale[14] and patent ductus arteriosus.[79] In severe cases some hypoxia may be due to a diffusion block.[59] Minimal maldistribution of ventilation has been demonstrated as well.[17] In meconium aspiration and transient tachypnea, both shunting and maldistribution of ventilation are causes of hypoxia. Shunts can be calculated clinically using the Berggren equation:

$$\frac{\dot{Q}_S}{\dot{Q}_T} = \frac{Cc'_{O_2} - Ca_{O_2}}{Cc'_{O_2} - C\bar{v}_{O_2}}$$

It should be understood that many assumptions are made when the equation is used and that the number derived is a "ball park" figure at best. After an FI_{O_2} of 1.00 has been administered for 10 to 15 minutes, Pa_{O_2} may fail to rise above 300 mm Hg. This measurement is a gross clinical method for determining the presence of a right-to-left shunt (see Fig. 2-2).

RECOGNITION

Hypoxia is first suggested when cyanosis is present. It appears when deoxyhemoglobin concentration exceeds 5 mg/100 ml. Cyanosis in the newborn may be central or peripheral (acrocyanosis). Acrocyanosis is limited to the hands, feet, and circumoral area and is most often of no consequence. However, since the condition is not present in all "normal" infants, acrocyanosis may indicate that some poorly understood physiologic adaptation has occurred. In addition, acrocyanosis may be prominent in congenital heart disease. Central cyanosis reflects a serious cardiopulmonary disturbance. The infant has generalized cyanosis over the entire body, sometimes best seen in the tongue and often associated with extreme greyish pallor.

Because of individual variations in the ability to detect cyanosis, indicators in the history and physical are also important in detecting hypoxia. Respiratory distress, meconium aspiration, and fetal distress should alert the physician to look for hypoxemia. When the clinical history and signs suggest hypoxia, an arterial blood oxygen tension and/or saturation should be measured. In newborn infants this measurement should be obtained from the radial, brachial, or temporal arteries. The normal full-term infant achieves a Pa_{O_2} of 60 mm Hg in the first hour and an adult value greater than 80 mm Hg in 2 to 3 days. Premature infants without distress have a lower Pa_{O_2} dependent on gestational age[92] (see Fig. 1-42B). Some non-distressed premature infants have a Pa_{O_2} less than or equal to 50 mm Hg for days or weeks without apparent harm. This low Pa_{O_2} has been shown to be due to right-to-left cardiopulmonary shunting.

Does a critical Pa_{O_2} exist in the newborn, and if so, what is the level and how can it be determined for a given patient? One approach might be to measure the level of Pa_{O_2} at which lactic acidosis occurs. Huckabee has shown that a lactacidemia occurs in adults with Pa_{O_2} between 26 and 32 mm Hg.[55] On the other hand, infants with transposition of great vessels, for example, grow and develop normally with Pa_{O_2} in the range of 25 to 30 mm Hg without metabolic acidosis indicating that factors other than absolute Pa_{O_2} are important. Distribution of cardiac output and the presence or absence of shock are as important as Pa_{O_2} in defining tissue hypoxia. Because no absolute index exists, hypoxia is generally considered to be present when Pa_{O_2} is lower than 45 to 50 mm Hg, and therapy is indicated at this time. Metabolic acidosis is frequently present when Pa_{O_2} is less than this value. However, in using this level of Pa_{O_2} as an index, it is important to be aware of the site of arterial sampling. Occasionally, great differences in Pa_{O_2} exist between temporal artery and descending aorta (because of right-to-left shunting through the ductus arteriosus). For this reason, in assessing need for oxygen therapy and avoiding the consequences of overoxygenation, such as retrolental fibroplasia (RLF), temporal or right radial or brachial artery samples are preferred. Continuous monitoring of O_2 tension has shown a considerable variation in Pa_{O_2} related to crying, feeding, and even routine care.

TREATMENT

The goal of treatment in the long run is to normalize tissue oxygenation. Consequently, methods to improve both lung function and tissue perfusion may be required. Having established that hypoxia is present on the basis of either central cyanosis or Pa_{O_2} less than 45 to 50 mm Hg, oxygen therapy must be given. Oxygenation may be improved by simply increasing the FI_{O_2} by providing warm, humidified gas through a mask or head box. However, some infants may require constant distending airway pressure (CDAP) or even assisted ventilation before achieving a satisfactory Pa_{O_2}. Because of potential toxicity (see also Chapters 16 and 18) the concentration of oxygen in inspired air (FI_{O_2}) should be regulated to maintain Pa_{O_2} between 50 and 70 mm Hg. Frequent monitoring and recording of FI_{O_2} and Pa_{O_2} are essential during oxygen therapy. Indiscriminate administration of 100% oxygen (because it is the only concentration available) must be avoided. FI_{O_2} may be varied by mixing air and 100% oxygen through a "Y" connection or with an oxygen blender.

Oxygen should be given only by written order that specifies indications, method of administration, route, and conditions for discontinuation. Pa_{O_2} should be measured frequently, especially in the early course of the illness and always in response to a change in FI_{O_2}. The FI_{O_2} should be recorded hourly.

When an emergency exists or when Pa_{O_2} is unavailable, the presence of cyanosis must be used to assess oxygenation. Oxygen should be given at an FI_{O_2} that will abolish central cyanosis, and its continuance should be based on the presence of this sign. In other words, FI_{O_2} must be frequently decreased to establish that cyanosis and thus the continuing need for oxygen exist.

The Use of CDAP in the Treatment of Hypoxia. In 1971, Gregory and co-workers demonstrated that FI_{O_2} could be reduced and Pa_{O_2} maintained at or above 50 mm Hg in infants with HMD by the use of CDAP.[44] Previously, Thibeault, Poblete and Auld had demonstrated that constant negative extrathoracic pressure could increase FRC and improve oxygenation in premature infants.[93] Distending airway pressure has been administered in a number of different ways, e.g., by endotracheal tube (Fig. 14-16), nasal prongs (Fig. 14-17), bag and mask, head box, and constant negative extrathoracic pressure (CNEP) (Fig. 14-18). This method is effective in improving oxygenation and lowering FI_{O_2} in the spontaneously breathing patient. Nasal continuous positive airway pressure appears most useful in patients being weaned from assisted ventilation, but otherwise may not be as effective as other methods.

Indications for use of CDAP have varied with different authors. Complications are common, particularly pneumothorax, and the risk : benefit ratio must always be considered. Proponents of minimal indications (when Pa_{O_2} is less than 60 mm Hg in FI_{O_2} greater than 0.40) for usage point to the toxic effects

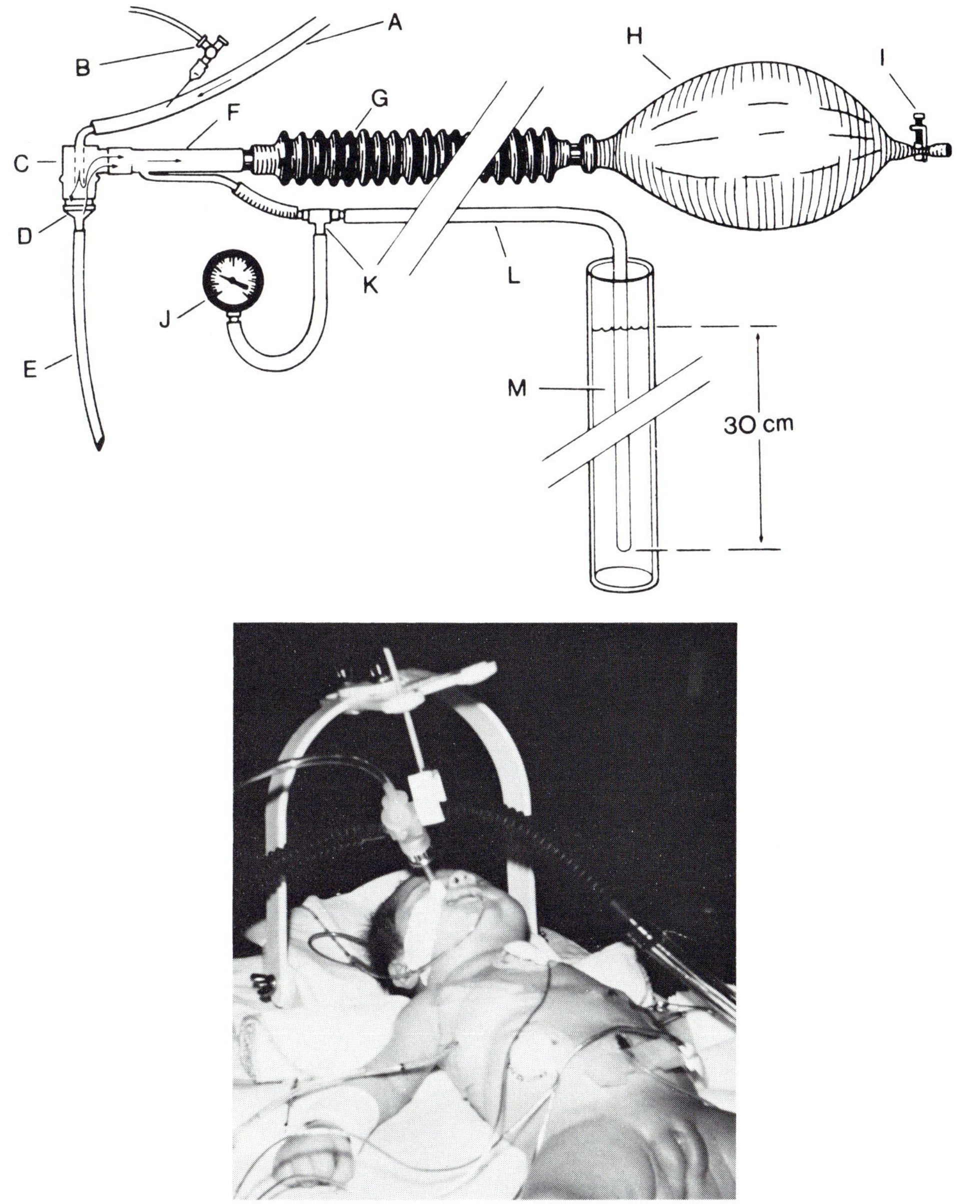

FIG. 14-16. Continuous distending airway pressure applied by endotracheal tube. (Reprinted, by permission from *N. Engl. J. Med. 284*:1333, 1971.)

of oxygen on the lung for justification of this approach. Many infants, particularly the larger more vigorous infants, can tolerate FI_{O_2} 0.70 to 0.80 without CDAP for several days and survive with no ill effects. It is recommended here that CDAP be applied when Pa_{O_2} is less than 50 and FI_{O_2} is greater than 0.60, particularly in infants under 1500 g. These levels should be a general guide for larger infants but clinical judgment

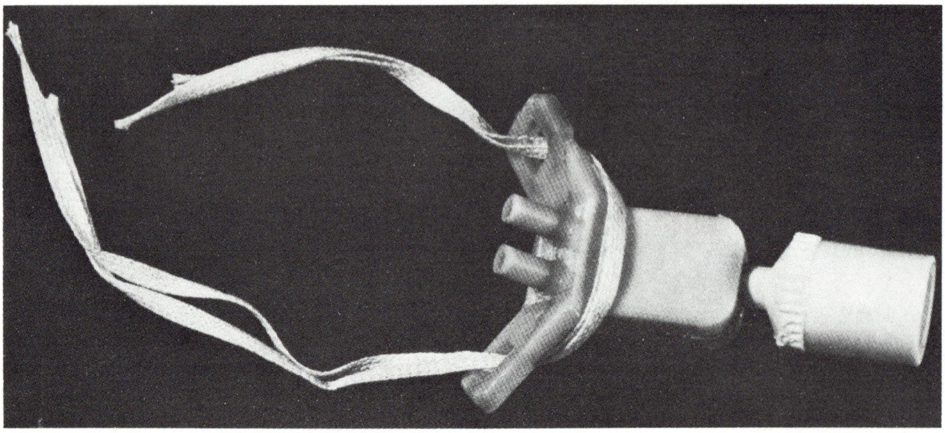

FIG. 14-17. Silicone-rubber nasal cannula for delivery of continuous positive airway pressure. (From Kattwinkel, J. et al.: A device for administration of continuous positive pressure by the nasal route. *Pediatrics 52*:130, 1973.)

must be used as well. Initially, 2 cm H_2O should be applied and titrated upward in increments of 2 cm H_2O to a maximum of 8 cm H_2O if lower values fail to achieve satisfactory oxygenation. CDAP is indicated only to improve oxygenation, never as primary treatment when respiratory acidosis is present.

An absolute indication for removal of CDAP is difficult to determine, but it should include an attempt to answer the following questions. When does the risk : benefit ratio of oxygen alone exceed the risk : benefit ratio of CDAP and oxygen combined? When $F_{I_{O_2}}$ is .40 and CDAP is 4 cm H_2O, would the infant be better served by removing CDAP and raising the $F_{I_{O_2}}$ to .50? In general CDAP should be reduced in a stepwise fashion along with $F_{I_{O_2}}$, maintaining a Pa_{O_2} above 50 mm Hg. Berman et al.[6] have demonstrated an improved Pa_{O_2} and FRC when endotracheal CDAP is held at 2 cm H_2O rather than allowing CDAP to be reduced to zero end-expiratory pressure (ZEEP) in the

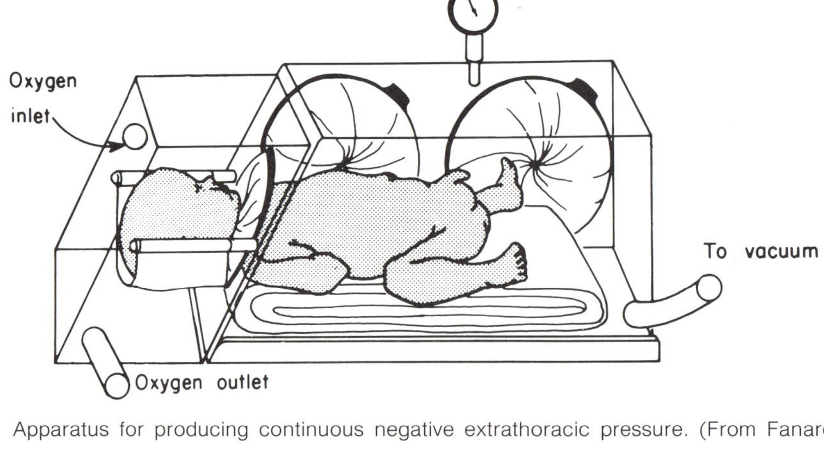

FIG. 14-18. Apparatus for producing continuous negative extrathoracic pressure. (From Fanaroff, A. A.[38])

process of weaning. This finding suggests that the glottis is an important factor to be considered in the weaning process.

CDAP may also be useful prophylactically to prevent increasing alveolar collapse. Advocates of this view recommend that CDAP be administered to most infants with HMD with this mechanism of action in mind. This routine approach is not recommended here because its efficacy has not been proven and the risk of developing a pneumothorax is increased. Since not all infants require this treatment, prophylactic CDAP is indicated as a routine only when it is possible to determine which infants will deteriorate if it is not administered. Currently this determination is not possible, and the risk : benefit ratio does not justify this routine approach.

CDAP has been shown to be useful in the treatment of primary apnea in premature infants. This technique is indicated when simple stimulation fails. However, CDAP is often not totally successful in these cases and other treatments may be indicated.

What has been achieved since the introduction of CDAP in 1971? CDAP has been shown to reduce oxygen requirement and to reduce the time in an increased $F_{I_{O_2}}$. It has not been shown to reduce mortality or incidence of chronic pulmonary disease.[38] Clearly the technique is useful, but because of complications such as air leak and a tendency to increase P_{CO_2}, it must be administered by strict indication only.

The proposed mechanisms by which CDAP improves Pa_{O_2} are basically as follows: (1) by increasing lung volume and preventing alveolar collapse, (2) by shifting interstitial pulmonary water into capillaries, (3) by increasing the diameter of large and small airways with a resultant decrease in airway resistance and improved distribution of ventilation, and (4) by improving $\dot{V}_A/\dot{Q}$ ratio.[56,62,98] With respect to mechanism (1) it has been shown that FRC is increased when CDAP is applied in HMD but lung compliance is decreased.[5] This latter result suggests that CDAP may actually be acting on already open alveoli and possibly overdistending them. It is not proven that CDAP opens atelectatic alveoli, and the improvement in chest roentgenogram cited by those who feel atelectasis is overcome could be due to overdistention of airways. With regard to mechanism (2) evidence exists that increased airway pressure favors the accumulation of fluid in extravascular spaces rather than the movement of interstitial pulmonary water into capillaries.[11]

Complications. Complications of CDAP are related both to effects of pressure on the heart and lungs and to the methods of delivery. Nasal prongs can erode the nose, the head box has been noted to restrict cerebral venous return, and endotracheal tubes can produce tracheal erosion and stenosis. Pressure effects result in pneumothorax, pneumomediastinum, and interstitial emphysema, and they have the potential of affecting venous return to the heart and seriously limiting cardiac output.

In certain instances, it may be necessary to provide assisted ventilation to maintain oxygenation. Typically these patients are larger infants with HMD whose principal problem is oxygenation and who are able to maintain a normal P_{CO_2} because of vigorous respiratory efforts. For the most part these infants can be managed with CDAP, but when the pressure level exceeds 8 cm H_2O, the physician must decide that an unfavorable risk : benefit ratio is present and assisted ventilation with or without positive end expiratory pressure (PEEP) should be begun. Successful assisted ventilation in these larger infants may require the elimination of asynchronous spontaneous respirations. This may be achieved using a neuromuscular blocking agent such as pancuronium bromide. It is desirable to use multiple small doses given as frequently as necessary to obtain the desired degree of relaxation.

The Use of PEEP in the Treatment of Hypoxia. PEEP is the provision of a constant distending airway pressure during assisted ventilation with a respirator. The technique has essentially the same indications and complications as CDAP and offers the same advantages. PEEP allows for maintenance of an acceptable Pa_{O_2} at a lower FI_{O_2} and may prevent alveolar collapse. Reduced dangers of oxygen damage to the lung may also result. As in the case of CDAP, a practical method to regulate PEEP to ensure maximal effectiveness is required. Suter et al.[91] have proposed the term "best" PEEP to describe that amount of distending airway pressure resulting in maximal oxygen transport and the smallest dead space fraction. In adults, they noted that this amount occurred at the point of maximal static compliance. Various additional indices have been suggested for the evaluation of PEEP effectiveness, including alveolar-arterial oxygen gradient (AaD_{O_2}), pulmonary shunt ($\dot{Q}S/\dot{Q}T$), and volume of oxygen transported per unit of tissue.[91] None of these proposed indices is easily obtainable in a clinical setting so that the level of PEEP must be regulated by trial and error, starting at a low pressure and slowly increasing to obtain optimum oxygenation. PEEP should rarely be increased over 8 to 10 cm H_2O in newborn infants.

Proposed mechanisms of action for PEEP are the same as those for CDAP. In fact, the most advantageous level of PEEP is determined by titrating its good effects against potential bad effects. Thus, Pa_{O_2}, blood pressure, urine output, and central venous pressure must be closely monitored. The harmful effects are concerned mainly with the changes in cardiac output and the production of pneumothorax, pneumomediastinum, and interstitial emphysema.

Complications of Oxygen Therapy. Little doubt exists about whether excessive Pa_{O_2} can result in RLF. However, the length of time of exposure necessary to produce RLF is unknown. With a more rational approach to oxygen therapy the condition is less common but still present. It is unlikely that RLF will be completely eradicated because of limitations of oxygen monitoring when treatment is required for prolonged periods of time. The decreased incidence of RLF is as much related to the awareness of its relationship to oxygen as to the efficacy of currently available methods of monitoring Pa_{O_2}.

Much more difficult to prevent or modify are the toxic effects of oxygen on the lung. Bronchopulmonary dysplasia (BPD) is a condition that is associated with oxygen and respirator therapy of HMD. A detailed discussion of the condition is presented in Chapter 16. Suffice it to say that BPD is related to the effects of oxygen and/or pressure on the lung. BPD is identified by its typical appearance on a chest roentgenogram. One of the goals of therapy must be to eliminate the recognized associated factors as soon as possible.

Some authors claim that CDAP or PEEP can reduce BPD. Reynolds and co-workers report a marked decrease in BPD by lowering the airway pressure during assisted ventilation (see p. 421) and reversing the usual I:E ratio.[47]

FAILURE OF TISSUE OXYGENATION—SHOCK

Shock is a frequent occurrence in infants with respiratory distress, particularly in HMD. The problem is considered under the treatment of hypoxia because of its implication for tissue oxygenation. Shock occurs in premature infants due to blood loss, e.g., intracranial hemorrhage, and factors associated with failure of autonomic control. (These latter factors are poorly understood.) Furthermore, one can identify a state perhaps best described as pre-shock, which is characterized by an initial increase in blood pressure followed by a lower than normal blood pressure and a metabolic acidosis, in the face of a well-maintained Pa_{O_2}. Treatment with plasma or blood at this time can often reverse the trend and prevent the development of true shock. When shock occurs, the renal failure that may develop often persists in the form of acute tubular necrosis after the initial event is successfully treated.

The diagnosis of shock is made difficult in premature infants because of the lack of standards for blood pressure (see Chapters 1 and 16). Clinically an infant in shock shows extreme pallor of the skin, cold extremities, and poor capillary filling. When a diagnosis is made, treatment should be commenced with plasma expanders or whole blood if available. Initial treatment should be given in volumes of 10 ml/kg. Cardiac failure is an ever-present problem, and care should be taken in administering large volumes of fluid rapidly.

Acute Problem II—Acidosis

Respiratory distress in the newborn from whatever cause must be evaluated in terms of its effect on pH. If acidosis is present, it must be categorized in terms of its metabolic and respiratory components. Because of the potentially devastating consequences of acidosis, immediate evaluation of every infant with respiratory distress to determine its presence or absence is mandatory. Therapy must then be instituted as soon as the determination is made. A normal pH for newborn infants is between 7.35 and 7.45. Any pH values below this level result in decreased responsiveness to catecholamines, with resultant poor temperature regulation and reduced control of blood flow. Pulmonary vascular resistance increases with acidosis, urine production is reduced, and glucuronide conjugation is decreased. At pH less than 7.0 heart muscle glycogen metabolism ceases and myocardial contractility is decreased.[12,13,21] The net effect is to diminish cardiac output and reduce oxygen delivery to tissues, especially the brain.

Acidosis can arise from either respiratory or metabolic causes. Often both are present simultaneously. Therapy begins with a blood determination of pH and $P\text{CO}_2$ as well as calculation of HCO_3^- to assess severity and determine the primary cause. A pH lower than 7.30 warrants treatment and a $P\text{CO}_2$ above 50 mm Hg identifies significant respiratory component. The basic approach to therapy is to provide improved ventilation for respiratory acidosis and alkali for metabolic acidosis while attempting to identify and treat any ongoing problem contributing to either. In combined acidosis that is not severe, it is usually best to provide assisted ventilation for 15 to 30 minutes to correct the respiratory component and then administer an appropriate dose of alkali to correct the remaining metabolic portion. In cases of severe acidosis that occurs with asphyxia, studies in animals indicate that best results are obtained with immediate adminstration of alkali and simultaneous ventilation and oxygenation with cardiovascular support as necessary.[18,21]

METABOLIC ACIDOSIS

In infants with respiratory distress, metabolic acidosis occurs as a consequence of hypoxia resulting in anaerobic metabolism and an accumulation of lactic acid. Hypoxia in this instance may occur because of failure to adequately oxygenate the blood in the lungs or may be secondary to poor tissue perfusion because of decreased cardiac output or shock.

Therapy for metabolic acidosis begins with an assessment of the extent of the metabolic component. This determination is accomplished by measurement of pH and $P\text{CO}_2$ and calculation of HCO_3^- from the Henderson-Hasselbalch equation directly or from nomograms, e.g., Siggaard-Andersen (Fig. 14-19). $NaHCO_3$ is the treatment for metabolic acidosis. Dosage is based on the HCO_3^- deficit, assuming a bicarbonate space of 0.6. One-half the calculated dose should be administered slowly over 15 to 20 minutes, using a 50% dilution of USP $NaHCO_3$ $7\frac{1}{2}$% with sterile H_2O. No further bicarbonate should be ad-

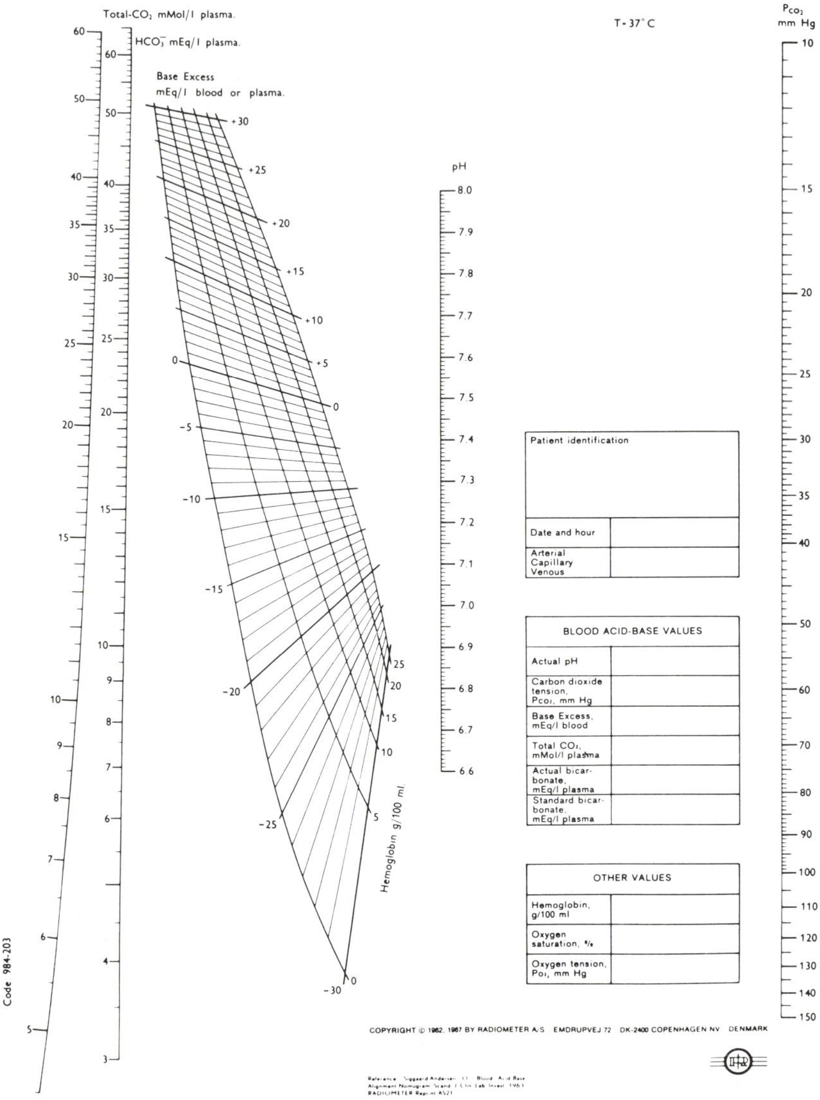

FIG. 14-19. The Siggaard-Andersen Alignment Nomogram (Radiometer, A/S, Copenhagen, Denmark).

ministered until a reassessment of the need has been made by repeating pH and Pco_2 measurement and recalculating HCO_3^-.

Great care must be exercised in administering sodium bicarbonate because of the risks of hyperosmolality and hypernatremia. In addition, some researchers have suggested that the acute hyperosmolality produced by $NaHCO_3$ may result in intracranial hemorrhage.[39,85] Infiltration of solutions containing $NaHCO_3$ can produce serious skin sloughs.

When it is no longer safe to administer $NaHCO_3$ and therapy for metabolic acidosis is still indicated, it is appropriate to use 0.3 M tromethamine (THAM). THAM functions as a proton acceptor converting an amino group to an ammonium ion. Its side effects are respiratory depression and/or hypoglycemia.

It is safest to use this drug when the patient is receiving assisted ventilation. THAM is administered intravenously in 5% glucose as a 0.3 M solution at a rate of 2 to 5 ml/kg/hr until the pH is normalized.

RESPIRATORY ACIDOSIS

In physiologic terms, respiratory acidosis represents a failure of the lung to compensate for large numbers of alveoli with low $\dot{V}A/\dot{Q}$ ($\dot{V}A/\dot{Q}$ less than 1) and thus indicates respiratory failure. Pulmonary disease frequently produces alveoli with a low $\dot{V}A/\dot{Q}$ but because of ease of diffusion of CO_2, accumulation may not occur due to compensatory diffusion through normal alveoli. The presence of these alveoli with low $\dot{V}A/\dot{Q}$ is identified by the presence of the arterial-alveolar CO_2 gradient (aAD_{CO_2}). The development of respiratory acidosis represents a failure of compensation. It may also occur as a result of hypoventilation, in which case minute volume of ventilation is insufficient to remove CO_2 produced (see also Chapter 2). In this case, poorly ventilated alveoli function as increased dead space. This condition can result from central nervous system factors such as hemorrhage, infection, or "immaturity" of the respiratory center. In this regard, it has been demonstrated that the ventilatory response to CO_2 is related to gestational age, with the more immature infant being the least responsive. It is not clear to what extent this lack of CO_2 responsiveness in the smaller infants is due to central nervous system factors and to what degree it is due to peripheral pulmonary factors.[60]

Characterization of the respiratory components of acid-base metabolism by determination of pH and P_{CO_2} is best performed on arterial blood. However, if this type is not available, a useful evaluation may be obtained from measurements of free-flowing venous blood or arterialized capillary blood. Again plasma bicarbonate concentration should be calculated using the Henderson-Hasselbalch equation or its graphic equivalent, the Siggaard-Andersen nomogram (see Fig. 14-19). In acute respiratory acidosis, HCO_3^- is unchanged, but in compensated respiratory acidosis it is increased.

Treatment of Respiratory Acidosis—Assisted Ventilation. Hypercapnea without acidosis does not require treatment. Once it has been determined that a particular patient has a significant respiratory component of acidosis, the choice of therapy should be guided by severity. In mild respiratory acidosis, e.g., pH 7.25 and P_{CO_2} 55 mm Hg it may be unwise to begin assisted ventilation. Experience has shown that in these cases intravenous infusion of small amounts of $NaHCO_3$ may correct the pH and improve $\dot{V}A/\dot{Q}$ relationships with normalization of P_{CO_2}. Here also, frequent blood gas and pH determinations must be made to guarantee that the expected result has occurred and the physician must be ready to provide assisted ventilation. $NaHCO_3$ can increase serum osmolarity, and if a significant limitation in CO_2 excretion exists, it may also increase P_{CO_2}. However, this effect is unlikely with mild respiratory acidosis. If CO_2 retention occurs with $NaHCO_3$, assisted ventilation must be instituted. When a moderate to severe respiratory acidosis exists, assisted ventilation must be undertaken immediately and $NaHCO_3$ should not be given. If a combined respiratory and metabolic acidosis exists, assisted ventilation should be begun first and alkali therapy for the metabolic component provided later.

Respiratory acidosis should be treated with assisted ventilation because it eliminates the immediate underlying cause of the infant's problem. No form of assisted ventilation is without complications. For this reason, it is necessary to select the most benign form compatible with the degree of underventilation seen in the individual patient. Basically three forms of intervention may improve ventilation: (1) stimulation, (2) bag and mask ventilation by hand, and (3) mechanically assisted ventilation.

Stimulation. Infants with mild acidosis resulting from elevation of P_{CO_2} may increase their minute volume as a result of gentle stimulation; e.g., the physician may gently stroke the bottom of the infant's foot or sides of the thorax. This technique is most effective in infants who are experiencing either exaggerated periodic breathing or short apneic episodes. This technique should not be used in circumstances of severe acidosis or marked CO_2 retention as it would only postpone definitive treatment.

Manual bag and mask ventilation. Effective assisted ventilation may be achieved through the use of a valveless bag equipped with a pressure gauge and a face mask of appropriate size. Such a setup is shown in Figure 14-20. An appropriate humidified gas mixture is provided at a continuous rate sufficient to keep the bag distended when the mask is placed over the infant's face (usually 10 to 12 liters/min.). The mask is held over the infant's nose and mouth with one hand. The neck is maintained in an extended position by means of a roll of linen under the neck to ensure that the tongue does not interfere with the airway. Gas is allowed to leak from the mask at a rate sufficient to keep the pressure between breaths from going above 5 cm H_2O. Ventilation is achieved by squeezing the bag with the free hand until the infant's chest is seen to rise. Ordinarily this procedure will produce a pressure reading on the gauge of 25 to 35 cm H_2O. If the gas leak around the mask is properly controlled, the bag will promptly refill with gas and breaths may be provided by repeated gentle squeezing of the bag at rates up to 70 breaths/min.

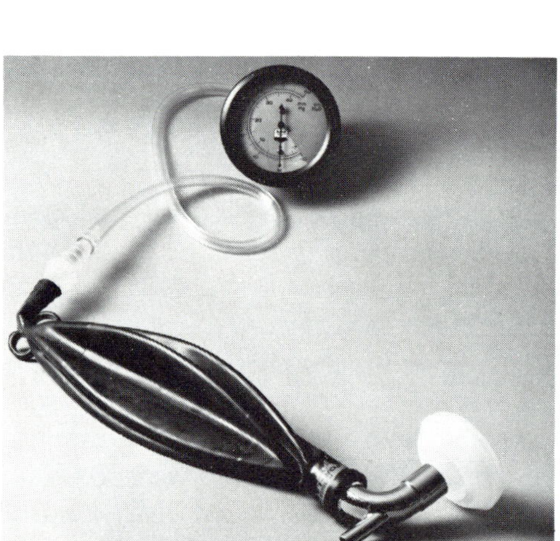

FIG. 14-20. A bag, face mask, and pressure gauge for giving either mask CDAP or assisted ventilation.

Since squeezing the bag forces air under pressure into the oropharynx and not just into the trachea, some provision must be made for avoiding overdistention of the stomach and bowel. Overdistention is ordinarily prevented by inserting a nasogastric tube that is left open to the atmosphere. The most difficult aspect of this type of manual ventilation is usually the control of the seal around the face mask. Controlling the seal is facilitated by cutting an aperture in a Telfa dressing to expose the infant's nose and mouth. The dressing material remains between the mask and the face, however. This technique provides a uniform slow leak as opposed to the abrupt intermittent type of leakage that occurs if the rubber rim of the mask is in direct contact with the skin.

Advantages of this type of ventilation are the avoidance of endotracheal intubation with its attendant hazards and the opportunity for close observation of the infant's condition. It is also possible to provide only intermittent assistance allowing spontaneous respiration as well. This technique is best adapted to infants under 2000 g and has the added advantage of requiring minimal equipment (as well as being highly portable). It provides lifesaving capability in a community hospital where prolonged therapy cannot be carried out.

Mechanical ventilation. Three different types of ventilators are available for use in newborn and premature infants: volume cycled, pressure cycled, and negative pressure ventilators. Each offers particular advantages, and if a choice is available, consideration should be given to selection of the most appropriate type.

Volume-cycled ventilators allow precise control over minute volume and require the selection of both tidal volume and respiratory rate as individual adjustments. Regulation of the flow rate in combination with the tidal volume and respiratory rate establishes the I:E ratio. On some machines, however, inspiratory hold is available and can be used to delay expiration, allowing additional time for all parts of the lung to respond to the distending pressure. This feature may be useful in circumstances where compliance and resistance are not uniform throughout the lung and alveolar time constants may be markedly different. Most ventilators of this type allow for limitation of peak airway pressure at the expense of tidal volume. In addition, pressure fluctuations in the ventilation circuit are measured with each breath. This feature is useful since rising pressures may suggest acute obstruction of the endotracheal tube.

Pressure-cycled ventilators, in contrast, deliver an unknown tidal volume at a preset peak inspiratory pressure and rate allowing easy adjustment of the I:E ratio. It is possible in some machines to obtain I:E ratios as high as 4:1. In these machines, tidal volume may be regulated by adjusting the peak inspiratory pressure since higher pressures result in higher tidal volumes. Adequate ventilation may be achieved ordinarily at a peak pressure of 25 cm H_2O with an I:E ratio of 1:1. The pressure gauge always indicates the preset pressure regardless of the status of the airway and consequently cannot be relied upon to indicate endotracheal tube obstruction, increased airway resistance, decreased compliance, or pneumothorax—all of which could raise airway pressure at a fixed tidal volume. The importance of airway pressure as a factor in respiratory management has been well established. It is generally known that elevated airway pressures are associated with increased incidence of pneumothorax. Reynolds has also suggested that pressure in combination with elevated oxygen concentrations may be responsible for increased incidence of bronchopulmonary dysplasia.[47] Both of these factors place a premium on low pressure ventilation, which is easily accomplished on the pressure-cycled ventilator.

Negative-pressure ventilators offer the advantage that endotracheal intubation is not required. They operate by enclosing the infant's thorax in a chamber where pressure can be reduced while his oral pharynx is exposed to atmospheric pressure. This setup necessitates some sort of pressure seal, most commonly at the neck. Because this seal must be loose, the pressure gradient established during inspiration forces a large flow of air from outside the body chamber to rush in through this seal as well as through the trachea. The problem thus created is chilling of the infant as a result of constant convection losses since the sources of prewarmed air are seldom sufficient. In addition, access to the infant for any procedure is severely restricted.

Indications and procedure for mechanical ventilation. The indication for mechanically assisted ventilation is most often the failure of either stimulation or manual bag and mask ventilation to correct the patient's blood gas status. Once the decision to place the baby on a respirator is made, special effort should be made to ensure that this transition is as smooth as possible. Provision must be made for ventilation of the patient both with and without an endotracheal tube. Medications ($NaHCO_3$ and epinephrine 1:10,000) should be available in the event that prolonged bradycardia occurs. A ventilator should be in position and set for operation at the time the infant is intubated. It is preferable to do this procedure on an open table under an infrared warmer.

Necessary equipment includes a valveless bag and mask; endotracheal tubes (sizes 12 Fr, 14 Fr, and 16 Fr); a laryngoscope with fresh batteries and the penlight size handle with a Miller speculum (size 0 (Premature) or 1); a valve bag of the Hope Infant Resuscitator type, which fits onto the endotracheal tube; benzoin; cloth adhesive tape; a nasogastric tube in place; and a small container filled with water.

Before any attempt is made to intubate the infant, the respirator should be correctly set and thoroughly checked. The most important setting on a volume-controlled respirator is the tidal volume. It is not possible to generalize about the correct setting because of differences from one manufacturer's product to another and because of differences in dead space and connecting tube compliance. The more flexible the tubing, the greater will be the loss of tidal volume at a given ventilating pressure. An infant's tidal volume is approximately 7 cc/kg. Loss due to tubing expansion is measured in cc/cm H_2O. This loss is interpreted by assuming a normal ventilating pressure of 25 to 35 cm H_2O and multiplying the loss number by 30. Thus, for example, if the loss is $\frac{1}{2}$ cc/cm H_2O and pressure is assumed to be 30, the total loss to the tubing would be 15 cc. The correct setting for the machine in this situation would be (7 cc/kg) × (weight in kg) + 15 cc. This setting should be made before intubation to avoid accidental overventilation and a possible pneumothorax.

The remaining settings include rate, flow rate, sigh interval, and pressure limits. Ventilatory rate is ordinarily started at 40 to 50 breaths/min. for the correction of hypercapnea. The flow rate depends on the tidal volume and the desired I:E ratio. Ventilator manufacturers usually provide nomograms or charts for determining correct settings of this ratio. At the time of intubation, it is most important to set pressure limits. For example, if the endotracheal tube has been improperly placed in the right main stem bronchus (the most common complication of assisted ventilation), the entire tidal volume would be delivered to the right lung. However, once the pressure limit is reached, the remaining air will be lost through an escape valve rather than being forced into one lung under high pressure.

Pressure-cycled ventilators require setting of the pressure limit before connection to the patient to ensure that overinflation will not occur. In addition, the mode of ventilation, PEEP, IPPB, or intermittent mandatory ventilation (IMV) must be selected and the respiratory rate, I:E ratio, gas flow rate, and $F_{I_{O_2}}$ set. It is usually appropriate to set the pressure limit at 25 cm H_2O for an infant. IMV may be used at any respiratory rate (usually 40 to 50 for respiratory acidosis), and I:E ratio should be set initially at 1:1 until further blood gas determinations are made. The gas flow rate determines the rate at which gas passes over the top of the endotracheal tube removing exhaled gas and preventing rebreathing. This setting may also influence the I:E ratio achieved on some machines. The operator should be thoroughly familiar with the manufacturer's instructions before attempting to use any mechanical ventilator. Once ventilation has been begun with a pressure-cycled ventilator, it is particularly important to monitor blood gases closely since no measurement is made of tidal or minute volume delivered. Underventilation may result from partial airway obstruction or increased lung stiffness. Without repeated blood gas assessment, this problem may be undetected until severe symptoms develop.

Intubation. Any physician providing intensive care to newborns must have the skill of intubation. Consequently, the technique selected must be easily mastered, minimally traumatic, and rapidly accomplished. Both nasotracheal and orotracheal intubation are widely practiced. House staff on rotation or other personnel without extensive experience should perform orotracheal intubation for tube replacement. This technique is easily learned and can be performed quickly in emergencies with the least manipulation. Nasotracheal intubation offers the advantage of more secure tube fixation and somewhat fewer accidental extubations. It is more difficult to perform and should therefore be used only by individuals experienced in airway management.

Numerous types of tubes are available. For ease of placement, straight tubes appear the most desirable. Cole tubes, though larger in diameter, do not offer a clinically useful reduction in airway resistance and add dead space. Their large size also makes them more difficult to place. Care should be taken to select a tube made of a material that remains patent when bent. Kinking is a serious problem since it occurs at the back of the pharynx and may not be seen. It is also desirable to mark the tubes in some way that allows the distance from any point to the tip to be determined. The selection of an endotracheal tube may not be reliably based on infant size. Endotracheal tubes should be No. 12 Fr or larger to avoid excessive airway resistance (Fig. 14-21) and ordinarily do not exceed No. 16 Fr in premature infants. Tubes that are too small produce excessive leaks and less effective ventilation. Large tubes cause damage to tracheal mucosa and cartilage and may erode into the esophagus. A snug fit is desirable but the tube should enter the trachea easily.

Orotracheal intubation sometimes requires the use of a stylet. If so, it is important to assure that the stylet cannot protrude beyond the tip of the tube. It is usually unnecessary to bend or curve the stylet. The airway will be nearly straight at the time the tube is introduced. Curvature increases the likelihood of trauma to the trachea, larynx, or vocal cords.

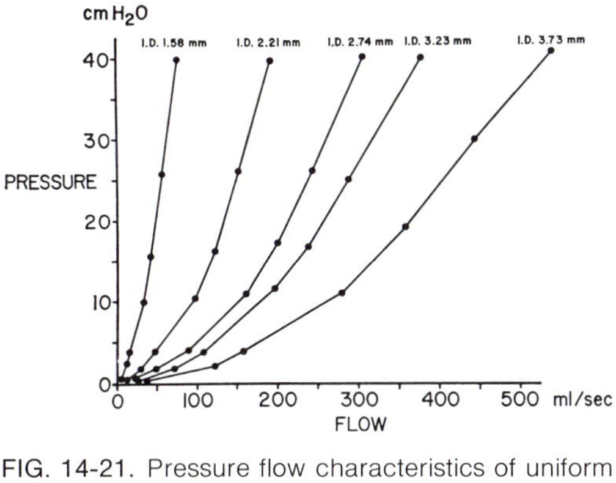

FIG. 14-21. Pressure flow characteristics of uniform diameter endotracheal tubes of various diameters. (From Glauser, E. M. et al.: Pressure flow characteristics and dead spaces of endotracheal tubes used in infants. *Anesthesiology* 22:339, 1961.)

Laryngoscopy for intubation of infants is not the same as for adults or older children. Special care is necessary to avoid laceration or other trauma to the hypopharynx, epiglottis, vocal cords, and dental ridge. The best instrument for most premature and newborn infants is a penlight-handle laryngoscope with a size 0 Miller blade. The light should appear bright white. Good illumination is essential. The infant should be in the supine position with the neck extended. The blade of the scope should be introduced gently until the tip is between the base of the tongue and the epiglottis. The glottis should now be directly visible. If the epiglottis is seen, the scope should be inserted a bit further. Slight pressure on the larynx by an assistant may be necessary to see the glottis. Do not attempt to insert an endotracheal tube unless the glottis is clearly visible. The tube should be straight, positioned so that the bevel is down (or posterior). Insert it so that the tip passes the glottal opening while still in direct view. From this point on, vision is obstructed. Gentle pressure should be maintained on the tube to prevent it from dislodging and passing into the esophagus. If it does not advance easily, do not apply force. Gentle side-to-side movement may be necessary to position the tip between the vocal cords. It may also be necessary to reorient the tube so that it is aimed posteriorly. All of this action happens rather quickly, and as the tube begins to advance, a sensation of mild resistance ordinarily occurs. If the tube suddenly advances very easily with no resistance, be suspicious. It may be in the esophagus. After passing the glottis, the tube should be advanced about 3 cm. Once in position, it may be secured with two pieces of adhesive tape, which go around the tube twice. Benzoin may be used where tape is to be attached to the skin.

The position of the tube should be checked before it is secured by ventilating the infant through the tube and placing the open end of the nasogastric tube under water. If the endotracheal tube is in the esophagus, bubbles will rapidly appear. Breath sounds are also a good guide to the position of the tube. Sounds should be absent or faint over the stomach and equal bilaterally over the lung fields unless known pathology would explain any asymmetry. The presence of breath sounds on the right only requires immediate repositioning of the tube by withdrawing it slightly while auscultating until sounds occur on the left as well. Once the tube appears to be in correct position by physical examination, it should be secured as described and a roentgenogram taken to verify its location.

Respirator operation. The extent to which a patient is allowed to participate in his own ventilation is controlled by the operator on most ventilators. These settings or modes of ventilation offer particular advantages in several different clinical settings. Although designations may vary, the most common terms are control or IPPB, assist, assist/control, and IMV.

Control mode is the most basic type of ventilator operation. With the machine set on "control," breaths of a set volume are given at a predetermined rate. The patient may not breathe between "machine" breaths since no source of air is connected to the endotracheal tube.

Assist mode is the exact opposite. Breaths are given only when the patient makes a sufficient inspiratory effort to trigger the machine. At this time a full tidal volume is delivered. Some machines are designed with a built-in safety factor so that the machine responds to a predetermined period of apnea or insufficient effort with several full breaths.

Assist/control mode permits the patient to trigger the respirator to give full breaths at a rate determined by the patient until this rate falls below the rate set on the machine. If this situation occurs, the machine gives several "unsolicited" breaths until the average rate is again above the preset rate when it again operates as in assist mode.

IMV differs from any of the three described modes. It provides a reservoir of humidified gas under slight pressure so that, regardless of what the respirator is doing, a continuous flow of air goes past the endotracheal tube. This mode permits the patient to take breaths at his own rate and depth. Intermittently (at a predetermined rate) the patient is ventilated with a full tidal volume that is mandatory. In effect, the machine operates as if in the control mode to provide assisted ventilation at a preselected rate. Because of the presence of the reservoir, changes in airway pressure can no longer be sensed and the assist mode will not operate. The patient breathes on his own from the reservoir, and the machine provides a fixed number of breaths at full tidal volume. This procedure permits the patient to assume whatever part of his minute volume he can, while the machine provides the remainder. The rate at which the machine is set should be governed by serial blood gas determinations after the process is begin. Ordinarily the only necessary response is to speed up or slow down the mandatory rate if the patient has become either acidotic or alkalotic respectively on a respiratory basis. The advent of this technique has almost completely obviated the need for either assist or assist/control mode ventilation.

I:E ratio. During spontaneous respirations, an infant's I:E ratio is approximately 1:3. With a volume-cycled respirator, short inspiratory periods result in higher peak airway pressures. Initially I:E ratios should be set at 1:1 to avoid these high pressures and the risk of pneumothorax and yet provide ventilation that is as nearly "physiologic" as possible. When the indication for assisted ventilation is hypoxemia and if a ratio of 1:1 is not successful, the ratio may be inverted to 1.5:1 or 2:1. A higher mean airway pressure is achieved with less time for alveolar collapse. It may be necessary to change to a pressure-cycled machine in order to achieve these inverted ratios.

Tracheal toilet. The presence of an endotracheal tube results in increased secretions and eliminates the patient's ability to clear his own airway. Suctioning is necessary, and when mucus is particularly tenacious, it may be necessary to instill 2 to 3 cc of 5% $NaHCO_3$ solution to dissolve mucus. After the solution is directly injected into the endotracheal tube, the tube should be reconnected to the ventilator for several breaths. Following this step, a suction catheter should be passed through the tube to remove residual mucus and bicarbonate. This type of lavage may be necessary every 2 hours depending on the quantity and viscosity of secretions obtained.

Viscous secretions may result from ventilation with unhumidified air, infection, or poor hydration. All ventilators should be equipped with either nebulizers or heated humidifiers.

Mucus plugging of the endotracheal tube is a serious complication and requires careful observation of the infant. Volume-cycled ventilators with pressure alarms immediately indicate tube plugging by a sharp increase in ventilation pressure. Pressure-cycled machines are not able to provide this type of alarm. Symptoms of mucus plugging are those of underventilation and may produce hypercapnea, acidosis, and cyanosis. Prompt replacement of the tube is the best treatment.

Assisted ventilation therapy. Immediate indications for mechanical ventilation include: diaphragmatic hernia, pneumothorax, surgery, respiratory acidosis, tracheoesophageal fistula, severe acidosis (pH less than 7.10 and P_{CO_2} greater than 75), or respiratory acidosis in an infant with a birth weight over 2 kg. Bag and mask ventilation is frequently difficult or impossible in large, struggling infants, and immediate intubation and mechanically assisted ventilation avoids delay in effective treatment.

Bag and mask assisted ventilation is often useful in infants weighing less than 2000 g and should be attempted when respiratory acidosis of mild or moderate severity exists. Mechanically assisted ventilation is also indicated when other methods of oxygenation fail (see p. 412). Most commonly this condition is accompanied by CO_2 retention. However, occasionally respiratory therapy is required for oxygenation alone.

Therapeutic plan. The initial goal of treatment is the correction of blood gas and pH abnormalities. The complications of mechanically assisted ventilation, however, are severe enough that every effort should be directed at withdrawing support as rapidly as possible. This support withdrawal is best achieved by allowing the patient to breathe spontaneously, while providing only enough assistance to normalize pH and P_{CO_2}. Intermittent mandatory ventilation is the most adaptable mode of ventilation for this purpose. It permits continuous opportunity for spontaneous respiration as well as assisted ventilation at any rate down to zero with complete control over I:E ratio and end-expiratory pressure. Initially blood gas tensions and pH should be determined at least every 4 hours. When the patient has spontaneous respirations and normal blood values, the ventilator rate should be reduced slightly to permit the patient to assume more of the burden of respiration. These challenges should be followed by repeat blood gas determinations after no more than 1 hour. Although individual patients vary, an infant may tolerate three or four of these rate reductions successfully in any 24-hour period. It is quite common after many successful rate reductions to find an infant who requires between 1 and 5 assisted breaths/min. and will not tolerate further reduction or extubation. This situation may persist for days or even weeks before the infant is able to breathe completely spontaneously. Repeated challenges are necessary but this condition is not well understood, and it is only by trial and error that the infant is finally successfully weaned from mechanically assisted ventilation.

Extubation should be attempted when an infant is breathing well spontaneously and requires no mechanical assistance. If distending airway pressure has been used to improve oxygenation, evidence by Berman et al.[6] indicates that reduction of this pressure below 2 cm H_2O is associated with decreased functional residual capacity and lower Pa_{O_2} measurements. Consequently, if a patient requires no mechanically assisted ventilation and less than 2 cm H_2O to obtain a Pa_{O_2} greater than 50 mm Hg with an FI_{O_2} less than 0.4, extubation should be attempted. Following extubation, blood gas surveillance is especially important, and determinations should be made after 15 minutes and 1 hour, and as appropriate thereafter.

The ongoing and acute problems discussed in this chapter comprise most of the medical conditions seen in the infant with respiratory distress. Occasionally, however, other abnormalities that require treatment are recognized. These defects may occur as isolated conditions with unknown cause, as in the case of congenital malformations or inborn errors of metabolism. Occasionally maternal conditions may influence the infant's hospital course. Drug addiction or maternal infection either at delivery or during gestation are two common examples of such situations. Unfortunately it is not uncommon for complications of "intensive care" to produce further problems.

The successful management of the high risk infant with respiratory distress requires knowledge and experience with the many potentially complicating conditions that may arise. However, it is beyond the scope of this section to provide further discussion of these conditions, but the interested reader may refer to a rapidly proliferating number of general texts on neonatology. It is to be hoped that the problem-oriented approach to management presented here will prove a useful cornerstone for the care of all infants regardless of their problems.

REFERENCES

1. Adamsons, K. Jr.: Role of thermal factors in fetal and neonatal life. *Pediatr. Clin. North Am. 13*:599, 1966.
2. Altman, R. P. and J. G. Randolph: Application and hazards of total parenteral nutrition in infants. *Ann. Surg. 174*:85, 1971.
3. Andrew, G., G. Chan and D. Schiff: Lipid metabolism in the neonate. II. The effect of Intralipid on bilirubin binding in vitro and in vivo. *J. Pediatr. 88*:279, 1976.
4. Auld, P. A. M., P. Bhangananda and S. Mehta: The influence of early calorie intake with IV glucose on catabolism of premature infants. *Pediatrics 37*:592, 1966.
5. Bancalari, E., O. L. Garcia and W. J. Jesse: Effects of continuous negative pressure on lung mechanics in idiopathic respiratory distress. *Pediatrics 51*:485, 1973.
6. Berman, L. S., W. W. Fox, R. C. Raphaely and J. J. Downes: Optimal levels of CPAP for tracheal extubation of newborn infants. *J. Pediatr. 89*:109, 1976.
7. Borresen, H. C., A. G. Coran and O. Knutrud: Metabolic results of parenteral feeding in neonatal surgery. *Ann. Surg. 172*:291, 1970.
8. Brueck, K., M. Brueck and H. Lemtis: Temperature regulation in newborn and premature infants after spontaneous and pathological delivery. *Beburtshilfe Frauenheilkd. 20*:461, 1960.
9. Brueck, K.: Temperature regulation in the newborn infant. *Biol. Neonatorum 3*:65, 1961.
10. Buetow, K. C. and S. W. Klein: Effect of maintenance of "normal" skin temperature on survival of infants of low birth weight. *Pediatrics 34*:163, 1964.
11. Caldine, P., J. D. Heith and M. J. Brennan: Effect of continuous positive pressure ventilation (CPPV) on edema formation in dog lung. *J. Appl. Physiol. 36*:672, 1975.
12. Cheek, D. B. and R. D. Rowe: Aspects of sympathetic activity in the newborn including the respiratory distress syndrome. *Pediatr. Clin. North Am. 13*:863, 1966.
13. Chrispin, A. R., D. Hull, J. G. Lillie and R. A. Ridison: Renal tubular necrosis and papillary necrosis after gastroenteritis. *Br. Med. J. i*:410, 1970.
14. Chu, J., J. A. Clements, E. K. Cotton, M. H. Klaus, A. Y. Sweet and W. H. Tooley: The pulmonary hypoperfusion syndrome. *Pediatrics 35*:733, 1965.
15. Coran, A. G. and R. Nesbakken: The metabolism

of intravenously administered fat in adult and newborn dogs. *Surgery 66*:922, 1969.
16. Coran, A.: Total intravenous feeding of infants and children without the use of a central venous catheter. *Ann. Surg. 179*:445, 1974.
17. Corbett, A. J. S., J. A. Ross, P. H. Beaudre and L. Stein: Ventilation-perfusion relationships as assessed by aAD$_{N_2}$ in hyaline membrane disease. *J. Appl. Physiol. 36*:74, 1974.
18. Corner, B. D.: Resuscitation in the newborn. *Abst. Br. Med. J. III*:228, 1967.
19. Dahm, L. S. and L. S. James: Newborn temperature and calculated heat loss in the delivery room. *Pediatrics 48*:504, 1972.
20. Davison, A. N. and J. Dobbing: The developing brain. In *Applied Neurochemistry.* A. N. Davison and J. Dobbing (Eds.). Blackwell Scientific Publications, Oxford, 1968.
21. Dawes, G. S., E. Hibbard and W. F. Windle: The effect of alkali and glucose infusion on permanent brain damage in Rhesus monkeys asphyxiated at birth. *J. Pediatr. 65*:801, 1964.
22. Dawkins, M. J. R. and J. W. Scopes: Non-shivering thermogenesis and brown adipose tissue in the human newborn infant. *Nature 206*:201, 1965.
23. Day, R. L., L. Caliguiri, C. Kamenski and F. Ehrlich: Body temperature and survival of premature infants. *Pediatrics 34*:171, 1964.
24. Delivoria-Papadopoulos, M., L. D. Miller, R. E. Forster II and F. A. Oski: The role of exchange transfusion in the management of low-birthweight infants with and without severe respiratory distress syndrome. I. Initial Observations. *J. Pediatr. 89*:273, 1976.
25. Dobbing, J.: Undernutrition and the developing brain. The relevance of animal models to the human problem. *Am. J. Dis. Child. 120*:411, 1970.
26. Dobbing, J.: Vulnerable periods in the developing brain. In *Applied Neurochemistry.* A. N. Davison and J. Dobbing (Eds.). Blackwell Scientific Publications, Oxford, 1968.
27. Dobbing, J.: Vulnerable periods of brain development. In *Lipids, Malnutrition and the Developing Brain.* Ciba Foundation Symposium. New York Assoc. Scientific Publishers, New York, p. 9, 1972.
28. Dobbing, J. and J. Sands: The timing of neuroblast multiplication in developing human brain. *Nature (Lond.) 226*:639, 1970.
29. Driscoll, J. M., Jr. and W. C. Heird: Maintenance fluid therapy during the neonatal period. In *The Body Fluids in Pediatrics,* R. W. Winters (Ed.). Little, Brown and Co., Boston, 1973.
30. Driscoll, J. M., Jr., W. D. Heird, J. N. Schullinger, R. D. Gongaware and R. W. Winters: Total intravenous alimentation in low-birth-weight infants: A preliminary report. *J. Pediatr. 81*:145, 1972.
31. Duc, G. and K. Engel: Hemoglobin oxygen affinity and erythrocyte 2,3,diphosphoglycerate (DPG) content in hyaline membrane disease (HMD) and cardiac malformations (CM). *Abst. Proc. Soc. Pediatr. Res.* p. 79, 1970.
32. Duc, G.: Assessment of hypoxia in the newborn: suggestions for a practical approach. *Pediatrics 48*:469, 1971.
33. Dweck, H. S. and G. Cassady: I. Incidence of hyperglycemia in infants of birthweights 1,100 grams or less. *Pediatrics 53*:189, 1974.
34. Dweck, H. S., Y. W. Brans, R. Milstead and G. Cassady: Glucose intolerance in infants less than 1000 gms. The effects of a double dose of glucose. *Abst. Pediatr. Res. 7*:158, 1973.
35. Edelmann, C. M., Jr. and H. L. Barnett: Role of the kidney in water metabolism in young infants. *J. Pediatr. 56*:154, 1960.
36. Erkan, V., W. Blankenship and M. T. Stahlman: The complications of chronic umbilical vessel catheterization. *Abst. Pediatr. Res. 2*:317, 1968.
37. Fanaroff, A. A., M. Wald, H. S. Gruber and M. H. Klaus: Insensible water loss in low birth weight infants. *Pediatrics 50*:236, 1972.
38. Fanaroff, A. A., C. C. Cha, R. Sosa, R. S. Crumrine and M. H. Klaus: Controlled trial of continuous negative external pressure in the treatment of severe respiratory distress syndrome. *J. Pediatr. 82*:921, 1973.
39. Finberg, L., C. Luttrell, and H. Redd: Pathogenesis of lesions in the nervous system in hypernatremic states. II. Experimental studies of gross anatomic changes and alterations of chemical composition of the tissues. *Pediatrics 23*:46, 1959.
40. Fomon, S. J.: *Infant Nutrition.* W. B. Saunders Co., Philadelphia, 1974.
41. Glass, L., W. A. Silverman and J. C. Sinclair: Effect of the thermal environment on cold resistance and growth of small infants after the first week of life. *Pediatrics 41*:1033, 1968.
42. Goldman, D. and D. G. Maki: Infection control in total parenteral nutrition. *J.A.M.A. 223*:1360, 1973.
43. Goldman, H. I., O. B. Liebman, R. Freudenthal and R. Reuben: Effects of early dietary protein intake on low-birth-weight infants: evaluation at 3 years of age. *J. Pediatr. 78*:126, 1971.
44. Gregory, G. A., J. A. Kitterman, R. H. Phibbs, W. H. Tooley and W. K. Hamilton: Treatment of the idiopathic respiratory-distress syndrome with continuous positive pressure. *N. Engl. J. Med. 284*:1333, 1971.
45. Gupta, J. M., N. R. C. Roberton and J. S. Wigglesworth: Umbilical artery catheterization in the newborn. *Arch. Dis. Child. 43*:382, 1968.
46. Heird, W. C., J. F. Nicholson, J. M. Driscoll, Jr.,

J. N. Schullinger and R. W. Winters: Hyperammonemia resulting from intravenous alimentation using a mixture of synthetic L-amino acids: a preliminary report. *J. Pediatr. 81*:162, 1972.

47. Herman, S. and E. O. R. Reynolds: Methods of improving oxygenation in infants mechanically ventilated for severe hyaline membrane disease. *Arch. Dis. Child. 48*:612, 1973.
48. Hey, E. N. and B. O'Connell: Oxygen consumption and heat balance in the cot-nursed baby. *Arch. Dis. Child. 45*:335, 1970.
49. Hey, E. N. and G. Katz: The range of thermal insulation in the tissues of the new-born baby. *J. Physiol.* (*Lond.*) *207*:667, 1970.
50. Hey, E.: Thermal neutrality. *Br. Med. Bull. 31*:69, 1975.
51. Huch. A. and R. Huch: New method for arterial blood sampling in infants and others. *Arch. Dis. Child. 48*:982, 1973.
52. Huch, R., D. W. Lubbers and A. Huch: Reliability of transcutaneous monitoring of arterial PO_2 in newborn infants. *Arch. Dis. Child. 49*:213, 1974.
53. Huch, R., D. W. Lubbers and A. Huch: Quantitative continuous measurement of partial oxygen pressure on the skin of adults and newborn babies. *Pfluegers Arch. 337*:185, 1972.
54. Huch, R., A. Huch and D. W. Lubbers: Transcutaneous measurement of blood PO_2 ($tcPO_2$)—method and application in perinatal medicine. *J. Perinat. Med. 1*:183, 1973.
55. Huckabee, W. E.: Relationship of pyruvate and lactate during anerobic metabolism. III. Effects of breathing low-oxygen gases. *J. Clin. Invest. 37*:264, 1958.
56. Hutch, J. S. and J. F. Murray: Continuous positive pressure ventilation. Effects on systemic oxygen transport and tissue oxygenation. *Ann. Intern. Med. 76*:193, 1972.
57. Kelly, H. J., R. E. Sloan, W. Joffman and C. Saunders: Accumulation of nitrogen and six minerals in the human foetus during gestation. *Hum. Biol. 2*:61, 1950.
58. Krauss, A. N., S. Waldman and P. A. M. Auld: Personal communication.
59. Krauss, A. N., D. B. Klain and P. A. M. Auld: Carbon monoxide diffusion capacity in newborn infants. *Pediatr. Res. 10*:771, 1976.
60. Krauss, A. N. and P. A. M. Auld: Diminished response to carbon dioxide in premature infants. *Biol. Neonate 30*:216, 1976.
61. Krieger, I.: The energy metabolism in infants with growth failure due to maternal deprivation, undernutrition, or causes unknown. *Pediatrics 38*:63, 1966.
62. Kumar, A., K. J. Falke, B. Geffin, C. F. Aldredge, M. B. Lauer, E. Lowenstein and H. Pontoppidan: Continuous positive pressure ventilation in acute respiratory failure. Effects on hemodynamics and lung function. *N. Engl. J. Med. 283*:143, 1970.
63. Larroche, J. C.: Umbilical catheterization, its complications. *Biol. Neonate 16*:101, 1970.
64. Mann, T. P. and R. I. K. Elliott: Neonatal cold injury due to accidental exposure to cold. *Lancet 1*:229, 1957.
65. Mann, T. P.: Hypothermia in the newborn: a new syndrome? *Lancet 1*:613, 1955.
66. Mann, T. P.: Observations on temperatures of mothers and babies in the perinatal period. *J. Obstet. Gynaecol. Br. Commonw. 75*:316, 1968.
67. Mestyan, J., M. Fekete, G. Bata and I. Jarai: The basal metabolic rate of premature infants. *Biol. Neonatorum 7*:11, 1964.
68. Mestyan, J., I. Jarai, G. Bata and M. Fekete: The significance of facial skin temperature in the chemical heat regulation of premature infants. *Biol. Neonate 7*:243, 1964.
69. Miller, R. and J. B. Grogan: Incidence and source of contamination of intravenous nutritional infusion systems. *J. Pediatr. Surg. 8*:185, 1973.
70. Moore, F. D. and M. R. Ball: *The Metabolic Response to Surgery.* Charles C Thomas, Springfield, p. 131, 1952.
71. Murdoch, A. I., B. S. L. Kidd, M. A. Leuwellyn, M. McC. Reid and P. R. Swyer: Intrapulmonary venous admixture in the respiratory distress syndrome. *Biol. Neonate 15*:1, 1970.
72. Nicolopoulos, D. A. and C. A. Smith: Metabolic aspects of respiratory distress (hyaline membrane syndrome) in newborn infants. *Pediatrics 28*:206, 1961.
73. Oh, W. and H. Kavecki: Phototherapy and insensible water loss in the newborn infant. *Am. J. Dis. Child. 124*:230, 1972.
74. Oski, F. A. and M. Delivoria-Papadopoulos: The red cell, 2,3,-diphosphoglycerate and tissue O_2 release. *J. Pediatr. 77*:941, 1970.
75. Oski, F. A.: The unique fetal red cell and its function. *Pediatrics 51*:494, 1973.
76. Perlstein, P. H., N. K. Edwards and J. M. Sutherland: Apnea in premature infants and incubator-air-temperature changes. *N. Engl. J. Med. 282*:461, 1970.
77. Rudolph, A. M. and M. A. Heymann: The circulation of the fetus in utero. Methods for studying distribution of blood flow, cardiac output and organ blood flow. *Circ. Res. 21*:163, 1967.
78. Rudolph, A. M. and M. A. Heymann: Circulatory changes with growth in the fetal lamb. *Circ. Res. 26*:298, 1970.
79. Rudolph, A. M., J. E. Drorbaugh, P. A. M. Auld, A. J. Rudolph, A. S. Nadas, C. A. Smith and J. P. Hubbell: Studies on the circulation in the respiratory distress syndrome. *Pediatrics 27*:551, 1961.

80. Salle, B., G. W. Chance and M. Ruiton-Ugliengo: Glucose assimilation in neonates of very low birth weight. In *Current Concepts of Neonatal Intensive Care,* Stetson and Swyer (Eds.). Warren H. Green, St. Louis, 1974.
81. Shaw, J. C. L.: Parenteral nutrition in the management of sick low birthweight infants. *Pediatr. Clin. North Am. 20*:333, 1973.
82. Shennan, A. T., A. G. Cherian, A. Angel and M. H. Bryan: The effect of Intralipid on the estimation of serum bilirubin in the newborn infant. *J. Pediatr. 88*:285, 1976.
83. Silverman, W. A., J. W. Fertig and A. P. Berger: The influence of the thermal environment upon the survival of newly born premature infants. *Pediatrics 22*:876, 1958.
84. Silverman, W. A., J. C. Sinclair and F. J. Agate, Jr.: The oxygen cost of minor changes in heat balance of small newborn infants. *Acta Paediatr. Scand. 55*:294, 1966.
85. Simmons, M. A., E. W. Adcock, III, H. Bard and F. C. Battaglia: Hypernatremia and intracranial hemorrhage in neonates. *N. Eng. J. Med. 291*:6, 1974.
86. Sinclair, J. C., J. M. Driscoll, Jr., W. C. Heird and R. W. Winters: Supportive management of the sick neonate. *Pediatr. Clin. North Am. 17*:863, 1970.
87. Snyderman, S. E., L. E. Holt, Jr., P. M. Norton and S. V. Phansalkar: Protein requirement of the premature infant. *Am. J. Clin. Nutri. 23*:890, 1970.
88. Snyderman, S. E.: Amino acid requirements. In *Intravenous Nutrition in the High Risk Infant,* R. Winters (Ed.). John Wiley & Sons, New York, p. 205, 1975.
89. Stegink, L. D.: Amino acid metabolism. In *Intravenous Nutrition in the High Risk Infant,* R. Winters (Ed.). John Wiley & Sons, New York, p. 181, 1975.
90. Strauss, F. W., M. Escabedo and D. Goldring: Continuous monitoring of arterial oxygen tension in the newborn infant. *J. Pediatr. 85*:254, 1974.
91. Suter, P. M., H. B. Fairley and M. D. Isenberg: Optimum end-expiratory airway pressure in patients with acute pulmonary failure. *N. Engl. J. Med. 292*:284, 1975.
92. Thibeault, D. W., B. C. Clutario and P. A. M. Auld: Arterial oxygen tension in premature infants. *J. Pediatr. 69*:449, 1966.
93. Thibeault, D. W., E. Poblete and P. A. M. Auld: Alveolar-arterial O_2 and CO_2 differences and their relation to lung volume in the newborn. *Pediatrics 41*:574, 1967.
94. Thibeault, D. W., B. Clutario and P. A. M. Auld: The oxygen cost of breathing in the premature infant. *Pediatrics 37*:954, 1966.
95. Travis, S. F., H. J. Sugerman, R. L. Ruberg, S. J. Dudrick, M. Delivoria-Papadopoulos, L. D. Miller and F. A. Oski: Alterations of red-cell glycolytic intermediates and oxygen transport as a consequence of hypophosphatemia in patients receiving intravenous hyperalimentation. *N. Engl. J. Med. 285*:763, 1971.
96. Usher, R. H.: Clinical and therapeutic aspects of fetal malnutrition. *Pediatr. Clin. North Am. 17*:169, 1970.
97. Van Leeuwen, G. and M. Patney: Complications of umbilical vessel catheterization: peritoneal perforation. *Pediatrics 44*:1028, 1969.
98. Wayne, K. S.: Positive end-expiratory pressure (PEEP) ventilation. *J.A.M.A. 236*:1394, 1976.
99. Widdowson, E. M. and R. A. McCance: Some effects of accelerating growth. 1. General somatic development. *Proc. R. Soc. Lond.* (*Biol.*) *152*:188, 1960.
100. Widdowson, E. M. and G. C. Kennedy: Rate of growth, mature weight and life span. *Proc. R. Soc. Lond.* (*Biol.*) *156*:96, 1962.
101. Widdowson, E. M. and J. W. T. Dickerson: In *Mineral Metabolism,* Vol. II, C. L. Comar and F. Bronner (Eds.). Academic Press, New York, 1961.
102. Widdowson, E. M.: Growth and composition of the fetus and newborn. In *Biology of Gestation, Vol. II: The Fetus and Neonate,* Assali (Ed.). Academic Press, New York, 1968.
103. Williams, P. R. and W. Oh: Effects of radiant warmer on insensible water loss in newborn infants. *Am. J. Dis. Child. 128*:511, 1974.
104. Wilmore, D. W. and S. J. Dudrick: Growth and development of an infant receiving all nutrients exclusively by vein. *J.A.M.A. 203*:860, 1968.
105. Winick, M. and P. Rosso: The effect of severe early malnutrition on cellular growth of the human brain. *Pediatr. Res. 3*:181, 1969.
106. Winick, M.: Cellular growth in intrauterine malnutrition. *Pediatr. Clin. North Am. 17*:69, 1970.
107. Wu, P. Y. K. and J. E. Hodgman: Insensible water loss in preterm infants: changes with postnatal development and non-ionizing radiant energy. *Pediatrics 54*:704, 1974.

Developmental Anomalies of the Lung

PAUL SYMCHYCH

15

Respiratory distress is by far the most frequent clinical problem in neonatology. Although disorders of alveolar collapse are the most prevalent within this group, the clinician and radiologist must constantly be aware of a differential diagnosis that includes malformations.

Recognition of respiratory malformations is vital in the diagnosis of the cause of respiratory distress, and may be important as a clue to some extrapulmonary malformations. Conversely, apparently extrapulmonary clinical problems occasionally have associated pulmonary malformations that may alter or affect the clinician's management of the neonate.

With the exceptions of cleft palate, tracheoesophageal fistula, diaphragmatic hernia, and lung hypoplasia, clinically significant malformation of the respiratory tract cannot be considered common. This relative rarity undoubtedly accounts for most of the errors in diagnosis or recognition of these malformations when they are encountered.

Underdevelopment of the Lungs

Underdevelopment of the lungs has generally been discussed according to the 1909 classification of Schneider, who proposed three groups: agenesis, aplasia, and hypoplasia. The three groups represent a continuum of degrees of underdevelopment. The hypoplasias are a broad, heterogeneous group of disorders that will be considered separately.

Agenesis and aplasia are technically distinct, but their differentiation is not always clear-cut and there is no practical need for their separation. For these reasons they will be considered together.

BILATERAL AGENESIS AND APLASIA

Bilateral agenesis and aplasia are extraordinarily rare.[12,59] Agenesis of the lungs is the complete absence of lungs, bronchi, and vascular structures. Aplasia is absence of lungs and vascular structures with small, rudimentary bronchi. Both conditions originate at a very early stage of development, at the time of appearance of the primary bronchial buds (the 4-mm stage). The malformations correspond to developmental arrest at approximately the 5-mm stage (fourth and fifth week of fetal life). Although neither bilateral agenesia nor aplasia is compatible with postnatal life, maintenance of pregnancy to term is possible.

UNILATERAL AGENESIS

Agenesis of one lung is more frequent. In contrast to bilateral agenesis, unilateral agenesis is compatible with postnatal life. However, a high association with other malformations (many of which are not necessarily lethal by themselves) contributes to an increased incidence of early death.

The defect is an asymmetric arrest of bronchial bud development at approximately the fifth week of gestation. Cause is unknown, and the majority of cases are sporadic. Experimentally, the lesion has been produced in the offspring of vitamin A deficient rats.[60] It has been described in identical twins: in one instance both showed the same anomaly; in another each had the anomaly but in contralateral lungs; and in four instances only one twin showed the anomaly. The lesion has no consistent association with chromosomal anomalies, although it has been noted in trisomy 18 and in trisomy of a C-group chromosome.[7,57]

Where stated, the agenesis occurs roughly equally on the right and left side. Females tend to predominate in a ratio of 3:2.

Anatomically, these patients demonstrate a voluminous single lung supplied by a single bronchus and pulmonary artery. The heart and mediastinum are displaced to the side of the agenesis. The developed contralateral lung is best described by Ryland and Reid, who studied the lung of a 3-month-old infant.[50] The lung was considerably increased in volume, with the upper lobe accounting for the enlargement. Bronchial branches (generations) were reduced, but the single lung contained nearly twice the normal number of alveoli. Individual alveoli were slightly smaller than normal. Pulmonary artery branches were reduced out of proportion to the reduction of bronchi that they usually accompany. Therefore, although an intrinsic, contralateral deficit in bronchial and vascular development occurs, the stimulus for alveolar generation to fill the available intrathoracic space seems to be independent.

Clinical presentation of unilateral agenesis is highly variable, and to a large extent it may be dominated by the associated extrapulmonary malformations. The chest is not necessarily asymmetric. Physical findings referable to the lungs may be absent. Severe cyanosis or stridor suggest the presence of an additional anomaly. Chest roentgenogram is often the first clue to the diagnosis, with opacity of one hemithorax and marked mediastinal shift. Bronchography and angiography are helpful.

There is a very high incidence of associated anomalies. Approximately one-half of the patients have extrapulmonary anomalies, often ipsilateral.[36,41] Table 15-1 is a condensed list of anomalies modified from the detailed list of Maltz and Nadas.[36]

The prognosis of *isolated* agenesis may be said to be good, with pneumonia in infancy being the major threat to survival. No documentation shows a tendency towards emphysema or to pulmonary hypertension in later life as a result of agenesis, unless cardiovascular or other anomalies are present.

In spite of the high association with other anomalies, the overall survival of cases reported between 1954 and 1968 was 66%.[36] Present-day survival rate should be expected to be even better.

HYPOPLASIA (GENERAL CONSIDERATIONS)

Hypoplasia is common and is frequently overlooked as a cause of respiratory distress in the newborn. As a category, it includes all gradations of underdevelopment between aplasia and normality. Hypoplasia is most often regarded as the effect on the developing lung of a diverse number of pathologic processes, the common end point of which is the failure of the lung to attain expected normal development.

Hypoplasia may be unilateral or bilateral, depending upon the underlying cause, and may vary in degree from a subtle decrease in size to a lung weighing only a few grams. Most often, an entire lung or pair of lungs is affected, but hypoplasia of only a portion of one lung may be encountered.

The largest group of known etiologic factors is characterized by a reduction of intrathoracic volume available for lung growth. The most dramatic of these causes is diaphragmatic hernia. Other readily demonstrable causes are cysts, tumors, gross cardiomegaly, pleural effusions as seen in hydrops fetalis, elevations of the diaphragm due to abdominal masses (renal or enteric cysts), and eventration of an intact hemidiaphragm. Bony anomalies of vertebrae and ribs with consequent decrease in thoracic volume include anencephaly, asphyxiating thoracic dystrophy, achondroplasia, thanatophoric dwarfism, and other rare skeletal diseases.

A syndrome of musculoskeletal deformity with marked lung hypoplasia has recently been described.[42,47] These infants are of particular interest because they had no apparent

TABLE 15-1. Agenesis of Lung (156 Cases) and Associated Anomalies

Anomaly	No. Anomalies	Anomaly	No. Anomalies
Cardiac (22 patients)		Skeletal (19 patients)	
Ventricular septal defect	10	Spinal anomalies	14
Atrial septal defect	3	Rib anomalies	3
Patent foramen ovale*	12	Digital-radial dysplasias	6
Other	3	Genitourinary (14 patients)	
Vascular (14 patients)		Absence of kidney(s)	2
Patent ductus arteriosus*	10	Polycystic kidney(s)	2
Other	17	Ureter anomalies	3
Gastrointestinal (22 patients)		Genitalia anomalies	3
Imperforate anus	8	Other	4
Tracheoesophageal fistula and/or atresia	8	Miscellaneous (28 patients)	
Other	8	Central nervous system anomalies	4
		Ear anomalies	3
		Cleft lip, palate, uvula	3
		Ptosis	2
		Other	10

*Most of these patients were newborns, and their pathophysiologic significance is suspect.

deformity of the thorax, but they did have polyhydramnios. Such examples of what appears to be "primary" or isolated hypoplasia (i.e., without other thoracic pathology) are rare or at least are rarely reported.

RENAL AGENESIS

Bilateral pulmonary hypoplasia is the rule in renal agenesis. Bilateral renal agenesis with oligohydramnios and/or placental amnion nodosum, characteristic facies, limb deformities, and pulmonary hypoplasia is commonly referred to as Potter syndrome.[45] The syndrome is more frequent than generally realized, occurring in approximately 1 to 3 per 1000 deliveries.[10,11] Males predominate in a ratio of 2:1. It is usually readily diagnosed at birth because of the typical external appearance, the respiratory distress, limb deformity, and anuria. The majority of infants die of asphyxia in the first 2 days. Uremia rarely supervenes because of the early pulmonary death.

Oligohydramnios secondary to lack of fetal urine production is the factor generally believed to be responsible for lung hypoplasia,[43,55] although it does not necessarily explain all of the features of the syndrome.[46] Fetal kidney function is not a requisite for fetal survival in the presence of a functioning placenta. Fetal urine, however, is a major source of amniotic fluid in the latter stages of pregnancy,[51] and "it appears that a normal volume of amniotic fluid is one of the conditions for normal lung development in the fetus."[43] An important supporting observation has been made in a set of monoamniotic twins. Although one twin had renal agenesis, he lacked the pulmonary hypoplasia and other stigmata of Potter syndrome except for low set ears, presumably because his twin was capable of producing urine.[38]

While a normal volume of amniotic fluid seems to be a requisite for lung growth, direct contact between amniotic fluid and lung bud (by way of a patent airway or fistula) does not seem to be necessary, as evidenced by the rare malformations of laryngeal or tracheal atresia,[20] the respiratory counterpart of esophageal atresia. These lungs grow normally, although they do have distal airway, mucous gland, and to a lesser extent alveolar dilatation with clear albuminous appearing mucoid secretion.[20,53] Similar observations have been made in animals.[8]

The role of oligohydramnios in pulmonary hypoplasia is now established. It is quite likely that the presence of amniotic fluid in the bronchi is not a major requirement for lung growth. Thoracic compression as a result of oligohydramnios remains the most attractive explanation of lung hypoplasia in Potter syndrome.

THORACIC DEFORMITY

Reduction of thoracic volume with associated lung hypoplasia is seen most commonly in association with the chest deformity of anencephaly, and is also present in a number of skeletal diseases. Many of these are clinically apparent as a skeletal developmental anomaly at the time of birth. Asphyxiating thoracic dystrophy of the newborn deserves special mention because extrathoracic manifestations may be minimal, and thoracic findings may be easy to overlook.

Asphyxiating thoracic dystrophy is a variety of chondrodysplasia, which is characterized by reduction of thoracic volume, with a cylindric and narrow (in both transverse and anteroposterior dimension) rib cage.[2,22,44] The chest is often elongated in the craniocaudal direction. The ribs are horizontal and short; their anterior portions are widened. Mobility of the ribs is restricted, and respiration is largely diaphragmatic. This syndrome may escape detection for a month or more, until cyanosis and tachypnea become evident. Clinical and radiographic examination of the chest should suggest the diagnosis, and pelvic roentgenograms are of great help in confirming it.

The syndrome is probably an autosomal recessive with a sibling recurrence risk of one in four.

Most patients die in infancy, but those who do not should show some improvement in respiratory symptoms even though the chest deformity persists. Patients should be observed for evidence of renal disease.[24]

DIAPHRAGMATIC HERNIA

Diaphragmatic hernia is the other common cause of hypoplasia, and is about as frequently encountered as renal agenesis. The defect occurs as a result of one hemidiaphragm's failure to close, with herniation of abdominal viscera into the hemithorax. The three different sites of herniation are the esophageal hiatus, the retrosternal foramina of Morgagni, and the posterolateral foramina of Bochdalek. Hernias at the esophageal hiatus or foramina of Morgagni account for 10% or less of diaphragmatic hernias, are usually small, and cause only minor respiratory symptoms. The typical site of herniation is through the posterolateral foramen of Bochdalek, with left-sided hernias predominating in a ratio of approximately 9 : 1. Males are affected twice as often as females.

Posterolateral hernias are usually large, with herniation of stomach, intestine, and often spleen and/or a lobe of the liver into the hemithorax. Pulmonary hypoplasia of varying degree on the side of the hernia is the rule. Dyspnea and cyanosis from birth or shortly after birth are a reflection of the pulmonary hypoplasia, the contralateral lung compression from mediastinal shift, and possibly the pneumothorax, which is frequently associated. Blood gas determinations and alveolar-arterial gradients are used as prognostic indicators, but they are not a reliable means of predicting the degree of hypoplasia.[48] Diaphragmatic hernias may also be associated with sequestered rather than hypoplastic lungs. The possibility should be kept in mind at the time of repair.

Pulmonary hypoplasia in diaphragmatic hernia is the result of displacement of abdominal viscera into the thorax, with developmental arrest of the lung. Whatever the timing of the actual herniation, its effect is to arrest, or at least limit, bronchial growth and development to a stage corresponding to that reached at 10 to 12 weeks of normal gestation.[1,5,29]

Experimental confirmation of the pathogenesis of this lesion is not available because of the technical difficulty of first trimester fetal surgery. Comparable but not absolutely identical lesions have been produced in fetal lambs operated upon in the middle and last trimester.[13,28] These experiments showed that the hernia's effect was principally one of alveolar rather than bronchial hypoplasia, because the hernias were created after bronchial development was complete or nearly complete.

HYPOPLASIA: EMBRYOLOGY AND PATHOLOGY

Discussion of the various anatomic appearances of hypoplastic lungs must take into account the embryology of the lung as well as the relevant extrapulmonary forces. An idealized premise is that the timing and/or nature of any disturbance of lung development will alter the ultimate structure in a predictable manner. This premise has been demonstrated best in diaphragmatic hernia. However, it should be noted that in many instances either the mechanism and the structural pathology of hypoplasia are unknown or the data are incomplete.

The pulmonary anlage appears at about 24 days after ovulation as a groove in the floor of the gut. Elongation of the laryngotracheal diverticulum in a caudal direction and separation from the foregut follows. By the fifth week (5.0-mm size), the trachea divides to form the main bronchi. Arrest at this stage is responsible for agenesis and aplasia of one or both lungs.

By the thirty-fifth day (8.0- to 10.0-mm size), secondary bronchial branches appear, followed in the next week by segmental and subsegmental branches. Bronchial growth and branching continue, with a growth spurt between 10 and 16 weeks. At 18 weeks (150-mm size) the lung consists only of branching bronchi sheathed by mesenchyme. By 16 to 18 weeks, the adult pattern and complement of bronchi have developed.

Interference with lung growth at the stage of bronchial development is characteristic of diaphragmatic hernia, which results from herniation of abdominal viscera into the thorax in early embryonic life. Total lung mass is decreased, with a pronounced hypoplasia on the side of the hernia.[49] Various components of both lungs are underdeveloped, but to varying degrees.[1,5,29] Bronchial and bronchiolar regions are both affected and, on occasion, the bronchiolar region is absent. Alveolar number per acinus is near normal, but because of deficient bronchial branching the total number of alveoli is markedly decreased. Alveolar size is also reduced. Cartilage is normally developed. Pulmonary arteries are abnormally small, possibly suggesting that their development is related to airway generation.[29]

The major impact of the hernia is on the bronchial tree, which is only developed to a late fetal stage. Following surgical correction of the hernia, pulmonary growth occurs, and the prognosis is favorable.[39] "All it needs is more time and more room."[5] It is thought to be unlikely that new bronchial or arterial branches would develop. Alveoli should multiply and grow with a normal number per bronchiolar unit but with a reduction of total number.[29]

Between 20 and 24 weeks (180 to 300 mm), clumps of cells in the most distal air passages begin to cannulate to form primitive alveoli. This action is accompanied by vascular proliferation and capillary invasion. Further alveolar differentiation and growth occur throughout pregnancy. A critical milestone is passed at about 26 weeks when the fetus weighs approximately 800 g. At this stage, alveolar surface area is sufficient to provide potential extrauterine survival if adequate surface active material is present.

Interference with lung development in the last half of pregnancy should have its major impact on alveoli, with a relatively minor effect on airway branching. Although these results may be shown experimentally,[13,28] they have not been clearly demonstrated in humans.

Body weight and lung weight increase proportionally by a factor of approximately 10 times in the last half of pregnancy. Any reduction of thoracic growth can theoretically be expected to accompany proportional reduction of pulmonary growth. In practice, a wide range of severity exists in the degree of hypoplasia found in situations known to be associated with lung underdevelopment. Lung weight : body weight ratios in anencephaly and Potter syndrome vary from severe hypoplasia to normal.[49] Radial alveolar counts, which are estimates of the numbers of airways in the secondary lobule, showed a range of 50 to 100% of normal in this study. Similar studies in asphyxiating thoracic dystrophy were interpreted as being comparable to the lung findings in diaphragmatic hernia.[18] No studies to date have quantified bronchial growth and branching in the preceding entities.

Standard histologic sections of severely hypoplastic lungs show an abnormally large number of bronchioles per microscopic field. This finding is probably a reflection of the degree of hypoplasia, regardless of the causes or associated malformations. Anatomic studies with the elegance of those reported in diaphragmatic hernia and the solitary lung in unilateral agenesis would be necessary to characterize the nature of the underdevelopment in lungs in this clinically miscellaneous group.

Conspicuously absent in this discussion of hypoplasia is mention of the concept of primary hypoplasia. Because of regularly recurring associations, it is convenient to view most hypoplasias as a result of an associated malformation. Although virtually no documentation exists, hypoplasia could be an intrinsic lung anomaly with or without associated anomalies in other organs.

Pulmonary Lymphangiectasia

Lymphatic dilatation with resultant respiratory distress is an uncommon but not extremely rare lesion. The first description is attributed to Virchow over a century ago. More than 60 cases have now been reported. That one group[17] has reported approximately one-quarter of all cases in the literature suggests that lymphangiectasia is more common than thought, and that "the condition is not rare, but unrecognized."[34]

Lymphangiectasia is a bilateral cystic dilatation of pulmonary lymphatics with bulky inelastic lungs and alveolar hypoventilation. Occurrence shows a slight male preponderance, no racial predilection, approximately a 30% incidence of prematurity, and an increased incidence of stillbirth.

Pulmonary lymphangiectasia has been classified into three major types:[40]

(1) A primary developmental defect with isolated pulmonary involvement.

(2) Associated with congenital heart disease (principally pulmonary venous obstruction).

(3) Associated with intestinal or generalized systemic lymphangiectasia.

Primary or isolated lymphangiectasia with no cardiac malformations accounts for approximately two-thirds of cases. The majority of patients are born with cyanosis and die within minutes to 24 hours. Chest roentgenograms may be nonspecific, may resemble atelectasis or hyaline membrane disease, or may be "normal." Approximately half of this group have polycystic or dysplastic kidneys.

The primary type has been further subdivided into a late onset clinical pattern.[17] This late onset variant is less common than the newborn variant. Patients become symptomatic days to a month or more after birth. The lungs are overexpanded with restricted movement due to the dilated lymphatics. Roentgenograms show a variable pattern of overaeration, infiltrates, and atelectasis, or they may be "normal." The blood gas values are those of alveolar hypoventilation. Prognosis is poor, with death in months to a few years.

One-third of the cases of lymphangiectasia is associated with congenital heart disease. It should be noted that this disorder is a massive cystic lymphangiectasia and not the minor dilatation of chronic passive congestion. Obstruction of pulmonary venous return is the common denominator in this group. Total anomalous pulmonary venous return with obstruction is the most frequent anomaly, with a small number of other cases showing normal venous return but obstruction of left ventricular outflow.

Clinically and radiologically, the cardiac-associated group is similar to the primary group, with the addition of the findings of congenital heart disease. Prognosis is very poor.

A small proportion of the pulmonary lymphangiectasias are a component of a generalized lymphangiectasia with principal manifestations in the intestine. Protein-losing enteropathy is the major clinical problem, although these patients may have intermittent pulmonary symptoms resembling asthma. Hemihypertrophy is a common somatic association.[40] Up to 10% of patients with intestinal lymphangiectasia have chronic respiratory disease with abnormal pulmonary lymphatics.[58]

Congenital pulmonary lymphangiectasia is a persistence of fetal proportions of lymphatics to lung parenchyma. Lymphatics grow into the lung bud in the ninth fetal week. By 14 weeks, they have formed large channels.

Normally, by the sixteenth week lymphatic growth has slowed, and after 20 weeks pulmonary septa and their lymphatics become progressively less conspicuous. Laurence has proposed that "congenital pulmonary lymphangiectasia represents continued growth of the lung, with tissue elements maintaining their 12 to 16 week proportions."[33] This explanation is generally accepted for the primary group. In the cardiac-associated group abnormal hemodynamic forces may contribute to maintenance of fetal lymphatic structure.[9]

The pathology of all types is similar. The lungs are bulky and inelastic, with pronounced lobulation (Fig. 15-1). Beneath the pleural surfaces is a network of markedly dilated, often cystic vessels containing clear, colorless, serous fluid. On section, the lungs are symmetrically honeycombed with irregular fluid-containing cysts in broad septa. Microscopically, the dilated lymphatics are in close proximity to vessels and bronchioles. They have a flat endothelium, and no true valves. Lymphatics are supported by immature "embryonic" connective tissue that is also edematous.

The largest source of confusion is the differentiation of lymphangiectasia from interstitial emphysema. Both may be somewhat similar grossly, and air may be present in lymphatics. Interstitial air can be shown to dissect along tissue planes but there is no endothelial lining. Most important, the spaces occupied by air do not have the rich endowment of immature connective tissue seen in lymphangiectasia.

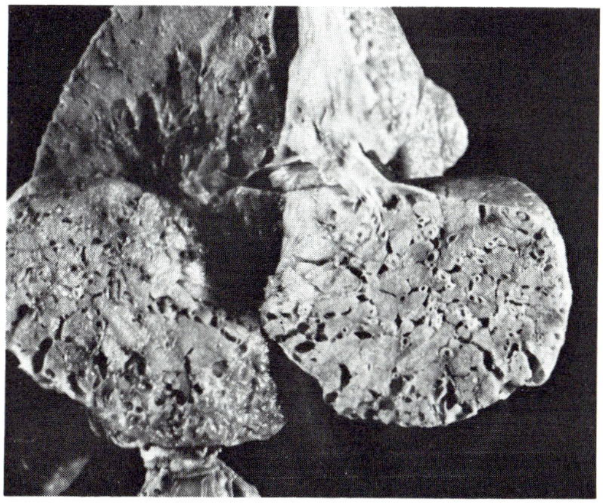

FIG. 15-1. Congenital Pulmonary Lymphangiectasia. Note the cystically dilated lymphatics in the peribronchial, perivascular, and interlobular connective tissue.

Lymphatic dilatation has been reported in the asplenia syndrome.[16] Although this syndrome is reminiscent of the typical lymphangiectasia syndrome, it may represent a milder form.

Cystic Lesions

Congenital pulmonary cystic lesions are not common. Their importance lies in the fact that they are often symptomatic in the newborn period (and occasionally in later life) and that the majority are potentially curable by resection. As a group, cystic lesions are perhaps the most disorganized subject in the thoracic literature, with nomenclature, criteria of diagnosis, and classifications almost as numerous as the authors who describe them. Several entities may be dissected out of this dazzling array of lesions, although many are still open to varying interpretations.

The congenital nature of cysts may be difficult to determine in patients past the neonatal period. Lesions identical to those observable in the newborn are usually regarded as being congenital if found in older patients. In the remainder, demonstration of a definite malformation with exclusion of an acquired pathogenesis is necessary to classify a cystic lesion as congenital. These criteria are contributory to the various interpretations and conflict in this literature.

Manifestations of cystic lesions vary greatly, and are related to the site and size of the lesion, the degree of compression of surrounding lung and other structures, and the presence of infection. In the newborn, clinical findings are usually those of dyspnea and cyanosis. In childhood, intermittent wheezing, cough, and recurrent pulmonary infections are more usual.

Clinical diagnosis of the various cystic lesions can be difficult. Chest roentgenograms are useful in differentiating cystic lesions from other lesions, although sequestered lobes are difficult to diagnose accurately. Angiography is useful in confirming sequestrations. Barium esophagograms are useful in delineating centrally located cysts, particularly bronchogenic cysts. Other radiologic contrast studies and bronchoscopy are of less value in establishing a preoperative diagnosis. A combination of thoracotomy with careful description of the vascular and bronchial connections and pathologic examination are frequently necessary to classify these lesions. In their comments on the accuracy of various diagnostic studies Buntain and colleagues conclude that at operation "the surgeon was almost always correct in his diagnosis of pulmonary sequestration, frequently correct in diagnosing bronchogenic cysts, and could not distinguish with acceptable accuracy between lobar emphysema and cystic adenomatoid malformation."[6]

BRONCHOVASCULAR FOREGUT ANOMALIES (SEQUESTRATIONS)

This grouping includes a malformation complex of dissociated or nonfunctional pulmonary tissue with aberrant arterial supply or venous drainage. Connection to the normal bronchial tree is not usually present, and in many cases the bronchial connection to enteric structures is abnormal. Traditionally, this group of malformations has been separated into distinct entities such as accessory lobes, extralobar sequestrations, and intralobar sequestrations (all subclassified according to bronchial connection). The distinction, for example, between accessory lobes and intralobar sequestrations was accepted as absolute by Spencer in the 1962 edition of *Pathology of the Lung,* while in the 1968 edition he states that ". . . the differences between the two conditions become increasingly blurred. . . ."[52] Current opinion seems to favor a common embryogenesis for these lesions.[19,21,37]

Theories on the genesis of these anomalies are reviewed by Spencer[52] and by Gerle and colleagues.[21] The theory that best explains the group of pulmonary, vascular, and foregut anomalies is the oldest one cited by both authors, the 1902 theory of Eppinger and Schauerstein. They postulated accessory foregut tracheobronchial budding distal to the normal tracheobronchial bud. This bud with its own blood supply migrates caudad, giving rise to "intralobar" sequestrations. As extended by Gerle's group, *all* forms of sequestration could be included, depending on the timing of the accessory foregut outpouching. Early development of this accessory diverticulum results in envelopment of accessory tissue by normally developing lung, resulting in intralobar sequestration. If the anomalous tracheal bud arose later, the elongation of the foregut would allow separation of normal lung and its pleura from anomalous lung and its pleura, giving rise to "extralobar" sequestration. Patent connections to the foregut are not present in the majority of sequestrations. This absence would have to be explained by involution of the original foregut connection. Fibrous nonpatent stalks and esophageal diverticulae have occasionally been demonstrated between foregut and sequestration. These stalks and diverticulae may be interpreted as evidence of partial involution of the connection.

Vascular supply to sequestrations is thought to be due to the persistence of portions of the intercommunicating capillary network that supplies the early tracheal bud from the sixth aortic arch (pulmonary artery system) and the fourth arch (aorta). As the pulmonary artery develops, the aortic connections to the lung bud normally disappear. True bronchial artery development from the aorta to normal lung is a much later phenomenon. The anomalous lung bud and its vessels (if they persist) will descend with the celiac axis and supply the lung from the aorta below the diaphragm or from the thoracic aorta. Venous drainage is variable, with connections to the pulmonary veins, azygos, hemiazygos, or portal veins.

The sequestrations traditionally classified as intralobar are found in the posterior basilar segments with a slight predominance of left lung over right. Arterial supply is said to be by a large vessel from the aorta either above or below the diaphragm. Venous drainage is to pulmonary veins. Foregut communication is uncommon.

In extralobar sequestration, the lung is said to be either above or below the diaphragm, is almost always on the left side, and is invested with its own pleural covering. Foregut communication is more common, and associated anomalies (particularly diaphragmatic hernia, diaphragmatic duplication, and pectus excavatum) are frequent. Arterial supply is by smaller vessels, either pulmonary or systemic. Venous drainage is to the azygos, hemiazygos, portal veins, or inferior vena cava.

In practice, these criteria for separation of sequestrations stand up in many cases, but sufficient variability and overlap suggest a common embryonic origin, and separation of types of sequestrations is artificial. Perhaps a more practical approach than the preceding classifications is emphasis on preoperative angiographic demonstration of abnormal vascular connections and determination of presence of enteric communication.

In addition to the frequently superimposed inflammatory changes, the abnormal lung may be atelectatic, but is usually cystic. It is composed of a mass of bronchial, bronchiolar, and alveolar tissue resembling a hamartoma. Fibrous tissue and abnormally distributed muscle are present in the interstitium. Rare cases with intestinal mucosa and pancreas have been described. The specimens are usually the size of a normal lung lobe or smaller, although similar lesions involving an entire lung have been studied.[27]

BRONCHOGENIC CYSTS

As an embryonic group, mediastinal bronchogenic and enteric cysts might be included as formes frustes of sequestrations. Bronchogenic cysts are relatively rare. They are usually found centrally, more often in a carinal, paratracheal, or paraesophageal location. The carinal location is most likely to produce respiratory obstruction in infancy.[15] These cysts are lined by respiratory epithelium and often have cartilage and bronchial glands in their wall. Aortic arterial supply similar to that seen in sequestrations has been recorded.[54]

Although bronchogenic cysts are occasionally noted in infancy, they are usually a clinical problem in older children and adults. They may be clinically silent, only to be diagnosed accidentally on routine chest roentgenograms. Approximately one-third of the patients come to the clinic with respiratory difficulty. Recurrent infection, cough, and chest pain are other presenting symptoms in decreasing frequency.[6]

The relationship between mediastinal bronchogenic cysts and the intrapulmonary cysts classified as "central" by Spencer is not proven. Sufficient morphologic similarities, however, suggest that they may represent varying locations of a similar if not identical process.

Intrapulmonary bronchogenic cysts are usually solitary and unilocular. Proximal communication with the bronchial tree is absent or difficult to demonstrate. Fibrous strings connecting cyst to proximal bronchus have been noted. They are lined by ciliated epithelium, and have cartilage and bronchial glands in the fibroelastic wall. Air may be present even though bronchial connection may not be demonstrated. Unless infected, the cyst contains mucoid material.

Bronchogenic cysts are frequently infected.

It is in the older patient with an infected intrapulmonary cyst that the argument of congenital bronchogenic cyst versus acquired localized cystic bronchiectasis arises. The components of the cyst wall resemble normal bronchus and have no dysplastic elements or anomalous vascular connections. If a patent connection to the bronchial tree is demonstrated, the distinction between infected congenital cyst and a post-inflammatory lesion becomes even more difficult. Simple excision is the treatment of choice.

CYSTIC ADENOMATOID MALFORMATION

This malformation is a focal pulmonary dysplasia characterized by a multicystic mass of terminal bronchiolar structures. The lesion may simulate infantile lobar emphysema, and may be one of the causes of lobar emphysema. Cause is unknown. Absence of abnormal vascular connections (as seen in sequestrations) has led to the proposal that the malformation originates later than sequestrations.[32] Absence of cartilage and seromucous glands is taken to mean that the lesion develops prior to the tenth week.[32,56]

Affected infants are often born prematurely, and become symptomatic in hours to weeks after birth. Symptoms are those of respiratory distress, with tachypnea and cyanosis. Although this lesion predominantly appears in stillborns and newborns, in one series of sugical cases 5 of 19 patients were over 5 years of age.[6] Radiologic features are those of an intrapulmonary mass with lucencies of various sizes and either mediastinal shift or herniation of affected lung into the contralateral hemithorax. Clinical and radiologic differential diagnosis includes the whole range of cystic lesions and is discussed by Belanger and colleagues.[3]

The lesion has been noted in all lobes of the lungs, with a tendency to be more common in the middle and upper lung fields. It is virtually always unilateral, but more than one lobe can be involved in the same lung.

The affected lobe is bulkier and heavier than normal, and no lobular septation or organized bronchial pattern exists. The cysts may contain air or liquid or both. Microscopic criteria are: (1) an "adenomatoid" increase of terminal respiratory structures with intercommunicating cysts of various sizes, and epithelium that is cuboid or bronchial; (2) polypoid mucosal proliferation and increased elastic fibers in walls of cysts; (3) absence of cartilage; (4) absence of inflammation; and (5) occasional alveoli with mucous epithelium.[32] Although the lesion is typically cystic, the proportion of its components varies. Almost solid lesions featuring mainly alveolar overgrowth have been described.[56] A variant with "cystic emphysema" and irregular intercommunicating cystically dilated bronchi, bronchioles, and alveolar ducts has also been described.[14] Cystic adenomatoid malformations and related pulmonary lesions are presented in Figures 15-2 through 15-6.

A frequent association, present in about half of the cases, is hydrops fetalis. Polyhydramnios is probably under-recorded, but is noted in about one-quarter of the cases. The anasarca has been postulated to be due to either compression of the right atrium and

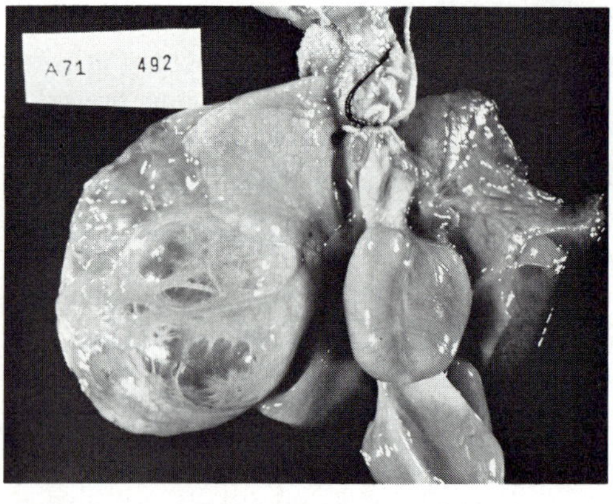

FIG. 15-2. Cystic Adenomatoid Malformation of the Lung. The right middle lobe is greatly enlarged and is composed of intercommunicating cysts of various sizes. Mediastinal structures are displaced, and the left lung is compressed.

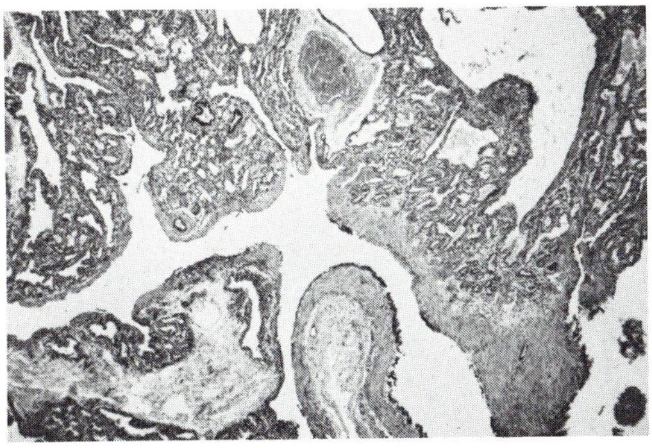

FIG. 15-3. Microscopic appearance of the middle lobe in Figure 15-2, illustrating the usual histology of cystic adenomatoid malformation.

inferior vena cava[56] or a decrease of pulmonary resorption of amniotic fluid.[30] A mechanism that seems more tenable than the latter would be a decrease in intestinal resorption of amniotic fluid because of esophageal compression. Cardiac anomalies are also frequently associated.

Management is surgical, with lobectomy the procedure of choice.

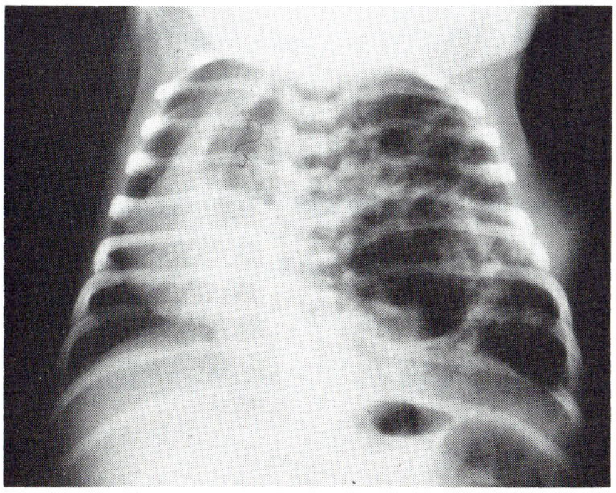

FIG. 15-4. Chest roentgenogram of an infant with respiratory distress from birth. The left hemithorax is filled with irregular cystic lucencies with intervening densities. The heart and other thoracic viscera are markedly displaced to the right. This patient was originally thought to have a diaphragmatic hernia. He was referred to this hospital where a left lower lobectomy was performed.

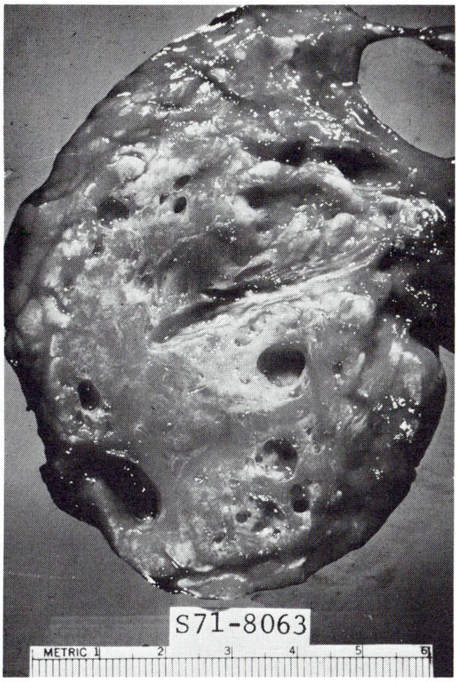

FIG. 15-5. Resection specimen from the patient in Figure 15-4. Although the lesion has cysts, the bulk of it is solid. (Photograph courtesy of Dr. George Gray, Laboratory of Surgical Pathology, The New York Hospital).

LOBAR EMPHYSEMA

Infantile lobar emphysema is a massive postnatal overinflation of one or more lobes of the lung. It is a disorder of infancy, with approximately one-quarter of patients developing symptoms at birth, approximately one-half in the first month, and only rare patients becoming symptomatic after 6 months. It may be found in any lobe of the lung, but is somewhat less common in the lower lobes. Cardiac anomalies are present in half or more of the cases.

Implicit in the word emphysema is a defect in the ability of the lung to deflate. In current use emphysema also implies dilatation of air spaces distal to terminal bronchioles *and* a destructive component. Whether infantile lobar emphysema is a true emphysema is

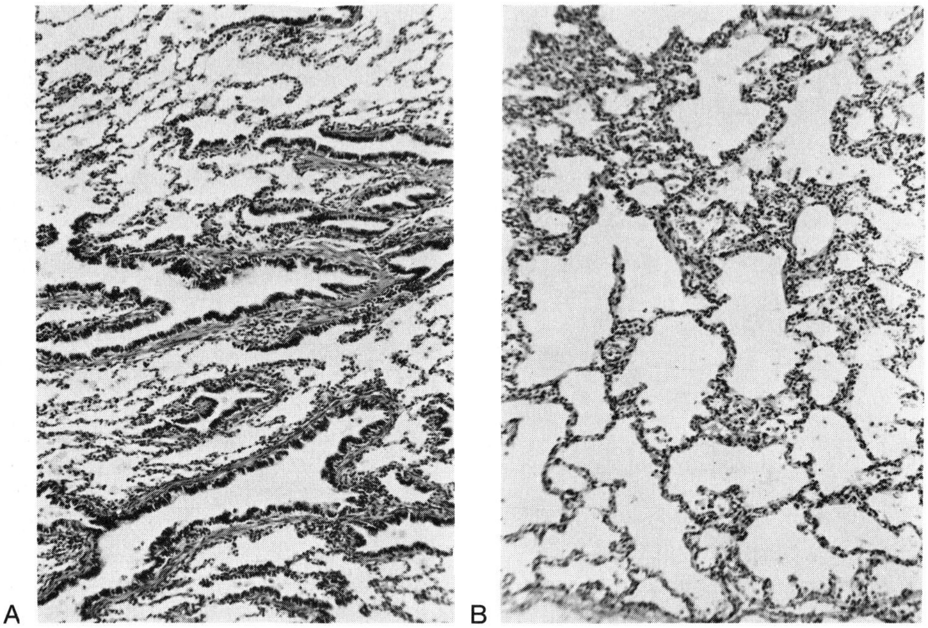

FIG. 15-6. Photomicrographs of the resected lobe show two distinct patterns.
A, Sections from the cystic areas have the histologic pattern of adenomatoid malformation.
B, The solid portions have the histology of lobar emphysema. Lesions such as this, composed of admixtures of cystic adenomatoid foci and solid purely alveolar areas resembling lobar emphysema, represent a morphologic and possibly embryonic link between the two lesions.

moot; however the term lobar emphysema is the one commonly used.

The cause of lobar emphysema is stated as unknown in more than half of the reported cases. Review of various mechanisms postulated shows sufficient diversity of opinion in the older literature to indicate that the lesion may have no single cause.[31] The most common suggestion is that a localized abnormality of bronchial cartilage permits a bronchial segment to collapse during expiration, thereby trapping air. This cartilage abnormality is variously described as absence, hypoplasia, or dysplasia. Internal obstruction by redundant mucosa, mucous plugs, or bronchial stenosis is the second most commonly cited cause. Extrinsic bronchial compression, principally by vascular structures and less commonly by lymph nodes or other regional masses, is also implicated.

An intriguing new approach to lobar emphysema arises out of a detailed quantitative study by Hislop and Reid.[25] They studied the resected lobe from three patients (aged 17 days, 3 months, and 8 months) who had typical infantile lobar emphysema on clinical and radiologic grounds. In all three cases, alveolar number was increased. The youngest patient had a five-fold increase in alveolar number, with normal alveolar size (i.e., no emphysema). The other two had approximately 50% more alveoli than expected, and slight degrees of true emphysema. They conclude that this condition represents a localized overgrowth of the alveolar region with alveolar "gigantism," and propose the term "polyalveolar lobe," further qualified as "with emphysema" and "without emphysema." Further quantitative studies from the same laboratory on clinically similar lesions indicate that lobar emphysema may have several different anatomic types. They describe a left upper lobe with normal arteries, bronchi, and alveolar number but with a four to five times increase in alveolar volume.[26] This condition was ascribed to torsion of the lobe about the lobar hilum, with a check valve mechanism of air trapping. Another patient had lung hypoplasia, with alveoli eight times normal volume on the left side, and a normally developed lung with increased alveolar volume (compensatory emphysema) on the right.[23] The authors propose that lobar emphysema may arise from a combination of anatomic features as observed in these cases: (1) a group with increased numbers of alveoli;[25] (2) a group with normally developed lung but overinflated alveoli;[26] and (3) a group with hypoplasia of all components of the lung, but with increased alveolar volume.[23]

An important question raised by these studies is: What proportion of emphysematous lobes (if studied in a detailed morphometric fashion) may be ascribed to a process of alveolar overgrowth? If this alveolar gigantism, present in three of the five lobes appropriately studied, can be shown to be important in infantile lobar emphysema as a group, a relationship (albeit embryonically a slightly later event) to cystic adenomatoid malformations would be implied. Possibly the adenomatoid malformations with alveolar overgrowth as the main feature are intermediate forms.[56] Absent or abnormal cartilage as implicated in the genesis of lobar emphysemas might then be related to absent cartilage as seen in adenomatoid malformations.

Symptoms depend on the size of the affected lobe, and may range from feeding difficulty, wheezing, and retractions to cyanosis. Hyperresonance on the affected side and decreased breath sounds may be difficult to appreciate in the neonate. Chest roentgenograms typically demonstrate a radiolucent lobe, mediastinal shift, and contralateral compression. Radiologic differentiation from other cystic lesions may be difficult.

Anatomically, the lobe (or lobes) are voluminous and air-filled, with focal interspersed areas of atelectasis. Routine microscopic examination usually shows normal alveolar septa, and dilated but normal alveoli, with or without areas of focal rupture (emphysema). Interstitial septal thickening with immature collagen has been noted.[4] Cartilaginous and mucosal abnormalities cited previously are mentioned, but in most cases these structures are normal.

Lobectomy is the treatment of choice for symptomatic lobar emphysema.[6,31] If a localized bronchial or peribronchial factor is to be implicated as the cause of the lesion, one should remember that it might have to be left in situ at the time of resection or distorted in such a way that pathologic confirmation is difficult.

PERIPHERAL CYSTS

There remains a group of cysts that are sometimes clearly congenital (having been noted in stillborns and neonates) and may represent a disorder of late pulmonary development, including postnatal development. Such lobes (and sometimes whole lungs) are composed of aggregates of thin-walled, large multilocular cysts of various sizes. The cysts intercommunicate, and often communicate with a parent bronchus. They have no mucous glands and usually have no cartilage, although a few cartilaginous plates may be present. The lining is variable and may be either ciliated or cuboid. The mucosal lining is folded and almost papillary in parts and in other areas is cribriform and reminiscent of abortive alveoli. These cysts have no immature or dysplastic appearing component, and vascular connections are normal. Symptoms arise from the potential for expansion due to air trapping, from rupture with pneumothorax, and from secondary infection.

As most cysts with these anatomic features are not resected until adolescence or later,[35] their nature is open to legitimate and heated debate. Unequivocal inclusion with the developmental cystic lesions is possible in only the small proportion of patients who present as stillborns and neonates. To classify the remainder as developmental anomalies resulting from postnatal derangement of pulmonary growth would be attractive but impossible to substantiate. Histologic criteria (mucosal cell type, cartilage, muscle, elastic tissue, mucous glands, and anthracotic pigmentation) are probably of limited value in proving the nature of such cysts in the adult. Infection is so frequently present that a post-inflammatory cause cannot be excluded. The relationship of this group of peripheral cysts to developmental disorders is confusing and contradictory.

In summary, an attempt has been made to discuss developmental anomalies of the lungs in a sequence relatable to the likely timing of growth disturbance during embryogenesis. Agenesis and aplasia are the earliest disturbances of lung development. The hypoplasias are a heterogeneous group of incomplete lung growth and development. The most dramatic hypoplasias are encountered in diaphragmatic hernia. The morphology of these lungs suggests early restriction of lung growth. The other (symmetric) forms of hypoplasia show considerable variability in severity. Since anatomic data are less complete in the symmetric hypoplasias, speculation as to the nature and timing of an embryonic insult is difficult.

Cystic pulmonary lesions are uncommon, but when encountered, they present tremendous difficulty in classification. I have grouped all sequestrations into a common embryonic group. The term, bronchovascular foregut anomalies (a slight modification of a previously proposed designation, bronchopulmonary-foregut malformation),[21] is introduced as a name for this embryonic group. Perhaps bronchogenic and thoracic enteric cysts can justifiably be appended as formes frustes of this group if anomalous tracheobronchial budding is indeed the mechanism of their formation.

Cystic adenomatoid malformation and infantile lobar emphysema are usually distinctive and separable. Mention has been made of the tantalizing possibility that these entities may represent related but temporally different disorders of intrinsic parenchymal overgrowth (see Figs. 15-5 and 15-6).

Further study and possibly reinterpretation of these lesions are necessary.

REFERENCES

1. Areechon, W. and L. Reid: Hypoplasia of lung with congenital diaphragmatic hernia. *Br. Med. J. 1*:230, 1963.
2. Bailey, J. A.: Jeune's asphyxiating thoracic dystrophy. In *Disproportionate Short Stature.* W. B. Saunders Co., Philadelphia, p. 174, 1973.
3. Belanger, R., L. R. LaFleche and J. L. Picard: Congenital cystic adenomatoid malformation of the lung. *Thorax 19*:1, 1964.
4. Bolande, R. B., A. F. Schneider and J. D. Boggs: Infantile lobar emphysema. *Arch. Pathol. 61*:289, 1956.
5. Boyden, E. A.: The structure of compressed lungs in congenital diaphragmatic hernia. *Am. J. Anat. 134*:497, 1972.
6. Buntain, W. L., H. Isaacs, V. C. Payne, G. G. Lindesmith and J. G. Rosenkrantz: Lobar emphysema, cystic adenomatoid malformation, pulmonary sequestration, and bronchogenic cyst in infancy and childhood: a clinical group. *J. Pediatr. Surg. 9*:85, 1974
7. Butler, L. J., N. E. France, A. Russell and L. Sinclair: A chromosomal aberration association with multiple congenital anomalies. *Lancet 1*:1242, 1962.
8. Carmel, J. A., F. Friedman and F. H. Adams: Fetal tracheal legation and lung development. *Am. J. Dis. Child. 109*:452, 1965.
9. Congenital pulmonary lymphangiectasis. Editorial, *Br. Med. J. 1*:395, 1972.
10. Davidson, W. M. and G. I. M. Ross: Bilateral absence of kidneys and related congenital anomalies. *J. Pathol. Bacteriol. 68*:459, 1954.
11. De, N. C. and J. R. Harper: Renal agenesis and pulmonary hypoplasia. *Br. Med. J. 3*:696, 1972.
12. De Buse, P. J. and G. Morris: Bilateral pulmonary agenesis, oesophageal atresia, and the first arch syndrome. *Thorax 28*:526, 1973.
13. de Lorimer, A. A., D. F. Tierney and H. R. Parker: Hypoplastic lungs in fetal lambs with surgically produced congenital diaphragmatic hernia. *Surgery 62*:12, 1967.
14. Enrile, F. T., L. M. Jourdain and A. Mathur: Con-

genital diffuse bronchio-alveolectasis: a variant of congenital cystic disease of the lung. *Chest 61*:507, 1972.

15. Eraklis, A. J., N. T. Griscom and J. B. McGovern: Bronchogenic cysts of the mediastinum in infancy. *N. Engl. J. Med. 281*:1150, 1969.
16. Esterly, J. and E. Oppenheimer: Lymphangiectasis and other pulmonary lesions in asplenia syndrome. *Arch. Pathol. 90*:553, 1970.
17. Feldman, A. H., R. M. Rhatigan and K. K. Pierson: Pulmonary lymphangiectasia—observation in 17 patients and proposed classification. *Am. J. Roentgenol. Radium Ther. Nucl. Med. 116*:548, 1972.
18. Finegold, M. J., H. Katzew, N. B. Genieser, and M. H. Becker: Lung structure in thoracic dystrophy. *Am. J. Dis. Child. 122*:153, 1971.
19. Flye, M. W. and R. J. Izant: Extralobar pulmonary sequestration with esophageal communication and complete duplication of the colon. *Surgery 71:*:774, 1972.
20. Fox, H. and J. Cocker: Laryngeal atresia. *Arch. Dis. Child. 39*:641, 1964.
21. Gerle, R. D., A. Jaretzki, C. A. Ashley and A. S. Berne: Congenital bronchopulmonary-foregut malformation. *N. Engl. J. Med. 278*:1413, 1968.
22. Hanissian, A. S., W. W. Riggs and D. A. Thomas: Infantile thoracic dystrophy—a variant of Ellis-van Creveld syndrome. *J. Pediatr. 71*:855, 1967.
23. Henderson, R., A. Hislop and L. Reid: New pathological findings in emphysema of childhood: 3. Unilateral congenital emphysema and hypoplasia—and compensatory emphysema of contralateral lung. *Thorax 26*:195, 1971.
24. Herdman, R. C. and L. O. Langer: The thoracic asphyxiant dystrophy and renal disease. *Am. J. Dis. Child. 116*:192, 1968.
25. Hislop, A. and L. Reid: New pathological findings in emphysema of childhood: 1. Polyalveolar lobe with emphysema. *Thorax 25*:682, 1970.
26. Hislop, A. and L. Reid: New pathological findings in emphysema of childhood: 2. Overinflation of a normal lobe. *Thorax 26*:190, 1971.
27. Hislop, A., M. Sanderson and L. Reid: Unilateral congenital dysplasia of lung associated with vascular anomalies. *Thorax 28*:435, 1973.
28. Kent, G. M., P. M. Olley, R. E. Creighton, T. Dobbinson, M. H. Bryan, P. Symchych, W. Zingg and J. H. Cummings: Hemodynamic and pulmonary changes following surgical creation of diaphragmatic hernia in fetal lambs. *Surgery 72*:427, 1972.
29. Kitigawa, M., A. Hislop, E. A. Boyden and L. Reid: Lung hypoplasia in congenital diaphragmatic hernia. *Br. J. Surg. 58*:342, 1971.
30. Kohler, H. G. and B. A. Rymer: Congenital cystic malformation of the lung and its relation to hydramnios. *J. Obstet. Gynaecol. Br. Commonw. 80*:130, 1973.
31. Kruse, R. L. and H. B. Lynn: Lobar emphysema in infants. *Mayo Clin. Proc. 44*:525, 1969.
32. Kwittken, J. and L. Reiner: Congenital cystic adenomatoid malformation of the lung. *Pediatrics 30*:759, 1962.
33. Laurence, K. M.: Congenital pulmonary cystic lymphangiectasis. *J. Pathol. Bacteriol. 70*:325, 1955.
34. Laurence, K. M.: Congenital pulmonary lymphangiectasia. *J. Clin. Pathol., 12*:62, 1959.
35. Lichtenstein, H.: Congenital multiple cysts of the lung. *Thorax 24*:646, 1953.
36. Maltz, D. L. and A. S. Nadas: Agenesis of the lung. Presentation of eight new cases and review of the literature. *Pediatrics 42*:175, 1968.
37. Marks, C., S. N. Wiener and M. Raydman: Pulmonary sequestration. *Chest 61*:255, 1972.
38. Mauer, S. M., R. S. Dobrin and R. L. Vernier: Unilateral and bilateral renal agenesis in monoamniotic twins. *J. Pediatr. 84*:236, 1974.
39. Morris, J. J., F. O. Black and H. E. Stephenson: The fate of the unexpanded lung in congenital diaphragmatic hernia. *Dis. Chest 48*:649, 1965.
40. Noonan, J., L. R. Walters and J. T. Reeves: Congenital pulmonary lymphangiectasia. *Am. J. Dis. Child. 120*:314, 1970.
41. Oyamada, A., B. M. Gasul and P. H. Hollinger: Agenesis of the lung. Report of a case and review of all previously recorded cases. *Am. J. Dis. Child. 85*:182, 1953.
42. Pena, S. D. J. and M. H. K. Shokeir: Syndrome of camptodactyly, multiple ankyloses, facial anomalies, and pulmonary hypoplasia: a lethal condition. *J. Pediatr. 85*:373, 1974.
43. Perlman, M. and M. Levin: Fetal pulmonary hypoplasia, anuria and oligohydramnios. *Am. J. Obstet. Gynecol. 118*:1119, 1974.
44. Pirnar, T. and E. B. D. Neuhauser: Asphyxiating thoracic dystrophy. *Am. J. Roentgenol. 98*:358, 1966.
45. Potter E. L.: Bilateral renal agenesis. *J. Pediatr. 29*:68, 1946.
46. Potter, E.: Oligohydramnios, further comment. *J. Pediatr. 84*:931, 1974.
47. Punnett, H. H., M. L. Kistenmacher, M. Valdes-Dapena and R. T. Ellison: Syndrome of ankylosis, facial anomalies and pulmonary hypoplasia. *J. Pediatr. 85*:375, 1974.
48. Raphaely, R. C. and J. J. Downes: Congenital diaphragmatic hernia—prediction of survival. *J. Pediatr. Surg. 8*:815, 1973.
49. Reale, F. R. and J. R. Esterly: Pulmonary hypoplasias: a morphometric study of the lungs of infants with diaphragmatic hernia, anencephaly, and renal malformations. *Pediatrics 51*:91, 1973.
50. Ryland, D. and L. Reid: Pulmonary aplasia—a

quantitative analysis of the development of the single lung. *Thorax 26*:602, 1971.

51. Seeds, A. E. Jr.: Water metabolism of the fetus. *Am. J. Obstet. Gynecol. 92*:727, 1965.
52. Spencer, H.: *Pathology of the Lung* (2nd ed.). Pergamon Press, Elmsford, N.Y., p. 81, 1968.
53. Symchych, P. S.: Unpublished observations, tracheal atresia with no fistula.

53a. Symchych, P. S. and P. W. Winchester: Animal model: amniotic fluid deficiency and fetal lung growth in the rat. *Am. J. Pathol. 90*:779, 1978.

54. Tilson, M. D. and R. J. Toulokian: Mediastinal enteric sequestration with aberrant pancreas. *Ann. Surg. 176.*:669, 1972.
55. Thomas, I. T. and D. W. Smith: Oligohydramnios, cause of the nonrenal features of Potter's syndrome. *J. Pediatr. 84*:811, 1974.
56. van Dijk, C. and C. A. Wagenvoort: The various types of congenital adenomatoid malformation of the lung. *J. Pathol. 110*:131, 1973.
57. Voorhees, M. L., T. Vahard and L. I. Gardner: Trisomy 16-18 syndrome. *Lancet 2*:992, 1962.
58. Waldman, T. A.: Intestinal lymphangiectasia. In *Birth Defects, Atlas and Compendium,* D. Bergsma, (Ed.). The National Foundation-March of Dimes, The Williams & Wilkins Co., Baltimore, 1973.
59. Warkany, J.: *Congenital Malformations.* Year Book Medical Publishers, Chicago, p. 604, 1971.
60. Wilson, J. G. and J. Warkany: Aortic arch and cardiac anomalies in the offspring of vitamin A deficient rats. *Am. J. Anat. 85*:115, 1949.

Respiratory Distress Syndromes of the Newborn

PETER A. M. AULD

16

The major causes of morbidity and mortality in the immediate newborn period are conditions in which the initial manifestation is respiratory distress. As used in this book, the term, respiratory distress, includes tachypnea, cyanosis, apnea, and subcostal retractions as the presenting sign or signs. Various disease entities or congenital malformations may underlie these presenting signs so that a wide variety of clinical and diagnostic techniques may be necessary to identify the specific problem. Frequently a specific disease entity cannot be identified precisely, but by excluding conditions for which curative (usually surgical) therapy is available, the remainder, which fall under the broad category of medical respiratory distress syndromes, can be managed using the basic principles of supportive therapy. In the latter situations, appropriate supportive care can be provided only if the physician has a thorough understanding of the pathophysiologic processes. For these reasons, this chapter attempts to provide an approach to the patient with respiratory distress (including emergency management), as well as a detailed discussion of diagnosis, pathophysiology, and treatment of the various disease entities. Emergency care is included as a separate section which, it is hoped, will help those practicing in community hospitals who will subsequently transfer patients to a tertiary center.

Part I: *Approach to the Newborn Infant with Cardiorespiratory Disease*

The physician or other health professional charged with the care of newborn infants first must diagnose whether the infant has respiratory distress. Having determined that respiratory distress is present, a cause must be sought immediately, excluding first those conditions for which definitive treatment exists. Every hospital must develop a strategy for ensuring that the distressed infant is recognized and treated immediately. This strategy involves having personnel on-site who can diagnose and treat neonatal emergencies. In community hospitals the pediatrician may not be available for emergency care so that these prerogatives must be delegated to other trained personnel until he arrives. Failure to develop an efficient "hospital strategy" may cause distressed infants to deteriorate irretrievably.

Diagnosis of Cardiorespiratory Distress in the Newborn

The infant with cardiorespiratory distress is easily identified because of *tachypnea* and *cyanosis*. A respiratory rate greater than 40 breaths/min. after the first hour of life is regarded as tachypnea. Frequently, cyanosis is masked by extreme pallor due to the presence of shock. A normal baby in the first few hours after birth is lobster pink. *Subcostal retractions* are frequently present in infants with cardiorespiratory distress. An *expiratory grunt* is abnormal. *Apnea* is also a sign of respiratory distress although its significance is often different from the other signs mentioned. An infant with any or all of these signs should be regarded as having cardiorespiratory distress and immediate systematic efforts begun to diagnose and treat the cause.

FETAL AND MATERNAL FACTORS

Often hints in the maternal history can alert the physician to the possible cause of the respiratory distress.

The presence of diabetes mellitus, either prenatal or gestational, may suggest a major congenital abnormality of the heart as a cause for respiratory distress. Infants of diabetic mothers are reported to be at increased risk to develop hyaline membrane disease (HMD). However, the literature is somewhat confusing in terms of whether the presumed susceptibility of these infants is related to maternal diabetes mellitus or to current programs of obstetric management. Early delivery of infants of diabetic mothers was the general rule in the past and is still indicated in some circumstances. However, the induced delivery of a very large but immature infant may explain the conjecture that maternal diabetes predisposes to HMD. A recent retrospective analysis of 805 diabetic pregnancies and 10,152 nondiabetic pregnancies from the Boston Hospital for Women showed the relative risk for HMD to be 23.7 times greater in the diabetic woman and, when factors such as gestational age are removed, 5.6 times more likely.[117] Because of the problems of accurately dating diabetic pregnancies, it is likely that a prospective study will be needed to determine whether the infant of a diabetic mother is at increased risk to develop HMD.

An infant born of a mother with renal disease, hypertension, or toxemia of pregnancy may have intrauterine growth retardation due to relative placental insufficiency. These infants are at risk for fetal distress during labor, and respiratory difficulty may occur due to meconium aspiration. When these conditions are diagnosed, the maternal-fetal unit must be monitored by techniques such as ultrasound and by determination of estriols and human placental lactogen (HPL) concentrations.

Accurate knowledge of gestational age is important in determining whether the low birth weight infant is either premature or small for gestational age. Frequently, only a detailed physical examination can be relied on to distinguish between the two. Premature infants have a high incidence of HMD, and small-for-dates infants may have respiratory distress from meconium aspiration. Unfortunately, it is very common that an infant is delivered by repeat elective cesarean section, is presumed to be at term, but actually is premature and proceeds to develop HMD. This confusion should no longer exist because, by the use of amniocentesis and examination of the fluid by either L/S ratio or foam test, lung maturity can be determined in cases where the gestational age is not accurately known. On the other hand, the postmature infant may suffer fetal distress during labor because of placental insufficiency and may then develop respiratory distress due to meconium aspiration.

When maternal polyhydramnios exists, the infant may be suffering from atresia of the upper gastrointestinal tract. In this case aspiration of contents of the atretic segment by the infant may cause respiratory distress.

Maternal infection with rubella during pregnancy may produce an infant with congenital heart disease and respiratory distress due to heart failure. If the mother is known to be colonized with β hemolytic streptococcus group B in her vagina or uterus, respiratory distress may be due to streptococcal pneumonia.

Certain events during labor and delivery may provide a clue to the cause of respiratory distress. Thus a difficult labor associated with fetal distress may result in meconium aspiration and its complications, pneumothorax and pneumomediastinum. Respiratory distress associated with prolonged rupture of membranes should suggest the possibility of pneumonia and sepsis. Instrumentation during resuscitation may be traumatic and result in tracheal perforation and respiratory distress due to pneumothorax or pneumomediastinum.

Infants delivered by cesarean section or who deliver precipitously may have transient tachypnea of the newborn, thought to be associated with insufficient removal of pulmonary fluid. These infants lack the "chest squeeze" provided by uterine contractions, which play a role in removing this fluid during vaginal delivery. Considerable discussion still revolves around the relationship between a cesarean section and the development of HMD. Does the section itself predispose to the disease, or is it the indication for section (e.g., placenta previa, abruptio placentae)? As infants are rarely delivered prematurely by cesarean section without cause (unless gestational age is misdiagnosed in an elective section), it would seem that any relationship between the operation and development of HMD is related to the indication for which the section is required. A contrary conclusion has been reached by Usher and co-workers.[136]

During labor and delivery excessive maternal analgesia and anesthesia are still factors in producing respiratory depression. Knowledge of the dose and time of administration of these drugs in relation to delivery must be available to determine whether respiratory distress is due to these causes.

If the physician has considered all these factors in the maternal and fetal history, the cause of respiratory distress is often obvious before detailed diagnostic studies are undertaken.

NEONATAL HISTORY

As has been emphasized, maternal and fetal history prior to birth can be very useful in arriving at a specific diagnosis. Of greatest value is historic information relating to the time of onset of respiratory distress and the condition of the infant at birth. A premature infant with severe perinatal asphyxia is more likely to have HMD than one without asphyxia. Thus information about the presence of intrauterine asphyxia as well as determination of condition at birth by Apgar score can be useful. Premature infants with respiratory distress due to HMD are most often diagnosed before they leave the delivery room, as evidenced by grunting, retractions, and cyanosis. It is most unusual for HMD to present after 2 to 3 hours of age in a well-observed infant. On the other hand, infants with meconium aspiration may not develop respiratory distress for many hours after birth. Similarly, infants with severe congenital heart disease may be well for many hours after birth and then suddenly develop severe cardiorespiratory difficulty. Severe progressive respiratory distress that is unresponsive to any therapeutic measures should suggest neonatal pneumonia and sepsis. Respiratory distress developing in small premature infants after 3 to 4 days suggests chronic pulmonary insufficiency (CPIP) or sepsis. Increasing respiratory distress in an infant in stable condition with HMD may signify the development of congestive heart failure due to patent ductus arteriosus.

Cyanosis that occurs only with crying in an infant with respiratory distress is more often due to congenital heart disease than to a pulmonary problem.

PHYSICAL EXAMINATION

Observation is the most important part of the examination of the infant with cardiorespiratory distress. The distressed infant is easy to recognize because of tachypnea or apnea, suprasternal or subcostal retractions, cyanosis or pallor, and expiratory grunting.

Full-term and premature infants without distress have a prominent chest cage, which decreases in size over the subsequent several days. This appearance is due to pulmonary gas trapping, a normal event in the adaptation to extrauterine life. In the premature infant with HMD the chest may initially appear of normal size, but as the condition worsens, the chest appears to collapse, most conspicuously in the axilla. This picture is most apparent after the second day of life. Collapse of the chest reflects the progressive alveolar collapse in a patient with a highly compliant chest wall. Infants who have aspirated meconium or who have transient tachypnea of the newborn have a barrel-chested appearance reflecting the underlying hyperaeration. When the chest appears overinflated, both intercostal muscle and diaphragmatic activity are obvious during breathing, whereas when chest volume is small, the breathing appears to be almost entirely abdominal.

Acrocyanosis, while often seen in the first several days in infants who are otherwise normal, is also present as an early sign of cardiorespiratory difficulty. Acrocyanosis is most likely a compensatory circulatory adjustment, and as it is not a universal finding in normal newborn infants, it must develop in response to some unrecognized insult.

Subcostal and substernal retractions are much more noticeable in infants with a collapsed chest and atelectasis than in the barrel-chested patient. This latter group of infants, while not showing retractions, have tachypnea, frequently with respiratory rates over 100 per minute, in contrast to the slower rate in infants with alveolar collapse. In observing the infant, the presence of excessive secretions should suggest esophageal atresia and tracheoesophageal fistula. A scaphoid abdomen indicates diaphragmatic hernia. Severe distress relieved by an oral airway may indicate imperforate nares. Meconium staining of the skin, cord, and nares should raise concerns about meconium aspiration pneumonitis. When respiratory distress is present together with signs of postmaturity, such as loss of subcutaneous tissue (baggy pants appearance), long fingernails, and parchment skin, meconium aspiration may be the cause. Similar considerations should exist in the presence of intrauterine growth retardation. With these factors in mind, every low birth weight infant should have a physical examination to assess gestational age.

Infants who appear edematous may have hydrops fetalis. A peculiar facial appearance suggestive of the trisomic syndrome points to congenital heart disease as the cause of the respiratory difficulty. Potter's syndrome (renal agenesis) frequently demonstrates profound respiratory distress due to pulmonary hypoplasia and a tendency to develop spontaneous pneumothorax (Fig. 16-1).

Clinical-Physiologic Correlates. Tachypnea and/or apnea are generally the first indications that cardiorespiratory difficulty is present in the newborn. Tachypnea results from low Pa_{O_2} and decreased lung compliance with the requirement for increased work of breathing. Tachypnea is more prominent in full-term or larger premature infants (over 1200 g). Very immature infants (less than 1200 g) with severe respiratory embarrassment are more likely to show apnea than tachypnea in response to pulmonary disease.

Apnea may be central in origin due to poor respiratory drive or peripheral, arising in the lungs, in which case mechanical deficiencies (low compliance and low functional residual capacity (FRC)) make it too difficult to breathe. Whether one or both factors are operating in any given case is difficult to determine. Causes suggested for apnea of the premature include hypoxemia, neurologic immaturity, altered sensitivity of central or peripheral chemoreceptors to O_2 or CO_2, or pulmonary insufficiency. Whatever the cause, apnea is most common in the more immature infants and occurs in them progressively more frequently in the first 2 weeks after birth. It is important to recognize that apnea is a common accompaniment of HMD, but that it is also frequently noted in sepsis, intracranial hemorrhage, and metabolic disturbance such as hypoglycemia. The latter conditions must be excluded before concluding that the response is the apnea of prematurity.

Subcostal retractions are prominent in infants with respiratory distress, particularly the premature infant. They occur as a result of collapse of the compliant chest wall as the infant attempts to generate high intrathoracic pressures in response to very low lung compliance. Full-term infants with meconium aspiration are less likely to demonstrate retractions because of underlying emphysema.

The expiratory grunt is a common feature of respiratory distress and generally occurs early in the clinical course of the disease, disappearing as the condition worsens. The expiratory grunt is an accompaniment of respiratory distress in larger infants and generally is absent in those who are very small. Several suggestions have been advanced to explain the expiratory grunt. Some workers have noted that the grunt disappears following endotracheal intubation, suggesting that the sounds occur during expiration to overcome a closed glottis.[64] These same authors noted that Pa_{O_2} fell when intubation was performed and the grunt was abolished, suggesting that the phenomenon served a function of maintaining FRC and secondarily sustaining Pa_{O_2}. Another theory relates the grunt to airway closure. This explanation recognizes that the high intrathoracic pressure of the distressed infant is transmitted to the very compliant smaller airways, causing airway collapse especially at low FRC. The grunt may be an attempt to overcome the effect of high intrathoracic pressure. Whatever the cause, the grunt while present serves a protective function and is the infant's attempt to maintain FRC and Pa_{O_2}.

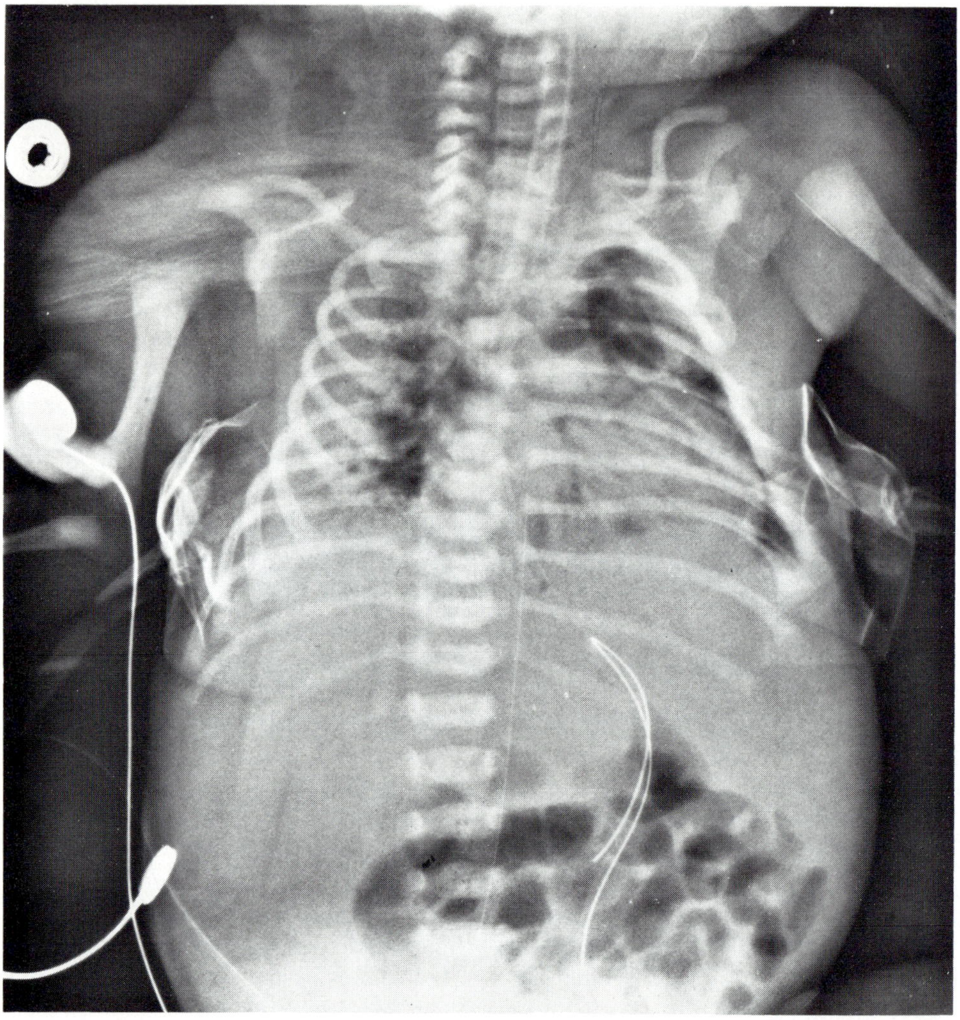

FIG. 16-1. Chest roentgenogram of an infant with Potter's syndrome (renal agenesis). Bilateral pneumothoraces are treated with indwelling catheters. Only a residual pneumomediastinum exists. Note continued collapse of the chest wall suggesting underlying hypoplasia of the lungs. The infant's condition was not improved by treatment of the pneumothorax.

Generally the cyanosis of the distressed newborn is the result of right-to-left shunting in either the heart (congenital heart disease) or lungs (respiratory distress syndrome). Attempts to relate cyanosis (low Pa_{O_2}) to diffusion barrier or maldistribution of ventilation have indicated that these physiologic abnormalities are rarely a major factor. A diffusion barrier may exist in the most severely ill infant with HMD. Maldistribution of ventilation has been noted in meconium aspiration and is claimed to exist to a degree in HMD as well.

The administration of high concentrations of oxygen (FI_{O_2} 1.00) for a short period of time can frequently be of great use in determining the extent of the right-to-left shunt (see also Chapter 2). Especially in the early stages of HMD, high oxygen breathing may remove cyanosis and significantly increase Pa_{O_2}, whereas in cyanotic congenital heart disease, cyanosis and Pa_{O_2} will not be substantially improved. This lack of improvement results from the relative size of the shunts, which, when expressed in terms of percent of cardiac output, at least at the outset, is smaller in HMD than in congenital heart disease.

Acrocyanosis must be distinguished from central cyanosis. Acrocyanosis is limited to the hands, feet, and perioral areas. It is related to peripheral vascular responses and as such is less significant than central cyanosis. Attempts should nevertheless be made to determine whether a pathologic process exists or has existed before considering acrocyanosis "normal."

Cyanosis is frequently masked by pallor in the distressed newborn. Pallor may indicate the presence of shock, and it should be excluded by appropriate measurement of blood pressure. Pallor also may reflect that the infant is under stress and has redistributed blood flow away from the skin to more vital organs. This change may occur in response to a difficult delivery or acidemia.

Palpation and Auscultation of the Chest. Palpation of the chest is most useful when the physician is attempting to determine the significance of a cardiac murmur in association with respiratory distress. Hyperactivity of the precordium particularly over the sternum suggests significant cardiac overload. Occasionally, a thrill can be palpated in cases of pulmonic stenosis or ventricular septal defect. Palpation of femoral and radial pulses is part of the physical examination, and pulses are poorly felt when shock is present. Infants with hypoplastic left heart syndrome have poor peripheral pulses. Bounding pulses suggest the presence of a patent ductus arteriosus. Frequently a shift in the point of maximal impulse (PMI) of the heart may be detected when mediastinal shift occurs secondary to atelectasis or pneumothorax.

Auscultation of the chest is seldom as rewarding in an infant with respiratory distress as in an older child. Bowel sounds in the chest signify diaphragmatic hernia. Breath sounds are widely transmitted and thus cannot be relied on to identify a pathologic state. In general breath sounds are decreased or absent in conditions associated with significant alveolar collapse. Differences in breath sounds from one side of the chest to the other suggest pneumothorax or diaphragmatic hernia. Rales and rhonchi are heard when a pneumonic process is present. Because of the difficulties of auscultation of the chest in the newborn, the physician must rely on chest roentgenograms to determine pulmonary status.

Examination of the heart by auscultation on the other hand is extremely important and useful. Infants may have respiratory distress as a result of a primary cardiac abnormality, or certain cardiac lesions may complicate the pulmonary problems so that the detection of murmurs is important in differential diagnosis.

Patent ductus arteriosus (PDA) may be a normal finding in full-term infants in the first 48 hours of life and is frequently present in premature infants for a week or two after birth. In these instances the condition may be recognized by only a short ejection murmur maximal along the left sternal border. In otherwise non-distressed premature infants, a continuous machinery murmur may be present. It may be difficult to determine whether a previously heard systolic murmur along the left sternal border was due to a PDA or a closed ventricular septal defect. Failure to hear the classic machinery murmur of the PDA reflects the fact that the pulmonary vascular resistance is still elevated. PDA is a frequent accompaniment of HMD, generally becoming significant when the pulmonary problem is abating. Congestive heart failure may result from this lesion, and if not recognized and treated, it can complicate management of the pulmonary condition. Thus, it is important to understand that a cardiac murmur in the presence of respiratory distress does not necessarily mean that a structural congenital heart defect exists, but rather that a significant complicating factor may have been added.

Sometimes when pneumomediastinum or pericardial effusion are present, a diagnosis can be made by noting distant heart sounds. Percussion of the chest of the newborn is not useful and is best not performed. Heart sounds may be heard in an abnormal position in the presence of mediastinal shift due to atelectasis or pneumothorax.

INITIAL LABORATORY EVALUATIONS

The following laboratory studies must be performed as soon as it is recognized that the infant has respiratory distress. The studies are done both to help in diagnosis and to determine whether supportive care is indicated.

Chest Roentgenogram. Because of the limitations of physical examination previously mentioned, chest roentgenograms in the anteroposterior and lateral projections should be obtained immediately on any infant with respiratory distress. The chest roentgenograms can diagnose or exclude conditions that require urgent surgical attention, such as an emphysematous lobe, diaphragmatic hernia, or tension pneumothorax. The inexperienced physician must be careful not to overinterpret the chest roentgenogram of infants. Streaks and densities that in the older child may indicate pneumonia may in the infant signify atelectasis, blood vessels, or lymphatics and may possibly be of little significance.

The chest film of the normal newborn or non-distressed premature infant appears overaerated with multiple streaks. A repeat film in several days may show that these characteristics have disappeared. These changes are thought to parallel the disappearance of intrapulmonary gas trapping. Portable chest roentgenograms taken by an experienced technician are usually adequate for most purposes.

Several types of neonatal respiratory distress have specific patterns on chest roentgenogram. In HMD, for example, the typical picture is a reticulogranular pattern and air bronchograms in the lung parenchyma. This picture reflects the underlying pathology of atelectasis and, when contrasted with the air-filled bronchi, allows them to stand out. It is important to recognize that the typical picture of HMD may not be present in the early stages of the disease, but develops only as the atelectasis becomes progressively more severe over the first 24 hours. It is possible to have an infant with a typical clinical picture who never develops a classic roentgenographic appearance.

Physicians have a tendency to perform repeated chest roentgenograms in order to eventually achieve a typical roentgenographic pattern of HMD. This approach should be avoided. When it is determined initially that a surgical emergency does not exist, repeat chest roentgenograms should be performed only when there is a clinical change (e.g., sudden or progressive increase in O_2 requirement, shock).

Infants with meconium aspiration syndrome show a pattern of hyperaeration and coarse parenchymal streaks on chest roentgenograms. These changes may not be present right after birth and may take 12 to 24 hours to become fully developed. Cardiomegaly is frequently present as well, adding confusion to the diagnostic efforts. Transient tachypnea of the newborn has a typical chest roentgenographic picture, at least in retrospect, characterized by overaeration of the lung parenchyma, thickening of fissures, an apparent blunting of the right costovertebral angle, and increased hilar markings. The changes, however, are not specific and may be confused with meconium aspiration or overcirculation of the lungs.

Assessment of heart size and pulmonary vasculature is an important part of the chest roentgenographic examination. While cardiomegaly generally implies a congenital heart lesion, it may be present as well in infants with meconium aspiration or birth asphyxia and in infants of diabetic mothers. On the other hand, lack of cardiomegaly does not exclude a congenital heart lesion, total anomalous pulmonary venous drainage being a case in point. Assessment of pulmonary vasculature with respect to overcirculation or venous congestion is difficult and confusing in the newborn because of the common presence of atelectatic streaks. In instances where cardiac disease cannot be excluded, an ECG is mandatory.

Acid-Base and Blood Gas Determinations. A determination of pH, Pa_{O_2} and Pa_{CO_2} is essential in evaluating an infant with respiratory distress. These measurements should be made as soon as the infant is noted to be in distress in order to determine the effectiveness with which the infant is compensating for the abnormality, and to act as a guide to therapy. This initial assessment is best obtained from a peripheral artery such as the temporal, radial, or brachial. If arterial blood is unavailable for technical reasons, free-flowing venous blood must be used to determine pH and P_{CO_2}. Blood from free-flowing venous and arterial samples has a similar pH and P_{CO_2} (except in shock) so that this method does not represent a significant compromise. In this instance, oxygenation must be assessed by observation, and regulation of increased oxygen requirements is determined by color.

If repeated blood gas evaluation seems likely, consideration must be given to the placement of an umbilical artery catheter or an indwelling peripheral arterial needle.

Blood Pressure. Infants in respiratory distress should have determination of blood pressure as part of the initial evaluation. This determination can be accomplished by noninvasive technique using the Doppler principle (Arteriosonde) or by a pressure transducer and umbilical artery catheter. Shock is indicated clinically by pallor and poor capillary filling.

Other Laboratory Tests. An hematocrit is an essential part of the initial care of the infant with respiratory distress. Blood loss due to intracranial hemorrhage or intrapartum bleeding may be sufficient to produce shock. Blood sugar and serum electrolytes should be measured as soon as the infant is stable enough for further tests.

In certain instances more extensive diagnostic studies are indicated. These should be carried out only after the preceding tests have been performed. A barium swallow may be required to rule out a vascular ring. If tracheoesophageal fistula is suspected, barium solution should be put into the blind pouch to confirm the diagnosis. Direct laryngoscopy may be required to determine the presence of tracheal occlusion due to webs or tumors. Respiratory distress relieved by an oral airway or worsened by feeding is an indication to determine patency of the nares.

Emergency Care

Each obstetric-pediatric service must have a well-defined approach to emergency care for the distressed newborn infant. Each hospital must clearly establish who will be responsible for initiating emergency care and what techniques are to be used. This plan requires the designation of persons on-site around the clock to deliver this care. Private physicians are not always in attendance when the emergency is recognized so that the medical board of each hospital must provide personnel with the ability and authority to begin emergency care.

The following approach is suggested.

(1) *Ensure a clear airway.* Blockage of

the upper airway is a very rare cause of respiratory distress in the newborn infant. However, it is imperative to ensure a clear airway by gentle suction of any secretions from the nose and mouth. Rule out imperforate nares at this time. Mucous plugs are an unlikely initial cause of respiratory distress in the newborn, although they are common when an endotracheal tube has been in place for several days.

(2) *Administer oxygen.* Oxygen should be administered in sufficient concentration to abolish central cyanosis, and the concentration recorded. When the condition of the infant is stabilized, it is essential to provide oxygen therapy based on the Pa_{O_2}. Certainly prolonged oxygen administration (over 4 hours) requires that the dosage be administered on the basis of monitored parameters to maintain Pa_{O_2} between 50 and 70 mm Hg. This recommendation recognizes that no completely acceptable method exists for monitoring blood oxygen. Indwelling arterial catheters have their hazards and cannot be used indiscriminately by untrained personnel. In these situations it is best to adjust the infant's oxygen to abolish cyanosis and arrange for early referral to an intensive care unit. Noninvasive methods of oxygen monitoring currently being developed may be useful in the future. However, as distressed infants frequently have impaired peripheral blood flow, these methods may not be completely acceptable in the very ill infant.

(3) *Assist ventilation.* This practice is necessary in the emergency care of the distressed infant. It is indicated for sustained apnea, respiratory acidemia, and hypoxemia uncorrected by high O_2 administration. Because of the low compliance of the lungs in infants with respiratory distress, the method used to provide emergency assisted ventilation must be capable of administering high pressures. Initially, assisted ventilation should be applied with an anesthesia bag and mask (Fig. 16-2). If valves are present, they must allow for administration of high pressures, but unfortunately most commercially available systems do not offer this capability. If oxygenation and respiratory acidemia are not corrected by this form of assisted ventilation, endotracheal intubation and a mechanical respirator may be necessary. If endotracheal intubation is necessary, assisted ventilation must be provided with a bag equipped with a valve or a respirator.

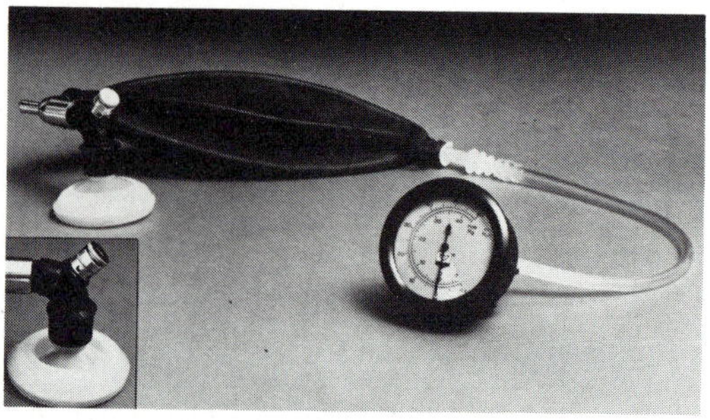

FIG. 16-2. Anesthesia bag and mask with Rovenstine angle. A pressure gauge is attached for use when giving constant distending airway pressure. When using this system, a high liter flow (15 liters/min.) is necessary to keep the bag inflated and allow escape of gas at the mouth to avoid accumulation of CO_2. A tube must be placed in the stomach for decompression as well. Bleeder valve should be used when the system is connected to an endotracheal tube.

When pulmonary disease is present and impaired oxygenation is the major problem without respiratory acidemia, constant distending airway pressure (CDAP) may be used to improve oxygenation at lower inspired oxygen concentrations. CDAP is capable of improving oxygenation and at a lower FI_{O_2}, thus reducing the risk of pulmonary oxygen toxicity. CDAP should be considered when an FI_{O_2} greater than 0.60 is required to maintain a Pa_{O_2} of 50 mm Hg. Although CDAP can be administered by a number of methods, in the emergency situation a simple anesthesia bag and mask (without valves) with an attached pressure measuring device is adequate (see Fig. 16-2). Positive airway pressures greater than 5 cm H_2O should be avoided because of the danger of alveolar rupture and pneumothorax. Use of CDAP may not be indicated when respiratory acidemia is present. (For detailed discussion see page 479.)

(4) *Correct acid-base disturbances.* Assisted ventilation is the therapy of choice for respiratory acidemia. When both respiratory and metabolic acidosis exists, begin ventilation and correct the respiratory component first, repeat blood gases, and then correct the residual metabolic component. When metabolic acidemia is present, the physician must determine whether it is due to lactic acid accumulation as a result of shock, impending shock, or hypoxemia. Metabolic acidemia secondary to shock must be corrected by appropriate therapy for shock. Attempts to correct hypoxemia by increasing FI_{O_2} may improve metabolic acidemia due to this cause. Frequently, metabolic acidemia persists even after attention to these details in which case sodium bicarbonate may be useful.

Sodium bicarbonate should be administered by dilution of a 7.5% solution at a dosage based on the calculated bicarbonate deficit obtained by the Siggaard-Andersen nomogram from measurements of pH and PCO_2. To calculate sodium bicarbonate dosage, measure the pH and PCO_2 in the blood and determine HCO_3^- from the nomogram. Then from the nomogram determine the HCO_3^- that would be present at pH 7.35 using the previously measured PCO_2. The difference between the two values is the HCO_3^- deficit in mEq/1. The infant's bicarbonate space is assumed to be 0.6 × total body weight. Then $0.6 \times HCO_3^-$ deficit × body weight = total body HCO_3^- deficit. Initially, give half of the calculated bicarbonate deficit intravenously. Repeat blood gas determinations are necessary in 15 to 20 minutes to determine the need for further therapy. If metabolic acidemia persists, give the other half of the calculated dose. When possible, sodium bicarbonate should be diluted in an equal volume and administered over 5 to 10 minutes to minimize complications that occur as a result of an acute increase in serum osmolarity.

(5) *Treat shock.* The diagnosis of shock is complicated by the lack of well-recognized standards for blood pressure in infants of different gestational ages. The normal blood pressure of full-term infants is higher than the blood pressure of a non-distressed small premature infant. In the emergency situation, infants frequently look "shocky." They are very pale, ashen, and underperfused, and capillary filling is poor. In this case plasminate (10 cc/kg) or blood, if available, should be administered. Shock may be due to blood loss from an intrapartum event or intracranial hemorrhage, while at other times no obvious bleeding has occurred. In the latter instances shock appears to be related to poor autonomic control because of immaturity, hypoxemia, and acidemia.

(6) *Administer fluid therapy.* In the emergency situation, fluid, calories, and electrolyte therapy can be most important. An intravenous infusion of 5% glucose and water should be provided in order to treat hypoglycemia as well as to provide for the increased glucose needs of the hypoxic infant. Infants in distress frequently have renal disturbances secondary to shock and hypoxemia, and glycosuria may occur even when blood sugar levels are normal. This condition may result in increased loss of fluid and electrolyte because of the osmotic effects of the glycosuria. For this reason 5% glucose only is recommended until it can be established that glycosuria is absent and 10% glucose can be tolerated.

Differentiation of Pulmonary and Cardiac Disease

The physician is frequently required to determine whether the infant is suffering from a primary pulmonary condition for which supportive care may suffice or whether a congenital cardiac condition exists for which definitive therapy, including cardiac catheterization and operation, is required.

This problem occurs more commonly in the full-term infant than in the premature one. Cyanotic congenital heart lesions such as transposition of great vessels, total anomalous pulmonary venous drainage, hypoplastic left heart syndrome, and pulmonary atresia can sometimes be confused with pulmonary disorders, particularly HMD and meconium aspiration. *Some differential points are:*

(1) The infant with cyanotic congenital heart disease often has a greyish blue pallor due to poor peripheral perfusion from the outset, which is only a late finding in pulmonary disorders.

(2) Palpation of the precordium may reveal hyperactivity of the heart in cyanotic congenital heart disease.

(3) The breath sounds are generally decreased or absent in infants with HMD, whereas in heart disease they are well transmitted.

(4) Peripheral pulses may be poorly felt in congenital heart disease from the outset.

The physical examination may provide points of confusion in that infants with heart disease may not have murmurs and the hepatomegaly of congestive heart failure may be difficult to distinguish from the liver pushed down as a result of emphysema.

The chest roentgenogram and laboratory studies frequently aid in the differential diagnosis. In the early stages administration of oxygen to the infant with pulmonary disease improves color and raises Pa_{O_2}, whereas no improvement is seen in infants with cyanotic congenital heart disease. An elevated Pa_{CO_2} indicates respiratory failure, whereas respiratory alkalemia with low Pa_{CO_2} occurs frequently in heart disease (it also occurs sometimes in meconium aspiration). A severe uncorrectable metabolic acidemia is often due to poor cardiac output secondary to a severe congenital heart disease.

Whereas cardiomegaly may be an accompaniment of both congenital heart lesions and meconium aspiration, more detailed examination by cardiac series may distinguish specific chamber enlargements in the former whereas the overall cardiomegaly is the rule in the latter. ECG examination and echocardiography can be of great value in determining the existence of and type of cardiac condition.

Emergency Care in Special Circumstances

When *pneumothorax* is present, the physician must judge whether it is contributing to the morbidity of the patient. Tension pneumothorax sufficient to produce mediastinal shift results in shock and hypoxemia, and is an emergency. The air must be evacuated immediately with a syringe connected to a needle and stopcock or intracatheter inserted in the chest and connected to underwater-seal drainage. Lesser degrees of pneumothorax can be compensated for with oxygen; those that produce no signs should be observed closely.

When respiratory failure secondary to a *diaphragmatic hernia* is diagnosed, infants must be treated by endotracheal intubation. In addition, a tube should be placed in the stomach for decompression. These infants should not be ventilated with bag and mask because gas will fill the stomach and herniated intestine, thereby further compromising respiratory function.

Esophageal atresia commonly is associated with *tracheoesophageal fistula.* Aspiration of the contents into the lung can produce severe chemical pneumonitis, which can delay definitive surgical procedure. Emergency care requires that the blind pouch not be allowed to accumulate secretions, so constant suction should be applied to a soft rubber catheter placed in the pouch.

Cardiopulmonary Physiology in Non-distressed Infants

An extensive description of neonatal cardiopulmonary adaptation to extrauterine life has been presented in the companion volume to this text.[121A] However, as the approach to neonatal respiratory distress to be outlined next is essentially a physiologic one, a brief review of the main points is provided.

ADAPTATION TO EXTRAUTERINE LIFE (FULL-TERM INFANT)

Adaptation to extrauterine life with respect to pulmonary function requires the exchange of a liquid-filled lung for an air-filled lung and appropriate adjustment of ventilation and perfusion to ensure regulation of blood gases. Liquid within the fetal lung is produced by the lung itself and is generally not contaminated with amniotic fluid. During vaginal delivery a considerable portion of this liquid is expelled by the force of uterine contractions squeezing on the infant's chest. Liquid not removed by this mechanism is removed by absorption into lung lymphatics and circulation after birth.

Gas Trapping. During the period in which lung liquid is present, gas trapping occurs in the newborn lung.[89] This phenomenon gives the prominent chest wall appearance normally seen at birth but resolved in several days. It is presumed that air is trapped in alveoli and bronchioles distal to the liquid and in bubbles in the liquid itself.

Establishment of Functional Residual Capacity (FRC). FRC is rapidly established soon after birth, with little change in the first week. This pattern is in contradistinction to that for thoracic gas volume (TGV), which is much increased at birth and decreases to approach FRC in 2 to 4 days. The difference between these two volumes is a measure of trapped gas. In the full-term infant, FRC averages 1.3 ml/cm in the first week of life, and TGV is 2.0 ml/cm on day 1 and 1.5 ml/cm on day 9. Lung compliance averages 4.9 ml/cm H_2O, and specific compliance is 0.04 to 0.06 ml/cm H_2O/ml. Total pulmonary resistance in the full-term newborn is high, averaging 34.1 cm H_2O/l/min. in one study.[114] The major portion of the resistance is in the airways particularly at the nose.

Ventilation-Perfusion Relationships ($\dot{V}A/\dot{Q}$). In the process of adaptation to extrauterine life the infant must match ventilation and perfusion as closely as possible to assure transport of gases into and out of the lung. These relationships can be evaluated by measurement of the alveolar-arterial oxygen gradient (AaD_{O_2}) and the arterial-alveolar carbon dioxide gradient (aAD_{CO_2}). Both these gradients are increased for several days after birth indicating that both right-to-left cardiopulmonary shunting and maldistribution of perfusion (areas of high $\dot{V}A/\dot{Q}$) occur during adaptation. These abnormalities are of little clinical significance and in the case of the shunting could be due to gas trapping. Ventilation is evenly distributed in the newborn as determined by measurement of nitrogen washouts and arterial-alveolar nitrogen gradients.

Blood Gases and pH Changes at Birth. During early normal labor, pH has been reported to be 7.28 to 7.33; P_{CO_2} 45 mm Hg, and O_2 saturation 30 to 40%.[121] P_{O_2} measured from fetal scalp blood during labor averaged 20 mm Hg. Normal infants in good condition at birth (Apgar 8 to 10) have a mild metabolic and respiratory acidemia (pH 7.25 P_{CO_2} 76 mm Hg, Pa_{O_2} 19.5 mm Hg). With the establishment of extrauterine breathing these values rapidly normalize within the first postnatal hour.[141] Pa_{O_2} approaches 60 mm Hg at 1 hour and is generally over 80 mm Hg within 2 to 3 days.

Circulatory Changes at Birth. With the onset of extrauterine breathing, the intracardiac circulation of blood changes dramatically. Expansion of the lungs with air lowers pulmonary vascular resistance and pulmonary blood flow increases dramatically. Return of this blood to the left atrium raises left atrial pressure, resulting in functional closure of the foramen ovale, and obliterates the previous right-to-left shunting through this structure. Blood flow through the ductus arteriosus, which during intrauterine life had been right-to-left, now becomes left-to-right as pulmonary vascular resistance falls. The ductus arteriosus is functionally closed within 12 to 24 hours. Pulmonary vascular resistance falls rapidly in the first week, but does not reach adult levels until 3 to 6 months.

Effective pulmonary blood flow has been determined by a number of methods in the full-term newborn, averaging 138 ml/kg/min. before 24 hours and rising to 166 ml/kg/min. by 81 hours in one study[33] and 175 ml/kg/min. in another.[73]

ADAPTATION TO EXTRAUTERINE LIFE (PREMATURE INFANT)

The completeness of extrauterine cardiopulmonary adaptation in the premature infant at any time is related to size and maturity. Large premature infants approaching term gestation adapt much as the full-term infant, whereas smaller but non-distressed infants of lesser gestation have abnormal pulmonary function. Furthermore, many aspects of the adaptation process are less well studied in the premature infant than in the full-term infant (e.g., pulmonary vascular resistance change). In this section, only differences between the full-term and premature infant have been mentioned.

Gas Trapping. When gas trapping occurs in premature infants, it persists longer than in full-term infants. Some smaller premature infants can be shown to have gas trapping for prolonged periods. In these cases, the gas trapping may be due to airway closure in infants with low lung volumes rather than associated with lung fluid.

Establishment of FRC. This capacity is related to body size. However, in the premature infant, FRC is smaller per unit of body size than in the full-term infant. This difference suggests that even in the non-distressed infant more areas of atelectasis are present at any one time. The reasons for this difference are not established. FRC averages 0.9 ml/cm. Lung compliance in the premature infant depends on size, ranging from 0.41 to 3.4 ml/cm H_2O; specific compliance ranges from 0.012 to 0.052. The chest wall in the premature infant is relatively compliant. Total pulmonary resistance is very high due in part to resistance at the nose and smaller airways. Average values in small premature infants are 83 cm $H_2O/l/min$. Because of these mechanical factors a tenuous balance exists in small premature infants between alveolar collapse and maintenance of FRC. The mechanical efficiency of breathing in the premature is much lower than in the adult.

$\dot{V}_A/\dot{Q}$ Relationships. Because of the relative mechanical instability mentioned previously, it is not surprising that premature infants do not adjust ventilation and perfusion as appropriately and rapidly as the full-term infant. Right-to-left cardiopulmonary shunts and areas of high $\dot{V}_A/\dot{Q}$ are prominent and persistent features of the pulmonary adaptation of the non-distressed premature infant.

Effective Pulmonary Blood Flow. Cardiac output and pulmonary blood flow may be important limiting factors in the newborn. The large variations in reported values are a testimony to the difficulty of measurement. Values for effective pulmonary flow ranging from 50 to 100 ml/kg/min.[86] to 214 ml/kg/min.[73] have been reported.

BREATHING PATTERNS IN THE NEWBORN

It is important that the physician be aware of the patterns of breathing in the newborn as they are normally quite distinct from those of the child or adult. Irregularity of respiration is the rule for even the full-term infant. The sleeping infant breathes first rapidly then slowly depending on the state of central nervous system activity.

Several characteristic breathing patterns have been identified for the premature infant. Very immature infants show apneic breathing characterized by breathing movements of irregular rate and depth interposed between long apneic pauses (Fig. 16-3). Lesser degrees of apnea are common. Attempts to relate apnea and other breathing patterns to the state of the premature infant, e.g., rapid eye movement (REM) versus non-REM sleep, have been inconclusive and conflicting at best. Clearly no single state of the infant relates to a specific breathing pattern in all cases.

Apnea is considered serious when it produces bradycardia because bradycardia in this instance is thought to reflect underlying hypoxemia. Repeated apneic episodes with bradycardia and hypoxemia can seriously jeopardize the developing brain of the premature infant. It is of interest that in some cases infants with apnea show immediate bradycardia as soon as breathing stops, but that in other instances many seconds elapse before bradycardia occurs. The literature on the subject of apnea is confused by the fact that each author has his own definition of significant apnea. Thus, the frequency of apnea depends on how the spells are defined. The approach to treatment of apnea is detailed on page 499.

Apnea also occurs in infants who are distressed with HMD, sepsis, and intracranial hemorrhage. Frequently, the sudden development of apnea is the sign that alerts the physician to the presence of sepsis in the infant. When apnea develops in a previously stable infant, sepsis should be considered and appropriate cultures taken and treatment begun.

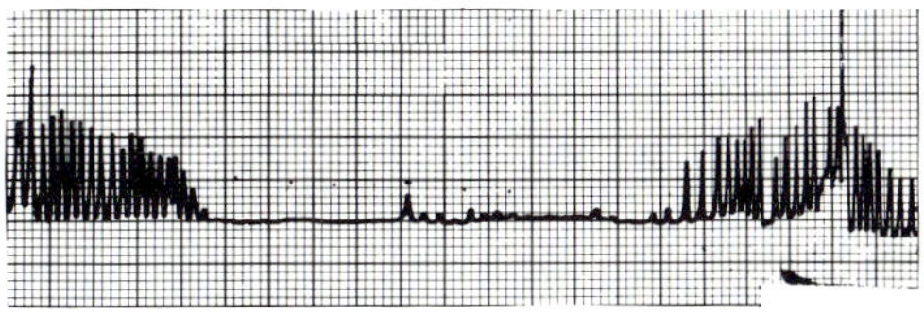

FIG. 16-3. Pneumogram of apneic breathing pattern in an immature infant. Note irregular rate and depth as well as apneic pause.

Periodic breathing occurs in most premature infants at some time (Fig. 16-4). In this condition, the apneic pauses are regularly interspersed between periods of rapid breathing. Infants slip into and out of periodic breathing for no apparent reason. Fenner et al. have observed that periodic breathing is more common during REM sleep.[50] It is uncommon that the apneic pauses during periodic breathing are of sufficient length to cause bradycardia and cyanosis. Like apnea the cause of periodic breathing is not known. Thibeault et al. showed that the patterns of periodic breathing could be abolished by increasing FRC by constant negative pressure around the chest and that measures that decrease FRC, such as application of positive pressure to the chest wall, provoked periodic breathing.[132] These studies suggested that

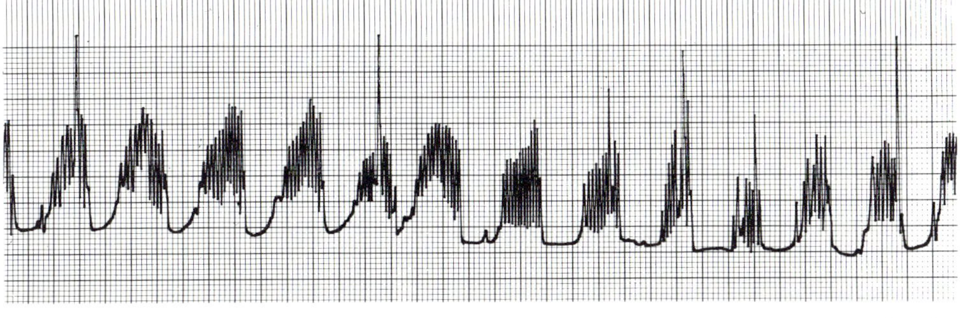

FIG. 16-4. Typical pneumogram pattern of periodic breathing in a premature infant. Note regularity of apneic pauses. Large inspiratory gasps or sighs are prominent.

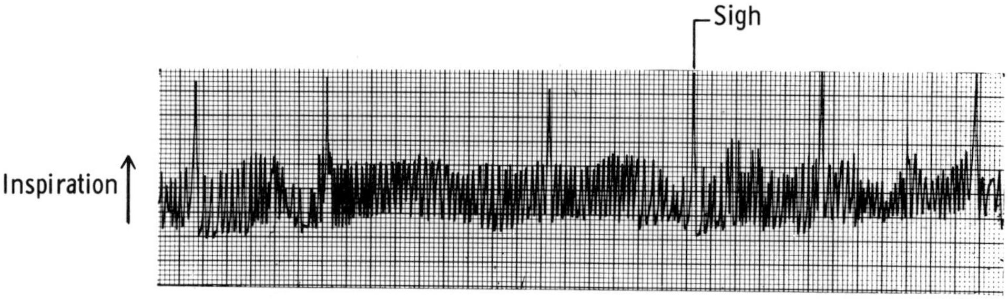

FIG. 16-5. Pneumogram tracing showing frequent sighs.

periodic breathing arises from factors in the lungs rather than primarily in the central nervous system respiratory control. Rigatto and Brady have suggested that hypoxemia initiates periodic breathing in pre-term infants.[115] Krauss et al. initiated periodic breathing in infants when oxygenation of mildly hypoxic infants was improved.[83] Periodic breathing requires no treatment and in fact reflects general well-being in a premature infant.

Frequent inspiratory gasps or sighs are observed in most premature infants (Fig. 16-5). Sighs can be abolished by increasing FRC, suggesting that they are caused by stimulation of deflation receptors in the lung in response to recurrent alveolar collapse.

Part II: *Pathologic States in the Newborn*

The care of the infant with respiratory insufficiency is an exercise in teamwork, and at no time is this more imperative than in the resuscitation of the newborn at birth.

Resuscitation in the Delivery Room

Not only must standard medical procedures be developed in each hospital, but also organizationally it must be clear who will be charged with resuscitation in every given instance. Too often after the resuscitation is completed, the infant is transferred to the nursery and no further observation is provided. Frequently during this time continuing respiratory insufficiency is unrecognized, to the detriment of the infant. It is anticipated that, with improved methods of monitoring the fetus in utero, the need for resuscitation will be lessened.

PATHOPHYSIOLOGY

An infant who requires resuscitation at birth has obviously failed to make an appropriate cardiopulmonary adaptation. As a result, extrauterine respiration is not established, and the minor physiologic disturbances that occur normally become seriously accentuated. Such an infant is suffering from hypoxemia, acidemia, and shock, and treatment must be directed toward these disturbances. Frequently, the obstetrician attempts to treat the apparently asphyxiated infant in utero by administering oxygen to the mother. This practice is not effective, may be detrimental, and delays more appropriate action. It should be emphasized that the need for resuscitation has quantitative aspects in that not all infants are asphyxiated to the same degree, so varying degrees of assistance are required. Milder degrees of asphyxia and acidemia may require only the administration of oxygen. Close clinical and laboratory monitoring dictates the need.

The following physiologic events with regard to cardiopulmonary adaptation are important in considering the principles of resuscitation.

Intrauterine State. The realization that the fetus in utero makes respiratory movements has drastically changed the thinking in regard to extrauterine breathing. Although not all the factors concerned with intrauterine fetal breathing, such as its intermittent nature, are understood, it appears that extrauterine breathing is a continuation of a previously established function. Although intrauterine breathing may be rapid, it results in little if any flow of lung liquid.

Lung liquid fills the lung so that intrauterine lung volume is approximately the same as FRC after birth. During the birth process a portion is removed by the pressure of uterine contractions on the chest wall, and the remainder is removed by the circulation and lymphatics in the first few days after birth.

Onset of Breathing. When the infant is born and the chest wall is released from the birth canal, elastic recoil results in entry of air up to one-third of the FRC before any respiratory movements are observed. Karlberg and co-workers have determined the pressure changes required for initial expansion of the lungs at birth.[78] Maximum inspiratory pressures varied between -45 to -75 cm H_2O in many instances (Fig. 16-6). High pressure is necessary to overcome surface forces at the air-liquid interface. No studies of this nature have been carried out in the premature infant where it may be expected that the presence of a more compliant chest wall might impose an additional mechanical disadvantage to aeration of the lung. This need for a high pressure should be remembered when resuscitation is required.

No single factor can be identified as a prime stimulus for extrauterine breathing. Rather a combination of factors is involved, including low pH, high P_{CO_2}, low P_{O_2}, thermal and cutaneous stimuli.

A mild combined respiratory and metabolic acidemia is present at birth due to an accumulation of CO_2 and lactate. Thus, for infants in good condition, the average pH is 7.25, average P_{CO_2} is approximately 70 mm Hg, and average P_{O_2} is approximately 20 mm Hg. In the infant who requires resuscitation, blood gases are worsened to the point where a severe combined respiratory and metabolic acidemia exists. The infant's pH may be as low as 6.8, P_{CO_2} as high as 100 mm Hg, and P_{O_2} approximately 0 mm Hg.

Cardiovascular Responses. During the birth process peripheral blood flow is thought to be regulated to provide maximum circulation to the vital organs such as the heart and brain. In the presence of hypoxemia and aci-

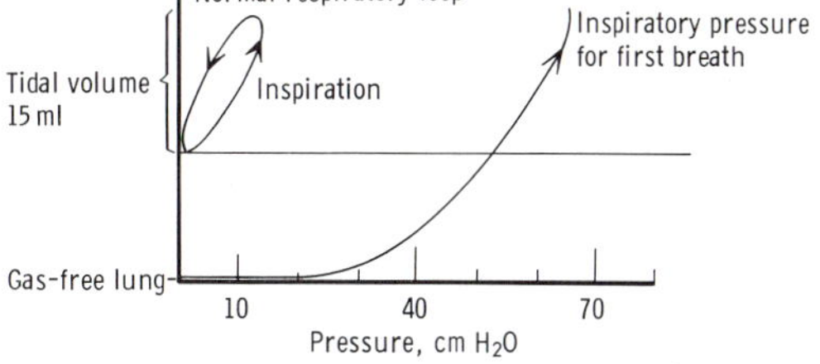

FIG. 16-6. Schematic pressure-volume loop of the first breaths. A normal P-V curve is included for contrast. Note high opening pressure of approximately -20 cm H_2O and high peak inspiratory pressure.

demia, more profound changes occur, with virtually complete diversion of blood flow from peripheral organs. In extreme cases, lung, renal, and bowel ischemia may occur. In the most hypoxic and acidotic infants compensatory mechanisms fail and shock intervenes, with resultant cardiac and brain hypoxemia as well. Infants who have required resuscitation and have made these circulatory adjustments show skin pallor for several days after birth. Large amounts of lactate accumulate in the blood in these circumstances, confirming the severity of hypoxemia and shock. The events associated with adaptation in the normal heart have been detailed previously. In the infant with asphyxia and acidemia, ductus closure may not occur and pulmonary vascular resistance remains high. These events result in a persistence of the fetal circulatory pattern.

CAUSES OF CARDIORESPIRATORY FAILURE AT BIRTH

An infant will fail to breathe at birth because of suppression of the intrinsic central nervous system respiratory drive caused by hypoxemia and acidemia or drugs. Maternal factors such as tumultous labor, placenta previa, and abruptio placentae interfere with fetal oxygenation and result in an asphyxiated fetus and infant. The placental insufficiency that produces uterine growth retardation or that occurs in postmaturity may be sufficient to cause hypoxemia and acidemia during labor. The likelihood of developing the latter condition may be evaluated by use of the oxytocin challenge test in suspected cases.[54] If the test is positive, labor and thus the risk of hypoxemia should not be allowed to occur, and the infant should be delivered by cesarean section. Excessive maternal anesthesia and analgesia are classic causes of cardiorespiratory insufficiency at birth and should be preventable.

Infants may also fail to establish normal cardiorespiratory function at birth for mechanical reasons that occur because of airway occlusion. Thus, imperforate nares, tracheal webs, or diaphragmatic hernia should be excluded as soon as possible.

A STRATEGY FOR INFANT RESUSCITATION

Approximately 1 to 2% of deliveries result in an infant with a severe resuscitation problem at birth. In many instances, knowledge of pregnancy and labor allows anticipation of a problem.

Anticipation of the Problem. Anticipation is important in order to ensure that personnel are available to provide resuscitation and subsequent observation for the infant. A partial list of risk situations includes premature birth, intrauterine growth retardation, prolapsed cord, placenta previa, abruptio placentae, primiparous breech delivery, cesarean section, polyhydramnios, oligohydramnios, postdatism, infants of diabetic mothers, twins, evidence of intrauterine asphyxia from fetal heart monitoring, or passage of meconium.

Identification of the Problem. The Apgar score performed at 1 minute is useful in documenting that a problem exists (Fig. 16-7). However, it is generally apparent before 1 minute whether the infant is having difficulty. In these instances pallor and apnea are sufficient evidence. Progress of extrauterine adaptation should be documented by an Apgar score at 5 minutes. Infants with low scores at 5 minutes may have a higher incidence of neurological deficit on subsequent follow-up.

Rough correlations can be made between Apgar score and pH of the infant, and because blood gas data are unavailable in the emergency situation, the Apgar score becomes particularly useful when considered as a reflection of pH (Fig. 16-8). If the Apgar score is to be used in this way, an objective

FIG. 16-7. The Apgar scoring system.

Sign	0	1	2
Heart rate	Absent	Slow (below 100)	Over 100
Respiratory effort	Absent	Slow, irregular	Good, crying
Muscle tone	Flaccid	Some flexion of extremities	Active motion
Reflex irritability	No response	Grimace	Vigorous cry
Color	Blue, pale	Body pink, extremities blue	Completely pink

evaluation of each infant is required. It is undesirable to have the Apgar score performed by the person who delivers the baby.

Apgar Score	*Approximate pH*
0, 1-3	6.90
4-7	7.10
8-10	7.25

Procedure for Resuscitation. Non-distressed infants require minimal nasopharyngeal suction and should be kept warm in an incubator or under a radiant heater. Infants with an Apgar score of 4 to 7 have initiated respiration and require only an increased oxygen environment until cyanosis is relieved. As a general principle a newborn infant should be transferred from the delivery room as soon as possible. Unnecessary procedures such as circumcision should not be carried out at this time.

The severely asphyxiated infant is suffering from hypoxemia, acidemia, and shock. It is generally obvious immediately that these factors are present because of extreme pallor and flaccidity, so these conditions should be treated without delaying to perform an Apgar score at 1 minute.

The following procedures are indicated. At least two persons are required to resuscitate the infant.

(1) *Maintain body temperature.* The infant should be placed on a table under radiant warmer to avoid chilling.

(2) *Provide a clear airway.* Unless meconium is present in the mouth and trachea, gentle nasopharyngeal suction is all that is required. Appropriate therapy should not be delayed because of excessive suctioning. In some instances vagal stimulation from too vigorous suctioning can produce severe brad-

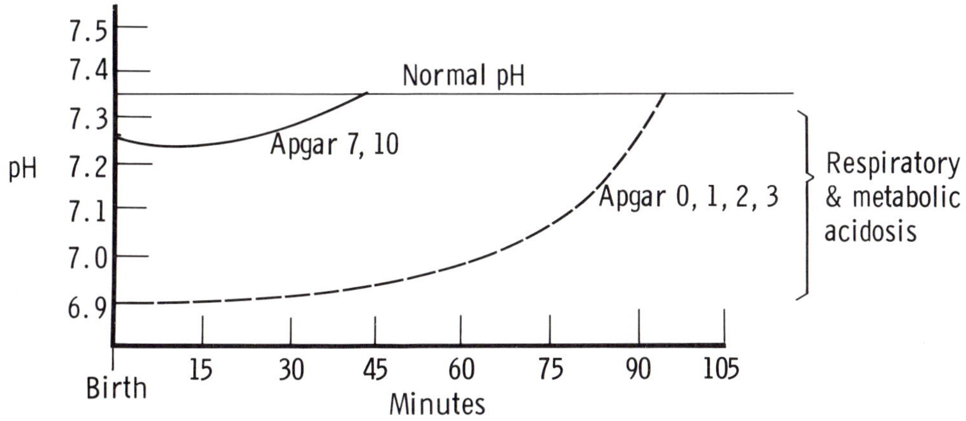

FIG. 16-8. Approximate relationships between pH and Apgar score at birth.

ycardia. Attempts should be made to clear meconium from the upper airway and trachea. However, prolonged efforts to remove meconium must be balanced against the urgent requirement for treatment of hypoxemia and acidemia.

(3) *Oxygenation.* Severely asphyxiated infants must be oxygenated by assisted ventilation. The method used should depend on the operator's expertise with a particular technique. Endotracheal intubation is desirable but requires repeated practice to maintain the skill. Because of the infrequent occurrence of the problem this skill may not be readily available in many delivery rooms. When the intubation has been performed, the operator must breathe through the tube providing sufficient pressure to elevate the chest at 40 breaths/min. A bag and mask with a valve can be adapted to the endotracheal tube. However, care must be taken to assure that the valves allow sufficient pressure to be applied to the airway to ventilate the lungs.

The use of an anesthesia bag and mask without valves is a simple effective technique that all personnel can learn with a minimum of training. This method can replace endotracheal intubation in most cases and is recommended as the initial approach particularly in community hospitals. It should not be used to provide assisted ventilation for a diaphragmatic hernia. When this technique is used, a feeding tube should be placed in the stomach to avoid overdistention. Under certain circumstances mouth-to-mouth resuscitation may be the method of choice.

(4) *Correction of acidemia.* Respiratory acidemia is rapidly corrected by assisted ventilation. Metabolic acidemia due to an accumulation of lactate is more profound and requires treatment. The lactic acidemia is due to both hypoxemia and shock. Currently alkali therapy with sodium bicarbonate is recommended; however, in certain circumstances it may be more appropriate to provide anti-shock treatment. Replacement with blood or plasma is obviously desirable if the condition is due to blood loss. Careful volume expansion may be indicated in shock due to asphyxia as well; however, this procedure is not presently the conventional therapy.

Sodium bicarbonate, $7\frac{1}{2}\%$, is administered into the umbilical vein by either catheter or small-bore needle. Dosage is empirical because blood gases and pH cannot be available for an accurate calculation of requirements. The basis for the use of alkali in this circumstance comes from work with asphyxiated monkeys in which it was shown that alkali and glucose infusions delayed complete cardiopulmonary collapse.[2] It is not necessary to completely correct metabolic acidemia by alkali therapy. Because of potential complications of sodium bicarbonate therapy, every attempt should be made to minimize the amount administered. Thus, initial therapy should restore pH to approximately 7.25, and if this therapy is followed closely with acid-base determinations, the infant can be allowed to provide the complete correction himself.

While the dosage of sodium bicarbonate is empirical, it is based on values of acid-base status known to exist in the asphyxiated infant. With assisted ventilation a portion of the base deficit is corrected. Approximately one-half of the remaining base deficit is due to metabolic acidemia and should be corrected by administration of sodium bicarbonate. For a full-term infant of 3 kg birth weight this amount is approximately 10 ml of $7\frac{1}{2}\%$ $NaHCO_3$ (1 mEq/ml). Because of the high osmolality of this solution some authors recommend diluting this dose with equal parts of 5% glucose and water. However, because the situation is an emergency and because large fluid volumes need to be avoided, the preceding doses of $NaHCO_3$ can be given once without dilution. Premature infants should receive an initial dose of 3 to 5 ml (1 mEq/ml) of $NaHCO_3$ depending on weight.

After the initial dose no further alkali therapy should be given until acid-base status is assessed by direct blood measurement. Further administration of sodium bicarbonate should be based on these values. During the correction of metabolic acidemia and subsequently, glucose stores must be replenished by the provision of 5% glucose and water until calories can be provided by oral feedings.

(5) *Cardiac massage.* Provision of adequate oxygenation and correction of acidemia generally result in improvement in heart rate and cardiac output. If bradycardia persists under 30 beats/min., cardiac massage should be begun. Massage is accomplished by compressing the sternum with the index and middle fingers at a rate of 80 beats/min.

Treatment of Infant Depression from Maternal Sedation. Morphine-like substances, particularly Demerol, used for maternal analgesia can result in respiratory depression at birth. This condition is most likely when the drug has been administered between ½ and 1 hour prior to birth. When this diagnosis is a possibility, nalorphine hydrochloride (0.1 to 0.2 ml/kg) should be administered through the umbilical vein.

Infant Follow-up. When sustained respiration has been achieved and the infant is no longer in shock and when the condition is stable, transfer from the delivery room area to an observation nursery should be expedited. Acid-base status should be followed until normal. Continued assisted ventilation and alkali therapy may be indicated based on these observations. The infant should be observed for the possible development of meconium aspiration or, if premature, HMD. It is during this post-resuscitation period that physiologic abnormalities may go unrecognized unless close clinical observation and biochemical evaluation are carried out.

Sequelae of Perinatal Asphyxia. The kidneys and the brain may suffer as a result of the shock and hypoxemia attendant on perinatal asphyxia. Shock can be so severe and prolonged under these circumstances as to produce acute tubular necrosis and renal shutdown.[36] Urinalysis frequently shows kidney damage as evidenced by the presence of albumin and red blood cells. Creatine is frequently elevated and creatinine clearance is low. It is most important to anticipate the renal problems in these cases to avoid the complications of overhydration and hyponatremia. This complication occurs when 5% glucose and water is being administered and anuria or oliguria is unrecognized. Urine collections should be carried out in all asphyxiated infants to determine whether oliguria or anuria is present.

Infants who have suffered perinatal asphyxia frequently have severe hypoglycemia and hypocalcemia. Blood sugar and calcium should be followed closely in these cases.

In the post-resuscitation period, infants are frequently flaccid. In the ensuing 6 to 12 hours and maybe as long as 24 hours after birth, increased tone advancing to jitteriness and convulsions may occur. Occasionally, these signs are related to hypoglycemia or hypocalcemia, but more often they reflect significant central nervous system damage. These problems must be anticipated and treated with appropriate anticonvulsant therapy, generally phenobarbital and Dilantin.

Hyaline Membrane Disease (Idiopathic Respiratory Distress Syndrome)

The commonest nonsurgical cause of respiratory distress in the premature infant is characterized pathologically and physiologically by alveolar collapse. Two clinical pictures (HMD and chronic pulmonary insufficiency) have been recognized although from the pulmonary physiologic viewpoint the conditions are similar.

HMD is the most common respiratory disorder of the newborn, occurring commonly in the premature infant and rarely in the truly full-term infant (2%). The precise cause of the condition is unknown so that specific therapy is not available. However, the pathophysiology of the condition is established in sufficient detail to allow for rational supportive care that saves lives and reduces morbidity.

INCIDENCE

In no precise way can the incidence of HMD be established because a definitive diagnosis can be established only at autopsy. However, the clinical description of the disease is sufficiently well developed to allow for reasonable estimates of frequency of the condition. Wood and Farrell, using data available for 1968 from the National Center for Health Statistics, showed that HMD or respiratory distress syndrome (RDS) accounted for 8237 deaths and was a contributing factor in 2624, a total of 19.3% of all neonatal deaths for that year.[146] Assuming that 75 to 80% of infants with HMD survived, these data could be extrapolated to show an incidence of 40,000 to 50,000 cases per year. In a more recent study these authors report similar findings over a 5-year period (1968–1973).[49] It is estimated that a considerable portion of the incidence of HMD is due to repeat elective cesarean section in pregnancies in which gestational age is inaccurately assessed.

HMD is more likely to occur in the more immature infant. Mortality is greatest in the most immature infants, with improvement in outcome occurring as gestational age increases. Over 90% of deaths occur by the fourth day of life, decreasing exponentially from a high point in the first 24 hours.[49]

RISK FACTORS

A number of factors have been implicated in an attempt to explain the presence of HMD in a particular infant. These factors are:

(1) Prematurity
(2) Cesarean section
(3) Maternal diabetes
(4) Perinatal asphyxia and shock
(5) Second twin

The importance of some of these factors is controversial, particularly the relationship between HMD and maternal diabetes and between HMD and cesarean section. The controversy with respect to the relationship of maternal diabetes and HMD is stimulated by the way these patients were handled by obstetricians in the recent past. Induction and delivery, sometimes by cesarean section prior to term, of infants of diabetic mothers was the favored method of management in the past decade. The delivery of a large but immature infant to avoid intrauterine demise was the rule. Thus, it is not clear whether the induced prematurity or the related maternal diabetes mellitus was the risk factor. In support of diabetes mellitus itself being a risk factor is the suggestion that the high insulin in the infant may inhibit surfactant production,[144] although a contrary study also exists.[76] Diabetic mothers with severe vascular changes frequently have small growth retarded infants who are not at risk to develop HMD but sometimes do develop meconium aspiration.

The confusion with regard to cesarean section centers around the relative risk caused by the reason for the section, e.g., maternal bleeding, and the operation itself. The picture is further confused by the fact that many infants who develop HMD after elective cesarean section are at what is incorrectly presumed to be term. Thus, these infants are at risk because of undiagnosed prematurity. Furthermore, infants with recognized prematurity should not be delivered by cesarean section except for cause, so that collection of appropriate data for the comparison is difficult if not impossible. Last, it is not clear what role intrauterine growth retardation may have played in the assessment of data in various studies.

On the other hand, the relation between prematurity and HMD does exist, and the condition is more common in the least mature infant. Male patients with HMD have an increased mortality for unknown reasons. The second-born twin is at greater risk for development of HMD than is the first-born. HMD is rare in the full-term infant, but does occur.

The relationship between perinatal asphyxia, shock, and HMD is less apparent. Many infants who develop the disease have low Apgar scores at birth, suggesting perinatal asphyxia as a risk factor. In other cases no evidence of asphyxia can be determined. It can be hoped that, with more sophisticated fetal monitoring techniques, methods can be applied to clarify this point.

FACTORS THAT MAY REDUCE RISK

A number of factors have been suggested as playing a role in reducing the risk of developing HMD. These factors generally can be classified as those that produce stress in the at-risk infant, and the protective effect is possibly exerted through a steroid mechanism.

Factors that have been mentioned as reducing risk are: (1) prolonged rupture of membranes, (2) prenatal steroid administration, (3) intrauterine growth retardation, and (4) maternal heroin addiction.[58] Items (3) and (4) are closely related in that intrauterine growth retardation may be the factor in patients with heroin addiction as well. In all instances the difficulty in accurately assessing gestational age complicates the evaluation of which factors have protective effect.

Studies are available that both confirm and deny a relationship between prolonged rupture of membranes and HMD.[150,75] Krauss and co-workers measured pulmonary function in premature infants with and without premature rupture of membranes and showed no difference between the groups.[88] Because of the well-identified abnormalities of pulmonary function in premature infants, if a protective effect were exerted by ruptured membranes, this non-rupture group would be expected to have more mature lungs in the physiologic sense. Bauer and colleagues observed a correlation between plasma cortisol levels and duration of ruptured membranes and suggested a protective effect through this mechanism.[14]

With regard to prenatal steroid administration, Liggins and Howie have shown that glucocorticoids given prior to 32 weeks' gestation and for more than 24 hours prior to delivery decrease the likelihood of HMD.[99] This effect is thought to be due to a specific effect of cortisol on lung maturation. However, the safety of this technique has not been established to date, and it should be considered to be in a research stage at present. That this approach may be useful is supported by the study of Spellacy et al., which showed an improved amniotic fluid L/S ratio in mothers to whom corticoid was administered.[127]

CLINICAL DIAGNOSIS

Infants with HMD are invariably premature although this fact may not be obvious from calculation of estimated date of confinement. However, examination of the infant using well-established physical and neurologic criteria usually establishes prematurity when doubt exists. The infant with a classic clinical picture has a birth weight between 1200 and 2000 g and gestational age of 30 to 36 weeks, although smaller and larger infants are affected. In the latter category is the infant of a diabetic mother who, when affected, is large in weight but immature by dates and physical criteria.

In cases of HMD, respiratory distress is generally obvious before transfer from the delivery room, and the condition is well developed by 3 to 4 hours after birth. The infant may have suffered perinatal asphyxia documented by fetal blood sampling, fetal heart rate monitoring, or Apgar score, or more commonly no evidence of perinatal insult can be detected.

Perhaps the most characteristic sign of

HMD is expiratory grunt, which, together with other signs such as tachypnea, cyanosis, and subcostal retractions, is frequently present prior to leaving the delivery room. The clinical course is variable in terms of severity, with a peak between 48 to 72 hours, although some infants are so seriously affected as to die within 6 to 12 hours if not properly treated. Increasing severity of the disease is manifest clinically by an increasing oxygen requirement, more obvious retractions, and the development of frequent apneic spells. The expiratory grunt becomes less obvious as the disease worsens. A decrease in volume of the chest, most apparent with the appearance of concavity in the axilla, can often be noted clinically. This sign is a reflection of the decrease in FRC that occurs as the disease worsens. On auscultation of the chest, breath sounds decrease to the extent that they are generally absent in moderate and severe cases. It is unusual to hear a cardiac murmur in the early stages of HMD, but it is common to hear a left sternal systolic murmur from the fourth to the tenth day. This murmur is indicative of left-to-right shunt through the patent ductus arteriosus, and right-to-left shunt is often present as well.

In the mild to moderate case of HMD, that is, when only a minimal amount of assisted ventilation is required, the clinical signs improve after the fourth or fifth day and clinical recovery is complete in 10 days to 2 weeks. Complications (such as oxygen toxicity) that are secondary to the treatment of the most severely affected infants may prolong respiratory insufficiency for varying periods of time, frequently many months.

LABORATORY DIAGNOSTIC STUDIES

As pointed out previously, as soon as respiratory distress is apparent in the infant, a chest roentgenogram in the anteroposterior and lateral projections should be obtained. The typical case of HMD shows a reticulogranular pattern with air bronchograms in the lung parenchyma (Fig. 16-9). Air bronchograms are a normal finding in the hilum radiating to the left lower lobe, but in HMD they are apparent throughout the lung. Initially, the heart size is normal in the typical case. It

A

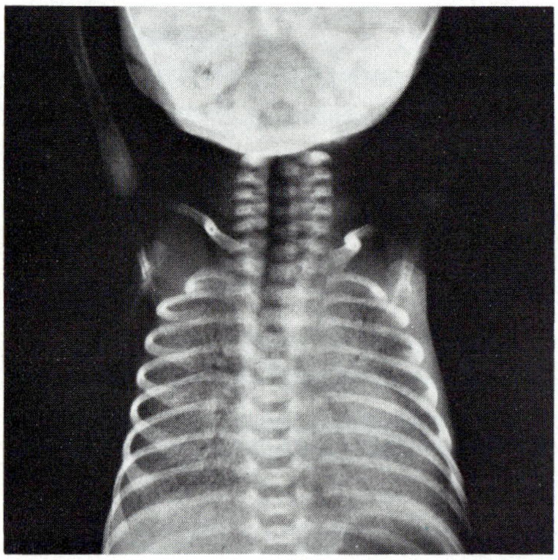

B

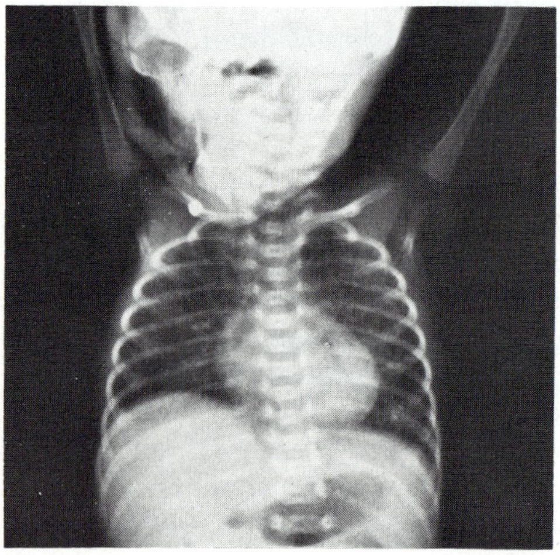

FIG. 16-9. Typical roentgenographic appearance of HMD.

A, Note reticulogranular appearance and air bronchograms. A chest roentgenogram of a non-distressed premature infant is shown as well for comparison.

B, Note streaks of atelectasis.

is common to have no abnormality in the chest roentgenogram when the respiratory distress is first apparent, only to have the typical pattern appear in the ensuing 12 to 24 hours. The air bronchograms occur because alveolar atelectasis makes the air-filled bronchi more apparent in contrast. The delayed appearance of the typical picture attests to the progressive nature of the atelectasis. In the most severe case no recognizable pulmonary parenchyma is seen on chest roentgenograms. In such cases the pattern is described as a "white-out" and reflects virtually total alveolar collapse (Fig. 16-10). The prognosis in these instances is grave. Not all infants with presumed HMD have a diagnostic chest roentgenogram. In general infants of larger birth weight may not have a sufficient degree of alveolar collapse to provide the contrasting densities.

Other clinical laboratory tests merely support the diagnosis of respiratory insufficiency and are not definitive for HMD. If perinatal asphyxia is present, early evaluation of blood gases and acid-base status may reflect this condition by showing a combined respiratory and metabolic acidemia. Clinical cyanosis confirmed by a low Pa_{O_2} in room air or oxygen is a constant feature of HMD. The presence of respiratory acidemia documents respiratory failure. An increased PCO_2 may not always be present in the early stages of the disease, and in certain infants who are capable of vigorous respiratory movements may not occur at all. However, most infants with HMD have a sufficiently disturbed physiology to develop an increased PCO_2. Metabolic acidemia related to either hypoxemia or poor cardiac output is a frequent occurrence. Recently, determination of L/S ratios in pharyngeal or tracheal secretions has been suggested as a method of definitively diagnosing HMD. Presently this technique is more useful in predicting outcome in that the severest cases have the lowest ratios.[18,142]

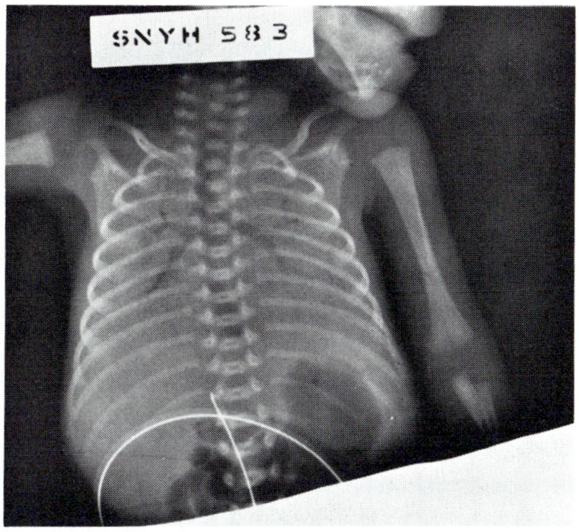

FIG. 16-10. Chest roentgenogram of severe HMD showing a "white-out."

CARDIOPULMONARY PATHOPHYSIOLOGY

As therapy of HMD is principally supportive, a thorough knowledge of the pathophysiology of the primary disease and its complications is essential.

The progressive alveolar collapse can be documented by serial measurements of FRC.[134] In general, two patterns are seen. In the most severely ill infant, FRC is maximally compromised almost from the beginning and can fall little thereafter (Fig. 16-11). In other less severe cases, FRC can be shown to fall progressively as the condition worsens (Fig. 16-12). It is in these cases that therapy directed toward prevention of alveolar collapse by constant distending airway pressure may be useful. In this group FRC may still be in the normal range even though the clinical disease is well developed. Other lung volumes are similarly decreased, particularly total lung capacity (TLC).[6] Vital capacity falls in infants with HMD as the disease worsens.[93] Some workers have used measurements of FRC and crying vital capacity to aid in diagnosis and as objective indices of severity of the disease (Fig. 16-13). Lung compliance is markedly decreased in HMD,[41]

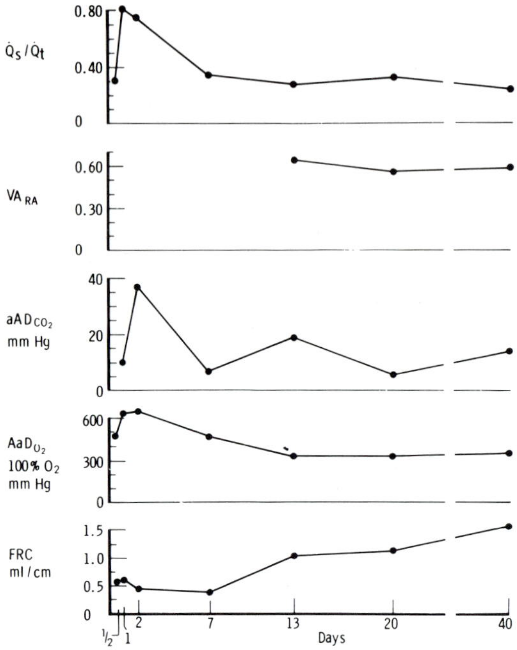

FIG. 16-11. Serial determinations of FRC and V̇A/Q̇ relationships in an infant with HMD. FRC is decreased from the outset.

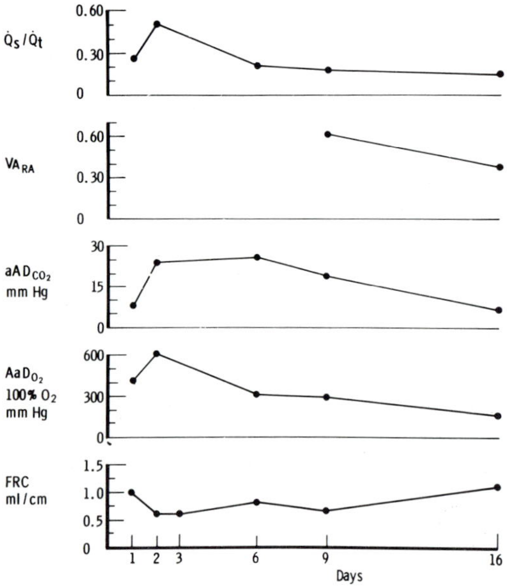

FIG. 16-12. Serial determinations of FRC and V̇A/Q̇ relationships in an infant with HMD. FRC initially normal decreases as the clinical and physiologic condition worsens.

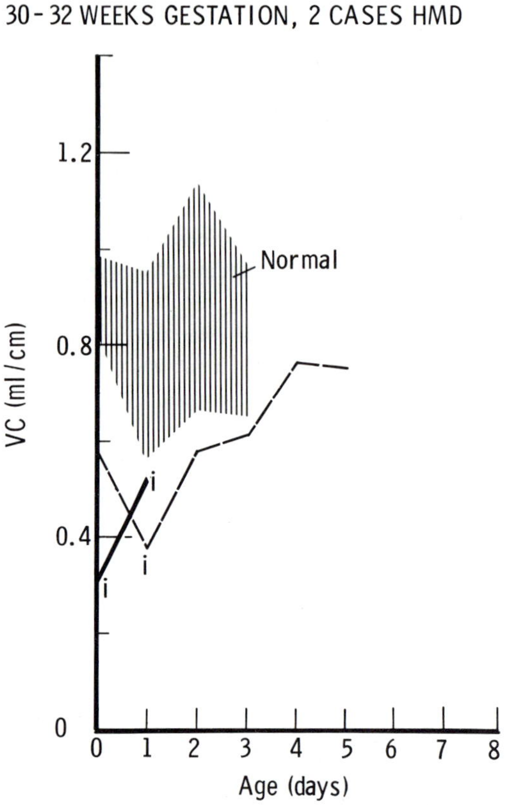

FIG. 16-13. Vital capacity (VC) in milliliters per centimeter in non-distressed infants at 30 to 32 weeks and in two infants with severe HMD. Note decreased VC in the infants with HMD.

and airway resistance is normal. The work of breathing is much increased.[32]

Significant abnormalities of ventilation-perfusion relationship have been documented in HMD. Most apparent is the right-to-left cardiopulmonary shunting,[109] which is thought to be the major reason for arterial oxygen unsaturation. Shunts occur through the foramen ovale,[27] ductus arteriosus,[105] and areas of the lung that are unventilated (collapsed) but perfused and may be as great as 80% of cardiac output (Fig. 16-14). In addition, significant degrees of maldistribution of perfusion (areas of high V̇A/Q̇) exist (Fig. 16-15), which results in the eventual increase of Pa_{CO_2} in most cases.[110] Attempts to docu-

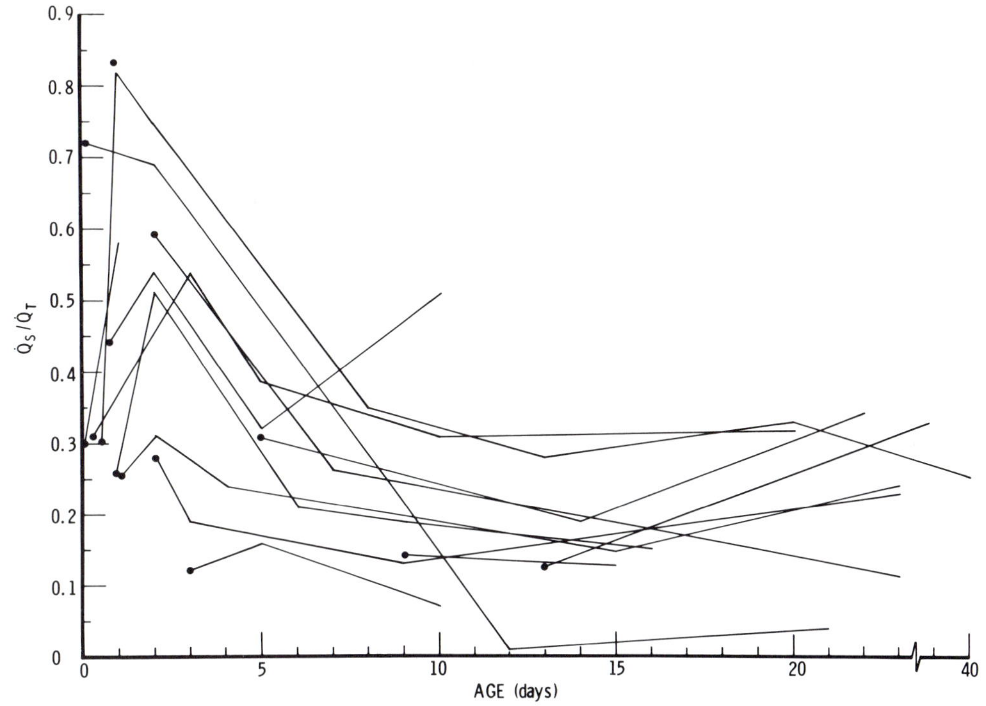

FIG. 16-14. Serial determinations of $\dot{Q}s/\dot{Q}t$ (shunt as percent cardiac output) in infants with HMD.

ment other forms of ventilation-perfusion abnormality, such as diffusion barrier or maldistribution of ventilation, have not revealed abnormalities extensive enough to be a major cause of arterial unsaturation. Krauss et al. have shown diffusion abnormality only in the most severe case.[90] During the recovery period, the low FRC returns to normal much before the abnormalities of ventilation and perfusion. However, these latter abnormalities are not of great clinical significance after FRC is normal.

Evaluation of the cardiovascular system in HMD has been much more difficult than evaluation of the pulmonary system. Cardiac catheterization studies have demonstrated right-to-left shunting through the foramen ovale and bidirectional shunt through the ductus arteriosus.[120] The much-needed assessments of cardiac output and distribution of peripheral blood flow in infants with HMD are not presently available. A number of workers have measured cardiac output in the normal premature infant and have found a value considerably below that of the full-term infant. Peripheral limb blood flow tends to be decreased in HMD and peripheral resistance increased as an attempt to redistribute blood flow to more vital areas[81] (Fig. 16-16A,B).

Blood pressure must be closely monitored as hypotension and shock are frequent occurrences during the early course of the disease[80,107] (Fig. 16-17). Infrequently, shock is due to blood loss either within the infant as in disseminated intravascular coagulation (DIC) or intracranially or from excessive blood sampling. The tendency of the distressed infant to hypotension and shock may also be due to the stress of the disease itself on a background of poor autonomic control in the premature infant in general.[140] It is important to recognize shock in its early stages, so-

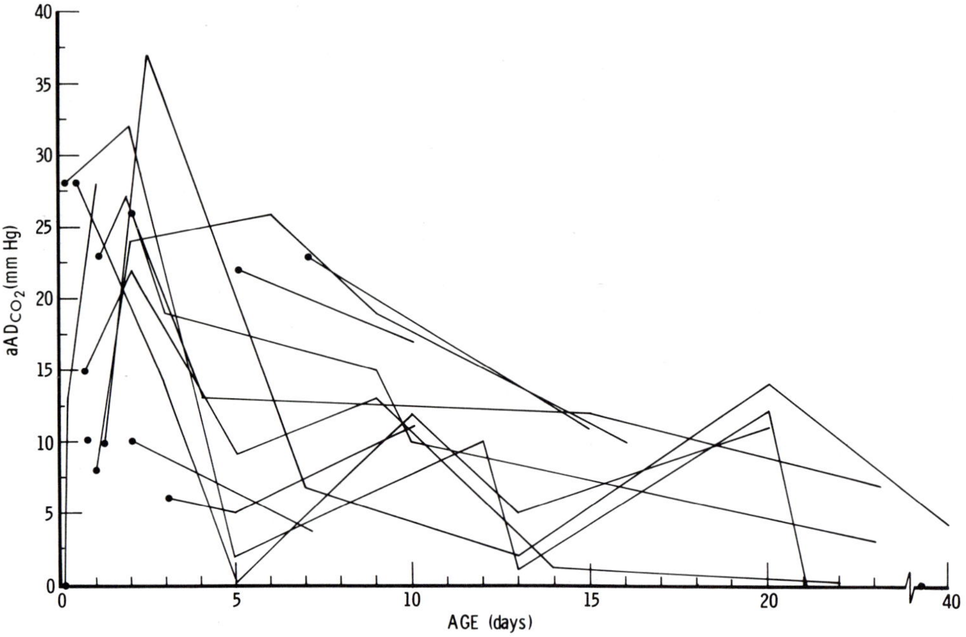

FIG. 16-15. Serial studies of aAD$_{CO_2}$ in infants with HMD. aAD$_{CO_2}$ indicates the presence of alveoli with increased $\dot{V}A/\dot{Q}$, i.e., underperfused with respect to ventilation.

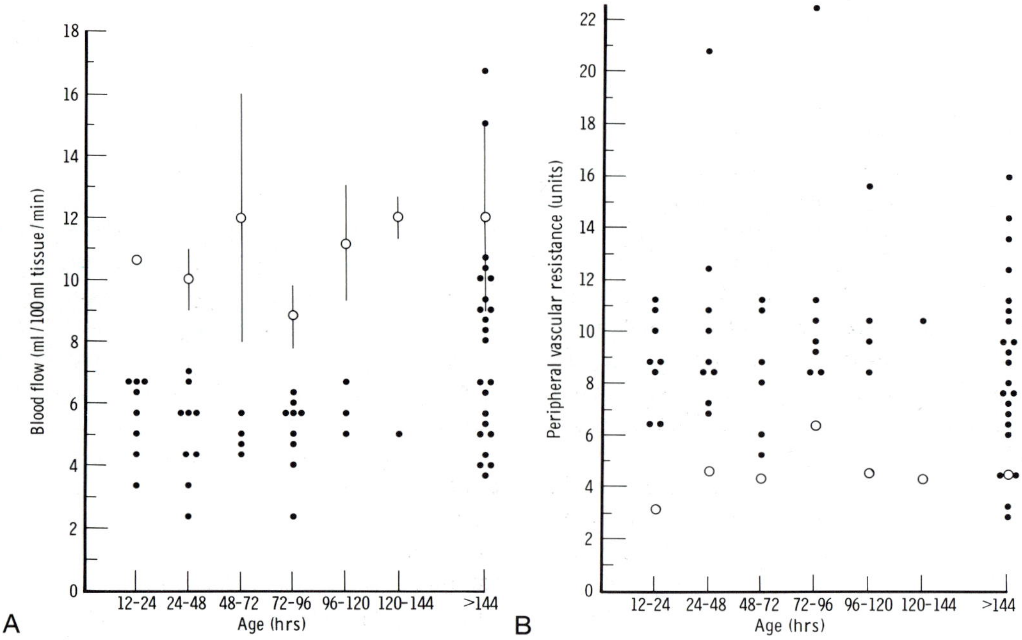

FIG. 16-16. *A*, Blood flow (ml/100 ml tissue/min.) in normal infants (open circles) and infants with HMD (closed circles). (From Kidd et al.[81])

B, Peripheral vascular resistance in normal infants (average value) (open circles) and infants with HMD (closed circles). (Adapted from Kidd et al.[81])

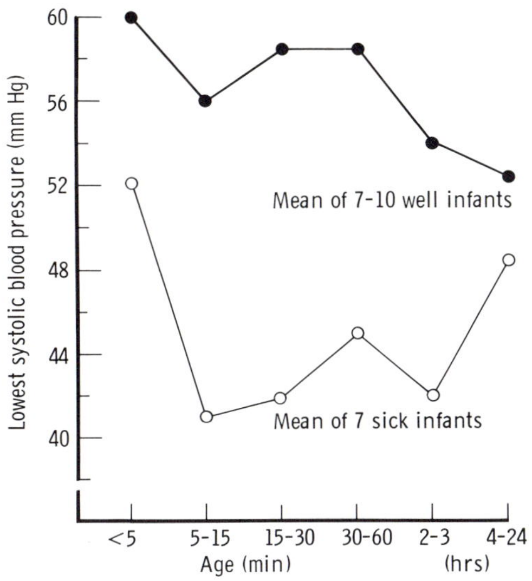

FIG. 16-17. Systolic blood pressure in sick versus well infants. (Adapted from Neligan and Smith.[107])

called impending shock. This identification is difficult sometimes because normal blood pressure values are so variable and generally are lower in the smallest infants (Fig. 16-18A,B). The presence of skin pallor, delayed capillary filling time, and oliguria are obvious clinical findings. Metabolic acidemia due to lactic acid in the absence of hypoxia should be regarded as evidence of decreased cardiac output to peripheral tissues. Grassi and coworkers have shown that hypotension in the distressed infant can be equated with decreased peripheral blood flow and lactic acidemia.[60] Treatment of shock by volume expansion reversed these findings (Fig. 16-19).

Infants ill from a wide variety of conditions lose the normal beat-to-beat variation of monitored heart rate, as is the case in HMD (Fig. 16-20). Clinically this loss of beat-to-beat variation is recognized as a fixed pulse rate.[119,137] With recovery, beat-to-beat variation is again noted. The reason for the phenomenon is poorly understood but is further evidence of autonomic dysfunction in HMD.

A reversible impairment of renal function occurs in the infant with HMD,[63] due to perinatal asphyxia and shock either before or after birth. Glomerular filtration rate determined by clearances of para-aminohippuric acid (PAH) and inulin were markedly reduced compared to non-affected infants in one study, whereas renal function was determined to be normal in another.[125] The difference may be related to severity of disease and clinical stability of blood pressure at the time of the study. Electrolyte abnormalities such as hyponatremia and hyperkalemia and increased blood urea may result from disturbed renal function. Hyponatremia occurs from overhydration particularly when decreased renal function is unrecognized. Hypernatremia may be secondary to excessive sodium bicarbonate administration. Hyperkalemia also may be due to tissue catabolism occurring when inadequate calories are provided to spare protein.

MONITORING THE INFANT'S COURSE

Detailed monitoring of cardiopulmonary function is the cornerstone on which the therapy of HMD is based. In addition, monitoring of parameters that may reflect involvement of other organs secondary to the effects of cardiopulmonary failure and to the effects of treatment is most important.

The first priority is to stabilize the infant and, for this, acid-base balance, blood gases, and blood pressure must be obtained. When this step has been accomplished, continued monitoring of cardiopulmonary function on a minute-by-minute basis is necessary. The frequency of blood gas and acid-base monitoring is often a matter of experience. Too frequent blood sampling is inadvisable and may result in excessive blood loss. In general, acid-base and blood gas sampling is needed at half-hourly intervals until the patient is stable by these parameters, after which it may be done much less frequently. Constant monitoring of Pa_{O_2} by indwelling electrode can be useful in this regard.[31] Transcutaneous Po_2 monitoring is in its infancy but may be lim-

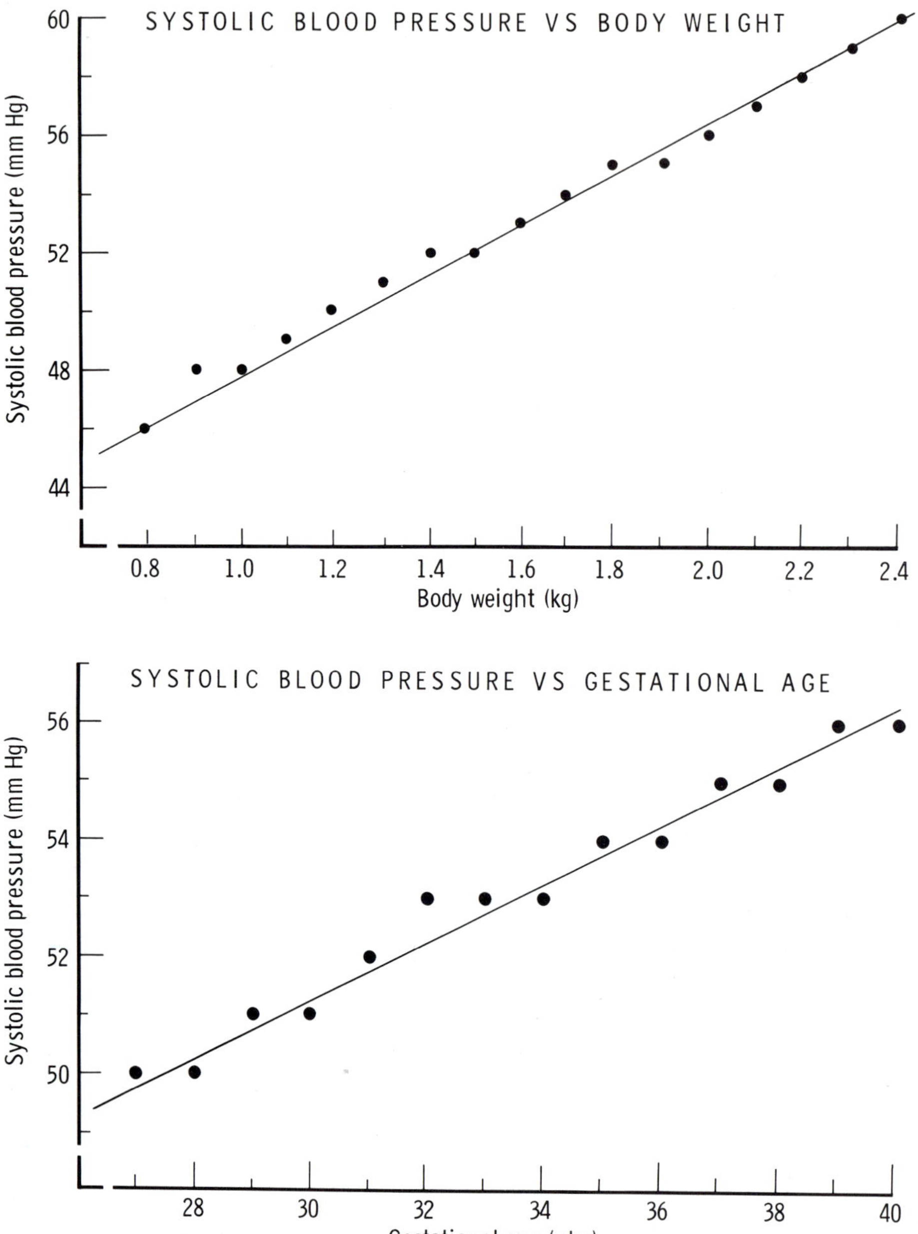

FIG. 16-18. Systolic blood pressure in non-distressed infants with respect to birth weight (*A*) and gestational age (*B*). (Data from Bucci et al.: The systemic blood pressure of newborns with low weight. *Acta Paediatr. Scand.* Suppl. 229, 1972.)

ited by poor peripheral perfusion in sick infants.[72]

The methods for cardiopulmonary monitoring are outlined in detail in Chapter 14. Blood gas and acid-base balance are most conveniently monitored by blood samples from the umbilical artery. Because of the risks involved considerable judgment is nec-

PHYSIOLOGIC PAMAMETERS OF SHOCK VS TIME

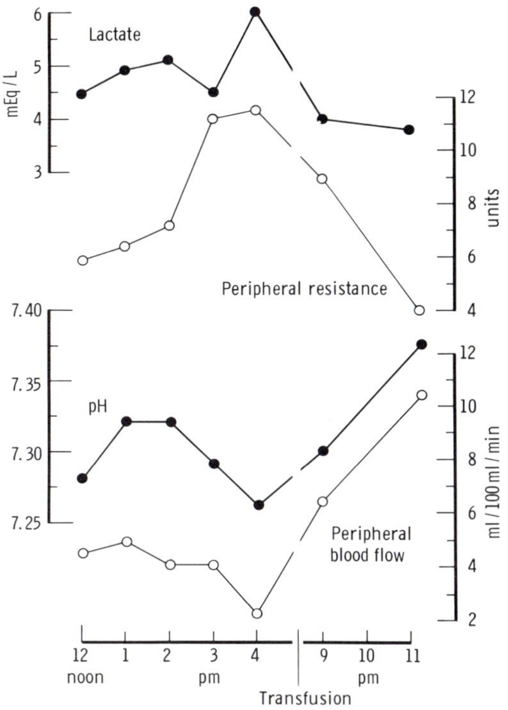

FIG. 16-19. Serial studies of pH, lactate, peripheral blood flow, and peripheral resistance in an infant with HMD. Note development of progressive lactic acidosis, fall in flow and rise in resistance reversed by transfusion.

essary to determine which patients require umbilical artery catheterization; when used, catheters should be removed as soon as possible. Mild to moderate cases of HMD may be better managed by less frequent peripheral arterial sampling and close clinical evaluation. Frequently, technical difficulties make arterial sampling impossible. In these cases, pH and P_{CO_2} measured in free-flowing venous blood may be used provided the infant is not in shock. Needless to say, P_{O_2} measured in venous blood is not useful.

Continuous blood pressure monitoring is mandatory. If an umbilical arterial catheter is in place, blood pressure monitoring through this site is preferred. Indirect determination of blood pressure by the Doppler technique or palpation must be used when an arterial line is not available, but these techniques are not as reliable.

Both heart rate and respiratory rate monitoring can be accomplished in the newborn. Techniques for determining respiratory rates continuously are less reliable than heart rate monitoring. For this reason, plus the fact that significant hypoxemia is reflected by bradycardia, many workers have relied principally on heart rate monitoring for a minute-by-minute assessment of overall cardiopulmonary status. Chest roentgenograms are useful in monitoring the cardiopulmonary status but should not be overused. Pneumothorax and pneumomediastinum may develop spontaneously or as a result of therapy, and they are best documented by chest roentgenograms. A pneumothorax can be diagnosed by transillumination as well.[95] An infant whose clinical condition worsens suddenly may have developed these complications. The chest roentgenogram is also useful to monitor cardiac size to determine the significance of PDA.

Other monitoring methods are required to determine the progress of specific therapeutic measures and to alert the physician to the complications of treatment. Thus, blood sugar, blood urea nitrogen (BUN), serum osmolarity, and electrolytes should be determined frequently to assess fluid and electrolyte balance and to act as a guide for fluid therapy. Urinalysis with attention to specific gravity and detection of glycosuria and hematuria are essential to determine the management of fluid and caloric requirements.

Because of potential central nervous system complications in high risk infants, assessment of head circumference and transillumination should be carried out on a weekly basis. When a neurologic problem develops, these measurements may provide guidance as to whether the problem existed from the outset or could be a complication of the disease. Evaluation of brain structure by computerized axial tomography is indicated in infants with prolonged respiratory insufficiency and may indicate development of cystic changes or other complications.

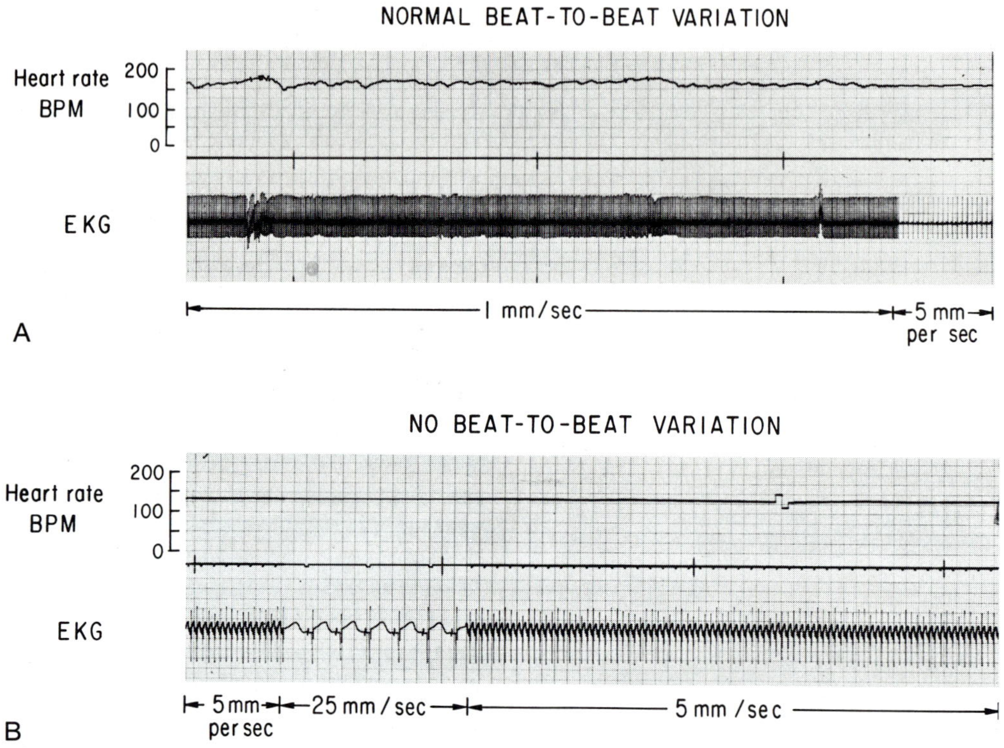

FIG. 16-20. *A*, Normal infant showing beat-to-beat variation in heart rate. has lost beat-to-beat variation.

In general as the infant improves as determined from the various monitored parameters, less frequent observations are necessary. Attempts must be made to avoid prolonging the monitoring process, and in this regard clinical judgment is important.

TREATMENT

Infants with HMD have a short well-defined list of problems and potential problems to which therapy must be directed. First, all patients have varying degrees of cardiopulmonary insufficiency for which treatment can be lifesaving. Then fluid, electrolyte, and caloric requirements must be met. Last, one must continually be aware of complications of the disease (pneumothorax, PDA, intracranial hemorrhage, and DIC) or complications of therapy (bronchopulmonary dysplasia) so that they may be diagnosed and given appropriate therapy as soon as possible. Because of the considerable likelihood of complications from therapy, management of each infant must be continually evaluated to determine that a need continues to exist for potentially harmful therapies.

General Supportive Measures. The well-known general principles of care of the premature infant must not be forgotten in the rush to apply cardiorespiratory therapy. Particularly important is the maintenance of body temperature. This regulation can be accomplished in either a modern incubator or infrared heater. The infrared heater is recommended particularly for the more immature infants for whom it is difficult to preserve temperature in an incubator, and for infants requiring extensive therapy. Body temperature should be maintained between 36 and 37° C. Similarly, for transport between hospitals, special incubators are available to maintain body temperature. Some hospitals have equipped vans with infrared heaters for this purpose. No predetermined incubator setting can guarantee maintenance of body temperature for a particular infant.

Gentle handling of the infant to minimize metabolic needs is an important aspect of treatment. Included here is the avoidance of unnecessary laboratory tests such as repeated chest roentgenograms for no cause. Considerable attention must be paid to maintenance of infection control procedures. In a busy unit in which doctor, nurses, and other personnel have many demands on their time, good handwashing technique should not be forgotten. Antibiotic therapy should never be a routine in an infant with HMD, but opinions differ as to the circumstances in which antibiotics are given prophylactically. Conditions for use refer particularly to the use of prophylactic antibiotics for indwelling catheters. Antibiotics are not recommended for this use. If antibiotic therapy is given for a presumed infection with an unknown bacteria, the particular agents used in therapy should be based on the circumstances of the situation (e.g., maternal amnionitis) as well as the predominant pathogens in a particular nursery. On the other hand, it is difficult to exclude a primary pneumonic process in an infant with respiratory distress. For this reason, antibiotic therapy should be provided for all infants with respiratory distress until pneumonia and sepsis can be excluded by cultures.

Infants with HMD frequently have excessive hyperbilirubinemia. Premature infants with HMD and hyperbilirubinemia are at increased risk to develop kernicterus because of a decreased amount of albumin available for binding in the premature infant as well as the presence of factors that interfere with the albumin binding of bilirubin, such as hypoxemia and acidemia. The anticipatory use of phototherapy is indicated in premature infants under 1500 g birth weight when indirect bilirubin levels approach 7 to 10 mg/100 ml and may be indicated from the outset in badly bruised and distressed infants. Every effort should be made to keep the indirect bilirubin level below 12 mg/100 ml in infants under 1500 g birth weight. Indices that measure the amount of unbound or free bilirubin may be useful in determining the safe limit of hyperbilirubinemia in a particular case (Sephadex Test).[77] Exchange transfusion should be performed to prevent excessive hyperbilirubinemia. At present, the level of indirect bilirubin at which exchange transfusion is performed is arbitrary, but most would agree that the level should be kept below 12 mg/100 ml. With careful attention to detail, exchange transfusion is well tolerated by very sick infants.

Management of the Respiratory Problem. The respiratory and cardiovascular insufficiency and the resultant acid-base disturbances are the major life-threatening problems of the infant with HMD, and immediate appropriate therapy can be lifesaving.

The hallmarks of respiratory insufficiency are hypoxemia and hypercarbia (retention of CO_2) and respiratory acidosis. Hypoxemia is a consequence of right-to-left cardiopulmonary shunting, and hypercarbia is due to alveoli with maldistribution of perfusion (high $\dot{V}_A/\dot{Q}$). Thus from the physiologic viewpoint three types of alveoli exist in HMD: (1) normal, (2) alveoli causing a shunt, and (3) alveoli with high $\dot{V}_A/\dot{Q}$ (Fig. 16-21).

Treatment of Hypoxemia. Oxygen therapy is required for almost every infant with HMD. The goal is to maintain a Pa_{O_2} of 50 to 70 mm Hg and minimize the toxic effects of oxygen (bronchopulmonary dysplasia and retrolental fibroplasia). Thus, the FI_{O_2} should be adjusted to maintain Pa_{O_2} within this range. Arterial blood gas monitoring is essential for this purpose. The umbilical artery is most frequently used, although temporal artery and right radial or brachial artery bet-

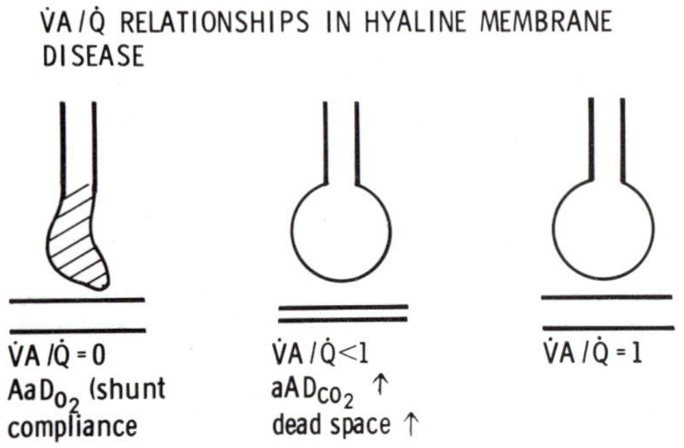

FIG. 16-21. Schematic representation of V̇A/Q̇ associated with HMD.

ter reflect oxygenation of the retina (because the source of these vessels is proximal to a right-to-left ductal shunt). All currently available methods of monitoring Pa_{O_2} are limited by the fact that Pa_{O_2} varies from minute to minute, and frequently apneic spells and other phenomena cause wide fluctuations. It is important to remember when administering increased FI_{O_2} to premature infants that, because of active oxygen chemoreceptor tone, an initial apneic response may be precipitated. During recovery from HMD the oxygen requirement may drop quickly, and the physician must be particularly aware of avoiding oxygen toxic effects at this time. Some workers report satisfactory results using an indwelling arterial oxygen electrode.[31] Noninvasive methods currently being tested may obviate the need for indwelling catheters.

Constant Distending Airway Pressure. When maintenance of a Pa_{O_2} greater than 50 mm Hg requires high FI_{O_2} (greater than 0.60) for prolonged periods of time, the use of constant distending airway pressure (CDAP) is indicated to maintain Pa_{O_2} at a lower FI_{O_2}.[61] This technique can be applied in a number of ways, either by applying a constant positive airway pressure (CPAP) through the airway or by applying a constant negative extending pressure to the airway (CNEP).[25] It should be appreciated that CDAP is indicated only when FI_{O_2} must be lowered because of risks of pulmonary O_2 toxicity. It should be used with great caution when hypercarbia and respiratory acidemia (high V̇A/Q̇ alveoli) complicate hypoxia as CDAP can produce high V̇A/Q̇ alveoli, which results in more CO_2 retention.[92]

The method by which CDAP raises Pa_{O_2} in HMD is not clear. Two possibilities have been suggested: (1) that CDAP opens up atelectatic alveoli and removes shunting from this cause, or (2) that CDAP distends the still patent alveoli, thus creating a greater surface area for diffusion. The fact that compliance falls even though FRC increases with CDAP suggests the latter explanation.[12] Unequal time constants of the lung (different areas of the lung with different resistance and compliance) with subsequent overdistention of relatively normal areas of the lung by CDAP has been postulated.

Currently the pressure used in CDAP is determined by trial and error, the goal being to establish a compromise between a minimal FI_{O_2} and an acceptable Pa_{O_2} and to avoid complications. Generally, airway pressures between 2 and 7 cm H_2O are recommended. Pneumothorax is the ever-present complication occurring as much as three times as often in infants receiving this therapy. Specific methods for applying CDAP appear in Chapter 14. The "best" CDAP is the one that maintains Pa_{O_2} between 50 and 70 mm Hg at minimal FI_{O_2} without complication.

Because HMD is a progressive disease characterized by a steadily diminishing FRC, the technique of CDAP has been recommended for use early in the disease to prevent the decrease. Several studies claim to have demonstrated the value of early CDAP in the treatment of HMD for this purpose.[46] However, controls are difficult to determine and more work clearly is indicated. In animals CDAP minimizes surfactant destruction;[148] if CDAP has the same effect in the human infant with HMD, early use is clearly indicated. The problem then is to determine early in the course of the disease who will be sick enough subsequently to warrant the risks of early CDAP.

The physician frequently must balance whether to allow an infant to be maintained in a high FI_{O_2} (greater than 0.70) for an anticipated short period (24 to 36 hours) or to institute CDAP and thus lower FI_{O_2} but run the risk of pneumothorax. As well as being concerned with the hazard of pneumothorax, CDAP has cardiovascular effects that must be recognized. CDAP will on occasion impede venous return to the heart, which results in decreased cardiac output with the risk of peripheral vascular collapse.

While many claims have been made for this technique, certain facts have emerged.

(1) CDAP improves Pa_{O_2} at a lower FI_{O_2} to a greater extent than when no pressure is applied.

(2) CDAP may be useful in preventing progressive alveolar collapse when applied early. (No experimental proof exists for this claim.)

(3) Pneumothorax and cardiovascular complications can be produced and must be weighed in any decision to use the treatment.

(4) As an example of one of the cardiovascular effects, CDAP may result in increased Pa_{CO_2} by increasing numbers of high $\dot{V}A/\dot{Q}$ alveoli.

While an immediate beneficial effect in improving oxygenation is evident when CDAP is used, it has not been clearly established that increased survival can be definitely ascribed to the technique,[43] although duration of oxygen therapy and intermittent positive pressure ventilation is shortened when started early.[46]

CDAP may be administered in the course of providing assisted ventilation. This mode is called positive end-expiratory pressure or PEEP. Many respirators have a PEEP mode, and the technique can also be used during hand-bagging. The same considerations apply to PEEP as for CDAP.

Complications of CDAP in addition to pneumothorax are related to specific methods of application and include excoriation of neck, obstruction of venous return from the head and neck, and excoriation of the nasal septa (nasal CPAP).

Treatment of hypercarbia. Vigorous infants with HMD may adequately ventilate their lungs to the extent that hypercarbia and respiratory acidemia do not occur. In these infants hypoxemia due to right-to-left shunts is the major pulmonary problem. However for the most part infants with HMD have hypercarbia sufficient to tax compensatory mechanisms and this disorder leads to respiratory acidemia (respiratory failure).

When respiratory failure occurs, assisted ventilation is indicated. Infants that need only minimal support can frequently be managed with hand-bagging. Whatever technique is used must allow the delivery of a pressure sufficient to ventilate noncompliant lungs. Patients with hypercarbia and respiratory acidemia that cannot be controlled by an intermittent schedule of hand-bagging must be intubated and placed on a respirator. Some authors have suggested use of negative pressure respirators to avoid complications of endotracheal intubation and respirator lung damage. Presently, the reputed good results in minimizing complications with negative pressure respirators may reflect only a selection factor in which the technique fails with the most severely ill infants.

Respiratory acidemia should be treated when pH is less than 7.30 and P_{CO_2} is greater than 50 mm Hg. The treatment of choice is assisted ventilation. Mild degrees of respiratory acidemia should be treated with intermittent hand-bagging. If ineffective, it may be necessary to intubate the infant and use a respirator. While buffering with sodium bicarbonate is generally contraindicated in respiratory acidemia, it may be useful in mild cases. In the process of buffering with sodium bicarbonate, CO_2 is produced and theoretically could worsen respiratory acidemia. However, in mild cases the resultant improvement in pH and secondarily the distribution of pulmonary blood flow may be sufficient to avoid this effect. If this approach is used, repeated blood gas monitoring is essential, and assisted ventilation must be used if the blood gas picture worsens.

Complications of Respiratory Therapy. The use of oxygen and assisted ventilation is a two-edged sword. While necessary to save life and avoid morbidity, both these treatments have potential complications.

Retrolental fibroplasia (*RLF*). Because of legal implications, pediatricians are particularly sensitized to the relationship between O_2 and retrolental fibroplasia. Fortunately, infants with HMD seldom are at risk for this condition because of the nature of the physiologic defect, namely shunting, which makes over-oxygenation difficult to obtain. During recovery a rapid decrease in oxygen requirement occurs, and infants are then at the most risk for RLF. Presently available methods of monitoring oxygen will not completely avoid the development of RLF in every case.

Pulmonary oxygen toxicity (*POT*). It is not clearly established whether bronchopulmonary dysplasia (BPD)[111] is due to the toxic effects of oxygen, the pressure effects generated by respirators on the lung, or both. Nor are the duration of exposure to oxygen and the concentration that produces the condition clearly determined. In addition, the relationship between BPD and Mikity-Wilson disease is not clear. Nevertheless, this complication, whatever its cause, is a major factor in morbidity and mortality in HMD. Clinically, the condition is suggested when after 3 to 5 days of severe respiratory distress requiring high concentrations of O_2 and respirator care, the infant fails to improve; in fact the condition may actually worsen. Chest roentgenograms, which previously had shown air bronchograms, reticulogranular appearance, or a "white-out" (stage II) now begin to show coarse streaks throughout. As the condition develops, roentgenograms show atelectasis, emphysema, and cystic changes (stages III and IV) (Fig. 16-22). The radiologic stages of BPD have been described by Northway et al.[111]

Pathologically the condition is characterized initially by increased vascular permeability and resultant interstitial edema. This lesion occurs principally in the peribronchiolar region in the first 2 days. Subsequently, hyaline membranes develop, and in 4 to 5 days peribronchiolar fibroplasia and squamous metaplasia in the terminal bronchioles develop. These lesions are associated with bronchiolar dilatation. It is not clear whether the cystic changes seen on chest roentgenogram are due to compensatory emphysematous changes or dilatation of terminal bronchioles secondary to destruction. All these lesions are reversible. Oxygen is also known to destroy pulmonary surfactant, impede ciliary activity, produce vascular damage, and inhibit DNA so that a vicious cycle is created.

Every effort must be made to avoid the development of POT by using only appropriate amounts of oxygen and discontinuing it as soon as possible. CDAP may be useful in this regard in minimizing oxygen usage; on the other hand, the added pressure on the airways may produce damage. Herman and Reynolds have suggested that the development of POT may be minimized by reversing the usual I:E ratio from 1:3 to 2:1 during respirator therapy and ventilating at low peak pressures and at low respiratory rates.[68] Rationale for this approach is based on the assumption that the lung of the infant with HMD has areas of different time constants and that a slow prolonged inspiration can better aerate those areas where time constants are prolonged and thus reduce complications. Diuretics such as furosemide may be useful in therapy of POT in the early stages, when edema is the dominant pathologic process.[104]

Infants who develop POT require prolonged periods of respiratory support and may not recover. Infants who do recover have a tendency to develop recurrent respiratory problems during early infancy. The roent-

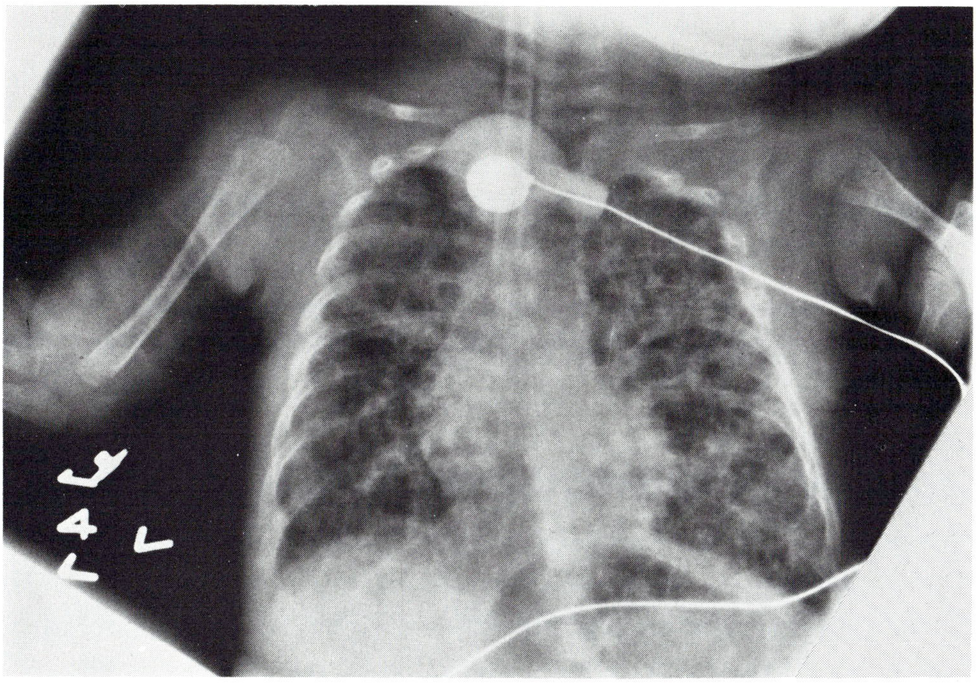

FIG. 16-22. Typical case of bronchopulmonary dysplasia showing cystic changes.

genographic abnormalities may persist for months.

Pneumothorax and pneumomediastinum. These two conditions may occur spontaneously in HMD or as a complication of respiratory therapy. Infants with HMD who develop pneumothorax and pneumomediastinum spontaneously (8% of patients in one series[30]) are generally the larger, more vigorous infants who have deep chest retractions and produce large pressure changes during respiration. This group of infants must be observed carefully for these complications; also these complications occur during therapy with CDAP and assisted ventilation with or without PEEP.

Early recognition of pneumothorax is imperative and can be achieved only by a high index of suspicion. An increasing O_2 requirement or a sudden deterioration in clinical condition should suggest the diagnosis and be an indication for chest roentgenogram to confirm the diagnosis. Transillumination of the chest can be used for diagnosis. Dissection of air into the tissues of the neck is rare in infants.

After diagnosis a decision regarding the significance of the pneumothorax must be made as not all require treatment. If a tension pneumothorax is present, emergency evacuation must be accomplished by needle aspiration using a stopcock and syringe or by placement of an indwelling catheter with underwater seal drainage. Occasionally the breathing of 100% O_2 for a short period of time will free the blood of nitrogen and create a gradient for N_2 between the pneumothorax and blood so that the gas is resorbed. This technique should not be used for large pneumothoraces.

Pneumomediastinum does not require treatment. Its importance lies in the confusion that the lesion can create in interpreting the chest roentgenogram.

Pneumothorax is caused by alveolar rupture. Pneumomediastinum occurs when the air leak produced by alveolar ruptures allows the gas to track through the interstitium along bronchi and blood vessels into the mediastinum.

Interstitial emphysema. Interstitial emphysema occurs most often as a complication of therapy in very sick infants with very stiff lungs. In these cases high airway pressures cause alveolar and bronchiolar rupture into the interstitial tissues with formation of bullae. Diagnosis is made by observing the typical picture on chest roentgenogram (Fig. 16-23).

Tracheal stenosis. Various lesions of the airways are produced by trauma and fibrosis in the course of treatment. Thus, nasal septum erosion occurs with nasotracheal intubation and nasal CPAP. Tracheal erosion with underlying esophageal erosion may occur from prolonged endotracheal intubation. Ste-

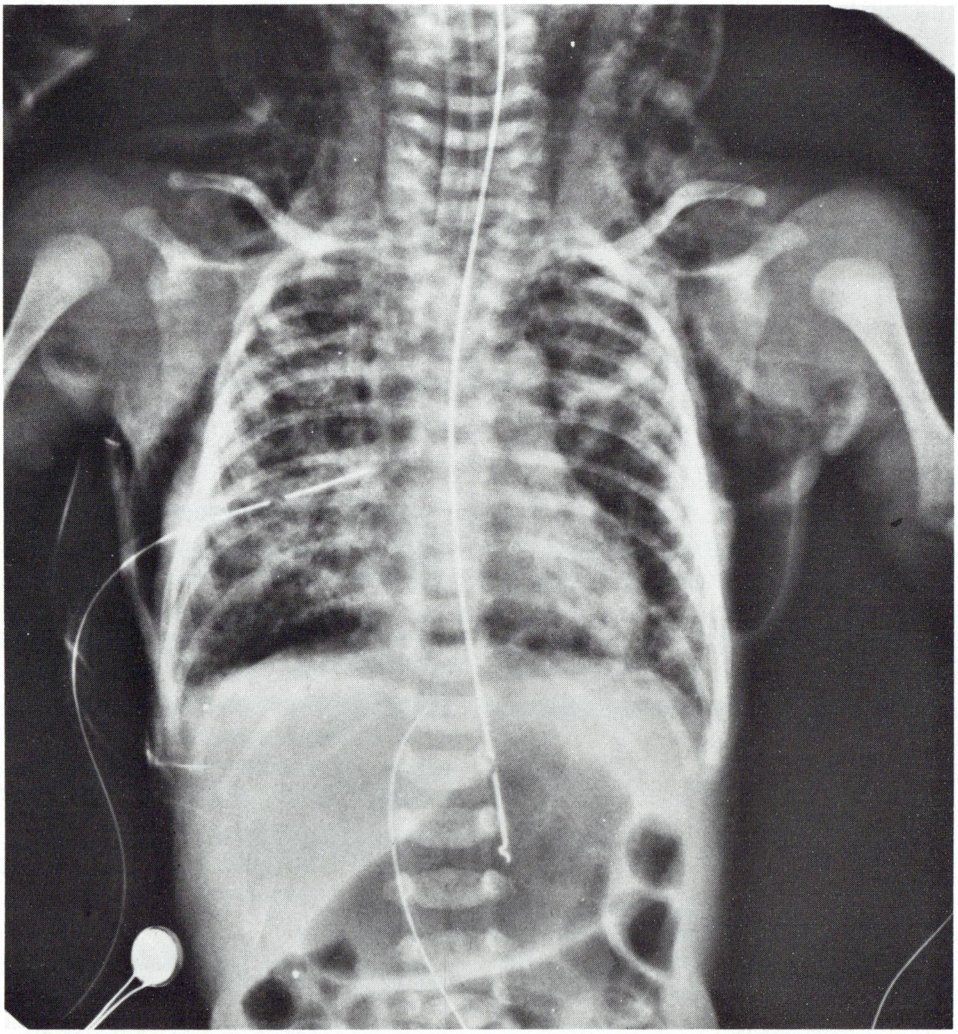

FIG. 16-23. Interstitial emphysema in a patient with HMD. Note dissection of air into the neck and axillae.

nosis of the trachea may be a secondary effect. Great care must be observed to fix endotracheal tubes firmly to minimize traumatic damage to the trachea. Tracheotomy may be necessary after prolonged endotracheal intubation because of the presence of tracheal stenosis.

Pneumopericardium. This disorder may occur spontaneously or as a complication of various forms of assisted ventilation[149] (Fig. 16-24). It generally occurs in association with pneumothorax and pneumomediastinum. Air probably enters the pericardium along the pulmonary vessels. Cardiac tamponade is frequently present. Muffled or distant heart sounds may be the only clue. Surgical aspiration by indwelling catheter is indicated.

The Acid–Base Problem. The treatment of metabolic acidemia is discussed in this section; respiratory acidemia has been considered under management of the pulmonary problem. Metabolic acidemia occurs in HMD due to hypoxemia (Pa_{O_2} less than 40 mm Hg) or shock or impending shock. Lactic acid accumulates in response to these factors. If hypoxemia is the cause, appropriate treatment is administered. If it can be determined that shock is the cause, the condition should be treated with either plasma or blood. As the importance of shock in the etiology of metabolic acidemia has become more clearly identified, anti-shock measures have replaced the use of buffering with sodium bicarbonate or THAM in many instances.

Difficulty can be encountered in deciding whether the infant is in shock because of variations in "normal" blood pressure in premature infants. Clinical measures such as capillary filling time and urinary output should be used in the assessment. If the blood pressure is low (systolic less than 40 mm Hg or diastolic less than 20 mm Hg), and Pa_{O_2} is greater than 50 mm Hg and metabolic acidemia is present, impending shock should be suspected.

Buffering with sodium bicarbonate or tris-hydroxymethyaminomethane (THAM) is indicated when metabolic acidemia is present and cannot be clearly related to shock or hypoxemia. In these instances dosage of $NaHCO_3$ ($7\frac{1}{2}$%) should be calculated from pH and P_{CO_2} using the Siggaard-Andersen nomogram. Base deficit is calculated assuming a bicarbonate space of 0.6 body weight, as in the following example in a 2 kg infant, e.g., pH 7.20, P_{CO_2} 60 mm Hg HCO_3^- (from nomogram) = 23 mEq/1. Correcting pH to 7.35 and assuming P_{CO_2} is unchanged, HCO_3^- should be 32 mEq/l. HCO_3^- deficit = $(32 - 23) \times 0.6 \times 2.0$ kg = 13 mEq/l (desired correction). Give one-half the calculated dose (6 mEq/l) diluted in an equal volume of 5% glucose and water over 20 minutes. The decision to give the remainder should be based on subsequent acid base determinations.

In certain instances THAM may be a more desirable buffer, particularly when hypernatremia and hypercapnia are a concern. The drug acts by binding H^+ ions to form NH_3^+. It does not contribute to CO_2 build-up. Dosage of THAM 0.3 M = base deficit (from nomogram) × body weight (kg) × 0.3 = ml THAM.

Complications of Acid Base Therapy. Both $NaHCO_3$ and THAM therapy have potential complications, which must be considered when utilizing the drugs.

Complications of $NaHCO_3$. $NaHCO_3$ can cause serious sloughs when infused into peripheral tissues. This sloughing can occur with an infiltrated intravenous needle. Moderate rises in serum osmolarity can occur and may predispose to intracranial hemorrhage.[51] Serum sodium can be raised to excessively high levels by excessive use of sodium bicarbonate. Theoretically when CO_2 is released from $NaHCO_3$, its rapid transfer into the cerebrospinal fluid could produce acidemia in that fluid before compensation with bicarbonate can occur.

Complications of THAM. This drug can produce respiratory center depression and hypoglycemia. It should not be administered

A

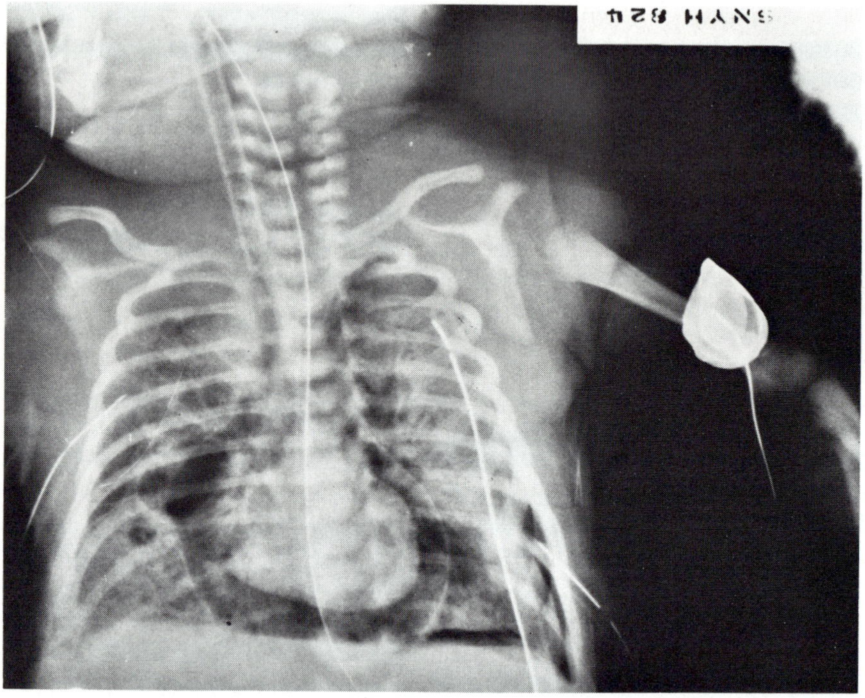

FIG. 16-24. Pneumopericardium in a patient with HMD in posteroanterior (*A*) and lateral (*B*) view (next page).

unless capability for respiratory support is available. When using THAM, the blood sugar should be measured at frequent intervals.

The Cardiovascular Problem. Close monitoring of blood pressure either indirectly by Doppler method or directly through an arterial line is essential to identify hypotension and shock as soon as possible. The cause of shock in HMD is not well understood. Blood loss due to intracranial hemorrhage, occult bleeding in the liver or elsewhere, or DIC is the explanation in some cases. Frequent measurement of hematocrit and, when appropriate, determination of clotting factors can aid in identifying these problems.

Frequently shock or hypotension develops when excessive blood loss has not occurred. In this case autonomic control of the circulation may be impaired. Waldman et al. have shown that in many instances small premature infants are unable to make the appropriate cardiovascular response to a stimulus such as tilting to 45 degrees (baroreflex stimulation).[140] In addition, they found that infants with HMD are more likely to lack the appropriate responses. These workers have also shown that the dive reflex is absent in some distressed premature infants. Theoretically this reflex can be viewed as a protective mechanism causing redistribution of blood flow from the periphery to central vital organs in response to stress. Absence of the reflex is further evidence of lack of autonomic control. On the other hand, other workers have shown decreased peripheral blood flow and increased vascular resistance in HMD indicating some capacity to respond to stress appropriately at least in mild cases of HMD.[81]

Shock and hypotension may also occur in infants with HMD who are receiving assisted ventilation because of inappropriately high I:E ratios or excessive use of CDAP. Both these techniques can reduce venous return, with a resultant decrease in cardiac output,

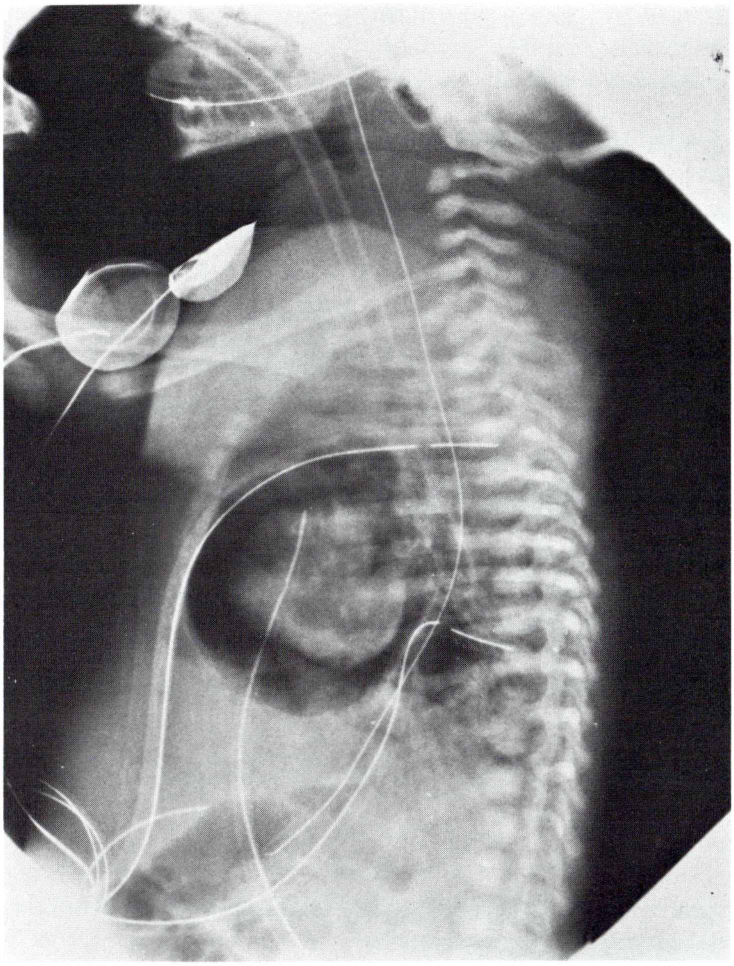

B

FIG. 16-24. Continued.

and these factors combined in an infant with poor autonomic control (inability in this case to vasoconstrict appropriately) can lead to shock.

Confusion exists as to what constitutes shock in a premature infant. The average blood pressure according to weight and age in normal infants is presented as a guide (Fig. 16-18A,B). When the blood pressure falls below 40 mm Hg systolic and/or 20 mm Hg diastolic, shock or impending shock should be considered. A fall in diastolic pressure frequently occurs prior to total cardiovascular collapse. Oliguria, poor peripheral perfusion clinically, and metabolic acidemia in the presence of a normal Pa_{O_2} must be used in addition. Current treatment is volume expansion with 10 ml/kg of plasma, plasminate, or blood after the possibility of respirator-induced shock has been excluded. Initially, this therapy is effective, but care must be taken to avoid excessive volume expansion subsequently.

Patent Ductus Arteriosus (*PDA*). Cardiac catheterization studies have demonstrated that patients with HMD have PDA from the outset. Both left-to-right and right-to-left shunting occurs through this structure. PDA is seldom clinically evident by murmurs in HMD until day 4 or 5 when pulmonary vascular resistance falls and sufficient flow develops through it. The murmur is systolic in character over the left sternal border or pulmonic area. A typical continuous murmur is unusual until 2 to 3 weeks of life. Most premature infants have a murmur of PDA at some time, generally at 2 to 3 weeks, and this characteristic applies to the infant with HMD. The reason for the PDA in premature infants is not clearly understood. The ductus is known to respond to oxygen, and hypoxemia can open a previously physiologically closed ductus arteriosus. Autonomic control and hormonal factors may also be involved. Prostaglandins of the E series have been shown to dilate an already constricted ductus,[29] and the role of inhibitors such as indomethacin in promoting ductus closure is presently under study.[69]

The problem presented by the PDA in HMD is not one of diagnosing PDA, but rather of determining its significance in the patient with HMD, particularly when pulmonary oxygen toxicity is beginning to occur. The two problems often appear simultaneously. The increased pulmonary blood flow of the PDA can worsen lung compliance, and thus require greater pressures from the respirator, which in turn worsens the lung disease.

Diagnosis of PDA is made by detecting a systolic murmur along the left sternal border or pulmonic area. Peripheral pulses are bounding in character. S_2 may be increased, and cardiomegaly may or may not be present. Pulmonary vascularity may or may not be increased. ECG sometimes shows a predominance of leftward forces, but this characteristic may be normal for a small premature infant (Fig. 16-25). The more usual predominance of rightward forces may also occur.

Having determined the presence of PDA, how does one proceed to determine its significance, particularly in the patient in congestive heart failure? Cardiomegaly and hepatomegaly together with tachycardia and gallop rhythm suggest congestive heart failure. The problem of its significance occurs most frequently when the infant is receiving respiratory support. If congestive failure or incipient failure is present, the infant should be digitalized and receive diuretics (furosemide). If no response to medical management is obtained within 48 hours, surgical closure of the PDA should be carried out. In general it is not necessary to perform a cardiac catheterization to confirm the diagnosis. The results of surgery, however, are not always favorable because of the presence of underlying BPD.

Echocardiography has been used in an attempt to determine the significance of PDA.[15,126] A significant PDA has an increased LA/AO ratio by this technique. Silverman et al. noted that all patients with LA/AO ratio greater than 1.15 require surgical closure (control value was 0.86 ± 0.10). Not all agree that an absolute value of LA/AO ratio for operation exists, but the echocardiogram is of great value in managing patients. Left ventricular end diastolic volume can also be determined by echocardiography, and this parameter is useful in evaluating the effect of the shunt on cardiac dynamics. Less clear cut is the approach to therapy when the child has a large left-to-right shunt and is not in congestive failure. Can closure of the shunt surgically, improve lung compliance sufficiently to allow the infant to be removed from the respirator? In some cases this approach is successful.

Certain authors report a much higher incidence of significant PDA in HMD than others.[44,79,151] The reasons for this discrepancy are not clear. More aggressive use of CDAP and fluids have been suggested as possible explanations.

Complications of catheterization. As the principal complications of umbilical artery and vein and peripheral vascular moni-

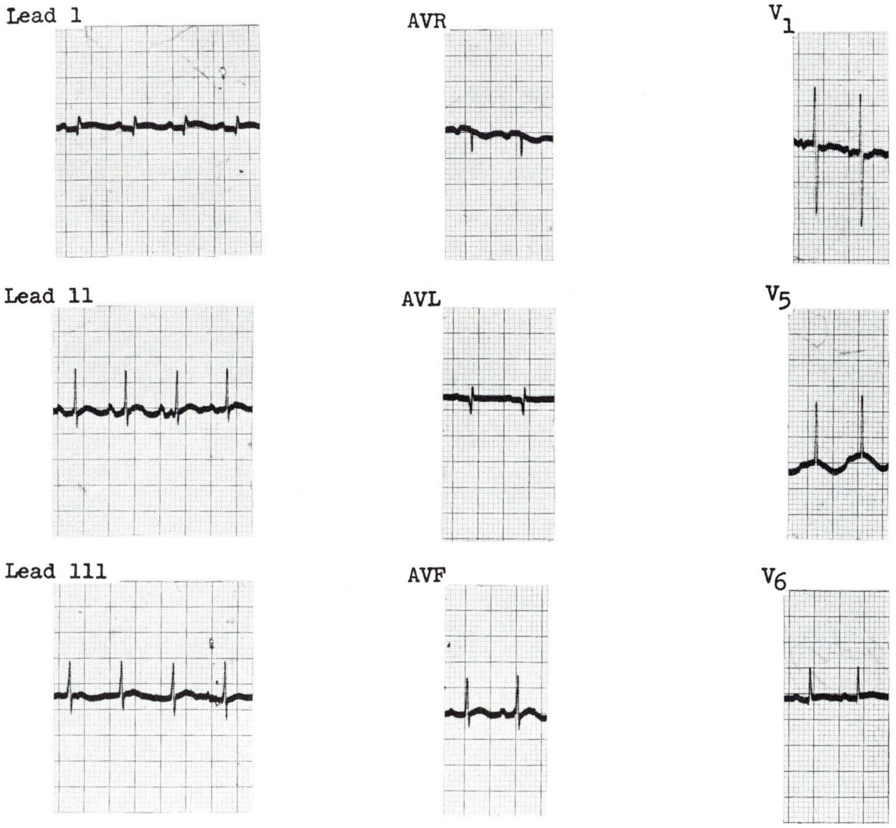

FIG. 16-25. EKG in a premature infant showing a predominance of leftward forces.

toring occur in the vascular system, it is appropriate to discuss them at this point. Because complications of umbilical artery and vein usage are common, they should be used only for proper indication.[98,133] Many mild cases of HMD can be managed without using these vessels for sampling.

Indwelling catheters, either peripheral or central, can be a source of sepsis. Careful attention to asepsis during placement of catheters and removing them as soon as possible can reduce the problem. It is not clear that prophylactic antibiotics can reduce catheter complications, perhaps because in many cases thrombi are produced around the catheter tip and become unreachable by antibiotics. If sepsis is present, the catheter should be removed.

Catheters in the umbilical vein may produce necrosis of the liver because of thrombosis and the effects of hypertonic solutions. This complication can be minimized by placing the umbilical venous catheters through the ductus venosus into the inferior vena cava at the right atrial junction. The catheter should not be allowed to remain in the heart because of the dangers of endocarditis (Fig. 16-26).[130] Catheters in the umbilical artery can produce peripheral ischemia in the toes, and obstruction to the renal arteries.[106] Thrombi can form around the catheter (end-hole catheters should be used) and produce emboli to the legs. To minimize these complications, the catheter must be placed low in the aorta (around L_2). Blanching or cyanosis of an extremity are indications for

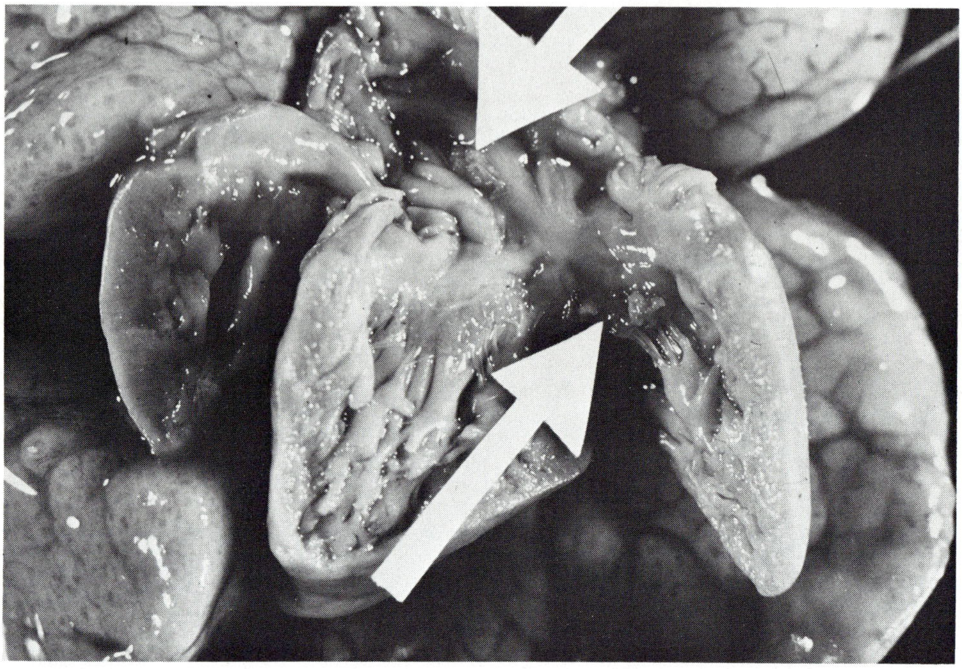

FIG. 16-26. Endocardial lesions in the right heart. The upper arrow points to a vegetation 2 mm in diameter attached to the anterior rim of the fossa ovalis. The lower arrow points to a similar lesion on the atrial surface of the tricuspid valve.

removal of the catheter. Assuring a continuous flow of fluid through the catheter can minimize thrombus formation. Some authors recommend a heparin-lock to avoid formation of thrombi in the catheter. The replacement of polyvinyl chloride catheters with silastic catheters may minimize this complication.[20] Skin sloughs can occur when hypertonic solutions infiltrate from peripheral veins.

Fluid Therapy and the Metabolic Problem. Infants with HMD are generally not able to receive fluid and calories by mouth using conventional techniques for the care of premature infants. However, as in all severely ill subjects, these considerations are often a determinant of life or death. The provision of adequate fluid and calories is complicated by two facts, namely, that renal function may be compromised in the distressed infant, and that metabolic needs are increased above normal by both the disease and methods of treatment.

Fluids and electrolytes. In the first 3 to 4 days of acute stage of the disease, fluid and electrolyte requirements should be provided entirely intravenously. Fluid requirements in sick infants depend to a large degree on particular modes of treatment, specifically whether the infant is being nursed in an incubator or open infrared heater and whether a respirator is being used. In addition, varying degrees of renal malfunction may be present in the form of acute tubular necrosis so that the likelihood of over- or underhydration is constantly present. For these reasons, fluid and electrolyte status must be reevaluated every 8 to 12 hours. Initially an evaluation of blood electrolytes, osmolarity, sugar, and calcium should be carried out. Urinalysis should be performed as soon as urine is available. Urine volume, urine sugar, and specific gravity should be monitored throughout the acute course.

If the infant is mild to moderately ill with HMD and being nursed in an isolette, fluid requirements are approximately 100 to 125 ml/kg/day. This fluid should be infused through a peripheral vein or properly positioned umbilical artery or vein catheter. The peripheral vein is preferred for this type of fluid therapy. The fluid is administered as 5 or 10% glucose and water depending on whether glycosuria is present. Electrolytes should be added on the second or third day in amounts determined by blood values and approximating daily requirements. Adequacy of fluid therapy can be assessed by determination of serum osmolality and urine osmolarity. A normally hydrated premature infant has a urine specific gravity of 1.005 and serum osmolality of 285 mOsm/l.

Infants with severe HMD are generally receiving respirator therapy and often are nursed under an infrared heater. This latter device may increase fluid requirements to as much as 300 ml/kg/day as a result of increased insensible loss through the skin.[47,147] Phototherapy also increases insensible losses. Respirator therapy reduces fluid requirements because of the necessity to humidify gases. Because all these effects on fluid therapy are different in any individual case, close monitoring of fluid and electrolyte status is necessary to avoid over- or underhydration. Every effort should be made to provide fluid and calories by mouth as soon as possible. If acute tubular necrosis and anuria occur, therapy must be adjusted to this complication. Of importance among other things is close evaluation for the presence of hyperkalemia.

Calories. Infants with HMD have increased caloric requirements, particularly as a result of the increased work of breathing. Premature infants in general have an increased oxygen cost of breathing. In addition, the nursing of infants in open infrared heaters may increase metabolic requirements. Basal caloric needs for a premature approach 50 cal/kg/day.[87] Provision of sufficient calories to prevent catabolism and to satisfy metabolic needs is one of the most important and difficult aspects of supportive care. Hypoglycemia (i.e., blood sugar less than 30 mg/100 ml) is common in distressed premature infants and must be monitored for and treated when it occurs.

Mild to moderately ill infants with HMD frequently can be maintained for several days by administering calories in the form of 10% glucose given at 100 cc/kg/day as 10% glucose in water. Forty calories per kilogram is provided, and this amount is often sufficient to prevent catabolism. However, this caloric intake is insufficient for longer than a day or so. Recently, amino-acid solutions and fat in the form of Intralipid have become available for use when prolonged intravenous therapy is required. In addition, many small infants are unable to handle 10% glucose infusions and develop glycosuria. If this complication is allowed to go unrecognized, body water and electrolytes are depleted by osmotic diuresis. Thus, glucose should be given only in concentrations that will not cause glycosuria. In some cases 1 or 2% glucose may be all that is tolerated.

Infants who require prolonged assisted ventilation have special caloric needs that can be difficult to fulfill. Total parenteral nutrition with glucose, amino acids, and Intralipid is often effective.[24,67] Great success has been achieved by some workers using milk feedings (formula or human milk) administered through a catheter passed into the stomach or the jejunum.[143] Both these techniques can produce complications. Total parenteral nutrition requires a well-established venous line either peripheral or central. Infection is a constant hazard. Amino-acid mixtures are variable in their composition and can produce metabolic acidosis. Intralipid has not been thoroughly evaluated in very sick infants, so the possibility of undiscovered side effects exists. The substance should not be given to jaundiced infants. Nasojejunal catheters can perforate the bowel[19] although, by using a silastic catheter with a mercury weight, this complication has not occurred.

Complications of therapy. Necrotizing enterocolitis (NEC) is a condition to be considered although it has not been established as a complication of therapy. The condition apparently has become common with the advent of neonatal intensive care. The disease frequently occurs in epidemic form, pointing to a bacterial or viral cause, but none has been consistently found. NEC occurs in the sickest infants, suggesting that shock, acidemia, and asphyxia are involved. Since infants with umbilical artery and venous catheters frequently develop it, these techniques may play an etiologic role. Animal studies have shown a protective effect when breast milk (of low osmolarity) is fed instead of cow's milk, which has a higher osmolarity.[13] The protective effect of breast milk may be due to the presence of macrophages and other immunologic factors that protect the bowel. In our own experience feeding of fresh breast milk has failed to prevent NEC.

The diagnosis of NEC is suggested when abdominal distention appears. Bloody diarrhea is an important accompaniment. The presence of air in the bowel wall (pneumatosis intestinalis) or portal vein radicals is diagnostic. Therapy at this stage consists of eliminating oral feedings and giving antibiotics by mouth and systemically. If perforation of the bowel occurs, surgical procedure is indicated. However, frequently the necrosis is so extensive at this time that surgical resection of the diseased segments is not feasible. Bowel stricture is often a late complication in the milder cases.

Problems of the Circulation and Blood. Problems related to hemorrhage and blood coagulation frequently complicate the course of infants with HMD and in certain instances influence outcome.

Very small premature infants frequently show excessive bruising over their entire body, related to increased capillary fragility and hypoxemia. These hemorrhages can frequently be so severe as to produce significant drops in hematocrit. Premature infants are known to have a decrease in most of the hemostatic factors compared to the full-term infant. In the smaller infants the decrease in hemostatic factor is greater, and in the presence of respiratory distress with its attendant problems of acidemia and hypoxemia, failure of these homeostatic mechanisms can be life-threatening. When excessive bleeding occurs, most often evident from puncture sites, appropriate studies of the coagulation mechanism should be carried out.

Intracranial hemorrhage. For the reasons mentioned previously, the premature infant is at great risk to develop intracranial bleeding, most particularly intraventricular hemorrhage. This problem is particularly common in infants with respiratory distress. The underlying susceptibility to bleeding may be accentuated by therapy such as sodium bicarbonate administration and hemodynamic factors related to assisted ventilation.

Disseminated intravascular coagulation (DIC). Infants with sepsis and infants with HMD frequently develop a disorder in which intravascular thrombus formation occurs causing the consumption of coagulation factors and their eventual depletion in the circulating plasma.[65] The condition commonly presents as excessive bleeding at venipuncture sites. When an infant with HMD develops this sign, screening tests such as platelet count, partial thromboplastin test (PTT), and prothrombin time (PT) should be performed. In DIC, platelets are reduced and PTT and PT are prolonged. PTT screens for most plasma coagulation factors except factors VII and XIII. PT is sensitive to deficiencies in the vitamin K dependent factors.

Current treatment of DIC is directed toward initial therapy of the etiologic factor and exchange transfusion. Replacement of factors is indicated when a non-consumption coagulopathy exists but in the presence of DIC may only be adding fuel to the fire.

ETIOLOGY AND PATHOGENESIS

The report by Avery and Mead demonstrating that the lungs of babies who died from HMD had abnormally high surface tension was a turning point in understanding the pathogenesis of HMD.[9] Previously, Von Neergaard had postulated that surface forces in the lung were important determinants of alveolar stability,[139] and Pattle had demonstrated that the mammalian lung contained surfactants that could lower surface tension in alveoli to nearly zero.[112] Pattle even suggested that abnormality of the surfactant system was involved in the cause of HMD. This pulmonary surface active material forms an alveolar surface film and, because of its low surface tension, acts as an anti-atelectatic factor. Thus in terms of current thinking, the decreasing FRC and histologically evident atelectasis in HMD are physiologic and pathologic correlates of the high alveolar surface tension, which results because of inhibition, destruction, or failure of production of surfactants.

The pulmonary surfactant system is rich in disaturated lecithin. Two pathways of de novo lecithin synthesis have been delineated, the choline pathway and the phosphatidyl ethanolamine pathway. At present, the choline pathway is considered to be the predominant one. Lecithin synthesis is presumed to occur in the type II alveolar pneumocytes. Lecithin can be demonstrated in large amounts in the human lung as early as 22 to 24 weeks of gestation, although if birth occurs at this time, the infant will die of respiratory distress. Furthermore, the concentration of lecithin in the premature infant's lung is less than that in the full-term infant's; it is lower still in the infant with HMD although the estimated amount exceeds that theoretically necessary to provide the alveolar lining. This apparent paradox has not been resolved.

At the present time, surfactant deficiency appears to explain most of the physiologic and pathologic changes in HMD.[48] Thus surfactant deficiency creates alveolar instability due to high surface tension and promotes alveolar collapse. Less well understood are the factors that produce surfactant deficiency. It is unlikely that immaturity is the sole factor, as evidenced by the greater occurrence of HMD in the second twin, absence of the disease in some obviously immature infants, and its occasional presence in documented full-term infants. These factors suggest that another insult added to a background of surfactant insufficiency may also be important. Such a factor could be perinatal asphyxia. Furthermore, the development of alveolar collapse (chronic pulmonary insufficiency of the premature[91]) in some immature infants after a period of relatively normal respiration suggests that it is possible to consume surfactant in excess of the ability of the lung to replenish it.

The many theories of causes of HMD have been reviewed by Nelson.[108] He concludes that shock as the initiating event appears to be the explanation that best encompasses all of them. Theories that have received varying degrees of popularity over the years include those related to pulmonary hypoperfusion,[26] PDA and left ventricular failure,[101] depression of the autonomic nervous system,[39] insufficient placental transfusion,[53] low serum proteins,[40] disturbances of coagulation,[65] fibrinolytic system,[4] as well as a primary surfactant problem.[9] More recently, the demonstration that in newborns with HMD the cord serum T_3 and the T_3 index are low and cord serum TSH is increased suggests an endocrine role in the cause.[34] In many instances factors that have been suggested as having an etiologic role in the disease have proven to be associated with usual findings in premature infants or are secondary phenomena.

The role of pulmonary surfactants in the

pathogenesis of the disease is clearly established although it is not necessarily the only factor.

PRENATAL DIAGNOSIS AND PREVENTION

When it is necessary to deliver a fetus prior to term, it is important to determine the risk of the infant developing HMD. This risk can be evaluated by examination of amniotic fluid for L/S ratio or shake test (see also Chapter 1). The L/S ratio is based on the fact that sphingomyelin (S) in the amniotic fluid is relatively constant throughout gestation, whereas lecithin (L) increases in concentration in the latter part of gestation (Fig. 16-27). The test assumes that these phospholipids enter the amniotic fluid from the lung and that the rising lecithin concentration is an index of lung maturation. Gluck and coworkers, who developed the L/S ratio test, state that, if the ratio is greater than 2.0, HMD is for all practical purposes unlikely to develop, although a few exceptions do exist.[59] On the other hand, when the L/S ratio is less than 2.0, the development of HMD is more likely but is not a certainty. Using the L/S ratio as an index, biochemical maturity of the fetal lung occurs at approximately 35 ± 2 weeks.[59]

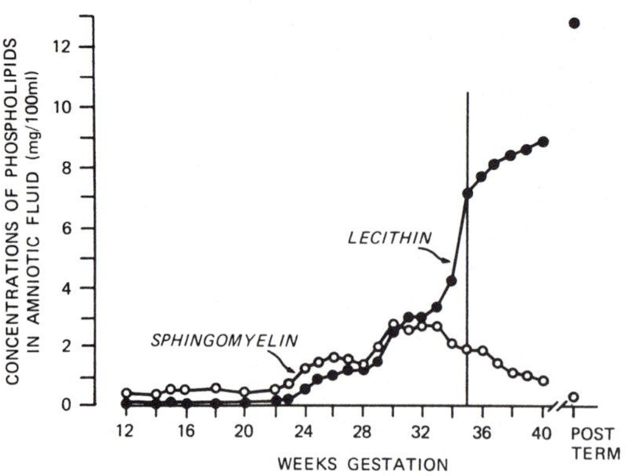

FIG. 16-27. L/S ratio in the amniotic fluid versus gestational age. (From Gluck.[59])

The shake test developed by Clements and associates takes advantage of the fact that the surfactant containing amniotic fluid produces stable bubbles on shaking.[28] This semiquantitative test is carried out by preparing serial dilutions of amniotic fluid in 47.5% alcohol and determining foam stability after shaking. A positive shake test (stable bubbles at 1:2 dilution) virtually excludes the possibility of HMD. A negative shake test has the same interpretation as an L/S ratio less than 2.0, but a greater number of false negatives apparently occur. Only a small number of affected infants have an intermediate reaction. These tests have revolutionized the assessment of risk for developing HMD.

Studies are currently under way around the country to confirm that antepartum glucocorticoids given more than 24 hours before delivery can prevent HMD in at-risk infants. It has previously been shown that glucocorticoids can accelerate lung maturation (surfactant synthesis and secretion) in a number of mammals.[37,38] The possible beneficial effect of this approach in the human is supported by the fact that cortisol concentrations in amniotic fluid increase in late gestation, and also by the observations of Spellacy et al.,[127] showing increased L/S ratio after maternal corticoid administration. Liggins and Howie were unable to show such an effect,[100] but did demonstrate a beneficial effect in reducing the incidence of HMD when betamethasone was administered at least 24 hours prior to delivery in infants under 32 weeks' gestation.[99] However, sufficient concern exists about the design of this study as well as possible side effects of maternal corticoid administration to advise that this approach be considered an area for further research. Furthermore, there are very few conditions associated with premature birth in which any therapy is a consideration, because of insufficient time or maternal considerations. Administration of corticoids to infants with established HMD has not been useful.[10]

PATHOLOGY

On gross examination the lungs of the infant with HMD are uniformly airless, red, and liverlike. Under light microscopy, atelectasis is the most striking feature, associated with dilatation of alveolar ducts. The eosinophilic "hyaline" membrane appears in the alveolar ducts overlying areas of epithelial necrosis (Fig. 16-28). If death occurs after 2 or 3 days, the membranes are fragmented and undergoing macrophage ingestion. The musculature of the pulmonary arterioles is thickened. Dilated lymphatics are a prominent feature. Electron microscopy reveals damage and disruption of alveolar epithelial cells.

Chronic Pulmonary Insufficiency of the Premature Infant (CPIP)[91]

Commonly, small premature infants (less than 1200 g birth weight after 28 to 30 weeks' gestation) appear to be in good condition at birth, only to develop respiratory difficulty hours to days later. This clinical presentation is sufficiently different from HMD to suggest a somewhat different cause although to date none has been proven.

CLINICAL COURSE

Characteristically the infant who develops CPIP is in good condition at birth as determined by Apgar score and need for increased oxygen. At birth physical examination of such an infant shows the usual overexpanded chest cage and breath sounds are normal. The favorable clinical condition is confirmed by studies of acid-base balance and blood gases. Arterial P_{O_2} ranges between 40 and 60 mm Hg in room air. At varying periods of time after birth but generally within 24 hours to 5 days the patient's condition gradually deteriorates. Respiratory difficulty characterized by prolonged apneic spells is noted. Tachypnea and subcostal retractions are minimal. Cyanosis is a prominent feature during the apneic spells. Chest volume becomes vis-

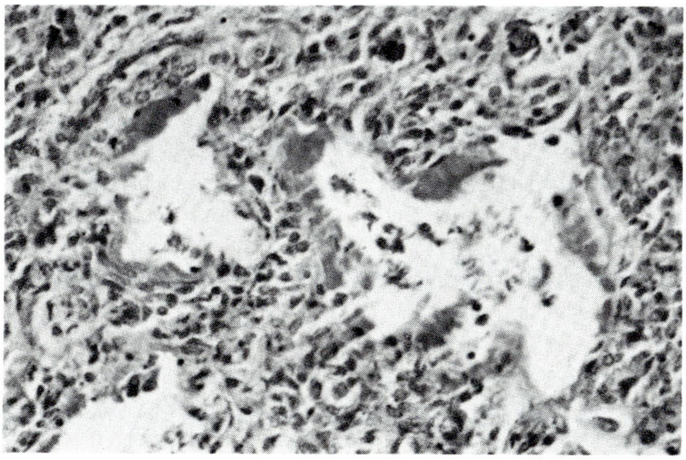

FIG. 16-28. Massive atelectasis and hyaline membranes in lung of infant who died at 2 days (HMD). Hale colloidal iron stain reveals membranes in blue. ×290 (From Scarpelli, E. M.: The Surfactant System of the Lung.[92])

ibly decreased. Hyperbilirubinemia is frequently a complicating factor.

Laboratory tests performed at this time show increasing respiratory acidemia and hypoxemia. Metabolic acidemia and hypotension are frequently present. Chest roentgenograms show a general haziness, and air bronchograms are reflections of the underlying severe atelectasis.

Infants with this condition require the same supportive measures as in classic HMD. Recovery is gradual over many weeks and complications of therapy are frequent. Because of the extensive period of time in which oxygen therapy must be provided, the development of various grades of RLF is a real possibility. Intraventricular hemorrhage is commonly the cause of death.

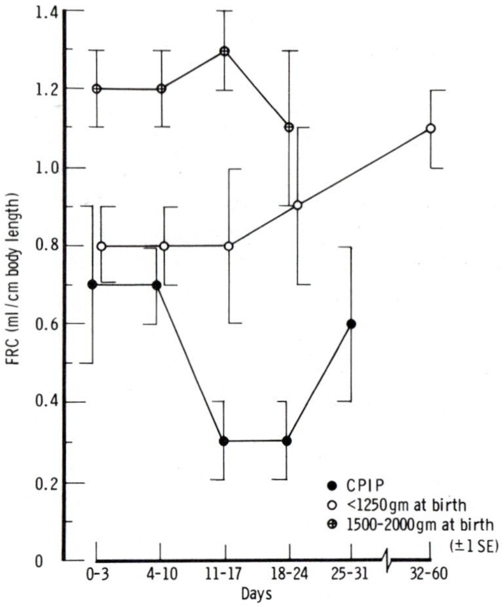

FIG. 16-29. Serial studies of FRC in non-distressed premature infants over various gestational ages and in CPIP.

PATHOLOGIC AND PHYSIOLOGIC CORRELATES

Atelectasis is the important finding in the lungs of these infants at autopsy. Unlike patients with HMD it is unusual for patients with CPIP to show the hyaline membrane. The pathologic changes of intracranial hemorrhage and NEC frequently complicate the clinical course in these infants. Krauss and Auld have reported on the abnormalities of pulmonary physiology in these infants.[91] FRC decreases in the first week (Fig. 16-29) associated with decreasing Pa_{O_2} and increasing Pa_{CO_2}. Changes in blood gases are due to abnormalities of $\dot{V}A/\dot{Q}$, which include right-to-left cardiopulmonary shunting (low Pa_{O_2}) and areas of high $\dot{V}A/\dot{Q}$ (high P_{CO_2}). Lung compliance is markedly decreased. These physiologic abnormalities persist for long periods of time even when clinical recovery is apparent. Krauss and co-workers have shown that immature prematures do not show the appropriate hyperventilatory response to carbon dioxide.[82] The presence of apnea in these infants often when P_{CO_2} is markedly elevated correlates with this observation, although the cause of the apnea is unknown.

TREATMENT

As in the case of HMD, supportive care is the only method of therapy for CPIP, and the reader is referred to this section for details. However, certain points in approach to treatment must be modified for these very small infants. Pediatricians frequently are lulled into a false sense of security when a very immature baby appears to be in good clinical condition. These circumstances frequently delay referral from a community hospital to a neonatal intensive care unit. Clearly, these small infants should be transferred as soon as possible. The good clinical condition may also delay the placement of umbilical arterial and venous catheters so that, when these catheters are required for monitoring, placement is technically difficult or impossible.

For these reasons infants under 1200 g birth weight should have an umbilical artery and vein catheter placed as soon as possible in anticipation of problems. Monitoring of blood gases, respiratory rate, and heart rate are extremely important. If no problems develop, the catheters can be removed in several days.

Perhaps the major problem in management of these infants as distinct from HMD is presented by the prolonged episodes of apnea. Apnea becomes significant when bradycardia is associated. The cause of apnea in these infants is unknown. Both central nervous system factors and peripheral pulmonary factors appear to be involved. Thus, unresponsiveness of the respiratory center to the usual stimuli as well as the extremely low compliance of the lungs, making breathing extremely difficult, are factors. Treatment directed toward both these deficiencies has been advocated. In the early stages of the disease cutaneous stimulation frequently terminates apnea. Increased FI_{O_2} (0.25 to 0.35) often makes apneic spells less frequent. Measures that increase FRC (such as CPAP or constant negative expiratory pressure (CNEP)) may secondarily affect stretch receptor reflexes and abolish or lessen apnea in many cases. More recently theophylline has been suggested for apnea although the details of safe dosage are not well established. This therapy for apnea is still under investigation and is not recommended for the routine therapy of apnea. Infants with CPIP may eventually require assisted ventilation. The progressive fall in FRC suggests that early CPAP could prevent alveolar collapse in these infants although the risk of pneumothorax must be weighed.

Supportive care of the metabolic problem in these infants frequently poses difficult technical problems. Maintenance of venous catheters is difficult, and the size of the infants limits the number of sites for intravenous therapy. In addition, NEC is a frequent complication. PDA can complicate the course of CPIP, and the same considerations about this problem obtain as for HMD.

ETIOLOGY AND PATHOGENESIS

The progressive decrease in FRC noted in CPIP and the presence of atelectasis at autopsy suggests the possibility of a surfactant insufficiency. The progressive nature of the condition raises the possibility that the surfactant supply is adequate initially but utilization outpaces the lung's ability to replenish the substance. The delayed appearance of respiratory distress noted in this condition may be related to the disappearance of trapped gas, as the clinical signs appear at this time. It could be theorized that trapped gas keeps alveoli open and producing surfactant and that resolution of trapped gas allows collapse to occur by a mechanism similar to that described by Wyszagradski et al.[148]

Apnea of the Premature Infant

As has been mentioned in other sections, apnea is a prominent feature of a number of the respiratory distress syndromes of the newborn. No theory of causes fully explains all the facts that have been accumulated. Interest in the subject arises because of the obvious relationship between apnea, hypoxemia, and neurologic damage.

PHYSIOLOGIC CONSIDERATIONS

While conventional wisdom might suggest that apnea of prematurity is directly related to the mechanisms of respiratory control, no unitarian theory has been developed to explain the process. Within this context one must explain that apnea is more common in the most immature and on the second or third day of life rather than on the first. It appears more likely that multiple factors can produce apnea. No agreement exists on the length of time of cessation of breathing that constitutes apnea. Most authors have used an apneic pause of 20 seconds or apnea of any duration associated with bradycardia to define significant apnea. However pauses of shorter duration are common. Two patterns of apnea and bradycardia occur. One pattern occurs when bradycardia follows apneic pauses by 15 to 20 seconds, in which it would seem that bradycardia is directly related to hypoxemia (Fig. 16-30). The other pattern is seen when bradycardia occurs almost simultaneously with apnea, which would seem to favor a reflex mechanism.

Interest in apnea has stimulated research on the control of breathing in the premature infant. From these studies of premature infants as they may relate to apnea, it can be stated that:

(1) Prolonged hypoxemia (i.e., over 5 min.) increases the occurrence of apnea.[115]

(2) Short-term hypoxemia (3 to 4 breaths of 15% O_2) stimulates respiration.[83]

(3) 100% O_2 breathing initially depresses respiration and causes apnea, indicating good chemoreceptor tone.[50,83]

(4) Infants of low gestational age are less responsive to CO_2 measured in terms of minute volume increase than more mature premature infants and full-term infants.[82]

(5) At least some of the decreased response is related to lung mechanics (low FRC and compliance—it is literally too mechanically difficult to respond).[85]

(6) Attempts to determine respiratory center drive by measurement of $P_{0.1}$ (airway pressure in the first 0.1 second after airway occlusion at FRC) shows poor response in some apneic infants and a good response in others.[88]

Considerable attention has been directed toward studying the effect of state on breathing and apnea. Gabriel and co-workers report more apnea (10 seconds) during REM sleep.[55] Krauss and co-workers found this not to be true in their infants.[84] Environmental temperature changes, such as sudden reduction in heat loss, have been proposed as a cause of apnea in immature infants.[113]

Periodic breathing is common in the premature infant. Fenner et al. found it to be more common during REM sleep.[50] Thibeault et al. have shown that periodic breathing can be abolished by inflation of the chest and stimulated by chest wall compression.[132] Periodic breathing has been initiated in premature infants on return to room air after a short period of 10% O_2 breathing. Rigatto

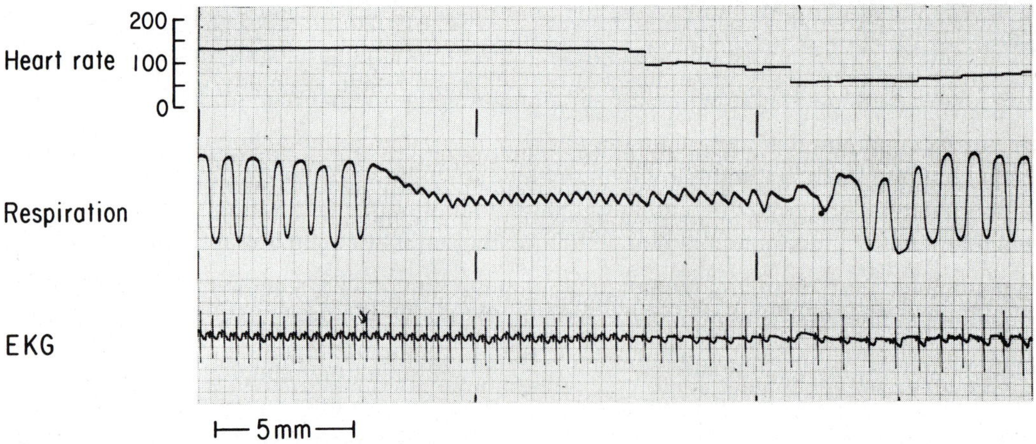

FIG. 16-30. Bradycardia occurring 15 to 20 seconds after the onset of apnea.

and Brady report that infants with periodic breathing hyperventilate, and they suggest hypoxia as a primary event.[115]

DIAGNOSIS

Apnea is detected by cardiorespiratory monitoring of low birth weight infants. The presence of bradycardia with apnea defines significant apnea. In a study of 22 premature infants Daily et al. noted that apnea of greater than 30 seconds occurred in 25% of infants in the first 10 days.[35] In contrast to apnea, periodic breathing is more common 3 to 4 days after birth than in the first day. Premature and full-term infants develop apnea in response to a wide variety of conditions. Thus, sepsis, intracranial hemorrhage, and hypoglycemia must be excluded before primary apnea can be diagnosed.

TREATMENT

When other disease processes have been excluded, a diagnosis of primary apnea can be made. Clinically physicians tend to wait for bradycardia (heart rate less than 100) with apnea before intervening. This approach may be unwise in that by this time significant metabolic changes may have occurred. Although not always technically perfect, monitoring of respiration should be used to determine the presence of apnea and cutaneous stimulation applied when it appears.

Treatment initially consists of cutaneous stimulation, which may be all that is necessary. By nursing infants in slightly increased oxygen environments, it is possible to reduce the number and severity of apneic spells. Constant distending airway pressure can reduce number of apneic spells presumably by increasing FRC, stabilizing blood gases, and in turn reducing the oscillations of blood gases affecting the respiratory center. Nasal prongs are a useful method of administration of CDAP. More recently aminophylline administered rectally or orally has been shown to reduce apnea.[96,123,135] This substance is a potent central nervous system stimulant. Theophylline has been shown to increase alveolar ventilation and increase sensitivity to CO_2 in adults, suggesting a direct effect on the respiratory center. On the other hand, some evidence suggests that the positive effect on apnea may be due to a general change of the central nervous system state. Theophylline can produce significant tachycardia and hypertension in premature infants, and dosage is difficult to predict. Administration of the drug must be monitored by frequent blood levels, as great variation in metabolism is common in premature infants.[5] At the moment this drug cannot be recommended for routine use.

Respiratory Problems Characterized by Hyperaeration

In contrast to the premature infant with HMD in which the prominent feature is alveolar collapse, the conditions to be discussed next have as their predominant characteristic a hyperaerated appearance of the chest, both clinically and radiographically. Within this group of disorders are meconium aspiration and transient tachypnea of the newborn. These conditions occur most commonly in the full-term infant.

MECONIUM ASPIRATION

Meconium aspiration pneumonitis is seen almost exclusively in the intrauterine growth retarded infant, the full-term infant with hypoxemia, and the postmature infant. Those who develop the condition have been subjected to an intrauterine insult, generally hypoxemia, which causes them to expel meconium into the amniotic fluid. The same hypoxic insult also provokes deep gasping movements in which the meconium stained fluid is aspirated into the lungs. The bronchiolitis that is produced by meconium is responsible for the clinical picture. Surprisingly the pathology of the lung in meconium aspiration often does not reflect the clinical picture. A true pneumonitis is seldom seen, often only squames and flecks of yellow meconium. Absence of pathologic change suggests that a chemically induced spasm produces the bronchiolitis. The frequency of meconium aspiration is related to obstetric practice.

Infants who have aspirated meconium are at risk to develop pneumothorax and pneumomediastinum presumably secondary to the alveolar overdistention from a ball-valve effect. Pneumothorax occurs when an emphysematous area ruptures into the pleura. Pneumomediastinum results when extra-alveolar air tracks through interstitial tissue to the mediastinum.

Disturbances of normal pulmonary physiology in these infants result in cyanosis and hypercarbia. In contrast to the infant with HMD, the low Pa_{O_2} is due to both the right-to-left cardiopulmonary shunting and the maldistribution of ventilation through areas of low $\dot{V}A/\dot{Q}$. This latter disturbance is similar to that produced by emphysema or asthma in the adult. Because in some cases cyanotic heart disease cannot be excluded, cardiac catheterization has been performed. The use of echocardiography may obviate the need for such studies.

Clinical Picture. Invariably, the infant with meconium aspiration pneumonitis has a history of intrauterine fetal distress and the amniotic fluid is meconium stained. Not all infants with this history develop the disease; however, they should all be observed carefully for 12 to 24 hours. Respiratory distress may develop immediately after birth, but more commonly it develops over the ensuing 12 to 24 hours. Tachypnea, sometimes to rates over 100 breaths per minute, together with a markedly overinflated appearance to the chest are the dominant clinical features. Cyanosis may or may not be obvious. Subcostal retractions are never as prominent as in HMD. This clinical picture should prompt the physician to review the birth history and examine the infant closely for evidence of meconium staining, particularly the fingernails, toenails, and umbilical cord. Aspiration of gastric contents for meconium can be a useful technique to confirm the diagnosis.

Physical examination reveals that the infant has the characteristics of intrauterine growth retardation (IUGR) or postmaturity, or he may even be a normal full-term infant. Meconium aspiration is exceedingly rare in a true premature infant. The characteristic barrel-chested appearance is noted. Breath sounds are generally well transmitted. Heart sounds may be difficult to hear when a pneumomediastinum is present. The clinical picture may be complicated by other effects of hypoxemia involving the brain and kidneys. Seizures, hypotonia, and hypertonia are frequent. Anuria and other evidence of renal involvement may be present. Most infants with meconium aspiration who survive recover within 7 to 10 days, although the most severely affected may have respiratory insufficiency for weeks or months as a result of respirator-induced complications.

Management. Can meconium aspiration be prevented or modified? If the condition results from an intrauterine insult, it would seem unlikely that anything short of prevention of insult could prevent the disease. On the other hand, removal of as much meconium as possible from the airway at birth is mandatory, and it is recommended that the trachea be visualized directly and meconium aspirated directly in every suspect case. This approach must be balanced against the urgent requirements of the infant for oxygenation.

Treatment is supportive and thus is problem oriented, as for HMD. A constant awareness of the possibility of pneumothorax developing is most important. As with all infants with respiratory distress an initial chest roentgenogram (posteroanterior and lateral) should be the initial immediate diagnostic test. Of particular interest will be whether pneumothorax or pneumomediastinum is present. If pneumothorax is suspected, a lateral decubitus film may be helpful in confirming the diagnosis. Typical chest roentgenogram in this condition is characterized by coarse streaks of atelectasis associated with a hyperaerated appearance, with increased anteroposterior diameter of the chest and flattened diaphragms (Fig. 16-31). This picture may take at least 12 hours to develop so that often initially a normal appearance may be seen. Frequently, cardiomegaly is noted on chest roentgenograms, sometimes to the extent that cyanotic congenital heart disease must be excluded.

As in all patients with respiratory distress, blood gases should be obtained. Severe hypoxemia and hypercarbia may occur in meconium aspiration. Generally, the first blood gases obtained reflect the intrauterine insult; thus hypoxemia, metabolic and respiratory acidemia, and shock may be present. Later, only hypoxemia may persist, and frequently a low P_{CO_2} is noted. Most infants with meconium aspiration require an increased $F_{I_{O_2}}$. Assisted ventilation is indicated when respiratory acidemia is present.

Meconium aspiration should be treated with antibiotics for two reasons. First, meconium is a good culture medium, and second, the condition cannot always be differentiated from a primary bacterial pneumonia.

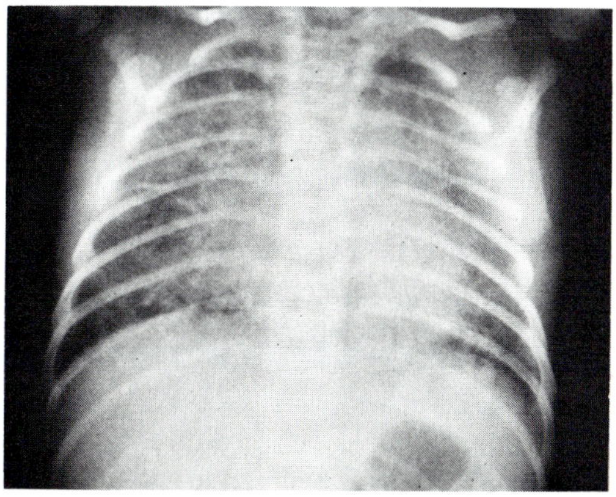

FIG. 16-31. Chest roentgenogram of infant with meconium aspiration pneumonia.

A change in clinical condition at anytime should suggest that a pneumothorax has occurred, and a chest roentgenogram should be taken. The poor clinical condition may dictate that aspiration of air should be performed before the roentgenogram can be taken. Transillumination of the chest can be useful in determining size and site of the pneumothorax.[95] The decision to treat a pneumothorax is based on severity of symptoms. A tension pneumothorax with mediastinal shift interferes with cardiac output and produces hypoxemia (Fig. 16-32). If shock or severe cyanosis and acidemia are present, surgical removal of the air is indicated. An asymptomatic pneumothorax can be observed provided surgical treatment is readily available. In some instances treatment of a small pneumothorax by having the patient breathe 100% oxygen for several hours can be successful, but this procedure should not be used unless the availability of surgical treatment is at hand.

Surgical treatment involves placement of a catheter in the chest with connection to underwater seal drainage. In an emergency, aspiration of air through a needle by a stopcock and syringe can be lifesaving. When the patient is receiving CDAP, the catheter should not be removed even though the pneumothorax appears to be closed. Pneumomediastinum rarely poses a threat to life. It is unusual in the newborn for air to track into the neck in spontaneous pneumomediastinum, but this complication is common in iatrogenic pneumomediastinum. A pneumomediastinum can produce a bizarre picture on the chest roentgenogram, but should not be mistaken for a pneumothorax (Fig. 16-33), and a lateral decubitus roentgenogram film can be helpful in clarifying the issue. Pneumomediastinum requires no treatment.

Differential Diagnosis. Cyanotic congenital heart disease frequently must be excluded in a meconium stained infant. Both conditions can

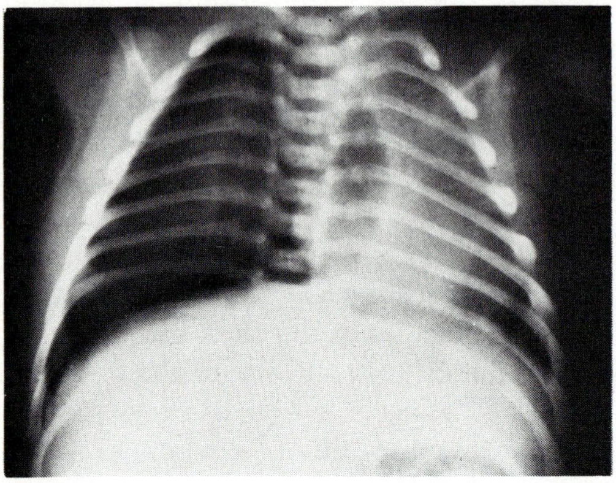

FIG. 16-32. Tension pneumothorax as seen on chest roentgenogram in an infant with meconium aspiration.

produce cyanosis and cardiomegaly on chest roentgenogram, and, of course, an infant with heart disease may be meconium stained. In general, the cyanosis of meconium aspiration responds readily to oxygen therapy, whereas it does not in transposition of the great arteries or hypoplastic left heart syndrome.

A recently recognized condition that may also provide confusion is the so-called "persistence of fetal circulation."[56,57] This condition can be idiopathic or associated with perinatal factors such as hypoxia,[124] hyperviscosity,[62] meconium aspiration, or polycythemia. Haworth and Reid report pathologic changes of three cases classified as idiopathic; one patient survived for 3 months.[66] These changes consisted of increased thickness of muscle in normally muscular pulmonary vessels and extension of muscle into vessels normally lacking it. In other cases the lungs are normal. Clinically, infants with this condition resemble meconium aspiration and many are meconium stained. Hypoxemia occurs due to right-to-left shunts through the foramen ovale and the patent ductus. Chest roentgenogram may show cardiomegaly, and ECG may reveal right ventricular hypertrophy (RVH), although both may be normal. Diagnosis can be made only by cardiac catheterization, which is performed to exclude cyanotic congenital heart disease. Presumably the cause relates to those factors that prevent the normal fall in pulmonary vascular resistance after birth. Apparently, these factors can be functional or represent pathologic change in vessels. Treatment is supportive. Some infants do recover. Attempts to relieve pulmonary vascular spasm with drugs have been difficult to control. It is not entirely clear whether most of these cases are really infants who have aspirated meconium.

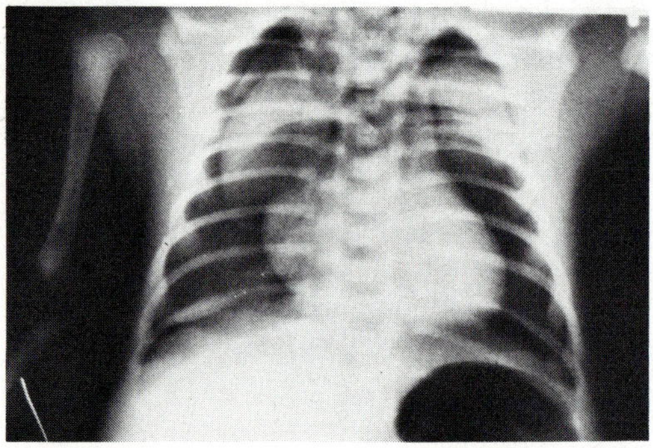

FIG. 16-33. Pneumomediastinum showing the "batwing" appearance of the thymic shadow.

TRANSIENT TACHYPNEA OF THE NEWBORN

Avery and co-workers described this syndrome, which occurs primarily in full-term infants and perhaps also in larger premature infants.[8] Overall prognosis for this condition is good although during the peak of the disease the infants appear desperately ill.

Clinical Picture. Many full-term infants have transient respiratory distress for several hours after birth. This distress is probably a result of excessive gas trapping. On the other hand, the designation, transient tachypnea of the newborn, should be reserved for a respiratory distress that persists for at least 12 hours after birth and more commonly for 3 to 5 days.[128] Both full-term and larger premature infants are affected. Clinically, the condition resembles meconium aspiration except that the infants are not meconium stained and the amniotic fluid is clear. The incidence of the condition is so variable that obstetric practice may play a role. Most often infants have been delivered by cesarean section or have had a precipitous delivery. Respiratory distress is apparent soon after birth, with worsening over the subsequent days and with a return to normal in 7 to 10 days. Some infants show only mild tachypnea and may never be cyanotic. In other cases, tachypnea is prominent, often with respiratory rates over 100 and considerable cyanosis.

A prominent feature of the examination of infants with this condition is a barrel-chested appearance, and because of this feature subcostal retractions are not prominent. As the infant improves, the chest assumes a more normal size. Breath sounds are well transmitted. Blood gases most frequently show a mild respiratory alkalemia with P_{CO_2} often less than 30 mm Hg. Chest roentgenograms show the so-called wet lung appearance, characterized by increased bronchopulmonary markings, liquid in interlobar fissures, and small collections of liquid particularly at the costophrenic angles (Fig. 16-34). Chest volume appears increased with increased antero-posterior diameters and flat diaphragms.

Management. The condition is self-limited and mild in most instances. Supportive care involves provision of increased oxygen to maintain Pa_{O_2}. Intravenous therapy should be provided during the height of the respiratory distress. Antibiotics should be given because of the possibility of pneumonia.

Etiology and Pathophysiology. The cause of transient tachypnea is only speculative. Because the presence of extra-alveolar liquid is a prominent feature, delayed clearance of lung

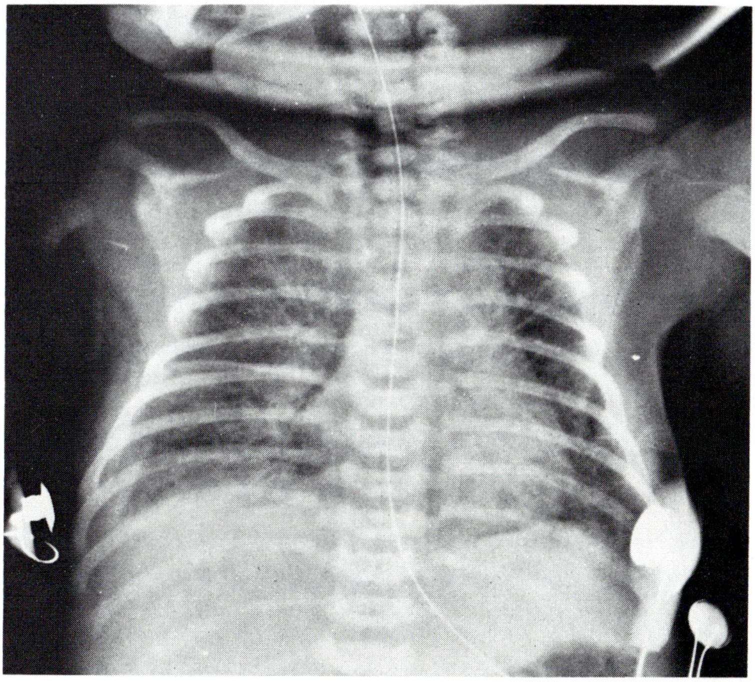

FIG. 16-34. Chest roentgenogram of infant with clinical diagnosis of transient tachypnea of the newborn. Note fluid in interlobar fissure on the right.

liquid has been suggested. An element of increased gas trapping because of retained liquid would explain the hyperaerated appearance. Physiologically the infants resemble those with meconium aspiration in that Pa_{O_2} is decreased because of both maldistribution of ventilation and shunting. Hyperventilation results in low Pa_{CO_2}.

Miscellaneous Pulmonary Conditions

PULMONARY HEMORRHAGE

Alveolar and interstitial pulmonary hemorrhage is rarely obvious clinically but is a frequent finding at autopsy in premature infants.[7] It is not clear whether pulmonary hemorrhage is a disease entity or merely secondary to a systemic process. However, on occasion the condition is seen in the absence of other bleeding, suggesting that it is a separate disease. In these cases the hemorrhage is generalized throughout the lungs. A relationship between increased intracranial pressure, anoxia, and pulmonary hemorrhage has been suggested.[102] Pulmonary hemorrhage is also a feature of generalized bleeding disorders such as disseminated intravascular coagulation. In these cases hemorrhage has a focal lobular distribution. Pulmonary hemorrhage is reported on occasion in association with hyaline membrane disease, pneumonia,[97] erythroblastosis fetalis and kernicterus,[3] and congenital heart disease. In one study Esterly and Oppenheimer reported massive pulmonary hemorrhage in 17.8% of autopsied newborns.[45]

Pulmonary hemorrhage is suspected clinically when obvious blood-stained liquid is seen arising from the trachea. Infants who have pulmonary hemorrhage at autopsy are usually in respiratory distress from birth. No specific laboratory tests exist although, if bleeding is noted, a coagulation work-up should be performed. Chest roentgenograms most frequently show total opacity of the lung fields although on occasion a reticulogranular appearance and air bronchograms are noted.

Treatment is supportive. If DIC or other coagulation defect is present, it should be treated. Problems are similar to those of infants with HMD. The usual monitoring procedures are indicated, including frequent determination of blood gases.

As much confusion exists about the cause and pathogenesis of pulmonary hemorrhage as exists about its place in the category of diseases. Hypoxemia and hyperoxia[122] have been suggested as etiologic factors. Infants with pulmonary hemorrhage frequently have received high concentrations of oxygen, and oxygen is capable of damaging capillaries to produce hemorrhage. In some instances an etiologic relationship between infection and hemorrhage has seemed apparent. Rowe and Avery noted a common association between HMD and pulmonary hemorrhage and suggested that high intralveolar surface tension could cause red blood cell transudation from capillaries into alveoli.[118]

WILSON-MIKITY SYNDROME

In 1960 Wilson and Mikity described a hitherto unrecognized form of respiratory distress in premature infants.[145] Time of onset of the condition was later than for HMD. A clinical picture of increasing tachypnea, cyanosis, and occasionally eventual cor pulmonale was described. However, the chest roentgenogram was considered to be the diagnostic feature. It was characterized by increased bronchovascular markings, atelectatic streaks and hyperaeration, and a typical multicystic appearance. At autopsy the lungs in their patients showed alveolar septal thickening and mononuclear cell infiltration. Recovery occurred in some cases. Numerous case reports and clinical studies have been presented since. The cause is unknown; in fact it is not clear that Wilson-Mikity syndrome is a distinct entity. In an extensive study of pulmonary function in premature infants, Burnard et al.[22,23] considered Wilson-Mikity disease at the extreme end of a spectrum of pulmonary insufficiency in premature infants.

Various causes have been suggested, including pulmonary dysmaturity[11] (developmentally, i.e., due to retarded and uneven maturation)[103] and oxygen toxicity.[131] The similarity in the chest roentgenogram to bronchopulmonary dysplasia suggests a relationship to oxygen. The presence of cor pulmonale in some cases also strengthens this hypothesis. On the other hand, the pathologic changes are different from those of POT in many instances with wide cellular septa, fibrotic and muscular alveolar septa, and mononuclear infiltration in a spotty distribution. On gross examination, the lungs have a characteristic appearance of uneven aeration.

Pathophysiology. Infants with this condition have increased oxygen requirements because of right-to-left cardiopulmonary shunting and maldistribution of ventilation. Carbon dioxide retention is due to alveoli with high $\dot{V}_A/\dot{Q}$ relationships. Mechanically, compliance is decreased markedly and airway resistance is increased. High pulmonary vascular resistance has been measured in the infants with cor pulmonale.[94] RVH is seen on the ECG. This high resistance is unresponsive to oxygen breathing suggesting a structural vascular change rather than spasm. Infants that have had cardiac catheterization show a PDA with minimal bidirectional shunting.

Clinical Picture and Diagnosis.[70,129] The condition most often affects premature infants in the lowest birth weight, although several cases have been identified in full-term infants following meconium aspiration. Onset of respiratory distress is variable from birth to 2 to 3 weeks of age. Respiratory distress is characterized by tachypnea, subcostal retractions, cyanosis, and apnea. The distress may persist for weeks and in some cases months. In the latter case cor pulmonale is generally present. Subsequent follow-up has shown complete healing of the lung and partial regression of cor pulmonale. Physical examination of the chest may be normal, although in many cases rales and wheezing are noted. When cor pulmonale develops, signs of RVH and congestive failure may be noted.

Diagnosis is made by the clinical picture plus a characteristic chest roentgenographic appearance. Early in the clinical course chest roentgenogram shows increased reticular markings, which are frequently noted in non-distressed infants as well. When the clinical picture is well developed, chest roentgenograms show a bilateral diffuse reticulonodular or reticular pattern with lucent foci giving a bubbly appearance (Fig. 16-35). Later, coarse streaks radiating from the hilum appear associated with areas of emphysema but disappearance of the bubbly appearance. Occasionally, fractures at the posterior rib angles are evident.

Treatment. Oxygen therapy is the cornerstone of treatment. Many of the infants who develop the classic roentgenographic appearance have had oxygen therapy from birth. Frequently, only little added oxygen is re-

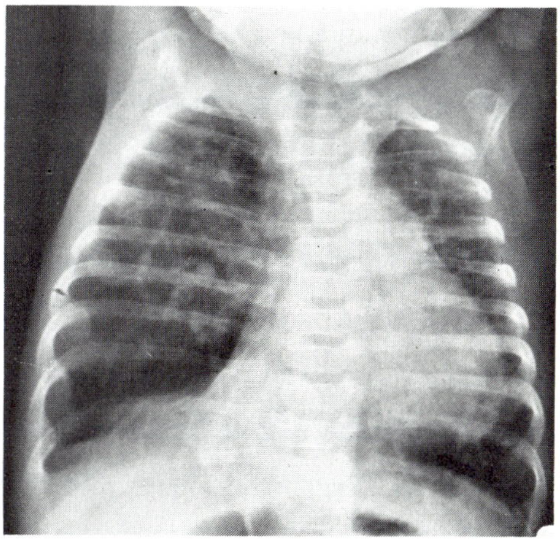

FIG. 16-35. Typical radiographic appearance of Mikity-Wilson disease showing translucent areas in lung parenchyma.

quired (e.g., FI_{O_2} of 0.25), and if it is removed, the patient deteriorates. Problems encountered in treatment are the same as for HMD. Acid-base and blood gas monitoring may be necessary for months. In these cases infrequent sampling from peripheral arteries (radial, brachial, and temporal) is necessary. Because of the prolonged requirement for oxygen therapy and difficulty in providing constant monitoring, these infants are at considerable risk for RLF. Assisted ventilation must be provided usually on an intermittent basis. Digitalis and diuretics may be required if congestive heart failure develops. These patients require considerable patience on the part of the staff and parents in that the need for a minimally increased oxygen environment is seemingly endless. However, most infants recover. The chest film returns to normal from 6 months to 1 year later. The first several years of life may be associated with an increased number of lower respiratory infections.

PNEUMOTHORAX AND PNEUMOMEDIASTINUM

These conditions have already been mentioned as complications of HMD and meconium aspiration. Frequently, they are the only presenting finding in an infant with respiratory distress, so it is appropriate to consider them as a disease entity. Early recognition and prompt treatment are mandatory and can be lifesaving. Both conditions generally occur together; however, pneumomediastinum is invariably benign and must not be confused on roentgenograms with a pneumothorax.

The following conditions are associated with pneumothorax and pneumomediastinum:

(1) Apparently spontaneous pneumothorax and pneumomediastinum.

(2) Trauma from intubation.

(3) Meconium aspiration pneumonitis.

(4) HMD. Pneumothorax and pneumomediastinum occur spontaneously in the larger vigorous infants with HMD who can produce large intrapleural pressure changes.

(5) Complications of CDAP or assisted ventilation with or without PEEP. With the exception of traumatic pneumomediastinum it is rare for air to track into the neck in the newborn.

Clinical Picture of Pneumothorax. Infants with this condition have signs that depend on the size of the pneumothorax and the presence or absence of a tension pneumothorax. It is likely that a considerable number of infants have the condition and are unidentified. A high index of suspicion in conditions that predispose to pneumothorax and pneumomediastinum is the best method of ensuring prompt diagnosis. The development of these lesions can occur acutely, in which case an abrupt change in clinical condition is apparent, or more gradually, in which case the most frequent sign is an increased environmental oxygen requirement. If a tension pneumothorax is present, cardiac output is decreased because of kinking of the great veins and the infant appears shocky. In addition, physical examination in tension pneumothorax shows deviation of cardiac apex away from the affected side, and breath sounds are absent as well.

Clinical Signs of Pneumomediastinum. Pneumomediastinum may be unrecognized because of its benign course. Distant heart sounds on auscultation are the only diagnostic sign.

Diagnosis. The chest roentgenogram taken in the anteroposterior and lateral projection (horizontal beam with patient supine) makes the diagnosis and allows assessment of size of the lesion. More recently, transillumination has been used for the diagnosis and is especially useful in emergencies. At least anteroposterior and cross-table lateral chest roentgenograms should be done in infants suspected for this lesion, and lateral decubitus films may also be needed. A single film is not sufficient to exclude other conditions such as lobar emphysema and lung cysts, which may confuse the diagnosis. Shift of the mediastinal structures should be sought to diagnose tension pneumothorax.

Pneumomediastinum frequently provides some of the most confusing chest roentgenograms. Free air in the mediastinum is evident on anteroposterior chest film as an area of hyperlucency around the heart border. On lateral films a hyperlucent area between the sternum and anterior heart border is noted (Fig. 16-36). Often the outline of the thymus can be seen in relief against the mediastinal air.

Treatment. No therapy is indicated for pneumomediastinum. A small pneumothorax producing only mild respiratory distress should be observed carefully, but only in places prepared to initiate emergency treatment. Breathing of 100% O_2 for several hours after can accelerate removal of the extrapulmonary air. In theory, this treatment serves to free the blood of nitrogen and to establish a nitrogen gradient between the pneumothorax and surrounding tissues, with subsequent resorption of gas. Large pneumothoraces producing signs such as hypoxemia and tachypnea should be aspirated and a tube left in place attached to underwater-seal drainage. Needle and syringe aspiration may be necessary in an emergency. The intrapleural tube can frequently be removed in 48 hours. The decision to remove the tube is made after bubbling through the tube has ceased for 12 hours or when clamping of the tube does not again result in pneumothorax.

Etiology and Pathogenesis. Alveolar rupture is the basis for both lesions, presumably as a result of gas trapping from overdistention due to occlusion of outflow of gas. In meconium aspiration alveolar distention occurs as a result of a chemical bronchiolitis. In HMD alveolar rupture occurs when high pressures are directed to still open (nonatelectatic) and often overinflated alveoli. Spontaneous rupture could also occur during the first breaths when high pressures are developed and act on alveoli overdistended and obstructed by lung fluid. Pneumothorax results when alveolar rupture occurs into the pleural cavity. When air enters the interstitial tissue along bronchioles and blood vessels, it tracks into the mediastinum.

A

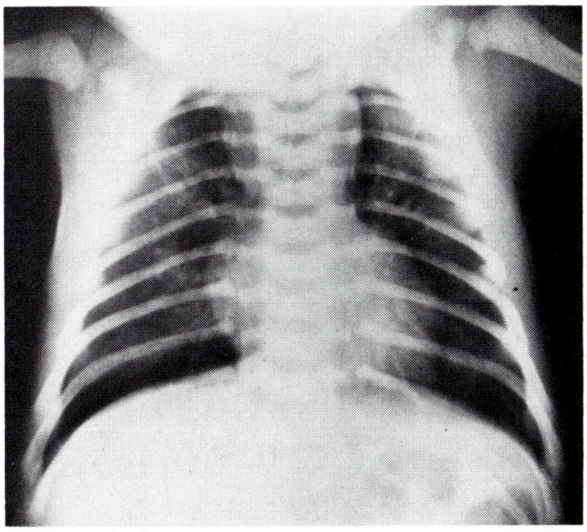

B

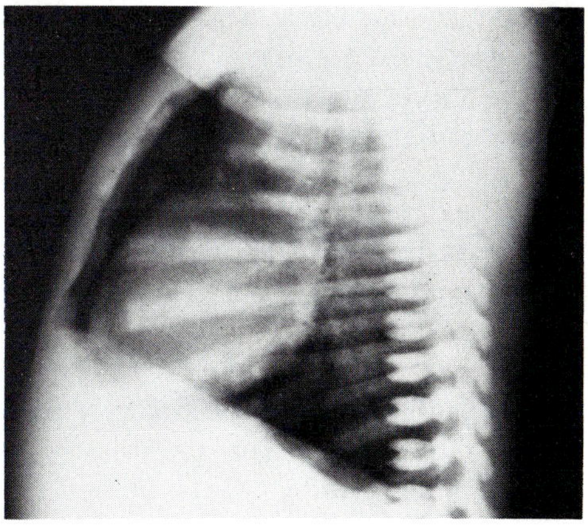

FIG. 16-36. Posteroanterior and lateral chest roentgenograms in an infant with pneumomediastinum.

A, On posteroanterior projection note area of hyperlucency around the heart.

B, On lateral note collection of air anterior to the heart. (There is also a small pneumothorax.)

PNEUMONIA AND SEPSIS

Although a detailed discussion of pneumonia appears in Chapter 12 and 13, it is mentioned here because the condition must be a consideration in every newborn infant with respiratory distress. Unlike most medical forms of neonatal respiratory distress in which therapy is supportive, treatment of pneumonia with antibiotics at least theoretically should result in cure. Neonatal pneumonia may be a primary cause of respiratory distress, or it may occur in association with HMD. In both these instances it frequently occurs as part of a generalized sepsis picture. Pneumonia may also occur in the sepsis that is a complication of indwelling catheters and other manipulations of intensive care.

The incidence of neonatal pneumonia has been difficult to determine. The diagnosis can be definitive only at autopsy so that the diagnosis in a recovered case is speculative at best. Thus it is important that the physician have a high index of suspicion for pneumonia and sepsis, and give treatment at the slightest suggestion of either. This approach by necessity leads to over-treatment, which may only become obvious in retrospect.

Source and Type of Infection. Infections in the newborn (including pneumonia) are acquired during the birth process or from personnel. Premature infants are most susceptible. Infants born after prolonged or premature rupture of membranes are at greatest risk, and increasingly so, the longer the condition has existed. Length of labor and obstetric manipulations on a background of ruptured membranes are added risk factors. In this setting, infection ascends from the vagina so that the organisms involved are common inhabitants of this area. At present, the commonest organism producing neonatal pneumonia is β-hemolytic streptococcus group B, and the infant who contracts the early-onset type in utero acquires the infection by this ascending route. Staphylococci and *E. coli* may enter the fetus by a similar pathway.

Other organisms may produce pneumonia and sepsis after entering the fetus by hematogenous spread from the mother through the placenta. Infections that are acquired by this route are *Listeria monocytogenes,* toxoplasmosis, and cytomegalic inclusion disease. Pneumonia may occur from a wide variety of organisms in association with atelectasis that may occur in relationship to endotracheal tubes. Viral pneumonia may also occur in the newborn, and the respiratory syncytial virus (RSV) has been implicated in epidemics in the premature nursery.[17]

Diagnosis. Infants who are subsequently proven to have primary pneumonia show the usual signs of respiratory distress. Thus, cyanosis, tachypnea, grunting, and retractions are common. Perinatal asphyxia may be present, and the infant can be a resuscitation problem at birth. Whereas HMD is generally obvious soon after birth, intrauterine pneumonia may not produce signs for hours after birth. Fever may be present, but hypothermia and difficulty in maintaining temperature are more common.

Recently, early-onset β-hemolytic streptococcus group B infection has been recognized as an important cause of neonatal respiratory distress and pneumonia. Howard and McCracken found an *E. coli* infection rate of 0.69 per 1000 deliveries and a group B infection rate of 1.35 per 1000 deliveries from 1969 to 1973.[71] The case fatality rate of early-onset β-hemolytic streptococcus group B in disease was 52% in a study by Vollman et al.[138] Pneumonia with this organism is a frequent accompaniment of HMD in premature infants. The clinical course differs from uncomplicated HMD by a rapid downhill turn, with apnea and shock common in the first 24 hours and requirement for lower pressures during mechanical ventilation.[1] A history of artificial, premature, or prolonged rupture of membranes, localized pulmonary infiltrates, and low neutrophil count have also been reported in this condition. The pathology of β-hemolytic streptococcus group B pneumonia shows alveolar polymorphonuclear infiltrates and frequently a prominent hemorrhagic component. The inflammatory reaction spreads to interlobular septa and pleura more readily than in other pneumonias.

Chest roentgenograms are less useful in the

newborn premature infant, particularly in the diagnosis of pneumonia because of the common finding of streaks of atelectasis in well infants. However, when localized infiltrates are seen, the likelihood is increased that penumonia is present. On occasion a chest roentgenogram indistinguishable from HMD is seen (Fig. 16-37).

Approach to Therapy. The previous considerations mandate that infants at risk for sepsis and pneumonia be managed in a manner that presumes they are infected. Thus a premature infant delivered after prolonged rupture of membranes should be cultured completely and treated with antibiotics. The antibiotics used should be broad spectrum and take into consideration diagnostic possibilities as well as the sensitivities of recently encountered organisms in a particular nursery. Ampicillin and gentamycin are currently used in many units.

Because it is difficult to exclude pneumonia in any infant with respiratory distress, it makes good sense to culture (e.g., nose, throat, ear canal, and blood) and treat these cases with antibiotics. Clinical course and culture results frequently dictate the time for discontinuance of antibiotics.

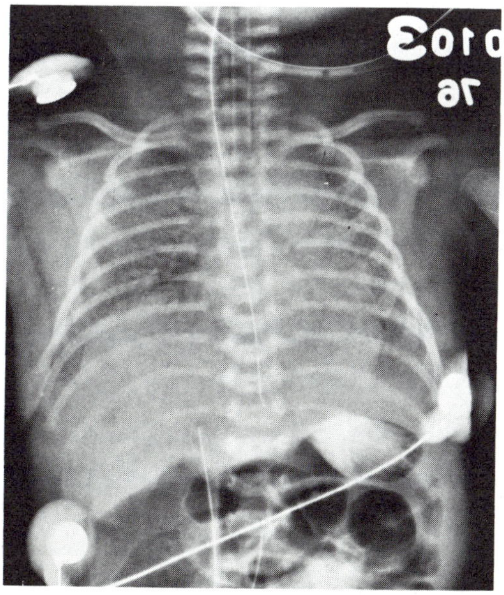

FIG. 16-37. Chest roentgenogram of infant with group B streptococcal pneumonia. Note typical air bronchogram.

Differential Diagnosis and Prognosis of Neonatal Respiratory Distress

While on a statistical basis a premature infant with respiratory distress is most likely to have HMD, other diagnoses must be considered at the outset. Most important, pneumonia should always be considered and appropriate therapy begun if this disease is a reasonable possibility. As pointed out at the beginning of this chapter, a chest roentgenogram must be obtained in every infant with respiratory distress, principally to exclude surgically treatable conditions. To be considered are pneumothorax, lung cysts (solitary and multiple), pleural effusions (chylothorax), diaphragmatic hernia, and congenital heart disease. Chest roentgenograms of representative cases are shown in Figures 16-38 through 16-42.

In the full-term infant with respiratory distress, three common diagnoses must be differentiated: meconium aspiration, transient tachypnea, and congenital heart disease.[116]

The prognosis for a particular infant with respiratory distress often depends on associated conditions. Thus, to a certain extent prognosis is related to prenatal factors such as degree of immaturity and evidence of perinatal asphyxia as well as severity of postnatal disease factors. Long-term outlook for these infants must be assessed in terms of neurologic, cardiopulmonary, and ophthalmologic sequelae. Neurologic sequelae are more common in the more immature infants as a general rule. Infants who require assisted ventilation have a higher incidence of neurologic disturbance. These associations are related to the effects of hypoxia on the brain and the development of intraventricular hemorrhage, which in turn produces hydrocephalus, spastic quadriplegia, and hemiplegia. In a recent

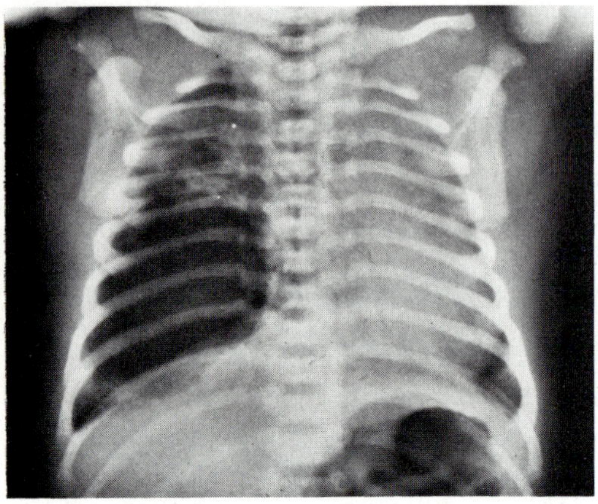

FIG. 16-38. Solitary lung cyst on the right.

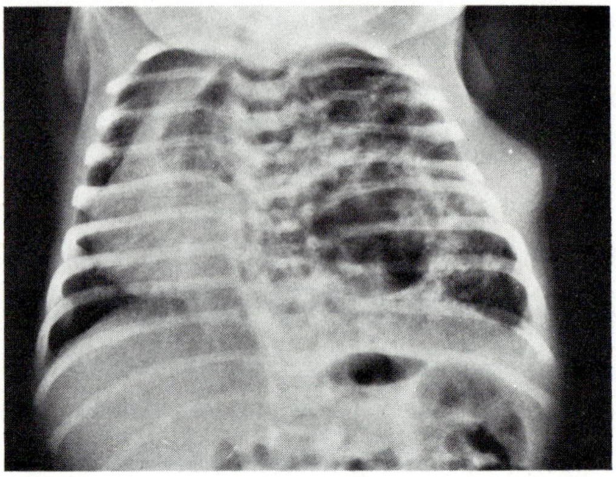

FIG. 16-39. Multicystic disease of the lung. Cystic adenomatoid malformation.

study on 73 low birth weight infants (less than 1501 g) treated with mechanical ventilation, Fitzhardinge and co-workers report 39% of males and 18% of females had major neurologic defects.[52] Other studies, which in-

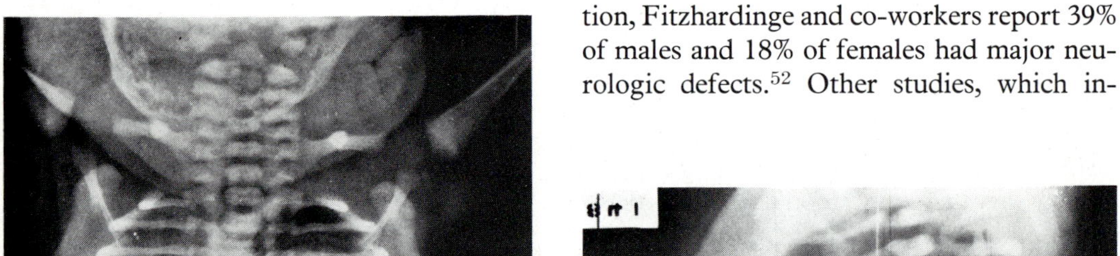

A B

FIG. 16-40. Diaphragmatic hernia through the foramen of Morgagni. This disorder can be confused with cystic disease of the lung.

A, posteroanterior view; *B*, lateral view.

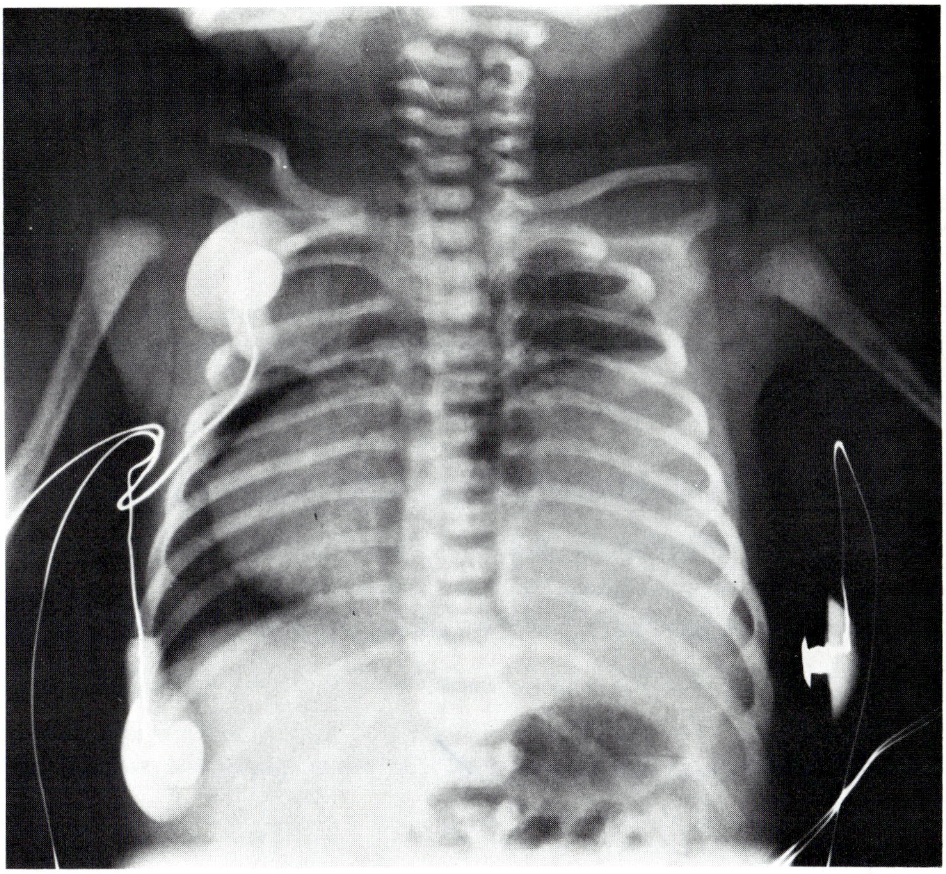

FIG. 16-41. Pulmonary sequestration on left. Right shift of the mediastinum is an unusual feature.

cluded a number of larger infants, have been more encouraging for both neurologic and intellectual outcome.[74] In the full-term infant severe neurologic abnormalities often are associated with meconium aspiration.

Cardiopulmonary problems, particularly an increased incidence of lower respiratory infections, occur in infants who have recovered from HMD.[21] In cases that require prolonged respiratory care bronchopulmonary dysplasia has its greatest incidence. Apparently, a locus minoris resistentiae is produced in the lung. The problem is most frequent in the first year of life, becoming less common thereafter.

RLF is an occasional complication of HMD. The complication most often occurs in infants who need prolonged oxygen therapy and have frequent apneic periods. In these instances it is impossible to monitor Pa_{O_2} with sufficient frequency to avoid over-oxygenation in every situation.

Many infants with subsequent neurologic or other disabilities are extremely ill at birth, and the problems are not preventable. On the other hand, improved ability to identify the high risk infant before birth as well as improved management immediately after birth could go a long way toward reducing these complications. It is probable that much of the poor outcome will be diminished when well-integrated regional perinatal programs

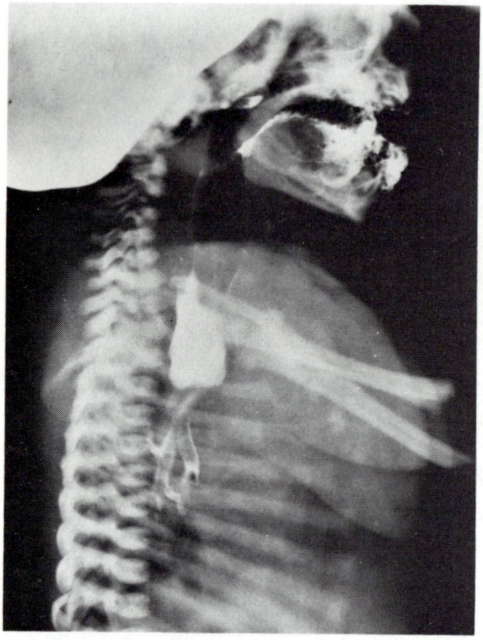

FIG. 16-42. Esophageal atresia and tracheoesophageal fistula. Roentgenograph showing blind esophageal pouch filled with barium with overflow into the bronchi.

are developed so that not a moment is wasted in the delivery of appropriate therapy. As it is at present, many infants languish undiagnosed and untreated in community hospitals, and as long as this condition is allowed to exist, many infants will have a poor outcome.

Teamwork between obstetricians, pediatricians, nurses, and social workers is the essence of the perinatal approach and can result in improved outcome for sick infants. Avoidance of unnecessary premature birth and delivery of high risk infants in specialized centers can go a long way toward preventing HMD, which is a subsequent problem.

REFERENCES

1. Ablow, R. C., S. G. Driscoll, E. L. Effmann, I. Gross, C. J. Jones, R. Uauy and J. B. Warshaw: A comparison of early-onset group B streptococcal neonatal infection and the respiratory distress syndrome of the newborn. *N. Engl. J. Med. 294*:65, 1976.
2. Adamsons, E., R. Behrman, G. S. Dawes, M. J. R. Dawkins, L. S. James and B. Ross: The treatment of acidosis with alkali and glucose during asphyxia in fetal rhesus monkey. *J. Physiol.* (*Lond.*) *169*:679, 1963.
3. Ahvenainen, E. K. and J. D. Call: Pulmonary hemorrhage in infants, a descriptive study. *Am. J. Pathol. 28*:1, 1952.
4. Ambrus, C. M., R. H. Weintraub, D. Dunphy, J. E. Dowd, J. A. Pickren, K. R. Niswander and J. L. Ambrus: Studies on hyaline membrane disease. I. The fibrinogen system in pathogenesis and therapy. *Pediatrics 32*:10, 1963.
5. Aranda, J. V., D. S. Sitar, W. D. Parsons, P. M. Loughnan and A. H. Neims: Pharmacokinetic aspects of theophylline in premature infants. *N. Engl. J. Med. 295*:413, 1976.
6. Auld, P. A. M., N. M. Nelson, R. B. Cherry, A. J. Rudolph, and C. A. Smith: Measurement of thoracic gas volume in the newborn infant. *J. Clin. Invest. 42*:476, 1963.
7. Avery, M. E. and B. D. Fletcher: *The Lung and Its Disorders in the Newborn Infant* (3rd ed.). W. B. Saunders Co., Philadelphia, 1974.
8. Avery, M. E., O. B. Gatewood and G. Brumley: Transient tachypnea of the newborn. *Am. J. Dis. Child. 111*:380, 1966.
9. Avery, M. E. and J. Mead: Surface properties in relation to atelectasis and hyaline membrane disease. *Am. J. Dis. Child. 97*:517, 1959.
10. Baden, M., C. R. Bauer, E. Colle, G. Klein, H. W. Taeusch, Jr. and L. Stern: A controlled trial of hydrocortisone therapy in infants with respiratory distress syndrome. *Pediatrics 53*:7, 1974.
11. Baghdassarian, O. M., M. E. Avery and E. B. D. Neuhauser: A form of pulmonary insufficiency in premature infants, pulmonary dysmaturity. *Am. J. Roentgenol. 89*:1020, 1963.
12. Bancalari, E., O. L. Garcia and M. J. Jesse: Effect of continuous negative pressure on lung mechanics in idiopathic respiratory distress syndrome. *Pediatrics 51*:485, 1973.
13. Barlow, B., T. V. Santulli, W. C. Heird, J. Pitt, W. A. Blanc and J. N. Schullinger: An experimental study of acute neonatal enterocolitis—the importance of breast milk. *J. Pediatr. Surg. 9*:587, 1974.
14. Bauer, C. R., L. Stein and E. Colle: Prolonged rupture of membranes associated with a decreased incidence of respiratory distress syndrome. *Pediatrics 53*:7, 1974.
15. Baylin, B. G., R. A. Meyer, S. Kaplan, W. E. Ringenberg and J. Korfhagen: The critically ill premature infant with patent ductus arteriosus and pulmonary disease—an echocardiographic assessment. *J. Pediatr. 86*:423, 1975.

16. Berg, T. J., R. D. Pagtakhan, M. H. Reed, C. Langston and V. Chernick: Bronchopulmonary dysplasia and lung rupture in hyaline membrane disease: influence of continuous distending pressure. *Pediatrics 55*:51, 1975.
17. Berkovich, S. and L. Taranko: Acute respiratory illness in the premature nursery associated with respiratory syncytial virus infections. *Pediatrics 34*:753, 1964.
18. Blumenfeld, T. A., J. M. Driscoll and L. S. James: Lecithin-sphingomyelin ratios in tracheal and pharyngeal aspirates in respiratory distress syndrome. *J. Pediatr. 85*:403, 1974.
19. Boros, S. J. and J. W. Reynolds: Duodenal perforation: a complication of nasojejunal feeding. *J. Pediatr. 85*:107, 1974.
20. Boros, S. J., T. R. Thompson, J. W. Reynolds, C. W. Jarvis and H. J. Williams: Reduced thrombus formation with silicone elastomere (silastic) umbilical artery catheters. *Pediatrics 56*:981, 1975.
21. Brown, J. K., F. Cockburn, J. O. Forfar, R. L. Marshall and G. W. Stephen: Problems in the management of assisted ventilation in the newborn and follow-up of treated cases. *Br. J. Anaesth. 45* (suppl.):808, 1973.
22. Burnard, E. D.: The pulmonary syndrome of Wilson and Mikity, and respiratory function in very small infants. *Pediatr. Clin. North Am. 13*:999, 1966.
23. Burnard, E. D., P. Grattan-Smith, C. G. Picton-Warlow and A. Grauaug: Pulmonary insufficiency in prematurity. *Aust. Paediatr. J. 1*:12, 1965.
24. Cashore, W. J., M. R. Sedaghatian and R. H. Usher: Nutritional supplements with intravenously administered lipid, protein hydrolysate and glucose in small premature infants. *Pediatrics 56*:8, 1975.
25. Chernick, V. and D. Vidyasagar: Continuous negative chest wall pressure in hyaline membrane disease. *Pediatrics 49*:753, 1971.
26. Chu, J., J. A. Clements, E. Cotton, M. Klaus, A. Y. Sweet and W. H. Tooley: The pulmonary hypoperfusion syndrome. *Pediatrics 35*:733, 1965.
27. Chu, J., J. A. Clements, E. K. Cotton, M. H. Klaus, A. Y. Sweet and W. H. Tooley: Neonatal pulmonary ischemia. Part I. Clinical and physiological studies. *Pediatrics 40*:709, 1967.
28. Clements, J. A., A. C. G. Platzker, D. F. Tierney, C. J. Hobel, R. K. Creasy, A. J. Margolis, D. W. Thibeault, W. H. Tooley and W. Oh: Assessment of the risk of the respiratory distress syndrome by a rapid test for surfactant in amniotic fluid. *N. Engl. J. Med. 286*:1077, 1972.
29. Coceani, F., P. M. Olley and E. Bodach: Lamb ductus arteriosus: effect of prostaglandin synthesis inhibitors on the muscle tone and response to prostaglandin E_2. *Prostaglandins 9*:229, 1975.
30. Cohen, D., W. Cochran, T. Griscom and G. B. C. Harris: Naturally occurring pneumothorax in hyaline membrane disease. *Pediatr. Res. 7*:400, 1973.
31. Conway, M., G. M. Durbin, D. Ingram, N. McIntosh, D. Parker, E. O. R. Reynolds and L. P. Soutter: Monitoring oxygen tension with catheter-tip polarographic electrode. *Pediatrics 57*:244, 1976.
32. Cook, C. D., J. M. Sutherland, S. Segal, R. B. Cherry, J. Mead, M. C. McIlroy and C. A. Smith: Studies of respiratory physiology in the newborn infant. III. Measurements of the mechanics of respiration. *J. Clin. Invest. 36*:449, 1957.
33. Cotton, E. K., J. J. Cogswell, B. Chir, G. J. A. Cropp and R. Losey: Measurements of effective pulmonary blood flow in the normal newborn infant. *Pediatrics 47*:520, 1971.
34. Cuestas, R. A., A. Lindall and R. R. Engel: Thyroid hormones and the respiratory distress syndrome of the newborn. *N. Engl. J. Med. 295*:297, 1976.
35. Daily, W., M. Klaus and H. Meyer: Apnea in premature infants: monitoring, incidence, heart rate changes and effect of environmental temperature. *Pediatrics 43*:510, 1969.
36. Dauber, I. M., A. N. Krauss, P. S. Symchych, and P. A. M. Auld: Renal failure following perinatal anoxia. *J. Pediatr. 88*:851, 1976.
37. DeLemos, R. A., D. W. Shermata, J. H. Knelson, R. Kotas and M. E. Avery: Acceleration of appearance of pulmonary surfactant in the fetal lamb by administration of corticosteroids. *Am. Rev. Respir. Dis. 102*:459, 1970.
38. DeLemos, R. A. and G. W. McLaughlin: Induction of the pulmonary surfactant in the fetal primate by the intrauterine administration of corticosteroids. *Pediatr. Res. 7*:425, 1973.
39. Desmond, M. D., J. L. Kay and A. D. Megarity: The phases of "transitional distress" occurring in neonates in association with prolonged postnatal umbilical cord pulsations. *J. Pediatr. 55*:131, 1959.
40. Domville Cooke, W. D.: Prognostic significance of serum protein content in premature babies and its relation to pulmonary hyaline membrane: preliminary communication. *Med. J. Aust. 1*:887, 1960.
41. Drorbaugh, J. E., S. Segal, J. M. Sutherland, R. B. Cherry, T. E. Oppe and C. A. Smith: A method for evaluating pulmonary function in newborn infants: measurement of lung compliance. *Am. J. Dis. Child. 90*:627, 1955.
42. Dubowitz, L. M., V. Dubowitz and C. Goldberg: Clinical assessment of gestational age in the newborn infant. *J. Pediatr. 77*:1, 1970.
43. Durbin, G. M., N. J. Huntir, N. McIntosh, E. O. R. Reynolds and P. D. Wimberley: Controlled trial of continuous inflating pressure for

hyaline membrane disease. *Arch. Dis. Child.* *51*:163, 1976.

44. Edmund, L. W. Jr., G. A. Gregory, M. A. Heymann, J. A. Kitterman, A. M. Rudolph and W. H. Tooley: Surgical closure of the ductus arteriosus in premature infants. *Circulation 48*:856, 1973.
45. Esterly, J. R. and E. H. Oppenheimer: Massive pulmonary hemorrhage in the newborn. I. Pathologic considerations. *J. Pediatr. 69*:3, 1966.
46. Fanaroff, A. A., C. C. Cha, R. Sosa, R. S. Crumrine and M. H. Klaus: Control trial of continuous negative external pressure in the treatment of severe respiratory distress syndrome. *J. Pediatr.* *82*:921, 1973.
47. Fanaroff, A. A., M. Wald, H. S. Gruber and M. H. Klaus: Insensible water loss in low birth weight infants. *Pediatrics 50*:236, 1972.
48. Farrell, P. M. and M. E. Avery: Hyaline membrane disease. *Am. Rev. Respir. Dis. 111*:657, 1975.
49. Farrell, P. M. and R. E. Wood: Epidemiology of hyaline membrane disease in the United States: analysis of national morbidity statistics. *Pediatrics* *58*:167, 1976.
50. Fenner, A., V. Schalk and H. Hoenicke: Periodic breathing in premature and neonatal babies: incidence, breathing pattern, respiratory gas tensions, response to changes in the composition of ambient air. *Pediatr. Res. 7*:174, 1973.
51. Finberg, L.: Danger to infants caused by changes in osmolar concentration. *Pediatrics 40*:1031, 1967.
52. Fitzhardinge, P. M., K. Pape, M. Arstikaitis, M. Boyle, S. Ashby, A. Rowley, C. Netley and P. R. Swyer: Mechanical ventilation of infants of less than 1501 gm birth weight: health, growth and neurologic sequelae. *J. Pediatr. 88*:531, 1976.
53. Frank, D. J. and M. Gabriel: Timing of cord ligation and newborn respiratory distress. *Am. J. Obstet. Gynecol. 97*:1142, 1967.
54. Freeman, R. K., U. Goebelsman, D. Nochimson and C. Cetrulo: An evaluation of the significance of a positive oxytocin challenge test. *Obstet. Gynecol. 47*:8, 1976.
55. Gabriel, M., M. Albani and F. J. Schulte: Apneic spells and sleep states in preterm infants. *Pediatrics* *57*:142, 1976.
56. Gersony, W. M., G. V. Duc and J. C. Sinclair: "P. F. C." syndrome (persistence of fetal circulation). *Circulation 40* (III):87, 1969.
57. Gersony, W. M.: Persistence of the fetal circulation: a commentary. *J. Pediatr. 82*:1103, 1973.
58. Glass, L., B. Rajegowda and H. Evans: Absence of respiratory distress syndrome in premature infants of heroin-addicted mothers. *Lancet 2*:685, 1971.
59. Gluck, L. and M. V. Kulovich: Lecithin/sphingomyelin ratios in amniotic fluid in normal and abnormal pregnancy. *Am. J. Obstet. Gynecol.* *114*:539, 1973.
60. Grassi, A., A. N. Krauss, S. Waldman and P. A. M. Auld: Personal communication.
61. Gregory, G. A., J. A. Kitterman, R. H. Phibbs, W. H. Tooley and W. K. Hamilton: Treatment of the idiopathic respiratory distress syndrome with continuous positive airway pressure. *N. Engl. J. Med. 284*:1333, 1971.
62. Gross, G. P., W. S. Hathaway and H. R. McGaughey: Neonatal hyperviscosity in the neonate. *J. Pediatr. 82*:1004, 1973.
63. Guignard, J. P., A. Torrado, S. M. Mazouni and E. Gautier: Renal function in respiratory distress syndrome. *J. Pediatr. 88*:845, 1976.
64. Harrison, V.C., H. deV. Hesse and M. Klein: The significance of grunting in hyaline membrane disease. *Pediatrics 41*:549, 1968.
65. Hathaway, W. E., M. M. Mull and G. S. Pechet: Disseminated intravascular coagulation in the newborn. *Pediatrics 42*:233, 1969.
66. Haworth, S. G. and L. Reid: Persistent fetal circulation: newly recognized structural features. *J. Pediatr. 88*:614, 1976.
67. Heird, W. C. and J. M. Driscoll, Jr.: Use of intravenously administered lipid in neonates. *Pediatrics* *56*:5, 1975.
68. Herman, S. and E. O. R. Reynolds: Methods of improving oxygenation in infants mechanically ventilated for severe hyaline membrane disease. *Arch. Dis. Child. 48*:612, 1973.
69. Heymann, M. A., A. M. Rudolph and N. H. Silverman: Closure of the ductus arteriosus in premature infants by inhibition of prostaglandin synthesis. *N. Engl. J. Med. 294*:530, 1976.
70. Hodgman, J. E., V.G. Mikity, D. Tatter and R. S. Cleland: Chronic respiratory distress in the premature infant, Wilson-Mikity syndrome. *Pediatrics* *44*:179, 1969.
71. Howard, J. B. and G. H. McCracken: The spectrum of group B streptococcal infections in infancy. *Am. J. Dis. Child. 128*:815, 1974.
72. Huch, A., R. Huch, E. Neumayer and G. Rooth: Continuous intraarterial p_{O_2} measurements in infants. *Acta. Paediatr. Scand. 61*:722, 1972.
73. Hutchison, A. A., A. M. W. Forbes and G. Russel: Effective pulmonary blood flow in preterm and light-for-dates infants. *Pediatrics 57*:187, 1976.
74. Johnson, J. D., N. C. Malachowski, R. Grobstein, D. Welsh, W. J. R. Daily and P. Sunshine: Prognosis of children surviving with aid of mechanical ventilation in the newborn period. *J. Pediatr.* *84*:272, 1974.
75. Jones, M. D. Jr., L. I. Burd, W. A. Bowes, Jr., F. C. Battaglia and L. O. Lubchencho: Failure of association of premature rupture of membranes with respiratory distress syndrome. *N. Engl. J. Med. 292*:1253, 1975.
76. Josimovich, J. B.: Lecithin secretion in infants of

diabetic mothers in respiratory distress syndrome. In *Respiratory Distress Syndrome*. Academic Press, New York, p. 219, 1973.

77. Kapitulnik, J., T. Vales, N. A. Kaufmann and S. H. Blondheim: Clinical evaluation of Sephadex gel filtration in estimation of bilirubin binding in serum in neonatal jaundice. *Arch. Dis. Child.* *49*:886, 1974.
78. Karlberg, P., R. B. Cherry, F. E. Escardo and G. Koch: Respiratory studies in newborn infants. II. Pulmonary ventilation and mechanics of breathing in the first minute of life, including the onset of respiration. *Acta Paediatr. Scand.* *1*:121, 1962.
79. Kitterman, J. A., L. H. Edmunds, Jr., G. A. Gregory, M. A. Heymann, W. H. Tooley and A. M. Rudolph: Patent ductus arteriosus in premature infants. *N. Engl. J. Med.* *287*:473, 1972.
80. Kitterman, J. A., R. H. Phibbs and W. H. Tooley: Aortic blood pressure in normal newborn infants during the first 12 hours of life. *Pediatrics* *44*:959, 1969.
81. Kidd, L., H. Levison, P. Gemmel, A. Aharon and P. R. Swyer: Limb blood flow in the normal and sick newborn. *Am. J. Dis. Child.* *112*:402, 1966.
82. Krauss, A. N., D. B. Klain and P. A. M. Auld: Ventilatory response to carbon dioxide in newborn infants. *Pediatr. Res.* *9*:46, 1975.
83. Krauss, A. N., C. A. Tori, J. Brown, J. Soodalter and P. A. M. Auld: Oxygen chemoreceptors in low birth weight infants. *Pediatr. Res.* *7*:569, 1973.
84. Krauss, A. N., G. E. Solomon and P. A. M. Auld: Sleep state apnea and bradycardia in premature infants. *Dev. Med. Child Neurol.* *19*:160, 1977.
85. Krauss, A. N. and P. A. M. Auld: Diminished response to carbon dioxide in premature infants. *Biol. Neonate* *30*:216, 1976.
86. Krauss, A. N. and P. A. M. Auld: Measurement of mixed venous oxygen tension in premature infants by a rebreathing method. *Pediatr. Res.* *6*:158, 1972.
87. Krauss, A. N. and P. A. M. Auld: Metabolic requirements of low birth weight infants. *J. Pediatr.* *76*:952, 1969.
88. Krauss, A. N. and P. A. M. Auld: Personal communication.
89. Krauss, A. N. and P. A. M. Auld: Pulmonary gas trapping in premature infants. *Pediatr. Res.* *5*:10, 1971.
90. Krauss, A. N., D. B. Klain and P. A. M. Auld: Carbon monoxide diffusing capacity in the newborn infant. *Pediatr. Res.* *10*:771, 1976.
91. Krauss, A. N., D. B. Klain and P. A. M. Auld: Chronic pulmonary insufficiency of the premature (CPIP). *Pediatrics* *55*:55, 1975.
92. Krauss, A. N., D. B. Klain and P. A. M. Auld: Letter to the editor. *Pediatrics* *49*:468, 1972.
93. Krauss, A. N., D. B. Klain, B. Dahms and P. A. M. Auld: Vital capacity in premature infants. *Am. Rev. Respir. Dis.* *108*:1361, 1973.
94. Krauss, A. N., A. R. Levin, H. Grossman and P. A. M. Auld: Physiologic studies in infants with Wilson-Mikity syndrome. *J. Pediatr.* *77*:27, 1970.
95. Kuhns, L. R., F. J. Bednarek, M. L. Wyman, D. W. Roloff and R. C. Borer: Diagnosis of pneumothorax and pneumomediastinum in the neonate by transillumination. *Pediatrics* *56*:355, 1975.
96. Kuzemko, J. A. and J. Paala: Apnoeic attacks in the newborn treated with aminophylline. *Arch. Dis. Child.* *48*:404, 1973.
97. Landing, B. H.: Pulmonary lesions of newborn infants; a descriptive study. *Pediatrics* *19*:217, 1957.
98. Larroche, J.: Umbilical catheterization; its complications. *Biol. Neonate* *16*:101, 1970.
99. Liggins, G. C. and R. N. Howie: A controlled study of antepartum glucocorticoid treatment for prevention of the respiratory distress syndrome in premature infants. *Pediatrics* *50*:515, 1972.
100. Liggins, G. C. and R. N. Howie: *The Prevention of RDS by Maternal Steroid Therapy in Modern Perinatal Medicine.* L. Gluck (Ed.). Year Book Medical Publishers, Chicago, 1974.
101. Lendrum, F. C.: The pulmonary hyaline membrane as a manifestation of heart failure in the newborn infant. *J. Pediatr.* *47*:149, 1955.
102. McAdams, A. J.: Pulmonary hemorrhage in newborn. *Am. J. Dis. Child.* *113*:255, 1967.
103. Mithal, A. and J. L. Emery: The postnatal development of alveoli in premature infants. *Arch. Dis. Child.* *36*:449, 1962.
104. Moylan, F. M. B., K. C. O'Connell, I. D. Todres and D. C. Shannon: Edema of the pulmonary interstitium in infants and children. *Pediatrics* *55*:783, 1975.
105. Murdock, A. I. and P. R. Swyer: The contribution to venous admixture by shunting through the ductus arteriosus in infants with respiratory distress syndrome of the newborn. *Biol. Neonate* *13*:194, 1968.
106. Neal, W., J. Reynolds, D. Jarvis and H. Williams: Umbilical artery catheterization: demonstration of arterial thrombosis by aortography. *Pediatrics* *50*:6, 1972.
107. Neligan, G. A. and C. A. Smith: The blood pressure of newborn infants in asphyxial states and in hyaline membrane disease. *Pediatrics* *26*:735, 1960.
108. Nelson, N. M.: On the etiology of hyaline membrane disease. *Pediatr. Clin. North Am.* *17*:943, 1970.
109. Nelson, N. M., L. S. Prod'hom, R. B. Cherry, P. L. Lipsitz and C. A. Smith: Pulmonary function in the newborn infant, the alveolar-arterial oxygen gradient. *J. Appl. Physiol.* *18*:534, 1963.
110. Nelson, N. M., L. S. Prod'hom, R. B. Cherry,

P. L. Lipsitz and C. A. Smith: Pulmonary function in the newborn infant. II. Perfusion-estimation by analysis of the arterial-alveolar carbon dioxide difference. *Pediatrics 30*:975, 1962.

111. Northway, W. H., Jr., R. C. Rosen and D. Y. Porter: Pulmonary disease following respiratory therapy of hyaline membrane disease—bronchopulmonary dysplasia. *N. Engl. J. Med. 276*:357, 1967.
112. Pattle, R. E.: Properties, function and origin of alveolar lining layer. *Proc. R. Soc. Lond. B148*:217, 1958.
113. Perlstein, P. H., N.K. Edwards and J. M. Sutherland: Apnea in premature infants and incubator-air temperature changes. *N. Engl. J. Med. 282*:461, 1970.
114. Polgar, G.: Airway resistance in the newborn infant. Preliminary communication. *J. Pediatr. 59*:915, 1961.
115. Rigatto, H. and J. Brady: Periodic breathing and apnea in preterm infants. II. Hypoxia as a primary event. *Pediatrics 50*:219, 1972.
116. Roberton, N. R. C., K. A. Hallidie-Smith and J. A. Davis: Severe respiratory distress syndrome mimicking cyanotic heart disease in term babies. *Lancet 2*:1108, 1967.
117. Robert, M. F., R. F. Neff, J. P. Hubbell, H. W. Taeusch and M. E. Avery: Association between maternal diabetes and respiratory distress in the newborn. *N. Engl. J. Med. 294*:357, 1976.
118. Rowe, S. and M. E. Avery: Massive pulmonary hemorrhage in the newborn. II. Clinical considerations. *J. Pediatr. 69*:12, 1966.
119. Rudolph, A. J., C. Vallbona and M. M. Desmond: Cardiodynamic studies in the newborn. III. Heart rate patterns in infants with idiopathic respiratory distress syndrome. *Pediatrics 36*:551, 1965.
120. Rudolph, A. M., J. E. Drorbaugh, P. A. M. Auld, A. J. Rudolph, A. S. Nadas, C. A. Smith and J. P. Hubbell: Studies on the circulation in the neonatal period. The circulation in the respiratory distress syndrome. *Pediatrics 27*:551, 1961.
121. Saling, E.: *Fetal and Neonatal Hypoxia.* The Williams & Wilkins Co., Baltimore, 1968.

121A. Scarpelli, E. M.: *Pulmonary Physiology of the Fetus, Newborn and Child.* Lea & Febiger, Philadelphia, 1975.

122. Shanklin, D. R. and S. L. Wolfson: Therapeutic oxygen as a possible cause of pulmonary hemorrhage in premature infants. *N. Engl. J. Med. 277*:833, 1967.
123. Shannon, D. C., F. Gotay, I. M. Stein, M. C. Rogers, I. D. Todres and F. M. B. Moylan: Prevention of apnea and bradycardia in low-birth weight infants. *Pediatrics 55*:589, 1975.
124. Siassi, B., S. J. Goldberg, G. C. Emmanouilides, S. M. Higashino and E. Lewis: Persistent pulmonary vascular obstruction in newborn infants. *J. Pediatr. 78*:610, 1971.
125. Siegal, S. E., D. A. Fisher and W. Oh: Renal function and serum aldosterone levels in infants with respiratory distress syndrome. *J. Pediatr. 83*:854, 1973.
126. Silverman, N. H., A. B. Lewis, M. A. Heymann and A. M. Rudolph: Echocardiographic assessment of ductus arteriosus shunt in premature infants. *Circulation 50*:821, 1974.
127. Spellacy, W. N., Buhi, W. C., Riggall, F. C. and Holsinger, K. L.: Human amniotic fluid lecithin/sphingomyelin ratio changes with estrogen or glucocorticoid treatment. *Am. J. Obstet. Gynecol. 115*:216, 1973.
128. Sundell, H., J. Garrott, W. J. Blankenship, F.M. Shepard and M. T. Stahlman: Studies on infants with type II respiratory distress syndrome. *J. Pediatr. 78*:754, 1971.
129. Swyer, P. R., M. Delivoria-Papadopoulos, H. Levinson, B. J. Reilly and J. W. Balis: The pulmonary syndrome of Wilson and Mikity. *Pediatrics 36*:374, 1965.
130. Symchych, P. S., A. N. Krauss and P. Winchester: Endocarditis following intracardiac placement of umbilical venous catheters. Submitted for publication, 1976.
131. Thibeault, D. W., H. Grossman, J. W. C. Hagstrom and P. A. M. Auld: Radiologic findings in the lungs of newborn infants. *J. Pediatr. 74*:1, 1969.
132. Thibeault, D. W., M. M. Wong and P. A. M. Auld: Thoracic gas volume changes in premature infants. *Pediatrics 40*:403, 1967.
133. Tooley, W. H.: What is the risk of umbilical artery catheter? *Pediatrics 50*:1, 1972.
134. Tori, C. A., A. N. Krauss and P. A. M. Auld: Serial studies of lung volume and $\dot{V}A/\dot{Q}$ in hyaline membrane disease. *Pediatr. Res. 7*:82, 1973.
135. Uauy, R., D. L. Shapiro, B. Smith and J.B. Warshaw: Treatment of severe apnea in prematures with orally administered theophylline. *Pediatrics 55*:595, 1975.
136. Usher, R. H., A. C. Allen and F. H. McLean: Risk of respiratory distress syndrome related to gestational age, route of delivery and maternal diabetes. *Am. J. Obstet. Gynecol. 111*:826, 1971.
137. Vallbona, C., A. J. Rudolph and M. M. Desmond: Cardiodynamic studies in the newborn. IV. Heart rate patterns in the non-distressed premature infant. *Pediatrics 36*:560, 1965.
138. Vollman, J. H., W. L. Smith, E. T. Ballard and J. I. Light: Early onset Group B streptococcal disease, clinical roentgenographic and pathologic features. *J. Pediatr. 89*:199, 1976.

139. Von Neergaard, K.: Neue auffassungen uber einen grundbegriff der Atemmechanik Die Retraktionskraft der Lunge abhangig von der Oberflachenspannung in den Alveolen. *Z. Gesamte. Exp. Med.* *66*:373, 1929.
140. Waldman, S., A. N. Krauss and P. A. M. Auld: Control of peripheral blood flow in newborn infants. Submitted for publication, 1976.
141. Weisbrot, I. M., L. S. James, C. E. Prince, D. A. Holaday and V. Apgar: Acid-base homeostasis of the newborn infant during the first 24 hours of life. *J. Pediatr.* *52*:395, 1958.
142. Weller, P. H., P. A. Jenkins, J. Gupta and J. D. Baum: Pharyngeal lecithin/sphingomyelin ratios in newborn infants. *Lancet* *1*:12, 1976.
143. Wells, D. M. and R. D. Zachman: Nasojejunal feedings in low birth weight infants. *J. Pediatr.* *87*:276, 1975.
144. Whitfield, C. R., W. B. Spinell and M. Brudenell: The amniotic fluid lecithin/sphingomyelin area ratio (LSAR) in pregnancies complicated by diabetes. *J. Obstet. Gynaecol. Br. Common.* *80*:918, 1973.
145. Wilson, M. J. and V. G. Mikity: A new form of respiratory disease in premature infants. *Am. J. Dis. Child.* *99*:489, 1960.
146. Wood, R. E. and P. M. Farrell: Epidemiology of respiratory distress syndrome (RDS). *Pediatr. Res.* *8*:452, 1974.
147. Wu, P. Y. K. and J. E. Hodgman: Insensible water loss in preterm infants: changes with postnatal development and non-ionizing radiant energy. *Pediatrics* *54*:704, 1974.
148. Wyszagradski, I., K. Kyli-Aboagye, H. W. Taeusch and M. E. Avery: Surfactant inactivation by hyperventilation; conservation by end-expiratory position. *J. Appl. Physiol.* *38*:416, 1975.
149. Yeh, T. F., D. Vidyasagar and R. S. Pildes: Neonatal pneumopericardium. *Pediatrics* *54*:429, 1974.
150. Yoon, J. J. and R. G. Harper: Observations on the relationship between duration of rupture of membranes and the development of the idiopathic respiratory distress syndrome. *Pediatrics* *56*:161, 1973.
151. Zachman, R. D., G. P. Steinmetz, R. J. Botham, S. N. Graven and M. K. Ledbetter: Incidence of and treatment of patent ductus arteriosus in the ill premature neonate. *Am. Heart J.* *87*:697, 1974.

Sudden Infant Death Syndrome

ALFRED N. KRAUSS

17

Sudden infant death syndrome (SIDS) is the leading cause of mortality for infants between 1 and 12 months old. It has been estimated to cause between 10,000 and 15,000 deaths yearly in the United States, and occurs with a frequency of 2 to 4/1000 live births.[4,23,24,31,59,61-63] SIDS is unusual within the first month of life, and rare after the first birthday. Its peak incidence is between the second and fourth month of life. As defined by the 1969 conference on SIDS, this syndrome consists of a sudden and unexpected infant death that cannot be explained after performance of a complete autopsy.[4,7,62,64] Since SIDS can be diagnosed only post mortem by exclusion of other possible causes of death, many theories exist regarding its cause. Because of its frequency SIDS is a medically important condition, and in recent years much research has been conducted in this and related fields.

Pathology

By definition, SIDS cases do not have an obvious "cause" of death. It must be realized that simply because an autopsy reveals an adequate pathologic cause for death, one may not assume that the particular lesion is the true or immediate cause of death. Thus, many explained deaths in infants and older adults may, in fact, be sudden and unexplained deaths with causes similar to those associated with SIDS. For example, an adult male found dead in bed in the morning, and on autopsy found to have significant coronary artery narrowing due to arteriosclerosis, could have his death ascribed to this lesion without any other proof that his death was actually due to coronary artery disease.

Although the definition of SIDS seems to deny the finding of any consistent pathologic lesion, pathologists agree that a constellation of lesions does occur in most cases of SIDS.[4,64] The body is generally that of a well-nourished, well-developed infant, most frequently male, between 2 and 4 months of age. External evidence of trauma is lacking. On examination of the thoracic contents, the lungs are seen to fill the thoracic cavity. They have a shiny exterior surface and are crepitant anteriorly. Posteriorly, this crepitance decreases. The thymus is large and the heart grossly appears normal. Closer examination of the surface of the intrathoracic organs reveals the presence of petechiae on the serosal surfaces. The blood in the heart is generally liquid. The nervous system is generally normal grossly. Other viscera, including the adrenals and parathyroids, are normal. The bowels and bladder are usually empty.

Microscopically, myocardial petechiae are observed in about 25% of cases. Lymphoid tissue throughout the body is normal, and no histologic evidence of massive anaphylaxis exists.[4,64] No consistent histologic evidence of massive viral infection, such as the presence of viral inclusion bodies, has been found in SIDS cases.[4] Examination of the conducting system of the heart reveals no evidence of myocarditis or hemorrhage, although some studies have reported evidence of "remodeling."[1,20,33,34,65] The carotid bodies of SIDS cases are smaller than those of control infants, while the lungs of SIDS infants demonstrate increased amounts of muscle in the pulmonary vasculature when compared to those of controls.[43,44] These changes suggest the presence of chronic mild hypoxemia in SIDS cases.[39-41]

Postmortem analyses of blood from SIDS victims have failed to reveal any consistent chemical abnormality. Thus, theories regarding anaphylactic reactions or biochemical abnormalities have not been confirmed. Postmortem levels of serum steroids and gamma globulins are normal.[4]

Viruses have been recovered in 23 and 42% of SIDS victims reported in different series.[4,7] With the exception of a temporal association between SIDS and influenza type A, reported in a 42-month period from Chicago,[22,27] SIDS has shown no consistent association with any viral infection.

The Susceptible Victim

Although none of the findings just reviewed are diagnostic of SIDS, their presence in the absence of other evidence of disease allows the pathologist to diagnose SIDS. In a similar fashion, although no one has diagnosed SIDS antemortem, its victims are generally similar in terms of personal history and other socioeconomic characteristics.

Most victims of SIDS are under 1 year of age. In the Washington study, over half were under 3 months of age and 90% of the cases had occurred in the first 6 months of life.[4,7,23,24,55,63] Male: female ratio is approximately 6:4. Although the overall risk of SIDS is about 2/1000 live births, this incidence varies considerably when different subgroups of infants are considered (Table 17-1).

SIDS shows a seasonal incidence. The peak period is January through March, the so-called respiratory season, when viral infections of the respiratory tract are most common.[22,46] Clustering of cases has been reported, and attributed to similar infections, changes in climate, and air pollution.[4,23] Al-

TABLE 17-1. Incidence* of SIDS in Various Groups of Infants

	Male	Female	Total
White	2.31	1.29	1.82
Non-white	4.51	5.38	5.01
Total	2.45	1.64	2.05

* Incidence figures represent the number of SIDS cases per 1000 live births.

though familial cases of SIDS have been reported, they are uncommon.[4]

SIDS occurs with increased frequency in infants of low birth weight.[4,23,24] When compared to a group of "advantaged" control infants, the SIDS victims were smaller at birth and grew more slowly in terms of weight, length, and head circumference. Their growth curves paralleled those of the reference population, but were below the median point.[50] A recent, retrospective study of the behavior of SIDS infants has also revealed behavioral differences with respect to a group of surviving sibling control infants. The SIDS victims were characterized as being less active, appearing more breathless with feeding, reacting less intensely to various environmental stimuli, and crying abnormally. These characteristics occur to some degree in a significant proportion of normal infants.[45]

Although some SIDS victims have died in their parents' arms, the most prominent characteristic of SIDS is that the victims expire during a sleep period.[4,7,23,29,59,62-64] Most victims are found dead in bed in the morning. Their bedclothes are frequently rumpled, and their bladder and bowels are empty, suggesting to some observers an agonal struggle for breath. None, however, are heard to cry out. Occasionally parents have noticed that their infant has stopped breathing. Following resuscitation, these infants comprise the group of "near-misses," who have been the subject of much recent research.[59]

Possible Causes of SIDS

The foregoing discussion has outlined the factors that render an infant susceptible to SIDS: age (below 1 year), low birth weight, poor socioeconomic status, male sex, viral infection, season of year, and sleep. In addition to these general factors, various specific causes of SIDS have been proposed. Few are mutually exclusive. In fact, it is reasonable to suppose that the combination of a susceptible infant and an external trigger event, acting through a final autonomic pathway, may be necessary to effect the cessation of breathing, asphyxia, and cardiac arrest associated with SIDS.

Infection has been a leading candidate for the external trigger event in SIDS. In favor of this hypothesis is the concurrence of SIDS with the viral respiratory season and the clustering of cases within this season.[22-24,27,46] Many parents relate a history of antecedent mild respiratory infection when they are questioned about their infants following a SIDS event.[4,7] Although up to 40% of infants in some series have positive cultures for viral agents, histologic evidence of viral infection is lacking in most cases, and only minor differences are reported pathologically when infants with this history are compared to those without such a history.

Anaphylaxis has also been suggested as a possible cause of SIDS.[4] Milk, viral and bacterial infections, and protein intoxication have been proposed as the underlying cause of this reaction. Although the rapid nature of SIDS is in favor of this hypothesis, histologic evidence is against it.[4]

A related hypothesis, "thymic dysfunction," has also been proposed in relation to SIDS. The thymus is, in fact, somewhat large in SIDS. Thymic atrophy, present in numerous forms of chronic disease, is absent.[64] Many cases of so-called status thymicolymphaticus were actually cases of SIDS.[10] At postmortem examination, the thymus is histologically normal with the exception of petechiae on the intrathoracic portions of the organ.

Suffocation has been another major theory related to SIDS.[4] Curds of gastric contents have been found in the larynx of victims. These curds may reach the larynx postmortem and are not regarded as a likely cause of death in most cases of SIDS.[4,64] While bedding may possibly be a cause of suffocation in some cases of SIDS, other cases are found with their faces free.[4]

Various metabolic theories,[4] such as rickets, parathyroid deficiency, magnesium deficiency, scurvy, and adrenal insufficiency have been proposed. They have not been independently confirmed in other series of SIDS cases. Similarly, theories that relate SIDS to climatic changes or hypothermia have not been confirmed. Respiratory obstruction with pharyngeal narrowing,[14,19,29] potentiated by infection, sleep, or abnormal reflex activity,[4,5,56,57] has also been suggested as a possible cause of SIDS. It has been hypothesized that SIDS victims suffer from chronic hypoxemia due to upper airway obstruction, which is similar to the condition seen in children with hypertrophied tonsils and adenoids.[38,40,41] Supporting this hypothesis are findings of increased musculature in the pulmonary arteries of SIDS victims.[43] Other investigators have found fatty changes in the brain in association with fat-laden macrophages in the cerebrospinal fluid in both SIDS victims and children with chronic hypoxemia, further supporting this hypothesis.[26]

Respiration During Sleep

Aserinsky's and Kleitman's electroencephalographic studies of sleep were among the first to reveal that sleep could be divided into several stages in normal adults.[2,6] One stage, associated with rapid eye movements and a characteristic low-voltage electroencephalogram, has been termed REM sleep. In adults, this stage has been highly associated with dreaming. Four other stages of sleep, all with characteristic EEG and EMG, but unassociated with rapid eye movements, have been termed non-REM sleep.[29,67] Fewer dreams are recalled following the various non-REM states, and they tend to be less elaborate than those associated with REM sleep.[67] After the onset of sleep, the normal adult passes through various stages of non-REM sleep and enters REM sleep after 70 to 90 minutes. Then cycles of non-REM and REM sleep regularly recur throughout the sleeping interval. In the adult it must also be remembered that sleep generally occurs once daily, usually at night.[67]

In the very premature infant, sleep/wake cycles and sleep stages are difficult to differentiate. By the time the infant is 30 to 33 weeks old, however, active sleep and quiet sleep (corresponding possibly to REM and non-REM sleep in the adult), transitional sleep (having characteristics of both active and quiet sleep), and a waking state can be recognized on the basis of physical and EEG criteria.[17,18,47-49,60,67] These stages become progressively more differentiated as development progresses throughout infancy. Compared to the adult, the infant spends much more time asleep, has more sleep periods during the course of a 24-hour day, and appears to spend more time in active sleep. Thus, sleep matures during the normal course of growth and development.

When compared with the awake state, respiration during sleep is depressed.[3,9,58,66] Oxygen consumption is reduced, presumably due to the reduced metabolic rate experienced during sleep. Alveolar ventilation is also reduced, but P_{CO_2} is elevated during sleep. In adults, the ventilatory response to carbon dioxide is diminished during sleep, although the response to hypoxia is not reduced.[5,58,67] Full-term infants have been shown to have higher respiratory rates and minute volumes during REM sleep as opposed to non-REM sleep.[3,28,30] This rise is associated with an elevated oxygen consumption during REM sleep and a greater central drive to breathe during this stage.[21]

Abnormalities of Autonomic Control

Respiratory irregularities are common during fetal life[8] and in premature infants;[9,11,14,16,32,42] these irregularities are absent in mature term infants[14,28,42] and during wakefulness.[16] Premature infants appear to be capable of responding appropriately to altered levels of O_2[37] and CO_2,[35,52-54] and to alterations of cerebrospinal fluid acid-base balance.[36] Thus, chemical control of ventilation is present from early life.

Abnormalities of respiratory rhythm have been associated with different sleep states.[66] Deuel, studying apnea in premature infants, found an increased frequency of apnea during non-REM sleep.[17] Gabriel and colleagues, however, found that their group of preterm infants had more apneic spells of longer duration during REM sleep.[25] Steinschneider, studying a group of SIDS near-miss infants, also reported more respiratory pauses during REM sleep.[59]

It is puzzling that REM sleep, a state associated with a greater central drive to breathe and a higher rate of minute ventilation, should also prove to be associated with higher apnea attack rates than other sleep states. Since all groups of infants so far reported have been small in number, some of these apparent conflicts may be resolved by improvements in methods, agreement on definitions, and subsequent study of larger groups of infants of various maturities. Another possibility, and one which is currently under investigation in several centers, is that these abnormalities of respiratory rhythm are maturational in origin. SIDS may therefore represent a persistence of immature respiratory control.

Several well-described sleep-apnea syndromes occur in adults,[29,51] but their relation to SIDS is not yet clear. They have been associated with cerebrovascular disease, bilateral cervical cordotomy, bulbar poliomyelitis, primary alveolar hypoventilation (Ondine's curse), and obesity (Pickwickian syndrome). A more recent classification divides these syndromes according to their presumed site of origin. *Upper airway apnea* consists of absence of airflow in the presence of respiratory movements, and is presumably due to reflex upper airway closure. *Central apnea* is absence of both respiratory movements and airflow, and is thought to have its origin in the central nervous system. A mixed type of apnea consists of absence of airflow in the absence of respiratory activity followed by unsuccessful attempts to reestablish airflow against a closed glottis. These various types of sleep apnea therefore involve peripheral reflex centers in the lungs, airways, and pharynx, as well as central respiratory areas and the chemosensitive areas of the autonomic nervous system.

The ability of infants to respond to respiratory stimuli is dependent on many factors. Immature infants with diminished ability to respond to carbon dioxide have abnormal lungs with a reduced mechanical response[35,37,52-55] as well as immature nervous systems, which may be insensitive to altered levels of CO_2.[54] Hypoxia appears to increase the frequency of apnea, presumably because of central nervous system depression.[52,53] Therefore, a spontaneously arising respiratory pause in an infant may result in hypoxemia, which may further impair the infant's ability to resume breathing.

Airway obstruction may also occur easily in infants. The nose accounts for a relatively higher proportion of the total airway resistance during infancy than during later life. This resistance may be increased by accumulation of mucus associated with feeding or infection.[13,28,38,40,41] The posterior pharynx may also be the site of reflex airway obstruction in infants.[14,28,61] Chemoreceptors in the posterior pharynx of several animal species respond to instillation of glucose solutions, distilled water, or cows' milk with reflex airway closure. This reflex appears to be mediated by the superior laryngeal nerve.[19]

Abnormalities of the cardiac innervation have also been proposed as a mechanism that might lead to SIDS.[56,57] The process by which cardiac innervation develops during infancy has been termed modeling by James.[33,34] This process involves redistribution of intracardiac conduction during growth and development of the infant heart, and is not accompanied by "pathologic" changes, such as fibrosis, inflammation, or gross hemorrhage. Although some workers deny the importance of modeling,[1,20,65] Schwartz has recently proposed that imbalance of cardiac innervation may lead to SIDS.[57] He theorizes that deficient innervation of the right side of the heart may result in the *long QT syndrome.* Individuals with long QT syndrome have lower thresholds for ventricular fibrillation. Any occurrence that could lead to a dysrhythmia might, therefore, result in a fatal arrhythmia in an infant with long QT syndrome due to a defect in autonomic innervation and intracardiac conduction. Bradycardia has been associated with apnea in premature infants, especially if apnea is prolonged beyond 30 seconds.[16,42]

Bradycardia has also been associated with vagal stimuli occurring in connection with feeding in premature infants.[13] Other arrhythmias have also been described in premature infants in connection with hypoxemia, and may arise from either myocardial hypoxia or reflex sites within the autonomic nervous system. Thus, it is possible for abnormalities in the development of the maturing cardiac conduction system to result in a situation that predisposes the infant to a fatal arrhythmia. The arrhythmia may develop during respiratory infection or during sleep, or in connection with autonomic stimuli, such as feeding or gastric distention.

A Synthesis

The SIDS victim is generally male and under 4 months of age. His autonomic nervous system is not yet fully developed, and various imbalances may be present. As a result of chronic upper airway obstruction, he may have suffered from hypoxemia through much of infancy, diminishing his drive to breathe. Familial factors may also result in a diminished drive to breathe. Like other members of his family, he may suffer from increased sleep apnea, especially during REM sleep. He is likely to have been premature at birth, and his growth since then, though within normal limits, has been slow. His living conditions are probably poor, although not necessarily so. During an early winter month, in the presence of a mild upper respiratory infection that further compromises his upper airway, he is put to bed. Sleep further diminishes his drive to breathe, and apnea increases. Hypoxemia depresses his central receptors. In this setting, either laryngeal closure or cardiac arrhythmia occurs. The infant does not cry. Terminal gasps against a closed glottis occur, causing intrathoracic petechiae. A final autonomic discharge causes emptying of the bladder and bowels. If other members of the household are asleep, the baby goes unheard and is discovered in the morning, a SIDS victim. If he is observed and promptly resuscitated, he becomes a near miss.

Counseling

In the past, the families of SIDS victims have been accused of neglect, abuse, and murder of their children. Needless to say, these attitudes have resulted in many broken lives and homes. As a result, parent groups have been organized in many communities to provide concerned sympathy and support for the parents of SIDS victims. According to most physicians, it is best to inform the parents as soon as possible that their child was a SIDS victim. Beckwith advises that parents be told early, even before complete autopsy findings have been reported.[4] If subsequent chemical or microscopic analysis reveals another cause of death, the parents may then be counseled appropriately. It is of utmost importance, however, to inform the parents that SIDS is a *real* disease and that their child's death was in no way their fault. For these reasons, an autopsy is of great importance in all infant deaths, and should be made available to all regardless of economic or social status.[15]

Of equal importance is the family's concern for subsequent siblings. Although a familial predisposition to SIDS may exist, and respiratory chemosensitivity may be at least partly hereditary, few instances of familial SIDS have been reported. In selected instances, determination of respiratory chemosensitivity, monitoring of respiration in a sleep laboratory, or home monitoring may be offered to siblings of SIDS victims.[12] As yet, no simple, rapid, noninvasive tests are available to determine the at-risk infant. It is in this direction that many workers are now moving. Until a screening test is possible, SIDS will remain a disease that is diagnosed too late.

The National Sudden Infant Death Syndrome Foundation, Suite 1904, 310 South Michigan Avenue, Chicago, IL (312)663-0650, will provide additional counseling and information to physicians and other concerned parties.

REFERENCES

1. Anderson, R. H., J. Bouton, C. T. Burrow and A. Smith: Sudden death in infants: a study of cardiac specialized tissue. *Br. Med. J. 2*:135, 1974.
2. Aserinsky, E. and N. Kleitman: Regularly occurring periods of eye mobility and concomitant phenomena during sleep. *Science 118*:273, 1953.
3. Ashton, R. and K. Connolly: The relation of respiration rate and heart rate to sleep states in the human newborn. *Dev. Med. Child Neurol. 13*:180, 1971.
4. Beckwith, J. B.: The sudden infant death syndrome. *Curr. Probl. Pediatr. 3*:1, 1973.
5. Bellville, J. W., W. S. Howland, J. C. Seed and R. W. Houde: The effect of sleep on the respiratory response to carbon dioxide. *Anesthesiology 20*:628, 1959.
6. Berger, R. J.: The sleep and dream cycle. In *Sleep Physiology and Pathology: A Symposium,* A. Kales (Ed.). J. B. Lippincott, Philadelphia, p. 17, 1969.
7. Bergman, A. B.: Sudden infant death syndrome in King County, Washington: epidemiologic aspects. In *Sudden Infant Death Syndrome,* A. B. Bergman, J. B. Beckwith and G. G. Ray (Eds.). Univ. of Washington Press, Seattle, 1970.
8. Boddy, K. and G. S. Dawes: Fetal breathing. *Br. Med. Bull. 31*:3, 1975.
9. Boutourline-Young, H. J. and C. A. Smith: Respiration of full term and of premature infants. *Am. J. Dis. Child. 80*:753, 1950.
10. Carr, J. L.: Status thymico-lymphaticus. *J. Pediatr. 27*:1, 1945.
11. Chernick, V., F. Heldrich and M. E. Avery: Periodic breathing of premature infants. *J. Pediatr. 64*:330, 1964.
12. Committee on Infant and Preschool Child. Home monitoring and sudden infant death. *Pediatrics 55*:144, 1975.
13. Cordero, L. and E. H. Hon: Neonatal bradycardia following nasopharyngeal stimulation. *J. Pediatr. 78*:441, 1971.
14. Cross, K. W.: *Sudden and Unexpected Deaths in Infancy* (*Cot Deaths*), F. E. Camps and R. G. Carpenter (Eds.). John Wright and Sons, Ltd., Bristol, England, p. 52, 1972.
15. Curran, W. J.: An enigma wrapped in swaddling clothes: Congress and "crib death." *N. Engl. J. Med. 287*:235, 1972.
16. Daily, W. J. R., M. Klaus and H. B. P. Meyer: Apnea in premature infants: monitoring, incidence, heart rate changes, and an effect of environmental temperature. *Pediatrics 43*:510, 1969.
17. Deuel, R. K.: Polygraphic monitoring of apneic spells. *Arch. Neurol. 28*:71, 1973.
18. Dittrichova, J.: Nature of sleep in young infants. *J. Appl. Physiol. 21*:1243, 1966.
19. Downing, S. E. and J. C. Lee: Laryngeal chemosensitivity: a possible mechanism for sudden infant death. *Pediatrics 55*:640, 1975.
20. Ferris, J. A.: Hypoxic changes in conducting tissue of the heart in sudden infant death syndrome. *Br. Med. J. 2*:23, 1973.
21. Finer, N., I. F. Abroms and H. W. Taeusch: Venti-

lation and sleep states in newborn infants. *J. Pediatr. 89*:100, 1976.

22. Foy, H. M. and C. G. Ray: Epidemiology of SIDS and lower respiratory tract illness in young children: a comparison. *Am. J. Epidemiol. 98*:69, 1973.
23. Froggatt, P.: The contribution of epidemiology to the study of the sudden infant death syndrome. In *Sudden Infant Death Syndrome,* A. B. Bergman, J. B. Beckwith and C. G. Ray (Eds.). Univ. of Washington Press, Seattle, p. 25, 1970.
24. Froggatt, P., M. A. Lynas and T. K. Marshall: Sudden death in babies: epidemiology. *Am. J. Cardiol. 22*:457, 1968.
25. Gabriel, M., M. Albani and F. J. Schulte: Apneic spells and sleep states in preterm infants. *Pediatrics 57*:142, 1976.
26. Gadsdon, D. R. and J. L. Emery: Fatty change in the brain in perinatal and unexpected death. *Arch. Dis. Child. 51*:42, 1976.
27. Greenberg, M. A., K. E. Nelson and B. W. Carnow: A study of the relationship between sudden infant death syndrome and environmental factors. *Am. J. Epidemiol. 98*:412, 1973.
28. Guilleminault, C., R. Peraita, M. Souquet and W. Dement: Apneas during sleep in infants: possible relationship with SIDS. *Science 190*:677, 1975.
29. Guilleminault, C., A. Tilkian and W. C. Dement: The sleep apnea syndromes. *Annu. Rev. Med. 27*:465, 1976.
30. Hathorn, M. K. S.: The rate and depth of breathing in new-born infants in different sleep states. *J. Physiol.* (*Lond.*) *243*:101, 1974.
31. Houstek, J.: Sudden infant death syndrome in Czechoslovakia: epidemiologic aspects. In *Sudden Infant Death Syndrome,* A.B. Bergman, J. B. Beckwith and C. G. Ray (Eds.). Univ. of Washington Press, Seattle, p. 55, 1970.
32. Illingworth, R. S.: Cyanotic attacks in newborn infants. *Arch. Dis. Child. 32*:328, 1957.
33. James, T. N.: Sudden death of babies. *Circulation 53*:1, 1976.
34. James, T. N.: Sudden death in babies: new observations in the heart. *Am. J. Cardiol. 22*:479, 1968.
35. Krauss, A. N., D. B. Klain, S. Waldman and P. A. M. Auld: Ventilatory response to carbon dioxide in newborn infants. *Pediatr. Res. 9*:46, 1975.
36. Krauss, A. N., D. W. Thibeault and P. A. M. Auld: Acid-base balance in cerebrospinal fluid of newborn infants. *Biol. Neonate 21*:25, 1972.
37. Krauss, A. N., C. A. Tori, J. Brown, J. Soodalter and P. A. M. Auld: Oxygen chemoreceptors in low birth weight infants. *Pediatr. Res. 7*:569, 1973.
38. Levy, A., B. Tabakian, J. Hanson and R. Narkewicz: Hypertrophied adenoids causing pulmonary hypertension and severe congestive heart failure. *N. Engl. J. Med. 277*:506, 1967.
39. Lie, J. T., H. S. Rosenberg and E. E. Erickson: Histopathology of the conduction system in the sudden infant death syndrome. *Circulation 53*:3, 1976.
40. Luke, M., A. Mehrizi, G. Folger and R. Rowe: Chronic nasopharyngeal obstruction as a cause of cardiomegaly, cor pulmonale, and pulmonary edema. *Pediatrics 37*:762, 1966.
41. Menashe, V., C. Farrehi and M. Miller: Hypoventilation and cor pulmonale due to chronic upper airway obstruction. *J. Pediatr. 67*:198, 1965.
42. Miller, H. C., F. C. Behrle and N. W. Smull: Severe apnea and irregular respiratory rhythms among premature infants. *Pediatrics 23*:676, 1959.
43. Naeye, R. L.: Pulmonary arterial abnormalities in the sudden infant death syndrome. *N. Engl. J. Med. 289*:1167, 1970.
44. Naeye, R. L. and R. S. Fisher: Carotid body abnormalities in the sudden infant death syndrome. *Am. J. Pathol. 82*:29a, 1976.
45. Naeye, R. L., J. Messmer, T. Specht and T. A. Merritt: Sudden infant death syndrome temperament before death. *J. Pediatr. 88*:511, 1976.
46. Nelson, K. E., M. A. Greenberg, M. A. Mufson and V. K. Moses: The sudden infant death syndrome and viral disease. *Am. J. Epidemiol. 101*:423, 1975.
47. Paul, K., J. Drittichova and E. Pavlikova.: The course of quiet sleep in infants. *Biol. Neonate 23*:78, 1973.
48. Parmelee, A. H., W. H. Wenner, Y. Akiyama, M. Schultz and E. Stern: Sleep states in premature infants. *Dev. Med. Child Neurol. 9*:70, 1967.
49. Parmelee, A. H., F. J. Schulte, Y. Akiyama, W. H. Wenner, M. A. Schultz and E. Stern: Maturation of EEG activity during sleep in premature infants. *Electroencephalogr. Clin. Neurophysiol. 24*:319, 1968.
50. Peterson, D. R., E. A. Benson, L. D. Fisher, N. M. Chinn and J. B. Beckwith: Postnatal growth and the sudden infant death syndrome. *Am. J. Epidemiol. 99*:389, 1974.
51. Plum, F.: Neurological integration of behavioral and metabolic control of breathing. In *Ciba Foundation Hering-Breuer Symposium: Breathing,* R. Porter (Ed.). J. and A. Churchill, London, p. 159, 1970.
52. Rigatto, H. and J. P. Brady: Periodic breathing and apnea in term infants: I. Evidence of hypoventilation possibly due to central respiratory depression. *Pediatrics 50*:202, 1972.
53. Rigatto, H. and J. P. Brady: Periodic breathing and apnea in preterm infants: II. Hypoxia as a primary event. *Pediatrics 50*:219, 1972.
54. Rigatto, H., J. P. Brady and R. de la Torre Verduzco: Chemoreceptor reflexes in preterm infants: I. The effect of gestational and postnatal age on the ventilatory response to inhalation of 100% and 15% oxygen. *Pediatrics 55*:604, 1975.

55. Rigatto, H., J. P. Brady and R. de la Torre Verduzco: Chemoreceptor reflexes in preterm infants: II. The effect of gestational and postnatal age on the ventilatory response to inhaled carbon dioxide. *Pediatrics 55*:614, 1975.
56. Salk, L., B. A. Grellong and J. Dietrich: Normal cardiac habituation and poor autonomic control. *N. Engl. J. Med. 291*:219, 1974.
57. Schwartz, P. J.: Cardiac sympathetic innervation and the sudden infant death syndrome: a possible pathogenetic link. *Am. J. Med. 60*:167, 1976.
58. Severinghaus, J. P. and C. P. Larson: Respiration in anesthesia. In *Handbook of Physiology, Section 3: Respiration,* Volume 2, H. Wofenn (Ed.). Rahn, Washington, D.C., p. 1219, 1965.
59. Steinschneider, A.: Prolonged apnea and the sudden infant death syndrome: clinical and laboratory observations. *Pediatrics 50*:646, 1972.
60. Stern, E., A. H. Parmelee and M. A. Harris: Sleep state periodicity in prematures and young infants. *Dev. Psychobiol. 6*:357, 1973.
61. Tonkin, S.: Sudden infant death syndrome: hypothesis of causation. *Pediatrics 55*:650, 1975.
62. Valdes-Dapena, M. A.: Sudden and unexpected death in infancy: a review of the world literature, 1954–1966. *Pediatrics 39*:123, 1967.
63. Valdes-Dapena, M. A.: Progress in sudden infant death research, 1963–1969. In *Sudden Infant Death Syndrome,* A. B. Bergman, J. B. Beckwith and C. G. Ray (Eds.). Univ. of Washington Press, Seattle, p. 3, 1970.
64. Valdes-Dapena, M. A.: Sudden death in infancy: a report to pathologists. *Perspect. Pediatr. Pathol. 2*:1, 1975.
65. Valdes-Dapena, M. A., M. Greene, N. Basavanand, R. Catherman and R. C. Truex: The myocardial conduction system in sudden death in infants. *N. Engl. J. Med. 289*:1179, 1973.
66. Webb, P.: Periodic breathing during sleep. *J. Appl. Physiol. 37*:899, 1974.
67. Weitzman, E. D. and L. Graziani: Sleep and the sudden infant death syndrome: a new hypothesis. *Adv. Sleep Res. 1*:327, 1974.

Uncommon Diseases, Extrapulmonary Diseases, Systemic Diseases, and Toxins

BELLA C. CLUTARIO AND BERNARD H. HOLZMAN

18

Part I: *Uncommon Pulmonary Diseases in Children*

Pulmonary fungous infections, hypersensitivity diseases, and a number of other pulmonary conditions are relatively uncommon in infants and children in the United States. Their occurrence can present a diagnostic dilemma and they must be considered in the evaluation of difficult problems.

Fungous Infections

Systemic fungous infections in previously healthy children are not common. For most of the fungi the rate of infection increases as the contact between the potential host and his community environment increases. Thus the rate of infection is low until adolescence and early adult life are reached—a fact that also generally holds for geographic areas in which specific fungous diseases are endemic. Superinfection or opportunistic infection by fungi is also relatively uncommon in children. Opportunistic infections may occur in subjects debilitated by a primary disease that seriously impairs host resistance (e.g., immunologic and metabolic disorders, constitutional diseases such as cystic fibrosis, blood dyscrasias, diseases of the lymphatic system), in which case common natural saprophytes such as Aspergillus and Candida may become the infecting agents. Iatrogenic predisposition to infection by these fungi may also be established, for example, by prolonged administration of antibiotics and corticosteroids. Diagnosis of pulmonary fungous infection rests on the isolation of the agent by culture or animal inoculation; direct microscopy of fresh specimens, such as properly collected sputum, pulmonary aspirates, and tissue, and serologic tests are important but secondary diagnostic aids (see also p. 62, Chapter 1).

HISTOPLASMOSIS[38,47,56,63,65,66]

Infection by *Histoplasma capsulatum* usually produces mild, acute illness and only infrequently progresses to chronic inflammatory disease of the lungs or to severe systemic infection. The more severe expressions of infection are generally seen in the very young (infants), the aged (over 60 years), and the debilitated. Infection is more common in males than females and in whites more than blacks. Its prevalence in the United States is indicated by the distribution of histoplasmin sensitivity on the mainland (Fig. 18-1).

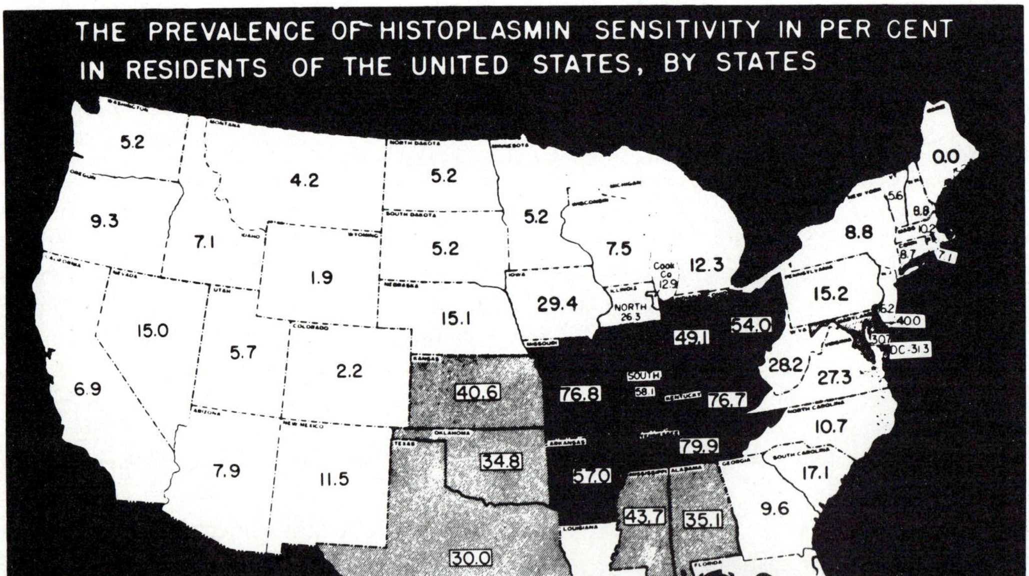

FIG. 18-1. Prevalence of histoplasmin sensitivity in residents of the United States, by states. (From Christie, A.: Histoplasmosis. In *Disorders of the Respiratory Tract in Children,* E. L. Kendig, Jr. (Ed.), W. B. Saunders Co., Philadelphia, 1972.)

Histoplasma infection can produce a number of pulmonary syndromes related, in part, to the dose and its distribution as acquired through the respiratory route, which is probably the essential mode of entry of the fungus into the body. Because of the protean expressions of Histoplasma infection of the lung, it should be included in the differential diagnosis of any cryptic pulmonary condition. The primary infection may occur as a single nodular lesion in the lung parenchyma or the lesions may be widespread throughout both lung fields. Constitutional symptoms, including fever, sweats, dyspnea, productive cough, weakness, and myalgia, may be prominent, or in surprising contrast to the roentgenographic appearance, symptoms may be few. Generally the lesions resolve slowly over a period of many weeks, leaving perhaps small residual areas of fibrosis or calcification. Rarely, the primary nodules may progress to serious systemic disease. Histoplasma infection may also begin as an apparent exudative process, which may be difficult to distinguish from acute bacterial or viral pneumonia. Signs of acute pneumonia are present (fever, cough, chills, sweats, anorexia, and chest pain), the pleura may be involved, and a positive blood culture for *H. capsulatum* may be obtained. The latter does not indicate active dissemination. Other, less common, manifestations of *H. capsulatum* infection include (1) "wandering pneumonia," in which new pulmonary infiltrates appear successively as the older lesions resolve; (2) infection apparently localized in the hilar lymph nodes without involvement of the pulmonary parenchyma; (3) potentially rapidly fatal disseminated histoplasmosis with miliary pulmonary lesions; and (4) chronic or reinfection histoplasmosis.

Diagnosis may be made in patients with overwhelming infection by histologic examination of the buffy coat of the blood or of bone marrow. Staining with Giemsa or Wright stain, or with fluorescein-conjugated antibodies[20] is preferred. Cultivation of the organism from sputum or tissues, or on occasion from blood, bone marrow, urine, or spinal fluid, may produce colonies as quickly as 2 days or may take as long as 3 weeks depending on the dose of the inoculum. Animal inoculation may also be helpful; cultures may be made of the liver and spleen 4 weeks after inoculation. The histoplasmin (mycelial antigen) skin test is positive in 75 to 90% of patients. Serologic tests[43,60,62] include complement-fixation (positive titers in over 80% of patients, including those with chronic pulmonary infection), collodion agglutination, and precipitin tests. Because a positive skin test may produce an increase in the complement-fixation titer, it should be reserved as a diagnostic measure until the serologic tests are completed. The most reliable serologic test for *H. capsulatum* infection is the agar gel precipitin test,[71] which may yield two bands: one (the "H band") denotes active infection and does not appear during infection with other fungi; the other (the "M band") may arise from positive skin tests and may persist after the acute infection.

Amphotericin B, given intravenously for 30 to 90 days or longer, is the most effective *therapy* for both acute pulmonary and severe disseminated infections, although no treatment may be needed for most patients who develop acute pulmonary histoplasmosis with benign symptomatology. A number of schedules for titration of the dose of amphotericin B have been recommended, including the regulation of blood concentration against the measured in vitro sensitivity of the *H. capsulatum* strain to the drug.[15] The toxicity of amphotericin B is well known:[59] its effects on renal function should be monitored especially carefully and the dosage reduced or the medication stopped in the face of a blood urea nitrogen over 40 mg/100 ml.

NORTH AMERICAN BLASTOMYCOSIS[24,41,61,64,67]

Pulmonary blastomycosis is caused by *Blastomyces dermatitidis*, which resides in the soil of many areas of the central and southeastern United States. Disease in humans generally involves the lungs and the skin. Although the lung is the principal portal of entry, initial symptoms are related to the lung in only half the patients and related to sites involved by hematogenous dissemination in the others. Respiratory signs and symptoms are not characteristic and may mimic the onset of bacterial pneumonia. Initially a single lobe or part of a lobe may be involved, but multilobar involvement has also been noted. Less frequently other patterns of respiratory tract involvement may be apparent: the spectrum is a wide one, which includes isolated mediastinal lymph node enlargement, perihilar roentgenographic densities, nodular densities, and granulomatous "coin" lesions. The lesions may resolve or they may alternately progress and regress or they may increase over a period of years. Chronic disease may produce fibrosis, cavity formation, and focal granulomas. Dissemination may take place to the skin, bones, and other viscera (including the joints, genitourinary tract, central nervous system, and, by direct extension, the heart and larynx). The skin lesions are papules, which form elevated granulomas that ulcerate and discharge purulent or sanguinopurulent material. Whereas mortality from untreated disseminated blastomycosis is probably greater than 90%, the estimated cure rate of patients with acute or chronic pulmonary disease and with disseminated blastomycosis is about 80% when amphotericin B is used.

Although a presumptive *diagnosis* of blastomycosis may be made by histologic examination of sputum and a tissue biopsy, confirmation by growing *B. dermatitidis* in culture should always be sought. Sputum, gastric washings, and bronchial aspirates may provide suitable material for culture.[37] Skin tests with filtrates of either the mycelial or yeast phase of *B. dermatitidis* may give falsely negative results in as many as 50% of the patients,[4] and patients with blastomycosis may also react to coccidioidin or histoplasmin antigen. The complement-fixation test for blastomycosis may be falsely negative in up to 60% of the patients, and significant cross reaction occurs with antigens from *Coccidioides immitis* and *H. capsulatum.*

Treatment of choice is intravenous amphotericin B.[36,48,74]

COCCIDIOIDOMYCOSIS

In the United States *C. immitis* seems to be limited to the soil of the southwestern states—Texas, Utah, New Mexico, Arizona, Nevada, and California.[53] Human infection takes place principally through the respiratory tract and the initial symptoms mimic the onset of influenza. Skin manifestations include subcutaneous swellings that resemble erythema nodosum of the extremities, lesions resembling erythema multiforme, and urticarial eruptions. Respiratory tract involvement ranges from apparent isolated hilar adenopathy through perihilar parenchymal densities or patchy pneumonia-like densities, to miliary lesions. Although the pleura is not often involved, large pleural effusions may be produced. Most patients with pulmonary coccidioidomycosis recover completely in a variable period lasting up to 4 months. Very few develop residual disease and pulmonary complications, including abscesses, fibrosis, persistent pleural effusion, empyema, pneumothorax, and cavity formation, which may require surgical intervention.[75] Death may result from severe pulmonary involvement or from spread to other viscera such as the heart, adrenals, and central nervous system.

Diagnosis is established by isolation of the fungus and by skin and serologic tests. *C. immitis* spherules may be seen in the sputum of infected patients, but this test is unreliable. The specific test is the growth in culture from tissue specimens or from exudates, blood, urine, pleural fluid, and cerebrospinal fluid. The intradermal test becomes positive in 99% of patients with acute nondisseminated disease within 3 weeks of the onset and reverts to negative in 6 months to 10 years. The skin test is a reliable tool, and despite cross reactions with histoplasmin and blastomycin, it virtually always produces the greater response. Serologic tests include a precipitin test and a complement-fixation test.[68,69] In about one-third the patients with primary pulmonary infection only the precipitin test is positive, although 90% of patients with acute coccidioidomycosis develop precipitins.

Most patients do not require specific antifungal *therapy*. Amphotericin B is the drug of choice for many patients with acute pulmonary disease and for some patients with disseminated disease. Louria's indications for instituting therapy include progressive pulmonary disease, evidence that the infection has become disseminated, skin anergy, or a complement-fixation titer greater than 1 : 16.[37,38]

CRYPTOCOCCOSIS[19,31,35]

Most cases occur in previously healthy individuals, although the incidence seems to be increasing in debilitated subjects, especially those with malignant disease of the reticuloendothelial system. *Cryptococcus neoformans* is found frequently in pigeon nests and pigeon droppings, and it enters man through the respiratory tract. The central nervous system is most often infected, but isolated pulmonary disease is not uncommon. The signs and symptoms of pulmonary disease may be minimal or may include cough (sometimes productive of purulent or blood-streaked sputum), chest pain, and signs of pleural disease. The pulmonary parenchyma may be affected in a number of ways including lobar or segmental densities with or without cavitation, single granuloma or abscess, one or more patchy parenchymal densities, and diffuse nodular lesions or miliary disease.

Diagnosis is made by culture of the organism from sputum, aspirates, or spinal fluid. Serologic or spinal fluid tests for the cryptococcol polysaccharide and for agglutinating antibody[10,21] are most helpful in establishing the specific diagnosis and in assessing the efficacy of therapy. Thus, if the polysaccharide is present, but agglutinating antibody is absent, infection is probably still active. Conversely, the presence of antibody and the absence of polysaccharide suggest that treatment has been successful.

Although isolated pulmonary disease may resolve without specific *therapy*, the danger of spread to the central nervous system dictates that pulmonary cryptococcosis should be treated with amphotericin B. The pulmonary response to this agent is excellent, whereas its effectiveness in the management of central nervous system disease is variable: thus approximately one-third the patients are cured, one-third improve, and the rest fail to respond or relapse.

THE OPPORTUNISTS

The following fungi are either classic opportunists or, as increasing evidence suggests, "secondary invaders."

(1) *Mucormycosis.* The fungi of the family Mucoraceae almost always produce infection in subjects with severe underlying disease such as leukemia, lymphoma, burns, and carcinoma.[42] The primary site of infection is probably the nasal sinuses with contiguous or hematogenous spread. Thus the eyes and central nervous system are often involved. As in other organs the fungus may invade the pulmonary vessels, producing infarcts, and grow into contiguous tissue, producing necrosis. *Diagnosis* is established by culture of sputum or exudates. (It should be noted, however, that patients with chronic, nonfungal pulmonary disease may have fungal spe-

cies in their sputum without evidence of pulmonary mucormycosis.) Amphotericin B is the only *therapy* that may be of help, although experience with it in the treatment of mucormycosis is not extensive.

(2) *Actinomycosis.* Since *Actinomyces israelii* may be isolated from the oronasal cavity but cannot be recovered from soil, it is suggested that actinomycosis arises endogenously after trauma to tissues that it inhabits. Thus, pulmonary actinomycosis is thought to arise from aspiration of infected material from the pharynx, for example, following tooth extraction. (Other forms of actinomycosis include cervicofacial and abdominal disease.) The pulmonary lesions progress to form abscesses, which may perforate the chest wall or the diaphragm, leaving chronically draining sinuses. When external perforation has not taken place, *diagnosis* may be difficult. Sputum and exudates may show the typical "sulfur granules," which are in fact collections of thin hyphae in dense networks that send projections out to the periphery. It should be noted that similar "granules" may be found in nocardiosis, staphylococcal infections, and some gram-negative bacterial infections. Since no reliable skin or serologic tests exist for actinomycosis, diagnosis must rest on the cultures. Penicillin is the drug of choice in the *treatment* of all forms of human actinomycosis.[25,50] It must be given in large doses for periods of 18 weeks to 18 months. Surgical excision and drainage of abscesses must be carried out, and together with appropriate antibiotic therapy, a recovery rate of at least 80% may be anticipated. Tetracycline may be used for patients sensitive to penicillin.

(3) *Nocardiosis.* Distributed worldwide, Nocardia spp. are readily isolated from the soil. Whereas nocardiosis may affect otherwise healthy people, it seems to be appearing more commonly in patients with underlying serious disease, such as alveolar proteinosis, lymphoma, leukemia, sarcoidosis, tuberculosis, and carcinoma,[13,45] and in patients receiving corticosteroid therapy. Pulmonary infiltration may present a variety of appearances, including "patchy" or "fluffy" densities, focal densities with evidence of abscess or cavity formation, and broad densities extending from the hilar region to the periphery. The pleura may be involved and the infection may extend into adjacent ribs or vertebrae. Nocardiosis originating in the lungs may spread to the central nervous system, in which case the disease is usually fatal. Spread may also be to the subcutaneous tissues; conversely, primary infections of the skin usually do not spread to other viscera. Since no reliable skin or serologic tests exist, *diagnosis* is established by culture of the organism from abscesses and sputum. Granules containing thin mycelia may be seen in exudates from abscesses or in sputum, and may be indistinguishable from the "sulfur granules" of actinomycosis. It is generally believed that sulfonamides are the drugs of choice in the *therapy* of nocardiosis, even if other agents appear to be more effective in vitro.[50] Either streptomycin or a broad spectrum antibiotic, in addition to sulfonamides, has been recommended.[50]

(4) *Candidiasis.* The diagnosis of systemic candidiasis, based on positive sputum and blood cultures for *Candida albicans,* has been made in a number of cases in which prolonged antibiotic and/or corticosteroid therapy seemed to be the predisposing conditions for establishment of the fungal infection. Whereas pulmonary candidiasis was present in some of the patients, the extrapulmonary disease was the dominant feature. Because Candida is often found in sputum, a positive sputum culture is not definitive, and the diagnosis of pulmonary candidiasis requires corroboration by cultures from other tissues or fluids, such as pulmonary tissue, exudates from pulmonary abscesses, and pleural fluid. Under such circumstances, or in the presence of positive blood cultures, treatment with amphotericin B is advised.

(5) *Aspergillosis.* Pulmonary aspergillosis is rare in previously healthy individuals, and

when it does occur, it is often associated with exposure to high concentrations of spores on grains or dust. Most often, pulmonary aspergillosis develops as a superinfection on a previously existing lung disease. For example, infections of the cavitary lesions of tuberculosis, histoplasmosis, bronchiectasis, and neoplasms by Aspergillus have been reported. In addition, an increasing number of patients seem to develop pulmonary aspergillosis following treatment with antibiotics and/or corticosteroids. Primary aspergillosis of the lung can be *diagnosed* with certainty only by culture from biopsied tissue. On the other hand, aspergillosis in a pre-existing cavity ("aspergilloma") gives a classic roentgenographic shadow, which may be diagnostic of the condition. In addition, over 90% of these patients give a positive serologic precipitin test. When opportunistic infection in antibiotic/steroid-treated patients is suspected, the diagnosis may be confirmed by repeated cultures of large numbers of aspergilli in sputum or by isolation from the blood stream. Aspergilloma are best *treated* by surgical removal, although some success may be had by medical treatment with potassium iodide. Amphotericin B may be of some benefit for the treatment of systemic aspergillosis and for pulmonary aspergillosis associated with antibiotic/steroid therapy. (See also allergic bronchopulmonary aspergillosis on page 536.)

RARE PULMONARY FUNGI

Pulmonary sporotrichosis has been reported. Skin tests, serologic tests, and sputum cultures establish the diagnosis, and amphotericin B is the therapeutic drug of choice. Pulmonary geotrichosis may be suspected if repeated positive cultures of the fungus occur in the sputum of a patient with unexplained pulmonary disease. Treatment with potassium iodide and autogenous vaccines is advocated. Allescheriasis may opportunistically complicate a pre-existing pulmonary lesion. Positive blood and sputum cultures are diagnostic; no effective therapy is known. South American blastomycosis (*B. brasiliensis*), endemic in certain areas of Latin America, may present as mucocutaneous, lymphangitic, or visceral disease. The latter, which includes pulmonary infection, is least common. Diagnosis may be made from cultures of sputum, blood, or tissue. Amphotericin B is probably the treatment of choice.

Hypersensitivity Diseases

A number of diseases of the lung appear to be caused by abnormal immunologic responses and hypersensitivity. For some diseases, the immunologic basis is fairly well established, whereas for others, it is inferred on the basis of identification of an offending antigen, antibody, or delayed hypersensitivity. Since certain histologic changes (including tissue eosinophilia, plasma cell infiltration, vasculitis, and granuloma) may be produced by immunologic means experimentally, their presence in pulmonary disease of unknown cause is often taken as presumptive evidence for abnormal immunologic response.[33]

GOODPASTURE'S SYNDROME

Goodpasture's syndrome is believed to be an autoimmune disease, generally characterized by recurrent pulmonary hemorrhages followed by progressive glomerulonephritis. It occurs predominantly in the 16- to 25-year-old group, with males outnumbering females. The disease begins insidiously, usually with pulmonary manifestations related to intrapulmonary hemorrhage. Hemoptysis may be the initial sign, at first manifested by blood-streaked sputum, then progressing to more extensive bleeding and anemia. Cough and dyspnea, related to irritation from bleeding and intra-alveolar filling with blood, are also common. Classically the second phase of the disease begins 1 to 9 months after the onset of pulmonary bleeding. This nephritic phase is characterized at first by albuminuria, microscopic hematuria, and cellular and granular casts in the urine. It is followed by uremia, which may develop rapidly and herald fatal renal failure. Most patients succumb to renal failure, but patients may die in respiratory failure from acute pulmonary hemorrhage and asphyxia.[3] Spontaneous remissions have been reported, but most individuals do not survive.

The histopathologic findings in Goodpasture's syndrome are limited to the lungs and kidneys, and may be associated with the presence of antibodies that are specific for glomerular and pulmonary basement membranes.[29,32] The ultrastructural lesion in the lungs[6] resembles the change that may be induced in the glomerular basement membranes of experimental animals by specific antibody.[72] The pulmonary basement membranes are thick with areas of irregular rarefaction. There is intra-alveolar hemorrhage, hemosiderin laden macrophages ("siderophages"), and development of interstitial fibrosis. Absence of pulmonary arteritis distinguishes this disease from the collagen diseases. Roentgenographically, the pulmonary densities involve the hilar regions and extend peripheralward. The densities are quite variable (coarse mottling, fine stippling, confluence) in relation to the magnitude and extent of bleeding, and they tend to disappear rapidly after bleeding has stopped. When pulmonary bleeding is recurrent, development of interstitial disease may become apparent.

Diagnosis is made on the basis of the typical clinical picture, involvement of the lungs and then the kidneys. Diagnosis of pulmonary bleeding is confirmed by identification of siderophages in sputum and gastric washings or by localization of radioactive chromium-labelled red blood cells over areas of pulmonary consolidation. The nephritic phase is characteristic of progressive glomerulonephritis. Interestingly, tests of blood coagulation and capillary fragility are normal; tests for lupus erythematosus and rheumatoid factor are negative; muscle biopsies are normal; and antistreptolysin O titers are usually normal. Treatment is symptomatic and includes ventilatory support and blood transfusion for the pulmonary disease. Although they are used frequently, corticosteroids appear to have no significant effect on ultimate survival, especially with regard to reversal of the renal disease. Prolonged maintenance by hemodialysis[29] and bilateral nephrectomy with successful renal allograft[9,40] may hold promise as effective therapeutic modalities.

IDIOPATHIC PULMONARY HEMOSIDEROSIS

This disease of unknown cause is usually seen in infants and children below the age of 16. It is characterized by recurrent pulmonary hemorrhage, the amount and frequency of which determines the acute pulmonary manifestations and the development of diffuse interstitial fibrosis. Like Goodpasture's syndrome, diagnostic features include the clinical picture of pulmonary hemorrhage with hemoptysis, the characteristic roentgenogram, the associated anemia, and hemosiderin-laden macrophages in sputum and gastric washings. Unlike Goodpasture's syndrome, there is no associated renal disease and death may occur in weeks or years during a course of illness characterized by remissions and relapses and ending in massive pulmonary hemorrhage. Occasionally, pulmonary hypertension, cor pulmonale, and right heart failure may occur. The histopathologic changes of idiopathic pulmonary hemosiderosis include widespread damage to pulmonary capillary basement membranes (similar to Goodpasture's syndrome), with interstitial iron deposits, swollen endothelium, and dense deposits of protein in the capillary basement membranes. The latter features distinguish idiopathic pulmonary hemosiderosis from Goodpasture's syndrome.[16,57] It has been suggested that this distinguishing characteristic indicates an immunologic mechanism as the basis for intrapulmonary hemorrhage, since the protein deposits are similar to those seen in glomeruli of patients with "immune complex" nephritis.[16]

Treatment of idiopathic pulmonary hemosiderosis by respiratory therapy and blood transfusion, as indicated, is mandatory. Corticosteroid therapy is recommended during episodes of hemorrhage, with tapering and discontinuance of the hormone during periods of remission.[26] Immunosuppression with azathioprine, in conjunction with corticosteroids, has also been recommended.[26] The possibility that pulmonary hemosiderosis may be related to milk allergy or allergy to other foods must always be considered, and meticulous efforts to identify possible allergens and to provide a hypoallergenic diet must be made. We have had particularly good success in the treatment of one child, who was sensitive to milk and cow meat allergens associated with pulmonary hemosiderosis, by removal of all milk and associated products. No pulmonary bleeding has recurred over a 4-year period, except for one occasion when he was inadvertently given milk chocolate to eat. The association between milk allergy and pulmonary hemosiderosis seems clear in some patients[27] and is typically manifested by recurrent pulmonary infiltrates (presumably hemorrhagic), siderophages, intermittent wheezing, eosinophilia, anemia, serum iron deficiency, failure to thrive, and elevated serum IgE.[5] Milk elimination and symptomatic therapy, including diet control, have been reported to be most effective.[5] Concomitant chronic rhinitis and enlargement of the adenoids may lead to significant upper airway obstruction (see later), which is effectively remedied by adenoidectomy.

(It should also be noted that "secondary" pulmonary hemosiderosis may be associated with myocardial disease *without* heart failure; it may occur as a consequence of chronic congestive heart failure; it may develop as part of a collagen-vascular or purpuric disease; and it may follow excessive parenteral administration of iron or repeated blood transfusions.)

LÖFFLER'S SYNDROME

This syndrome, as described originally, is a relatively benign disease characterized by blood eosinophilia with migrating pulmonary infiltrates. Clinical symptoms are mild, usually consisting of dry cough and fever. Löffler's syndrome has been termed "simple pulmonary eosinophilia,"[12] to distinguish it from other, more serious, pulmonary eosinophilic disease. Simple pulmonary eosinophilia resolves within a few weeks. Its cause is thought to be an allergic reaction to a variety of drugs such as para-aminosalicylic acid, penicillin, sulfonamides, aspirin, and nitrofurantoin.[8,14,18,49] Often, no cause is found and the condition regresses spontaneously. When a causative agent is found, regression follows withdrawal of the drug.

Other pulmonary eosinophilic syndromes include (1) "prolonged pulmonary eosinophilia," either idiopathic or in association with a wide spectrum of diseases (e.g., with sarcoidosis, psittacosis, primary atypical pneumonia, and farmer's lung); (2) "pulmonary eosinophilia with asthma," which is a prolonged eosinophilia associated with asthma or with allergy to Aspergillus (in bronchopulmonary aspergillosis) or Candida; (3) "tropical pulmonary eosinophilia," which is generally thought to be caused by microfilariae in the lung. In addition, various parasites are associated with cough, fever, pulmonary infiltrates, eosinophilia, and hemoptysis, including Ascaris, Strongyloides, and Ancylostoma species, and *Toxocara canis;* and (4) "pulmonary eosinophilia with periarteritis nodosa." This classification of pulmonary infiltrations with eosinophilia is based on that proposed by Crofton et al.[12]

Prolonged *idiopathic* pulmonary eosinophilia may be termed "chronic eosinophilic pneumonia."[7,54] Its roentgenographic characteristics include dense pulmonary shadows that progress with time and are more prominent peripherally than centrally. Eosinophilia of the peripheral blood is inconstant, whereas the pulmonary pathologic changes consist of eosinophilic exudation into the alveoli and interstitium. The disease has been reported in a 1-year-old child, who, like adults, responded dramatically to corticosteroid therapy and had no recurrence of the disease process after cessation of therapy.[54]

Prolonged pulmonary eosinophilia associated with an underlying disease, and pulmonary eosinophilia with periarteritis have the gross and microscopic morphologic pattern of the underlying disease. Superimposed on this condition is an increase in the number of tissue eosinophils. Treatment is directed against the underlying disease.

Tropical pulmonary eosinophilia is thought to be related to the phagocytic function of eosinophils, in which they ingest and presumably metabolize antigen-antibody complexes and occasionally organisms.[58] Analogously, it has been suggested that the eosinophil degrades histamine in tissues following degranulation of mast cells and basophils,[2] and that this function is the basis for the association between eosinophilia and allergic rhinitis and asthma. Indeed, pulmonary eosinophilia of a transitory nature has been described in asthmatics.[17] A subcategory of asthma with bronchopulmonary aspergillosis and with Candida hypersensitivity has been associated with pulmonary eosinophilia.[52] The so-called "allergic bronchopulmonary aspergillosis" syndrome consists of chronic asthma, superimposed acute febrile episodes of productive cough with pulmonary infiltrates and eosinophilia, and eventual development of focal bronchiectasis. It has been suggested that pathogenesis involves a unique combination of two immunologic mechanisms: reaginic hypersensitivity mediated by IgE and Arthus hypersensitivity mediated by IgG.[51] Treatment of this condition is only symptomatic. Corticosteroids during the acute episodes dramatically reverse the symptoms and pulmonary infiltrates, thus presumably preventing the development of bronchiectasis. Treatment of the fungus with amphotericin B is recommended, but it is not known how effectively recurrences can be prevented.

HYPERSENSITIVITY ALVEOLITIS

The term, hypersensitivity alveolitis, refers to the reaction produced by specific antigens inhaled in small particles that reach the distal lung parenchyma. Common clinical manifestations include acute respiratory and constitutional symptoms that appear several hours after exposure to the offending antigen and recurrent episodes that may lead to progressive pulmonary disability. At the time of the acute episode the roentgenographic appearance of the lung is characteristic of diffuse interstitial edema, which is followed by the appearance of miliary or patchy infiltrates. In the chronic phase there is typical interstitial fibrosis. All patients have precipitating antibodies to the offending antigen.

Histopathologic changes include (1) proliferation of epithelial cells, which cover the alveolar surface; (2) elaboration of reticulum fibers between the proliferated cells; and (3) lymphocytic and plasma cell infiltration. Ultimately, interstitial fibrosis develops if repeated exposures to the antigen are not avoided.

The diseases are named according to the offending antigen: farmer's lung (antigen produced by thermophilic actinomycetes, which grow under conditions produced by the fermentation of moist hay); bagassosis (antigen possibly produced by a thermophilic actinomycete in rough cane fiber, bagasse, a by-product of cane sugar refining); pigeon breeder's disease (antigen probably from pigeon excreta); maple bark disease (antigen from *Cryptostroma corticale* in maple bark); and similar diseases produced by a number of antigens that may be inhaled, for example, by mushroom growers, redwood sawyers, cheese washers, and people exposed to home humidifiers that are contaminated with fungi.

Progression of the disease resembles an Arthus type reaction with acute vasculitis of the alveolar capillaries and leukocytic infiltration. An obstructive bronchiolitis may develop with destruction of the bronchiolar walls. Granuloma formation, tissue destruction, and fibrosis result in the roentgenographic appearance of a honeycomb lung. Vital capacity and residual volume are low, flow rates are decreased, diffusing capacity is low, and pulmonary compliance may be increased (tissue destruction or "emphysema effect"). The abnormalities of pulmonary function may persist even after the roentgenogram returns to normal. Corticosteroid therapy is most effective in the acute episodes. Avoidance of exposure is the only effective treatment.

Diseases of Alveolar Filling

A number of diseases may be characterized as "occlusive diseases of the alveoli" in which alveoli become filled with foreign material and thus can no longer take part in gas exchange with blood. These diseases have been described in general in the section, Right-to-Left Shunts, of Chapter 2 and with regard to specific diseases (e.g., pulmonary hemorrhage, aspiration syndromes, pneumonias) in other sections of this book. The present section surveys some of the less common diseases that may be grouped together, perhaps for lack of a better understanding of their pathogenesis, according to this shared characteristic.

ALVEOLAR PROTEINOSIS

Pulmonary alveolar proteinosis is an uncommon disease in which large quantities of granular material, with a high content of protein and lipid, are deposited within the terminal air spaces of the lung. The alveolar walls and interstitial tissue are normal. Proteinosis (which is not properly descriptive, since the intra-alveolar material is as much lipid and phospholipid as it is protein) occurs most commonly between the ages of 20 and 50 years, and in males twice as frequently as in females. The lungs are involved bilaterally and symmetrically, so that the roentgenographic appearance may be confused with pulmonary edema. Whereas the "butterfly" appearance is common, the roentgenographic distribution of the lesions may be poorly defined.[22,30] Symptoms begin insidiously and progress slowly. Malaise, fatigue, weight loss, cough, chest pain, and dyspnea are common complaints. Clubbing is common, as is polycythemia. Death is usually due to respiratory failure or to superimposed infection, often with Nocardia.

Pulmonary function testing is consonant with restrictive pulmonary disease, low diffusing capacity, right-to-left shunting, and reduced vital capacity. No specific therapy exists, although improvement is reported following pulmonary lavage.

PULMONARY ALVEOLAR MICROLITHIASIS

In this disease, calculi are produced within the alveoli. Most cases are seen between the ages of 30 and 50 years, but about 20% of the cases occur in children. The process may even begin in utero, and in about half the cases there is a familial occurrence. The intra-alveolar concretions contain calcium and phosphorus on a base of apatite similar to bone. In the early stages alveolar walls are normal, but eventually there is formation of giant cells and of interstitial fibrosis leading to formation of bullae, especially at the apices of the lungs. The roentgenogram reveals diffuse involvement of the lungs and dense deposits of microliths on the pleural surfaces.

Spontaneous pneumothorax, pulmonary hypertension, and cor pulmonale may complicate the clinical picture. Clinical manifestations include dyspnea, hemoptysis, clubbing, and cyanosis. Diagnosis is confirmed by examination of a biopsied specimen. Survival beyond mid-adulthood is not expected.

DESQUAMATIVE INTERSTITIAL PNEUMONITIS

Desquamative interstitial pneumonitis may occur at any age, and in many cases it is a mild disease that responds to corticosteroid therapy. However, there are reports of the disease beginning in infancy with deterioration to death.[28,49] The disease is characterized by massive proliferation and desquamation of large alveolar cells into the terminal air spaces of the lungs.[34,55] There is infiltration of the alveolar septae by eosinophils, plasma cells, and lymphocytes, and the roentgenographic appearance is one of diffuse densities extending peripheralward from the hilar areas. Symptoms may begin with respiratory infections by viruses or by *Mycoplasma pneumoniae,* or there may be no obvious predisposing condition. Dyspnea, weight loss, clubbing, and cyanosis may occur. Lung volume progressively decreases and segmental atelectasis, pneumothorax, pleural effusion, and cor pulmonale may complicate the clinical picture.

Diffuse Idiopathic Interstitial Pulmonary Fibrosis

Diffuse idiopathic interstitial pulmonary fibrosis or Hamman-Rich syndrome[23] is a disease of the small pulmonary vessels and alveoli, which has characteristics of inflammation and hypersensitivity.[23] It affects both sexes equally and includes all age groups. Pulmonary changes are similar if not identical to those found in scleroderma, rheumatoid disease, and disseminated lupus erythematosus. Initially there is edema and fibrin deposition in alveolar walls, with cellular infiltration by lymphocytes, plasma cells, and eosinophils.[46] Subsequently, alveolar lining cells become hyperplastic and may undergo desquamation and necrosis. Fibroblasts appear and fibrous tissue proliferates in the interstices. The roentgenographic appearance reflects the coarse ("reticular" or "reticular-nodular") pattern of the lesions, especially in the lower pulmonary zones, and the development of degenerative cysts, which impart a honeycomb pattern. Lung volume decreases progressively.

Clinical manifestations include cough, weight loss, fatigue, and progressive dyspnea. Clubbing is very common and may antedate the other pulmonary symptoms.[70] Cyanosis and secondary polycythemia may develop. As the disease progresses, pulmonary hypertension, cor pulmonale, and cardiac failure ensue. Important clinical diagnostic features include clubbing, dyspnea on exertion without orthopnea, diffuse crackles especially in the lower pulmonary zones, and the associated roentgenographic appearance. Lung volumes are reduced, including vital capacity and functional residual capacity, and diffusing capacity is low, especially during exertion. In addition, significant inequality of ventilation and perfusion occurs, and pulmonary compliance is low.[73] The disease is usually fatal in 5 to 10 years. Corticosteroids may give some relief of symptoms, but apparently cannot reverse the course of the disease.

Chronic Nasopharyngeal Obstruction

The syndrome of chronic upper airway obstruction by hypertrophied tonsils and adenoids, associated with hypoventilation and cor pulmonale, was first detailed by Menashe et al.[44] The cardiopulmonary effects of obstruction from chronically enlarged tonsils and adenoids range from moderate cardiomegaly and right ventricular hypertrophy to severe right heart failure and pulmonary edema. A history of frequent respiratory infections may be elicited, but more commonly it is reported that the child is lethargic, tends to sleep for periods longer than usual, and has stridor especially when in the supine position. The consequence of chronic obstruction is chronic hypoventilation, which in turn produces alveolar and arterial hypoxemia and hypercapnia. The increased pulmonary vascular resistance in these children is due, most likely, to the sustained changes in blood gas tensions and perhaps also to the large swings in intrapleural pressure that are required to overcome the increased upper airway resistance. The electrocardiographic changes include right atrial and right ventricular hypertrophy, and right ventricular strain. The roentgenographic appearance is that of cardiomegaly, pulmonary arterial dilatation, and possibly pulmonary edema. Cardiac catheterizations, which have been performed in a number of these children, have revealed elevated right ventricular pressures (up to 50 mm Hg) that do not appear to be consonant with the severity of right heart failure. It has been suggested that this apparent discrepancy may be explained by the comparative rapidity with which the right ventricular pressure overload develops or by depression of myocardial performance as a consequence of hypoxemia and acidemia or, perhaps, that pulmonary arterial and right ventricular pressures may in fact be much higher during periods of sleep when the level of hypoventilation increases.[1,39]

Definitive treatment for this condition is tonsillectomy and adenoidectomy. Attempts should be made to reduce the cardiopulmonary strain prior to admission to the operating room. Relief of obstruction by endotracheal intubation with oxygen administration, if required, and increasing myocardial performance by digitalization may be indicated. Since the condition can be fatal, the physician should not hesitate to institute these palliative measures prior to surgery.

Upper airway obstruction from other causes can lead to cor pulmonale and right ventricular failure. Thus laryngotracheomalacia, which is usually a self-limited disease causing only noisy respiration, has produced severe pulmonary hypertension and heart failure in a 29-month-old child.[11] Marked clinical improvement occurred following tracheostomy (which was closed after 11 months), and pulmonary arterial pressure improved significantly. Significant upper airway obstruction may also occur in children in association with laryngeal granuloma of sarcoidosis, with infections or congenital malformations of the upper airways, and with stenoses following tracheostomy or endotracheal intubation. The possibility of developing hypoventilation syndrome with cor pulmonale must be recognized in these cases.

REFERENCES: PART I

1. Ainger, L. E.: Large tonsils and adenoids in small children with cor pulmonale. *Br. Heart J. 30*:356, 1968.
2. Archer, R. K.: *The Eosinophil Leukocytes.* F. A. Davis, Philadelphia, 1963.
3. Benoit, F. L., D. B. Rulon, G. B. Thiel, D. D. Doolan and R. H. Watten: Goodpasture's syndrome: A clinicopathologic entity. *Am. J. Med. 37*:424, 1964.
4. Blastomycosis Cooperative Study of the Veterans Administration. *Am. Rev. Respir. Dis. 89*:659, 1964.
5. Boat, T. F., S. H. Polmar, V. Whitman, J. I. Kleinerman, R. C. Stern and C. F. Doershuk: Hyperreactivity to cow milk in young children with pulmonary hemosiderosis and cor pulmonale secondary to nasopharyngeal obstruction. *J. Pediatr. 87*:23, 1975.
6. Botting, A. J., A. C. Brown, and M. B. Divertie: The pulmonary lesion in a patient with Goodpasture's syndrome as studied with the electron microscope. *Am. J. Clin. Pathol. 42*:387, 1964.
7. Carrington, C. B., W. W. Addington, A. M. Goff, I. M. Madoff, A. Marks, J. R. Schwaber and E. A. Gaensler: Chronic eosinophilic pneumonia. *N. Engl. J. Med. 280*:787, 1969.
8. Citro, L. A., M. E. Gordon and W. T. Miller: Eosinophilic lung disease. *Am. J. Roentgenol. Radium Ther. Nucl. Med. 117*:787, 1973.

9. Cleveland, R. J., H. M. Lee, G. R. Prout and D. M. Hume: Preservation of the cadaver kidney for renal homotransplantation in man. *Surg. Gynecol. Obstet. 119*:991, 1964.
10. Cohen, A. A., A. Davis and S. M. Finegold: Chronic pulmonary cryptococcosis. *Am. Rev. Respir. Dis. 91*:414, 1965.
11. Cox, M. A., G. L. Schiebler, W. J. Taylor, M. W. Wheat, Jr. and L. J. Krovetz: Reversible pulmonary hypertension in a child with respiratory obstruction and cor pulmonale. *J. Pediatr. 67*:192, 1965.
12. Crofton, J. W., J. L. Livingstone, N. C. Oswald, and A. T. M. Roberts: Pulmonary eosinophilia. *Thorax 7*:1, 1952.
13. Cross, R. M. and C. H. Binford: Is *Nocardia asteroides* an opportunist? *Lab. Invest. 11*:1103, 1962.
14. Cuthbert, R. T.: Loeffler's syndrome occurring during streptomycin and PAS therapy. *Br. Med. J. 2*:388, 1954.
15. Drutz, D. J., A. Spickard, D. E. Rogers and M. G. Koenig: Treatment of disseminated mycotic infections: a new approach to amphotericin B therapy. *Am. J. Med. 45*:405, 1968.
16. Elliott, M. L. and C. Kuhn: Idiopathic pulmonary hemosiderosis. Ultrastructural abnormalities in the capillary walls. *Am. Rev. Respir. Dis. 102*:895, 1970.
17. Ford, R. M.: Transient pulmonary eosinophilia and asthma: review of 20 cases in 5,712 asthma sufferers. *Am. Rev. Respir. Dis. 93*:797, 1965.
18. Glueck, M. A. and M. Janower: Nitrofurantoin lung disease—clues to pathogenesis. *Radiology 107*:818, 1969.
19. Goldstein, E. and O. N. Rambo: Cryptococcal infection following steroid therapy. *Ann. Intern. Med. 56*:114, 1962.
20. Gordon, M. A.: Fluorescent staining of *Histoplasma capsulatum. J. Bacteriol. 77*:678, 1959.
21. Gordon, M. A. and D. K. Vedder: Serologic tests in diagnosis and prognosis of cryptococcosis. *J.A.M.A. 197*:961, 1966.
22. Greenspan, R. H.: Chronic disseminated alveolar diseases of the lung. *Semin. Roentgenol. 2*:77, 1967.
23. Hamman, L. and A. R. Rich: Acute diffuse interstitial fibrosis of lungs. *Bull. Johns Hopkins Hosp. 74*:177, 1944.
24. Harell, E. R. and A. C. Curtis: The treatment of North American blastomycosis with amphotericin B. *Am. J. Med. 27*:750, 1959.
25. Harvey, J. C., J. R. Cantrell and A. M. Fisher: Actinomycosis: its recognition and treatment. *Ann. Intern. Med. 46*:868, 1957.
26. Heiner, D. C.: Pulmonary hemosiderosis. In *Diseases of the Respiratory Tract in Children. Vol. 1. Pulmonary Disorders.* E. L. Kendig, Jr. (Ed.). W. B. Saunders Co., Philadelphia, p. 336, 1972.
27. Heiner, D. C., J. W. Sears and W. T. Kniker: Multiple precipitins to cow milk in chronic respiratory disease. A syndrome including poor growth, gastrointestinal symptoms, evidence of allergy, iron deficiency anemia, and pulmonary hemosiderosis. *Am. J. Dis. Child. 103*:634, 1962.
28. Howatt, W. F., K. P. Heidelberger, D. P. Leglovan, and B. Schnitzer: Desquamative interstitial pneumonia. *Am. J. Dis. Child. 126*:346, 1973.
29. Koffler, D., J. Sandson, R. Carr and H. G. Kunkel: Immunologic studies concerning the pulmonary lesions in Goodpasture's syndrome. *Am. J. Pathol. 54*:293, 1969.
30. Kroeker, E. J. and S. Korfmacher: Pulmonary alveolar proteinosis. Report of a case with application of a special sputum examination as an aid to diagnosis. *Am. Rev. Respir. Dis. 87*:416, 1963.
31. Kuykendall, S. J., F. H. Ellis, Jr., L. A. Weed and F. E. Donoghue: Pulmonary cryptococcosis. *N. Engl. J. Med. 257*:1009, 1957.
32. Lerner, R. A., R. J. Glassock and F. J. Dixon: The role of anti-glomerular basement membrane antibody in the pathogenesis of human glomerulonephritis. *J. Exp. Med. 126*:989, 1967.
33. Liebow, A. A.: New concepts and entities in pulmonary disease. In *The Lung.* A. A. Liebow and D. E. Smith (Eds.). The Williams & Wilkins Co., Baltimore, p. 332, 1968.
34. Liebow, A. A., A. Steer and J. Billingsley: Desquamative interstitial pneumonia. *Am. J. Med. 39*:369, 1965.
35. Littman, M. L. and L. E. Zimmerman: *Cryptococcosis, Torulosis or European Blastomycosis.* Grune & Stratton, New York, 1956.
36. Lockwood, W. R., F. Allison, Jr., B. E. Batson and J. F. Busey: The treatment of North American blastomycosis: 10 years' experience. *Am. Rev. Respir. Dis. 100*:314, 1969.
37. Louria, D. B.: Fungus infections of the lungs. In *Textbook of Pulmonary Diseases.* G. L. Baum (Ed.). Little, Brown and Co., Boston, p. 219, 1974.
38. Louria, D. B. and N. Feder: Sulfonamides in experimental histoplasmosis. *Antibiotics 7*:471, 1957.
39. Macartney, F. J., J. Panday and O. Scott: Cor pulmonale as a result of chronic nasopharyngeal obstruction due to hypertrophied tonsils and adenoids. *Arch. Dis. Child. 44*:585, 1969.
40. Maddock, R. K., Jr., L. E. Stevens, K. Reemstma and H. A. Bloomer: Goodpasture's syndrome: cessation of pulmonary hemorrhage after bilateral nephrectomy. *Ann. Intern. Med. 67*:1258, 1967.
41. Martin, D. S. and D. T. Smith: Blastomycosis (American blastomycosis, Gilchrist's disease): a review of the literature. *Am. Rev. Tuberc. 39*:275, 1939.
42. McBride, R. A., J. M. Corson and G. J. Dammin: Mucormycosis: two cases of disseminated disease with cultural identification of Rhizopus: review of literature. *Am. J. Med. 28*:832, 1960.

43. McDearman, S. C. and J. M. Young: Development of positive serologic tests with *Histoplasma capsulatum* antigens following single histoplasmin skin tests. *Am. J. Clin. Pathol. 34*:434, 1960.
44. Menashe, V. D., C. Farrehi and M. Miller: Hypoventilation and cor pulmonale due to chronic upper airway obstruction. *J. Pediatr. 67*:198, 1965.
45. Murray, J. F., S. M. Finegold, S. Froman and D. W. Will: The changing spectrum of nocardiosis: a review and presentation of nine cases. *Am. Rev. Respir. Dis. 83*:315, 1961.
46. Nagaya, H. and H. O. Sieker: Pathogenic mechanisms of interstitial pulmonary fibrosis in patients with serum antinuclear factor. *Am. J. Med. 52*:51, 1972.
47. Palmer, C. E.: Nontuberculous pulmonary calcification and sensitivity to histoplasmin. *Public Health Rep. 60*:513, 1945.
48. Parker, J. D., I. L. Doto and F. E. Tosh: A decade of experience with blastomycosis and its treatment with amphotericin B: a national Communicable Disease Center cooperative mycoses study. *Am. Rev. Respir. Dis. 99*:895, 1969.
49. Patchegsky, A. S., H. Israel, W. S. Hoch and G. Gordon: Desquamative interstitial pneumonia: relationship to interstitial fibrosis. *Thorax 28*:680, 1973.
50. Peabody, J. W., Jr. and J. H. Seabury: Actinomycosis and nocardiosis: a review of basic differences in therapy. *Am. J. Med. 28*:99, 1960.
51. Pepys, J.: *Hypersensitivity Diseases of the Lungs Due to Fungi and Organic Dusts.* Karger, New York, 1969.
52. Pepys, J., R. W. Riddell, K. M. Citron, Y. M. Clayton and E. I. Short: Clinical and immunologic significance of *Aspergillus fumigatus* in the sputum. *Am. Rev. Respir. Dis. 80*:167, 1959.
53. Proceedings of a Symposium on Coccidioidomycosis, 1957. *Public Health Service Publication No. 575.* U.S. Department of Health, Education, and Welfare, Washington, 1957.
54. Rao, M., P. Steiner, J. S. Rose, E. G. Kassner, P. Kottmeier and M. Steiner: Chronic eosinophilic pneumonia in a one-year-old child. *Chest 68*:118, 1975.
55. Rhales, M. L.: Desquamative interstitial pneumonia: new ultrastructural findings. *Am. Rev. Respir. Dis. 108*:950, 1973.
56. Rubin, H., M. L. Furcolow, J. L. Yates and C. A. Brasher: The course and prognosis of histoplasmosis. *Am. J. Med. 27*:278, 1959.
57. Rusby, N. L. and C. Wilson: Lung purpura with nephritis. *Q. J. Med. 29*:501, 1960.
58. Samter, M. and D. Czarny: Secondary cells involved in the allergic reaction: eosinophils, basophils, neutrophils. In *Immunological Diseases,* 2nd ed. M. Samter (Ed.). Little, Brown and Co., Boston, p. 376, 1971.
59. Sanford, W. G., J. R. Rasch and R. B. Stonehill: A therapeutic dilemma: the treatment of disseminated coccidioidomycosis with amphotericin B. *Ann. Intern. Med. 56*:553, 1962.
60. Saslaw, S. and C. C. Campbell: The use of the yeast phase antigens in a complement fixation test for histoplasmosis. *J. Lab. Clin. Med. 33*:811, 1948.
61. Schoenbach, E. B., J. M. Miller, M. Ginsberg and P. H. Long: Systemic blastomycosis treated with stilbamidine: a preliminary report. *J.A.M.A. 146*:1317, 1951.
62. Schubert, J. H., L. Aiello, J. S. Cooper and L. C. Runyon: Evaluation of histoplasmin and yeast phase antigens derived from a single strain of *Histoplasma capsulatum* in the complement fixation test. *J. Bacteriol. 69*:558, 1955.
63. Schwartz, B.: Histoplasmosis of lungs. *Arch. Intern. Med. 94*:970, 1954.
64. Schwarz, J. and G. L. Baum: Blastomycosis. *Am. J. Clin. Pathol. 21*:999, 1951.
65. Schwarz, J., G. L. Baum and H. Floyd: The pathogenesis of "epidemic" histoplasmosis. *Ann. N.Y. Acad. Sci. 89*:47, 1960.
66. Silverman, F. N., J. Schwarz, M. E. Lahey and R. P. Carson: Histoplasmosis. *Am. J. Med. 19*:410, 1955.
67. Smith, J. G., Jr., J. S. Harris, N. F. Conant and D. T. Smith: An epidemic of North American blastomycosis. *J.A.M.A. 158*:641, 1955.
68. Smith, C. E. and M. T. Saito: Serologic reactions in coccidioidomycosis. *J. Chronic Dis. 5*:571, 1957.
69. Smith, C. E., M. T. Saito and S. A. Simons: Pattern of 39,500 serologic tests in coccidioidomycosis. *J.A.M.A. 160*:546, 1956.
70. Stack, B. H. R., I. W. B. Grant, W. J. Irvine and M. A. S. Moffat: Idiopathic diffuse interstitial lung disease: a review of 42 cases. *Am. Rev. Respir. Dis. 92*:939, 1965.
71. Tompkins, V. N.: Soluble antigenic constituents of yeast-phase *Histoplasma capsulatum. Am. Rev. Respir. Dis. 92*(*Suppl.*):126, 1965.
72. Unanue, E. R., F. J. Dixon and J. D. Feldman: Experimental immunologic diseases of the kidney. In *Textbook of Immunopathology.* P. A. Miescher and H. J. Muller-Ederhard (Eds.). Grune & Stratton, New York, p. 164, 1968.
73. West, J. R. and J. K. Alexander: Studies on respiratory mechanics and the work of breathing in pulmonary fibrosis. *Am. J. Med. 27*:529, 1959.
74. Wilson, J. W.: Therapy of systemic fungous infections in 1961: a symposium. *Arch. Intern. Med. 108*:292, 1961.
75. Winn, W. A.: A long-term study of 300 patients with cavitary-abscess lesions of the lung of coccidioidal origin: an analytical study with special reference to treatment. *Dis. Chest 54*(*Suppl.*): 268, 1968.

Part II: *Systemic and Extrapulmonary Systems Disease*

Following is an outline of pulmonary involvement in primary diseases of extrapulmonary systems and in systemic diseases that are of particular concern to pediatricians.

Extrapulmonary Systems

On occasion the respiratory system may be affected secondarily as a consequence of disease of extrapulmonary organ systems. In some cases the pulmonary involvement may be disabling or even life-threatening, whereas in others it may complicate diagnosis or simply add to the discomfort of the patient. This section presents some of the respiratory consequences of primary disease of other organs.

SKELETAL SYSTEM

Skeletal diseases that may alter pulmonary function are generally limited to those that involve the ribs, chest wall, or spine.

(*1*) *Ribs and Chest Wall.* Congenital abnormalities of the ribs, such as fusion of multiple ribs or bifid ribs, are of little clinical significance. However, an anomalous seventh cervical rib may compress the ipsilateral subclavian vein and produce pain and swelling of the arm. Although rib notching itself does not compromise pulmonary function, its presence is important, for example, as a sign of coarctation of the aorta or tetralogy of Fallot.[24] Asphyxiating thoracic dystrophy is a rare congenital anomaly of the rib cage in which the abnormally short and stubby ribs may extend no further than the mid-axilla.[136] Movement of the thoracic cage is seriously impaired, and recurrent infections and marked hypoventilation may ensue.

Fractures occur most commonly in ribs 4 through 10. When fracture is suspected, a roentgenogram is indicated because of the possibility of hemo-, pneumo-, or hemopneumothorax resulting from laceration by the bone or from contusion associated with impact. When possible, the roentgenogram should be taken or repeated several hours after the trauma is incurred, since development of roentgenographic signs may appear only after a period of several hours.[44,71] Fractures of the first two ribs are potentially even more serious, since greater force is required to break them, and their injury is often associated with major intrathoracic damage, such as torsion of the lung or tracheobronchial rupture. Fractures of several ribs may result in "flail chest." The paradoxic movements of the severed segment during respiration and possible injury of underlying viscera may lead rapidly to respiratory failure.[71]

Primary inflammatory disease of the ribs is unusual. Inflammation is more often associated with primary infections of the lungs (e.g., tuberculosis or fungal disease) or with empyema. Tietze's syndrome or costochondral osteochondritis is more common.[6] It is characterized by painful, nonsuppurative swelling of one or more costochondral or chondrosternal joints, often affecting the second rib. Pain, accentuated by the movements of respiration, is the chief symptom. In relapsing polychondritis,[132] which also affects costochondral joints, cartilage in many areas of the body undergoes destruction, probably secondary to abnormal release of lysosomal enzymes. When the process involves cartilages of the airways, the resultant flaccidity (due to lysis) of the airway(s) may lead to severe, even fatal, airway obstruction. Other manifestations of this disease include iritis, cataracts, myocarditis, aortic valvulitis, hepatic dysfunction, and anemia.[49]

(2) *Spine.* Deformities of the thoracic spine may be predominantly lateral (scoliosis), predominantly posterior (kyphosis), or a combination of the two (kyphoscoliosis). Kyphoscoliosis may be congenital (in association with neurofibromatosis, Friedreich's ataxia, muscular dystrophy, osteogenesis imperfecta, and Marfan's syndrome), paralytic (e.g., secondary to poliomyelitis), or idiopathic. The incidence in females is four times that in males. The major cardiopulmonary complication of kyphoscoliosis is pulmonary hypertension and cor pulmonale. It has been estimated that the external angle of scoliosis exceeds 100 degrees, that the kyphosis is greater than 20 degrees, and that vital capacity (in adults) is less than 1.0 liter, in those in whom cor pulmonale will develop.[16,177] Clinical signs and symptoms of cardiopulmonary difficulties usually do not appear before the fourth or fifth decade of life, but once they become apparent, progress may be rapid. Several surveys of patients with kyphoscoliosis reveal the following functional characteristics: normal airway resistance, decreased vital capacity and total lung capacity with normal residual volumes, and mismatching of $\dot{V}_A/\dot{Q}$.[50,163] Hypoventilation may also supervene (primarily as a consequence of reduced tidal volume), resulting in systemic hypoxemia and hypercapnia.

Ankylosing spondylitis, which is more common in males and has its peak incidence in the third and fourth decades, is characterized by synovitis, chondritis, and juxta-articular osteitis of the sacroiliac, apophyseal, and costovertebral articulations.[23] As the disease progresses, subchondral bone erodes, with cartilage destruction and, ultimately, bony ankylosis. The chest cage becomes fixed in an "inspiratory" position, and generalized overexpansion of the lungs occurs. Functional residual capacity and residual volume are high, whereas vital capacity is low. Flow rates and $\dot{V}_A/\dot{Q}$ are normal. Rarely, the disease is complicated by development of fibrosing interstitial pneumonitis with intra-alveolar exudates and inflammation.[41]

NEUROMUSCULAR SYSTEMS

Increased intracranial pressure, of any cause, can result in the production of pulmonary edema (neurogenic pulmonary edema). Although the mechanism for this response is not known, it has been noted that many of the patients so affected are comatose and develop frequent periods of apnea. Pulmonary edema has also been reported to follow epileptiform seizures either immediately or within several hours.

Neuromuscular disease generally results in hypoventilation and in repeated aspirations (due to muscle weakness, incoordination and difficulty in swallowing, and reduced ability to clear secretions by coughing). Examples of clinical conditions and the underlying pathophysiologic mechanisms are discussed in Chapter 2. Selected additional examples and complications are presented in this section.

Familial dysautonomia or Riley-Day syndrome is an autosomal recessive disease found in Jews; it appears to involve a dysfunction of both the somatic and autonomic nervous systems.[7] Patients have motor instability, incoordination, hyporeflexia, absence of corneal reflexes, indifference to pain, failure to produce tears, and lack of response to intradermal histamine. It is believed that the lungs produce an excess of viscid tracheobronchial secretions. Although the precise pathophysiologic process is not understood, these patients often suffer from chronic and recurrent pneumonia and atelectasis, with many exacerbations and remissions. Acute episodes are manifested by cough, fever, and shortness of breath, which virtually always require prompt pulmonary physical and inhalation therapy and, often, appropriate antibiotics.

Tuberous sclerosis is a familial disease

characterized by mental deficiency, epilepsy, angiomyolipomas of the kidney, intracranial calcifications, sclerotic lesions of the bone, rhabdomyomas of the myocardium, and sebaceous adenomas of the skin. The disease can be diagnosed most accurately by computerized axial tomography.[78] Pulmonary disease includes multiple cystic formations in the lung and an increase of bronchiolar smooth muscle.[30] Respiratory failure, with or without hemoptysis, is a frequent cause of death. Pulmonary laboratory findings reveal hyperinflation of the lungs, high compliance, and decreased diffusing capacity.[173]

Guillain-Barré syndrome, or acute polyneuritis, is a disease of unknown cause in which the ventral spinal nerve roots and cranial nerve roots are involved primarily. It usually begins a few days to 2 weeks after an upper respiratory or gastrointestinal infection and is characterized by acute ascending motor paralysis, sensory findings that follow peripheral nerve distribution, and cranial nerve involvement. Muscle weakness usually precedes sensory symptoms, often appearing first in the lower extremities. When the intercostal nerves become involved, vital capacity is reduced to a variable degree as respiration is sustained by diaphragmatic activity. The clinical course is variable and the paralysis tends to reach its peak within 7 to 10 days. (Complete recovery may take from 2 to 18 months.) Signs of respiratory muscle weakness with marked reduction of vital capacity and evidence for impending respiratory failure, obtained by direct measurement of vital capacity, Pa_{O_2}, and Pa_{CO_2} and estimation of minute volume (the latter, both while the patient is awake and while he is sleeping), will provide the determinants for institution of assisted or controlled respiratory therapy. With proper management and detailed attention to respiratory problems, the mortality should be less than 5%.

Werdnig-Hoffmann syndrome (progressive infantile spinal atrophy) is a lethal disease of infancy and early childhood in which there is progressive loss of anterior horn cells leading to paralysis of respiratory and other muscles.[121] Respiratory failure and death usually occur before the age of 5 years. Because intercostal muscles are more seriously involved than is the diaphragm, the chest wall retracts and the upper abdomen protrudes during inspiration, producing a paradoxic (seesaw) breathing pattern. The chest wall is characteristically flattened in the anteroposterior diameter. Symptomatic support during acute illness is recommended.

Other neuromuscular disorders in which significant weakness of the respiratory muscles and respiratory failure may develop include poliomyelitis, porphyria, myasthenia gravis, severe potassium deficiency, and muscular dystrophy.[88,159] Certain drugs have been reported to produce a syndrome like myasthenia gravis—neomycin, streptomycin, polymyxin B, and kanamycin,[53,64,104] whereas other drugs may depress respiration by their action on the central nervous system (e.g., the barbiturates, meprobamate, phenothiazine, and glutethamide).

ENDOCRINE SYSTEM

Alterations of pulmonary function have been reported in patients with acquired hypopituitarism. These changes include reduced lung volumes (residual volume and functional residual capacity) and reduced pulmonary compliance, which have been attributed to a deficiency of growth hormone.[92] Airflow rates and pulmonary gas exchange, however, are normal. As might be expected, lung volumes are high in patients with acromegaly, whereas compliance, airway resistance, and pulmonary gas exchange are normal.[29] Brody and Bukain have suggested that the lung continues to grow during adulthood under the influence of abnormally high levels of growth hormone.[28]

Hypothyroidism is often associated with small lung volumes, low diffusing capacity, and reduced alveolar ventilation.[16,183] Alveolar hypoventilation and occasionally respiratory failure have been reported in myxedema even in the presence of relatively normal lung volumes. Abnormal responses to increased arterial Pco_2 have been demonstrated in some of these patients,[116] so that both muscular weakness and impaired ventilatory control are thought to be responsible for the hypoventilation.[87] Hypoventilation may be reversed in myxedema and hypothyroidism by hormonal replacement therapy.[188] Hyperthyroidism may also be associated with low vital capacity, compliance, and diffusing capacity.[114,167] Although its pathophysiologic basis has not been defined, alterations of pulmonary flow, flow distribution, and blood volume must play a central role.

THE LIVER

Pulmonary effects of hepatic disease are often secondary to hypoproteinemia and its effects on alveolar, interstitial, and pleural liquid flux. The effects of hepatic failure on respiratory control and respiratory center activity have been presented (p. 44).

The coincidence of cyanosis, clubbing, and hepatic disease has been reported.[17,164] Whether primary or secondary pulmonary disease exists in all of these patients is not known. However, the association of chronic hepatic disease and pulmonary arteriovenous fistulas has been documented.[61,77,102,153] The pulmonary fistulas, which may in fact be anatomically well-defined communications between the pulmonary arterial and venous systems (Fig. 18-2), can result in significant right-to-left shunts, profound hypoxemia, systolic murmurs, and thoracic bruits that may at first suggest congenital heart disease. The hypoxemia and high shunt flow may lead to cardiac and/or pulmonary failure, but more often death results from chronic active hepatitis and hepatic failure. Of interest is that, whereas oxygen breathing may reverse the hypoxemia, cyanosis may persist.[102] The reason for this continuation of cyanosis is not clear: perhaps cutaneous shunts reduce perfusion in the true capillaries of the skin so that oxygen extraction is markedly increased—a mechanism suggested also for digital clubbing.[12] The development of shunts in some patients with chronic active hepatitis is also unexplained, although it has been speculated that a substance, such as reduced ferritin, may be released from the diseased liver and consequently lead to the establishment or opening of arteriovenous communications.[75,164]

Alpha-1-antitrypsin metabolism and function is an area in which hepatic and pulmonary function are related. Alpha-1-antitrypsin is synthesized in the parenchymal cells of the liver and secreted into serum. It may be found normally in cerebrospinal fluid, tears, human breast milk, colostrum, amniotic fluid, duodenal secretions, nasal secretions, saliva, and tracheobronchial secretions.[170] It is bound to the surfaces of human pulmonary alveolar macrophages[42] and neutrophils.[185] Alpha-1-antitrypsin is an "acute phase reactant," so that serum levels are elevated after surgery, during pregnancy, in inflammatory states, after estrogen and corticosteroid therapy, and after typhoid vaccination. In vitro it is a potent inhibitor of elastase and neutral protease activity, both enzymes being present in polymorphonuclear leukocytes and having the ability (along with other proteases) to disrupt human pulmonary tissue. The associations between alpha-1-antitrypsin deficiency and familial infantile cirrhosis, familial chronic pulmonary disease that usually begins in the third and fourth decades of life, and combinations of hepatic and pulmonary disease in siblings are well known. In addition, low levels of alpha-1-antitrypsin have been reported in patients with respiratory distress syndrome,[58] the significance of which—if any—has not been assessed.

Serum alpha-1-antitrypsin types are inherited through codominant alleles, the Pi system, which can be distinguished electrophoretically.[170] Pi type MM subjects have

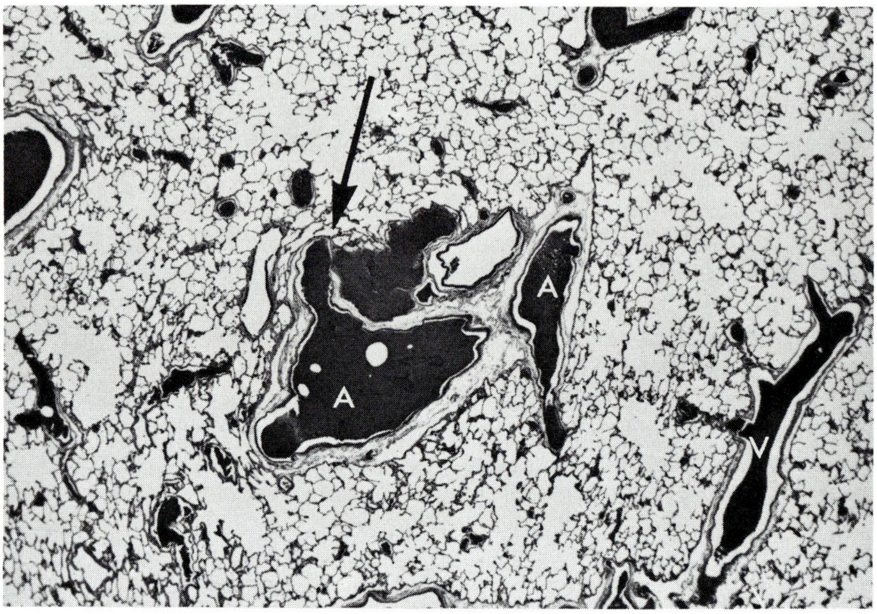

FIG. 18-2. Postmortem lung of 16-year-old girl with chronic active hepatitis, cyanosis, and pulmonary arteriovenous fistula. This photomicrograph was prepared after a barium-gelatin mixture was injected into the pulmonary artery. The pulmonary artery branches (A) are dilated and contain barium. One artery communicates (arrow) with congeries of thin-walled vessels. The interlobar veins (V) are also dilated and filled with barium (H&E × 13). (From Kravath, R. J. et al.[102])

normal amounts of alpha-1-antitrypsin, whereas type ZZ is associated with severe deficiency, often with manifestations of familial infantile cirrhosis or familial emphysema. Pi type MZ heterozygotes have reduced levels of alpha-1-antitrypsin and may be more susceptible to eventual development of pulmonary disease.

Dyspnea, related to familial emphysema, usually begins insidiously toward the end of the third decade. Progressive "hyperaeration" (due to emphysema) of the lung may be documented by serial roentgenographic studies, and progressive obstructive pulmonary disease by appropriate tests of pulmonary function. Recurrent bronchitis, other pulmonary infections, and bronchiectasis usually accelerate the progressive deterioration of the lungs. A few children with this disease have been described; in these children an initial severe pulmonary disease such as measles pneumonia[171] seems to have triggered the onset of chronic obstructive lung disease. In some children, progressive lung disease with alpha-1-antitrypsin deficiency coexisted with asthma or cystic fibrosis.[162]

The syndrome of familial infantile cirrhosis usually begins in the first month and is characterized by cholestatic jaundice and progressive hepatic failure. Most patients die, but some may be in remission for variable periods of time.[170] A few adults have been described with type ZZ alpha-1-antitrypsin, no detectable pulmonary disease, but chronic liver disease.[15] Current estimates indicate that 80% of individuals with Pi type ZZ will develop emphysema, 10% will have infantile cirrhosis, and the rest will have no apparent disease.[170]

GASTROINTESTINAL SYSTEM

Pulmonary effects of gastrointestinal disease generally result from aspiration into the respiratory tract or from masses (including air-distended stomach and bowels) that compromise thoracic space by pressure on the diaphragm or by herniation through the diaphragm.

Primary disease of the esophagus is uncommon in children. Neoplasms are rare. Diverticula may produce dysphagia and, more seriously, repeated aspirations. They can occur in the upper portion of the esophagus (pharyngeal or Zenker's diverticula) or in the lower esophagus. They may be detected by air-fluid levels in the conventional roentgenogram and by barium contrast studies. Megaesophagus or esophageal dilatation may be caused by inflammation (e.g., mediastinitis or regurgitant esophagitis), achalasia, scleroderma, or neoplasms. Symptoms include dysphagia, pain on swallowing, and in some cases aspiration with chronic cough.

Hernias through the foramen of Bochdalek are in the posterolateral portion of the diaphragm, more frequently on the left because of the protection provided by the liver on the right. Herniated organs may include any of the abdominal viscera, and the diagnosis may be apparent by examination of a conventional roentgenogram. Roentgenographic confirmation may be obtained by a number of studies determined by the clinical presumptive diagnosis as discussed in Chapter 19. Massive herniation may be fatal shortly after birth. The severe dyspnea associated with herniated viscera in the thoracic cavity is due to compression of the lungs and to the frequently associated pulmonary hypoplasia (see Chapter 15) and congenital heart disease.[14]

Gastroenteric cysts are unusual malformations (more frequent in males than females), which may occur in the paraspinal regions of the posterior mediastinum.[108] They may compress the upper airways and produce significant obstruction to airflow. Thoracic duct cysts are even more unusual. They are located in the posterior mediastinum, anywhere from the thoracic inlet to the diaphragm, and may produce symptoms by mechanical displacement of the mediastinal viscera.

THE KIDNEYS

Pulmonary edema may occur in association with acute and chronic glomerulonephritis and with nephrosis. In most instances it is the result of left ventricular failure, possibly exacerbated by an increased extracellular fluid volume. Pulmonary edema has also been observed in cases of chronic renal failure in the absence of significant elevations of the blood urea nitrogen. Pleural effusion is a rather common complication of acute glomerulonephritis;[99] it may be associated with segmental or lobar atelectasis, pneumonia, and pulmonary edema. A postmortem study of patients with nephrosis has revealed that some patients may also develop chronic interstitial pulmonary fibrosis.[43]

The possible interrelation between pulmonary and renal pathophysiology is discussed in this chapter under "Goodpasture's Syndrome."

IMMUNOLOGIC DEFICIENCIES

Most patients with immunologic deficiencies are infants and young children, and most succumb to infections prior to adulthood. Diseases of the immune system may be classified as either humoral deficiencies or deficiencies of delayed hypersensitivity.

Humoral deficiencies include transient hypogammaglobulinemia, congenital agammaglobulinemia, primary and secondary acquired agammaglobulinemia, and dysgammaglobulinemia.

(1) Transient hypogammaglobulinemia characterizes the normal infant from birth to about 9 to 15 months of age. Serum concentrations of IgM and IgA, which depend on the infant's ability to synthesize them and which do not cross the placenta from mother to fetus, attain adult levels by 1 to 2 years of age. On the other hand, since IgG does cross the placenta, its levels are relatively high at birth, then fall transiently and return to the higher levels by about 15 months of age. The apparent increased susceptibility of very

young infants to infection, especially from gram-positive bacteria, is probably related to the transient period in which immunoglobulin concentrations are low.

(2) Congenital agammaglobulinemia is a sex-linked recessive disease, usually manifested near the end of the first year, in which the subject is especially susceptible to infection by staphylococcus, streptococcus, pneumococcus, and Hemophilus organisms.[147] Lymph nodes contain no plasma cells, and nodes draining infected areas do not enlarge.

(3) Primary acquired agammaglobulinemia may occur at any age. These patients, who have an increased incidence of thymomas, often develop noncaseating granulomas of the skin, liver, spleen, and lung. Lymphoid tissue also contains no plasma cells.

(4) Secondary acquired agammaglobulinemia may occur in association with excessive loss of protein, leukemia, lymphoma, "M" component disease (such as multiple myeloma and Waldenström's macroglobulinemia), and immunosuppressive therapy.[57,80] These patients have high susceptibility to "opportunistic" infections, including fungi, *Pneumocystis carinii,* cytomegalic inclusion disease, and bacteria such as Pseudomonas. Bronchopneumonia, bronchiectasis, and chronic interstitial pneumonia may result.[57]

(5) The three types of dysgammaglobulinemia are (I) IgA and IgG deficiency with elevated IgM, (II) IgA and IgM deficiency or absence with normal IgG, and (III) isolated IgA deficiency. Type I may be congenital or acquired and may be manifested by increased susceptibility to infection, thrombocytopenia, neutropenia, renal disease, aplastic anemia, and hemolytic anemia. Types II or III may be seen in apparently normal people and also in association with ataxic telangiectasia,[119] wherein recurrent pulmonary and paranasal sinus infections may prove fatal.

Delayed hypersensitivity deficiencies include the Wiskott-Aldrich syndrome, hereditary thymic aplasia, and the DiGeorge syndrome.

(1) The Wiskott-Aldrich syndrome is a sex-linked recessive disease, characterized by increased susceptibility to infection, thrombocytopenia, and intractable eczema with or without "asthma." The defect seems to involve both humoral and cellular immune responses: IgM may be slightly decreased, IgA may be slightly increased, serum anti-A and B blood group titers are low, and the patient appears unable to recognize and metabolize antigenic polysaccharides such as the pneumococcal capsular antigen. Lymphopenia occurs in most cases, and thymic-dependent delayed hypersensitivity responses are diminished.[147]

(2) Hereditary thymic aplasia is an autosomal recessive disease with a high incidence of consanguinity. Patients fail to thrive and are susceptible to infection with Candida, *Pneumocystis carinii,* Pseudomonas, and viruses.[147]

(3) The DiGeorge syndrome or agenesis of the thyroid and thymus glands is characterized by malformations of the face, ears, and nose, neonatal tetany, cardiovascular abnormalities, and apparent failure to develop normal delayed hypersensitivity responses.

Malignancies

Lymphoreticular malignancies (of which Hodgkin's disease and lymphosarcoma account for about 8 to 10% of all childhood neoplasms), the leukemias, and metastatic tumors in the lungs comprise virtually all the pulmonary malignancies of childhood. Primary disease of the lung is rare. Pulmonary involvement in lymphoreticular malignancy may appear as (1) hilar lymphadenopathy with involvement of the mediastinum; (2) small, single or multiple foci within the lung parenchyma, which can be the apparent site of origin of the disease; and (3) pleural effusion including serous, chylous, or hemorrhagic fluid more common in Hodgkin's disease than in lymphosarcoma[151].

HODGKIN'S DISEASE

The first case of a child with the disease was reported by Hodgkin in 1832. The youngest patient in the Stanford series[51] was 21 months old. In the pediatric age group the frequency is higher in males than females, and the predominant histologic types of the disease are "nodal sclerosing" and "lymphocytic."[51,168] Cause is unknown, and theories have ranged from hormonal determinants (because of the higher incidence in males during the first decade of life) to origin related to infection. The clinical signs and symptoms as well as the laboratory findings are essentially the same in children and adults. The most common presenting sign is painless lymphadenopathy, commonly of the cervical nodes. Diagnosis must be based on histologic examination of excised lymph nodes or other tissues that may be involved. Management and prognosis of Hodgkin's disease are based on the histopathologic classification (Table 18-1), the clinical staging of the disease, which is an attempt to determine its extent (Table 18-2), and the extent and characteristics of systemic signs and symptoms (Table 18-2). In most centers a staging laparotomy is done; the procedure includes biopsy of the para-aortic, celiac, hepatic portal, splenic hilar, and iliac nodes and removal of the spleen.[96] Recent studies, however, suggest the possibility of increased risk to serious bacterial infection in splenectomized patients with Hodgkin's disease, who also receive radiotherapy and chemotherapy.[51]

Pulmonary involvement may be expected in 15 to 40% of patients with Hodgkin's disease.[181] The Stanford group reports a 14% incidence of parenchymal pulmonary involvement in the 11- to 15-year-old age group and an incidence of less than 3% in patients between 1 and 10 years. When the lungs are involved at the time of diagnosis, the disease is classified as stage IV. The pulmonary lesions, which have no characteristic distribution, include homogeneous, confluent, or fibronodular densities, discrete nodules, and true consolidations, by roentgenographic examination.[168] These lesions are usually of the nodal sclerosing type.[181] Kaplan and Rosenberg indicate that pulmonary parenchymal involvement is always associated with lymphadenopathy,[96] whereas Kern et al. have documented parenchymal disease without hilar or mediastinal nodal involvement.[98] This finding suggests that primary pulmonary disease is possible, but its significance is not understood.

Pulmonary involvement can appear at any

TABLE 18-1. Histopathologic Classification in Hodgkin's Disease*

Type	Features	Relative prognosis
Lymphocyte predominance (LP)	Abundant lymphocytic stroma; sparse Reed-Sternberg (R-S) cells†	Most favorable
Nodular sclerosis (NS)	Nodules of lymphoid tissue of varying size, separated by bands of collagen and containing "lacunar" cell variants of R-S cells	Favorable
Mixed cellularity (MC)	More numerous R-S cells in pleomorphic stroma rich in eosinophils, plasma cells, fibroblasts, and lymphocytes	Guarded
Lymphocyte depletion (LD)	Paucity of lymphocytes; diffuse, irregular fibrosis in some instances; bizarre, anaplastic R-S cells usually numerous	Least favorable

*From Kaplan, H. S. and S. A. Rosenberg.[96]

†R-S cells are essential for diagnosis of Hodgkin's disease, but are not pathognomonic; they may be seen in infectious mononucleosis, metastatic breast cancer, etc. It is therefore important to observe them in an appropriate stroma.

TABLE 18-2. Clinical Staging Classification in Hodgkin's Disease*

Stage	Definition
I	Involvement of a single lymph node region (I) or of a single extralymphatic organ or site (I_E)
II	Involvement of two or more lymph node regions on the same side of the diaphragm (II) or localized involvement of an extralymphatic organ or site and of one or more lymph node regions on the same side of the diaphragm (II_E)
III	Involvement of lymph node regions on both sides of the diaphragm (III), which may also be accompanied by involvement of the spleen (III_S) or by localized involvement of an extralymphatic organ or site (III_E) or both (III_{SE})
IV†	Diffuse or disseminated involvement of one or more extralymphatic organs or tissues, with or without associated lymph node involvement

* From Kaplan, H. S. and S. A. Rosenberg.[96]

† The presence or absence of fever, night sweats, and/or unexplained loss of 10% or more of body weight in the 6 months preceding admission are denoted by the suffix letters B and A, respectively. Biopsy-documented involvement of Stage IV sites is also denoted by letter suffixes: marrow = M^+; lung = L^+; liver = H^+; pleura = P^+; bone = O^+; skin and subcutaneous tissue = D^+.

time during the course of the disease. It is associated with better prognosis when it is present at the time of diagnosis than when it occurs afterward, probably as an expression of "escape" from therapy.[181] Thus, it is especially essential to rule out and treat other possible causes of pulmonary disease in a patient with Hodgkin's disease. Intrathoracic complications of Hodgkin's disease include pleural effusion, obstruction of the superior vena cava, phrenic nerve paralysis, paralysis of the recurrent laryngeal nerve, bronchoesophageal fistula, and atelectasis. High risk to infection is related to immunosuppression from therapeutic drugs, from hypogammaglobulinemia that may be associated with the disease and/or extensive irradiation, and from splenectomy.[51,181]

Treatment of choice is radiotherapy either alone or in combination with chemotherapy.[51,96] The estimated cure rate for all forms of Hodgkin's disease collectively is now about 50%, and the rate is significantly higher for certain stages and types (Table 18-3). Within the pediatric age group, the mean survival of all stages is now more than 10 years from diagnosis,[51] a notable improvement over expectations in the not too distant past.[59,93,168,187]

LYMPHOSARCOMA GROUP

The lymphosarcoma group of lymphoreticular malignancies includes lymphosarcoma, reticulum cell sarcoma, follicular lymphoma, and mycosis fungoides.

Lymphosarcoma is characterized by lymphocytic proliferation in lymph nodes and is spread either directly into surrounding tissues or via the blood and lymphatics to

TABLE 18-3. Relationship of Prognosis to Stage in Hodgkin's Disease*

Group	5-Year Survival (%)	5-Year Relapse-Free (%)†
All stages, all cases	81.3	61.5
Stage PS I (A & B)	86.0	72.5
Stage PS II (A & B)	93.6	69.0
Stage PS III (A & B)	81.3	61.1
Stage PS IV (A & B)	39.0	26.9

* From Kaplan, H. S. and S. A. Rosenberg.[96]

† At 10 years, the curve for relapse-free survival has flattened out at about 50%, suggesting that at least 50% of all cases may now be permanently cured of their once inevitably fatal disease by meticulous diagnostic evaluation and staging and the judicious selection and skillful administration of megavoltage radiotherapy and/or multidrug combination chemotherapy.

other nodes and viscera. The most common presenting sign is peripheral node enlargement involving a single or multiple groups of nodes. In contrast to lymphosarcoma, reticulum cell sarcoma is characterized by proliferation of reticulum cells rather than lymphocytes and by the additional involvement of bone, which results in osteolytic lesions. Follicular lymphoma is believed to be a stage in the development of either lymphosarcoma or reticulum cell sarcoma, although its prognosis is better than either of the others'. Mycosis fungoides is primarily a disease of the skin, which in its later stages may involve the lungs and other viscera.[1,21,27] When lymph nodes are involved, their histopathologic appearance closely resembles that of other lymphosarcomas or the lymph nodes in Hodgkin's disease.

Usually intrathoracic involvement in the lymphosarcoma group of diseases signifies widespread disease, although primary intrathoracic disease is estimated to occur in about 4% of patients.[148] Of these, about 80% involve the mediastinal nodes, 10% the lung parenchyma, and 10% the pleura. Primary pulmonary parenchymal disease may simulate lobar pneumonia; often the lesion is well circumscribed and produces no obstruction to airflow.[9] When the lungs are affected secondarily, the lesion(s) may be single or multiple, and usually appear in the lower pulmonary zones. They tend to coalesce progressively and produce bronchial obstruction with subsequent atelectasis and pulmonary infection.

Survival is about 24% in adults, whereas it is about 9% in children,[95] perhaps because leukemic transformation is more common in children.

LEUKEMIA

The acute leukemias predominate in children, and of these about 80% are of the acute lymphoblastic type.[174] Respiratory manifestations may be due to (1) enlargement of mediastinal lymph nodes leading to airway obstruction, (2) bleeding into the pulmonary parenchyma; and (3) susceptibility to infection. In addition, histologic analysis of the lung parenchyma indicates that leukemic infiltrations may be present in half the patients.[22] These lesions, located primarily in peribronchial tissue, are recognized infrequently by roentgenographic examination. They apparently produce no significant clinical abnormalities. On the other hand, significant interstitial leukemic infiltrations have been reported in adults; these infiltrations may lead to reduced lung volumes ("restrictive disease") and abnormal diffusing capacity.[72,140] Pleural effusion is more frequently found in chronic lymphatic leukemia (which itself is rare in children), where it is probably the result of infection, lymphatic obstruction, or myocardial failure rather than direct leukemic infiltration of the pleura.

Patients with leukemia are at high risk to pulmonary infections as a result of a number of factors that either suppress immunologic responsiveness or disrupt the normal balance of flora within the host. Thus hypogammaglobulinemia, which may develop in some patients, and immunosuppressive drugs, corticosteroid therapy, irradiation, and antibiotic therapy reduce resistance to infection. Bacterial infection is the major cause of death of children with leukemia. The incidence of fungal and viral infections is increasing,[85] and "opportunistic" infection by fungi (particularly systemic candidiasis), Pseudomonas, cytomegalovirus, and *Pneumocystis carinii* continue to be major problems. Treatment of pulmonary infections must be based on cultures and sensitivity tests. If antibiotics must be started before results of culture are available, it is recommended that combination therapy be used to cover resistant staphylococcus and gram-negative organisms, particularly Pseudomonas.[103]

METASTATIC PULMONARY LESIONS

Metastatic tumors in the lung are relatively rare in children. Whereas the incidence is over 85% in patients beyond middle age,[129] it is about 30% for malignant neoplasms in children.[94] The malignancies of childhood that may be expected to produce pulmonary metastases include the sarcomas such as Wilms' tumor, skeletal tumors (e.g., chondroma, osteogenic sarcoma, and Ewing's tumor), and soft tissue tumors such as lymphosarcoma and malignant neurilemmoma.

Metastatic lesions in the thorax may originate from any part of the body and be spread either by contiguous extension or via lymphatics and the blood stream. Tumors of the chest wall, mediastinum, and below the diaphragm (e.g., liver and spleen) may extend directly into the thoracic cavity. The most common route is the systemic veins, either directly from the primary site or by way of the thoracic duct. Seeding of metastatic tissue probably begins in the pulmonary capillaries.[34]

Metastases may appear as either single or multiple lesions in the roentgenogram. They may take on a miliary appearance or appear as large (cannonball) masses. In children, isolated metastasis is usually associated with sarcomas of the bone. Cavity formation is rare in children, as is calcification. The latter finding is usually associated with osteogenic sarcoma or chondrosarcoma.

Sarcoidosis (Boeck's Sarcoid)

Sarcoidosis is characterized by nonspecific, noncaseating granulomas that may appear in the lung, heart, eyes, liver, spleen, lymph nodes, skin, and bone. In a worldwide distribution, it is three times more common in females than males[89,172] and 10 to 17 times more common in blacks than whites.[105,117] Its peak incidence is between the ages of 20 and 40 years, but at least 2% of all cases are recorded in children under the age of 10 years.[97] It has been proposed[31,90,109-111] that the development of sarcoidosis is related to a deficiency of delayed hypersensitivity response to bacteriophage, in which the inability to produce appropriate neutralizing antibodies results in the formation of the typical sarcoid granuloma.[31]

The lesions in the lung are predominantly interstitial. The wide distribution of these lesions in the interstices of other viscera suggests that spread may be by the hematogenous route; blood vessel walls may be affected, whereas vascular endothelium remains intact. The lesions may either resolve or fibrose progressively. A small percentage of patients develop extensive pulmonary (interstitial) fibrosis and bronchiectasis with gross distortion of pulmonary architecture.

CLINICAL CORRELATIONS

Sarcoidosis may appear as diffuse enlargement of the lymph nodes or as diffuse pulmonary disease with little or no apparent involvement of the lymph nodes.[97] In some cases lymph node disease may precede involvement of the lung by several years. Pleural involvement in sarcoidosis is not common (its incidence probably does not exceed 10%), so that development of pleural effusion in a patient with sarcoidosis should lead to suspicion of superimposed disease or heart failure.

In 50% of the patients with sarcoidosis, the disease is limited to lymph node enlargement and the patient is asymptomatic. When the disease involves other systems, constitutional symptoms may include weight loss, fatigue, weakness, malaise, and fever. *Cardiac* involvement may be manifested by arrhythmias, Stokes-Adams attacks ("cardiac syncope"), myocardial infarction, and cardiac failure. *Ocular* lesions include uveitis and perhaps involvement of the conjunctiva, sclera, retina, and lens. Thus, cataracts, glaucoma, and blindness may result. *Cutaneous* manifestations, especially common in blacks, include slightly raised nodules of the face, neck, shoulders, and nasal mucosa, and erythema nodosum. (The constellation, erythema nodosum, hilar adenopathy, and arthralgia in association with the acute onset of sarcoidosis with fever, is Löfgren's syndrome). *Hepatic* involvement usually does not compromise function, whereas *splenic* disease may produce hypersplenism. Expressions of involvement of the *bones* and *joints* include migratory polyarthritis, single or repeated episodes of poly- or monoarticular arthritis, and persistent arthritis. *Uveoparotid fever* may occur in the presence of uveitis and parotid gland involvement. Abnormalities of *blood* may include chronic hypercalcemia (which can lead to nephrocalcinosis and nephrolithiasis), hypercalciuria, elevated serum globulins, leukopenia with relative eosinophilia, and positive latex fixation.

Approximately 25% of the patients with sarcoidosis have *pulmonary* symptoms including cough and shortness of breath. Hemoptysis and chest pain are rare. Auscultatory signs are unusual, although crackles associated with small lung volumes (see p. 51) may be heard. Pulmonary involvement may be detected even in the absence of roentgenographic abnormalities of the lung.[26] Significant pulmonary interstitial involvement may be detected as a defect of diffusion (low diffusing capacity, especially during exercise) and $\dot{V}_A/\dot{Q}$ abnormality, in the presence of "restrictive pulmonary disease," i.e., low functional residual capacity and low pulmonary compliance.

Characteristically, poor correlation exists between the roentgenographic signs of pulmonary involvement and the results of pulmonary function tests in patients with sarcoidosis. For example, when the disease appears to involve only the hilar lymph nodes, with the pulmonary parenchyma seemingly spared, it is not unusual to find that pulmonary compliance and diffusing capacity are abnormal[25,161,169] and that little improvement occurs in these functions either with or without therapy.[55,186] On the other hand, marked changes in pulmonary function are expected in the very small number of patients whose disease progresses to the state of diffuse interstitial fibrosis. The marked impairment of gas exchange and resultant hypoxemia expectedly lead to dyspnea and eventually to cor pulmonale.

DIAGNOSIS AND TREATMENT

Diagnosis of sarcoidosis rests on the clinical presentation, the associated clinical laboratory features, and histologic confirmation preferably from both a biopsy specimen and the Kveim test. The *Kveim* "antigen" is prepared from homogenized sarcoid tissue and injected intradermally. After 4 to 6 weeks a biopsy is performed at the injection site and the tissue examined histologically. The best "antigens" give a correct positive reaction in 85% of the cases and no more than 10% false negatives. The *biopsy* site of choice for direct diagnosis of sarcoidosis is an obvious skin lesion, which rarely is misleading. The lymph nodes of the right scalene fat pad provide an accurate diagnosis in about 85% of patients with hilar and mediastinal adenopathy. When sarcoidosis appears to be limited to the pulmonary parenchyma, the lung itself may be the tissue of choice, which is obtained by direct biopsy. It is recommended strongly that the diagnosis of sarcoidosis be withheld until the biopsied material has been *stained and cultured* for mycobacteria and fungi.

Most patients with sarcoidosis do not require treatment. It is generally agreed that systemic steroid therapy is to be used for patients with advanced disease, albeit no conclusive evidence supports its efficacy. With regard to pulmonary lesions, it cannot be agreed that steroids result in improved function, although the possibility has been raised that appropriate testing must include a number of parameters both while the patient is at rest and while he is exercising. Definite indications for the use of steroid therapy have to do with nonpulmonary manifestations of the disease. Thus, steroids may be most effective for the treatment of hypercalcemia, ocular disease, and myocardial disease. Steroids are also indicated for progressive and extensive pulmonary disease with compromised pulmonary function. It should be remembered that one is committed to continuing steroid therapy for a minimum of 1 to 3 years,[45] since interruption of therapy may produce severe exacerbations of the disease.

Diabetes Mellitus

The susceptibility of patients with diabetes mellitus to infection has not been explained. Possibilities include associated deficiencies of vitamins A and C, impaired phagocytic activity associated with diabetic ketoacidosis, depressed responsivity of polymorphonuclear leukocytes to infection, and decreased opsonizing capacity of serum.[35,112,123,134,151] Pulmonary disease in diabetes mellitus is not uncommon, and certain conditions are associated with it more frequently than would be expected in the general population.

(1) Aspiration syndromes, which were relatively common in diabetic patients, would often present as fulminating pneumonias or, more insidiously, as chronic lung abscesses. Contemporary use of antibiotic therapy has reduced the incidence of these complications significantly.

(2) The common association of diabetes mellitus and pulmonary tuberculosis is well known. Again, prompt and adequate use of antituberculous drugs is effective, and death due to pulmonary tuberculosis in diabetics is rare.[107,157,180] Preventive measures, including annual chest roentgenograms and tuberculin skin testing, are recommended. BCG immunization has also been recommended by some.

(3) Two forms of pulmonary candidiasis in diabetes have been described: In "bronchial candidiasis" the major lesions are plaques of Candida covering the airway mucosa which resemble the plaques of oral candidiasis. Cough, productive of mucoid-milky sputum, is the most prominent and distressing symptom. Bronchial involvement may be apparent in the chest roentgenogram, and heavy growths of Candida may be expected in sputum cultures. Pulmonary "parenchymal candidiasis," sometimes with pleural effusion, produces fever, cough, hemoptysis, chest pain, and respiratory distress. This serious complication is also discussed on page 532.

INFANTS OF DIABETIC MOTHERS

Infants of diabetic mothers have a significantly higher incidence of respiratory disease in the neonatal period. Whereas it has been suggested that this fact is associated with the higher incidence of premature birth and delivery by cesarean section, a recent report of Robert and her colleagues indicates that maternal diabetes per se predisposes the newborn to respiratory distress syndrome.[143] These authors examined, retrospectively, perinatal data on 805 infants of diabetic mothers and 10,152 infants of nondiabetic mothers, and showed that, in general, the syndrome occurred in 23.4% of the diabetic group and 1.3% of the nondiabetic group. When features associated with maternal diabetes, which are in themselves risk factors (e.g., gestational age and route of delivery), were taken into account, it was determined that infants of diabetic mothers were 5.6 times more likely to develop respiratory distress syndrome than infants of nondiabetic mothers (Fig. 18-3). Although respiratory distress syndrome was defined for the diabetic group as abnormal respirations (tachypnea, grunting, or retractions), administration of oxygen therapy, and diagnosis of the syndrome on the infant's data card—and therefore, perhaps, not confirmatory for respiratory distress syndrome in each case—it is clear that infants of diabetic mothers are at significantly higher risk than comparable infants of nondiabetic mothers. The authors suggest that the hyperinsulinism of the fetus may impair normal cortisol induction of surfactant synthesis during gestation.[143]

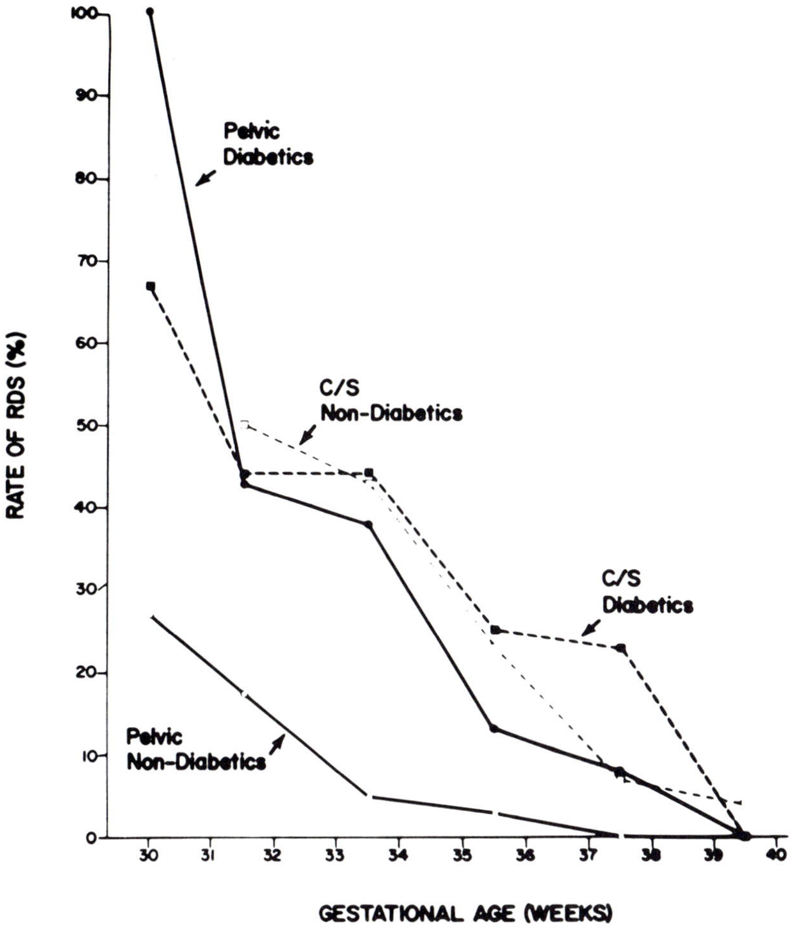

FIG. 18-3. Rate of respiratory distress syndrome versus gestational age according to route of delivery: pelvic (vaginal) or C/S (cesarean section). Each point represents the rate for all infants born in the week before and the week after the gestational age designated. (Reprinted, by permission, from *N. Engl. J. Med. 294*:357, 1976.)

Sickle Cell Disease

Sickle cell disease is a hereditary hemoglobinopathy (hemoglobin S) that occurs virtually exclusively in Negroes. The heterozygotic state is termed "sickle cell trait," and the homozygotic state is called "sickle cell disease." About 40% of those afflicted with sickle cell disease develop clinically apparent pulmonary abnormalities, including bacterial pneumonia and pulmonary vascular obstruction, and the majority reveal laboratory evidence of some degree of impairment of pulmonary function.

PNEUMONIA

Whereas it is often difficult to distinguish between acute vascular obstruction and pneumonia (or a concurrence of the two) in a child with sickle cell disease, it is generally believed that bacterial pneumonia is the more common pulmonary complication and that the infecting agents are the usual bacterial pathogens that produce disease in the general pediatric population.[46,175] The child with sickle cell disease may be predisposed to pulmonary infections on two counts: (1) debilitation in the presence of chronic anemia and (2) the possibility of co-existing functional splenic insufficiency, which has been documented as early as 5 months of age.[127,133,184] Although relevant data have not been compiled, in general experience *recurrent* bacterial pneumonias are not uncommon in those children who do develop pulmonary complications.

PULMONARY VASCULAR OCCLUSION AND INFARCTION

Circulatory stasis and vascular occlusion may follow intravascular sickling and thrombosis in situ or embolization to the lung from tissue such as the bone marrow or from a peripheral site of thrombophlebitis. The pulmonary vascular defect may be small and transient or it may involve large areas of the lung. Similarly, circulation may be re-established ultimately at the affected site without permanent tissue damage, or infarction may lead to replacement of normal lung parenchyma with fibrous tissue. Thus, the acute episode may be mild with few signs of pulmonary disease or it may be life-threatening with rapid development of cardiopulmonary failure.

Individuals with sickle cell disease are predisposed to pulmonary vascular occlusion in a number of ways.

(1) Local changes in the lung that may accompany airway or alveolar infection may lead to a fall in pH and Po_2 of the affected pulmonary parenchyma; this, in turn, may produce both the sickling deformation of red blood cells and constriction of the local blood vessels. The respective effects on the circulation, namely, increased blood viscosity and decreased size of the lumen of the vessels, may effectively reduce blood flow or stop it completely.

(2) Similarly, any other (noninfectious) change within the lung that may alter pH and Po_2 can result in vascular occlusion.

(3) Other viscera and tissues may suffer infarction in sickle cell disease and thereby become the source of emboli to the lung. Bone marrow is especially vulnerable and it is not uncommon for the spine, bony thorax, or extremities to be involved. Local bony pain is an important sign that always must be sought in a patient with pulmonary disease. Bone marrow emboli are particularly dangerous in that they produce a number of pathologic effects in the lung: directly they obstruct blood flow, and because of their high fat content, they may also disrupt normal surface tension and thereby produce alveolar collapse. The resultant changes in local pH and Po_2 may then establish a second process analogous to that described in (1).

DIFFERENTIAL DIAGNOSIS

The usual difficulties in making a clinical distinction between pneumonia and infarction are exaggerated in the presence of sickle cell disease. Barrett-Connor has listed points of difference between pulmonary infarction and bacterial pneumonia and compared these in patients with sickle cell disease and those without the hemoglobinopathy (Table 18-4).[10] About half the points listed are of limited practical value when dealing with a patient with sickle cell disease. Some points hold promise as potentially important diagnostic tools, but they await further documentation to establish their clinical usefulness. For example, the presence of "blister cells" (atypical red blood cells) in the blood of patients with pulmonary infarction and the elevation of fibrinogen levels in patients with infection and sickle cell disease are observations that need to be pursued.

SICKLE CELL LUNG DISEASE

This term is used to describe patients with sickle cell disease in whom there is radiographic evidence of chronic pulmonary par-

TABLE 18-4. Differential Diagnosis of Pulmonary Infarction Versus Bacterial Pneumonia

Finding	Condition Suspected in Patients Without Hemoglobinopathy	Condition Suspected in Patients With Sickle Cell Anemia
Age < 5 yrs	Pneumonia	Pneumonia
Previous upper respiratory infection	Pneumonia	No value
Preceding crisis	Does not apply	Infarction
Onset with chill	Pneumonia	Pneumonia
Temperature $> 39.4°C$	Pneumonia	No value
Purulent sputum	Pneumonia	Pneumonia
Hemoptysis	Infarction	No value
Thrombophlebitis	Infarction	No value
Previous episodes	Infarction	No value
Patient appears more ill than objective findings	Infarction	No value
Positive blood culture	Pneumonia	Pneumonia
Chest roentgenogram film negative at onset	Infarction	Infarction
Migratory infiltrates	Infarction	No value
Upper lobe infiltrates	Pneumonia	Pneumonia
Prominent pulmonary conus	Infarction	No value
Leukocytosis	Pneumonia	No value
Bilirubin > 5 mg/100 ml	No value	Infarction
Fever > 48 hours after antibiotics	Infarction	No value

enchymal lesions, thought to be caused by repeated episodes of infarction or pneumonia. In the series of adults discussed by Reynolds, less than 10% had evidence of permanent pulmonary damage.[141] The roentgenographic appearance of a finely mottled and reticular pattern is consonant with interstitial involvement, but without the classic features of pulmonary fibrosis.[141] In general, the lower lung fields are relatively radiolucent (perhaps a reflection of areas of oligemia). With time the upper pulmonary zones may appear to contain a proportionately larger blood volume than the lower zones, especially when pulmonary hypertension exists. Of significance, however, are studies which suggest that the prevalence of sickle cell lung disease may be much greater than indicated by roentgenographic criteria alone. Margolies reported that microscopic organized thromboemboli found post mortem in the lungs of patients with sickle cell disease may not be appreciated in the conventional chest roentgenogram,[113] and several studies of young adults suggest that most patients with sickle cell disease (even those with equivocal histories for pulmonary disease) have evidence of restrictive lung disease, i.e., low total lung capacity and low functional residual capacity.[63,122] The natural history of sickle cell lung disease, its progression or amelioration, and its relationship to clinical signs and symptoms of cardiopulmonary disease require additional investigation.

TREATMENT

Pneumococcal pneumonia is relatively frequent and comparatively virulent in patients with sickle cell disease.[158] Underlying responsible factors include functional asplenism, a reported deficiency in serum opsonizing activity for pneumococcus, and the possibility that alveolar macrophages are less active in this disease.[11] Because of the seriousness of pneumonia in sickle cell disease, its diagnosis or presumptive diagnosis demands prompt institution of antibiotic therapy as appropriate cultures are obtained.

Attempts have been made to prevent pneumococcal infections in sickle cell disease, and further studies are warranted. Thus, trials of antibiotic "prophylaxis" in African children with sickle cell disease were found to reduce the incidence of painful crises, but no firm conclusions could be drawn about prevention of lung disease.[179] The possibility that antipneumococcal vaccines may be of value has been considered;[5] especially relevant is the fact that only 14 of the 82 types of pneumococcus are responsible for 75% of pneumococcal disease.

Along with antibiotics, the treatment of pulmonary disease (vascular occlusive disease and pneumonia) in patients with sickle cell disease demands prompt correction of the hypoxemia, anemia, and acidemia to prevent further primary or secondary vascular obstruction and infarction. Anticoagulation therapy for the treatment of acute pulmonary infarction—which may be fatal in 10 to 20% of the cases—has not been demonstrated to alter the course of the infarction or to accelerate its resolution. Resolution usually is spontaneous in 7 to 10 days.

No direct therapy exists for the hemoglobinopathy. Maintenance of a total hemoglobin concentration of 12 g/100 ml, with a hemoglobin A to S ratio of 30:70, may help avert additional thromboembolic phenomena.[3] Attempts to prevent sickling by altering the hemoglobin S molecule are problematic: thus, reduction of the amount of S hemoglobin by binding with urea is feasible, but its effectiveness and safety have not been evaluated thoroughly.[118,126] Production of methemoglobin and carboxyhemoglobin has been explored, but these substances interfere with oxygen transport and have not been found useful.[18,138]

Collagen Diseases

The diseases that are classically grouped under this heading share the following characteristics: (1) probable hypersensitivity as an underlying etiologic factor; (2) involvement of connective tissue with inflammatory, degenerative, or granulomatous changes; and (3) widespread multiple organ disease. Pulmonary involvement is not unusual in each of these diseases, and pleural or pulmonary abnormalities may be the presenting condition.

POLYARTERITIS (PERIARTERITIS) NODOSA

This disease, which is uncommon in pediatrics but has been reported in both infants and children,[60,144] affects small arteries primarily and is characterized by segmental necrosis, by fibrinoid changes and inflammation of all layers of the arterial wall, and by acute inflammatory reactions with accumulations of polymorphonuclear leukocytes and eosinophils around the vessel walls. Adventitial fibrosis leads to the characteristic nodules, and intimal occlusion of the vessels produces thrombosis and infarction. Symptoms referable to the gastrointestinal tract, kidneys, and central nervous system are common. Cardiopulmonary symptoms may follow acute carditis, pericarditis, bronchial ulcerations, pneumonitis, and pleural disease. Cardiomegaly, pericardial effusion, and pleural effusion may occur, but pulmonary edema is not common.[68] Pulmonary parenchymal lesions may be discrete or confluent, progressive or evanescent. Large thromboses may produce serious infarctions, which rarely lead to cavity formation.[156] Serious pulmonary involvement is more common in those cases with ominous prognosis.

WEGENER'S GRANULOMATOSIS

This uncommon disease was first described as a variant of polyarteritis nodosa. Although widespread necrotizing damage occurs in the glomeruli, the basic granulomatous reaction that characterizes this disease permits differentiation from the primarily vascular involvement of polyarteritis. Necrotizing granulomas are produced primarily in the upper (including oronasal pharynx) and lower respiratory tract. Glomerulitis, angiitis, and granuloma are the hallmarks of the disease; but patients have been reported who have had no glomerulitis, limited angiitis, and granulomatosis of the lungs.[38] Granulomas and ulcerations leading to airway obstruction—from the pharynx and larynx to the lower respiratory tract—may produce a picture of hoarseness or stridor or bronchitis, with superimposed wheezing due to edema of the airways. Additional destruction of the pulmonary parenchyma by the underlying necrotizing process may lead to respiratory failure. Prognosis is poor, particularly in patients with significant glomerulitis, and death may result from renal failure, hemoptysis, or advanced pulmonary disease.

LUPUS ERYTHEMATOSUS

Systemic lupus erythematosus is considerably less frequent in children than adults, but bears the same clinical and laboratory manifestations in both.[76,101] Of all the collagen diseases, pulmonary and pleural involvement are most frequent in lupus.[32,68,84] Cardiopulmonary abnormalities include cardiomegaly, pericardial effusion, pleural effusion, and pneumonitis. The latter is seen in the roentgenogram as poorly defined parenchymal densities usually in the lower zones or at the periphery of the lung. Roentgenographic evidence also exists for the progressive decrease of lung volume as pulmonary involvement continues.[74] Clinical pulmonary manifestations include cough with or without the production of sputum, pleuritic pain, hemoptysis, and dyspnea. Pulmonary performance in the laboratory is often worse than might be anticipated on the basis of clinical and roentgenographic findings: lung volumes may be low, diffusing capacity is reduced, and Pa_{O_2} is usually low as is pulmonary compliance; Pa_{CO_2} may be low or normal.[26,69,74,81,83,84] The histopathologic correlations of pulmonary dysfunction in lupus include interstitial inflammatory lesions with atelectasis;[65,139] diffuse or focal interstitial alveolar exudates and swelling of the alveolar septae;[137] and "mucinous" edema of the peribronchiolar, perivascular, and interstitial connective tissue.[137] Bronchopneumonia, hemorrhages, and pleural effusion are relatively frequent complications. Although ultimate prognosis depends on the presence and severity of renal lesions and vascular thrombosis, previous morbidity and mortality from bronchopneumonia and pleural effusion have been improved significantly by appropriate antibiotic and corticosteroid therapy respectively. Two points should be noted in this regard: (1) pleural effusion may recur when corticosteroids are discontinued and (2) the danger of producing "opportunistic" infections occurs with prolonged use of corticosteroids, with or without concurrent antibiotics.

RHEUMATOID DISEASE

Pulmonary involvement is estimated to occur in 5% of patients with rheumatoid disease.[151] Pulmonary disease may take several forms, which may coexist in a given patient or may appear at different times during the course of the disease.

Diffuse interstitial pulmonary fibrosis (diffuse interstitial pneumonitis) may appear at first as nonspecific interstitial pneumonia with mononuclear cell infiltration. As the course progresses, inflammatory cells are replaced by mature fibrous tissue. In the early stages, the roentgenographic appearance is characterized by small ("punctate") or nodular lesions, which progress to a typical fibrotic stage and then to a stage of "honeycombing" when parenchymal destruction is produced. Small lung volume is apparent in the roentgenogram. Pulmonary function tests confirm this impression and reveal further the expected reduction of diffusing capacity.

Pleural disease (pleuritis and pleural effusion) is the most common manifestation of rheumatoid disease in the thorax, more common in males than females.[37,48,176,178] Pleural fluid has high protein content and low sugar, which does not increase with intravenous infusions of glucose as it does in tuberculosis. Pleural fluid may contain lymphocytes, has a lactic dehydrogenase level higher than that of serum, and produces latex fixation titers that parallel those of serum. The effusion is persistent and may remain for months or years.[37]

"Necrobiotic nodules" are well-circumscribed masses in the periphery of the lungs, pleura, or pericardium, which are identical to the subcutaneous rheumatoid nodules. They are generally associated with advanced rheumatoid disease and they may progress to formation of rather thick-walled cavities. It is of interest to note that in Caplan's syndrome (the association of pneumoconiosis with rheumatoid arthritis in some patients with nodular pulmonary fibrosis[36]), there may be an enhanced generation of the rheumatoid nodules in the lung, perhaps on the basis of antigen-antibody reactions[135] induced by the inhalation of industrial dusts such as silica.

Prognosis, in general, is poor. Antibiotic therapy is indicated for concurrent pulmonary infections, but does not reverse the course of rheumatoid pulmonary disease. Steroid therapy has been employed for the latter, but results have been disappointing. Healing may occur gradually, leaving residual fibrosis, which is unaffected by steroids and antibiotics.[54] Although penicillamine has been reported to reduce joint pain, after pulmonary infiltrations, and improve pulmonary function,[106] its value needs to be confirmed by additional trials.

SCLERODERMA (PROGRESSIVE SYSTEMIC SCLEROSIS)

This disease is characterized by atrophy and sclerosis of skin, gastrointestinal tract, musculoskeletal system, heart, and lungs. Most patients are in the fourth to sixth decade of life, and females outnumber males three to one.[47,70] About 90% of the patients have morphologic evidence of pulmonary fibrosis, which does not correlate with the degree of clinical or apparent roentgenographic involvement, but does correspond to abnormal measurements of pulmonary function. Vital capacity, lung volumes, pulmonary compliance, and diffusing capacity are low; interestingly, chest wall compliance is normal.[154,155] Systemic hypoxemia may be present at rest and virtually always develops during exercise.[19,39,182] The usual pulmonary findings include diffuse interstitial fibrosis with thickening of the basement membranes of alveoli and small vessels. As the disease progresses, there is gross distortion of the parenchyma and the formation of "cysts" that present a honeycomb appearance roentgenographically. The lower lung zones seem to be affected more than the upper zones, as is true for most pulmonary manifestations of collagen disease in general. Pleural involvement is not common.[68] The association of pulmonary disease, as described, with typical gastrointestinal and skin involvement is pathognomonic of scleroderma. Prognosis generally depends on the severity of cardiac or renal disease.[62,145,154] Of the many therapeutic drugs that have been used, corticosteroids continue to be preferred, albeit their effectiveness is rather limited.

DERMATOMYOSITIS-POLYMYOSITIS

These conditions are clinical variants of the same disease process, in which the fundamental abnormality is inflammation and degeneration within and around skeletal muscle fibers (polymyositis), which may or may not be associated with cutaneous manifestations (dermatomyositis). Females are affected twice as often as males, and overall incidence peaks during the first decade of life, then again during the fifth and sixth decades. The disease in children may be distinguished from that in adults by the prominence of vascular lesions, which produce a systemic angiopathy involving skin, gastrointestinal tract, adipose tissue, and the nervous system. In adults, the disease may be associated with malignancy.

Weakness of the muscles of respiration may lead to hypoventilation with respiratory failure and to complications such as atelectasis and pneumonia (see also Chapter 2). Small lung volumes may be the result of respiratory muscular weakness or parenchymal changes due to vascular lesions, i.e., interstitial fibrosis. Tests of pulmonary function demonstrate both the muscle weakness and fibrosis.[52,67,128,130] In addition, because of weakness of the pharyngeal muscles, these children may suffer repeated aspirations. Morphologic characteristics of the pulmonary disease reflect the fibrotic process (thickened alveolar septae, increased interstitial connective tissue), the inflammatory changes, and the effects of aspiration (infiltration of plasma cells and leukocytes, and hyaline membranes). Corticosteroid therapy is extremely successful as a palliative measure and may produce profound increases in muscle strength.

RHEUMATIC FEVER

Pulmonary involvement in patients with rheumatic fever can take several forms. Pulmonary edema may result from congestive heart failure secondary to rheumatic carditis. The classic manifestations of crackles, orthopnea, tachypnea, and roentgenographic abnormalities are reversed when cardiac therapy is successful. Rarely, the persistence of pulmonary edema fluid has been thought to contribute to the formation of chronic intra-alveolar fibrinous exudates.[66]

"Rheumatic pneumonia," a rare manifestation, is frequently fatal. It is characterized by extensive consolidation of the lungs—often without auscultatory crackles—and failure to respond to both corticosteroid and antibiotic therapy.[115] The histopathologic features of rheumatic pneumonia include marked congestion, alveolar exudate, hemorrhage, necrosis, marked interstitial infiltration by inflammatory cells, and proliferation of endothelial cells.[160] It is now believed that rheumatic pneumonia is caused by the hypersensitivity reaction that is responsible for rheumatic fever itself, rather than being the consequence of heart failure or pulmonary embolism. Pathologic changes are similar to those encountered in experimental hypersensitivity.[73,142]

Reticuloendothelioses

Nonlipid reticuloendothelioses are diseases that involve proliferation of typical "histiocytes" in various tissues, including the lung. This group of diseases, collectively known as histiocytosis X, is of unknown cause, probably not hereditary, not familial, and not infectious. High classifies these diseases in the following order of decreasing severity and mortality: the Letterer-Siwe syndrome, the Hand-Schüller-Christian syndrome, eosinophilic granuloma of bone, and histiocytic infiltrations of atypical distribution.[79] Each of these conditions, except eosinophilic granuloma of bone, may produce mononuclear histiocytic infiltrates in the alveolar septae and bronchial walls,[165] which may progress to deposition of collagen and ultimately marked fibrosis. Histiocytes are systemic macrophages, and it has been suggested that the "nonlipid reticuloendothelioses" should be included in the spectrum of diseases that involve abnormal differentiation and proliferation of histiocytes.[40] This classification of Cline and Golde is shown in Figure 18-4.[40] It differs from the one of High only in that the latter's "histiocytic infiltrations of atypical distribution" would be included in "eosinophilic granuloma" of Figure 18-4. In addition, Cline and Golde suggest that "histiocytic medullary reticulosis" is merely a variant of the well-differentiated form of reticulum cell sarcoma.

Letterer-Siwe syndrome occurs in children

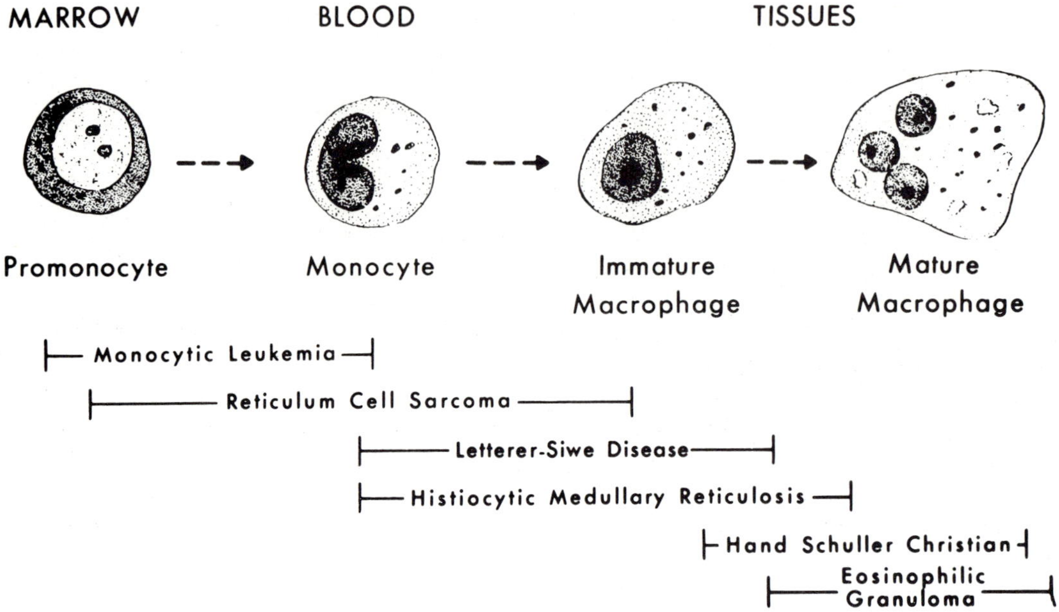

FIG. 18-4. A classification of the malignant histiocytic disorders based on mononuclear-macrophage differentiation. (From Cline, M. J. and D. W. Golde.[40])

predominantly. Lesions are disseminated widely (e.g., to lungs, lymph nodes, skin, central nervous system, liver, spleen, gastrointestinal tract, kidney and bone), and the course may be rapidly fatal. Hans-Schüller-Christian syndrome, which may appear during childhood and adolescence, takes a variable course that may be comparatively benign. Eosinophilic granuloma involves only the bone. The infiltrates of atypical distribution generally involve only one organ.

Pulmonary involvement in the nonlipid reticuloendothelioses may be widespread with nodular lesions developing especially in peribronchial and perivascular tissue and within the alveolar septae. Alveolar walls may become progressively involved, with fibrous tissue replacement of the "granulomas" and formation of parenchymal cysts.[125,165] Hilar adenopathy is rare, pleural effusion is uncommon, but as might be expected from the parenchymal destruction, spontaneous pneumothorax is frequent.[100,125,146] Patients usually present with constitutional symptoms, such as fatigue, weight loss, and fever. Nonproductive cough is common, but hemoptysis is rare. Children may fail to demonstrate serious respiratory symptoms even with pulmonary involvement.[56] Pulmonary function tests reveal a decreased vital capacity, decreased diffusing capacity, and increased physiologic dead space, which are consonant with the expected pathophysiologic processes, i.e., poor diffusion and $\dot{V}_A/\dot{Q}$ abnormality.

The so-called *lipid reticuloses* may involve the lungs and produce pulmonary disease. Gaucher's disease, which is a deficiency of catabolism of the cerebroside, glucosylceramide, affects females more often than males. About 95 % of the patients are Jewish. The disease has been classified according to the organ system primarily affected: in the "neurologic form" death usually occurs before the age of 2 years; the "visceral form," characterized by hepatosplenomegaly, affects children from 6 months of age to early adolescence and death is often due to intercurrent infection or hemorrhage; the "osseous form," which occurs in late adolescence or adulthood, includes splenomegaly and bone involvement. Rare involvement of the lungs is manifested by widespread infiltration of the parenchyma by granular cells, and respiratory failure may be fatal.[91] Niemann-Pick disease is a genetic deficiency of the enzyme needed to catabolize sphingomyelin. Lipid accumulates in virtually all viscera including the lung. Alveoli are dilated and filled with large "foam cells," which are also found in peribronchial and perivascular tissue. The disease is usually apparent in infants and is fatal before the age of 6 years.[151] Fabry's disease is another metabolic genetic defect in which the ceramide, trihexoside, accumulates in many tissues, with especially high concentrations in the glomeruli. Cutaneous lesions are usually the first to appear, followed in 5 to 10 years by progressive visceral involvement, which leads to myocardial or renal failure. Pulmonary involvement has been reported;[131] the clinical picture resembled that of pulmonary embolism.

Polycythemia and Anemia

Both polycythemia and anemia may result from and complicate the course of chronic pulmonary disease, and both may compromise the normal compensatory cardiopulmonary adaptations to acute disease.

POLYCYTHEMIA

Polycythemia vera is extremely rare in children. Its cause is not known. Its course is chronic and progressive and is characterized by marked plethora, splenomegaly, thrombosis, and hemorrhage. All of the formed elements of blood are elevated and the bone marrow is hyperplastic. Pulmonary function studies in adults indicate that lung volumes, maximum ventilatory capacity, and inert gas distribution are normal.[13,33] Arterial oxygen saturation may be low in some patients, whereas diffusing capacity is elevated before treatment but may become abnormally low when hematocrit is restored to normal,[33] perhaps as a consequence of pulmonary vascular thromboses.

Primary erythrocytosis is a benign, familial elevation of total red blood cell mass without an accompanying elevation of white blood cells and platelets. It is more common in children than polycythemia vera[2,4] and usually produces no symptoms, except for the ruddy appearance of the child.

Polycythemia secondary to chronic hypoxemia may develop in children with chronic pulmonary disease. In adults, secondary polycythemia often complicates chronic bronchitis and emphysema. A comparison of adults with secondary polycythemia and those with polycythemia vera indicates that patients with lung disease have a significant reduction of plasma volume, whereas red cell volume is twice as great in polycythemia vera.[86] Secondary polycythemia in children is more commonly associated with cardiovascular diseases that involve a right-to-left shunt (e.g., congenital heart disease and pulmonary arteriovenous malformation) or with pulmonary disease that involves parenchymal destruction, fibrosis, or chronic hypoventilation (see Chapter 2).

The functional significance of polycythemia and increased hemoglobin content is to increase the oxygen carrying capacity of blood. The limiting factor is the concomitant increase of blood viscosity, especially rapid at high hematocrits (Fig. 18-5), which may result in impeded flow, sludging of red blood cells ("thrombosis"), and consequent reduction of perfusion and oxygen delivery to tissues. Cyanotic children with polycythemia are hypervolemic, principally as a result of an increase in red blood cell volume with normal or decreased plasma volume.[149,150] Hypervolemia, which would tend to lower systemic vascular resistance and increase cardiac output, could counterbalance some of the opposite effects on blood flow associated with high

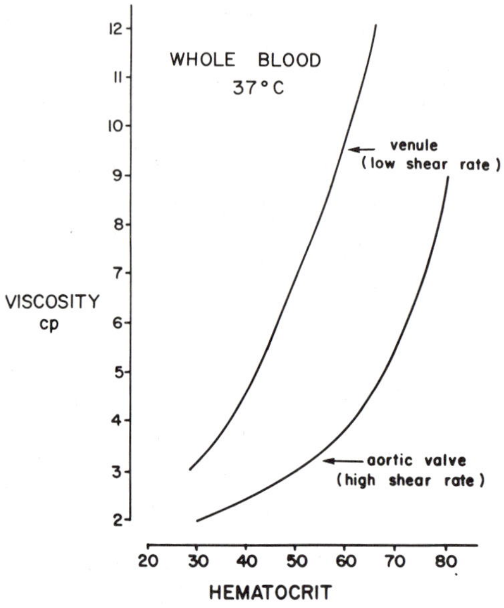

FIG. 18-5. Relationship between blood viscosity and blood hematocrit at 37° C. Note that in the venule the effective viscosity is higher because of low shear rate. (From Wells, R. In A. S. Nadas and D. C. Fyler.[124])

viscosity. With these facts in mind, Nadas and Fyler recommend that hematocrit should not exceed 60 to 70% in children with tetralogy of Fallot and appreciable arterial unsaturation.[124]

Whereas the hematocrit and hemoglobin concentration of newborn infants are normally generally higher than those of the adult and clinicians have accepted high hematocrits in the first days of life as physiologic and without clinical effect, it is important to note that unusually high neonatal polycythemia may have serious effects.[100a] For example, it is well known that intrauterine twin-to-twin transfusions may lead to death in utero of the plethoric twin or, if he is born alive, to the development of symptoms of congestive heart failure, respiratory distress, central nervous system disturbances, or hyperbilirubinemia. (Of course the donor infant may also be seriously affected, presenting with anemia and shock.) The possible causes of neonatal polycythemia include intrauterine hypoxia or infection, placental dysfunction (both dysmaturity and postmaturity), developmental defects (including small-for-gestational-age infants, intrauterine growth retardation, Down's syndrome, adrenal hyperplasia, oligohydramnios, trisomy D), and transfusions (twin-twin, maternal-fetal, placental-cord), or the polycythemia may be idiopathic.[100a] A hematocrit above 65% may be associated with clinical symptoms in these early newborn infants for whom the term "neonatal hyperviscosity syndrome" has been used.[73a,100a,108a] Symptoms are related to impaired perfusion of the particular organ. Thus, as the viscosity of blood increases, capillary flow is retarded and sludging of blood flow results in impairment of tissue oxygenation and a tendency to form microthrombi. Local ischemia and hypoxia may produce signs of respiratory and/or cardiovascular failure, and central nervous system disease, including seizures, lethargy, and vomiting. For the lung both pulmonary vascular hypoperfusion and the associated lowering of pulmonary compliance[127a] may contribute to respiratory distress. Treatment by hemodilution with exchange transfusion is generally effective in reversing clinical symptoms.

ANEMIA

Chronic anemia has a variety of causes. It is not unusual in children with chronic debilitating disease (with or without pulmonary involvement) or with nutritional deficiencies. Anemia associated with pulmonary disease may compromise cardiopulmonary function beyond the effects of the primary disease and to the point of cardiopulmonary exhaustion. Thus anemia must always be considered seriously in such patients and corrected. The principal effect of anemia is to reduce the oxygen carrying capacity of blood and to induce an increase in myocardial work (increased cardiac output) in order to sustain peripheral perfusion at a level at which optimal oxygen delivery to tissues may be restored. In addition, whereas arterial oxygen *saturation* may be "normal" in patients with chronic anemia,[120] the difference between alveolar and arterial oxygen tension is greater than normal, so that Pa_{O_2} may be lower than normal.[152] With stress or exercise, the difference may increase and oxygen-hemoglobin saturation may be significantly compromised.[20,166]

The parameter of pulmonary function that appears to be deranged in the presence of anemia is diffusing capacity, although it has been suggested that anatomic pulmonary shunts may also become functional.[82] Thus, the anemic patient's ability to respond to an exercise or other stressful load is seriously impaired. The respiratory adaptation to anemia consists in increasing alveolar oxygen tension by hyperventilation, which may be a response to the lowered oxygen carrying capacity of blood and to the increase of extracellular fluid volume that often accompanies chronic anemia.

Studies of the effects of acute blood loss are relatively few. It has been shown, however, that 1 hour after donation of 500 ml of blood by normal adult subjects, maximal oxygen uptake had fallen 10 %, pulmonary ventilation had increased by about the same amount, pulse rate had increased, and the level of maximal work possible was reduced.[8]

REFERENCES: PART II

1. Aach, R. and J. Kissane: Mycosis fungoides with pulmonary and neurologic complications. *Am. J. Med. 42*:129, 1967.
2. Abildgaard, C. F., J. A. Cornet and I. Schulman: Primary erythrocytosis. *J. Pediatr. 63*:1072, 1963.
3. Anderson, R., M. Cassell, G. L. Mullinax and H. R. Chaplin, Jr.: Effect of normal cells on viscosity of sickle cell blood. In vitro studies and report of six years' experience with prophylactic program of partial exchange transfusion. *Arch. Intern. Med. 111*:286, 1963.
4. Auerback, M. L., J. A. Wolff and S. R. Mettier: Benign familial polycythemia of childhood. Report of two cases. *J. Pediatr. 21*:54, 1958.
5. Austrian, R.: The current status of pneumococcal disease and the potential utility of polyvalent pneumococcal vaccine. In *Proceedings, International Conference on the Application of Vaccines Against Viral Rickettsial and Bacterial Disease of Man.* Pan American Health Organization, Washington, p. 359, 1971.
6. Ausubel, H., B. D. Cohen and J. S. Ladue: Tietze's disease of eight years' duration. *N. Engl. J. Med. 261*:190, 1959.
7. Axelrod, F. B., N. Branom, M. Becker, R. Machtigal and J. Dancis: Treatment of familial dysautonomia with bethanecol. *J. Pediatr. 81*:573, 1972.
8. Balke, B., G. P. Grillo, E. B. Konecci and U. C. Luft: Work capacity after blood donation. *J. Appl. Physiol. 7*:231, 1954.
9. Baron, M. G. and W. M. Whitehouse: Primary lymphosarcoma of the lung. *Am. J. Roentgenol. 85*:294, 1961.
10. Barrett-Connor, E.: Acute pulmonary disease and sickle cell anemia. *Am. Rev. Respir. Dis. 104*:159, 1971.
11. Barrett-Connor, E.: Pneumonia and pulmonary infarction in sickle cell anemia. *J.A.M.A. 224*:997, 1973.
12. Bashour, F. A.: Clubbing of the digits: physiologic considerations. *J. Lab. Clin. Med. 58*:613, 1961.
13. Bedell, G. N., R. F. Sheets, H. W. Fischer and E. O. Theilen: Polycythemia: a manifestation of heart disease, lung disease or a primary blood dyscrasia. *Circulation 18*:107, 1958.
14. Benton, C. and F. N. Silverman: Some mediastinal lesions in children. *Semin. Roentgenol. 4*:91, 1969.
15. Berg, N. O. and S. Eriksson: Liver disease in adults with alpha-1-antitrypsin deficiency. *N. Engl. J. Med. 287*:1264, 1972.
16. Bergofsky, E. H., G. M. Turino and A. P. Fishman: Cardiorespiratory failure in kyphoscoliosis. *Medicine 38*:263, 1959.
17. Berthelot, P., J. G. Walker, S. Sherlock, and L. Reid: Arterial changes in the lungs in cirrhosis of the liver-lung spider nevi. *N. Engl. J. Med. 274*:291, 1966.
18. Beutler, E.: The effect of methemoglobin formation in sickle cell disease. *J. Clin. Invest. 40*:1856, 1961.
19. Bianchi, F. A., A. R. Bistue, V. E. Wendt, H. E. Puro and M. K. Keech: Analysis of 27 cases of progressive systemic sclerosis (including two with combined systemic lupus erythematosus) and a review of the literature. *J. Chronic Dis. 19*:953, 1966.
20. Bishop, J. M., K. W. Donald and O. L. Wade: Circulatory dynamics at rest and on exercise in the hyperkinetic states. *Clin. Sci. 14*:329, 1955.

21. Block, J. B., J. Edgcomb, A. Eisen and E. J. Van Scott. Mycosis fungoides: natural history and aspects of its relationship to other malignant lymphomas. *Am. J. Med. 34*:228, 1963.
22. Bodey, G. P., R. D. Powel, Jr., E. M. Hersh, A. Yeterian and E. J. Freireich: Pulmonary complications of acute leukemia. *Cancer 19*:781, 1966.
23. Boland, E. W.: Ankylosing spondylitis. In *Arthritis and Allied Conditions*, S. L. Hollander (Ed.). Lea & Febiger, Philadelphia, p. 633, 1966.
24. Boone, M. L., B. E. Swenson and B. Felson: Rib notching: its many causes. *Am. J. Roentgenol. 91*:1075, 1964.
25. Boushy, S. F., R. S. Kurtzman, N. D. Martin and B. M. Lewis: The course of pulmonary function in sarcoidosis. *Ann. Intern. Med. 62*:939, 1965.
26. Boushy, S. F. and L. B. North: Pulmonary function in infiltrative lung disease. *Chest 64*:448, 1973.
27. Breaky, W. F.: A case of mycosis fungoides. *J. Cutan. Dis. 20*:316, 1902.
28. Brody, J. S. and W. J. Bukain: Hormone induced growth of the adult lung. *Am. J. Physiol. 223*:1444, 1972.
29. Brody, J. S., A. B. Fisher, A. Gorman and A. B. Dubois: Acromegalic pneumonomegaly. *J. Clin. Invest. 49*:1051, 1970.
30. Bruwer, A. J., R. R. Kierland and H. W. Schmidt: Pulmonary tuberous sclerosis: report of a case. *Am. J. Roentgenol. 75*:748, 1956.
31. Buckley, C. F., III, H. Nagaya and H. O. Sieker: Altered immunologic activity in sarcoidosis. *Ann. Intern. Med. 64*:508, 1966.
32. Bulgrin, J. G., E. L. Dubois and G. Jacobson: Chest roentgenographic changes in systemic lupus erythematosus. *Radiology 74*:42, 1960.
33. Burgess, J. H. and J. M. Bishop: Pulmonary diffusing capacity and its subdivisions in polycythemia vera. *J. Clin. Invest. 42*:997, 1963.
34. Burn, J. I., A. L. Watne and G. E. Moore: The role of the thoracic duct lymph in cancer dissemination. *Br. J. Cancer 16*:608, 1962.
35. Bybee, J. D. and D. E. Rodgers: The phagocytic activity of polymorphonuclear leukocytes obtained from patients with diabetes mellitus. *J. Lab. Clin. Med. 64*:1, 1964.
36. Caplan, A.: Certain unusual radiological appearances in chests of coal-miners suffering from rheumatoid arthritis. *Thorax 8*:29, 1953.
37. Carr, D. T. and J. G. Mayne: Pleurisy with effusion in rheumatoid arthritis with reference to the low concentration of glucose in pleural fluid. *Am. Rev. Respir. Dis. 85*:345, 1962.
38. Carrington, C. B. and A. A. Liebow: Limited forms of angiitis and granulomatosis of Wegener's type. *Am. J. Med. 41*:497, 1966.
39. Catteral, M. and N. R. Rowell: Respiratory function in progressive systemic sclerosis. *Thorax 18*:10, 1963.
40. Cline, M. J. and D. W. Golde: A review and reevaluation of the histiocytic disorders. *Am. J. Med. 55*:49, 1973.
41. Cohen, A. A., E. A. Natelson and R. F. Fecherer: Fibrosing interstitial pneumonitis in ankylosing spondylitis. *Chest 59*:369, 1971.
42. Cohen, A. B.: Interrelationships between the human alveolar macrophage and alpha-1-antitrypsin. *J. Clin. Invest. 52*:2793, 1973.
43. Cooke, R. E., G. S. Spears and J. P. Dorst: Nephrosis with cardiac and pulmonary complications. *J. Pediatr. 80*:881, 1972.
44. Craighead, C. C. and B. A. Glass: Management of non-penetrating injuries of the chest. *J.A.M.A. 172*:1138, 1960.
45. Daniel, T. M., P. B. Barlow and J. J. Picken: Sarcoidosis. In *Textbook of Pulmonary Diseases*. G. L. Baum (Ed.). Little, Brown and Co., Boston, p. 407, 1974.
46. Diggs, L. W.: Sickle cell crisis. *Am. J. Clin. Pathol. 44*:1, 1965.
47. Divertie, M. B.:Lung involvement in the connective tissue disorders. *Med. Clin. North Am. 48*:1015, 1964.
48. Dodson, W. H. and J. W. Hollingsworth: Pleural effusion in rheumatoid arthritis. Impaired transport of glucose. *N. Engl. J. Med. 275*:1337, 1966.
49. Dolan, D. L., G. B. Lemmon, Jr. and S. L. Teitelbaum: Relapsing polychondritis. Analytical literature review and studies on pathogenesis. *Am. J. Med. 41*:285, 1966.
50. Dollery, C. T., P. M. S. Gillam, P. Hugh-Jones and P. A. Zorab: Regional lung function in kyphoscoliosis. *Thorax 20*:175, 1965.
51. Donaldson, S. S., E. Glatstein, S. A. Rosenberg and H. S. Kaplan: Pediatric Hodgkins disease. II. Results of therapy. *Cancer 37*:2436, 1976.
52. Duncan, P. E., J. P. Griffin, A. Garcia and S. B. Kaplan: Fibrosing alveolitis in polymyosites. *Am. J. Med. 57*:621, 1974.
53. Editorial. Antibiotic-induced myasthenia. *J.A.M.A. 204*:164, 1968.
54. Ellman, P. and L. Cudkowicz: Pulmonary manifestations in the diffuse collagen diseases. *Thorax 9*:46, 1954.
55. Emirgil, C., B. J. Sobol and M. H. Williams, Jr.: Long-term study of pulmonary sarcoidosis: the effect of steroid therapy as evaluated by pulmonary function studies. *J. Chronic Dis. 22*:69, 1969.
56. Enriquez, P., D. C. Dahlin, A. B. Hayles and E. D. Henderson: Histiocytosis X: a clinical study. *Mayo Clin. Proc. 42*:88, 1967.
57. Essig, L. J., E. S. Timms, D. E. Hancock and G. C. Sharp: Plasma cell interstitial pneumonia

and macroglobulinemia. A response to corticosteroid and cyclophosphamide therapy. *Am. J. Med. 56*:398, 1974.
58. Evans, H. E., M. Levi and I. Mandl: Serum enzyme inhibitor concentration in respiratory distress syndrome. *Am. Rev. Respir. Dis. 101*:359, 1970.
59. Evans, H. E. and W. L. Nyhan: Hodgkin's disease in children. *Bull. Johns Hopkins Hosp. 114*:237, 1964.
60. Fager, D. B., J. A. Bigler and J. P. Simonds: Polyarteritis nodosa in infancy and childhood. *J. Pediatr. 39*:65, 1951.
61. Farber, S. and G. F. Vawter: The Children's Hospital Medical Center, Boston, Mass. (Clinical pathological conference) *J. Pediatr. 58*:126, 1961.
62. Farmer, R. G., R. W. Gifford, Jr., and E. A. Hines, Jr.: Prognostic significance of Raynaud's phenomenon and other clinical characteristics of systemic scleroderma: a study of 271 cases. *Circulation 21*:1088, 1960.
63. Femi-Pearse, D., K. M. Gazioglu and P. N. Yu: Pulmonary function studies in sickle cell disease. *J. Appl. Physiol. 28*:574, 1970.
64. Foldes, F. F., J. N. Lunn and H. G. Benz: Prolonged respiratory depression caused by drug combinations. Muscle relaxants and intraperitoneal antibiotics as etiologic agents. *J.A.M.A. 183*:672, 1963.
65. Foldes, J.: Acute systemic lupus erythematosus. *Am. J. Clin. Pathol. 16*:160, 1946.
66. Fraser, R. G. and J. A. P. Pare: *Diagnosis of Diseases of the Chest.* W. B. Saunders Co., Philadelphia, 1970.
67. Frazier, A. R. and R. D. Miller: Interstitial pneumonitis in association with polymyosites and dermatomyosites. *Chest 65*:403, 1974.
68. Garland, L. H. and M. A. Sisson: Roentgen findings in the "collagen" diseases. *Am. J. Roentgenol. 71*:581, 1954.
69. Gold, W. M. and D. B. Jennings: Pulmonary function in patients with lupus erythematosus. *Am. Rev. Respir. Dis. 93*:556, 1966.
70. Gondos, B.: Roentgen manifestations in progressive systemic sclerosis (diffuse scleroderma). *Am. J. Roentgenol. 84*:235, 1960.
71. Gracey, D. R., D. A. Solomon and D. W. Cugell: A case of post traumatic respiratory failure. *Chest 65*:323, 1974.
72. Green, R. A., W. J. Nichols and E. J. King: Alveolar capillary block due to leukemic infiltration of the lung. *Am. Rev. Respir. Dis. 80*:895, 1959.
73. Gregory, J. E. and A. R. Rich: The experimental production of anaphylactic pulmonary lesions with basic characteristics of rheumatic pneumonitis. *Bull. Johns Hopkins Hosp. 78*:1, 1946.
73a. Gross, G. P., W. E. Hathaway and H. R. McGaughey: Hyperviscosity in the neonate. *J. Pediatr. 82*:1004, 1973.
74. Gross, M., J. R. Esterly and R. H. Earle: Pulmonary alterations in systemic lupus erythematosus. *Am. Rev. Respir. Dis. 105*:572, 1972.
75. Hall, G. H. and C. D. Laidlaw: Further experimental evidence implicating reduced ferritin as cause of digital clubbing. *Clin. Sci. 24*:121, 1963.
76. Hanson, V. and H. Kornreich: Systemic rheumatic disorders in childhood: lupus erythematosus, anaphylactoid purpura, dermatomyositis, and scleroderma. *Bull. Rheum. Dis. 17*:435, 1967.
77. Hansoti, R. C. and N. J. Shah: Cirrhosis of liver simulating congenital cyanotic heart disease. *Circulation 33*:71, 1966.
78. Harwood-Nash, D. C. and D. L. Buckbill: Computed tomography in children. *J. Pediatr. 89*:343, 1976.
79. High, R. H.: Idiopathic histiocytosis (histiocytosis X). In *Pulmonary Disorders,* E. L. Kendig, Jr., (Ed.). W. B. Saunders Co., Philadelphia, p. 622, 1972.
80. Hill, R. B., Jr., D. T. Rowlands, Jr. and D. Rifkind: Infectious pulmonary disease in patients receiving immunosuppressive therapy for organ transplantation. *N. Engl. J. Med. 271*:1021, 1964.
81. Hoffbrand, B. I. and E. R. Beck: "Unexplained" dyspnoea and shrinking lungs in systemic lupus erythematosus. *Br. Med. J. 1*:1273, 1965.
82. Housley, E.: Respiratory gas exchange in chronic anaemia. *Clin. Sci. 32*:19, 1967.
83. Huang, C. T., G. R. Hennigar and H. A. Lyons: Pulmonary dysfunction in systemic lupus erythematosus. *N. Engl. J. Med. 272*:288, 1965.
84. Huang, C. T. and H. A. Lyons: Comparison of pulmonary function in patients with systemic lupus erythematosus, scleroderma and rheumatoid arthritis. *Am. Rev. Respir. Dis. 93*:865, 1966.
85. Hughes, W. T.: Fatal infections in childhood leukemia. *Am. J. Dis. Child. 122*:283, 1971.
86. Hume, R. and A. Goldberg: Actual and predicted normal red-cell and plasma volumes in primary and secondary polycythemia. *Clin. Sci. 26*:499, 1964.
87. Ingbar, S. H. and K. A. Woeber: The thyroid gland. In *Textbook of Endocrinology.* W. B. Saunders Co., Philadelphia, p. 95, 1974.
88. Inkley, S. R., F. C. Oldenburg and P. J. Vignus: Pulmonary function in Duchenne muscular dystrophy related to stage of disease. *Am. J. Med. 56*:297, 1974.
89. Israel, H. L. and M. Sones: Sarcoidosis: clinical observations on 160 cases. *Arch. Intern. Med. 102*:766, 1958.
90. Israel, H. L. and M. Sones: Immunologic defect in

patients recovered from sarcoidosis. *N. Engl. J. Med. 273*:1003, 1965.

91. Jackson, D. C. and G. Simon: Unusual bone and lung changes in a case of Gaucher's disease. *Br. Med. J. 38*:698, 1965.
92. Jain, B. P., J. S. Brody and A. B. Fisher: The small lung of hypopituitarism. *Am. Rev. Respir. Dis. 108*:49, 1973.
93. Jenkin, R. B., T. C. Brown, M. V. Peters and M. J. Sunly: Hodgkin's disease in children. *Cancer 35*:979, 1975.
94. Johnson, R. M. and G. E. Lindskog: 100 cases of tumor metastatic to the lung and mediastinum. *J.A.M.A. 202*:94, 1967.
95. Jones, B. and W. G. Klingberg: Lymphosarcoma in children. A report of 43 cases and a review of the recent literature. *J. Pediatr. 63*:11, 1963.
96. Kaplan, H. S. and S. A. Rosenberg: The management of Hodgkin's disease. *Cancer 36*:796, 1975.
97. Kendig, E. C.: The clinical picture of sarcoidosis in children. *Pediatrics 54*:289, 1974.
98. Kern, W. H., A. G. Crepeau and J. C. Jones: Primary Hodgkin's disease of the lung: report of four cases and review of the literature. *Cancer 14*: 1151, 1961.
99. Kirkpatrick, J. A., Jr. and D. S. Fleisher: The roentgenographic appearance of the chest in acute glomerulonephritis. *J. Pediatr. 64*:492, 1964.
100. Kittredge, R. D., A. Geller and N. Finby: The reticuloendothelioses in the lung. *Am. J. Roentgenol. 100*:588, 1967.
100a. Kontras, S. B.: Polycythemia and hyperviscosity syndromes in infants and children. *Pediatr. Clin. North Am. 19*:919, 1972.
101. Kornreich, H. K., E. Drexler and V. Hanson: Antinuclear factors in childhood rheumatic diseases. *J. Pediatr. 69*:1039, 1966.
102. Kravath, R. E., E. M. Scarpelli and J. Bernstein: Hepatogenic cyanosis: arteriovenous shunts in chronic active hepatitis. *J. Pediatr. 78*:238, 1971.
103. Lampkin, B. C., N. B. McWilliams and A. M. Mauer: Treatment of acute leukemia. *Pediatr. Clin. North Am. 19*:1123, 1972.
104. Lindesmith, L. A., D. Baines, A. B. Bigelow and T. L. Petty: Reversible respiratory paralysis associated with polymyxin therapy. *Ann. Intern. Med. 68*:318, 1968.
105. Longscope, W. T. and D. H. Friedman: A study of sarcoidosis. Based on a combined investigation of 160 cases, including 30 autopsies from the Johns Hopkins Hospital and Massachusetts General Hospital. *Medicine 31*:1, 1952.
106. Lorber, A.: Penicillamine therapy for rheumatoid lung disease: effects on protein sulfhydryl groups. *Nature 210*:1235, 1966.
107. Luntz, G. W.: The prognosis of tuberculosis in diabetic patients. *Tubercle* (London) *42*:379, 1961.
108. Lyons, H. A., G. L. Calvy and B. P. Sammons: The diagnosis and classification of mediastinal masses. I. A study of 782 cases. *Ann. Intern. Med. 51*:897, 1959.
108a. MacKintosh, T. F. and C. H. M. Walker: Blood viscosity in the newborn. *Arch. Dis. Child. 48*:547, 1973.
109. Mankiewicz, E.: The relationship of sarcoidosis to anonymous bacteria. (Proc. Third Internat. Conf. on Sarcoidosis). *Acta Med. Scand. 425*:68, 1964.
110. Mankiewicz, E. and J. Beland: The role of mycobacteriophages and of cortisone in experimental tuberculosis and sarcoidosis. *Am. Rev. Respir. Dis. 89*:707. 1964.
111. Mankiewicz, E. and M. Van Walbeek: Mycobacteriophages: their role in tuberculosis and sarcoidosis. *Arch. Environ. Health 5*:122, 1962.
112. Marble, A., H. J. White and A. T. Farnand: The nature of the lowered resistance to infection in diabetes mellitus. *J. Clin. Invest. 17*:423, 1938.
113. Margolies, M. P.: Sickle cell anemia. *Medicine 30*:357, 1951.
114. Massey, D. G., M. R. Becklake, J. M. McKenzie and J. V. Bates: Circulatory and ventilatory response to exercise in thyrotoxicosis. *N. Engl. J. Med. 276*:1104, 1967.
115. Massumi, R. A. and J. F. Legier: Rheumatic pneumonitis. *Circulation 33*:417, 1966.
116. Massumi, R. A. and J. L. Winnaker: Severe depression of the respiratory center in myxedema. *Am. J. Med. 36*:876, 1964.
117. Maycock, R. L., P. Bertrand, C. E. Morrison and J. H. Scott: Manifestations of sarcoidosis. Analysis of 145 patients with a review of nine series selected from the literature. *Am. J. Med. 35*:67, 1963.
118. McCurdy, P. R. and L. Mahmood: Urea therapy for sickle cell disease (abstract). *Blood 36*:841, 1970.
119. McKusick, V. A. and H. E. Cross: Ataxia-telangiectasia and Swiss-type agammaglobulinemia. *J.A.M.A. 195*:739, 1966.
120. Meakins, J. C. and H. W. Davies: *Respiratory Function in Disease.* Oliver and Boyd, Edinburgh, 1925.
121. Mellins, R. B., A. P. Hayes, A. P. Guld, N. E. Berdon and J. D. Bowdler: Respiratory distress as the initial manifestation of Werdnig-Hoffmann disease. *Pediatrics 53*:33, 1974.
122. Miller, G. U. and G. R. Sargeant: Lung function in sickle cell anemia. *Thorax 26*:490, 1971.
123. Mowat, A. G. and J. Baum: Chemotaxis of polymorphonuclear leukocytes from patients with diabetes mellitus. *N. Engl. J. Med. 284*:621, 1971.
124. Nadas, A. S. and D. C. Fyler: *Pediatric Cardiology.* W. B. Saunders Co., Philadelphia, 1972.
125. Nadeau, P. J., F. H. Ellis, Jr., E. G. Harrison, Jr. and R. S. Fontana: Primary pulmonary histiocytosis. *Dis. Chest 37*:325, 1960.

126. Nalbandian, R. M., G. Shultz, J. M. Lusher, J. W. Anderson and R. L. Henry. Sickle cell crisis terminated by intravenous urea in sugar solutions—a preliminary report. *Am. J. Med. Sci. 261*:309, 1971.
127. O'Brien, R. T., S. McIntosh, G. T. Aspens and H. A. Pearson: Prospective study of sickle cell anemia in infancy. *J. Pediatr. 89*:205, 1976.
127a. Oh, W., G. Wallgren, J. S. Hanson and J. Lind: The effects of placental transfusion on respiratory mechanics of normal term newborn infants. *Pediatrics 40*:6, 1967.
128. Olsen, G. N. and E. W. Swenson: Polymyositis and interstitial lung disease. *Am. Rev. Respir. Dis. 105*:611, 1972.
129. Paglicci, A.: Metastatic tumours of the lung: a study of 152 cases. *Radiol. Med. 42/2*:184, 1956.
130. Park, S. and W. L. Myhan: Fatal pulmonary involvement in dermatomyositis. *Am. J. Dis. Child. 129*:723, 1975.
131. Parkinson, J. E. and A. Sunshine: Angiokeratoma corporis diffusum universale (Fabry). Presenting as suspected myocardial infarction and pulmonary infarcts. *Am. J. Med. 31*:951, 1961.
132. Pearson, C. M., H. M. Kline and V. D. Newcomber: Relapsing polychondritis. *N. Engl. J. Med. 263*:51, 1960.
133. Pearson, H. A., R. P. Spencer and E. A. Cornelius: Functional asplenia in sickle cell anemia. *N. Engl. J. Med. 281*:923, 1969.
134. Perillie, P. E., J. P. Nolan and S. C. Finch. Studies of resistance to infection in diabetes mellitus. Local exudative cellular response. *J. Lab. Clin. Med. 59*:1008, 1962.
135. Pernis, B. and F. Paronetto: Adjuvant effect of silica (tridymite) on antibody production. *Proc. Soc. Exp. Biol. Med. 110*:390, 1962.
136. Pirnar, T. and E. B. D. Neuhauser: Asphyxiating thoracic dystrophy of the newborn. *Am. J. Roentgenol. 98*:358, 1966.
137. Purnell, D. C., A. H. Baggenstoss and A. M. Olsen: Pulmonary lesions in disseminated lupus erythematosus. *Ann. Intern. Med. 42*:619, 1955.
138. Purugganan, H. B. and A. E. McElfresh: Failure of carbonmonoxy sickle cell haemoglobin to alter the sickle state. *Lancet 1*:79, 1964.
139. Rakov, H. L. and J. S. Taylor: Acute disseminated lupus erythematosus, without cutaneous manifestations and with heretofore undescribed pulmonary lesions. *Arch. Intern. Med. 70*:88, 1942.
140. Resnick, M. E., R. D. Berkowitz and T. Rodman: Diffuse interstitial leukemia infiltration of the lungs producing the alveolar capillary block syndrome. Report of a case with studies of pulmonary function. *Am. J. Med. 31*:149, 1961.
141. Reynolds, J.: The thoracic viscera. In *The Roentgenologic Features of Sickle Cell Disease, and Related Hemoglobinopathies.* Charles C Thomas, Springfield, p. 183, 1965.
142. Rich, A. R. and J. E. Gregory: On the anaphylactic nature of rheumatic pneumonitis. *Bull. Johns Hopkins Hosp. 73*:465, 1943.
143. Robert, M. F., R. K. Neff, J. P. Hubbell, H. W. Taeusch and M. E. Avery: Association between maternal diabetes and the respiratory distress syndrome in the newborn. *N. Engl. J. Med. 294*:357, 1976.
144. Roberts, F. B. and G. H. Fetteman: Polyarteritis nodosa in infancy. *J. Pediatr. 63*:519, 1963.
145. Rodnan, G. P.: The natural history of progressive systemic sclerosis (diffuse scleroderma). *Bull. Rheum. Dis. 13*:301, 1963.
146. Roland, A. F.: Recurrent spontaneous pneumothorax. A clue to the diagnosis of histiocytosis X. *N. Engl. J. Med. 270*:73, 1964.
147. Rosen, F. S. and C. A. Janeway: The gamma globulins. III. The antibody deficiency syndromes. *N. Engl. J. Med. 275*:709, 1966.
148. Rosenberg, S. A., H. D. Diamond, B. Jaslowitz and L. F. Craver: Lymphosarcoma: a review of 1,269 cases. *Medicine 40*:31, 1961.
149. Rosenthal, A., L. N. Button, D. G. Nathan, O. S. Miettinen and A. S. Nadas: Blood volume changes in cyanotic congenital heart disease. *Am. J. Cardiol. 27*:162, 1971.
150. Rosenthal, A., D. G. Nathan, A. T. Marty, L. N. Button, O. S. Miettinen and A. S. Nadas: Acute hemodynamic effects of red cell volume reduction in polycythemia of cyanotic congenital heart disease. *Circulation 42*:297, 1970.
151. Rubin, E. H. and S. S. Siegelman: *The Lungs in Systemic Diseases.* Charles C Thomas, Springfield, p. 83, 1969.
152. Ryan, J. M. and J. B. Hickam: The alveolar-arterial O_2 pressure gradient in anemia. *J. Clin. Invest. 31*:188, 1952.
153. Rydell, R. and F. W. Hoffbauer: Multiple pulmonary arteriovenous fistulas in juvenile cirrhosis. *Am. J. Med. 21*:450, 1956.
154. Sackner, M. A.: *Scleroderma.* Grune & Stratton, New York, 1966.
155. Sackner, M. A., N. Akgun, P. Kimbel and D. H. Lewis: The pathophysiology of scleroderma involving the heart and respiratory system. *Ann. Intern. Med. 60*:611, 1964.
156. Sandler, B. P., J. H. Matthews and S. Bornstein: Pulmonary cavitation due to polyarteritis. *J.A.M.A. 144*:754, 1950.
157. Scott, R. A.: Tuberculosis and diabetes. *Am. Rev. Tuberc. Pulm. Dis. 77*:990, 1958.
158. Seeler, R., W. Metzger and M. Mufson: Diplococcus pneumonia infections in children with sickle cell anemia. *Am. J. Dis. Child. 123*:8, 1972.
159. Selecky, P. A. and I. Ziment: Prolonged respirator

support for the treatment of intractable myasthenia gravis. *Chest 65*:207, 1974.
160. Serlin, S. P., M. E. Rimsza and J. Gay: Rheumatic pneumonia: the need for a new approach. *Pediatrics 56*:1075, 1975.
161. Sharma, O. P., C. Colp and M. H. Williams, Jr.: Course of pulmonary sarcoidosis with and without corticosteroid therapy as determined by pulmonary function studies. *Am. J. Med. 41*:541, 1966.
162. Sharp, H. L.: Alpha-1-antitrypsin deficiency. *Hosp. Pract. 6*:83, 1971.
163. Shaw, D. B. and J. Read: Hypoxia and thoracic scoliosis. *Br. Med. J. 2*:1486, 1960.
164. Silverman, A., M. D. Cooper, J. H. Moller and R. Good: Syndrome of cyanosis, digital clubbing, and hepatic disease in siblings. *J. Pediatr. 72*:70, 1968.
165. Smith, M., L. J. McCormick, H. S. Vanordstrand and R. D. Mercer: Primary pulmonary histiocytosis X. *Chest 65*:176, 1974.
166. Sproule, B. J., J. H. Mitchell and W. F. Miller: Cardiopulmonary physiological responses to heavy exercise in patients with anemia. *J. Clin. Invest. 39*:378, 1960.
167. Stein, M., P. Kimbel and R. L. Johnson, Jr.: Pulmonary function hyperthyroidism. *J. Clin. Invest. 40*:348, 1961.
168. Strum, S. M. and H. Rappaport: Hodgkin's disease in the first decade of life. *Pediatrics 46*:748, 1970.
169. Svanborg, N.: Studies on the cardiopulmonary function in sarcoidosis: III. Cases with fibrosis of the lungs. *Acta Med. Scand. 170*:75, 1961.
170. Talamo, R. C.: Basic and clinical aspects of the alpha-1-antitrypsin. *Pediatrics 56*:91, 1975.
171. Talamo, R. C., H. Levinson, M. J. Lynch, A. Gercz, N. Hyslop, Jr. and H. W. Bain: Symptomatic pulmonary emphysema in childhood associated with hereditary alpha-1-antitrypsin and elastase inhibitor deficiency. *J. Pediatr. 79*:20, 1971.
172. Terris, M. and A. D. Chaves: An epidemiologic study of sarcoidosis. *Am. Rev. Respir. Dis. 90*:50, 1966.
173. Vadas, G., J. A. P. Pare and W. Thurlbeck: Pulmonary and lymph node myomatosis: review of the literature and report of a case. *Can. Med. Assoc. J. 96*:420, 1967.
174. Vaughan, V., R. J. McKay and W. Nelson: *Nelson Textbook of Pediatrics.* W. B. Saunders Co., Philadelphia, 1975.
175. Victor, A. B. and L. E. Imperial: The pulmonary and small bone changes in infants with sickle cell anemia. *N.Y. State J. Med. 57*:1403, 1957.
176. Walker, W. C. and V. Wright: Rheumatoid pleuritis. *Ann. Rheum. Dis. 26*:467, 1967.
177. Wanderman, K. L., M. S. Goldstein and J. Faber: Cor pulmonale secondary to severe kyphoscoliosis in Marfan's syndrome. *Chest 67*:2, 1975.
178. Ward, R.: Pleural effusion and rheumatoid disease. *Lancet 2*:1336, 1961.
179. Warley, M. A., P. J. S. Hamilton, P. D. Marsden, R. E. Brown, J. G. Merselis, and N. Wilks: Chemoprophylaxis of homozygous sicklers with antimalarials and long-acting penicillin. *Br. Med. J. 2*:86, 1965.
180. Warwick, M. T.: Pulmonary tuberculosis and diabetes mellitus. *Q. J. Med. 26*:31, 1957.
181. Whitcomb, W. E., M. I. Schwarz, A. R. Keller, E. P. Flannery and J. Blom: Hodgkin's disease of the lung. *Am. Rev. Respir. Dis. 106*:79, 1972.
182. Wilson, R. J., G. P. Rodman and E. D. Robin: An early pulmonary physiologic abnormality in progressive systemic sclerosis (diffuse scleroderma). *Am. J. Med. 36*:361, 1964.
183. Wilson, W. R. and G. N. Bedell: The pulmonary abnormalities in myxedema. *J. Clin. Invest. 39*:42, 1960.
184. Winkelstein, J. A. and R. H. Drachman: Deficiency of serum opsonizing activity in sickle cell disease. *N. Engl. J. Med. 279*:459, 1964.
185. Wintraub, B. U., E. J. Goetzl and K. F. Austin: A neutrophil dependent pathway for the generation of a neutral peptide mediator. *J. Exp. Med. 140*:812, 1974.
186. Young, R. C., C. Carr, T. G. Shelton, M. Mann, A. Ferrin, J. R. Laurey and K. A. Harden. Sarcoidosis: relationship between changes in lung structure and function. *Am. Rev. Respir. Dis. 95*:224, 1967.
187. Young, R. C., V. T. DeVita and R. E. Johnson: Hodgkin's disease in childhood. *Blood 42*:163, 1973.
188. Zwillich, C. W., D. J. Pierson, F. D. Hefeldt, E. G. Lufkur and J. V. Weel: Ventilatory control in myxedema and hypothyroidism. *N. Engl. J. Med. 292*:662, 1975.

Part III: *Toxins*

Pulmonary toxins are either inhaled as gases, vapors, airborne particles, bulk liquid, or solids, or they may be ingested. If ingested, they may be absorbed into the blood stream or regurgitated and inhaled, or both. Pulmonary toxins are substances foreign to that organ, from the obvious, such as industrial distillates and automobile fumes, to the cryptic, such as 100% oxygen. Some have not seen the respiratory system up to the time of the first intoxication (e.g., gastric secretions), whereas others have been there once but cannot return as natural residents (e.g., water, which is the solvent of fetal pulmonary fluid). Then some toxins gain access to the respiratory system quite by accident (e.g., fire and smoke), others by mistake and accident (e.g., salicylates), and still others by necessity (e.g., oxygen) or irrational design (e.g., the air pollutants).

Of all poisonings in the United States, about 90% involve children—most often in the kitchen and bathroom—and most often the offending agent is a medicine. Aspirin is the champion medicine in this category. When medicines are not involved, the odds are that the poison is a hydrocarbon. Of all accidents in the United States, fire, smoke, and drowning are the most serious hazards after the automobile. When common medications are prescribed, the most dangerous are salicylates again, oxygen, sedatives, and depressants, all of which may poison the respiratory system.

The common pulmonary toxins are reviewed in this section. First those that are inhaled as gases, vapors, or airborne particles (oxygen and smoke being the exemplars), then those that are inhaled—aspirated—as solids or liquids (water, hydrocarbons, and gastric secretions being the exemplars), and finally toxins that are ingested and absorbed (salicylates).

Oxygen

One hundred percent oxygen at atmospheric pressure* is toxic to the lung. As the concentration of O_2 in inspired gas is reduced below 100%, a concentration is reached at which pulmonary toxicity is no longer apparent. For adult humans this point is generally accepted to be 50%, i.e., $FI_{O_2} = 0.5$, primarily on the basis of studies in which impairment of pulmonary function could not be detected in men during multi-day exposures to O_2 pressures ranging from 0.23 to 0.55 atmosphere (Fig. 18-6).[18] However, Clark has noted that this limit may not be precisely applicable to patients because of many factors that may modify the rate of oxygen poisoning (Table 18-5).[16] These modifying factors, with the exception of CO_2 inhalation and intermittent exposure to normal inspired PO_2, have been demonstrated in animal experiments. Nonetheless, each bears serious consideration when oxygen therapy is used in humans. It is also important to note that analogous studies have not been conducted in infants and young children exposed to high concentrations of oxygen and that, despite animal experiments, which indicate that some newborn animals are more resistant,[72] oxygen toxicity may play a central, if not etiologic role in the development of "chronic respiratory insufficiency" or bronchopulmonary dysplasia in the newborn infant (see also Chapters 14 and 16). It is also pertinent to note that the extrapulmonary effects of hyperoxia, particularly effects on the central nervous system and on circulation of the retina, are determined directly by the oxygen tension in arterial blood (Pa_{O_2}) and not by the FI_{O_2}. It is also relevant that a large alveolar-arterial oxygen gradient often occurs in severely ill infants and children, so that very high and potentially toxic concentrations of inspired oxygen may be required to maintain a minimally acceptable arterial oxygen tension.

The *clinical signs* of pulmonary oxygen toxicity may be deduced from studies of adult volunteers. In evaluating the effects of oxy-

*One hundred percent oxygen at atmospheric pressure is expressed as $FI_{O_2} = 1.0$ (fraction of inspired oxygen); $PI_{O_2} = 760$ mm Hg (pressure of inspired oxygen at sea level, neglecting water vapor pressure). Under these conditions $PA_{O_2} = 673$ mm Hg (alveolar oxygen pressure = 760-40-47 mm Hg, i.e., atmospheric pressure minus alveolar CO_2 and water vapor pressures).

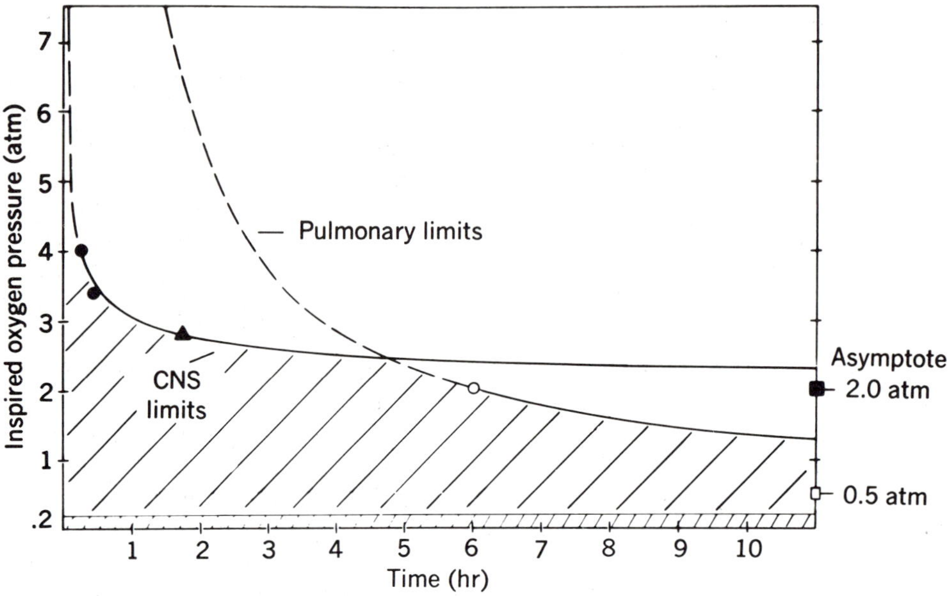

FIG. 18-6. Pulmonary and central nervous system tolerance of normal men at rest to 100% O_2 breathing at various levels of ambient pressure. These curves are rectangular hyperbolas constructed using available data and assuming that (1) at infinitely high inspired Po_2, duration of pulmonary or central nervous system O_2 tolerance will be nearly zero (this provides one common asymptote for central nervous system and pulmonary tolerance curves) and (2) at some sufficiently low inspired Po_2 there will be no detectable limit to O_2 tolerance. Po_2 that will produce borderline pulmonary toxicity is here considered to be 0.5 atm, since 0.5 atm of O_2 did not cause a problem in 14 days. Central nervous system tolerance to O_2 toxicity is assumed to be borderline at 2 atm of inspired Po_2 since exposure of subjects to O_2 for between 10 and 11 hrs has produced no detectable central nervous system effects. Important findings that further determine character of central nervous system tolerance curve are shown at 4.0, 3.5, and 2.8 atm. These represent the time a 10% incidence of central nervous system symptoms developed in normal subjects.

Pulmonary tolerance curve, best studied at low levels of inspired Po_2, is determined by information concerning time required to produce symptoms and 5% reduction of vital capacity at 1 and 2 atm. Choice of hyperbolic relationship between O_2 pressure and duration of tolerance is based on demonstrations that toxicity of O_2 in small organisms and mice closely follows such a pattern. (From Lambertson, C. J.[56])

gen, the physician must take into account both concentration in inspired air and duration of exposure. Thus continued exposure to an FI_{O_2} of about 0.34 produced no apparent toxic effects for periods as long as 30 days.[88] However, when an FI_{O_2} of 0.80 is breathed at sea level for periods of more than 12 hours, symptoms of irritation of the respiratory passages may develop, including substernal distress or soreness, cough, nasal congestion, and sore throat.[21] Human subjects are not usually exposed to oxygen for more extended periods. However, exposure to an FI_{O_2} of 1.0 at sea level for up to 110 hours has produced serious consequences, including persistent severe cough, bronchopneumonia in some subjects, and pleural effusion in others.[29,57]

The development of pulmonary oxygen toxicity in humans may be assessed more accurately by repeated measurements of selected parameters of *pulmonary function,* a requirement that would be difficult and sometimes impossible to meet in infants and young children. The studies of Clark and Lambertson show the following parameters significantly altered early in the progression

TABLE 18-5. Factors That Modify Rate of Development of O_2 Poisoning*

Hasten Onset or Increase Severity	Delay Onset or Decrease Severity
Adrenocortical hormones	Acclimatization to hypoxia
Adrenocorticotropic hormone	Adrenergic blocking drugs
CO_2 inhalation	Anesthesia
Convulsions	Antioxidants
Dextroamphetamine	Chlorpromazine
Epinephrine	Gamma-aminobutyric acid
Hyperthermia	Ganglionic blocking drugs
Insulin	Glutathione
Norepinephrine	Hypothermia
Paraquat	Hypothyroidism
Thyroid hormones	Immaturity
Vitamin E deficiency	Intermittent exposure
X-irradiation	Reserpine
	Starvation
	Tris-aminomethane
	Vitamin E

*Data from Clark, J. M.[16]

of pulmonary oxygen toxicity: respiratory rate, vital capacity, inspiratory flow rate, functional residual capacity, pulmonary compliance, and diffusing capacity.[19] In these studies adult males were exposed to oxygen ($FI_{O_2} = 1.0$) at 2 atmospheres pressure (PI_{O_2} is about 1520 mm Hg), and in this sense they are not comparable to patients receiving respiratory therapy. Nonetheless the investigators found that reduction of vital capacity was the most useful index of the onset and rate of development of pulmonary oxygen toxicity in trained, normal men. These and other studies of normal men breathing oxygen at 2 atmospheres pressure indicate that exposure for as long as 9 hours produces only minimal decrease of diffusing capacity and increases of alveolar-arterial oxygen gradient, airway resistance, and pulmonary compliance.[17,35,83] Perhaps, more pertinent is the study of 11 healthy young men exposed to oxygen at 1 atmosphere ($FI_{O_2} = 1.0$, PI_{O_2} is about 760 mm Hg) for 6 to 12 hours: No significant changes were found in alveolar-arterial oxygen gradient, physiologic pulmonary shunt, pulmonary arterial pressure, total pulmonary vascular resistance, cardiac output, and pulmonary extravascular water volume.[100] The important parameters of pulmonary function, including vital capacity, were not measured. Extrapolation from these studies to the ill infant and child is tenuous, and the authors look forward to the development of clinical tests that may permit early diagnosis, especially in the young patient, of actual or pending pulmonary oxygen toxicity.

Chemical and morphologic studies of the lungs of humans and animals exposed to oxygen provide insights to the pathogenesis of pulmonary injury. Postmortem examination of the lungs of adult patients exposed to 60 to 100% oxygen indicates that exposure to 70% oxygen for 14 hours results in marked dilatation of the pulmonary capillaries and swelling of capillary endothelial and type I alveolar epithelial cells.[51] Thus, cellular manifestations of oxygen toxicity begin soon after exposure, in agreement with a number of controlled studies in animals. With continued exposure to oxygen there appears to be progressive decrease of alveolar gas volume and increase of pulmonary tissue volume, as capillary volume at first increases then falls considerably (Fig. 18-7). The increased volume of interstitial tissue, and also epithelial hyperplasia, appear to be responsible for the considerable increase in thickness of the alveolar gas-blood barrier that is apparent after prolonged exposure to oxygen. On the basis of these studies,[51] it was postulated that diffusing capacity should be very much reduced in patients given 60 to 100% oxygen for periods longer than 3 days.

A number of theories have been proposed to explain the metabolic basis of pulmonary oxygen toxicity. Collectively they provide a basis for continued research in this area, since a definitive explanation is not now available.

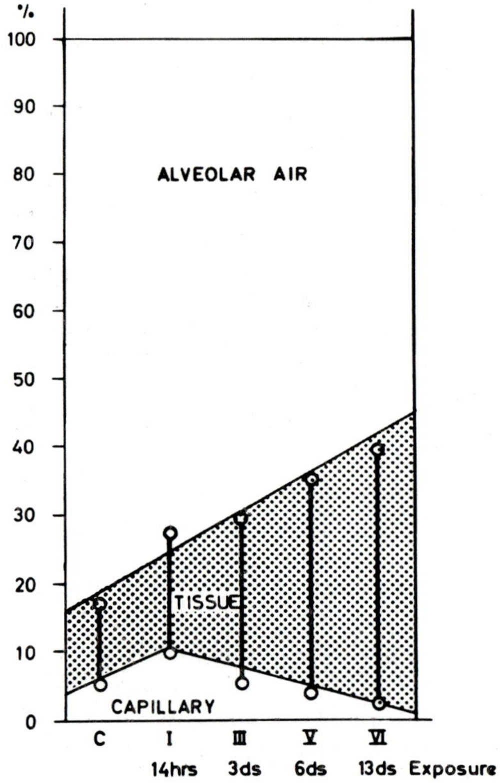

FIG. 18-7. Subdivision of lung volume in four patients exposed to oxygen and one control case. Derived from electron microscopic analyses. (From Kapanci, Y. et al.[51])

Among the more recent discoveries may be included the following five aspects.

(1) It is possible that inactivation or deficiency of pulmonary surfactants is one of the earliest pathogenic alterations[52] and that impairment of surfactant synthesis plays a central role in oxygen toxicity.[99]

(2) It has been observed that the first ultrastructural abnormality in lungs of rats exposed for 10 days to oxygen at an $F_{I_{O_2}}$ of 0.70 is irregular widening of the alveolar-capillary basement membrane and development of pulmonary edema, which may not be dependent on a primary deficiency of surfactants.[85]

(3) A number of studies have demonstrated that hyperoxia is a potent inactivator of several enzymes involved in the early stages of hydrogen transfer (including a number of dehydrogenases), in pyruvate oxidation, or in the formation of high energy phosphate bonds.[27,48]

(4) It has been reported that production of the free radical superoxide (O_2^-) contributes to the pulmonary toxicity of oxygen, that the enzyme superoxide dismutase provides an in vivo defense against this radical, and that development of oxygen tolerance (a phenomenon observed in many animals during experimentally controlled exposure to oxygen) parallels an increase in the activity of pulmonary superoxide dismutase.[24]

(5) It has similarly been observed that the enzyme system for the reduction of the peroxy free radical (a product of the reaction of O_2^- with hydrogen peroxide) may play a central role in both the induction of toxicity and the adaptation to it.[53]

The characteristic pulmonary lesions of oxygen toxicity resemble those of "shock lung"[79] (see also Chapter 2). They include thickening and congestion of the alveolar septae, formation of hyaline membranes, epithelial and endothelial cell damage followed by hyperplasia of type II epithelial cells, and ultimately interstitial cell hyperplasia with severe septal edema and fibrosis.[51,79] These findings are consonant with the alterations of pulmonary function previously presented.

Prevention of oxygen toxicity is the primary consideration. To this end one must regulate oxygen therapy to provide the minimal $F_{I_{O_2}}$ that results in a minimally acceptable Pa_{O_2}. The use of positive end-expiratory pressure and related modalities has permitted better blood oxygenation (Pa_{O_2}) with less oxygen ($F_{I_{O_2}}$), but this improvement has been at the expense of introducing other complicating factors into the treatment program (see also Chapter 14). Whenever possible, one should intermittently expose the patient to normal $F_{I_{O_2}}$ as this action is probably the most practical method for extending oxygen tolerance in man.[55] No known medication is effective for oxygen toxicity.

ADDENDA

A note should be made on the cause of the "local irritant" effects of oxygen. Whereas symptoms of local irritation, such as sore throat, nasal congestion, cough, and substernal soreness, were once attributed to the dryness of oxygen as obtained from its source, it is now apparent that these symptoms are induced even when the gas is properly humidified. The irritant effect is definitely related to the abnormally high oxygen pressure and not due to the delivery systems, dryness, or denitrogenation.[21,56]

Finally, a complication of oxygen therapy that must be kept in mind is the effect of absorption of oxygen from gas-containing viscera both during therapy and after the patient is returned to ambient air. Thus, during oxygen breathing significant amounts of nitrogen are removed (denitrogenation) from the alveoli, paranasal sinuses, and middle ear cavity, as oxygen becomes the principal gas of these structures. If communication to the outside is blocked (e.g., by inflamed or edematous tissue, or by mucous plugs), the isolated "pocket" of oxygen will be absorbed into the blood stream (see also Chapter 2). The effect in the lungs is alveolar collapse, which can be diffuse, and the effect in the sinuses and middle ear may be exudation or hemorrhage into the cavity and pain. Thus one should remember to "wash-out" oxygen after a course of therapy or when oxygen breathing is used to estimate right-to-left shunting. This procedure may be effected by encouraging the patient to breathe deeply and to make swallowing or yawning movements, which aid in equilibrating gas tensions in the middle ear with ambient air.

Fire and Smoke

In the United States, automobile accidents, drownings, and burns are the most common causes of accidental death in childhood.[1] Involvement of the respiratory tract, either directly by thermal injury or by inhalation of smoke, is one of the major causes of mortality of burn victims. Thus it is standard procedure not to move the victim from the site at which first aid is administered until any respiratory difficulties are relieved and control of the airway is obtained.[49] When the patient arrives at the treatment center, the first order of business is to check the adequacy of the airway, provide oxygen and ventilatory assistance as indicated, and establish a proper airway by endotracheal intubation or tracheostomy if necessary.[49] Surface burns of the oronasal cavity, the larynx, and trachea should always be suspected, especially when the face or neck has been burned; and what may appear as only minimal when seen soon after the injury may develop into serious edema, with swelling and exudation, and fatal obstruction of the upper airways. Thus frequent examinations against which the signs of upper airway obstruction must be weighed (i.e., inspiratory and expiratory stridor, posterior pharyngeal stridor and "snoring," retractions of the chest wall, and alterations of Pa_{O_2} and Pa_{CO_2}) are essential. The physician should not hesitate to provide an airway for patients with apparent surface burns of the upper airways.

More frequent than direct thermal injury to the upper respiratory tract is injury to the airways and lungs by inhalation of smoke. Severe injury can be sustained even in the absence of surface burns, so that one's suspicion of possible serious respiratory tract involvement must rest only on the fact that the subject has been exposed to fire or smoke. Smoke inhalation may produce injury as a consequence of its heat content (thermal injury), carbon monoxide content (carbon monoxide poisoning), and high concentration of irritant gases (chemical injury).[59,61]

THERMAL INJURY

Whether thermal injury can occur below the carina, because of the efficient heat exchange that takes place in the upper airways, is a moot question. Nonetheless, since certain vapors such as steam have an extremely high heat content and since continued oxidation of incompletely burned material may persist in the bronchi,[104] direct thermal injury to airway mucosa remains a distinct possibility.

CARBON MONOXIDE POISONING

Carbon monoxide is produced in all fires, and smoke contains variable concentrations of the gas. The pathologic effects of carbon monoxide are related to its association with hemoglobin.[61]

(1) The affinity of carbon monoxide for hemoglobin is many times greater than that of oxygen, so that once combined the binding site is no longer available to oxygen.

(2) Carbon monoxide produces a shift of the oxyhemoglobin dissociation curve to the left so that delivery of oxygen to tissues requires very low tissue Po_2.

(3) Carbon monoxide changes the shape of the oxyhemoglobin dissociation curve so that it resembles more the curve of fetal hemoglobin, which, in turn, further retards the delivery of oxygen to tissues. Thus, for example, whereas hemoglobin is half-saturated with oxygen (P_{50}) when the Po_2 is 30 mm Hg under normal conditions, the P_{50} may fall to 0.12 mm Hg when carboxyhemoglobin is present. The total effect is a marked fall of tissue oxygenation in spite of the fact that the blood may appear "cherry red," the color of carboxyhemoglobin.

Since carbon monoxide poisoning occurs during inhalation of smoke, it must be suspected as soon as the patient is seen. The toxicity of carboxyhemoglobin in relation to its concentration has been summarized.[78,91] Its chief manifestations are related to tissue hypoxia within the central nervous system: headache and some diminution of visual acuity and higher cerebral functions may be experienced at carboxyhemoglobin concentrations below 20%; between 20 and 40%, irritability, nausea, dimness of vision, impaired judgement, and rapid fatigue may occur; levels of 40 to 60% produce confusion, hallucinations, ataxia, collapse, and coma; and concentrations over 60% are usually fatal. Carboxyhemoglobin may also be a serious threat to myocardial function leading to conduction abnormalities (T wave and S-T segment changes, atrial fibrillation, intraventricular block) or tissue death resembling myocardial infarction. Other tissues, including the skin (with lesions resembling frostbite), liver, and kidney, may be similarly affected.

The concentration of carboxyhemoglobin is determined by the duration of exposure and by the concentration of carbon monoxide in smoke, both of which are difficult to assess in fire victims. This, and the fact that carbon monoxide poisoning has its effects rapidly after exposure to fire and smoke, require a high index of suspicion and early laboratory determination of carboxyhemoglobin concentration.

CHEMICAL INJURY

A number of irritant gases may be generated during fires.

(1) SO_2 and NO_2 combine with water in the lung to form corrosive acids or alkalis.

(2) Aldehydes, which denature proteins, can cause cellular damage, pulmonary edema, and hemorrhage.

(3) Phosgene and other products of burning plastics can produce hydrochloric acid when in contact with tissues leading to tissue destruction, edema or hemorrhage, alveolar collapse, and pulmonary hypertension.

(4) Soot particles may be responsible for inducing reflex bronchoconstriction and for carrying other noxious gases adsorbed at their surfaces into the alveoli.

(5) Other toxins include ammonia and acrolein.

Mellins and Park have noted that it is still not clear to what extent the pathologic changes in the lung are produced by direct chemical injury on the one hand and by secondary complications of surface burns (circulatory, metabolic, infectious) or of therapeutic maneuvers (oxygen administration, mechanical ventilators, aggressive intravenous therapy) on the other hand.[61] Postmortem studies of the 13 infants who died in the Dellwood fire give some insight into the effects of smoke inhalation since only 2 of the 13 victims sustained any surface burns.[23] Exposure to smoke lasted 20 to 30 minutes, and the victims died in 1 to 3 days. The bronchial walls were highly congested and edematous, and the epithelium of the larger bronchi was extensively destroyed, with fused necrotic cells forming dense membranes, which contributed to obstruction of the airways. The bronchioles had fewer membranes, and in a few cases, acute bronchiolitis and the appearance of bronchopneumonia were evident. Alveoli contained carbonaceous material; they were congested, edematous, and hemorrhagic. Large quantities of mucus were retained in the airways, perhaps as a consequence of obstruction by the membranes and destruction of most of the ciliated epithelium. Thus, the effects of chemical injury to the lung from smoke inhalation may range from obstruction and epithelial damage of airways (large and small) to alveolar epithelial damage and occlusion by edema, hemorrhage, and foreign particles.

Attempts to simulate the pulmonary damage produced by smoke in animals made to inhale steam may have limited relevance,[61] whereas the known effects of inhalation of toxic gases such as phosgene, chlorine, or oxides of nitrogen may be more pertinent. These gases produce airway and alveolar epithelial damage, widespread obstruction, and hemorrhagic edema, analogous to the pathologic changes observed in the unfortunate Dellwood babies.

TREATMENT

Immediate cardiopulmonary resuscitation, as described in Chapter 3, must be provided the victim of fire and smoke. A patent airway must be assured, and oxygen must be provided with assisted or controlled ventilation if necessary. The upper airway should be assessed by direct or indirect laryngoscopy as soon as possible in order to determine whether the pharynx and larynx have been injured directly and therefore may require endotracheal intubation. Adequate alveolar ventilation must be established rapidly in order to reverse asphyxia secondary to smoke and obstruction, and to begin elimination of carbon monoxide. Humidified 100% oxygen is most effective in that it accelerates carbon monoxide removal from the body significantly and provides maximal levels of oxygen to reverse alveolar and tissue hypoxia.

The indications for endotracheal intubation include: (1) severe burns of the nose, face, or mouth in which pharyngeal or glottic-epiglottic obstruction are likely to develop; (2) laryngeal obstruction or increasing edema and immobility of the vocal cords on direct laryngoscopy; (3) difficulty handling tracheobronchial secretions; and (4) progressive respiratory insufficiency requiring mechanical assistance to ventilation.[61] Nasotracheal intubation is preferred, especially when the anticipated need is for a relatively short period.[49] Although the question of tracheostomy is controversial,[58] it may be reasonable to replace an endotracheal tube with tracheostomy when intubation is required for excessive periods of time. (See also Chapter 3.) Mechanical ventilatory assistance may be required when there are signs of marked obstruction (e.g., retractions and decreased breath sounds) or evidence of alveolar hypoventilation or respiratory failure, i.e., a rising Pa_{CO_2}.

The clinical manifestations of serious smoke inhalation may be delayed for several hours. For example, auscultatory evidence of respiratory tract damage was noted within 12 to 15 hours in the 14 infants who survived for at least 1 day after the Dellwood fire.[23] In addition, roentgenographic evidence of pulmonary injury usually lags several hours or more behind the appearance of auscultatory signs.[77,96] Thus one must rely on observation of breathing pattern and frequency, and on laboratory determinations (Pa_{CO_2}, Pa_{O_2}, pH, carbon monoxide concentration) in assessing possible lower respiratory tract involvement shortly after exposure and in determining appropriate ventilatory therapy.

Once the decision is made to support or control ventilation mechanically, one must consider the possible additional benefit of maintaining positive end-expiratory pressure. In light of the actual or potential instability of small airways and alveoli following smoke inhalation and considering the evidence that zero end-expiratory pressure may compromise functional residual capacity and alveolar-capillary gas exchange,[9] maintenance of 2 cm H_2O PEEP would seem appropriate. The need for higher pressures would have to take into account the ease with which Pa_{O_2} is maintained and the inspired oxygen concentration required to maintain it. Any decision to increase PEEP must be made with recognition of its effects on venous return and cardiac output, and with understanding of the friability of pulmonary tissue that is injured by smoke and is thus at risk to the complications of PEEP (see Chapters 3 and 14).

Sedatives and other respiratory center depressants are contraindicated in the treatment of smoke victims. Although corticosteroids in large doses have been recommended, their efficacy in counteracting inflammatory changes in the lung has not been established and their long-term use would seem ill-advised because of the possibility of promoting opportunistic infections. Bronchodilators may be tried when evidence for bronchospasm exists, and chest physical therapy should be encouraged, when possible, since airway obstructive debris and mucociliary dysfunction are major problems.

Other "Inhalants"

The "air pollutants" include a number of gases and volatilized liquids. They are a product of our industrialized society, which may cause acute and chronic toxicity. The principal source of *carbon monoxide* pollution is the motor vehicle, which contributes about 60% of the total 66,000,000 tons of the gas that is placed into the environment each year.[3] Acute poisoning may result from exposure to auto fumes in a poorly ventilated area, to waste fumes in steel-processing plants, and to smoke from fires. The acute effects of carbon monoxide poisoning and treatment are discussed in the preceding section. It may be noted here that chronic or low-grade poisoning is a hazard faced in a variety of ordinary circumstances, e.g., living in a city where automobile exhausts and power plants contaminate the air; smoking cigarettes and cigars, which can increase the concentration of carboxyhemoglobin up to 10%; and using coal gas and "water gas" for illumination—natural gas contains little or no carbon monoxide. The symptoms of chronic exposure may be subtle (e.g., headache and lassitude), but can be aggravated by exercise, strain, anemia, or mild intercurrent respiratory illnesses.

Nitrogen oxides (which may be converted to the yellow, pungent nitrogen dioxide in the atmosphere and which is present in automobile exhausts and produced by the burning of soft coal), *sulfur dioxide* (from coal and oil combustion), and *phosgenes* (from chemical and dye manufacturing) are potent irritants of the respiratory tract that may inhibit mucociliary activity and thus airway clearance, stimulate nerve endings and induce cough, induce bronchospasm, destroy airway and alveolar epithelial cells, produce submucosal and interstitial edema, induce pulmonary vasoconstriction and hypertension, and result in pulmonary edema or hemorrhage. *Hydrogen sulfides* (from refineries and chemical industries), *aldehydes* (emitted during thermal decomposition of fats and oils), *chlorines* and *ammonia* (from a number of chemical industrial processes), and *hydrogen fluoride* (from refineries and aluminum and fertilizer production) are highly irritating and corrosive, but usually provide sufficient warning by the intense reaction produced in the oronasal passages. Acute toxicity following exposure to large concentrations can result, in effect, in corrosion of the lower respiratory tract.

Pulmonary toxicity due to *inhaled particles* may be classified as an occupational hazard and does not usually involve infants and children. Chronic exposure may result in pulmonary fibrosis or in so-called hypersensitivity alveolitis. The latter topic is presented in this chapter (Uncommon Pulmonary Diseases in Children) and the former is discussed in Chapter 2. Offending agents are listed in Table 1-6.

Commercial *aerosol sprays* (e.g., hair sprays) are potential pulmonary toxins. The components of aerosol sprays are their propellant (most commonly fluorochlorohydrocarbons—Freon), solvent, and active ingredients. The propellent is a gas at room temperature, whereas 90% of the solvent and ingredients are emitted as nonvolatile droplets or particles greater than several microns in diameter.[37] The remaining 10% or less are submicronic particles. The larger particles, once inhaled, deposit principally in the oronasal cavity and central airways, whereas the smaller particles may reach the terminal airways and alveoli. Presumably the latter cause granulomatous lesions of the lungs, for example, following prolonged and excessive exposure to hair sprays,[42] or cause acute airway constriction immediately after exposure.[105] Much controversy exists concerning the nature of the chronic lesion induced by hair sprays, and it has been suggested that the term "thesaurosis" (storage disease) be discarded since precise cause and effect have not been established.[37] Nonetheless, it seems rather positive that hair sprays cause infiltrative lesions of the lung, that allergic persons are particularly susceptible, and that the lesions are heterogeneous and probably not related to a single chemical cause.[37]

It should also be noted that the propellant fluorocarbons of commercial aerosol sprays may affect cardiovascular function. They may depress myocardial contractility, disturb myocardial conduction, and sensitize the myocardium to sympathomimetic amines. These effects, combined with the effects of bronchodilators and hypoxemia in asthmatic children who use hand nebulizers, could produce serious, even fatal, cardiovascular effects.[10,30] Thus, it has been recommended that these nebulizers be used "sparingly and (then) only as a supplement to appropriate oral bronchodilator therapy." It is unsettling however that the "physician's voice is small,"[37] while the sale of bronchodilator nebulizers without prescription is promoted by intense advertising.[10]

Water

Whereas it was commonly held that the primary cause of death after sea water drowning was respiratory and after fresh water drowning, cardiovascular (secondary to electrolyte changes and fluid shifts), now firm evidence, based mainly on the work of Modell and colleagues, demonstrates that the primary problem of the near-drowning victim—after both sea water and fresh water aspiration—is respiratory insufficiency.[63-69]

When a conscious subject is submerged, breath-holding, swallowing, and laryngospasm are the initial reaction.[43] Thus asphyxia is the first insult. However, when a human is submerged, a reflex is triggered (probably by somatic inputs through the trigeminal nerve as the head enters the water), which results in bradycardia and peripheral vasoconstriction everywhere except in the heart, brain, and lungs—the "diving reflex."[41] This reflex is typical of diving vertebrates,[2] where it results in a greatly reduced cardiac output while perfusion of the vital organs is maintained. It permits survival for extended periods under water. The reflex is much less pronounced in man, but may be useful, to some degree, in protecting against asphyxia initially. In this regard the report of a 5-year-old boy who survived after 40 minutes' submersion in ice-cold fresh water may be pertinent.[93] When seen at hospital, the boy had a rectal temperature of 24°C; he was apneic and no clinical signs of cardiovascular activity were present. Cardiopulmonary resuscitation, rewarming, correction of severe metabolic acidemia (arterial pH was about 6.8), and positive end-expiratory pressure ventilation with oxygen were successful. Thirteen months after the accident there were no sequelae; cardiopulmonary and central nervous systems were normal. The successful outcome was attributed to rapid cooling of the body during submersion in cold water (thereby reducing oxygen requirement of the brain) and possibly to the "diving reflex." This case emphasizes the importance of attempting resuscitation, even after lengthy submersion.

The initial period of breath-holding during submersion is often followed by aspiration of small amounts of liquid. Such aspiration may play a part in the initial phases of drowning in man, and is therefore relevant to intelligent maneuvers for resuscitation.[43] The effects of aspiration of small amounts of liquid have been demonstrated in animals:[46] thus, introduction of 1 to 3 ml/kg body weight of fresh or sea water into the trachea of sheep resulted in a gross fall of pulmonary compliance (probably related to widespread closure of terminal airways as a consequence, perhaps, of local and central reflex mechanisms and local humoral effects), a variable increase of airflow resistance (probably due to blocking of airways by fluid and foam), and pulmonary hypertension with reduction of effective pulmonary blood flow (the former being independent of and the latter related to the changes in pulmonary mechanics). The resultant severe systemic arterial hypoxemia was due to large intrapulmonary right-to-left shunts and $\dot{V}_A/\dot{Q}$ abnormality. Resuscitation by intermittent positive pressure breathing, up to 30 cm H_2O pressure, with 100% oxygen effectively restored arterial oxygen saturation to normal. (Further discussion of therapy is presented below.)

Recent suggestions that *therapeutic lavage* of the lung may be of value in the care of patients with asthma, bronchiectasis, cystic fibrosis, and alveolar proteinosis,[54,60,84,89] although not sufficiently convincing to establish the procedure for general or routine use in pediatrics, have provided information relevant to the effects of bulk liquid in the lung. The pulmonary lavage procedure is generally carried out by endotracheal insertion of a Carlens catheter (which has separate orifices leading to each lung through which each lung may be ventilated separately), inhalation of oxygen for about 20 minutes (to remove nitrogen from the lungs), occlusion of the orifice to one lung (which will then collapse as oxygen is absorbed), and introduction of saline solution unbuffered or buffered with $NaHCO_3$ into the collapsing or collapsed lung to a volume roughly equivalent to the estimated functional residual capacity of that lung. The lung is then ventilated with tidal volume of liquid at a frequency of 10 to 18 per minute. After lavage, the liquid-filled lung is allowed to drain by gravity and ventilated (about half the total liquid containing phospholipid surfactants is ultimately recovered from the lung). Thereafter, total ventilation is assisted by intermittent positive pressure breathing with 40 to 80% oxygen.

Thus the procedure is in effect a controlled drowning of one lung, with careful monitoring of cardiopulmonary function and respiratory assistance until the patient is able to sustain normal cardiopulmonary function independently. Cardiopulmonary function was most compromised in the immediate post-lavage period, which may be comparable to the status of an individual after near-drowning. During this period Pa_{O_2} may fall to 40 mm Hg (due primarily to intrapulmonary right-to-left shunting), but it is controlled by intermittent positive pressure breathing, which often requires no more than 40% oxygen. Arterial hypercapnia may develop in association with bronchospasm, and metabolic acidemia may occur. Roentgenographic resolution of the pulmonary densities usually takes place within 24 hours.

The animal experiments and human studies presented thus far give some insight into the pathophysiologic processes induced by near-drowning.

(1) There is a (reflex) fall of pulmonary compliance and possible closure of terminal airways.

(2) Resistance to airflow is increased.

(3) Pulmonary hypertension and reduced effective pulmonary blood flow may develop.

(4) Surfactants may be displaced from their normal position in the alveolar lining layer, which itself may be disrupted.

(5) Pulmonary right-to-left shunts and $\dot{V}_A/\dot{Q}$ abnormalities develop.

(6) Arterial hypoxemia, which may be severe, hypercapnia, and acidosis may result.

(7) Intermittent positive pressure breathing with oxygen is effective therapy.[20]

SEA WATER AND FRESH WATER

Whereas the list just presented is applicable to near-drowning in both fresh and sea water and whereas general principles of therapy are the same for both, one difference in the pulmonary effects of the two is outlined here. Introduction of water into the alveoli disrupts the normal topography of pulmonary surfactants in the alveolar lining layer and even removes surfactants from the lungs. Thus, successful therapy includes restoration of the surfactants and the normal alveolar lining layer. The former is probably taken care of by continued synthesis and secretion of surfactants by alveolar epithelium; the latter is influenced by the nature of the aspirated water.[40] It has been demonstrated in vitro that distilled water (analogous to fresh water) seriously alters the normal surface tension properties of pulmonary surfactants, whereas normal saline solution and solutions of higher osmolarity sustain these properties.[90] Thus alveolar instability on this basis would be an added problem in the management of victims of near-drowning in fresh water.[40]

Another difference between fresh and sea water near-drowning is the expected more rapid transfer of the low osmolarity liquid into the blood stream[45] and the consequent hemodilution. The very simple and elegant experiments in dogs of Modell et al. seem to have clarified this point.[67] These studies showed that rapid intravenous infusion of 44 ml/kg of distilled water (which exceeds the volume that might be transferred in near-drowning*) produces only a mild decrease of serum electrolyte concentrations and pH, and a transient increase of pulmonary artery pressure. No significant changes in cardiac output, arterial blood pressure, Pa_{O_2}, Pa_{CO_2}, or hemolysis occurred. *However,* when the hypervolemia was combined with hypoxia, hypercapnia, and acidemia, hemolysis, hypotension, hyperkalemia, hypochloremia, hyponatremia, and decreased cardiac output (all potential effects of near-drowning in fresh water) ensued. These changes suggested that in the face of hypoxia the circulation is not capable of redistributing the water load, so the effects of acute hemodilution become more profound. The authors concluded that the important consideration when treating a near-drowning victim is respiratory insufficiency with hypoxemia and acidemia, and if these complications are rapidly and effectively treated, it is unlikely that death will occur from electrolyte imbalance, hemolysis, or acute circulatory insufficiency.

If fresh water enters the circulation rapidly from the lungs, the converse problem with sea water, i.e., prolonged retention in the lungs, may also be expected. Again, Modell

*It has been estimated that only 15% of human *drowning* victims aspirate a sufficient volume of liquid to cause severe electrolyte changes.[65] Animal studies indicate that this volume is 44 ml/kg distilled water.[65,68]

et al. have provided insight into this problem in studies of animals and humans.[64,70] They demonstrated that when dogs aspirated 11 ml/kg of sea water and no attempt was made to drain the liquid and/or to resuscitate the animal, 80% succumbed. In contrast, when animals aspirated twice that volume and were treated with gravity drainage and intermittent positive pressure breathing, more than 90% survived at least 24 hours. In further studies, which were confirmed by successful treatment of two nearly drowned adults, it was shown that positive end-expiratory pressure, with or without mechanical ventilation, significantly increases Pa_{O_2} after aspiration of sea water and that this mode of therapy is indicated for the treatment of sea water near-drowning victims.

The efficacy of positive end-expiratory pressure for treatment of sea water near-drowning makes it a preferred mode of treatment. It is also preferred for treatment of fresh water near-drowning with one stipulation based on the effects of fresh water on pulmonary surfactants. Since alveoli are presumably less stable after fresh water near-drowning, they and perhaps the distal airways would tend to collapse (either spontaneously or with high intrapleural pressures during spontaneous breathing) so that large opening pressures might be needed for inspiration. Thus high inspiratory pressures, as generated by a mechanical ventilator, in addition to positive end-expiratory pressure, would be useful when indicated in the treatment of victims of fresh water drowning, as the studies of Modell et al. suggest.[64]

TREATMENT

The immediate goal of therapy is to drain the lungs, especially in near-drowning in sea water, when the victim is seen shortly after submersion and, most importantly, to establish ventilation. Prevention or reversal of hypoxemia, hypercapnia, and acidemia are the immediate goals, and they must be accomplished rapidly to prevent potentially fatal sequelae. Thus sufficient concentrations of inspired oxygen must be provided immediately, and the basic principles of cardiopulmonary resuscitation (Chapter 3) must be followed. Positive end-expiratory pressure seems to be very useful for all near-drowning victims, supplemented by ventilator support with positive pressure breathing when indicated especially for near-drowning in fresh water. Acidemia should be corrected rapidly with $NaHCO_3$.

Additional therapy, determined by development of secondary effects of near-drowning, includes cardiovascular support for low cardiac output and/or low systemic blood pressure, sedation with appropriate respiratory control for restlessness or convulsions, red blood cell transfusion for significant hemolysis, and rewarming if there is hypothermia. "Secondary" pulmonary edema should not be a problem if pulmonary resuscitation and support have been successful.[93] The principles of cardiopulmonary therapy, as outlined in Chapter 3, should be followed strictly.

Hydrocarbons

In their study of 1057 cases of poisoning in children through the age of 8 years, Deeths and Breeden found that, after aspirin poisoning, hydrocarbons accounted for more childhood poisoning (18.4%) than any other agent.[26] The peak incidence of poisoning by these agents occurs between 1 and 2 years of age and involves a significant preponderance of males over females, which the authors suggest may be due to the boys' greater resourcefulness in play.[26] The incidence of hydrocarbon poisoning falls sharply after 3 years of age. In the years 1951 through 1958, 763 persons died in the United States after accidental ingestion of hydrocarbons, with children under the age of 5 years accounting for 90% of the total.[34] Perhaps because of hydrocarbons' decreased use in households and increased public awareness of the dangers, nine hydrocarbon fatalities were reported in children under 5 years in 1972.[71]

The hydrocarbons to which children are exposed most frequently are distillates of petroleum (e.g., gasoline, kerosene, mineral seal oil), coal tar (e.g., benzene, naphthalene), or pinewood (turpentine). Gasoline and kerosene have the lowest surface tensions and viscosities of the petroleum distillates. Kerosene is used extensively in the southern United States for curing tobacco, heating, cooking, and, in some places, for lighting.[3] Mineral seal oil is composed principally of saturated hydrocarbons, is "heavier" (vis à vis surface tension and viscosity) than kerosene, and is used especially in furniture polishes. Red furniture polish may contain from 20 to 90% mineral seal oil to which may be added kerosene, turpentine, camphor, and oil of cedarwood. Benzene is used widely as a commercial solvent and in certain motor fuels. Turpentine is used as a solvent in paints, polishes, and varnishes; "hexol" is related to turpentine and is commonly used as a household disinfectant. These substances are included collectively in the term "hydrocarbons" as used in this section. Naphthalene is a highly volatile *powder* used in the house in the form of moth balls, moth flakes, and deodorant "cakes."[3] Toxicity following ingestion of naphthalene is due to the development of what can be a severe and rapidly progressive hemolytic anemia. In addition, naphthalene vapors may be inhaled or absorbed from the skin and produce severe hemolytic anemia.[3]

Inhalation of the vapors of many of these toxins is an occupational hazard for some adults, and severe toxicity can result. Thus inhalation of high concentration of vapors of gasoline, kerosene, and benzene can produce acute toxicity usually referable to the central nervous system. The central nervous system manifestations may begin as euphoria and motor hyperactivity, then progress to profound depression, coma, and death.[3,97] Inhaled vapors of other hydrocarbons may also produce signs of central nervous system toxicity and, in addition, severe hemolytic anemia (naphthalene) or nephritis (turpentine). Primary toxicity to extrapulmonary organs in these cases is probably explained by acute inhalation of high concentrations and rapid delivery of the toxin by the blood stream, so that direct pulmonary toxicity is of secondary importance.

Press and Done have reviewed the problem of solvent (or "glue") sniffing among adolescents and children in the United States.[81,82] Of the wide variety of organic solvents that are inhaled for the intentional induction of intoxication, all produce toxic effects in the central nervous system. Among the more common solvents sniffed are those containing toluene, acetone, benzene, petroleum naphtha, and gasoline, in addition to a number of other lipid solvents. Toxicity is most often associated with the central nervous system effects. Less frequently, the blood, liver, and kidney may also be affected seriously. Although acute toxicity to the lung is apparently unusual, it may be significant to note that the postmortem examination of some fatalities reported by Press and Done indicated that intrapulmonary hemorrhage and edema played a central role in the terminal event.[82]

Ingestion of hydrocarbons is by far the most common route of intoxication by these agents. Whereas the organ systems affected include the lungs, central nervous system, heart, gastrointestinal tract, liver, and kidneys, symptomatic involvement of the respiratory tract is the most common complication,[6,58,74,80] and death is almost always due to pulmonary rather than central nervous system involvement.[25] Eade et al. present four lines of evidence which demonstrate convincingly that pulmonary involvement is due to aspiration and not to gastrointestinal absorption of the hydrocarbons.[34]

(1) Direct instillation of sublethal doses

into the stomach of an animal whose esophagus has been ligated is followed by little or no pulmonary damage.[102]

(2) Animal studies indicate that the LD_{50} ratio of oral to intratracheal kerosene is 140 : 1,[38] which makes it highly unlikely that children will swallow[50] large enough quantities to produce pulmonary lesions after gastrointestinal absorption.[87]

(3) The pulmonary roentgenographic appearance in children is consonant with aspiration, rather than with diffuse involvement, which would probably result from blood-borne toxicity.[38]

(4) The rapidity with which pulmonary symptoms and lesions develop also suggests aspiration. Aspiration is also favored by the physical properties of hydrocarbons. Their low surface tension promotes surface spreading over mucosae and thus would facilitate entrance through the glottis and into the airways. Their low viscosity favors movement of the bulk liquid into the respiratory tract, since resistance to flow is related directly to viscosity. Their high volatility would promote high vapor concentrations at body temperature and thus effectively increase the amounts that may enter the lung and, at the same time, reduce the pressures of the normal respiratory gases.

The *clinical picture* of hydrocarbon aspiration is very much the same regardless of the specific agent involved. Eade et al. describe the typical picture:[34] initially there is a burning sensation in the mouth and throat, followed by gagging, choking, grunting respirations, and cough. Cough, which is probably induced by direct irritation of the airway mucosa, reflects the extent of airway involvement, so that continued nonproductive cough is often prognostic of severe pulmonary damage. Cyanosis may appear rapidly (perhaps as a reflection of the high concentration of hydrocarbon vapors in the alveoli), and intercostal retractions (due to airway irritation with edema or smooth muscle contraction) and fever may appear within 30 minutes. Tachycardia, tachypnea, and auscultatory findings may be present, indicating diminished ventilation.

Signs and symptoms of respiratory involvement usually progress during the first 24 hours after aspiration, reach a plateau, then subside between the second and fifth days.[36] With severe pulmonary injury, edema and hemorrhage occur, increasing cyanosis appears, and death may follow usually within 24 hours of aspiration.[92] The chest roentgenogram may be abnormal within 30 minutes of aspiration and is virtually always positive within 12 hours where pulmonary involvement exists.[25,36] Initially, the roentgenogram may reveal punctate or mottled perihilar densities that extend into the midlung region. Densities may become confluent, and involvement of the lower lung zones is common. Atelectasis is diagnosed frequently, hyperaeration is often evident, and pleural effusion may develop.[58,86] Roentgenographic abnormalities are usually maximal at 72 hours and clear within a few additional days, although they may persist for weeks or months on occasion, and pneumatoceles or cysts may form.[15] Poor correlation exists between clinical symptoms and roentgenographic abnormalities: Whereas 75% of patients who ingest hydrocarbons have radiographic evidence of lung involvement, only 25 to 50% of these develop respiratory symptoms.[12,25] Conversely, respiratory symptoms without roentgenographic abnormality also occur.[92]

Postmortem examination of the lung reveals (1) inflammatory response in the interstices; (2) hyperemia and vascular thromboses; (3) intra-alveolar hemorrhage and edema, alveolar cell necrosis, polymorphonuclear exudates, hyaline membranes, and atelectasis; and (4) bronchial and bronchiolar epithelial necrosis and polymorphonuclear exudation.[11] Thus the entire pulmonary parenchyma may be involved; (1) the interstices, (2) the small vessels, (3) the alveoli, and (4) large and small airways.

The *pathophysiologic derangements* that may be expected as a result of the pulmonary lesions include right-to-left shunts (in association with atelectasis, alveolar filling, and thromboses) and diffusion and $\dot{V}A/\dot{Q}$ abnormalities (in association with interstitial and airway lesions). The rare report of blood gas tensions in a child[34] and the study in dogs,[95] which show arterial hypoxemia and normal to low Pa_{CO_2}, are consonant with these expectations. Pathogenesis has not been defined, but several reasonable inferences may be made. First, the high vapor concentrations of hydrocarbons may initiate hypoxemia by proportionately reducing alveolar Po_2.[34] The first contact between vaporized and liquid hydrocarbons on the one hand and pulmonary tissue on the other hand would be at the lining layers of the airways and alveoli. Since the former contain surfactants (at least in the terminal airways) and modulate ciliary activity, it may be expected that small airway instability and impaired mucociliary clearance would result (the beginning of $\dot{V}A/\dot{Q}$ imbalance); and since the latter contains the pulmonary surfactant system, it may be expected that alveolar instability and disruption of normal alveolar-capillary liquid balance would result (the beginning of right-to-left shunt). Indeed, the work of Giammona in dogs and rats shows that hydrocarbons are potent direct inhibitors of pulmonary surfactants. This observation led him to the conclusion that the initial pulmonary injury was determined by the interaction of hydrocarbons and the pulmonary surfactants.[39] Following disruption of airway and alveolar surfaces, as described, it is expected that the hydrocarbons would attack the epithelial cells of these structures. Cell membranes could be disrupted by these lipid solvents, leading to necrosis and sloughing, and then to disruption of the underlying capillaries (which is consonant with the findings of epithelial necrosis, polymorphonuclear exudation, edema, hemorrhage, and hyaline membrane formation). With progression, vascular thromboses and interstitial inflammation could result.

With regard to the *management* of children following hydrocarbon ingestion, the advice and warning of Eade et al. bear enforcement: "Since large volumes of hydrocarbon in the gut can apparently generally be tolerated without severe systemic changes and aspiration is the principal hazard, it is apparent that *vomiting should not be induced by syrup of ipecac* or any other means. Vomiting when it occurs is frequently associated with repeated gagging, choking and coughing and could contribute to the damage. The value of mineral oil or olive oil lavage is controversial and in our opinion is not to be recommended."[34]

Therapy should include the following considerations.

(1) Maintenance of an acceptable Pa_{O_2} by administration of humidified oxygen (see Chapter 3). Since surfactants are disrupted by hydrocarbons, one may consider the use of constant distending airway pressure (CDAP) or positive end-expiratory pressure (PEEP) if oxygen supplementation at atmospheric pressure does not sustain an acceptable Pa_{O_2} or if high—and potentially toxic—concentrations of inspired oxygen are required for prolonged periods. However, parenchymal tissue damage puts the patient at risk to pneumothorax, and vascular lesions may compound the cardiovascular effects of CDAP, so that this therapy should be used with caution.

(2) Maintenance of normal arterial pH is especially important since acidemia (for example, due to hypoxemia) may further compromise pulmonary cellular metabolism and bronchovascular muscle tone.

(3) Bronchodilators may be tried in order to reverse any bronchospastic component in the pulmonary response to aspiration.

(4) Antimicrobial therapy is not advised routinely or for "prophylaxis." When there is underlying illness upon which aspiration is superimposed or when the patient seems to have severe pulmonary involvement, antibiotics should be considered after careful diagnostic microbiologic studies.

(5) Both animal and human studies have failed to demonstrate an effective therapeutic or prophylactic role for adrenal corticoste-

roids in hydrocarbon ingestion. It is noted that the children studied had mild to moderate pulmonary involvement.[11,44,95]

Sequelae and long-term complications following hydrocarbon ingestion have not been evaluated extensively, although it has been suggested that these patients may be at greater risk than normal to upper respiratory tract infection and perhaps also to pneumonia.[36] A recent study by Bergeson et al. indicates that the incidence of pneumatocele development may be greater than previously realized.[8] Pneumatoceles may develop 3 to 15 days after mild to severe pulmonary involvement, and resolve in days to months leaving no apparent pleural or parenchymal residua.

Gastric Secretions

Aspiration of gastric contents into the lungs may occur in a variety of circumstances: in states of impaired consciousness, in conditions of debilitation, during resuscitation, as a complication of general anesthesia, in association with neurologic disease, in conditions that involve gastroesophageal reflux, and in association with the use of nasogastric tubes and tracheostomy.[4] Although the term, aspiration pneumonia, is used generally to designate the effects of aspiration of stomach contents into the lung, it is apparent that the composition of the aspirate varies according to the material ingested and the length of time it has been in the stomach prior to aspiration. Thus aspiration of stomach contents may deliver to the lung a variety of solid material, especially dangerous because it may obstruct large airways, and liquids, which may produce effects analogous to those described in the section entitled "Water." The toxicity of liquids is determined by their chemical nature and by the volume aspirated. Thus, in an animal study designed to test the idea that a solution of 5% glucose in water is preferred for the first feeding of newborn infants (on the assumption that, if aspirated, it would be less injurious to the lungs than milk), Olson showed that glucose and milk had equally deleterious effects on the lung (including changes in pressure-volume characteristics, reduction of resting lung volumes, consolidation and "interstitial pneumonia," and hypoxemia) and that water produced significantly less damage.[73]

Aspiration of material from a previously "empty" or non-fed stomach is itself extremely dangerous, and focus, in this section, is on the effects of aspiration of gastric acid. The aspiration of liquid gastric contents, primarily gastric acid, has been called Mendelson's syndrome.[62] Initially acute respiratory distress occurs due primarily to severe bronchospasm, in which frothy, nonpurulent sputum may be seen.[7] Many patients may become hypotensive, perhaps due to an immediate reflex reaction[75] or to subsequent intravascular volume depletion as liquid accumulates in the lungs. Profound hypoxemia may develop as a consequence of $\dot{V}_A/\dot{Q}$ abnormality (related to airway response) and also, right-to-left shunting (related to alveolar filling and alveolar collapse) may occur. Pulmonary compliance is reduced as a consequence of edema, hemorrhage, and atelectasis. This general sequence of events has been reproduced in animals by intratracheal instillation of sterile hydrochloric acid.[5,13,98] Conversely, instillation of saline solution, saliva, and neutralized gastric acid produced only transient respiratory distress and no roentgenographic changes.

The pulmonary toxic effects of gastric acid are related to the dose aspirated and its pH. Apparently, no severe effect occurs when the pH is above 2.4,[98] and the extent of the toxic effect is inversely related to pH below this level. Toxicity studies in animals have generally utilized an inoculum of gastric acid of 1 to 4 ml/kg, which is equivalent to the water inoculum used in animal studies as discussed in the section entitled "Water." Experimental studies of the isolated, perfused animal lung show that the effects of aspirated acid are immediate and extensive: When gastric secretions were mixed with methylene blue, the dye was detected at the surface of the lungs 12 to 18 seconds after it was instilled, and extensive atelectasis occurred within 3 minutes.

Clinical distress is usually maximal 2 to 12 hours after aspiration, with evidence of both airway and alveolar involvement. The right lower lobe is most often involved, but in severe cases both lungs are affected. Wheezing and crackles, tachypnea, tachycardia, and hypoxemia occur. The presence of pink, frothy sputum may suggest acute pulmonary edema. The morphologic changes include atelectasis, edema, hemorrhage, and tissue necrosis. Mortality ranges from 30 to 70%. Prognosis is significantly better when only one lobe is involved.[14,28]

Immediate therapy is directed at support of ventilation and correction of the hypoxemia. Oxygen and positive pressure ventilation are indicated. Because of the corrosive effect of acid and the induced hypersecretion and transudation, special care must be taken to maintain the airways as clear as possible. Correction of acidemia with $NaHCO_3$ and hemoconcentration by appropriate intravenous fluid therapy is essential. The use of systemic steroids, especially if initiated within 12 to 24 hours after aspiration, probably helps reduce extravasation into the lungs and is generally recommended,[7,33] whereas endotracheal instillation of steroids has no effect.[32] Bartlett advised *against* intratracheal instillation of buffering solutions,[7] since aspirated acid is neutralized within minutes by the tracheobronchial tree.[5] He also warns that preliminary lavage is futile (since the full extent of injury has usually occurred by the time diagnosis is made) and that instillation of diluents is contraindicated (since this procedure would add mechanical obstruction to an already compromised airway). Generally, antibiotics should be reserved until there is evolving evidence for infection, such as significant fever, purulent sputum, leukocytosis, and progressive infiltrates. There is little evidence that early use of antibiotics prevents subsequent infection.[7]

The sequelae of gastric aspiration in those who survive the acute episode may not be as benign as has been described.[47] One patient who was followed closely for more than 5 months after aspiration continued to show abnormalities of $\dot{V}_A/\dot{Q}$ and physiologic dead space to tidal volume ratio, in association with roentgenographic evidence of interstitial fibrosis.[94]

Salicylates

Acetylsalicylic acid (aspirin), sodium salicylate, and methyl salicylate are referred to collectively as the "salicylates." They act generally by virtue of their salicylic acid content, and their effects can be discussed, in general, as a class. The two most commonly used preparations for systemic effects are aspirin and sodium salicylate; methyl salicylate (oil of wintergreen), because of its relatively poor absorption from the gastrointestinal tract, is reserved for use in salves and liniments for the skin. Toxic ingestion of salicylates occurs by accident (especially in children below 5 years of age and especially with candy-flavored products), by therapeutic overdose, or by deliberate overdose in adolescents. It should be noted that preparations of methyl salicylate contain more salicylate than other remedies (1 teaspoonful is equivalent to about 21 aspirin tablets containing 325 mg each),[3] and that gastrointestinal absorption of methyl salicylate may be delayed for hours: Hence, its relatively greater toxicity and the rationale for gastric lavage even hours after ingestion. Aspirin is probably the single most common accidental poison for children,[22,26] with a peak incidence between 1 and 4 years of age. Diagnosis of salicylate intoxication is confirmed, but not necessarily established, by determination of the serum salicylate concentration (Fig. 18-8), which Done has related to clinical symptomatology and time from ingestion.[31] Salicylate poisoning may be classified, for purposes of presentation, into two phases: (1) respiratory alkalosis and (2) combined acidosis. It has been noted that the pediatrician may not see the child during the first phase, since often the patient is not examined soon enough.

RESPIRATORY ALKALOSIS

The initial event in salicylate poisoning is intracellular and extracellular respiratory alkalosis, by both direct and indirect stimulation of respiratory center activity.[103] The indirect effect is mediated by an uncoupling of oxidative phosphorylation in which the terminal phosphorylation step concerned

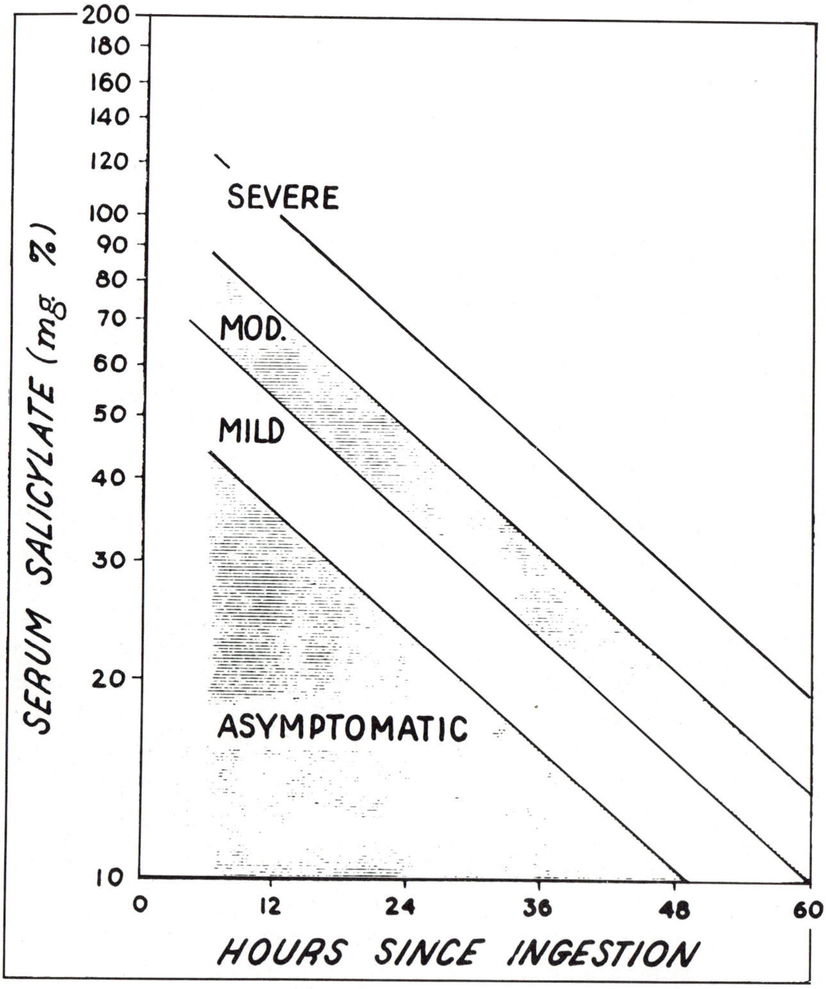

FIG. 18-8. Nomogram relating serum salicylate concentration and expected severity of intoxication at varying intervals following the ingestion of a single dose of salicylate. (From Done, A. K.[31])

with the oxidation of cytochrome C appears to be especially sensitive. As a result, a number of adenosine triphosphate-dependent reactions are inhibited, and enhanced oxidation compensates for the relative inefficiency of the phosphorylating mechanism. Thus oxygen uptake ($\dot{V}O_2$) is increased, as is the production of carbon dioxide ($\dot{V}CO_2$). The latter increases respiratory activity, which tends to balance the increased CO_2 production and prevent Pa_{CO_2} from rising. As salicylate gains access to the medulla, it stimulates the respiratory center directly and results in an increased depth and, more profoundly, in an increased rate of breathing. Minute ventilation may be increased as much as tenfold, and PA_{CO_2} and Pa_{CO_2} may fall to very low levels. The central effect seems to be due directly to the action of salicylates on the respiratory centers in the medulla and pons and not to concomitant local changes in hydrogen ion concentration or PCO_2.[76] At this point, there is classic respiratory alkalosis, i.e., low Pa_{CO_2}, low serum $[HCO_3]$, and high pH. Renal compensation begins rapidly. HCO_3^- excretion, along with sodium and potassium, is increased, plasma HCO_3^- is reduced further, and pH tends to return toward normal (compensated respiratory alkalosis—see also Chapter 2). This phase is seen most often in adults given high doses of salicylates therapeutically.

COMBINED ACIDOSIS

As serum salicylate levels increase after ingestion of toxic doses, the stage of combined acidosis is entered as two additional effects take hold. One of these effects may be termed "respiratory" and the other "metabolic."

The "respiratory effect" is due to (1) direct *depression* of the respiratory centers by high serum levels of salicylate and (2) the continued high production of carbon dioxide. As a consequence, Pa_{CO_2} increases from its previously low levels and may return to normal or nearly normal levels, which in the face of the low serum $[HCO_3^-]$ represents a relative respiratory acidemia; i.e., the ratio $[HCO_3^-] : [H_2CO_3]$ is less than the normal 20 : 1. As respiratory center depression deepens, Pa_{CO_2} may increase to levels above 40 mm Hg, i.e., absolute hypercapnia. Other central and local effects of salicylates may aggravate the condition seriously. These include (1) induction of pulmonary edema (probably due to a central effect of salicylates), which would reduce alveolar-capillary gas exchange ("shunt effect."), reduce Pa_{O_2}, and promote metabolic acidemia, and (2) the hypersensitivity to salicylates, which could induce bronchospasm, $\dot{V}A/\dot{Q}$ abnormality, and further reduction of Pa_{O_2} and elevation of Pa_{CO_2}.

The "metabolic effect" is the result of three processes:[103] (1) Salicylic acid derivatives dissociate at plasma pH and may displace significant amounts of HCO_3^-; (2) vasomotor depression caused by toxic doses of salicylate impairs renal function with consequent accumulation of metabolic acids; and (3) organic acids (e.g., pyruvic, lactic, and acetoacetic acids) accumulate secondary to salicylate-induced derangement of carbohydrate metabolism.

The pathophysiologic processes discussed are outlined in Figure 18-9.

Other complications of salicylate poisoning include hyperpyrexia (due to the high metabolic rate with high $\dot{V}O_2$); hypoglycemia (due to disturbances of carbohydrate metabolism); dehydration (due to vomiting, sweating, hyperventilation, and increased rate of urine production); "toxic encephalitis" manifested as chorea, delirium, hallucinations, and convulsions, which may be replaced—as toxicity progresses—by depression, stupor, and coma; gastrointestinal symptoms including nausea, vomiting, anorexia, and occasionally abdominal pain; and, infrequently, hemorrhagic phenomena associated with a prolonged

SALICYLATE INTOXICATION: STAGES OF INCREASING SEVERITY

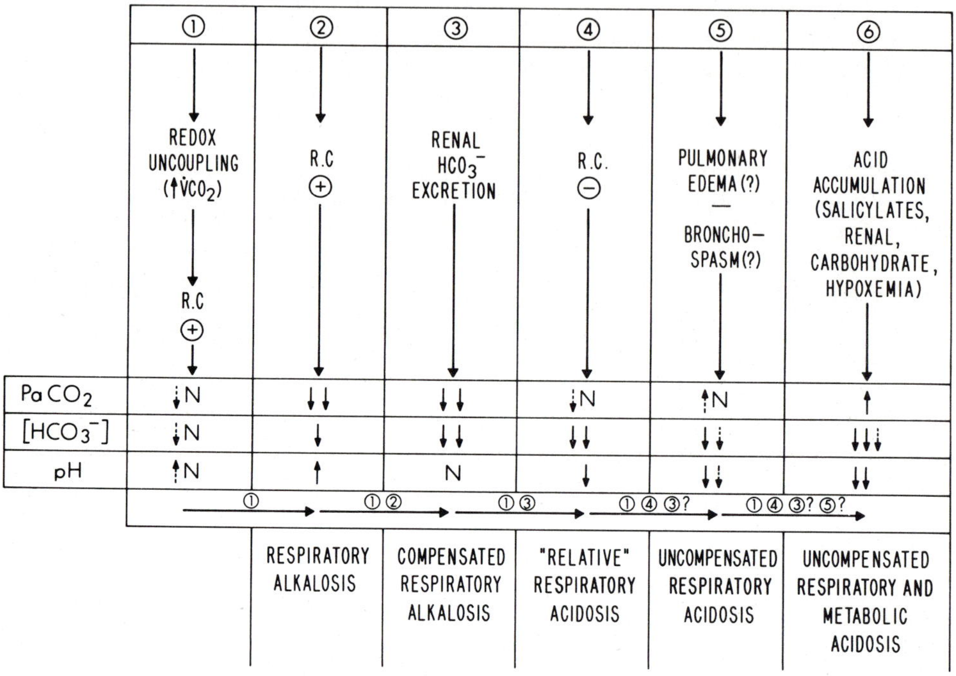

FIG. 18-9. Salicylate intoxication: stages of increasing severity.

bleeding time (due perhaps to aspirin-induced inhibition of platelet aggregation in situ).

DIAGNOSIS AND TREATMENT

Most often the patient's history points to the diagnosis of salicylate intoxication. If history is not reliable, the diagnosis can be confused with pneumonia, encephalitis, or diabetic acidosis, in which case measurement of serum salicylate concentration permits differentiation. Salicylate levels should be extrapolated back to time zero using Done's nomogram (Fig. 18-8) in order to estimate the probable degree of toxicity. Thus patients with time zero values above 40 mg/100 ml probably require hospitalization, and patients with values between 30 and 40 mg/100 ml require hospitalization only if symptoms of salicylate intoxication are noted. It should be noted that in chronic poisoning, little relationship exists between serum concentration and severity of poisoning. In this case patients with serious and even fatal reactions may have relatively low levels of salicylate in the blood.

Arena recommends that, if the patient is seen within 4 to 6 hours of ingestion, the stomach should be emptied by thorough emesis or lavage followed by maximal doses of activated charcoal by mouth or gastric tube, which will absorb large quantities of salicylates and greatly decrease blood levels.[3] He also recommends fever reduction by cold or tepid sponging, large quantities of parenteral fluids to offset dehydration and to augment salicylate excretion in urine, vitamin K to reduce the possible bleeding tendency, glucose in the presence of hypoglycemia and fixed acidemia, appropriate electrolytes to correct electrolyte imbalance, and $NaHCO_3$ to increase blood pH and to improve urinary excretion (since optimal excretion of salicylates requires an alkaline urine).

No attempt should be made to depress respiratory center activity when hyperventilation exists, because of the potentially hazardous effects of such therapy should salicylate-induced central depression develop. Similarly, it is generally held that attempts to increase Pa_{CO_2} by increasing inspired PCO_2 are ill-advised.

The seriously ill patient, for example, the patient with fever above 103° F or convulsions, coma, or pulmonary edema, may require additional therapeutic measures to accelerate the rate of removal of salicylates from the body. Thus attempts may be made to accelerate renal clearance and to increase urinary pH above 7.5. This may be achieved by administration of (1) $NaHCO_3$, which, however, Winters feels may present a serious threat to the patient because of the concomitant alkaline pH produced in blood;[101] (2) acetazolamide, which increases urinary excretion of salicylates and lowers serum $[HCO_3^-]$, an effect that can be remedied by administration of exogenous HCO_3^-, and (3) tromethamine (THAM), which requires additional clinical testing before it can be recommended categorically. Of the "extrarenal" methods for salicylate removal (exchange transfusion, peritoneal dialysis, and hemodialysis), hemodialysis is the most efficient for life-threatening salicylism in older children, and exchange transfusion is the treatment of choice for young infants.

REFERENCES: PART III

1. American Public Health Association: Accident Prevention. McGraw-Hill Book Co., New York, p. 51, 1961.
2. Andersen, H. T.: Physiological adaptations in diving vertebrates. *Physiol. Rev. 46*:212, 1966.
3. Arena, J. M.: *Poisoning—Toxicology, Symptoms, Treatments.* Charles C Thomas, Springfield, 1963.
4. Arms, R. A., D. E. Dines and T. C. Tinstman: Aspiration pneumonia. *Chest 65*:136, 1974.
5. Awe, W. C., W. S. Fletcher and S. W. Jacob: The pathophysiology of aspiration pneumonitis. *Surgery 50*:232, 1966.
6. Baldachin, B. J. and R. N. Melmed: Clinical and therapeutic aspects of kerosene poisoning: a series of 200 cases. *Br. Med. J. 2*:28, 1964.
7. Bartlett, J. G. and S. L. Gorbach: The triple threat of aspiration pneumonia. *Chest 68*:560, 1975.
8. Bergeson, P. S., S. W. Hales, M. D. Lustgarten and H. W. Lipow: Pneumatoceles following hydrocarbon ingestion. *Am. J. Dis. Child. 129*:49, 1975.
9. Berman, L. S., W. W. Fox, R. C. Raphaely and J. J. Downes: Optimum levels of CPAP for tracheal extubation of newborn infants. *J. Pediatr. 89*:109, 1976.
10. Bierman, C. W. and W. E. Pierson: Hand nebulizers and asthma therapy in children and adolescents (editorial). *Pediatrics 54*:668, 1974.
11. Bolande, R. P.: *Cellular Aspects of Developmental Pathology.* Lea & Febiger, Philadelphia, 1967.
12. Cachia, E. A. and F. F. Fenech: Kerosene poisoning in children. *Arch. Dis. Child. 39*:502, 1964.
13. Cameron, J. L., P. Caldini and J. K. Toung: Aspiration pneumonia: physiologic data following experimental aspiration. *Surgery 72*:238, 1973.
14. Cameron, J. L., W. H. Mitchell and G. D. Zuidema: Aspiration pneumonia: clinical outcome following documented aspiration. *Arch. Surg. 106*:49, 1973.
15. Campbell, J. B.: Pneumatocele formation following hydrocarbon ingestion. *Am. Rev. Respir. Dis. 101*:414, 1970.
16. Clark, J. M.: The toxicity of oxygen. *Am. Rev. Respir. Dis. 110*(No. 6, part 2): 40, 1974.
17. Clark, J. M. and C. J. Lambertsen: The rate of development of pulmonary oxygen toxicity in man. In *Proceedings of the Third Symposium on Underwater Physiology.* Williams & Wilkins Co., Baltimore, 1967.
18. Clark, J. M. and C. J. Lambertsen: Pulmonary oxygen toxicity: a review. *Pharmacol. Rev. 23*:37, 1971.
19. Clark, J. M. and C. J. Lambertsen: Rate of development of pulmonary O_2 toxicity in man during O_2 breathing at 2.0 Atm. *J. Appl. Physiol. 30*:739, 1971.
20. Colebatch, H. J. H. and D. F. J. Halmagyi: Lung mechanics and resuscitation after fluid aspiration. *J. Appl. Physiol. 16*:684, 1961.
21. Comroe, J. H., Jr., R. D. Dripps, P. R. Dumke and M. Deming: Oxygen toxicity. The effect of inhalation of high concentrations of oxygen for twenty-four hours on normal men at sea level and at a simulated altitude of 18,000 feet. *J.A.M.A. 128*:710, 1945.
22. Corsa, L., Jr. and R. A. Stallones: Epidemiologic

study of childhood poisonings in two California counties. *Pediatrics 28*:480, 1961.
23. Cox, M. E., B. F. Heslop, J. J. Kempton and R. A. Ratcliff: The Dellwood fire. *Br. Med. J. 1*:942, 1955.
24. Crapo, J. D. and D. F. Tierney: Superoxide dismutase and pulmonary oxygen toxicity. *Am. J. Physiol. 226*:1401, 1974.
25. Daeschner, C. W. Jr., R. J. Blattner and V. P. Collins: Hydrocarbon pneumonitis. *Pediatr. Clin. North Am. 4*:243, 1957
26. Deeths, T. M. and J. T. Breeden. Poisoning in children—a statistical study of 1,057 cases. *J. Pediatr. 78*:299, 1971.
27. Dickens, F.: The toxic effect of oxygen on nervous tissue. In *Neurochemistry*, A. C. Elliott (Ed.). Charles C Thomas, Springfield, 1955.
28. Dines, D. E., J. L. Titus and A. D. Sessler: Aspiration pneumonitis. *Mayo Clin. Proc. 45*:347, 1970.
29. Dolezal, V.: The effect of long lasting oxygen inhalation upon respiratory parameters in man. *Physiol. Bohemoslov. 11*:145, 1962.
30. Dollery, C. T., F. M. Williams, G. H. Draffan, G. Wise, H. Sahyoun, J. W. Paterson and S. R. Walker: Arterial blood levels of fluorocarbons in asthmatic patients following use of pressurized aerosols. *Clin. Pharmacol. Ther. 15*:59, 1974.
31. Done, A. K.: Salicylate intoxication. *Pediatrics 26*:800, 1960.
32. Downs, J. B., R. L. Chapman, Jr., J. H. Modell and C. I. Hood: An evaluation of steroid therapy in aspiration pneumonitis. *Anesthesiology 40*:129, 1974.
33. Dudley, W. R. and B. E. Marshall: Steroid treatment for acid-aspiration pneumonitis. *Anesthesiology 40*:136, 1974.
34. Eade, N. R., L. M. Taussig and M. I. Marks: Hydrocarbon pneumonitis. *Pediatrics 54*:351, 1974.
35. Fisher, A. B.: Effect of oxygen at two atmospheres upon the pulmonary mechanics of normal man. *J. Appl. Physiol. 24*:529, 1968.
36. Foley, J. C., N. B. Dreyer, A. B. Soule, Jr. and E. Woll: Kerosene poisoning in children. *Radiology 62*:817, 1954.
37. Frank, R.: Are aerosol sprays hazardous? *Am. Rev. Respir. Dis. 112*:485, 1975.
38. Gerarde, H. W.: Toxicological studies on hydrocarbons: V. kerosene. *Toxicol. Appl. Pharmacol. 1*:462, 1959.
39. Giammona, S. T.: Effects of furniture polish on pulmonary surfactant. *Am. J. Dis. Child. 113*:658, 1967.
40. Giammona, S. T. and J. H. Modell: Drowning by total immersion. Effects on pulmonary surfactant of distilled water, isotonic saline and sea water. *Am. J. Dis. Child. 114*:612, 1967.
41. Gooden, B. A.: Drowning and the diving reflex in man. *Med. J. Aust. ii*:583, 1972.
42. Gowdy, J. M. and M. J. Wagstaff: Pulmonary infiltration due to aerosol thesaurosis, a survey of hairdressers. *Arch. Environ. Health 25*:101, 1972.
43. Greene, D. G.: Drowning. In *Handbook of Physiology, Section 3: Respiration*, Volume 2, W. O. Fenn and H. Rahn (Eds.). American Physiological Society, Washington, 1965.
44. Gross, P., J. M. McNerney and M. A. Babyak: Kerosene pneumonitis: an experimental study with small doses. *Am. Rev. Respir. Dis. 88*:656, 1963.
45. Halmagyi, D. F. J.: Lung changes and incidence of respiratory arrest in rats after aspiration of sea and fresh water. *J. Appl. Physiol. 16*:41, 1961.
46. Halmagyi, D. F. J. and H. J. H. Colebatch: Ventilation and circulation after fluid aspiration. *J. Appl. Physiol. 16*:35, 1961.
47. Hartzell, H. C. and E. P. Mininger: Bronchopneumonia following ether anesthesia in obstetrics. *Surg. Gynecol. Obstet. 82*:427, 1946.
48. Haugaard, N.: Poisoning of cellular reactions by oxygen. *Ann. N.Y. Acad. Sci. 117*:736, 1965.
49. Herrin, J. T. and J. D. Crawford: Care of the critically ill child: major burns. *Pediatrics 45*:449, 1970.
50. Jones, D. V. and C. E. Work: Volume of a swallow. *Am. J. Dis. Child. 102*:427, 1961.
51. Kapanci, Y., R. Tosco, J. Eggermann and V. E. Gould: Oxygen pneumonitis in man. Light- and electron-microscopic morphometric studies. *Chest 62*:162, 1972.
52. Kennedy, J. H.: Hyperbaric oxygenation and pulmonary damage. The effects of exposure at two atmospheres upon surface activity of lung extracts in the rat. *Med. Thoracalis 23*:27, 1966.
53. Kimball, R. E., K. Reddy, T. H. Peirce, L. W. Schwartz, M. G. Mustafa, and C. E. Cross: Oxygen toxicity: augmentation of antioxidant defense mechanisms in rat lung. *Am. J. Physiol. 230*:1425, 1976.
54. Kylstra, J. A., D. C. Rausch, K. D. Hall and A. Spock: Volume-controlled lung lavage in the treatment of asthma, bronchiectasis, and mucoviscidosis. *Am. Rev. Respir. Dis. 103*:651, 1971.
55. Lambertsen, C. J.: Respiratory and circulatory actions of high oxygen pressure. In *Proceedings of the Underwater Physiology Symposium*, L. G. Goff (Ed.). National Academy of Sciences—National Research Council Publ. 377, Washington, p. 25, 1955.
56. Lambertsen, C. J.: Effects of excessive pressures of oxygen, nitrogen, carbon dioxide, and carbon monoxide: implications in aerospace, undersea, and industrial environments. In *Medical Physiology*, V. B. Mountcastle (Ed.). The C. V. Mosby Co., St. Louis, Chapter 66, 1974.

57. Lee, W. L., Jr., P. B. Caldwell and H. S. Schildkraut: Changes of lung volume, diffusion capacity, and blood gases in oxygen toxicity in humans. *Fed. Proc. 22*:395, 1963.
58. Lesser, L. I., H. S. Weens and J. D. McKey: Pulmonary manifestations following ingestion of kerosene. *J. Pediatr. 23*:352, 1943.
59. Lloyd, E. L. and W. R. Macrae: Respiratory tract damage in burns. *Br. J. Anaesth. 43*:365, 1971.
60. Mazyck, E. M., J. T. Bonner, H. M. Herd and P. N. Symbas: Pulmonary lavage for childhood pulmonary alveolar proteinosis. *J. Pediatr. 80*:839, 1972.
61. Mellins, R. B. and S. Park: Respiratory complications of smoke inhalation in victims of fires. *J. Pediatr. 87*:1, 1975.
62. Mendelson, C. L.: The aspiration of stomach contents into the lungs during obstetric anesthesia. *Am. J. Obstet. Gynecol. 52*:191, 1946.
63. Modell, J. H.: *The Pathophysiology and Treatment of Drowning and Near-Drowning.* Charles C Thomas, Springfield, Ill. 1971.
64. Modell, J. H., H. W. Calderwood, B. C. Ruiz, J. B. Downs and R. Chapman, Jr.: Effects of ventilatory patterns on arterial oxygenation after near-drowning in sea water. *Anesthesiology 40*:376, 1974.
65. Modell, J. H. and J. H. Davis: Electrolyte changes in human drowning victims. *Anesthesiology 30*:414, 1969.
66. Modell, J. H., J. H. Davis, S. T. Giammona, F. Moya and J. B. Mann: Blood gas and electrolye changes in human near-drowning victims. *J.A.M.A. 203*:337, 1968.
67. Modell, J. H., E. J. Kuck, B. C. Ruiz and H. Heinitsh: Effect of intravenous vs. aspirated distilled water on serum electrolytes and blood gas tensions. *J. Appl. Physiol. 32*:579, 1972.
68. Modell, J. H. and F. Moya: Effects of volume of aspirated fluid during chlorinated fresh water drowning. *Anesthesiology 27*:662, 1966.
69. Modell, J. H., F. Moya, E. J. Newby, B. C. Ruiz and A. V. Shoers: The effects of fluid volume in seawater drowning. *Ann. Intern. Med. 67*:68, 1967.
70. Modell, J. H., F. Moya and H. D. Williams: Changes in blood gases and $A\text{-}aD_{O_2}$ during near-drowning. *Anesthesiology 29*:456, 1968.
71. National Clearing House for Poison Control Centers. Tabulation of 1972 reports, bulletin. May-June 1973.
72. Northway, W. H., Jr., L. Rezeau, R. Petriceks and K. G. Bensch: Oxygen toxicity in the newborn lung: reversal of inhibition of DNA synthesis in the mouse. *Pediatrics 57*:41, 1976.
73. Olson, M.: The benign effects on rabbits' lungs of the aspiration of water compared with 5% glucose and milk. *Pediatrics 46*:538, 1970.
74. Olstad, R. and R. M. Lord, Jr.: Kerosene intoxication. *Am. J. Dis. Child. 83*:446, 1952.
75. Pamintuan, R. L., R. E. Brashear, J. C. Ross and R. E. Deatley. Cardiovascular effects of experimental aspiration pneumonia in dogs. *Am. Rev. Respir. Dis. 103*:516, 1971.
76. Pentiah, P., R. Reilly and H. L. Borison: Interactions of morphine sulfate and sodium salicylate on respiration in cats. *J. Pharmacol. Exp. Ther. 154*:110, 1966.
77. Phillips, A. W., J. W. Tanner and O. Cope: IV. Respiratory tract damage (an account of the clinical, x-ray and postmortem findings) and the meaning of restlessness. *Ann. Surg. 158*:799, 1963.
78. Polson, C. J. and R. N. Tattersall: *Clinical Toxicology.* J. B. Lippincott Co., Philadelphia, p. 578, 1969.
79. Pratt, P. C.: Pathology of pulmonary oxygen toxicity. *Am. Rev. Respir. Dis. 110* (No. 6, part 2):51 1974.
80. Press, E.: Co-operative kerosene poisoning study: evaluation of gastric lavage and other factors in the treatment of accidental ingestion of petroleum distillate products. *Pediatrics 29*:648, 1962.
81. Press, E. and A. K. Done: Solvent sniffing. Physiologic effects and community control measures for intoxication from the intentional inhalation of organic solvents. I. *Pediatrics 39*:451, 1967.
82. Press, E. and A. K. Done: Solvent sniffing. Physiologic effects and community control measures for intoxication from the intentional inhalation of organic solvents. II. *Pediatrics 39*:611, 1967.
83. Puy, R. J. M., R. W. Hyde, A. B. Fisher, J. M. Clark, J. Dickson and C. J. Lambertsen: Alterations in the pulmonary capillary bed during early O_2 toxicity in man. *J. Appl. Physiol. 24*:537, 1968.
84. Ramirez-R, J. and W. H. Obenour, Jr.: Bronchopulmonary lavage in asthma and chronic bronchitis: clinical and physiologic observations. *Chest 59*:146, 1971.
85. Redding, R. A., T. Arai, W. H. J. Douglas, H. Tsurutani and J. Overs: Early changes in lungs of rats exposed to 70% O_2. *J. Appl. Physiol. 38*:136, 1975.
86. Reed, E. S., S. Leikin and H. D. Kerman: Kerosene intoxication. *Am. J. Dis. Child. 79*:623, 1950.
87. Richardson, J. A. and H. R. Pratt-Thomas: Toxic effects of varying doses of kerosene administered by different routes. *Am. J. Med. Sci. 221*:531, 1951.
88. Robertson, W. G., J. J. Hargreaves, J. E. Herlocher and B. E. Welch: Physiologic response to increased oxygen partial pressure. II. Respiratory studies. *Aerosp. Med. 35*:618, 1964.
89. Rogers, R. M., J. P. Szidon, J. Shelburne, J. L. Neigh, J. F. Shuman, and K. R. Tantum: Hemodynamic response of the pulmonary circulation to

bronchopulmonary lavage in man. *N. Engl. J. Med.* *286*:1230, 1972.
90. Scarpelli, E. M., K. H. Gabbay and J. A. Kochen: Lung surfactants, counterions, and hysteresis. *Science* *148*:1607, 1965.
91. Schulte, J. H.: Effects of mild carbon monoxide intoxication. *Arch. Environ. Health* *7*:524, 1963.
92. Skirkey, H. C.: Treatment of petroleum distillate ingestion. *Mod. Treat.* *4*:697, 1967.
93. Siebke, H., T. Rod, H. Breivik and B. Lind: Survival after 40 minutes' submersion without cerebral sequelae. *Lancet* *1*:1275, 1975.
94. Sladen, A., P. Zanca and W. H. Hadnott: Aspiration pneumonitis—the sequelae. *Chest* *59*:448, 1971.
95. Steele, R. W., R. H. Conklin and H. M. Mark. Corticosteroids and antibiotics for the treatment of fulminant hydrocarbon aspiration. *J.A.M.A.* *219*:1434, 1972.
96. Stone, H. H., D. W. Rhame, J. D. Corbitt, K. S. Given and J. D. Martin, Jr.: Respiratory burns. A correlation of clinical and laboratory results. *Ann. Surg.* *165*:157, 1967.
97. Swinyard, E. A.: Noxious gases and vapors. In *The Pharmacological Basis of Therapeutics,* L. S. Goodman and A. Gilman (Eds.). Macmillan Publishing Co., Inc., New York: p. 900, 1975.
98. Teabeaut, J.: II. Aspiration of gastric contents: an experimental study. *Am. J. Pathol.* *28*:51, 1952.
99. Valimaki, M., T. Pelliniemi and J. Ninikoski: Oxygen-induced changes in pulmonary phospholipids in the rat. *J. Appl. Physiol.* *39*:780, 1975.
100. Van de Water, J. M., K. S. Kagey, I. T. Miller, D. A. Parker, N. E. O'Connor, J. Sheh, J. D. MacArthur, R. M. Zollinger, Jr., and F. D. Moore: Response of the lung to six to 12 hours of 100 per cent oxygen inhalation in normal man. *N. Engl. J. Med.* *283*:621, 1970.
101. Winters, R. W.: Salicylate intoxication. In *Pediatrics,* H. L. Barnett (Ed.). Appleton-Century-Crofts, New York, p. 552, 1972.
102. Wolfe, B. M., A. E. Brodeur and J. B. Shields: The role of gastrointestinal absorption of kerosene in producing pneumonitis in dogs. *J. Pediatr.* *76*:867, 1970.
103. Woodbury, D. M. and E. Fingl: Analgesic-antipyretics, anti-inflammatory agents, and drugs employed in the therapy of gout. In *The Pharmacological Basis of Therapeutics,* L. S. Goodman and A. Gilman (Eds.). Macmillan Publishing Co., Inc., New York, p. 325, 1975.
104. Zikria, B. A., W. Q. Sturner, N. K. Astarjian, C. L. Fox, Jr. and J. M. Ferrer, Jr.: Respiratory tract damage in burns: pathology and therapy. *Ann. N.Y. Acad. Sci.* *150*:618, 1968.
105. Zuskin, E. and A. Bouhuys: Acute airway responses to hair spray preparations. *N. Engl. J. Med.* *290*:660, 1974.

Pediatric Pulmonary Radiology

HAROLD S. GOLDMAN

19

The explosive development of newer modalities in the field of radiology during the last several years has caused the radiologist to think of his expanding field more in terms of "diagnostic imaging" than in terms of the more restrictive historic concept of roentgenography. It behooves all physicians to become acquainted with the techniques of nuclear medicine, ultrasonography, and computerized tomography as they find their way into our diagnostic armamentarium alongside plain film roentgenography, conventional tomography, contrast studies of the esophagus and major airways (esophagogram and bronchogram), venography, and angiography.

It would be wise to keep in mind, however, that the plain roentgenographic examination still accounts for nearly all diagnostic studies. This situation is not likely to change because the nature of the common diagnostic problems of chest disease in childhood, namely pneumonia and aspiration, leads to questions that are mostly answerable by conventional roentgenology. For this reason, the first consideration of this chapter is the most simple of the methods by which diagnoses can be made; additional techniques are to be used only to gain critical information not otherwise obtainable. Availability of the tools and expert personnel as well as cost in terms of radiation, invasiveness, and money are included among those factors that determine our choice of approach.

The Roentgenographic Method

The diagnostic utility of the conventional roentgenographic examination depends on the presence of contrasting film densities; in ordinary clinical practice, these densities are related to air, water (soft tissues), bone, fat, and certain metals (usually contrast agents).

The lung is well suited to the needs of roentgenography because of the presence of air everywhere—in the airways and in the alveoli. Air is the natural contrast medium against which the blood vessels can be seen. The conventional roentgenogram defines only these two constituents in the normal lung, the thin walls of the intrapulmonary airways remaining generally unseen.

Departure from established norms in the appearance of the vessels in terms of size, contour, and position is the basis for making certain diagnoses. For example, an appearance of "increased radiolucency" may be due to a decrease in vessel size because of embolus, or it may be due to spreading apart of vessels because of increased lung size. Disease and deformity announce their position in the lung by means of added soft tissue density, making them easy to identify against surrounding air. This agreeable circumstance in the lung is lost, for instance, in the abdomen where the contrasting density of air is to be found only sometimes and then often not really in a suitable position to evaluate organs other than the bowel. Fat, though sometimes useful because of its contrasting density, is not nearly as dependable since it is often sparsely represented and since the difference from soft tissue density is less pronounced. Partly because of this relative deficiency in contrasting roentgenographic densities, the more recently developed modalities alluded to in the opening paragraph of this chapter have found greater favor for use in the abdomen than for the evaluation of pulmonary disease.

The melding soft tissues of the mediastinum and its structures present a situation similar to that of the abdomen, in which it becomes necessary to introduce opaque media to provide contrasting densities for diagnosis. Recently, ultrasound, nuclear medicine, and especially computerized tomography are also being used in this area, chiefly to identify and characterize tumors and cysts. Still, the air-filled lungs and the large mediastinal airways (as well as the air-filled esophagus) provide enough contrast to enable the radiologist to make diagnoses without resorting to these other methods.

The one, often vitally important, area that defies easy radiologic exploration is the intrapulmonary airway. Unless the lung surrounding the bronchus is airless, or the bronchial "wall" is thickened, the bronchogram is the only method available to study the bronchus. However, because of its dangers in children, bronchography can be recommended only for the exceptional case in which the essential information, vital to management, cannot be obtained in any other way. This statement will be amplified later in the chapter.

The basic roentgenographic examination of the chest is accomplished by inspection of frontal and lateral films. These films are ordinarily obtained with the child in the standing position, chest against the film cassette, x-ray beam pointing at the child's back (posteroanterior or PA position). The distance from the focus (x-ray source) to the film is 72 in. (the x-rays are essentially parallel at this distance and divergent at shorter distances). The lateral projection is conventionally made with the left side against the film.

The child who is too young to stand or maintain a position voluntarily is examined in the supine position. At this age, a nonrotated roentgenogram is more easily and predictably obtained when the child is restrained or immobilized while lying down. Devices that purport to immobilize the child in the erect position have generally not proven to be of value with the "difficult" child. The erect position, usually sitting in these children, is used often in an attempt to obtain a film with the diaphragms low; surprisingly, this result is more often achieved with the child supine.[63] Indeed, "high diaphragms" frequently result when the child's film is made in the sitting position. This situation probably occurs because the abdominal organs, which protrude and cause the "pot belly" of the young child, are forced upward in the sitting position, elevating the diaphragms.

The heart of a large child or adult is magnified when the patient is in the supine position, because the film-focus distance must be shortened to 40 in. or less. Since the x-rays, directed at the anterior chest wall, are divergent, and the heart is positioned at a considerable distance from the film placed behind the patient, the cardiac image is enlarged on the film. On the other hand, since the magnification factor is directly related to the distance between the heart and the film and this distance is very much reduced with infants and small children, magnification is negligible.[63]

Interestingly, shortening the film-focus distance significantly reduces the radiation to the patient. The radiation dose is inversely related to the square of the distance from the source of radiation to the patient. Therefore, using a film-focus distance of 36 in. instead of 72 in. would result in a fourfold reduction in radiation.

It must be emphasized that, though these positions are recommended as appropriate in most cases, the type of examination required is determined by the problem at hand. One should use the various combinations of patient position (erect, supine, prone, decubitus, oblique) and x-ray tube orientation (vertical, horizontal, or angled beam) in a well-calculated, efficient manner. The argument that centers around the necessity for either one or two films or more must be answered ultimately by careful definition of the object of the examination.

Organization

Abnormalities that disturb lung size and shape are dealt with first. Following this, attention turns to those that "infiltrate" the lung without significantly altering lung size (as estimated by radiologic means). This decision is arbitrary; clearly considerable overlap exists. Nonetheless, this framework has been chosen since it serves to emphasize the great importance of determining the lung size and shape in the roentgenologic diagnosis of childhood chest disease.

Obstruction

MOUTH, NOSE, AND PHARYNX

The relative proportions of the tongue and mandible can be assessed radiographically (Fig. 19-1). *Hypoplasia of the mandible* may force the tongue to impinge on the airway. The position and the movements of the tongue in relation to surrounding bone and soft tissue landmarks can be determined fluoroscopically. This determination may become important in the dynamic evaluation of the airway during swallowing. Fluoroscopic study is useful in speech pattern evaluation during normal as well as abnormal development.[56] If barium paste is spread over key landmarks, radiographic visualization is improved. Recording these events for later inspection can be done by: (1) magnetic tape or disc recording (the information can be transposed to movie-type film); (2) 70 mm or 105 mm film, usually programmed at 1 to 6 frames per second; or (3) 16 or 35 mm cine film from about 6 to 60 frames per second. Since many factors enter, the choice of a

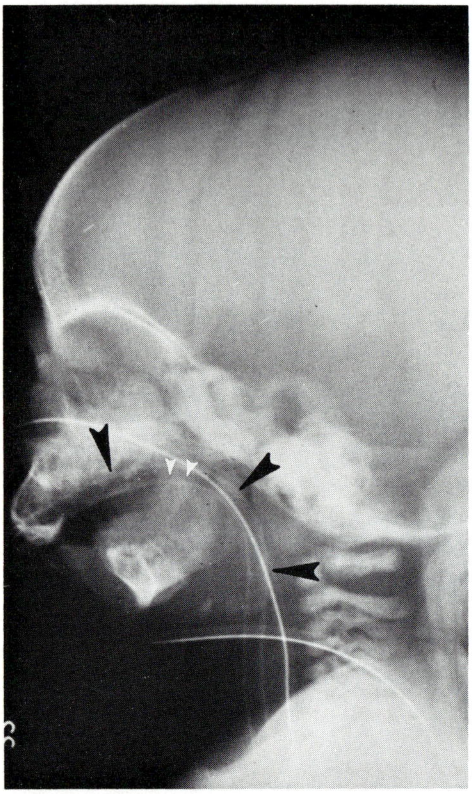

FIG. 19-1. Mandibular hypoplasia in an infant causing the tongue (white arrows) to press against the posterior wall of the pharynx (in this case, an orotracheal tube has been inserted, black arrows).

system would depend on the circumstances in any given instance. However, for ordinary general usage in a pediatric unit, magnetic tape and 70 mm film provide a satisfactory system in terms of visual detail, motion analysis, radiation exposure, and cost.

Nasal airway obstruction due to *choanal atresia* in the newborn infant, diagnosed by the inability to pass a feeding tube through the nose, can be confirmed anatomically by the placement of a few milliliters of thin, milk-like barium through an infant feeding tube into the nose one side at a time. It is done under fluoroscopic control with the child's head in the submento-vertex position (head hanging back and down position, shoulders elevated from the x-ray table). Films are made in the anteroposterior and lateral (cross-table) positions (Fig. 19-2, A and B). The obstruction characteristically is

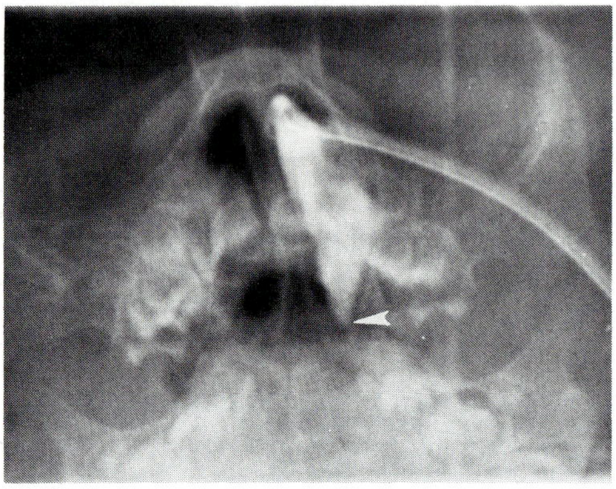

A

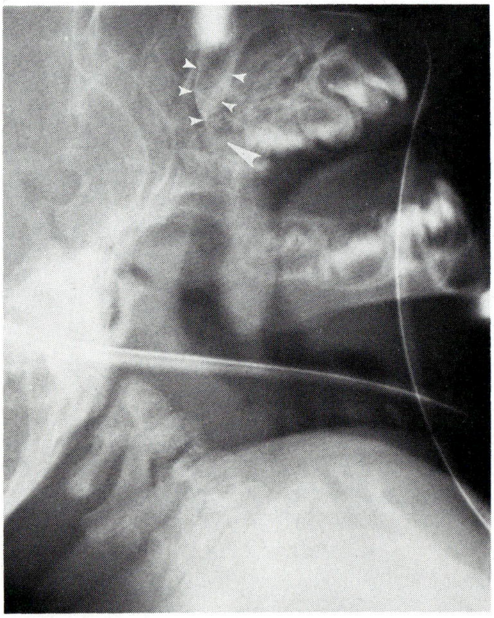

B

FIG. 19-2. *A*, Frontal view of an infant with choanal atresia. The barium column is obstructed after nasal injection through feeding tube. Point of obstruction (arrow) is typically conical in appearance.

B, Lateral view shows that point of obstruction is at the level of the posterior margin of hard palate (large arrow).

at the level of the posterior edge of the hard palate, is usually not ossified at birth, and often presents a somewhat conical posterior edge to the contrast material in both views. The obstruction may be complete or incomplete, and may involve the two sides asymmetrically.

Obstruction to the nasal passageway may be caused by foreign body or tumor. An interesting example (Fig. 19-3, A and B) of encroachment on the nasal and nasopharyngeal airway by blood-forming tissues in the sinuses of this 5-year-old child with *thalassemia* is one of the unusual causes for such obstruction.

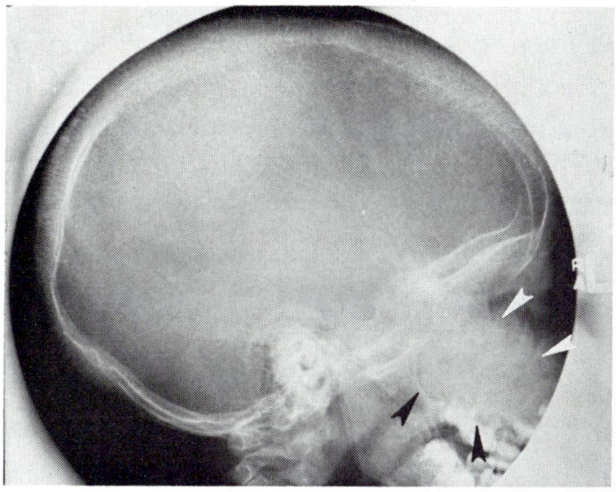

A

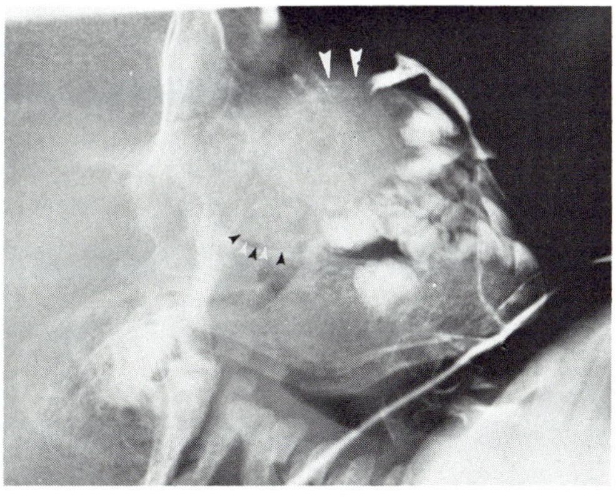

B

FIG. 19-3. *A*, Lateral view of the skull of a 5-year-old child with thalassemia exhibiting massive opacity of the maxillary sinuses.

B, Coned lateral view shows obstruction to the passage of barium into the nasal passageway by the mass of hemopoietic tissue in the sinus (large arrows). Small arrows mark the posterior edge of the mass that obstructs the nasopharyngeal airway.

While examining the lateral film, one should not mistake a prominent inferior turbinate for a tumor mass just above the posterior margin of the hard palate. The clinical diagnosis of *adenoid hypertrophy* and obstruction of the nasopharynx is commonly an indication for radiographic examination. The adenoid shadows often appear quite large on the lateral view of the nasopharynx without clinical abnormality; the submento-vertex view is complementary, showing the region at right angles to the lateral view. The most important contribution of the radiologist is to identify the unusual lesion causing the obstruction if it is not simply enlarged adenoid tissue. By using the criterion of a lobular shadow in the posterior nasopharynx whose anterior edge is at the level of the pterygoid processes (just behind the posterior edge of the hard palate), one can usually accurately identify the shadow as adenoids. The comfortable diagnosis of "adenoid tissue" may be comfortable only because of the exceedingly rare occurrence of tumors such as lymphoma and epithelial tumor. However, the possibility of tumor should not be disregarded, and if the shape and/or position varies from the criteria set forth, one should inspect the lesion directly.

Tomography is sometimes an asset in terms of evaluating the integrity of the base of the skull to rule out bony destruction. Because of the presence of overlying bony structures, the soft tissue-air interfaces are sometimes hard to see. The high kilovoltage technique (125 to 140 kv, properly filtered)[39,50] is useful since it tends to reduce the visibility of the osseous structures. (The coefficient of x-ray absorption of bone and soft tissue approaches equality at kilovoltage levels in this range and above.) The high kilovoltage technique is mentioned again with regard to the examination of the trachea and bronchi.

Tonsillar and adenoid enlargement has been shown to produce significant airway obstruction (see Chapter 18). Although the tonsils are easily evaluated by direct inspection, their diagnostic importance to the radiologist is that the tonsillar shadows must be recognized for what they are. Seeming to "hang" from the soft palate on the lateral film (Fig. 19-11), the shadow could be misinterpreted as a tumor, e.g., angiofibroma or rhabdomyosarcoma.[37] The size of the palatine and lingual tonsils, as well as that of prevertebral lymph tissues, varies considerably within the normal range. Except in the case of extreme enlargement, they cannot often be diagnosed as normal or abnormal by radiographic means.

LARYNX, LARYNGEAL PHARYNX, EXTRATHORACIC TRACHEA

When radiographic assessment of the larynx, laryngeal pharynx, and extrathoracic trachea is required, it is often in an emergency situation due to airway obstruction. It should be determined first that it is safe to delay treatment (e.g., endotracheal intubation) in order to obtain roentgenograms for diagnostic purposes. Since a specific diagnosis, e.g., epiglottitis, can be made or ruled out with a single lateral film, the physician may decide to obtain this film using a mobile (portable) x-ray unit if the situation warrants it. The usefulness of the ordinary mobile unit for the examination of the airway is, however, limited. For example, it is not well suited for magnification films with high kilovoltage technique (though it could be adapted for that purpose), and one may not be able to obtain very fast exposure in order to avoid motion artefact. Therefore, it is suggested that the study be done in the radiology department whenever possible.

Laryngeal Anatomy, Epiglottitis, Croup. The radiographic *anatomy of the larynx* can be defined on the lateral film as a triangle (Figs. 19-4, 19-6 and 19-7). The apex of the triangle is the tip of the epiglottis (e); the descending limbs are the posterior edge of the epiglottis (Fig. 19-7, black arrows) and the posterior edge of the aryepiglottic folds (a); and the cords are the base. The ovoid lucency of the laryngeal ventricle (V), representing the space between false and true cords (its longest diameter lying in the plane of the cords), enables one to identify the base of the triangle. The cords then join the base of the epiglottis to the arytenoid cartilage (A), which is seen as a somewhat conical mass of soft tissue density. To find the apex or tip of the epiglottis, one follows the curve of the tongue backward to the valleculae (v), the air-filled pocket just anterior to the tip of the epiglottis (Fig. 19-4). Normally, one should be able to define all of these structures if the film is taken during inspiration and if the patient is not swallowing. Swallowing, occurring at end-expiration, tends to obscure

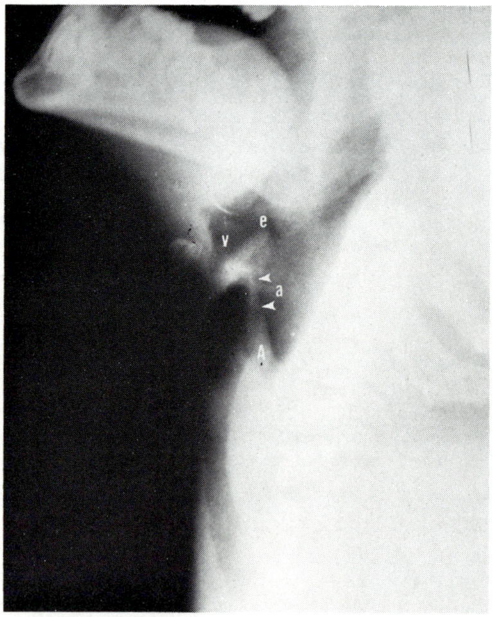

FIG. 19-4. Normal larynx of a 3-year-old child: valleculae (v); epiglottis, tip (e); aryepiglottic folds (a); and arytenoid cartilage (A).

the laryngeal structures: the larynx is elevated so that it is positioned against the base of the tongue and the epiglottis is curled backwards and downwards over the glottis. If not recognized, it is possible to confuse this picture with that seen in the patient with *epiglottitis,* where all of the normal landmarks are obliterated by the swelling of all of the laryngeal structures. With epiglottitis, however, the pharynx is invariably distended with air, and the radiographic picture (Fig. 19-5) is characteristic, even pathognomonic.[15]

In the case of *croup,* the supraglottic landmarks are normal, except for the ventricle (Fig. 19-6), and the infraglottic area is described as hazy.[16] However, the latter is not a necessary criterion for diagnosis since it may simply be a manifestation of the phase of ventilation, i.e., when the film is taken in expiration. The frontal or AP view may show subglottic narrowings in both croup and epiglottitis; this view does not make the differential diagnosis definitively as does the lateral view.

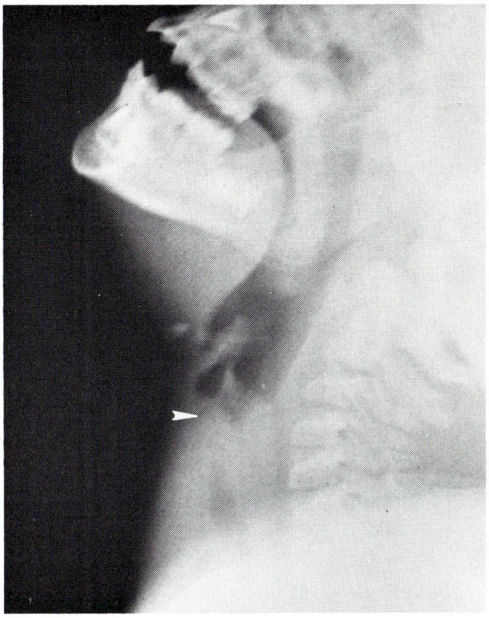

FIG. 19-6. Croup. The laryngeal triangle appears normal. The ventricle is filled with air (arrow). The subglottic airway is hazy and the trachea dilated inferiorly (probably due to expiration).

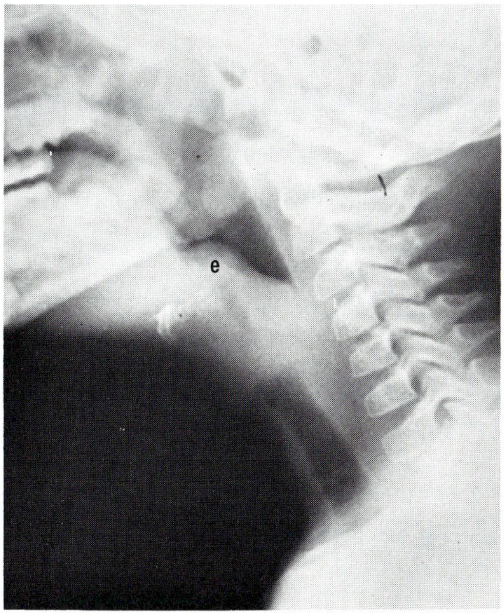

FIG. 19-5. Epiglottitis. All of the laryngeal landmarks are obscured by the swelling. The tip of the epiglottis is marked (e).

UPPER AIRWAY OBSTRUCTION, METHODOLOGY

The diagnostic problem of upper airway obstruction due to factors other than those mentioned to this point may be clarified by careful attention to radiologic method. Conventional roentgenography in AP and lateral views, followed if necessary by the use of properly filtered high kilovoltage films,[39] using 2 : 1 or 3 : 1 magnification, increases the accuracy of diagnosis. Xeroradiography has been suggested for diagnostic use in the study of airway disease in the neck, and the method as published appears impressive.[55,73] We have no personal experience and do not know of any work to compare its accuracy with the methods mentioned here. Tomography plays little or no role here. Fluoroscopy, using one or more of the permanent recording methods mentioned previously, is occasionally an aid in diagnosis. For example, Dunbar has shown[5] anterior "prolapse" of the aryepiglottic folds and backward "collapse" of the epiglottis during inspiration in children with congenital laryngeal stridor during quiet breathing (Fig. 19-7). Fluoroscopic examination of the airway of the infant is done best in the supine position with the infant being fluoroscoped "cross-table" laterally. To do this, the fluoroscopic table is turned vertically and the footstool is raised to eye level. The infant is then laid crosswise on it. For certain purposes (examining for H-type tracheoesophageal fistula) the infant may be placed in the prone position. An esophagogram is sometimes used to look for a diverticulum of the esophagus,[48] to show an indentation due to an aberrant vessel, or to aid in localization of a prevertebral mass. It can identify an esophageal foreign body as a rare cause for airway obstruction. Whereas an esophagogram is only sometimes necessary as a diagnostic aid for disease in the neck, it is almost routine for the evaluation of intrathoracic airway problems.

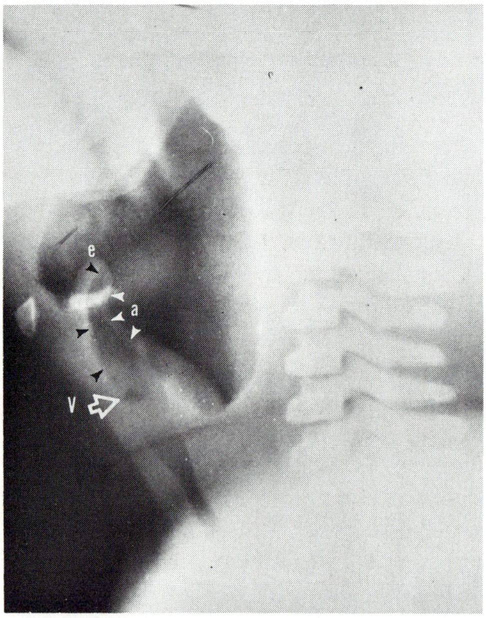

FIG. 19-7. Congenital laryngeal stridor. Notice the forward bowing of the aryepiglottic folds (a) and the epiglottis (black arrows). The ventricle (V) is wide open during inspiration.

Although it is too early to be sure of their role, ultrasound, computerized tomography, and radionuclide studies would likely be helpful in the evaluation of neck masses. Ultrasound and computerized tomography can define anatomic location as well as determine the presence of cystic or solid components of a mass. Radionuclide studies can be helpful in making an estimate of blood flow or, through the use of gallium, can locate abscesses and lymphomatous tumors. As with bronchography, tracheography carries with it the risk of using an iodized oily, viscid medium, which increases airway resistance considerably. Because of this, there is virtually no place for the procedure especially in the small airway of the infant and child. The use of powdered tantalum,[54] a superb contrast medium, which does not increase airway resistance, has not gained FDA approval for general use in children. If its safety in children is confirmed, it could become the penultimate examination of the airway before direct laryngoscopy.

The normal radiographic anatomy of the neck varies with phase of ventilation, deglutition, phonation, and patient position; knowledge of these various attitudes allows one to identify those abnormalities that cause obstruction.

For example, although the epiglottis of the child in Figure 19-8 seems swollen, the ability to identify landmarks such as valleculae, the lower posterior edge of the epiglottis, and the normal-appearing arytenoid cartilage mass serves to distinguish the abnormality from epiglottitis (Fig. 19-5) and to identify the problem as an epiglottic mass. In this case, a *congenital cyst of the epiglottis* was found (see also Fig. 6-64).

Likewise, an infraglottic mass, a *hemangioma* (Fig. 19-9),[11,38] is identified after locating the base of the laryngeal triangle.

Masses and swellings extrinsic to the airway narrow, stretch, and displace it. In Figure 19-10, the larynx is elevated, and the

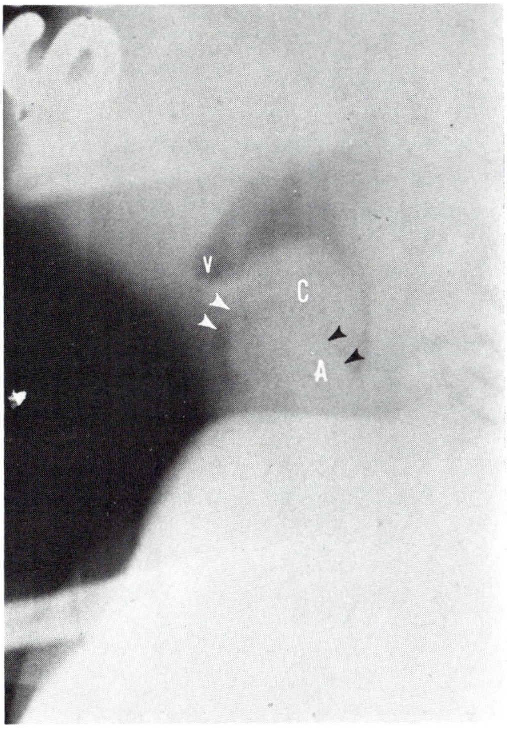

FIG. 19-8. Cyst (C) arising from the tip of the epiglottis. Identification of normal structures, valleculae (V), inferior posterior surface of the epiglottis (white arrows), and posterior surface of the arytenoid cartilage (black arrows), serves to distinguish them from epiglottis.

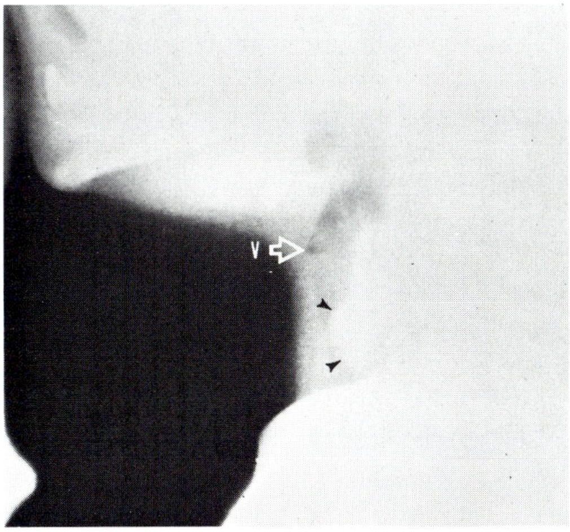

FIG. 19-9. Tracheal hemangioma (black arrows). The subglottic location is defined by the identification of the ventricle (V).

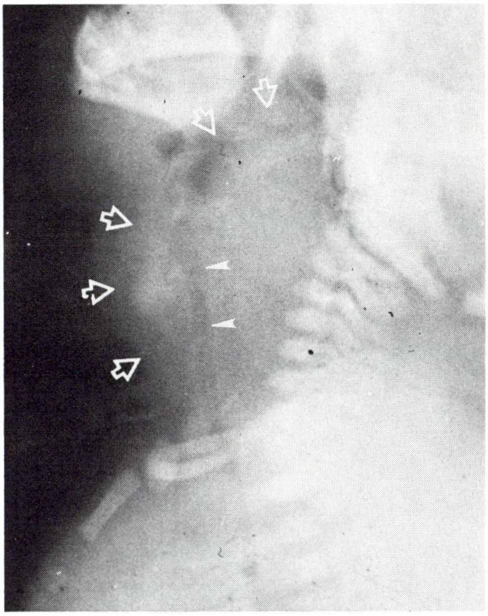

FIG. 19-10. Newborn child with displacement and narrowing of the trachea (solid arrows) due to a large thyroid goiter that encircles it. Open arrows indicate border of the thyroid mass.

trachea is elongated, narrowed, and displaced anteriorly by a *thyroid goiter* in a newborn child. Other tumors, such as cystic hygroma, may grow from behind and present a similar appearance. In addition, the latter must be distinguished from prevertebral masses, such as a retropharyngeal abscess, pharyngeal diverticulum, and anterior meningocele, and even from diffuse swellings as seen in myxedema. In the child, it is difficult to give a satisfactory guide to the normal width of the prevertebral space, as is done in the adult, because of variations in the extent of vertebral ossification as well as the other factors mentioned in the preceding paragraph. One can obtain a good idea of the "normal" prevertebral space by studying Figures 19-1 through 19-9. On the other hand, the apparent mass in the prevertebral area in Figure 19-11 occurs because the film was made in expiration. It is quite characteristic in appearance; the acute anterior buckling of the

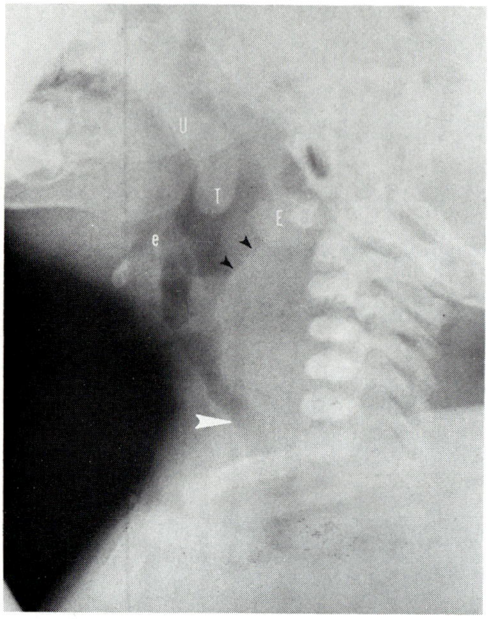

FIG. 19-11. Pseudotumor of the prevertebral space due to anterior buckling of the airway in expiration: uvula (U); tonsils (T); earlobe (E); epiglottis (e). White arrow shows typical location and appearance of acute angulation of trachea just above thoracic inlet.

trachea one to two vertebrae above the thoracic inlet, the slightly elevated position of the larynx close to the tongue base, and the posterior sloping of the upper edge of the apparent mass are the criteria for recognizing that this "mass" is normal. A repeat film in inspiration usually confirms normalcy. It is rarely necessary to do an esophagogram to prove normalcy.

TRACHEAL OBSTRUCTION WITHIN THE THORAX

When the clinical evidence points to major airway obstruction at the intrathoracic level, management decisions in terms of providing an airway become more complicated. Often emergency bronchoscopy is clearly indicated, for example, for foreign body aspiration with tracheal obstruction. However, in other situations, radiologic assessment is required to establish the presence of tracheal obstruction, define its location and its extent, and, whenever possible, identify the cause. The use of plain films, high kilovoltage films, and an esophagogram usually provides the information required to proceed with proper management. Tomography is rarely necessary; moreover, it cannot usually be carried out since exposure times are long and the patient must hold his breath for a minimum of a half second, usually longer. Exposure times for conventional chest roentgenograms are of the order of 1/100 sec. and never longer than 1/30 sec.: these short exposures are used in order to "stop motion" in the infant or older child with respiratory distress and tachypnea. Occasionally angiography can be helpful in the definition of unusual variations in vessel distribution that may cause obstruction (see Fig. 6-16 and 6-18).

Computerized tomography (CT), and ultrasonography are useful for the diagnosis of tumors and cysts of the mediastinum. CT has the advantage in the mediastinum since ultrasound does not "penetrate" air or the osseous structures of the chest wall. It shares with ultrasound the ability to distinguish cystic lesions from solid ones, but is uniquely able to diagnose the presence of fat in the solid mass.

The roentgenograms shown in Figure 19-12 are those of a child who was admitted because of suspected tracheal obstruction. The films give evidence of a large anterior mediastinal mass narrowing the airway. An endotracheal tube is in place. The "thymic appearance" given by an exaggerated "wave sign" suggests the correct diagnosis of non-Hodgkin's *lymphoma* infiltrating the thymus. High kilovoltage films would have improved visualization of the airway (see also Fig. 6-9). Although the normal thymus almost certainly does not cause tracheal obstruction, it has been seen to displace lung and intrapulmonary bronchi on bronchography. On the other hand, lymph node enlargement of a nonmalignant nature in the anterior mediastinum, mimicking

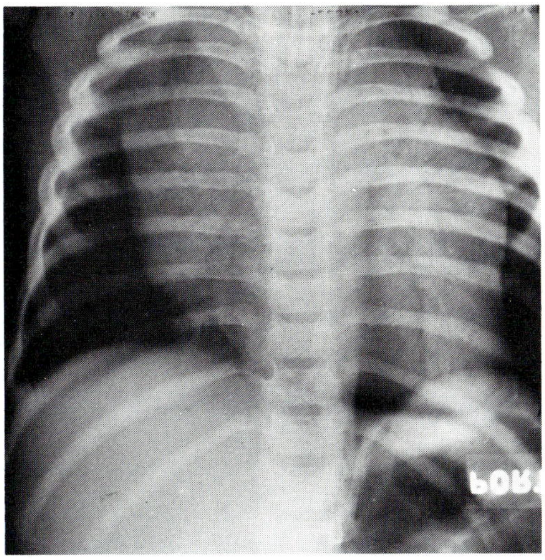

A

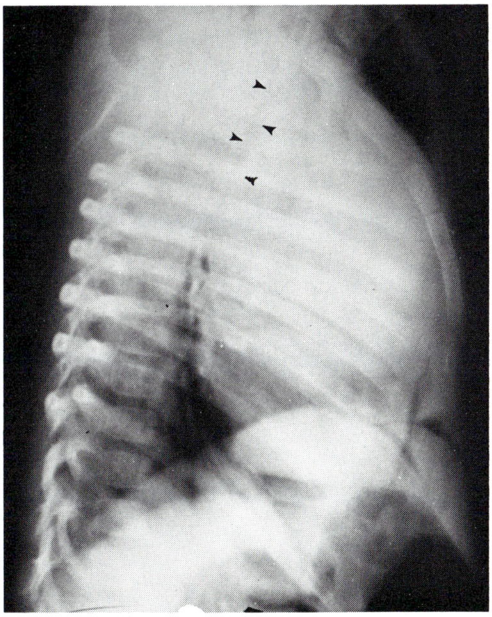

B

FIG. 19-12. *A*, Frontal projection shows large mediastinal image due to lymphomatous enlargement of the thymus.

B, Lateral projection shows anterior mediastinal mass causing narrowing of the trachea (arrows).

thymus, has been seen to cause tracheal compression.

Evaluation of the mediastinal shadow of the thymus, or what seems to be the thymus, is difficult, and interpretation sometimes must be made by the pediatric radiologist on the basis of his experience. However, changes seen after inspiration and after expiration as in Figure 19-13, A and B point strongly to a normal thymus. Figure 19-14, A and B shows that surprisingly much of the mediastinal shadow can in fact be due to a normal thymus. A thymus that is normal is frequently seen later in childhood and even in the early teens.

The esophagogram in Figure 19-15 established the diagnosis of *vascular ring.*[6] The important criterion of a bilateral indentation on the barium-filled esophagus in the frontal view is met. A lateral film showing a posterior indentation completes the study. The airway may narrow opposite this indentation. The need for aortography to define the exact anatomy of the ring is limited since surgical correction can usually be carried out successfully on the basis of plain film examination, high kilovoltage airway studies, and the esophagogram (see also Chapter 6). Tracheography is unnecessary for diagnosis and, as indicated previously, may be quite dangerous.

BRONCHIAL OBSTRUCTION

Obstruction of one lung or one of its divisions may be recognized on the plain film because of evidence of volume loss (atelectasis) or volume increase ("air-trapping"). Rarely, obstruction can be diagnosed in the absence of volume change; in this case the diagnosis of obstruction is suggested by the presence of homogenous opacity of the lung or lobe in question without evidence of an air bronchogram.

In general, inequality in the size of the lungs is immediately recognized by: (1) shift of the mediastinum toward the smaller side and (2) elevation of the diaphragm on the smaller side. A third classically described parameter, narrowing of the rib interspaces on the small side, is often more difficult to

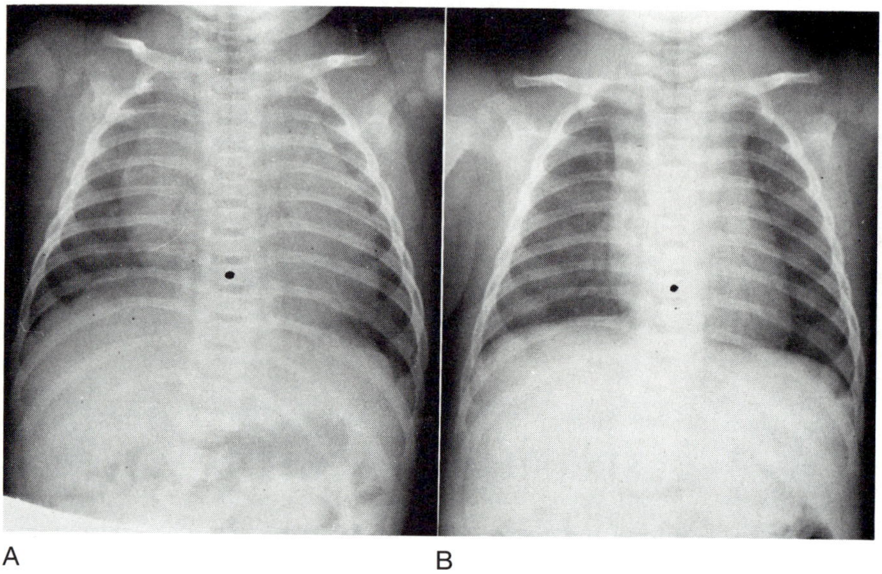

FIG. 19-13. Change in mediastinal shadow due to expiration (A) and inspiration (B). Black dot marks T-8 (eighth thoracic vertebra) on both roentgenograms.

appreciate. To avoid a mistaken diagnosis of unequal lung size, two points are emphasized. First, the infant's trachea normally buckles to the right; this buckling should not be taken to represent mediastinal shift. Tracheal buckling is most pronounced when the film is taken during expiration and when the child is less than a year of age; buckling may be seen through the third year of life. Second, rotation of the patient may either mimic lung size

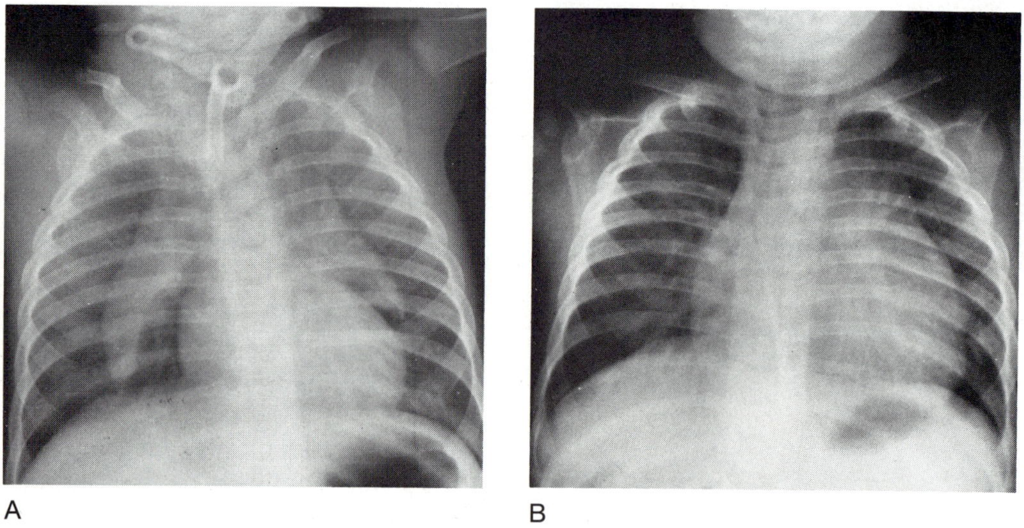

FIG. 19-14. Pneumomediastinum due to tracheostomy (A) shows that the right lobe makes up the entire right mediastinal border in (B) and that the left lobe forms most of the left mediastinal border in (B).

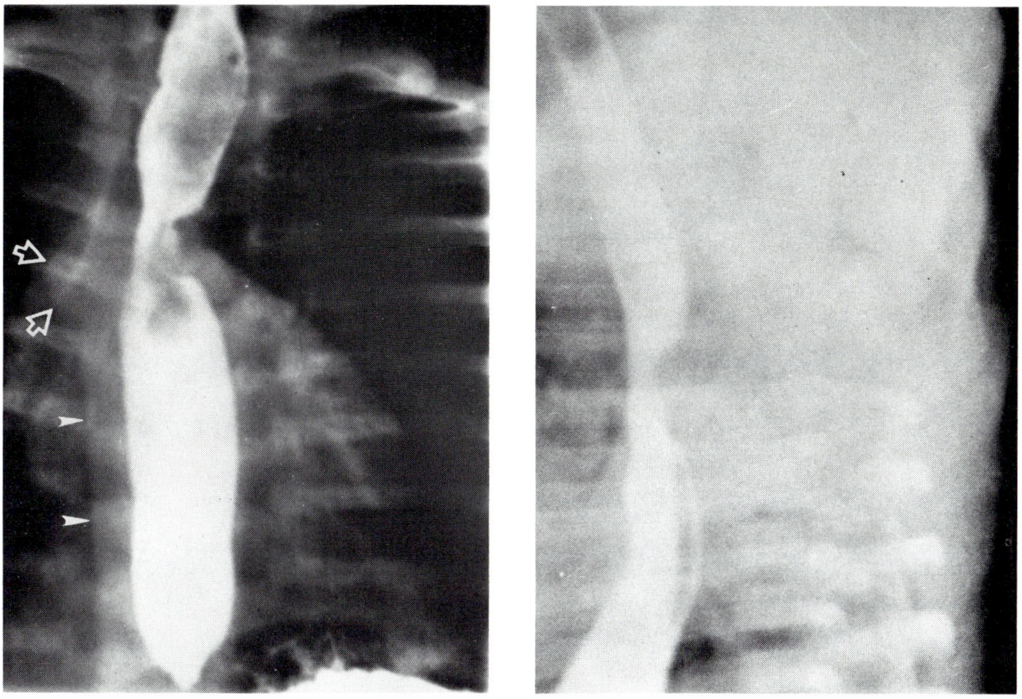

A B

FIG. 19-15. *A*, Aortic ring showing bilateral indentations on the esophagogram. The aorta arches (open arrows) and descends (solid arrows) on the right. A persisting ligamentum arteriosum indents the left side. *B*, Lateral view shows the posterior indentation on the esophagus.

inequality—or mask its presence. Infants, especially, tend to turn their heads and bodies to the right causing the mediastinum to appear shifted to the right and the right diaphragm to appear higher and slightly more rounded than the left. The difference is exaggerated during deep inspiration and minimized with expiration because the posterior part of the diaphragm descends and flattens when contracted, while the anterior part of the diaphragm changes very little. It is because the anterior part of the diaphragm is seen on the side toward which the child is turned, and the posterior part of the diaphragm on the other side, that the apparent inequality is produced. Since minor degrees of rotation may be overlooked, the following guidelines may be of help. When the child is straight, the medial end of the clavicles should be equidistant from the midline of the spine on the roentgenogram; the distance is lengthened on the side toward which the child is rotated. In the infant, it is usually enough to note that the medial end of the clavicle on one side is projected completely away from the spine (Fig. 19-16, A and B).

Reduced Lung Volume. If *agenesis* of a lung represents the ultimate expression of lung volume reduction (Fig. 19-17), atelectasis must represent the penultimate state (Fig. 19-18A). In both instances, mediastinal shift and rib interspace narrowing are clearly evident on the ipsilateral side. Because of the total lack of air, the outline of the diaphragm as well as the heart is lost in the opacity of the hemithorax. Evidence that the diaphragm is elevated (Fig. 19-17) is provided by the high position of the fundus of the stomach, which

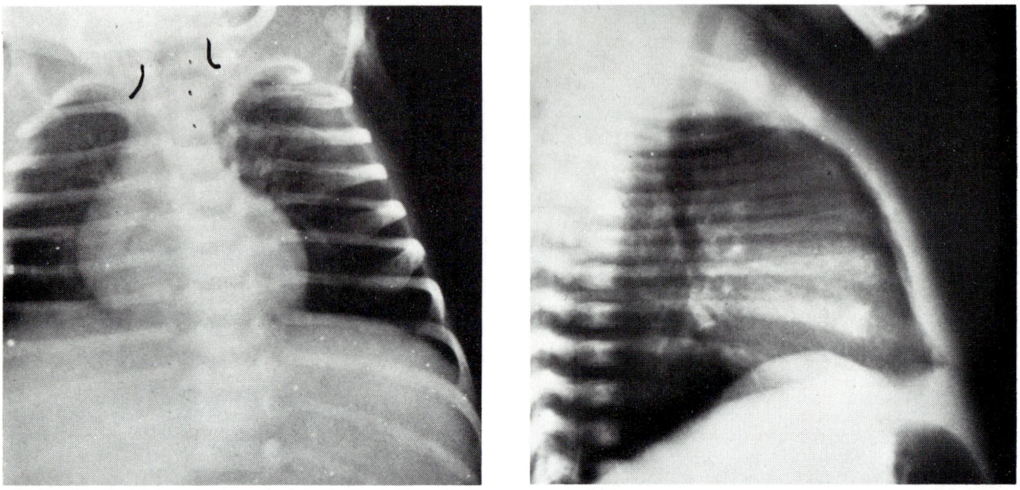
A B

FIG. 19-16. The medial end of the right clavicle is displaced away from the vertebral midline signifying patient rotation to the right (A). The anterior part of the diaphragm is high and rounded (B) while the posterior part is flat and lower (B). Rotation to the right causes the anterior diaphragm to be seen on the right (A) and the posterior part on the left (A) in the frontal roentgenogram.

is air-containing and presumed to be just beneath the diaphragm. The means for establishing the presence of a lung lies in the ability to demonstrate an ipsilateral bronchus and/or pulmonary artery (see also Chapter 15, p. 431).

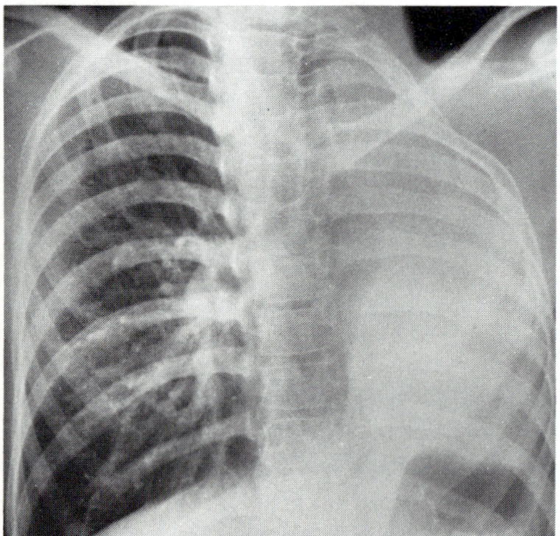

FIG. 19-17. Agenesis of the left lung. The rib anomalies are coincidental. Elevation of the stomach bubble suggests diaphragm elevation.

In Figure 19-18B, the origin of a bronchus of normal diameter, though "cut off," is shown by tomography. This 9-year-old girl was bronchoscoped and found to have a *bronchial adenoma causing atelectasis* of the right lung. A number of advantages are gained with the use of the high kilovoltage film technique over tomography with this kind of problem: it can be done in multiple views, with varied patient position, and with varying degrees of inspiration and expiration. Bronchography, done selectively, could also be helpful to define more clearly the abnormal anatomy. However, if any of the oily contrast material should gain access to the normal lung, it may have several undesirable effects, including (1) further compromise of pulmonary function by increasing major airway resistance and by blocking peripheral airways and alveolae (the former effect requires only a small amount of the contrast agent and is probably the more important factor) and (2) delay of surgery, since the oil

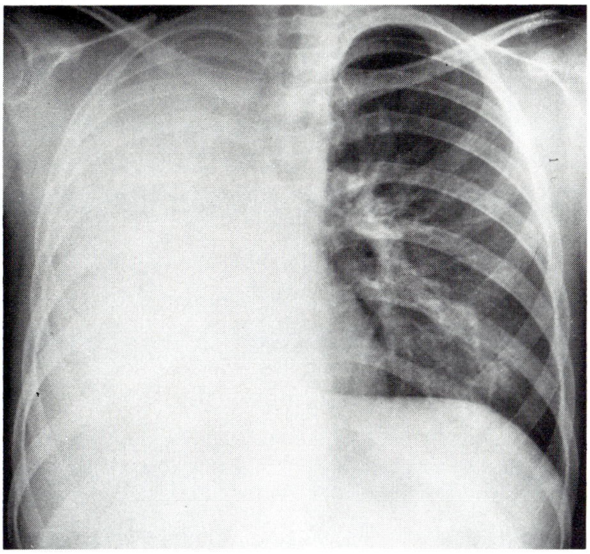

A

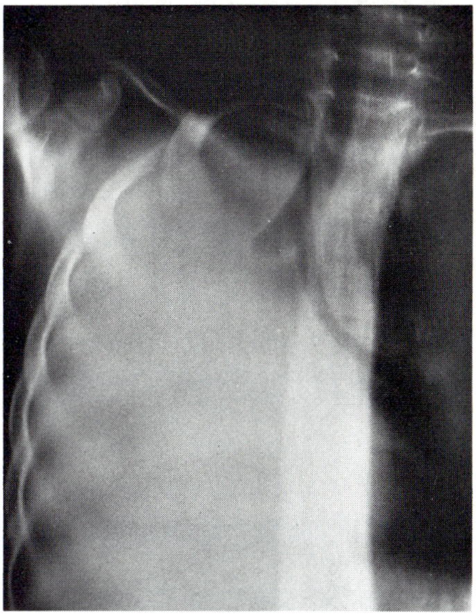

B

FIG. 19-18. *A*, A 9-year-old girl with a bronchial adenoma causing complete obstruction and atelectasis of the right lung.
B, Tomography shows cutoff of right main bronchus.

may not be cleared from the normal lung for as long as a month. The radiograph may show that the radiopacity of the contrast agent disappears in days, since the iodine is removed much more quickly than its oily carrier.

If one were unable to affirm the presence of a collapsed lung by a noninvasive technique designed to identify a bronchus, the next approach would be to establish the presence of a pulmonary artery. This determination may be made by use of a "lung scan." The term, lung scan, applies to procedures in which a linear scanner is used. When a gamma camera is the radiation detector, the appropriate terms are "radionuclide perfusion study," "lung scintigram," and "lung imaging." Currently, macroaggregated albumin or gelatin particles, about 30 μ in diameter, are tagged with technetium 99m, and are injected through a peripheral vein. The particles lodge in the pulmonary capillaries (10 to 15 μ). The chest should be "imaged" immediately after the injection, since the aggregated particles disaggregate. The method provides a reliable indication of blood flow and has been shown to be safe.[29,67] However, when blood flow is considerably reduced, as in atelectasis, the threshold for counting or imaging must be lowered over the suspect side, or slow flow may be mistaken for no flow. In any case, only evidence for flow, clearly distinguishable from background, is useful for the diagnosis of atelectasis. If no clear evidence of pulmonary arterial blood flow is demonstrated by this method, pulmonary arteriography is the definitive procedure. Bronchography, because of the risks in children and the need for anesthesia, is not recommended.

Complete *atelectasis* of a lung can also be sustained after *trauma to the thorax* with rupture of the bronchus and subsequent *scarring*. With the child shown in Figure 19-19, no evidence of pulmonary abnormality existed immediately after injury. However, 3

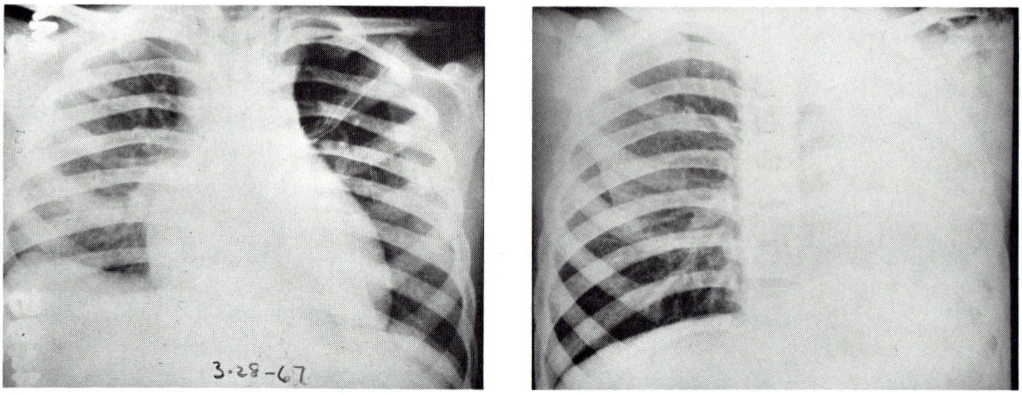

A B

FIG. 19-19. The chest roentgenogram was normal at the time of severe chest trauma due to an automobile accident (A) and showed complete atelectasis (B) 3 weeks later due to narrowing of the bronchus after scarring.

weeks later, the chest film showed atelectasis. At the time of bronchoscopy, a bronchogram (not shown) was done to delineate the exact location and length of the stenosis, essential information that was not otherwise obtainable.

The diagnosis of lobar and segmental atelectasis depends on the ability to recognize the features of volume loss unique to each lobe and to each segment separately or in combination. It is necessary to be familiar with these criteria in order to distinguish roentgenographic densities due to collapse from those of infiltrative lesions.[44,46] Although it is beyond the scope of this chapter to review these characteristics in detail, several cases of lower lobe atelectasis will serve to make certain basic points.

Lower lobe *atelectasis due to a mucous plug* in an asthmatic child is seen on the left of Figure 19-20A as a triangular density "through the heart shadow" with obliteration of the diaphragm, the vertebral-pleural line, and the aorta. The fact that the descending branch of the pulmonary artery is not seen, as it is in Figure 19-20B following clearance of the plug, serves to distinguish this density from an extrapulmonary mass or pleural fluid. The oblique sharp border of the density identifies it as atelectasis rather than pneumonia or other "infiltrate." Since the lower lobe collapses posteriorly, severe atelectasis may show no abnormality on the lateral roentgenogram.

Figure 19-21A is an example of *Kartagener's syndrome*[40] (situs inversus, bronchiectasis, and sinusitis), in which there is evidence of dextrocardia and bilateral lung disease, primarily of the lower lobes. The "right" lower lobe is typical of atelectasis while the "left" lower lobe shows a density that cannot be distinguished from pneumonia. The lateral film (not shown) gave clear evidence of "left" middle lobe involvement, i.e., a density with volume loss. The child's films were unchanged over a 2-year period, whether or not he had evidence of pneumonia clinically. Evidence of "clearing" appeared only after a period of excellent pulmonary physical therapy. At bronchoscopy, after a month of such therapy, there was no significant exudate. Bronchography (Fig. 19-21B) was done following this therapy, and the left lower and middle lobes were examined selectively with catheter positioning under fluoroscopic control. (Of note is the contrast material outlining the trachea and the left upper lobe (Fig. 19-21C), which points to the difficulty

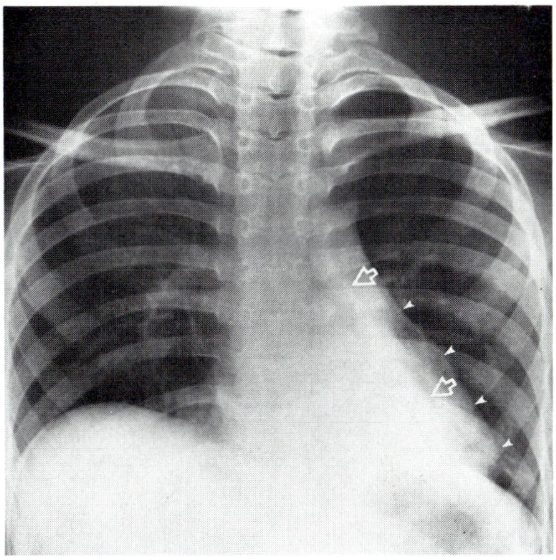
A

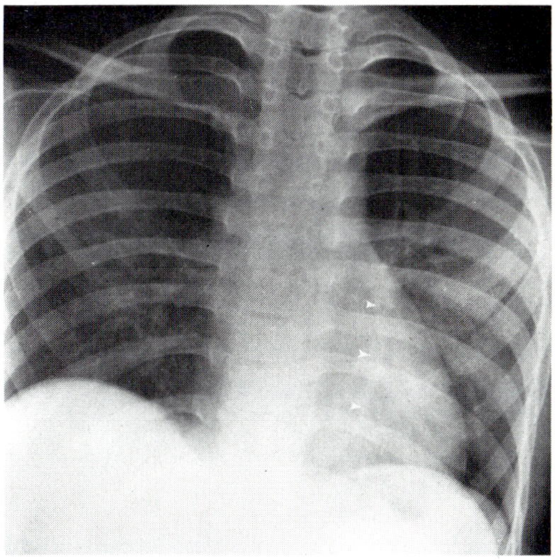
B

FIG. 19-20. *A*, Asthmatic child in whom a mucous plug caused left lower lobe atelectasis. Large open arrows indicate the border of the atelectatic lobe; small solid arrows indicate the cardiothymic border. *B*, After re-expansion of the lobe, the left lower branch of the pulmonary artery is easily identified (arrows).

in maintaining absolute control over the distribution of the contrast agent, as discussed previously.) On the spot film (Fig. 19-21B), the left lower bronchi are filled with contrast material. The bronchi are primarily cylindrically dilated though there does appear to be cystic dilatation in some. Bronchi are "bunched" together (atelectasis), and no obstructing lesion exists. One can easily appreciate the same findings in the right lower lobe, but this time because of the presence of an air bronchogram. One may also note on the lateral roentgenogram (Fig. 19-21C) that (1) the middle lobe is "pancaked" and consists chiefly of dilated bronchi and (2) the lower lobe bronchi are somewhat less dilated compared to those in Figure 19-21B. The change in caliber of these abnormally compliant bronchi is a function of the phase of ventilation.

On occasion, the nature of an abnormal radiodensity in the supine or erect frontal position can be clarified by placing the patient in the *decubitus position* with the side in question up. This position tends to enlarge the "up" lung. With the patient facing the technician, the "up" shoulder is brought forward slightly to visualize the entire lung. This maneuver is especially useful in children who cannot take a deep breath on command. The child whose film is shown in Figure 19-22A had an unspecified chronic neuromuscular disease (note the bell-shaped thorax and scoliosis). The nature of the ill-defined density in the right lower chest is clearly shown (Fig. 19-22B) to be due to atelectasis of both middle and lower lobes on the left decubitus film. It cleared with physiotherapy.

AIR-TRAPPING DUE TO INTRINSIC CAUSES

The phenomenon of air-trapping due to obstruction is widely appreciated. Conceptually, enlargement of the blocked lung or lung subdivision has been said to result from obstruction of the "ball-valve" variety. According to this theory, air enters during inspiration as the bronchus widens and air is trapped on expiration as the bronchus closes on the

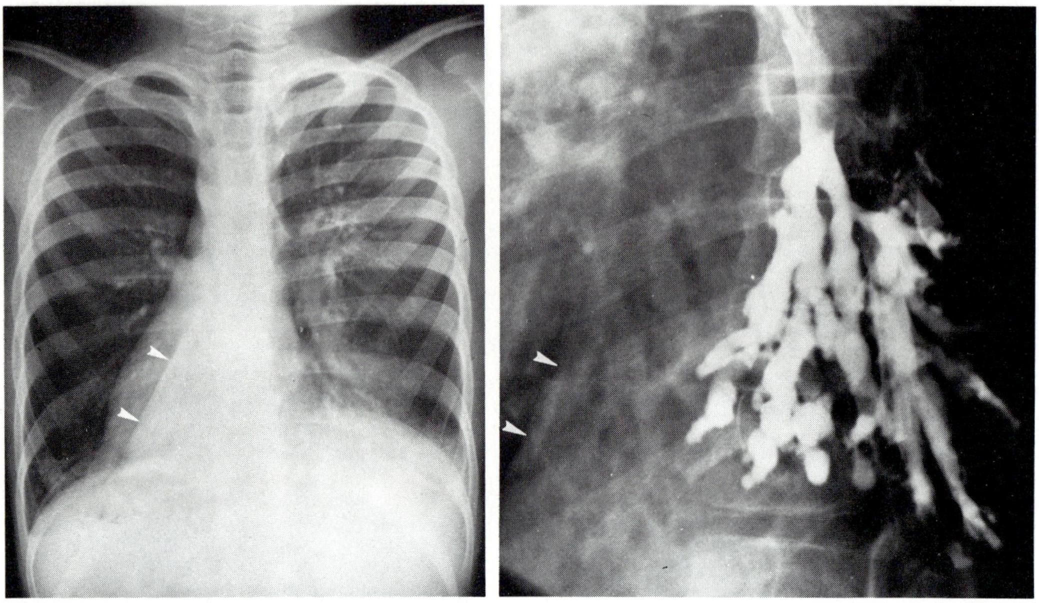

A B

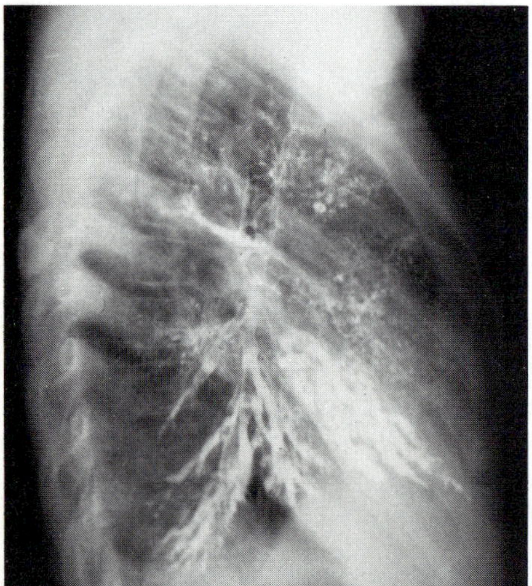

C

FIG. 19-21. *A*, Kartagener's syndrome showing situs inversus with stomach bubble below right diaphragm and dextrocardia. Compensatory enlargement of the upper lobe occurs because of lower lobe atelectasis on the right (arrows). Pneumonic density on the left is due to atelectasis and fluid-filled bronchi.

B, Fluoroscopic spot film of the lower lobes during selective bronchogram of the left-sided lower lobe showing bronchiectasis. Air-filled bronchi in right-sided collapsed lower lobe (arrows) are also bronchiectatic.

C, Post-bronchogram lateral roentgenogram showing contrast material scattered on left side with bronchiectasis of middle and lower lobes.

obstructing lesion (see also Chapter 2). The mechanism for reaching equilibrium may be explained in several ways, involving the acceptance of varying rates of airflow within the lung; however, since there are instances of complete obstruction with maintenance of the aerated lung, the mechanism of collateral ventilation has been invoked as an alternative explanation. The diagnosis of air-trapping is made on the roentgenogram because of the presence of (1) increased blackening on the film (radiolucency) in the abnormal area relative to comparable areas in the other lung and (2) relative enlargement of the suspect area (volume). The increased radiolucency is due to a decrease in size and number of blood vessels per unit area (volume), resulting in a

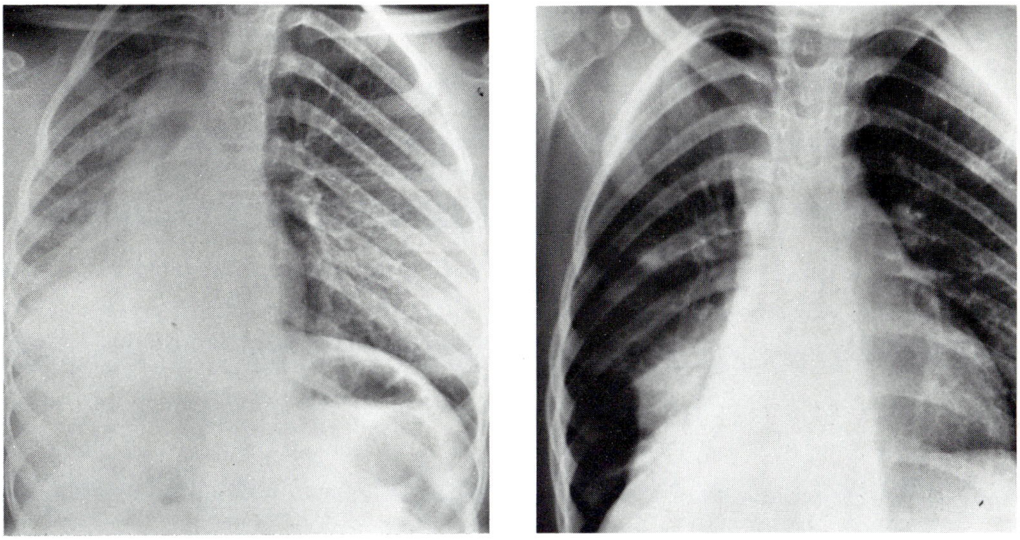

A B

FIG. 19-22. *A*, Right lower lung opacity in a child with unspecified neuromuscular disease. *B*, Left decubitus position shows the opacity to be atelectasis of right middle lobe and right lower lobe.

decrease of photon absorption and increased film blackening. Although spreading of vessels undoubtedly contributes to the appearance of radiolucency when the obstructed lung is quite large, the more important factor is the reflex constriction of the precapillary arterioles in the presence of decreased Po_2.[36] This factor results in decreased flow and smaller blood vessels to the part of the lung involved. Errors in the diagnosis of air-trapping are due to (1) poor film technique; (2) rotation, which in itself causes asymmetry in radiolucency; and (3) film exposure during inspiration or after a prolonged slow expiration.

There is clear evidence of obstruction with increased radiolucency and there is evidence of volume increase on the right in Figure 19-23. Bronchoscopy revealed a *mucous plug* in this $1\frac{1}{2}$-year-old child. Figure 19-24 shows a similar finding in another child, this time due to a *foreign body* in the left main bronchus (peanut). The diagnosis was easily made because the films were taken after expiration. On the other hand, when the film is

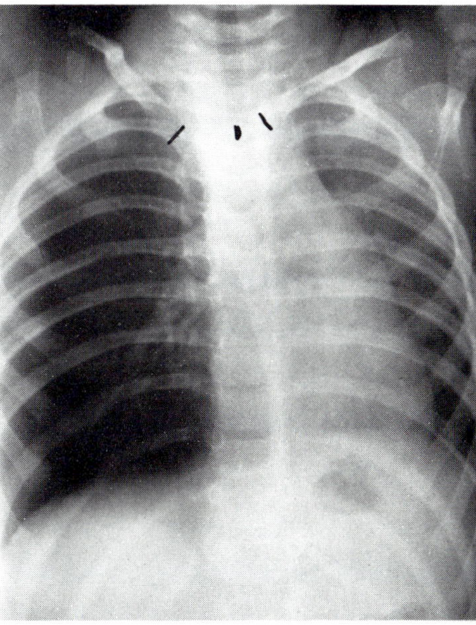

FIG. 19-23. Obstructed right lung due to a mucous plug in the right bronchus. Medial ends of the clavicles and posterior spinous process are marked and indicate the patient is rotated to the right.

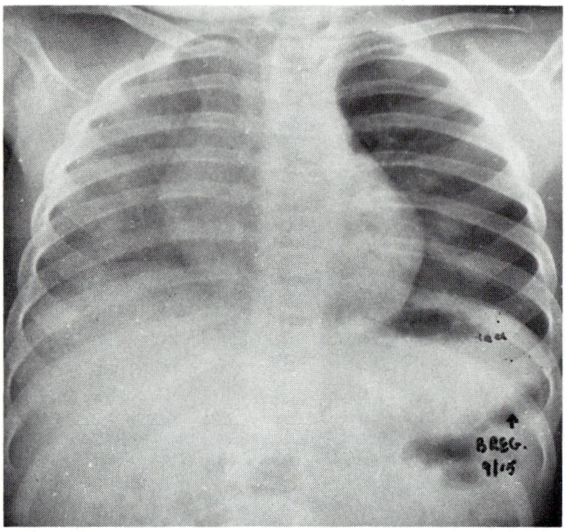

FIG. 19-24. Air-trapping on the left due to the aspiration of a peanut.

made in the same child after deep inspiration, the diagnosis of obstruction (to the left upper lobe in Fig. 19-25A) is less certain, since small degrees of rotation to the right may produce an apparent increase in lung size and increased lucency on the left. Figure 19-25B is made with the patient lying on the left side (left decubitus position). Volume of the left lower lobe is small as one would expect in this position; thus it casts the denser shadow seen there. Conversely the left upper lobe remains large and lucent, and the diagnosis of air-trapping is made.[10,30] This child was asymptomatic and had been followed for 1 year, with improvement seen on the film during the interval. Tentatively, he was diagnosed as having lobar emphysema.

Congenital lobar emphysema (see Chapter 15 for discussion of etiology) involving the middle lobe is shown in Figure 19-26. The first film on the first day of life is virtually normal; the small pneumothorax on the left medially cleared rapidly. On the tenth day of life, there is "compression" atelectasis of the right upper lobe and the right lower lobe. It should be noted that, when roentgenograms are a bit darker than shown, the lower lobe density due to downward but chiefly posterior displacement and compression is often missed. The distribution of ^{133}xenon, a radioactive gas, after it was inhaled and exhaled by this infant, is shown in Figure 19-26, C and D. There is a suggestion of a defect in the middle lobe region during the inhalation phase in Figure 19-26C and clear evi-

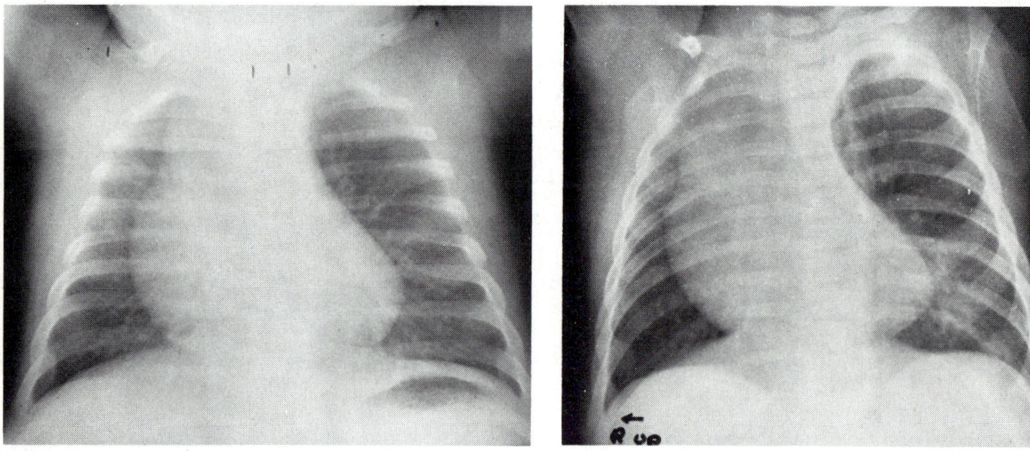

A B

FIG. 19-25. *A*, Essentially normal film in a child diagnosed as having left upper lobe emphysema. Apparent mediastinal shift is due to rotation.

B, With patient in the left decubitus position, air-trapping in the left upper lobe becomes evident.

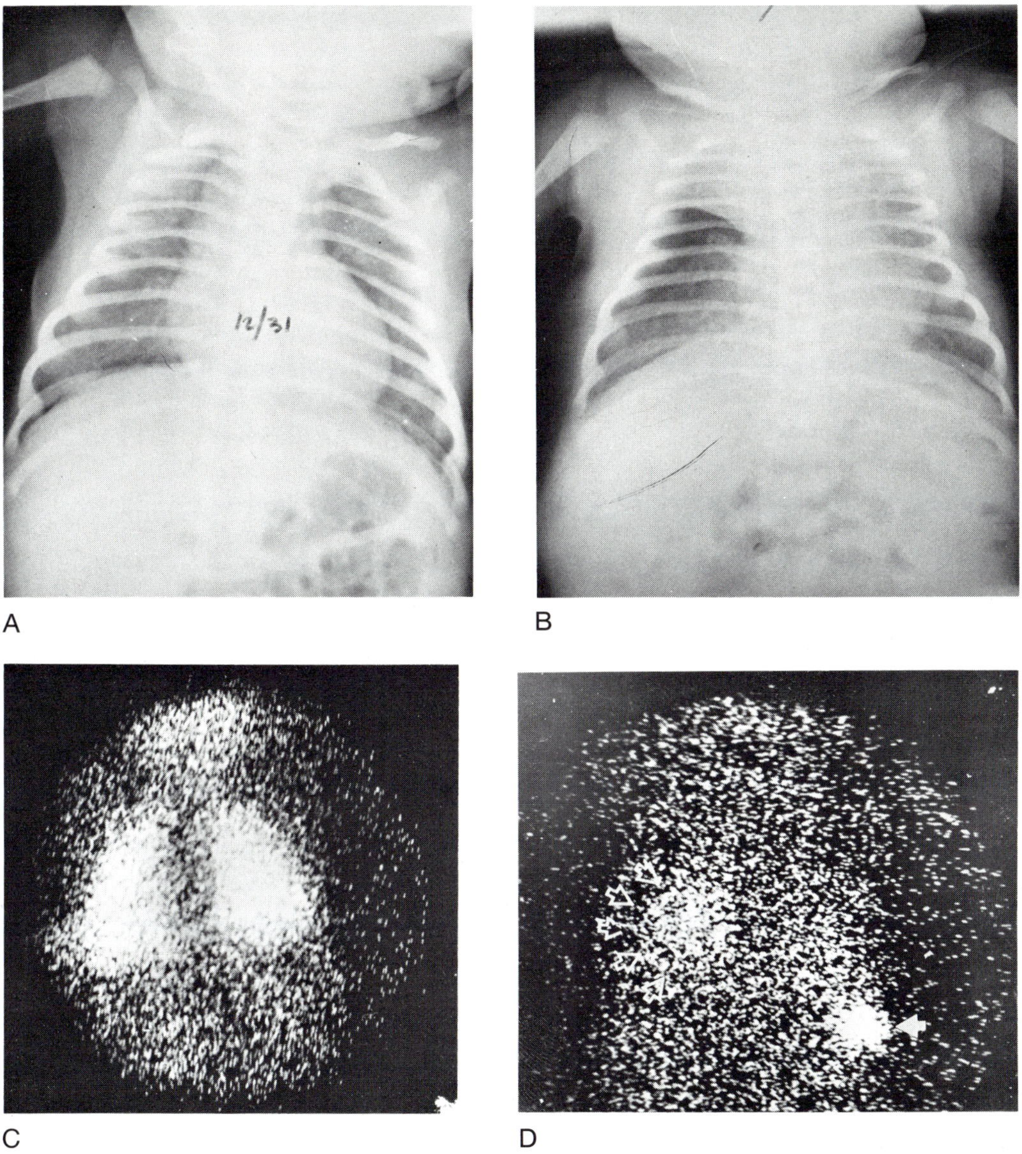

FIG. 19-26. *A*, Newborn on day 1 with essentially normal roentgenogram except for minimal pneumothorax on the left, which resolved quickly.

B, On day 10, with increasing respiratory distress, middle lobar emphysema is seen; air-trapping causes compression atelectasis of adjacent lobes.

C, With infant in the supine position, a posterior image during inhalation of ^{133}Xenon gas in air shows suggestion of delay of entry to the middle lobe (ordinarily studied better with anterior position).

D, After "washout," ^{133}Xenon was cleared from the lungs, except for the right middle lobe (open arrows). Radioactive source marks lower rib cage on the left (solid arrow).

dence of residual radioactivity after the remainder of the lung has cleared (Figure 19-26D). This situation indicates only that the middle lobe is ventilated less well than the rest of the lung. It does not indicate that ventilation is normal elsewhere, and it does not specify that the cause of the decreased ventilation is an obstruction. The usefulness of the method in the present state of its development would seem to be in the detection of regional abnormal ventilation where standard roentgenographic methods show no abnormality.[31,70] More experience and improved methods for interpretation of data are needed before the role of radioactive gases as a diagnostic tool in evaluating abnormalities of the lung in children is clearly defined.

On occasion, the presence of a right upper lobe atelectasis raises the question of compression by an enlarged middle or lower lobe that may be air-trapping. Although a radioactive gas study may resolve the problem, an even simpler mode can be used: the *decubitus film.* Left and right decubitus films (Fig. 19-27, A and B) show normal decompression of the right lower lung and indicate that the right upper lobe atelectasis is due to some other cause, in this case, a mucous plug in the upper lobe bronchus.

In another patient, an increase in radiolucency (Fig. 19-28A) again suggests loss of vascular markings, and a radionuclide microsphere (albumin) perfusion study indicated a marked decrease in blood flow to the area (not shown). A subsequent ^{133}xenon inhalation study indicated a primary problem of ventilation, as shown in Figure 19-28, B and C. Figure 19-28D shows data that are retrieved continuously from the left and right upper lung fields during the examination. Figure 19-28E, a tomogram of the bronchi, shows calcification in the bronchus to the upper lung, after division of the lingular branch. The calcification was in inspissated mucous behind a foreign body—a tooth. Neither this 7-year-old boy nor his parents remembered the episode in which the tooth was aspirated.

A similar picture is seen in Figure 19-29A

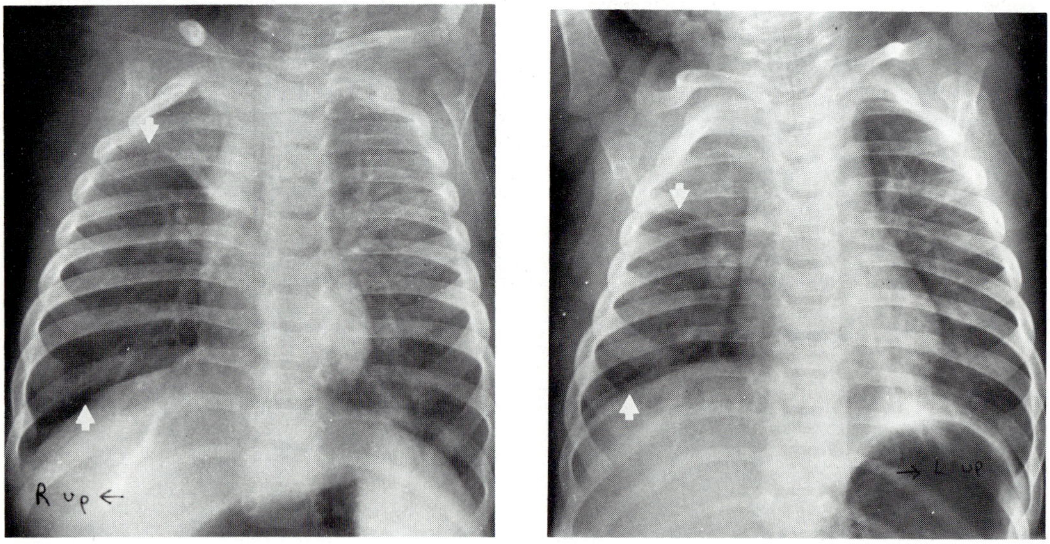

A B

FIG. 19-27. Left (A) and right (B) decubitus positions showing right upper lobe atelectasis. The marked change in volume of the region of the middle and lower lobe indicates that no air-trapping of either lobe accounts for right upper lobe atelectasis.

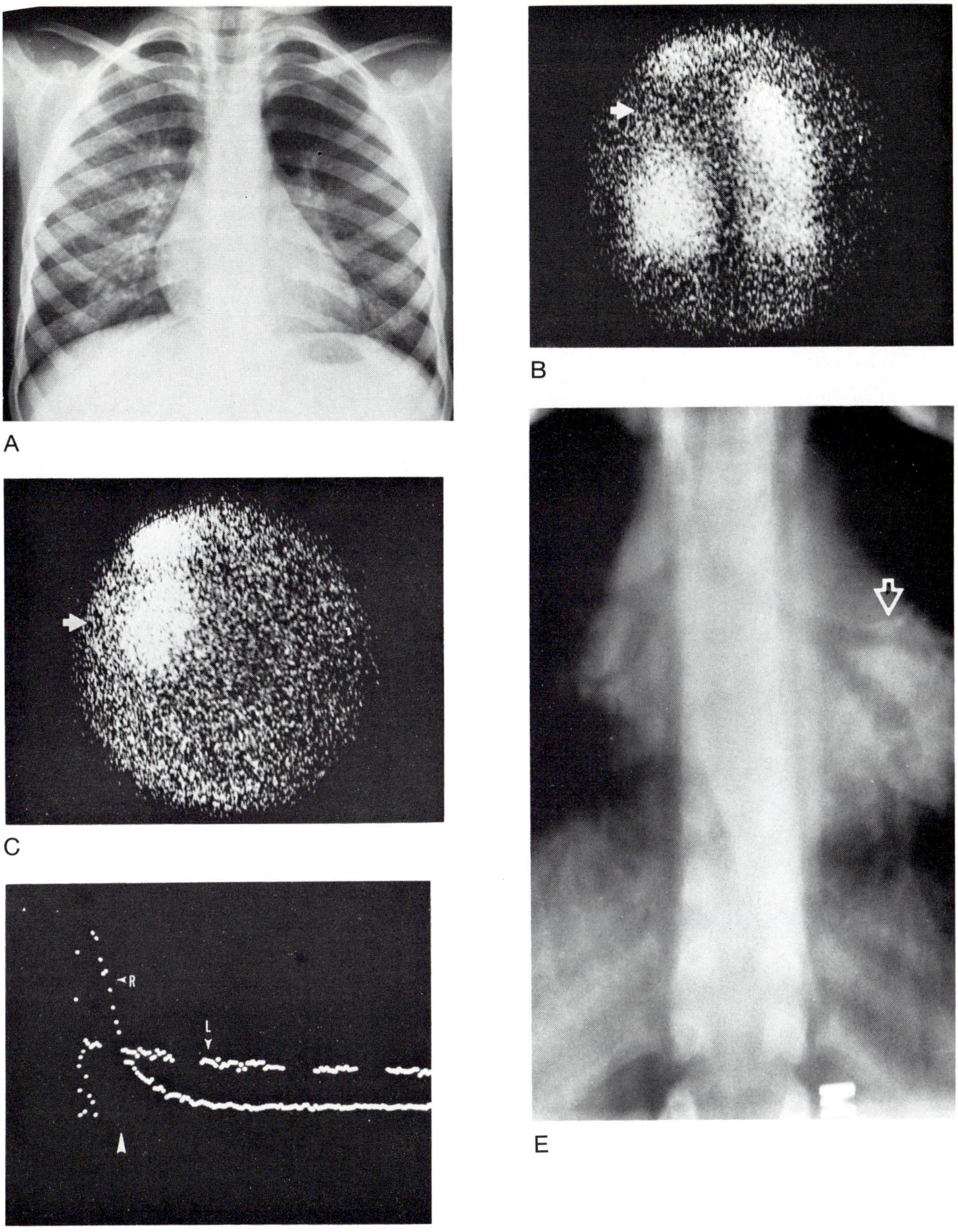

FIG. 19-28. *A,* Essentially asymptomatic 7-year-old boy, whose roentgenogram shows a relative increase in blackening of the left upper chest due to a decrease in vessels; radionuclide perfusion study showed a marked decrease in flow to the upper lung. Roentgenograms taken at end expiration showed no air trapping.

B, ^{133}Xenon is delayed in entering the left upper lung (arrow) during inhalation.

C, Residual radioactivity is present in the left upper lung (arrow) after washout indicating slow ventilation of the left upper lobe.

D, Demonstration of recording of relative level of radioactivity in the upper lung fields. Left upper lobe (L) shows less activity and slower clearance than right (R). Arrow indicates the beginning of washout.

E, Tomogram shows calcification in the upper lobe divisional bronchus (arrow); the lingular branch is not obstructed and the lower lobe division is normal.

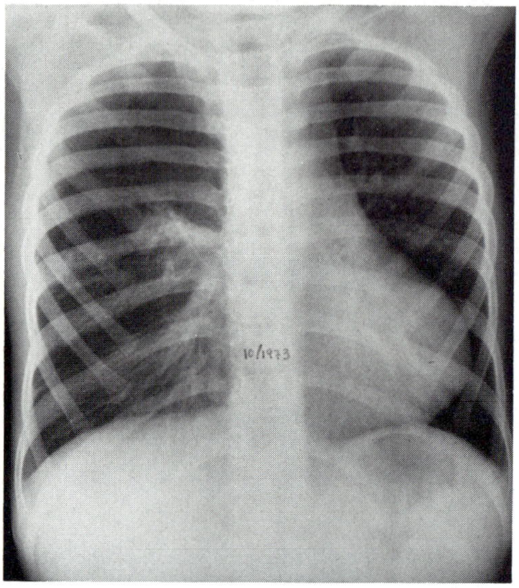

A

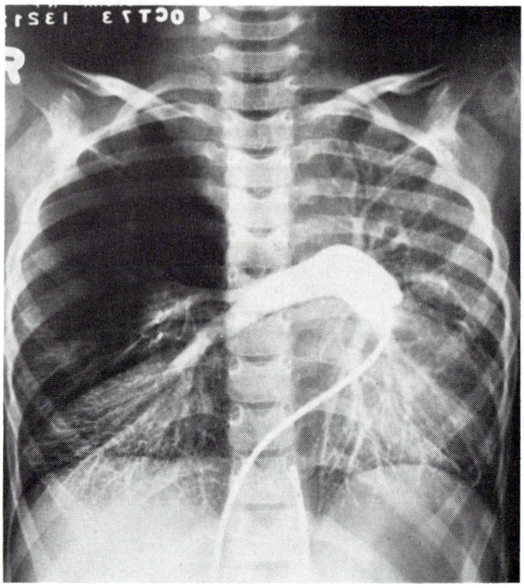

B

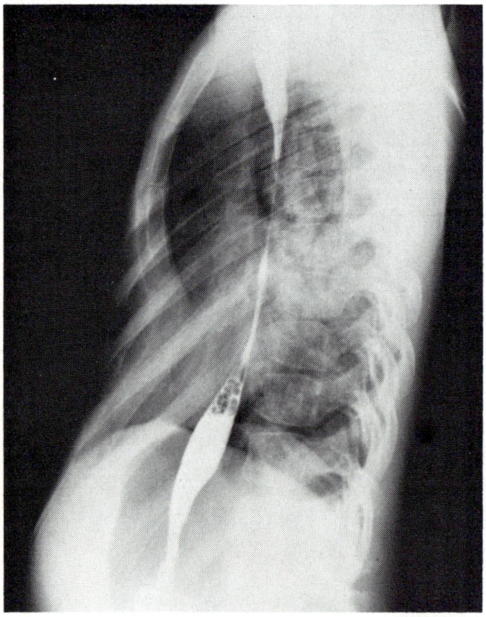

C

FIG. 19-29. *A*, *B*, Patient with stenosis of the right upper lobe bronchus shows a decrease in vascular markings in the right upper lung and expansion of the right upper lobe causing crowding of vascular markings in the middle and lower lobes. Pulmonary arteriogram confirms these observations.

C, Pectus excavatum is responsible for the shift of the heart to the left seen in A, B.

which shows loss of vascular markings due to *stenosis* of the right upper lobe bronchus. No foreign body was found however. A pulmonary arteriogram (Fig. 19-29B) demonstrates that the visible lung markings on the plain film are indeed vascular. Radionuclide studies (not shown) showed decreased blood flow and ventilation in the right upper lung. The shift of the heart to the left and the loss of the right heart border are due to severe pectus excavatum[25] (see Fig. 19-29). Note also the characteristic configuration of the ribs on the plain film.

AIR-TRAPPING DUE TO EXTRINSIC CAUSES

Although the child shown in Figure 19-30 also had severe pectus excavatum, the mediastinum paradoxically was shifted to the right. A thin-walled *bronchogenic cyst*[24] obstructed the bronchus to the apical-posterior segment of the left upper lobe, and this large incompressible lung segment shifted the heart to the right. The density seen at end-expiration in the left lower lung because of the crowded blood vessels is relieved in the right decubitus position (Fig. 19-30). Tomograms of the airway (not shown) showed that the upper lobe bronchus (before its segmental division) and the lower lobe bronchus were normal.

Plain film examination of the next case (Fig. 19-31) would suggest again a cyst with compression of a bronchus (without the chest deformity of a pectus excavatum). However, it is a case of *atresia of the bronchus* of the apical posterior segment of the left upper lobe. Presumably the segment remains "aerated" by means of collateral ventilation. The mass, which here contains a fluid level, is actually the widely dilated bronchus distal to the atresia. It is filled with mucus and secretions. A bronchogram (not shown) could not differentiate this lesion from others that produce complete obstruction since contrast material did not get into the segment. Bronchial atresia is most commonly found in the apical-posterior segment of the left upper lobe[61] but may occasionally be encountered in other segments.

An *esophagogram* should be done as part of the work-up when evidence of obstruction of the lung exists but the cause is unknown. In Figure 19-32, the esophagus is displaced to the right and posteriorly by a mediastinal bronchogenic cyst. The chest roentgenogram showed a decrease in vascular markings in the left upper lung and slight forward displacement of the trachea. Aberrant vessels may be discovered as shown in the case of right-sided origin of the left pulmonary artery.[6] The left pulmonary artery produces an anterior indentation on the esophagus as it courses from the right side to the left lung (see Fig. 6-18).

A unique presentation of the problem in the newborn (Fig. 19-33) is shown by the roentgenograms taken at 4 hours (Fig. 19-33A) and at 14 hours (Fig. 19-33B) of age. There is enlargement of the right lung on both films; the abnormal roentgen density seen at 4 hours is related to slow clearance of the fetal pulmonary fluid[32,62] resulting from obstruction of the right main bronchus by an *ectopic left pulmonary artery.* On occasion, the esophagogram is not diagnostic, and a pulmonary arteriogram may have to be done.

Another example of obstruction causing mediastinal shift and slow clearing of fetal pulmonary fluid is shown in Figure 19-34. This time the cause is compression of the bronchus by aneurysmal enlargement of the pulmonary artery associated with congenital *absence of the pulmonary valve.*

Hilar node enlargement due to *tuberculosis* caused a decrease in vascular markings and enlargement of the lung on the left in Figure 19-35, suggesting air-trapping.[69] These observations indicate encroachment on the bronchus and possibly endobronchial involvement. Radionuclide perfusion study (not shown) confirmed that blood flow was reduced. Radionuclide ventilation examination was not done until 3 months later, following treatment, at which time the ventilation study, the chest roentgenogram, and a repeat perfusion scintigram were all normal.

PERIPHERAL OBSTRUCTIVE DISEASE

Obliterative bronchiolitis with septal destruction due to infection may cause a lung or a lobe to appear enlarged in expiration (or in the decubitus position), and demonstrate a decrease in vascular markings. The condition is known as the *Swyer-James syndrome.*[26,49,66] The involvement is uneven. Distortion of the lung markings results from scarring. The child in Figure 19-36 demonstrates these roentgenographic changes. Although the radionuclide perfusion study shows reduction in blood flow, the pulmonary arteriogram is remarkably normal. The pulmonary artery anatomy appears normal because a pressure injection was made directly into the pulmonary artery. On the other hand, the radionuclide injection was

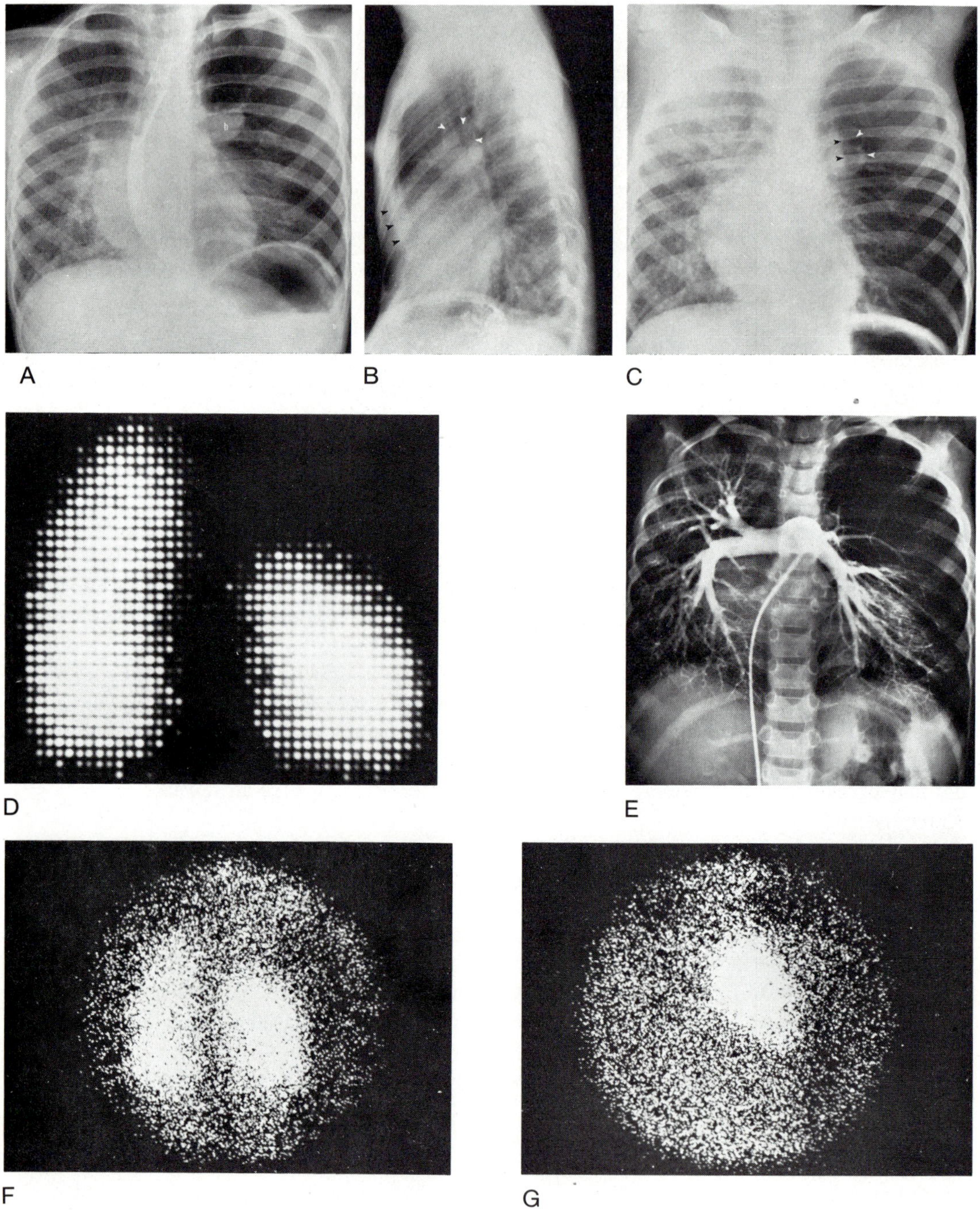

FIG. 19-30. *A*, Bronchogenic cyst (b) causing obstruction of the left upper lobe bronchus and "air-trapping" in the upper lobe. Compression atelectasis is present in the left lower lobe.

B, Thin wall of the cyst is demonstrated (white arrows). Pectus excavatum (black arrows), narrowing the chest, causes the shift of the heart to the right in this case because of the presence of the incompressible left upper lobe.

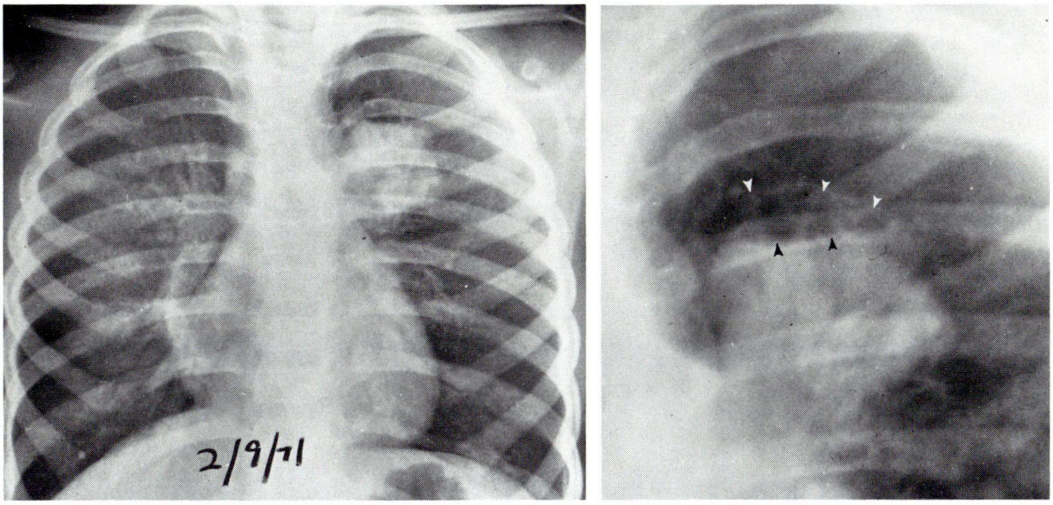

FIG. 19-31. *A*, Atresia of the bronchus of the apical posterior segment of the left upper lobe. The mass, which looks like a bronchogenic cyst, is the dilated bronchus distal to the atresia. It is filled with inspissated mucus.

B, Enlarged view shows the thin wall (white arrows) of the dilated bronchus, which also contains fluid (black arrows). Descending between the two black arrows is a tubular structure oriented vertically and representing a branch of the segmental bronchus packed with thick mucus. (Courtesy of Dr. George Kassner, State University of New York (S.U.N.Y.), Downstate Medical Center, Brooklyn, New York.)

made in a peripheral vein, and more accurately reflects the actual distribution of blood flow. A bronchogram was taken, and fluoroscopic spot films made during inspiration and expiration reveal marked tapering beyond the tertiary bronchi and lack of filling of the smaller radicles beyond the fifth generation. The major difference in inspiration and expiration is that the first three generations are cylindrically dilated during inspiration and compressed during expiration. Obstructive changes are peripheral to the bronchi, which are seen in Figure 19-36, D and E.

LARGE LUNGS

The diagnosis of "hyperaerated lungs" can be imprecise from the perspective of pathophysiology, though it carries fairly clear meaning because of common usage in terms of

---

C, Right decubitus position expands the left lower lobe. Bronchogenic cyst (white arrows) contains a fluid lever (black arrows).

D, Radionuclide perfusion study shows marked reduction in blood flow to the left upper lobe with no detectable difference in the lower lobes despite the presence of compression atelectasis of the left lower lobe.

E, Pulmonary arteriogram shows normal opacification of the arteries, which are diminished in size and spread in the left upper lobe while they are of normal size and crowded in the left lower lobe.

F, Radionuclide ventilation study (^{133}Xenon) shows a delay of entry of the radioactive gas into the left upper lobe during the inhalation phase; Notice that although the left lower lobe is reduced in volume, ventilation seems about the same as in the right lower lobe.

G, Residual radioactivity appears in the left upper lobe after washout. The study indicates decreased (slow) ventilation of the left upper lobe.

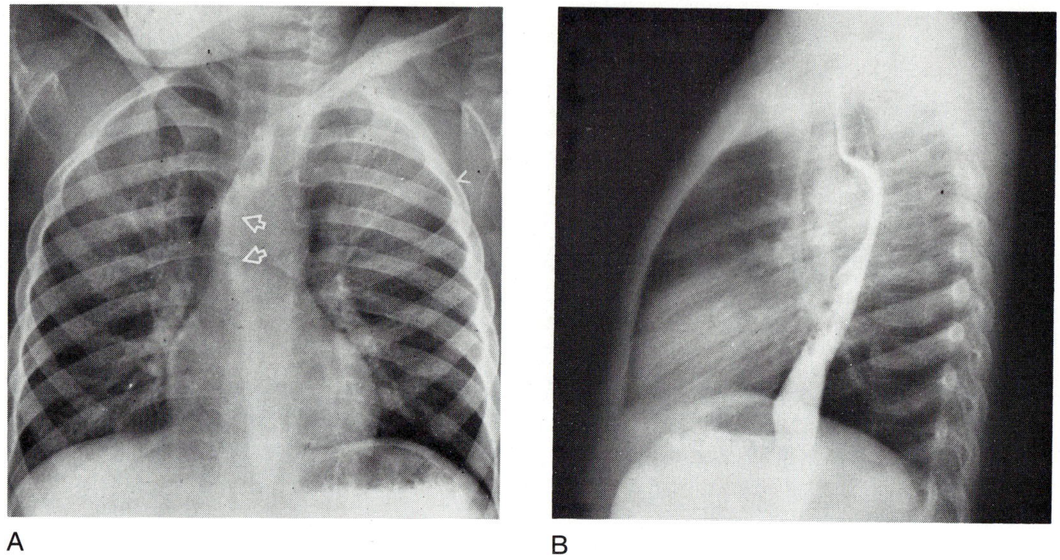

FIG. 19-32. *A*, Mediastinal bronchogenic cyst, not seen in frontal roentgenogram, displaces esophagus around it (arrows).

B, Lateral view in which the esophagus is displaced posteriorly with only minimal anterior displacement of trachea. Child was wheezing. (Courtesy of Dr. Walter Berdon, Babies Hospital, New York, New York.)

the roentgenogram. It means large and hyperlucent lungs. The diagnosis of "hyperlucency" is subject to error because of technical factors (e.g., high contrast films or overexposed films). Perhaps, a more useful classification would include the use of the terms "normal," "large," and "small" lungs. The definition of lung size should take into account the phase of ventilation, e.g., end-inspiration and end-expiration. For clinical purposes, the lung size is often assessed on the basis of experience, using the shape and position of the diaphragms and the position of the ribs as the essential landmarks. For example, normally, flattened diaphragms suggest that the diaphragm has contracted and that therefore the roentgenogram was made during inspiration, whereas the diaphragm exhibits a rounded, convex-upward configuration at end-expiration. Evaluation of the phase of respiration could be more objective and precise if, for example, film exposure were triggered electronically at some predetermined phase. Accurate measurements of lung size can be made from the conventional roentgenogram. These methods correlate well with other standard methods of lung volume measurement.[4,45]

Any discussion of the causes of "large" lungs invariably includes asthma, the most important chronic pulmonary disease of children. Ordinarily, roentgenograms are obtained in the acute situation in order to rule out the presence of a major area of localized obstruction due to a mucous plug and to exclude the possibility of clinically significant pneumothorax. When the patient is examined during or shortly after an acute attack, the lungs are usually symmetrically enlarged. The diaphragms are flattened, the anterior chest wall bulges, and the ribs are elevated. These changes result from peripheral airway collapse, obstruction, and constriction, which lead to air-trapping. Other changes may also be present.

(1) Segmental or subsegmental areas of atelectasis are peripherally located, and are wedge-shaped or linear in appearance in one of the views taken. Presumably, these areas

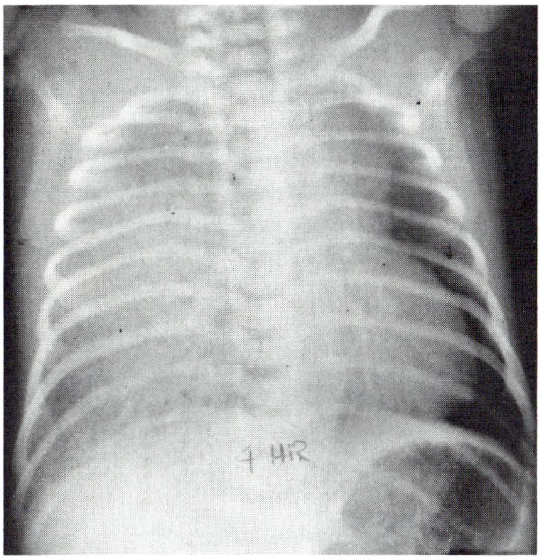

A

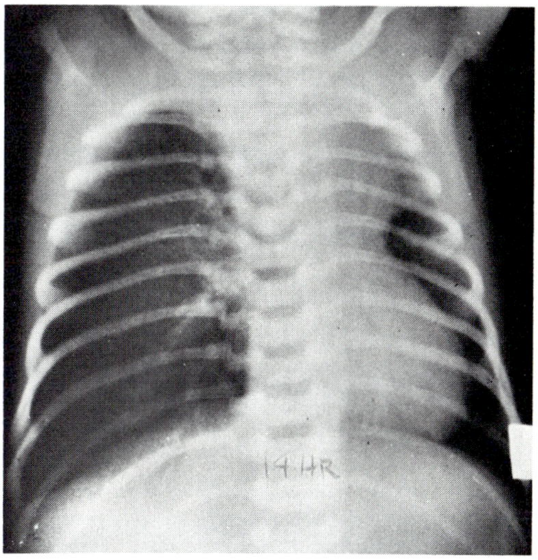

B

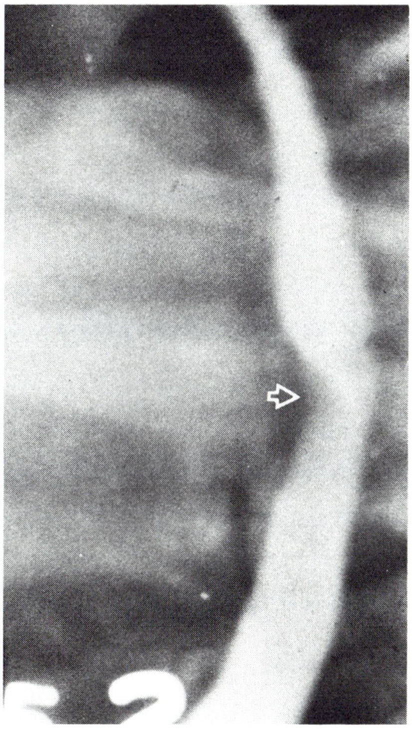

C

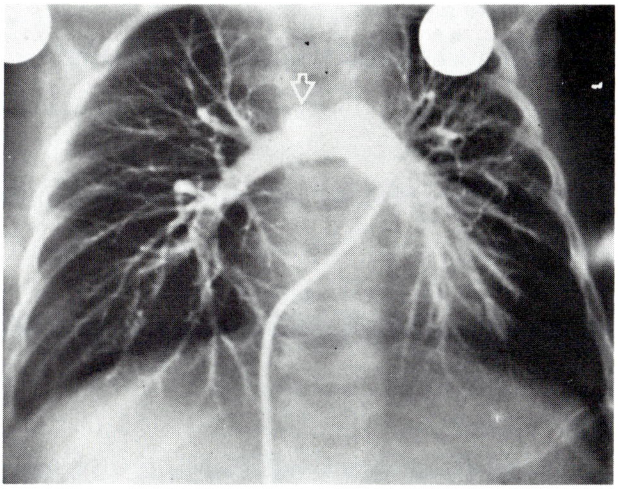

D

FIG. 19-33. *A*, *B*, Ectopic (right-sided) origin of the left pulmonary artery causes air-trapping of the right lung because the artery compresses the right bronchus. It also causes retention of fetal pulmonary fluid, seen to opacify the lung at 4 hours (A), then clear slowly so that the lung is both enlarged and hyperlucent at 14 hours (B).

C, Diagnosis is made by finding an indentation on the anterior aspect of the esophagus (arrow) caused by the left pulmonary artery as it courses from right to left.

D, Pulmonary arteriography shows the typical location of the origin of the ectopic artery (arrow). (Courtesy of Dr. Jack Korsower, Washington, D.C.)

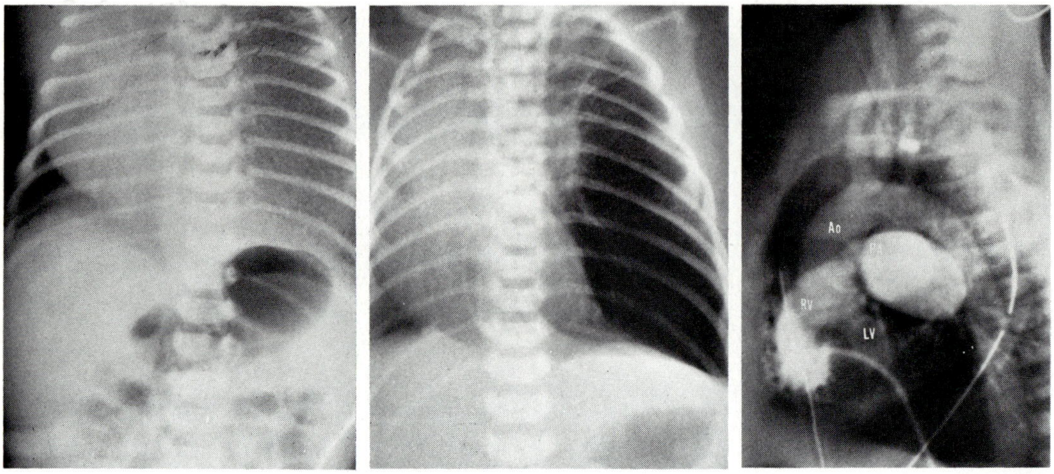

A B C

FIG. 19-34. Massive pulmonary artery dilatation due to congenital absence of the pulmonary valve caused obstruction of the left bronchus. Air-trapping and fetal pulmonary fluid "trapping" appear on the left (A) with clearance of the fluid after 24 hours (B).

C, Lateral roentgenogram made during angiocardiography. The injection was made into the right ventricle (RV) with immediate opacification of the left ventricle (LV) through a ventricular septal defect. With systole both the aorta (Ao) and a huge pulmonary artery (PA) are opacified. The position of the left main bronchus is just inferior to the pulmonary artery (left). (Courtesy of Dr. O. Robert Levine and Dr. James Marquis, Newark, N.J.) (From Levine, O., J. R. Antillon and B. Lauton: Fallot's tetralogy with pulmonary arterial aneurysm. J. Med. Soc. N.J. *72*:839, 1975.)

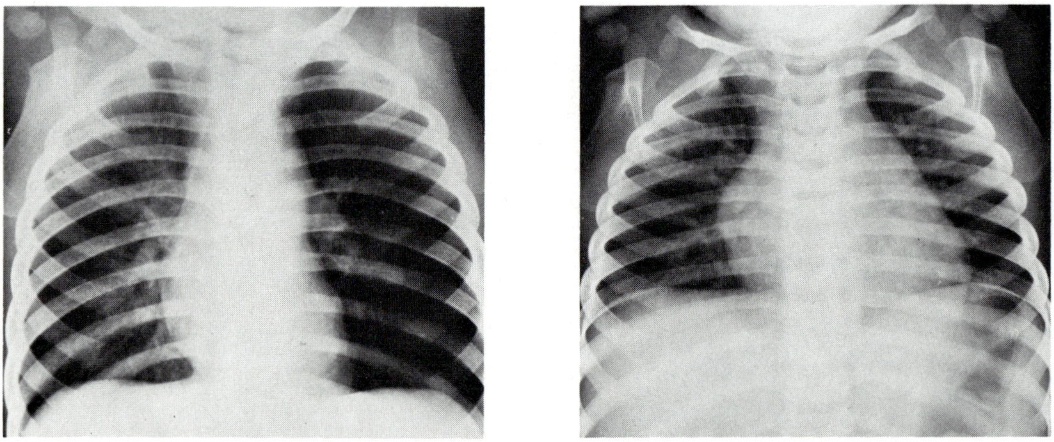

A B

FIG. 19-35. *A*, Primary tuberculosis with left hilar node enlargement causing compression of the left bronchus, resulting in enlargement of the left lung and a decrease in vascularity. Radionuclide perfusion study (not shown) showed a severe reduction in blood flow to the left lung.

B, After 3 months of appropriate therapy, the chest roentgenogram made at end-expiration was normal. Radionuclide perfusion and ventilation studies (not shown) were normal.

occur due to mucous plugging. They are usually present transiently and should not be diagnosed as areas of pneumonia.

(2) A mucous plug in a segmental bronchus, wherein aeration of the segment is sustained by collateral ventilation, may be mistaken for a blood vessel.

(3) Bronchial wall thickening, characteristically described as "tram-line" in appearance, is indicative of bronchial or peribronchial involvement in the disease. The association of peribronchial thickening with reticular pattern densities and septal lines in asthma supports the notion of an important interstitial component in this disease. It cannot be determined by roentgenographic means whether the interstitial process is due to infection or edema.

Figure 19-37, the roentgenogram of a child who had a chronic history of *asthma,* was made during an acute attack. The infant with acute *bronchiolitis* in Figure 19-38 has numerous areas of plate and wedge-shaped atelectasis, as well as large lungs, which bulge at the apex. Roentgenographically, pneumonia cannot be diagnosed though it may be presumed to be present on a clinical basis.

Figure 19-39 is a film of a 4-month-old child with *cystic fibrosis.*[71] The heart has enlarged and there is clinical evidence of cor pulmonale. The obstructive pulmonary disease could explain the large lungs on the basis of air-trapping. However, the child in Figure 19-40 is a 2-week-old infant with a left-to-right shunt due to a ventricular septal defect. The lungs are seen to have enlarged at 2 months of age at the time that the infant's heart decompensated. The large lung size is related to the respiratory distress of heart

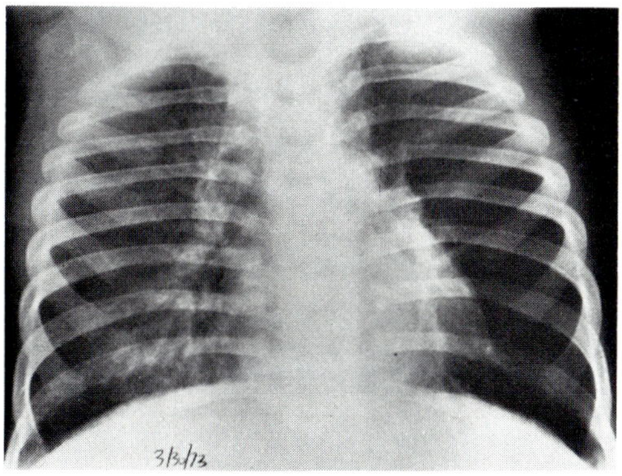

A

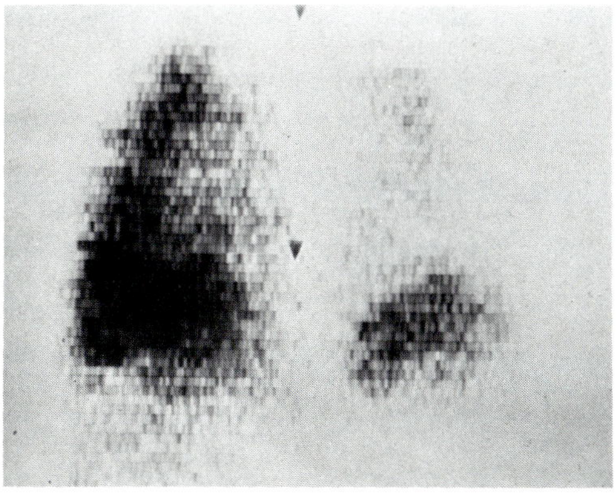

B

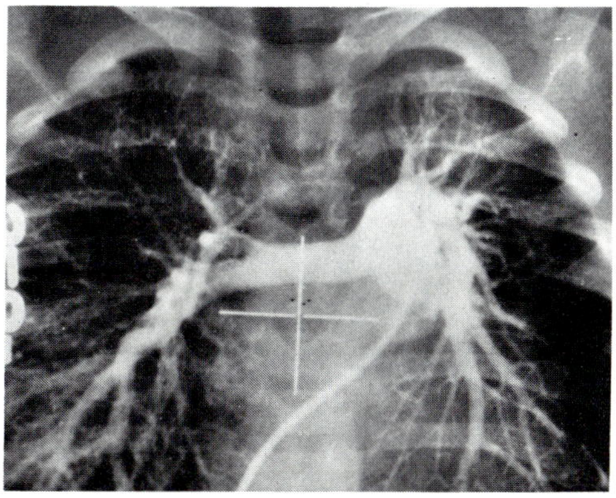

C

FIG. 19-36. *A*, The Swyer-James syndrome. The decrease in vascularity results in a hyperlucent lung. The lung is air-trapping and does not reduce in size after expiration.

B, Radionuclide perfusion study shows irregular reduction in blood flow. A ventilation study, if it were done, would show a marked reduction in ventilation.

C, Pulmonary arteriography shows opacification of the vessels because of the injection pressure into the pulmonary artery.

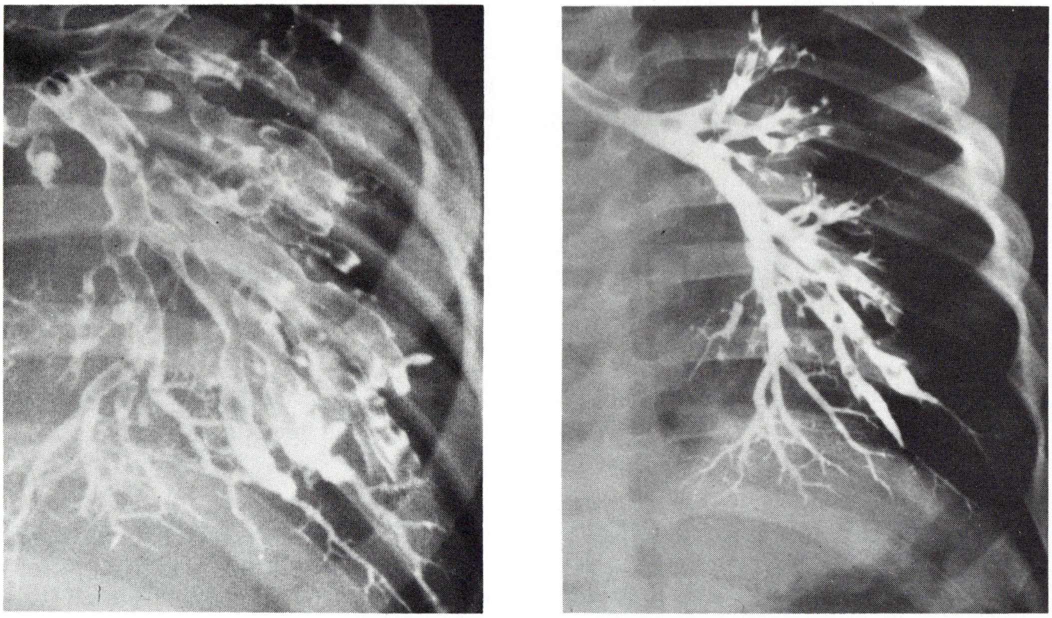

D E

D, *E*, Bronchogram. Inspiration (D) and expiration (E) films show the larger bronchi to alter markedly in size and contour due to an increase in compliance with bronchial wall injury. Beyond the fourth generation, the bronchi are relatively rigidly fixed by scarring. The more peripheral generations did not fill. (Courtesy of Dr. George Kassner, S.U.N.Y., Downstate Medical Center, Brooklyn, New York.)

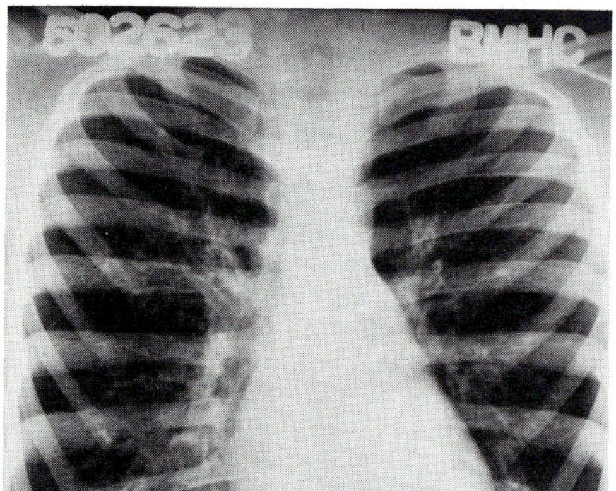

FIG. 19-37. Asthma. Large lungs with an increase in central markings and peribronchial thickening. Conical or wedge-shaped density in right lower lung is a typical finding and is probably related to mucous plugging of segmental bronchi. It usually disappears within 48 hours and is often mistaken for pneumonia.

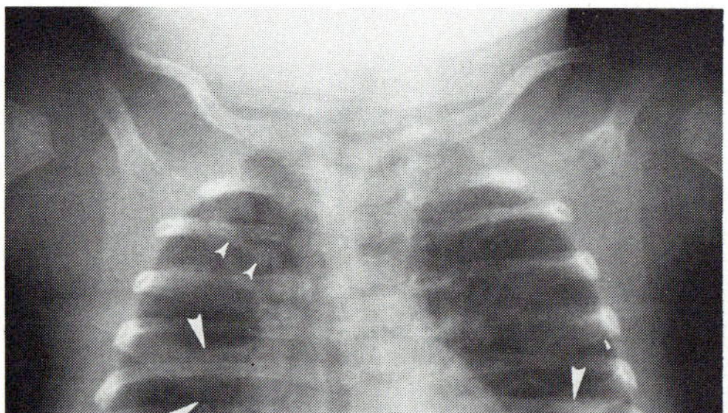

FIG. 19-38. Bronchiolitis. Large lungs with many areas of segmental atelectasis (large arrows) and subsegmental or plate atelectasis (small arrows).

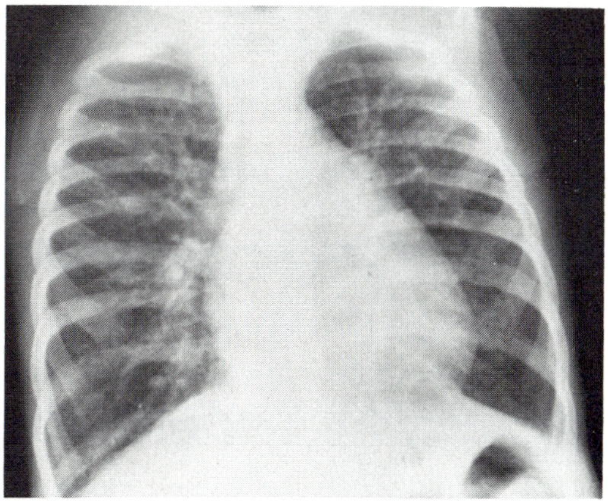

FIG. 19-39. Cystic fibrosis. Four-month-old child with cor pulmonale. The roentgenographic findings of large lungs, prominent hilar structures, and cardiomegaly are suggestive of the diagnosis at this age. The changes of hilar adenopathy and chronic infectious and obstructive lung disease are usually seen in an older child.

failure. The lateral roentgenogram in this child best illustrates the change in the contour of the diaphragm when it was normal (at 2 weeks) and when the lungs became large (at 2 months); the frontal film failed to exhibit this change. In the infant, the anterior third of the diaphragm does not move very much; it is the posterior part of the diaphragm that flattens obliquely downward when it contracts. Since it is the peak of the unmoving anterior part of the diaphragm that is seen in the frontal view, it is understandable that the lateral view would be best for assessing lung volume. Large lungs may be an expression of an altered pattern of breathing due to respiratory distress in the infant and often may exist for reasons other than air-trapping. Indeed, occasionally large lungs may be seen in the infant in respiratory distress with tetralogy of Fallot (Fig. 19-41) or metabolic acidosis due to kidney disease.

Nowhere, however, is this so clearly expressed as in the newborn with *respiratory distress syndrome* (i.e., hyaline membrane disease). This disease, in its most extreme form (Fig. 19-42A), causes such severe atelectasis that the lung is virtually airless; note that the stomach gas bubble has risen to the seventh rib, the diaphragm being above that. The same disease (a different child in Fig. 19-42B) in its milder form causes the lungs to appear significantly larger than normal. The roentgenographic evidence for respiratory distress syndrome in this child is the reticular pattern seen best in the right lower lung field with a suggestion of an air bronchogram associated. Whereas the lung enlargement is not a predictable result of a surfactant deficiency, it is probably related to an adaptive response of the child's breathing pattern to the respiratory distress produced by the basic defect.

On the other hand, the lung size of a newborn with benign *idiopathic slow clearing of fetal pulmonary fluid* is normal. The chest roentgenogram (Fig. 19-43) showed puffy and streaky densities, which cleared within a few days. The child whose chest roentgenogram is seen in Figure 19-44 had evidence of *meconium aspiration* on direct inspection of the larynx and was in severe respiratory distress; the lungs are large. This condition again illustrates that, whereas the presence of symmetrically enlarged lungs might suggest obstructive airway disease, one must consider this condition as an adaptive response to respiratory distress, particularly in the infant.

SMALL LUNGS

Congenital absence of the lung[22] (Fig. 19-45) must be differentiated from atelectases (see also p. 608–610 or 608ff). The diagnosis can be made by (1) the absence of a bronchus on proper airway films, (2) the absence of evidence of pulmonary arterial blood flow on a radionuclide perfusion study, and/or (3) the absence of a pulmonary artery on angiography (with the injection made into the pulmonary artery). All three conditions were met in this child (Fig. 19-45; see also Fig. 6-69). However, a very small lung that is poorly aerated may be a cause for confusion (Fig.

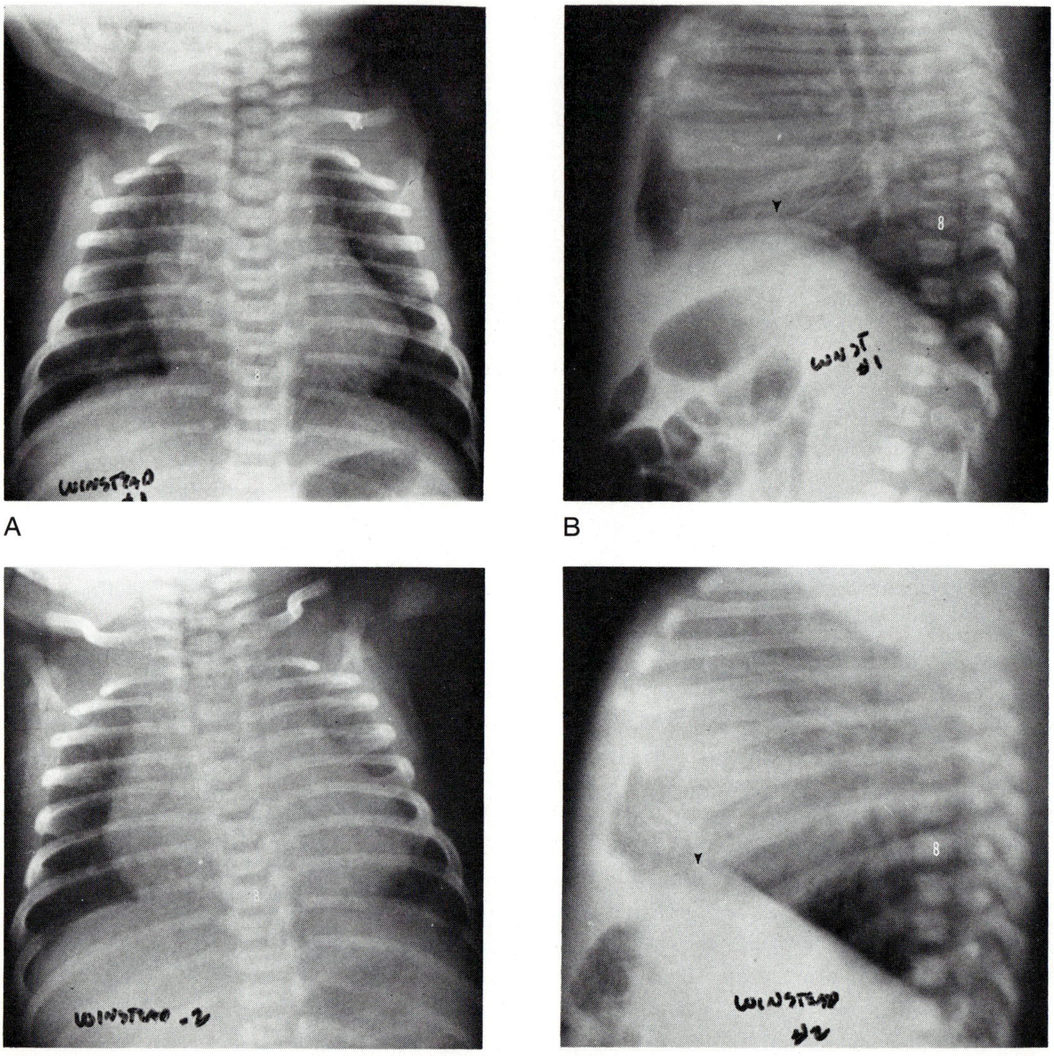

FIG. 19-40. Infant who, at 2 weeks of age (A, B), exhibits mild cardiomegaly because of a ventricular septal defect. At 2 months of age (C, D), heart failure ensues and cardiomegaly increases. In frontal view (A, C), diaphragms are at T-8; however in lateral views (B, D), the posterior part of diaphragm descends and flattens, thus enlarging the lungs. The anterior part of the diaphragm remains at about T-8. The lungs enlarge in response to the respiratory distress produced by heart failure.

19-46). In this case, a foregut malformation,[28] a very small lung originated from the lower esophagus. In other cases, both lungs may arise from the esophagus, and the size of these lungs can vary: the diagnosis can be suspected if one can demonstrate that the origin of the air-filled bronchi is lower than normal. In Figure 19-46, A and B the right main bronchus is missing at the level of the carina but a few air-filled bronchi can be detected in the right lower thorax. More commonly, this anomaly involves a single

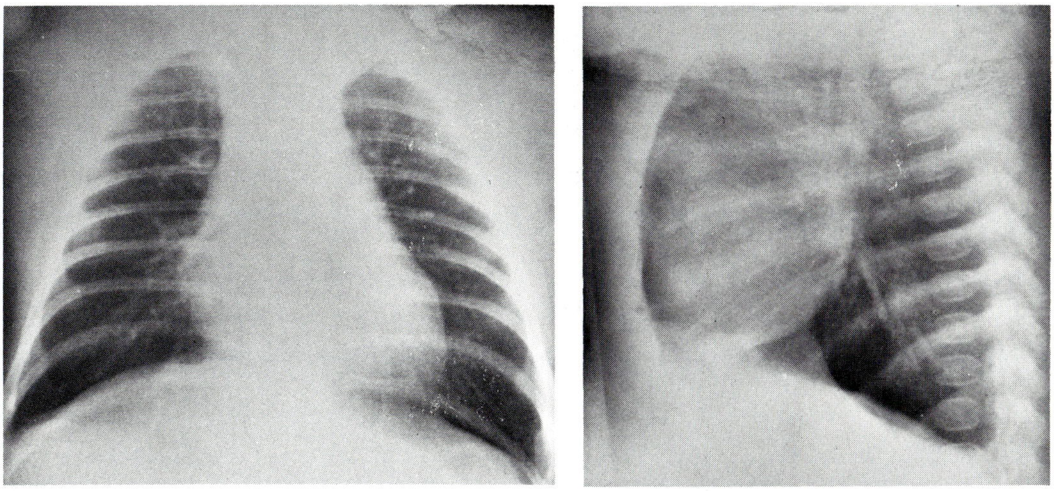

A B

FIG. 19-41. Infant with tetralogy of Fallot with large lungs. No clinical evidence of pulmonary disease was present.

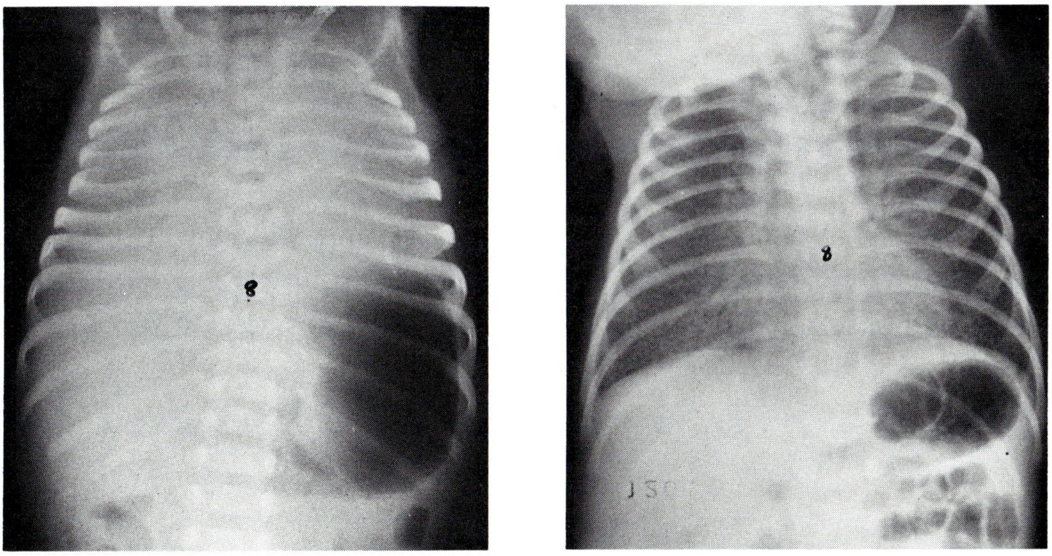

A B

FIG. 19-42. *A*, Respiratory distress syndrome, severe. The lungs are very small because of atelectasis. Note that the stomach bubble is at the seventh rib. The diaphragm is usually found at the eighth rib.

B, Respiratory distress syndrome, mild. The lungs are larger than those of the normal newborn. There is no evidence for atelectasis; the reticular pattern present is probably related to retained fetal pulmonary fluid due to the presumed surfactant deficiency.

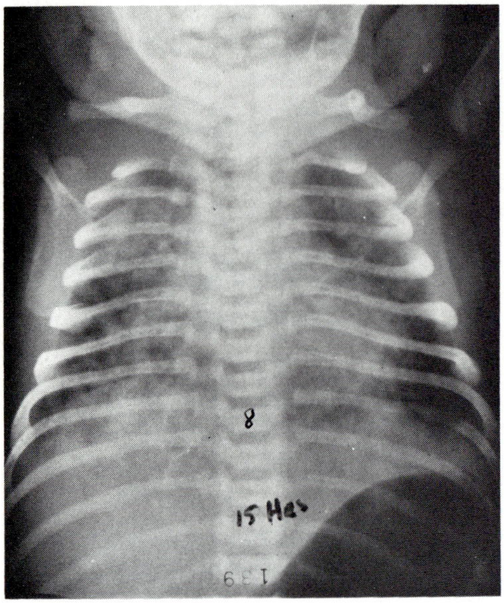

FIG. 19-43. Idiopathic retention of fetal pulmonary fluid. This 15-hour-old infant with transient tachypnea exhibits normal lung size and puffy and streaky lung densities. These densities cleared in 36 hours; improvement in tachypnea was noted at 24 hours of age.

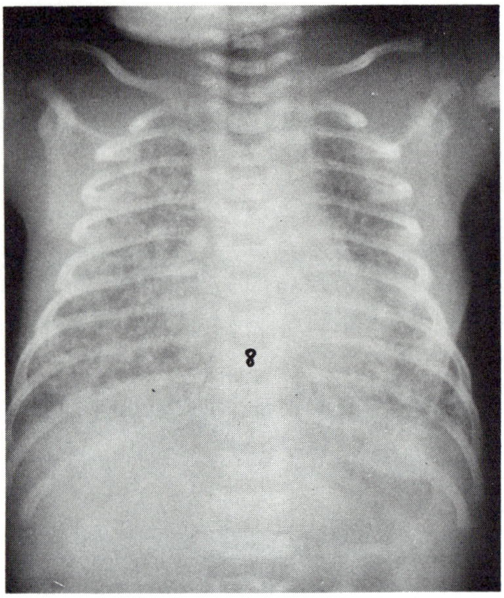

FIG. 19-44. Meconium aspiration syndrome. Typical picture of symmetrical opacification of the lungs with some linear components. Mild cardiomegaly exists, and the lungs are larger than normal; the diaphragms are down to the ninth rib. Much of the density is probably due to retained pulmonary fetal fluid.

lobe and presents as a localized density in the lower thorax since the other lobes are normal. The diagnosis in this case (Fig. 19-46) was made by serendipity: an esophagogram was done because of the "routine" procedure established for the investigation of obstruction of unknown etiology (see p. 619), and the bronchus to the *esophageal lung* filled with barium.

Congenital "smallness" of one lung may be due to hypoplasia of the whole lung or to abnormal development of the segments or lobes, with absence of a lobe or segment accounting for the diminished volume. The recognition of abnormal or unusual fissures in the presence of reduced lung volume would suggest a developmental abnormality of this kind. Hypoplasia (see p. 432) is an error in development that seems to be associated, in various combinations, with errors in blood vessel formation, with errors in airway formation, and possibly with errors in lymphatic

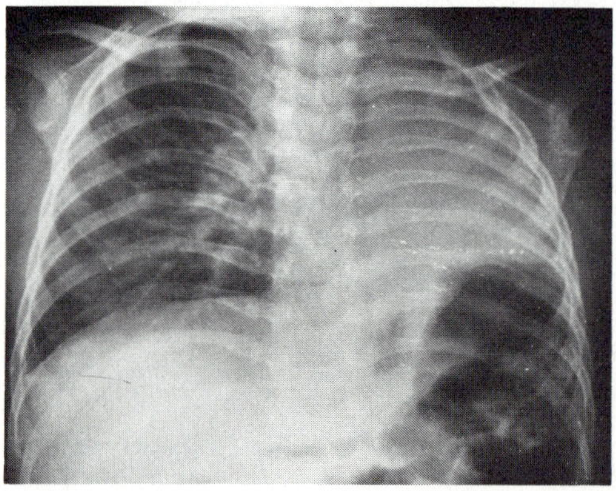

FIG. 19-45. Congenital absence of the lung. No left bronchus exists. Angiocardiography (not shown) showed no pulmonary artery on the left.

development. Recognition of an abnormal vascular pattern is of diagnostic value in this regard. An anomalous pulmonary vein draining to the inferior vena cava is seen in a child (Fig. 19-47) with a small right lung. This

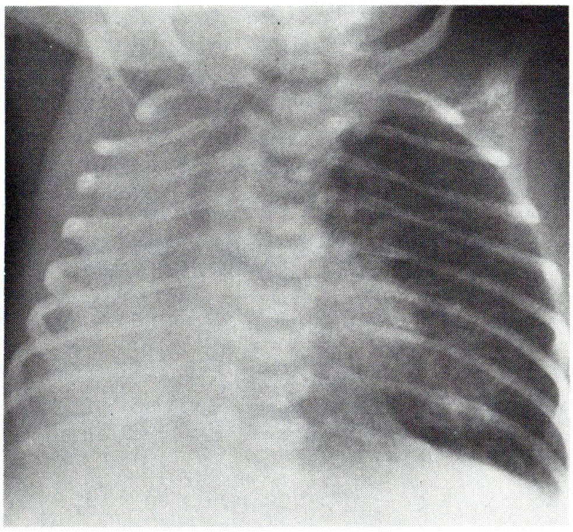

A

FIG. 19-46. *A*, Hypoplasia of the right lung with esophageal origin of the lung. The right bronchus is apparently absent.

B, Esophagogram. Barium was injected through a feeding tube (open arrow) in the esophagus (E). The trachea (T) becomes the left main bronchus (L) at the carina (C); the right bronchus is not present. Branching tubular structures resembling bronchi are filled with air to the right of the lower esophagus.

C, The hypoplastic lung bronchi opacify with barium through a connection to the esophagus.

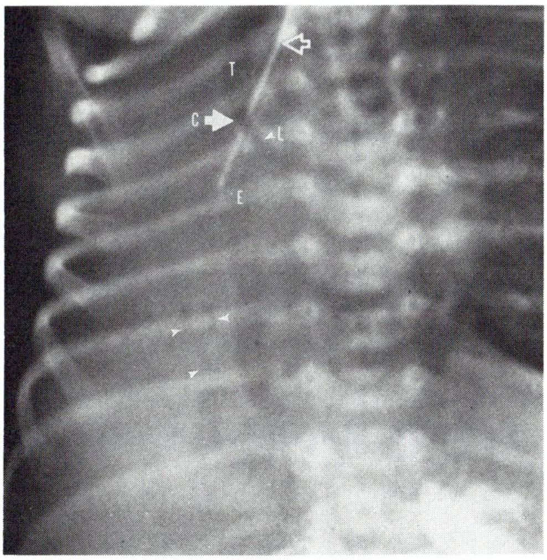

B

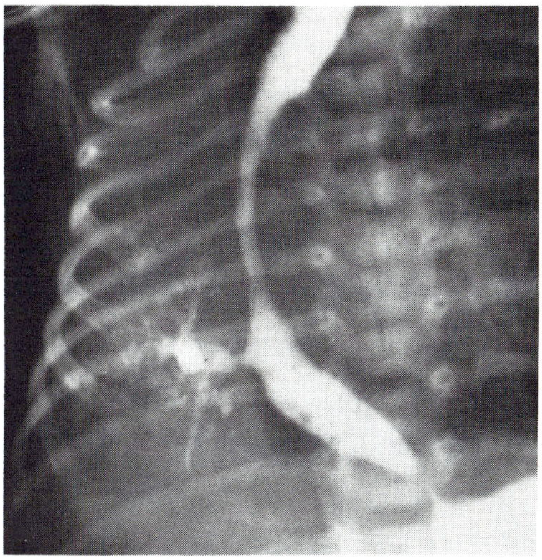

C

condition has been termed the *scimitar syndrome*[57] because of the shape of the roentgenographic shadow. It is one of the more common forms of the *hypogenetic lung syndrome.* This rare anomaly is associated with dextrocardia and mirror-image abnormalities of the bronchi. Systemic arteries supply the hypogenetic lung. Clinically, the occurrence of repeated infections as the child grows is probably related to an abnormally developed airway and occasionally the development of cystic changes.

On the lateral film of another case of lung hypoplasia (Fig. 19-48), an anterior band exists and has a relatively sharp air-interface on its posterior margin. This band represents the anterior edge of the small right lung abutting against soft tissue, mostly fatty, in the anterior compartment. This appearance is very similar to that seen in severe atelectases of the left upper lobe; it is not difficult to imagine that, instead of reduction in volume due to atelectasis, this problem really represents failure of formation of the upper lobe

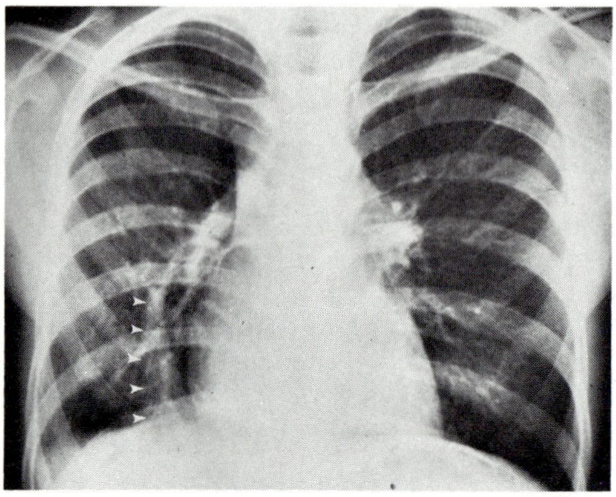

FIG. 19-47. Scimitar syndrome. The dextrocardia, and elevation (with flattening) of the right diaphragm define hypoplasia of the right lung. This condition, together with an anomalous pulmonary vein (arrows) draining to the vena cava, comprise the elements of the syndrome. The contour of the vein gives it its name.

and middle lobes. Because of the association of lung inversion (left to right), only the upper lobe need be postulated to be absent.

Not only does hypoplasia have to be distinguished from atelectasis, the entity of *accessory diaphragm*[14,20] (Fig. 19-49) with an excluded lobe has to be ruled out. Assuring against this possibility can be achieved only by angiography or bronchography.

One other variation of the hypoplastic lung syndrome is important since it may be confused with the Swyer-James syndrome (see Fig. 19-36): it is the anomaly of *absence of the right or left pulmonary artery* associated with a small, but well-aerated lung.[1,20] Distinction from the Swyer-James syndrome can be made easily since the Swyer-James patient shows evidence of air-trapping, which can be demonstrated on expiratory and decubitus films. Radionuclide perfusion study will show no flow in the absence of a main branch pulmonary artery in contrast to reduced, irregularly distributed flow in the Swyer-James patient; radionuclide ventilation study will be relatively normal in the former patient whereas gas distribution is slow and uneven in the Swyer-James patient. A pulmonary arteriogram is probably unnecessary.

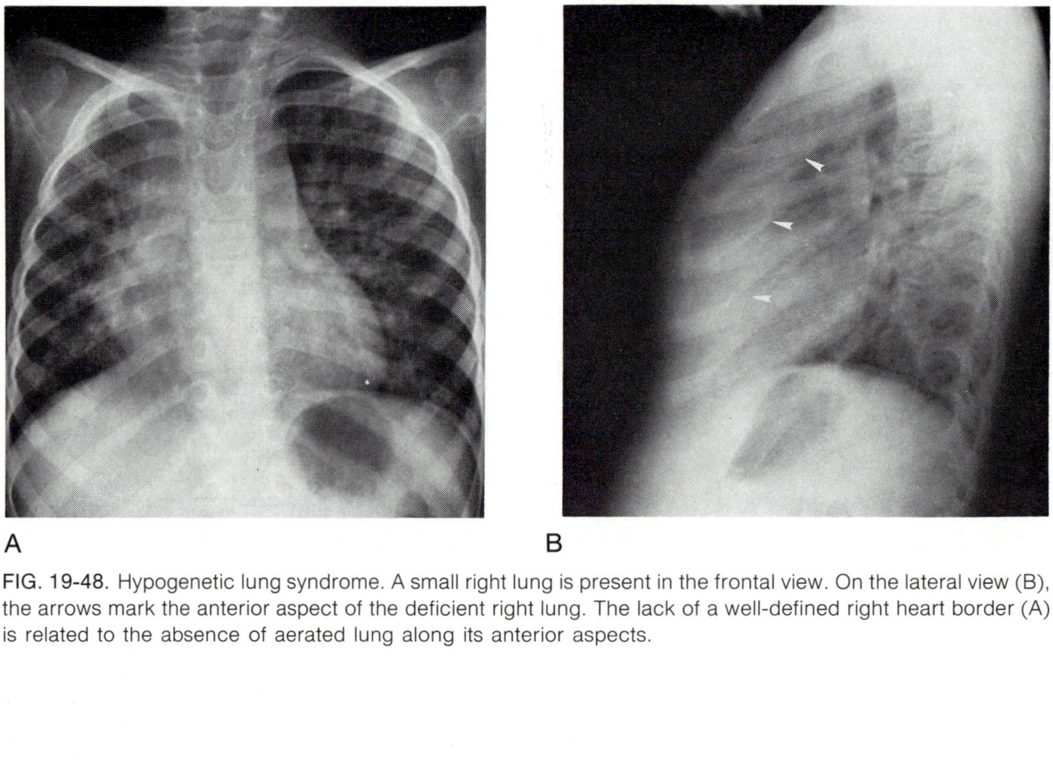

A B

FIG. 19-48. Hypogenetic lung syndrome. A small right lung is present in the frontal view. On the lateral view (B), the arrows mark the anterior aspect of the deficient right lung. The lack of a well-defined right heart border (A) is related to the absence of aerated lung along its anterior aspects.

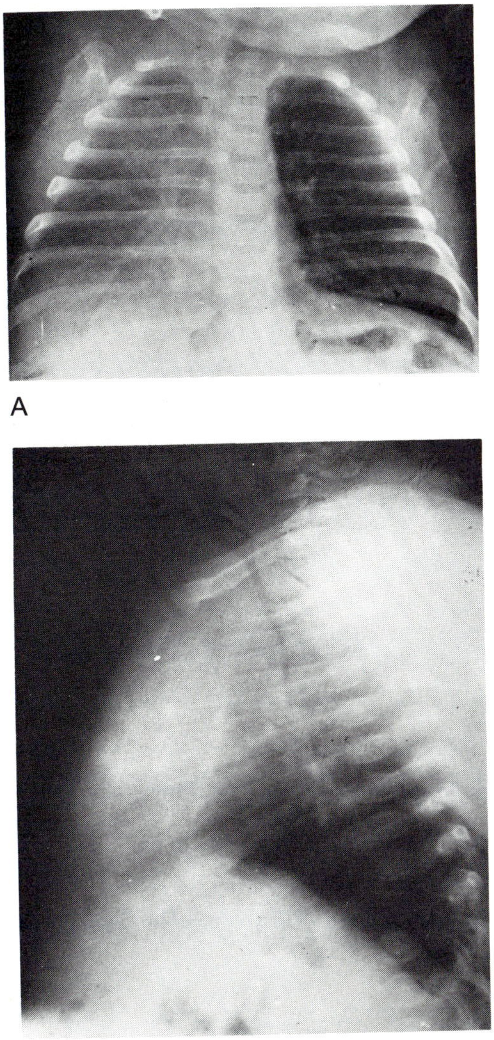

A

B

FIG. 19-49. Accessory diaphragm. The right lung is partitioned into two compartments by a diaphragm (B). Only the posterior compartment contains aerated lung. (Courtesy of Dr. George Kassner, S.U.N.Y., Downstate Medical Center, Brooklyn, New York.)

VOLUME LOSS BY COMPRESSION

Pleural effusions surround and compress the lung. In the infant particularly, an infected effusion due often to staphylococcus seems to entrap the lung within days.[64] Because the infection limits its ability to enlarge during inspiration, this lung appears smaller than the opposite lung (Fig. 19-50). Minimal change in size is seen fluoroscopically or on decubitus films (see also Fig. 6-40).

Dextrocardia (Fig. 19-51) may be mistaken for volume loss; however, normal volume may be determined by the normal position of the diaphragms and the ribs. Similarly, the leftward displacement of the heart due to pectus excavatum (Fig. 19-52) should not be ascribed to loss of lung volume when the following signs of pectus excavatum are present: haziness at the right paravertebral area above the diaphragm with loss of a sharp right heart border and an unusual configuration of the ribs, which slope downward rather sharply (see also Figs. 19-29 and 19-30). Paradoxically though, the child in Figure 19-53, whose lungs appear about normal size, has had his left lower lobe removed because of bronchiectasis. Compensatory enlargement of the upper lobe produces the "normal" appearance.

The mass effect of a pleural effusion is demonstrated in Figure 19-54 in a 1-day-old newborn infant. The heart is shifted to the right, returning to normal after needle and catheter drainage of the fluid. The air bubble

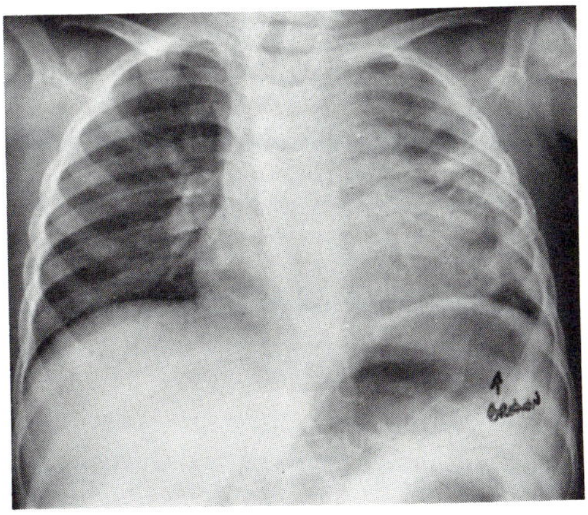

FIG. 19-50. Staphylococcal pneumonia with pleural reaction. Three days after therapy started, the pleural fluid is loculated and restricts the size of the lung and change in size during ventilation.

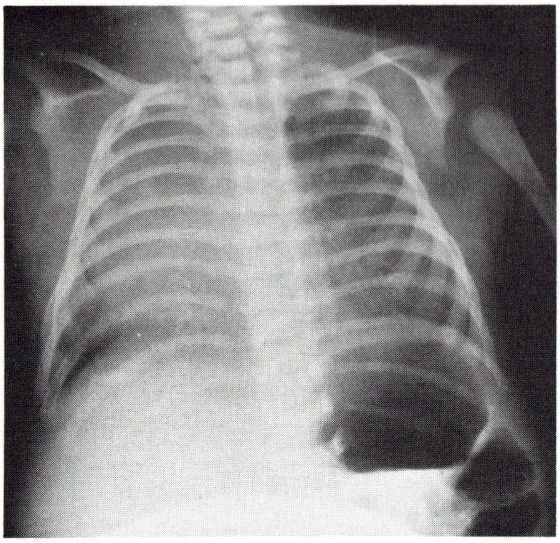

FIG. 19-51. Dextrocardia. No volume loss exists.

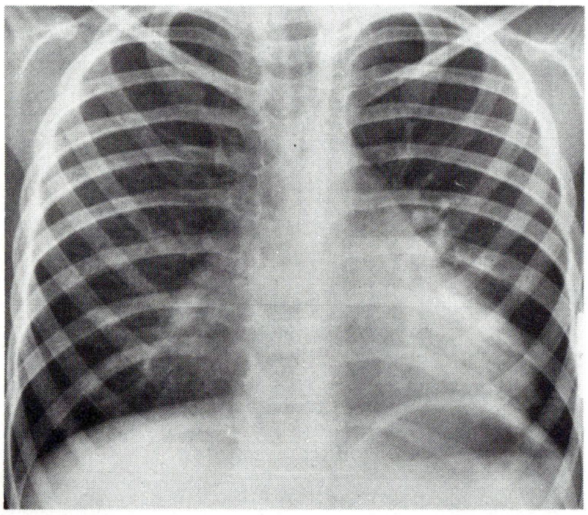

FIG. 19-52. Pectus excavatum. The shift of the mediastinum to the left should not be misdiagnosed as volume loss. Notice characteristic haziness at right cardiophrenic angle.

in the stomach is depressed and the ribs have widened. There would be no way that conventional roentgenography could be used to distinguish this condition from a large cystic or solid mass. In addition, the possibility of fetal pulmonary fluid trapped within the lung (see Figs. 19-33 and 19-34) by an obstructing mediastinal structure had to be considered. When the roentgenographic diagnosis of pleural effusion cannot be made definitively, ultrasonography is the method of choice.

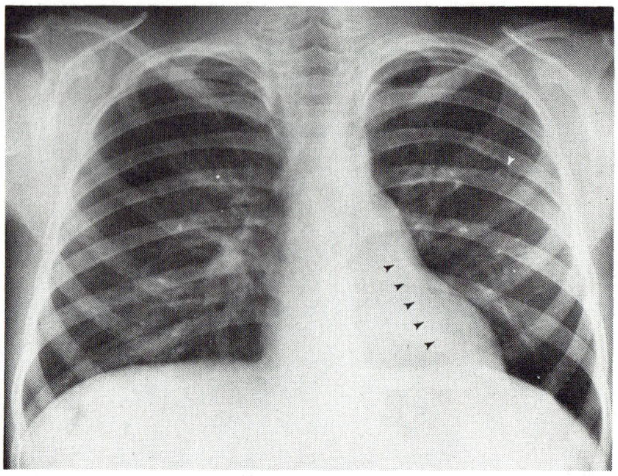

FIG. 19-53. Surgical resection of the left lower lobe. The lung volume appears normal. White arrow indicates the site of rib abnormality due to surgery. Black arrows point to "lower lobe artery" in abnormally oblique position; the normal artery is vertical.

Moreover, ultrasonography could have provided information to differentiate among a solid tumor, a fluid-filled bronchogenic cyst, an intrapericardial effusion or mass, and a fluid-filled lung.

Pneumothorax causes compression atelectasis, and in the older child and adult, the lung "clusters" around the hilum as it collapses. In the newborn period, however, pneumothorax is generally localized anteriorly and medially, with the lung compressed posteriorly. In the newborn child, a large pneumothorax does not necessarily cause the edge of the lung to be seen separated from the lateral wall of the thorax in the supine frontal view. When the pneumothorax exceeds about 30 ml, the lung edge does come into view, initially at the apex[52] (Fig. 19-55). Characteristically, the radiolucent edge is curved with the convexity outward. Beyond the perimeter of the radiolucency, the lung is often somewhat dense and may display an air bronchogram. The density of the lung may be due to atelectasis but is probably chiefly due to retained fetal pulmonary fluid. The density of the compressed lungs tends to curl around the edge of the anterior component of the pneumothorax. The blackened crescent,

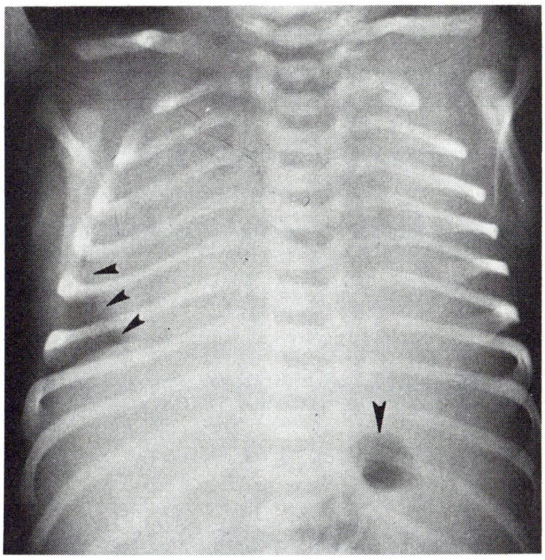

A

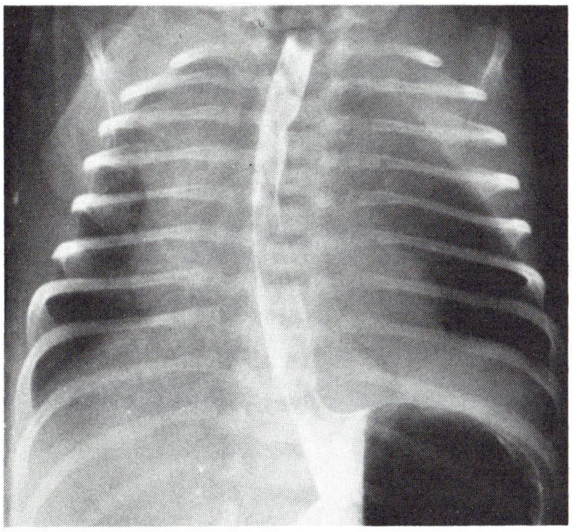

B

FIG. 19-54. *A*, Congenital pleural effusion. The heart is displaced to the right; arrows indicate convex cardiac border against aerated right lung. The effusion is so large that it also depresses the left diaphragm (arrow indicates depressed stomach bubble). This condition would have to be distinguished from a mass and an obstructed lung.

B, Right decubitus position. After drainage, the lung is aerated and the mediastinum returns to normal position. After the child began feeding, the fluid became chylous. After several weeks of drainage, the fluid disappeared and the child's condition was normal.

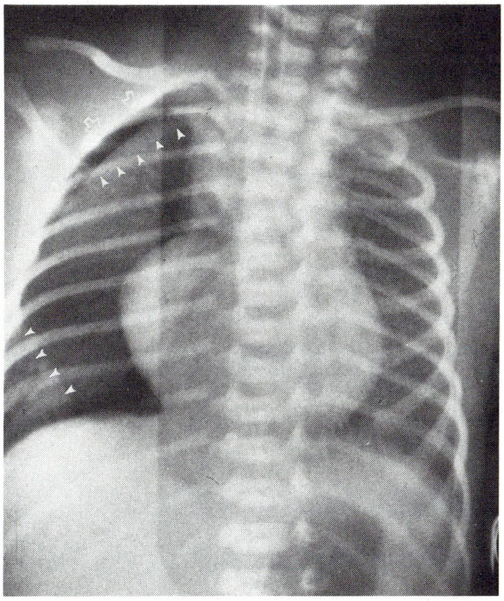

FIG. 19-55. Pneumothorax in the newborn infant. Though the lung is separated minimally from the chest wall at the apex (open arrows), the size of the pneumothorax is large. The pneumothorax is medially and anteriorly located; it presents as a radiolucency next to the mediastinum and has a curved edge (small white arrows).

which exposes the edge of the lung, is due to a component of the pneumothorax, which is laterally located. It would be a mistake to consider this a 5 or 10% pneumothorax; it is rather more like 50%. Using these criteria, the skin fold on the right in Figure 19-56 is easily recognized as such: the contour and position of the line, and the lack of a medial lucency indicate a skin fold rather than a pneumothorax. A moderate pneumothorax on the left in Figure 19-57 may be mistaken for lobar emphysema or a cyst, except that it meets the criteria for pneumothorax. The presence of air tracking from the mediastinum into the abdomen raises the question of *pneumomediastinum.* Differentiating pneumomediastinum from pneumothorax occasionally is a difficult problem; pneumomediastinum may be diagnosed if the thymus is elevated and surrounded by air. Notice that

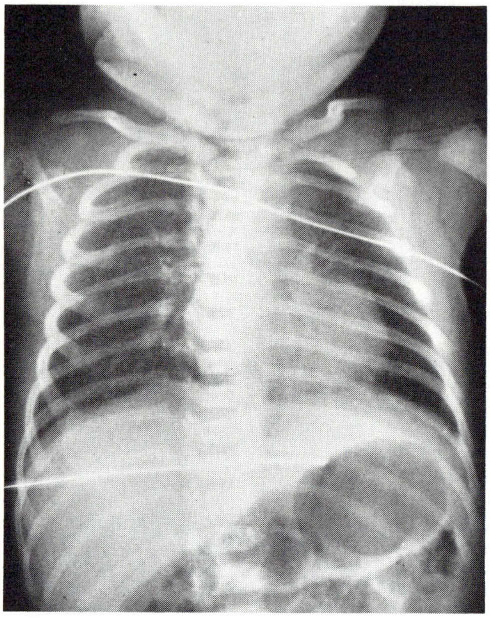

FIG. 19-56. Skin fold. This fold can be distinguished from a pneumothorax because it is not more radiolucent medially.

the thymus is flattened against the mediastinum (Fig. 19-57).

Because of faulty technique (high contrast), a pneumothorax (Fig. 19-58) can be over-

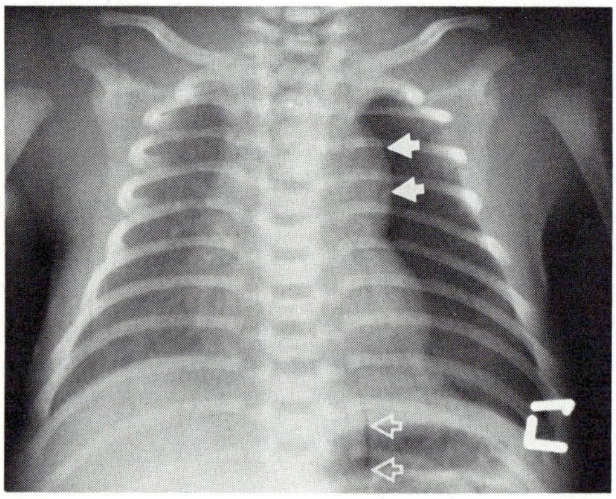

FIG. 19-57. Pneumothorax. Because of the strip of air dissecting into the abdomen (open arrows), the radiolucent area next to the mediastinum on the left must be distinguished from a pneumomediastinum. In this case, the thymus appears flattened against the mediastinum (solid arrows) instead of separated from it as in a pneumomediastinum.

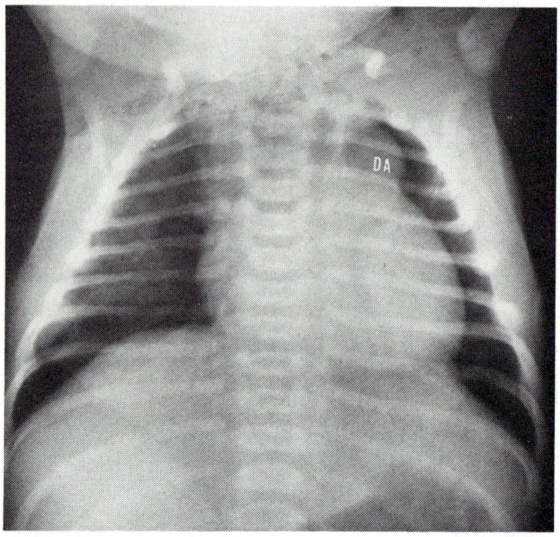

A

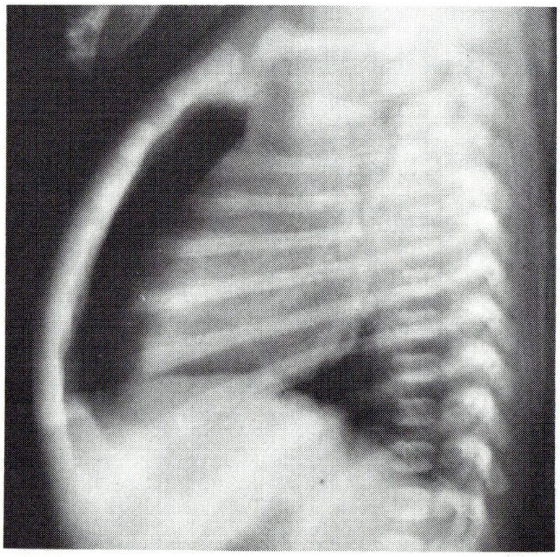

B

FIG. 19-58. Pneumothorax. Because of the faulty technique of the roentgenogram, the pneumothorax is not seen on the frontal view (A). DA-ductus arteriosus. On the lateral view (B) taken with the infant in the supine position, the anterior position of a large pneumothorax separating the heart from the chest wall is easily appreciated.

looked easily. However, if routine horizontal beam lateral roentgenograms (cross table lateral with patient lying in the supine position) are made at the same time, any clinically important pneumothorax can be easily seen anteriorly.[47] Decubitus films may also be of assistance in some cases; however, the change

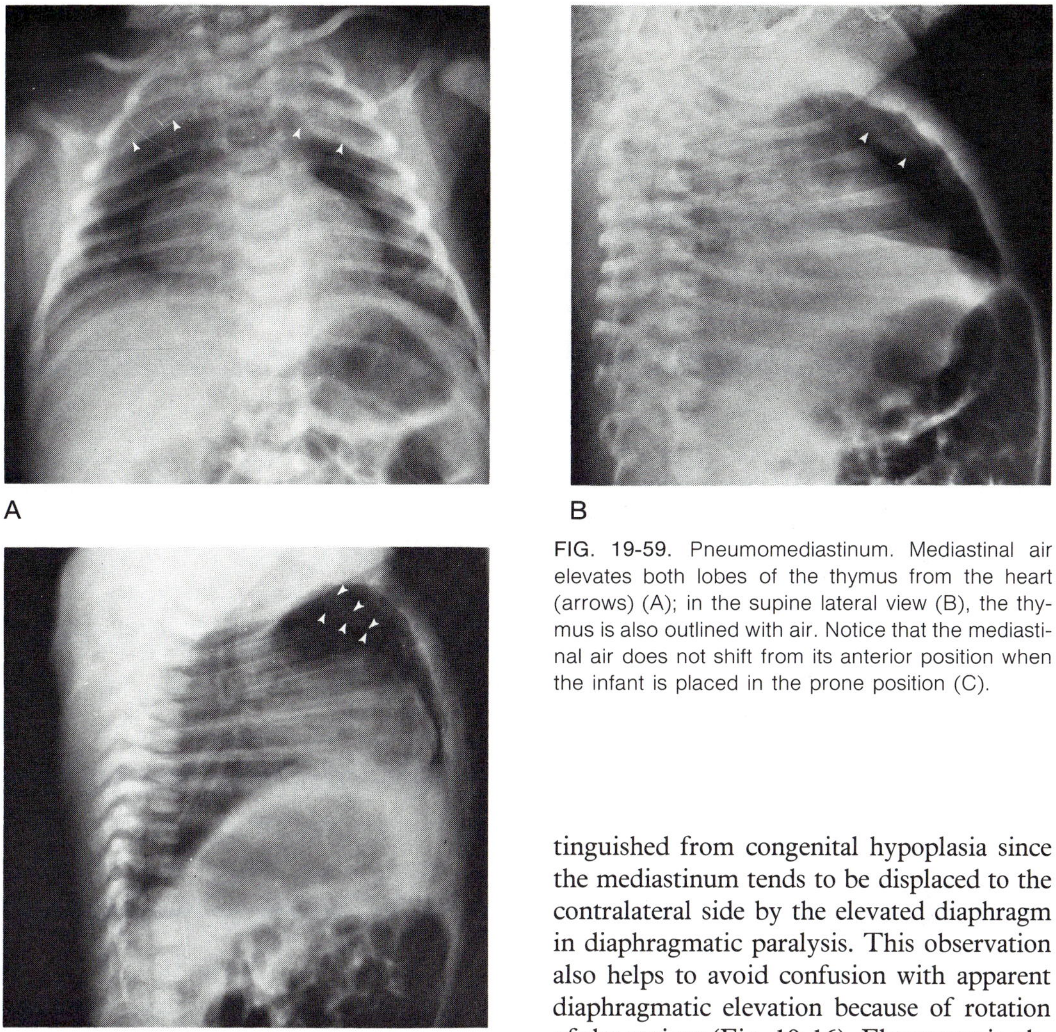

A

B

C

FIG. 19-59. Pneumomediastinum. Mediastinal air elevates both lobes of the thymus from the heart (arrows) (A); in the supine lateral view (B), the thymus is also outlined with air. Notice that the mediastinal air does not shift from its anterior position when the infant is placed in the prone position (C).

in the patient's position does not always change the location of the anterior pneumothorax and the lung may not separate from the chest wall as it usually does in older children.

The pneumomediastinum in Figure 19-59 is identified because it separates the thymic lobes from the heart in both views. Notice that the location of the air collection remains anterior to the heart whether the patient is in the supine or prone position.

Lung volume reduction because of *diaphragmatic paralysis* (Fig. 19-60) can be distinguished from congenital hypoplasia since the mediastinum tends to be displaced to the contralateral side by the elevated diaphragm in diaphragmatic paralysis. This observation also helps to avoid confusion with apparent diaphragmatic elevation because of rotation of the patient (Fig. 19-16). Fluoroscopic observation of movement of the heart back toward the midline during expiration with or without paradoxic motion of the diaphragm is helpful in the diagnosis of paralysis. Eventration usually cannot be distinguished from paralysis. The cross-table lateral view with the child placed in the supine position affords the best opportunity to diagnose paralysis fluoroscopically in the infant (p. 602). In this view, one is able to assess diaphragmatic motion best since the mobile posterior part of both diaphragms is seen in a single line of sight without having to shift the eye from left to right. Actually lateral fluoroscopy of the diaphragms is useful at any age and may be

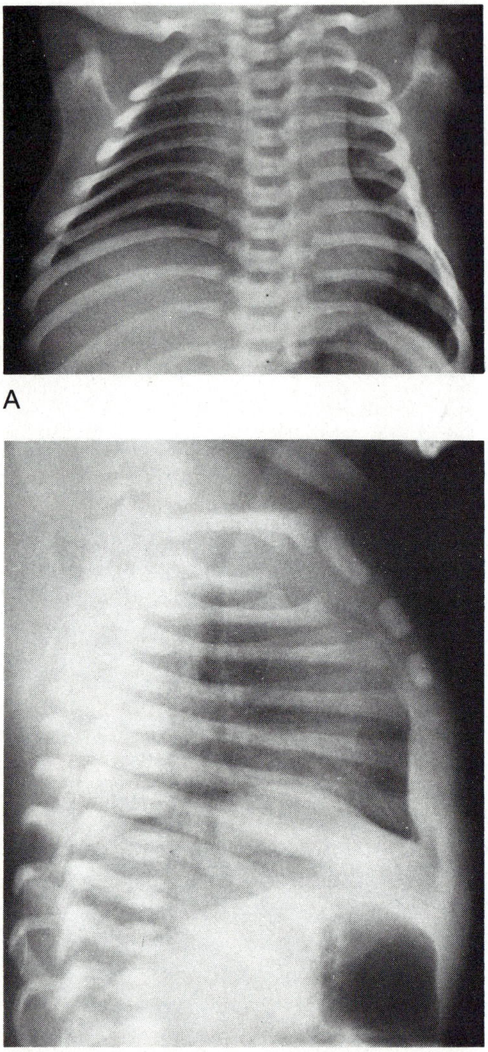

A

B

FIG. 19-60. Paralysis of the right diaphragm. Two-week-old infant who has Erb's palsy on the right. The lateral roentgenogram is made with the infant in the supine position since the decubitus position causes asymmetry of the height of the diaphragms.

done in the supine or erect positions. The decubitus position itself affects the contour of the diaphragms, causing the "downside" diaphragm to be higher and rounder and the "upside" diaphragm to be lower and flatter; thus, this position may not be used for the purpose of assessing diaphragmatic movement.

Partial *eventration of the diaphragm* is usually anteriorly located and may appear as a "mass" (Fig. 19-61) on the chest roentgenogram, obliterating the diaphragmatic contour and the heart border; through the "mass" the lower lobe vessels are seen. The clue to the diagnosis is the high level of the liver edge, which may even be absent to palpation. A diagnostic pneumoperitoneum using nitrous oxide (which is absorbed within minutes) shows the anatomy. For doubtful cases today, a radionuclide liver study or ultrasonography would replace the diagnostic pneumoperitoneum.

Herniation of the liver through the diaphragm may be present at birth but may occur suddenly later, even many weeks later.[3,27] The film of the premature infant in Figure 19-62 was taken on the second day of life because of sudden severe exacerbation of respiratory distress. The density in the right lower chest was thought not to be pneumonia or bleeding because the pulmonary vessels were visible behind the density. Comparison with an earlier film taken in the morning of the same day for the purpose of assessing the position of the umbilical arterial catheter shows the area to be clear and the liver edge lower by at least three vertebral bodies. In this case, because of the patency of the pleuroperitoneal canal, the nitrous oxide study caused a pneumothorax. The pneumothorax would have been avoided by the use of a radionuclide liver study or ultrasonogram.

On the left side of the chest, the most serious problem resulting from herniation of an abdominal organ through a persisting pleuroperitoneal canal is that caused by *bowel herniation.* The herniated bowel may appear initially as a solid mass because of the lack of time for swallowed air to pass into the bowel after birth (Fig. 19-63); the abdomen appears scaphoid and empty. Air may be administered through a nasogastric feeding tube as a contrast agent if the diagnosis is still in doubt.

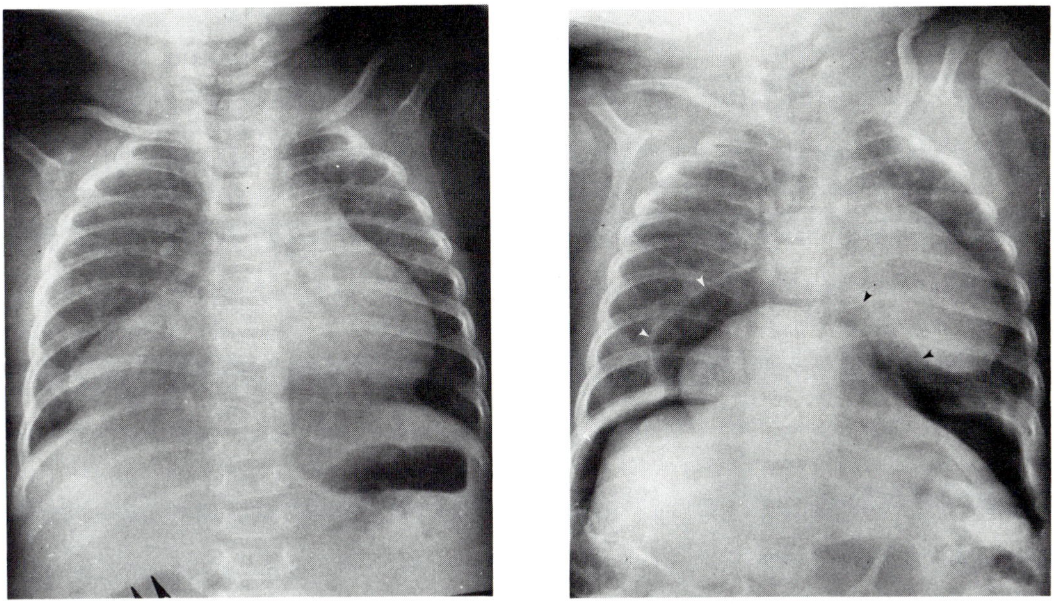

A B

FIG. 19-61. *A*, Anterior eventration of the liver. The diaphragmatic contour is obliterated by the "mass" in the right cardiophrenic angle. The liver edge (arrows) is higher than normal; this observation suggests the proper diagnosis. Incidentally, congenital malformations appear in the ninth and tenth vertebral bodies, a finding usually indicative of congenital neuroenteric abnormalities.

B, Diagnostic pneumoperitoneum shows that the diaphragm (arrows) is eventrated medially on both sides and that the liver mass actually extends across the midline (lateral views showed the eventration to be anteriorly located).

Clinical problems of lesser severity are incurred because of sliding hiatal hernias of the stomach, which frequently present to the right of the heart in the infant but may be seen on the left (Fig. 19-64). Differential roentgenographic diagnosis of a solid mass of the thorax must be considered when the stomach is fluid filled and therefore radiopaque; on the other hand, if the stomach is air containing, the differential diagnosis includes a cystic mass. An upper gastrointestinal tract series study quickly resolves the problem. In this case, the unusually high position of the colon suggests the diagnosis of volvulus of the stomach, i.e., the herniated stomach turns upside down. The transverse colon, attached to the greater curvature, is pulled up in the manner seen here. Other organs, e.g., kidney (Fig. 19-65) or spleen, may herniate and can be identified most easily by ultrasonography.

VOLUME LOSS DUE TO MASSES

Sequestration of the lung (see also Chapter 15) is defined and diagnosed by its arterial blood supply, which is of systemic origin.[68] The sequestration in Figure 19-66 appears as a rounded mass, irregular in outline, in the left lower lung. Tomograms demonstrate a structure related to the mass; this structure has the configuration of a blood vessel that is oriented toward the aorta. An aortogram shows that this shadow is a branch vessel from the aorta supplying the mass; the venous return flow was also to the systemic circulation (not shown). The diagnosis of an

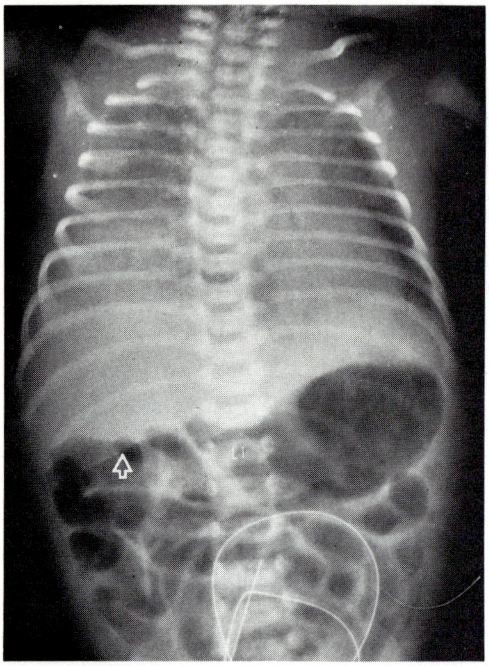

A

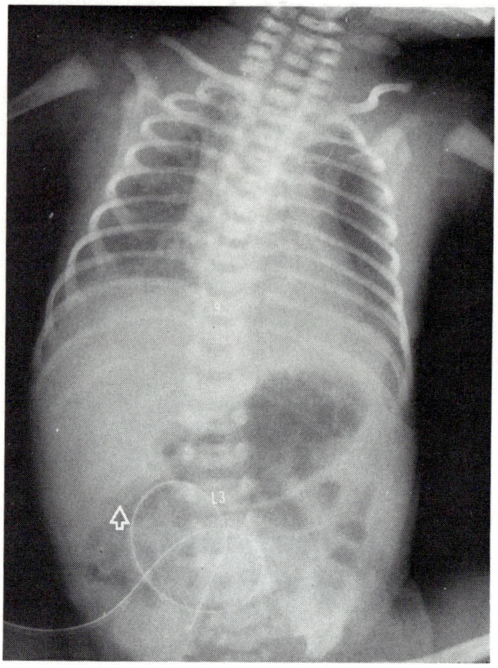

B

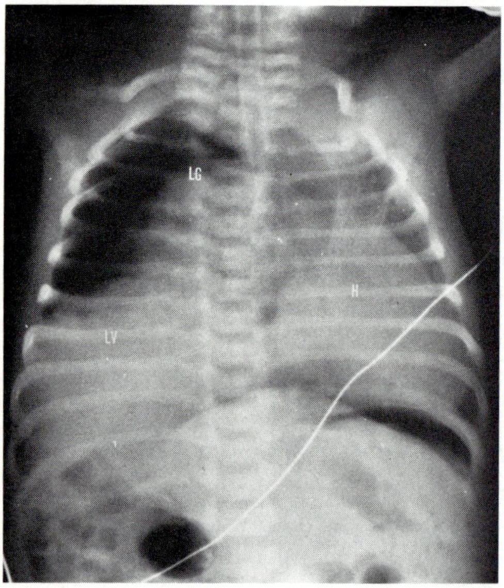

C

FIG. 19-62. *A*, Herniation of the liver occurred suddenly on the second day of life. The roentgenogram shows a right lower lung density through which vessels are seen. The liver edge is elevated (arrow) and is in a more horizontal position than normal.

B, Roentgenogram taken for umbilical catheter localization 8 hours earlier. The chest is essentially normal in appearance; the liver edge is lower and more vertically oriented.

C, A diagnostic pneumoperitoneum caused a pneumothorax because of an incomplete partition by a normal diaphragm. LV = liver; LG = lung; H = heart.

extralobar sequestration was made because both artery and vein were of the systemic circulation. Sequestered blood supply from the aorta may supply an area of otherwise normal lung (Fig. 19-67). The chest roentgenogram showed dextrocardia (not related to sequestration usually). The lung was apparently normal. The aortogram shows the

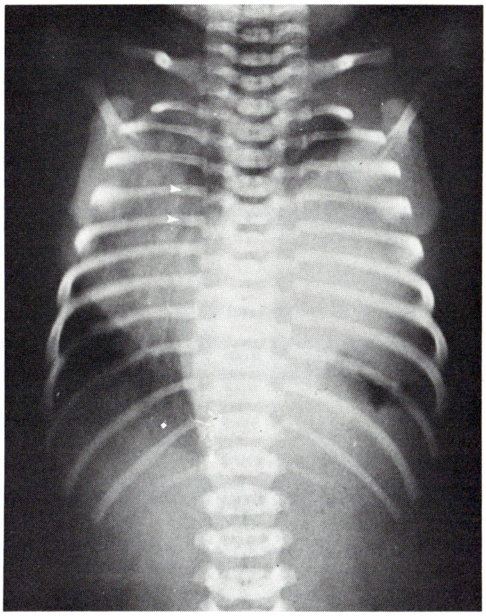

A

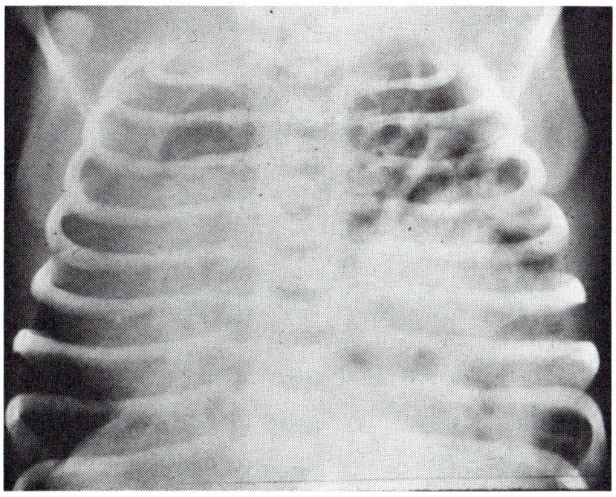

B

FIG. 19-63. *A*, Herniation of intestine through a persisting pleuroperitoneal canal. The roentgenogram, taken shortly after birth, shows that the trachea (arrows) and other mediastinal structures are shifted to the right by the mass of bowel, not yet filled with air, in the left side of the chest. Bowel gas is not present in the scaphoid abdomen.

B, The bowel in the chest filled with air.

blood supply to the lower lung to be from the aorta and the venous return to be through the pulmonary veins. Because of the latter, this condition can be classified as an intralobar

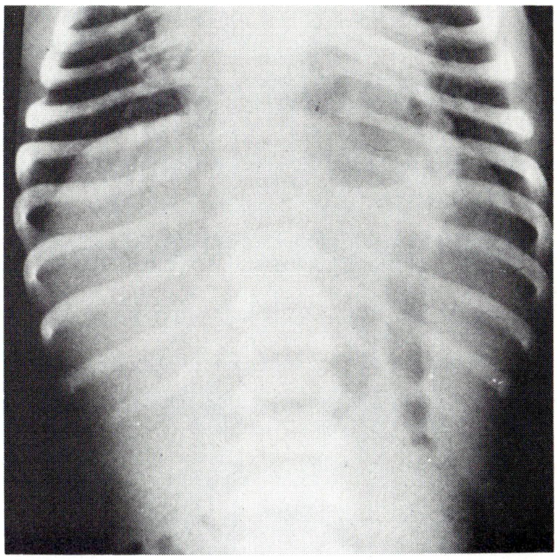

A

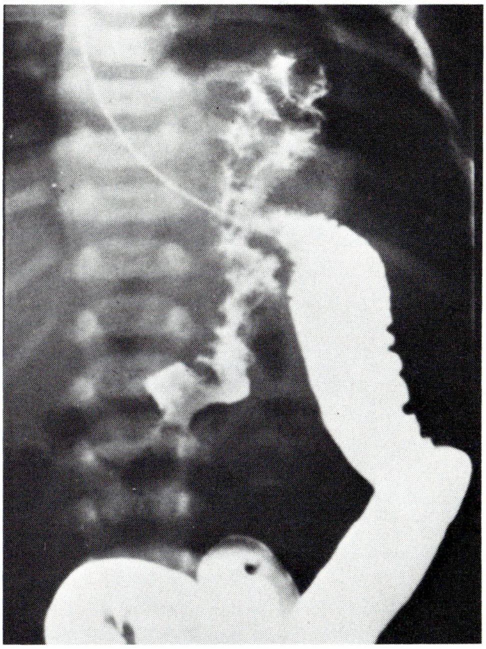

B

FIG. 19-64. Herniation of the stomach with volvulus. Since the colon is tethered by its mesenteric attachments to the greater curvature of the stomach, it is pulled upward in characteristic fashion when a volvulus of the stomach occurs. This condition can be seen on the plain roentgenogram (A) and on the barium enema (B). The large "cystic" lesion behind the heart is the herniated stomach (proven by upper gastrointestinal tract series, not shown).

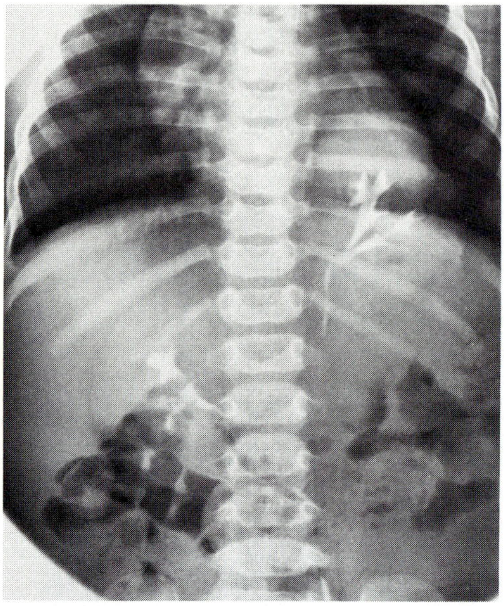

FIG. 19-65. Herniation of the kidney. Notice that the gas-filled splenic flexure of the colon is abnormally medially placed. This observation may be made when the kidney is absent or in ectopic position.

sequestration; such sequestrations are frequently associated with airway and alveolar abnormalities and become the site of multiple pneumonias later in life.[33]

The *neuroblastoma* in the left lower lobe in Figure 19-68 might be confused with a sequestration because it is a mass in the classic position in which sequestrations are found. An injection of radiopaque contrast material made in the pulmonary artery shows both the right and the left side of the central circulation excellently, and there is no evidence of systemic blood supply. However, the diagnosis of neuroblastoma can be made correctly because of the suggestion of paraspinal adenopathy indicated by a localized widening of the paraspinal line.[21] This widening is characteristic of the upward spread of neuroblastoma in the young child. When no evidence exists of vertebral bone destruction, a finding that would suggest infection or histiocytosis, neuroblastoma should be suspected. Localized bronchiectasis may appear (as in Fig. 19-69) as a mass, having a varicose appearance that suggests a vascular abnormality. Bronchography shows bronchiectasis and atelectasis of the lower lobe.[7] This 12-year-old boy had a positive response to purified protein derivative (PPD) of tuberculin and a large suprahilar lymph node. Of interest was the evidence of abnormal ventilation at both

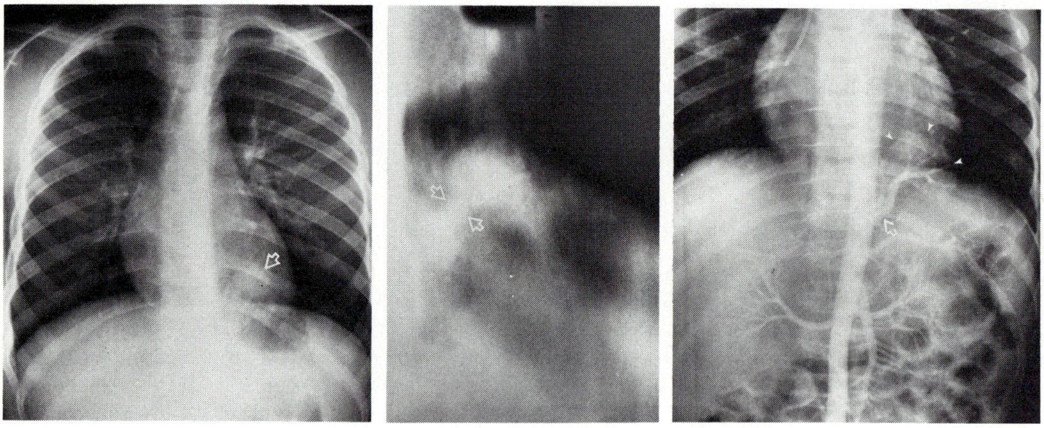

A B C

FIG. 19-66. *A*, Sequestration of the lung. A round density is seen through the heart (arrow).
B, Tomography shows a tubular, vessel-like structure leading from it toward the aorta.
C, Angiography shows that the mass is supplied by a large vessel arising from the aorta. The venous return was to the vena cava.

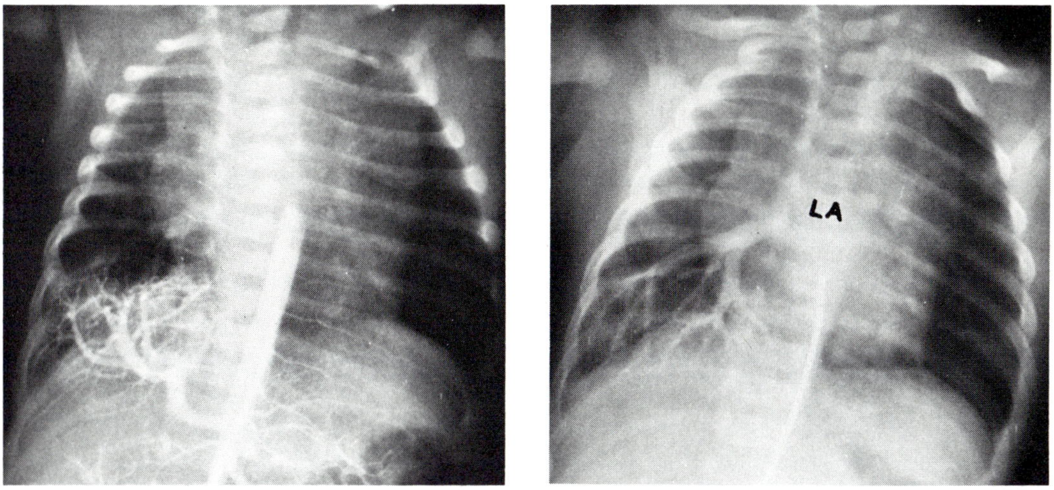

A B

FIG. 19-67. Sequestration of the lung. The plain roentgenogram was normal except for dextrocardia. Aortography shows that the lower lung is supplied by a large vessel from the aorta (A) and drains into the left atrium (LA) through a large pulmonary vein.

lung bases on the ^{133}xenon study; only minimal roentgenographic evidence of peribronchial thickening was present on the right.

The large mass on the left in Figure 19-70 is a *pulmonary abscess*; there is a large suprahilar lymph node. Tomography showed normal lobar bronchi. The pulmonary arteriogram was done to rule out the possibility of a sequestration and incidentally showed the typical arteriographic findings of an abscess: (1) pruning of the major branch pulmonary artery and (2) small irregular "new" vessels associated with infection. Bronchography was not done. A similar roentgenographic density in the patient in Figure 19-71 was produced by a sliding *hiatus hernia*. This patient had an unspecified neuromuscular disease.

A mass that might well raise suspicions of a tumor should always raise the question of a pulmonary *arteriovenous malformation*[53] (Fig. 19-72; see also Fig. 18-2). Tomograms showed a large draining vein and a radionuclide perfusion study using ^{99m}Tc pertechnetate showed that most of the flow was preferentially to the malformation as well.

Thymus can be distinguished from the large ganglioneuroblastoma in Figure 19-73 because the upper mediastinal border, which represents the anterior mediastinum, is obliterated by the thymus. The tumor is in a different plane, located posteriorly, and the border is seen very well.

Cysts of the lung in the child almost always are *post-infectious pneumatoceles*[8,35] (although some are post-traumatic),[19] appearing at the time of the infection and enlarging for a period well after the pneumonia is cured. They last for days or weeks, occasionally months, and rarely for years. The patient should be followed with care even though pneumatoceles ordinarily do not cause symptoms, since pneumothorax or secondary infection occasionally supervenes. Pneumatoceles also may become quite large and multiple (Fig. 19-74). This 5-month-old child had had a staphylococcal infection 1 month previous to the time of this film. Shortly thereafter, he developed a pneumothorax without experiencing respiratory distress. Gradually, over several weeks, his lung reexpanded, and 2 months later the chest roentgenogram was normal. On the third day

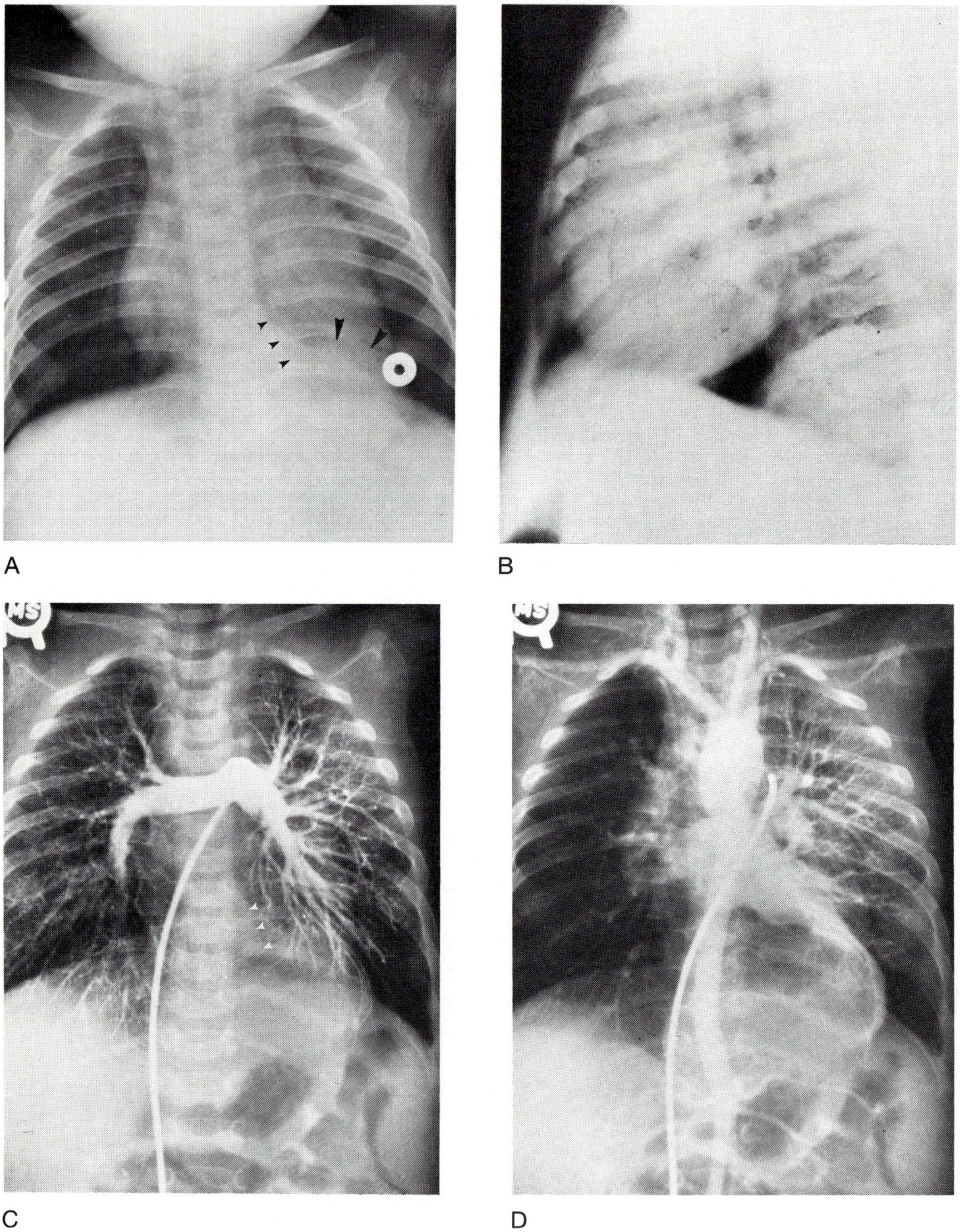

FIG. 19-68. Neuroblastoma. The large round mass in the posterior basilar region of the chest (A, B) is a neuroblastoma. The paravertebral shadow, somewhat triangular with its oblique edge marked with small arrows (A), suggests that this component is a mass of lymph nodes. The adjacent vertebral body is normal. In this setting, the diagnosis of malignancy (neuroblastoma) is most probable.

Pulmonary angiography shows that the lower lobe vessels are displaced around the mass (C). There is no systemic blood supply from the aorta (D). The thick band surrounding the mass is the pulmonary vein stretched over it.

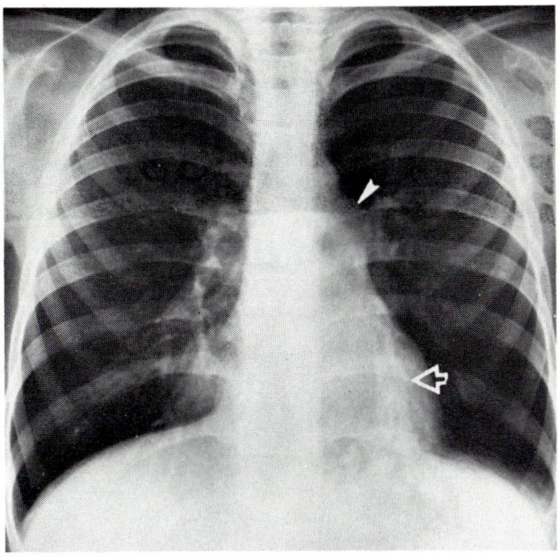

A

FIG. 19-69. Bronchiectasis in a 12-year-old boy appears as a localized density in the lower lobe (A). The linear component (open arrow) is due to crowded, thick-wall bronchi (B); the grape-like collection at the most inferior aspect represents bronchiectatic collections of infected secretions. Notice the enlarged lymph node (arrow) in the left suprahilar region (A). Selective bronchography of the left lung shows the abnormality to be confined to the left lower lobe (B). The upper lobe appears normal. The washout phase of a radionuclide ventilation study shows slow clearing of radioactivity from both lower lobes (C). The plain roentgenogram showed only minimal thickening of the bronchus; however, rales were heard in the area.

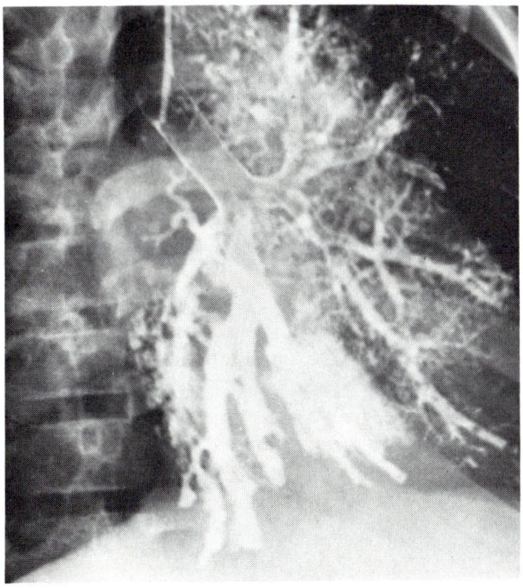

B

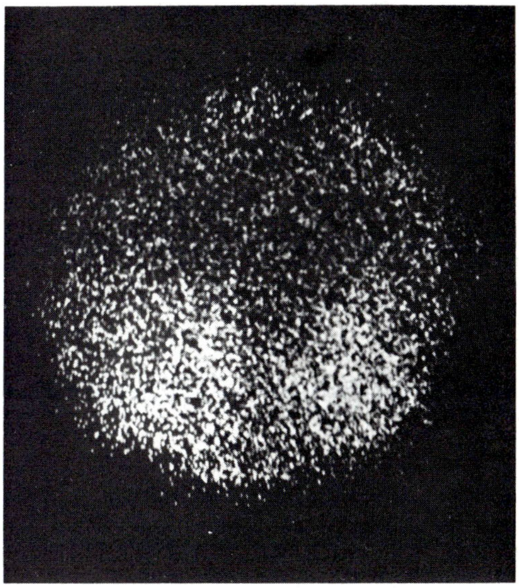

C

of life this child (Fig. 19-75) developed a pneumothorax. A cyst was already forming. The roentgenogram on day 1 was normal except for minimal evidence of fetal fluid retention. Because of the rapid enlargement of the cyst within 24 hours, it was decided to remove the cyst surgically. The pathologic diagnosis after removal was post-infectious pneumatocele.

Currently a second common cause of intrapulmonary air collections is that associated with the use of constant positive airway pressure in the treatment of severe RDS.[65] These interstitial collections vary considerably in the size of the bubbles, their number, and their distribution.[65] They may pack the lung or the lobe and, being essentially incompressible, crowd the lung tissue within the lung or lobe so that gas exchange is impaired and perfusion reduced. Indeed, the lung itself,

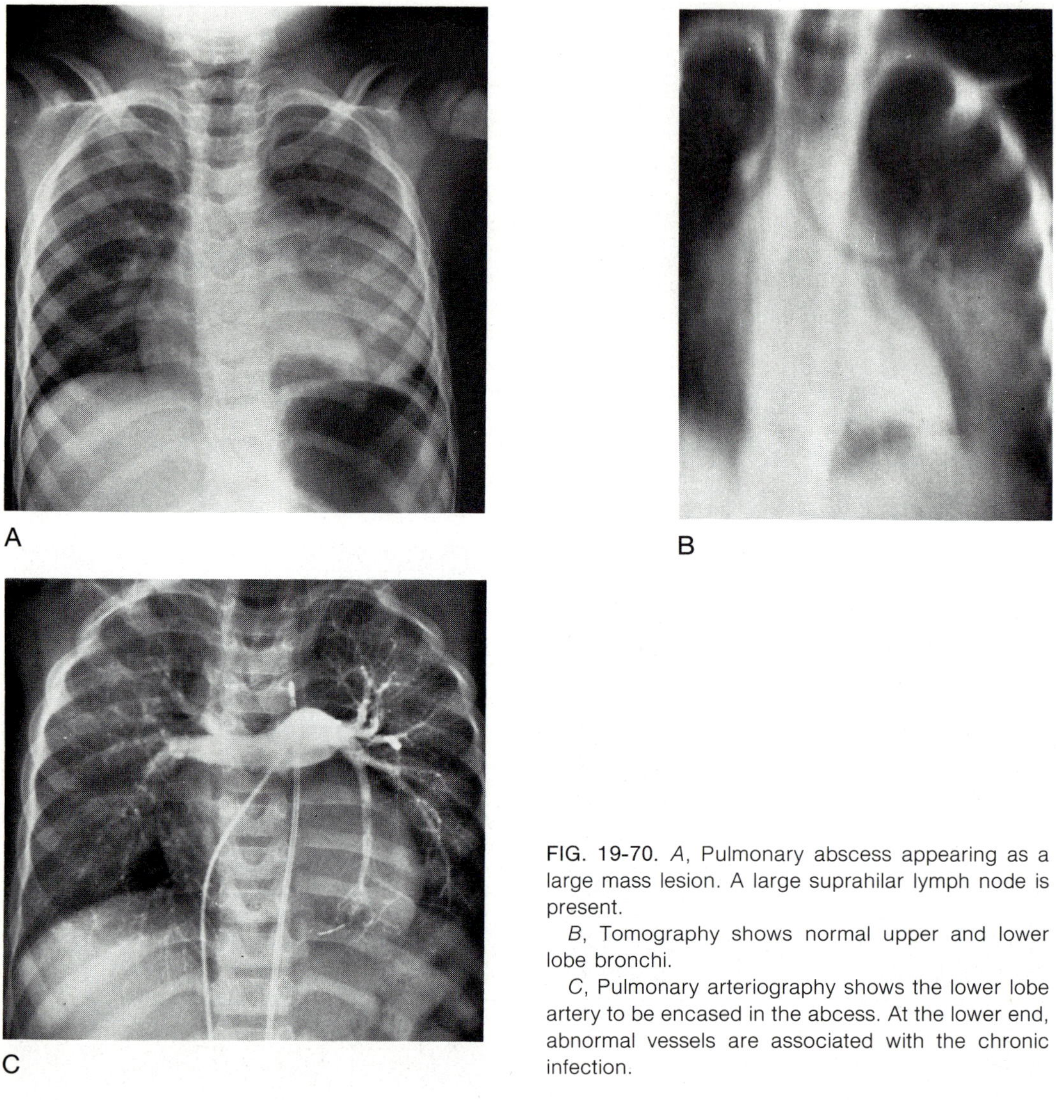

FIG. 19-70. *A*, Pulmonary abscess appearing as a large mass lesion. A large suprahilar lymph node is present.

B, Tomography shows normal upper and lower lobe bronchi.

C, Pulmonary arteriography shows the lower lobe artery to be encased in the abcess. At the lower end, abnormal vessels are associated with the chronic infection.

so packed, acts as a mass and may displace the structures around it. Figure 19-76 shows evidence of *interstitial air;* the lung between the bubbles is compressed, and in some areas, the compressed tissue looks almost like interstitial thickening. Figure 19-77 is a film of another child treated with protracted ventilator support for RDS; this child then developed bronchopulmonary dysplasia. At autopsy, large cystic collections of air were located in the interstitium of the lung, especially in the left upper lobe.

Congenital cysts[59] (see also Chapter 15) consist chiefly of two kinds. One is the *adenomatoid malformation,*[13] which, though solid at birth, enlarges and becomes "pneumatized" as it grows. Usually multilocular (Fig. 19-78), it may rarely appear as a single cyst on the film. Tne lower lobes are in the usual location. Usually diagnosed in the neonatal

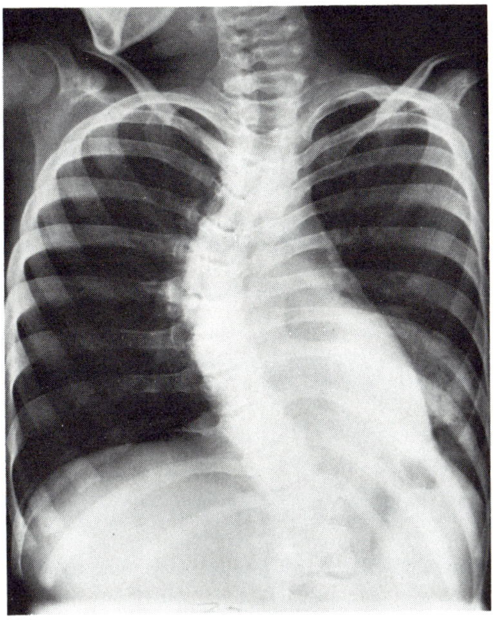

A

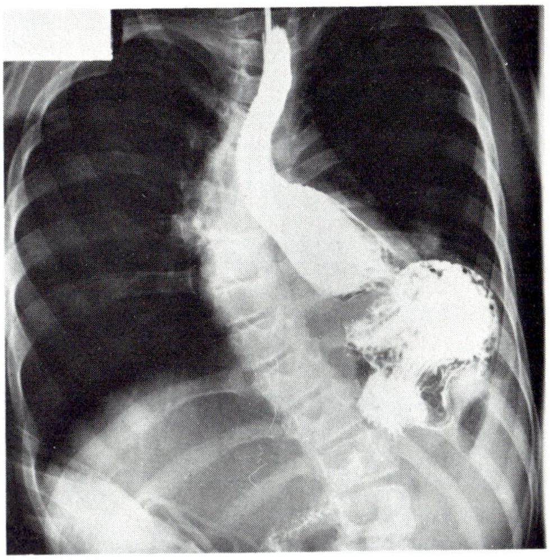

B

FIG. 19-71. A sliding hiatus hernia is seen in a patient with severe neuromuscular disease (B). The plain roentgenographic findings are those of an irregular mass (A).

period because of the respiratory symptoms produced by their rapid growth, they may be diagnosed later as shown in the 6-month-old child in Figure 19-79 (compare with Figs. 19-74 and 19-75).

A second type of congenital cyst is the

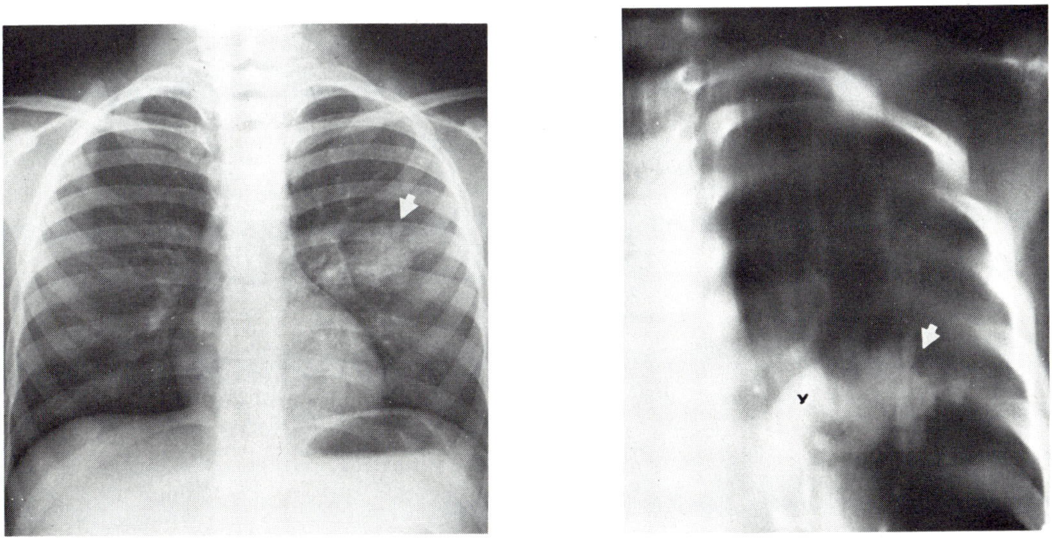

A B

FIG. 19-72. *A*, Pulmonary arteriovenous malformation. This 7-year-old girl was severely cyanotic. Her mother was known to have small pulmonary arteriovenous malformations.

B, Tomography shows a large draining vein (v) to the left atrium.

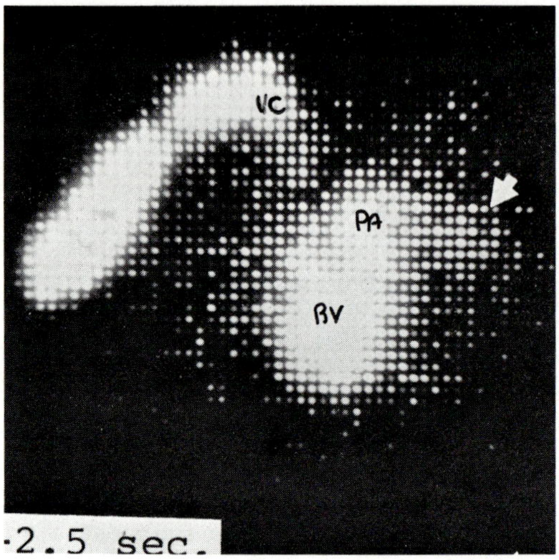

C

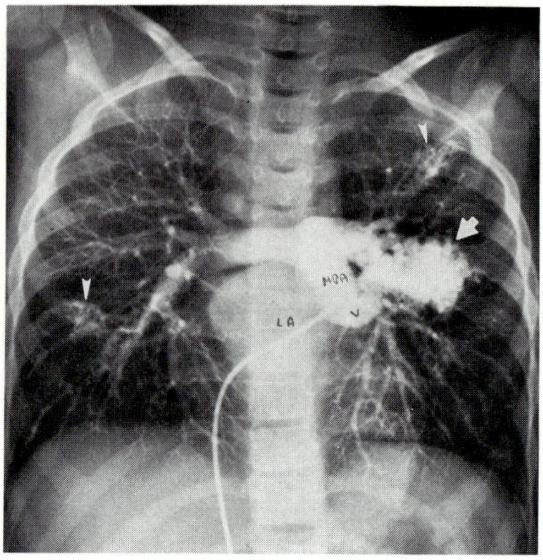

D

C, Radionuclide perfusion study using ^{99m}Tc pertechnetate showed that virtually all of the blood flow to the left lung was to the malformation (arrow). VC = vena cava; RV = right ventricle; PA = pulmonary artery.

D, Pulmonary arteriography shows the large malformation (arrow), the draining vein (V), the left atrium (LA), and the main pulmonary artery (MPA). Several other smaller malformations had not been seen previously (small arrows).

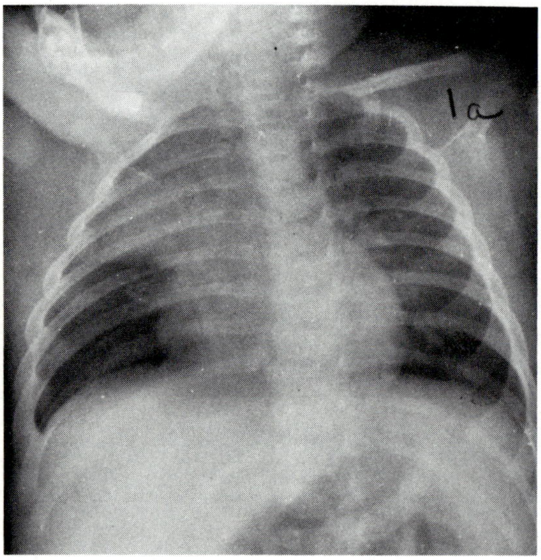

A

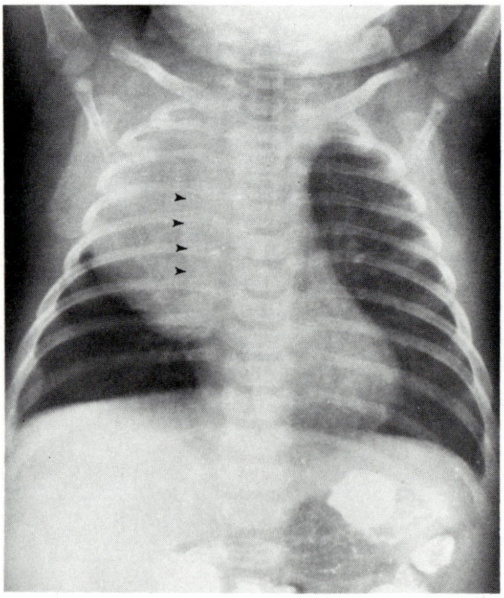

B

FIG. 19-73. *A*, Normal thymus. Notice that, because it is an anterior structure, the right upper mediastinal border is lost.

B, Ganglioneuroblastoma. In this case, because the mass is located posteriorly, the right upper mediastinal border is preserved (arrows).

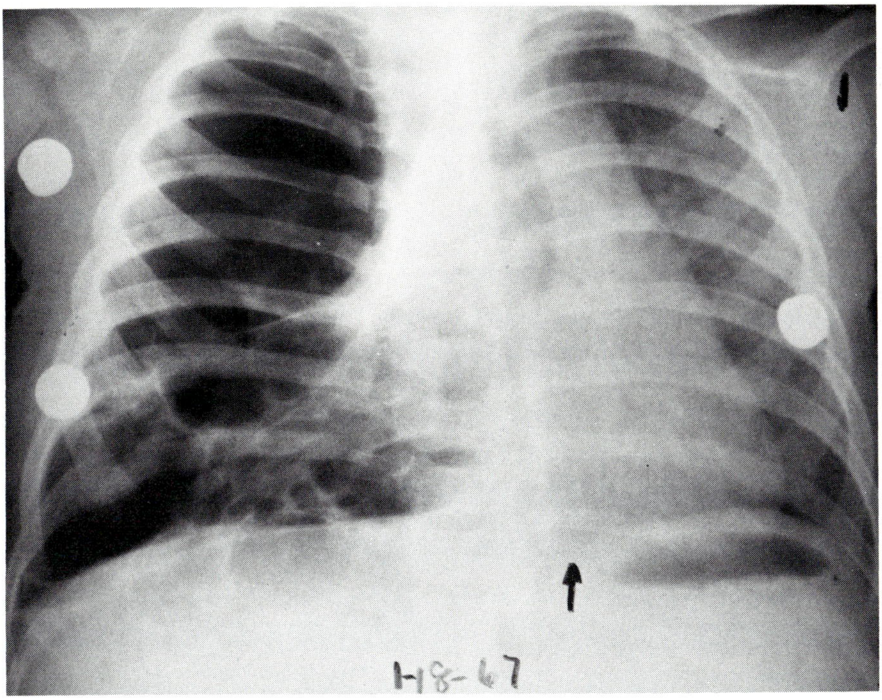

FIG. 19-74. Post-infectious pneumatoceles.

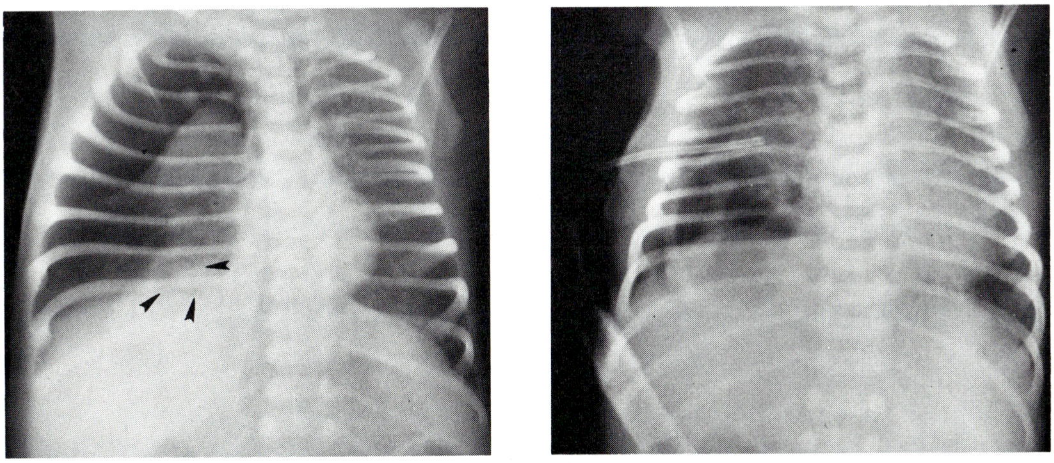

A B

FIG. 19-75. *A*, Pneumatocele. Spontaneous pneumothorax occurring on the third day of life. Arrows indicate the presence of a cyst. Roentgenograms on the first day of life were essentially normal.

B, The cyst enlarged rapidly after treatment of the pneumothorax was instituted. It was removed surgically and was a post-infectious pneumatocele by histologic criteria.

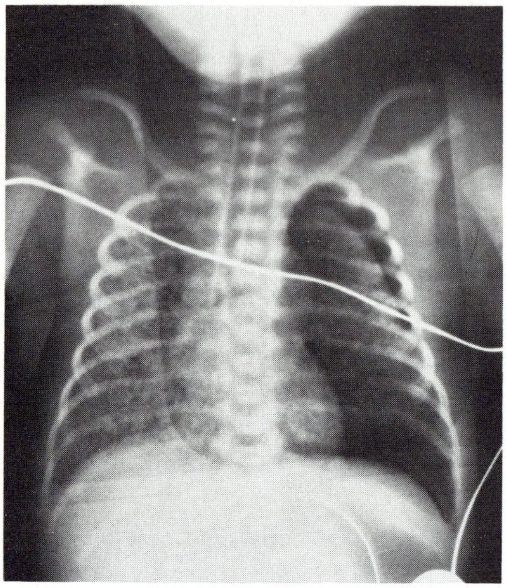

FIG. 19-76. Interstitial air. The small bubbles of air tend to compress the adjacent lung and this compression may produce a roentgenographic appearance that suggests an interstitial pattern. The lungs are large and tend to stay large. A large pneumothorax appears on the left.

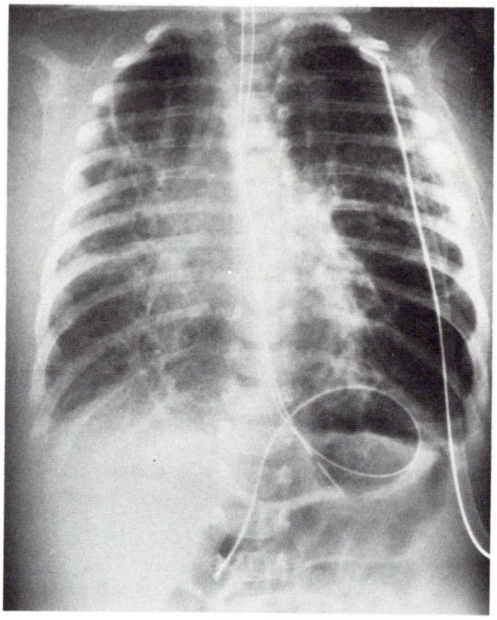

FIG. 19-77. Severe bronchopulmonary dysplasia. The autopsy showed, among other things, large interstitial collections of air. These collections compressed the lung around them and largely accounted for the appearance of the upper lobes on the roentgenogram.

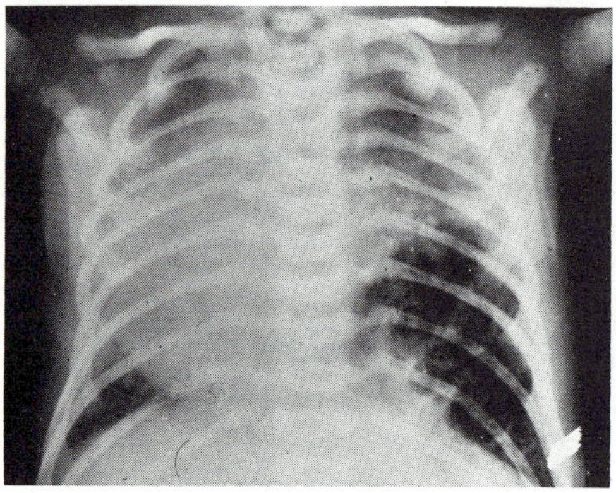

A

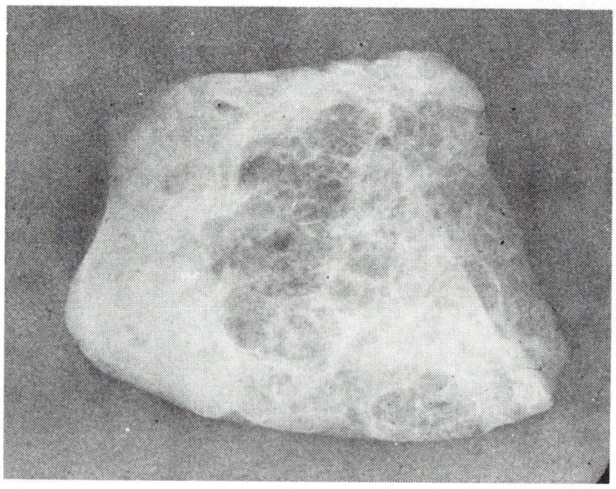

B

FIG. 19-78. *A*, Congenital adenomatoid malformation. The heart is displaced to the right and the left lung compressed upward by the multilocular cystic lesion in the left lower lung. It should be distinguished from hernia and from pneumatocele formation.

B, The resected specimen shows that it is partly solid. (From Babies Hospital, New York, New York.)

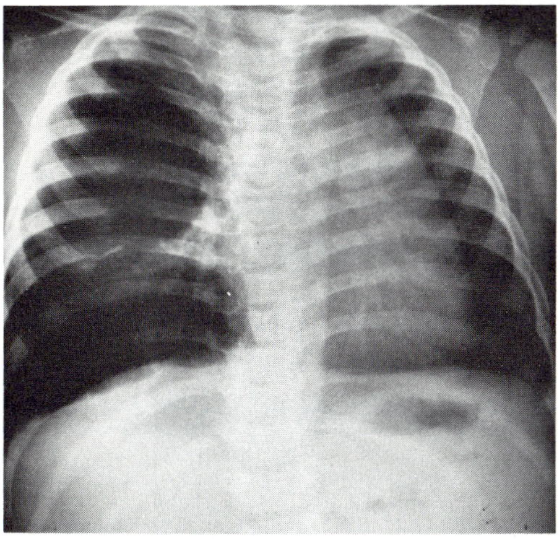

FIG. 19-79. Congenital adenomatoid malformation. This 6-month-old child had mild respiratory distress. Evidence exists for significant shift of the mediastinum. This condition had to be distinguished from an obstructed lung and from pneumatoceles (see Fig. 19-74).

bronchogenic cyst[58] (see also Chapter 15). Communication with the airway is inconstantly demonstrated. Figure 19-80 shows a bronchogenic cyst which changes size grossly and sometimes appears airless. The lack of demonstration of air within the cyst does not necessarily indicate that no airway communication exists. Figure 19-81 shows a bronchogenic cyst with a fluid level (the child is lying on the right side) and a thin wall. These two features enable one to distinguish this lesion from lobar emphysema (see Chapter 6).

A rare *pulmonary cyst* (Fig. 19-82), arising from the superior segment of the right lower lobe, is seen to fill the thorax, compressing the lung against the mediastinum and herniating anterior to the heart. It was initially confused with a pneumothorax but the child was virtually symptomless. It was removed and the lung reexpanded slowly to normal size. The wall of the cyst was found to have some cartilage in it.

Though the presence of cartilage would tend to speak for a congenital origin of the cyst, it is of interest that the remainder of the lung was of normal size. Evidence derived from newborn patients with large diaphragmatic hernias shows that the lung is hypoplastic as a result and does not grow to normal size. Consequently, one would guess that,

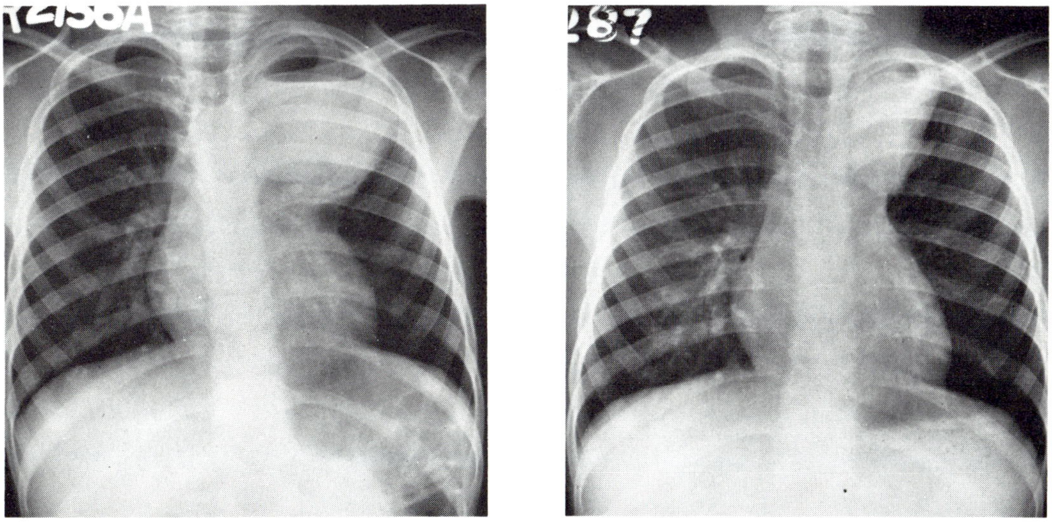

A B

FIG. 19-80. Bronchogenic cyst. An air-fluid level (A) indicates a communication with the airway. (B) A marked change in size appears and no obvious fluid level. This "diverticulum-like" action is unusual.

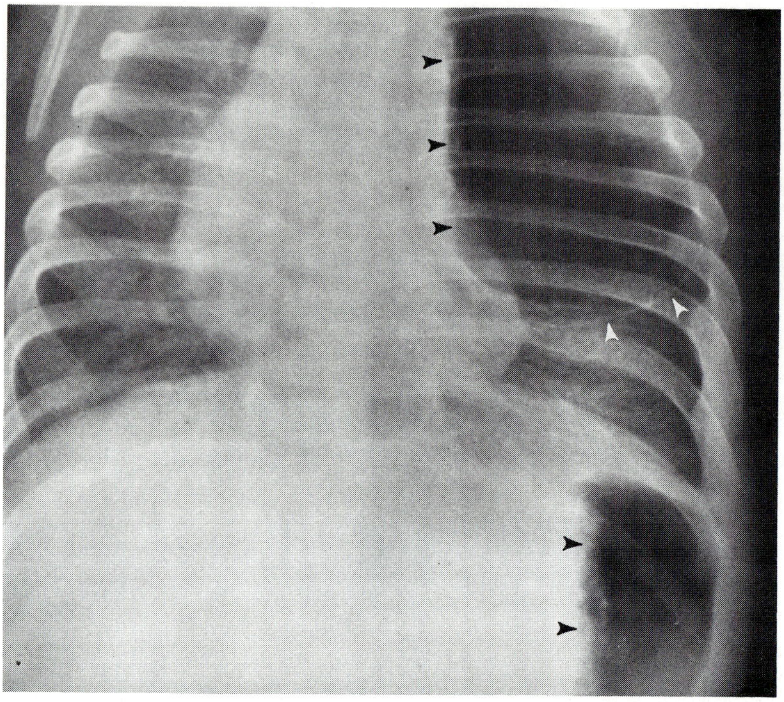

FIG. 19-81. Bronchogenic cyst. The patient is in the right decubitus position (see parallel fluid levels in the cyst and in the stomach, marked by black arrows). The thin wall (white arrows) and the long fluid level distinguishes this condition from lobar emphysema (see Fig. 19-25).

since the lung does not appear hypoplastic, the cyst grew to its present size rather recently.

Cavitation of masses in the lung is another means of cyst production. Among the causes are metastatic Wilms' tumor (Fig. 19-83),[41] metastatic sarcomas,[12] histiocytosis,[42] and fungal infections. The latter have a special

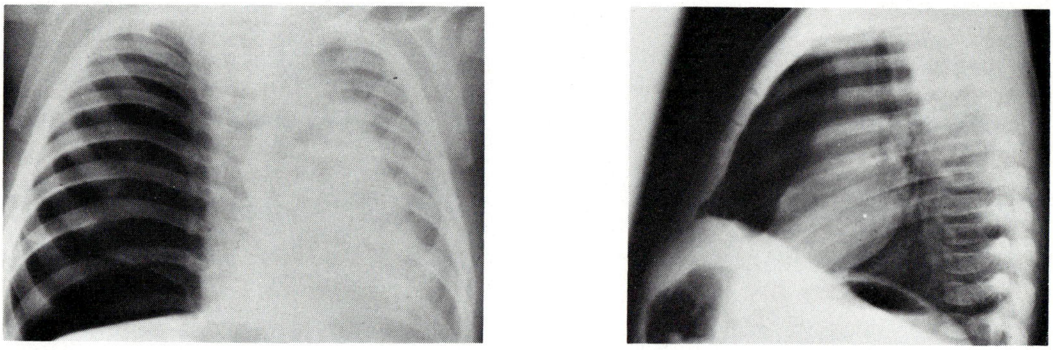

A B

FIG. 19-82. Pulmonary cyst. A large cyst arising from the periphery of the superior segment of the right lower lobe filled the right chest and compressed the remainder of the lung against the heart. It changed size in the decubitus positions. It was removed and contained cartilage in the wall.

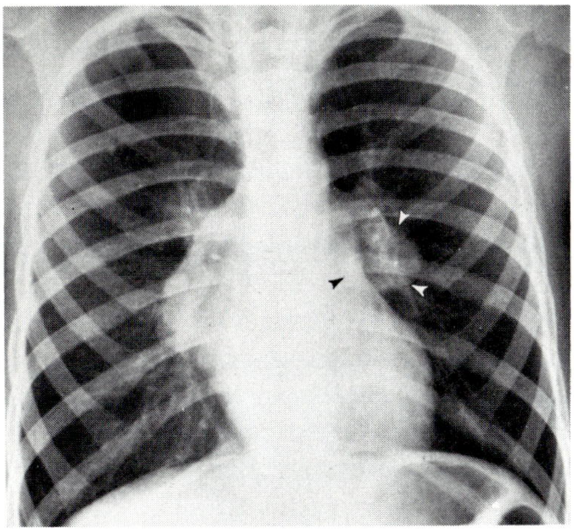

A

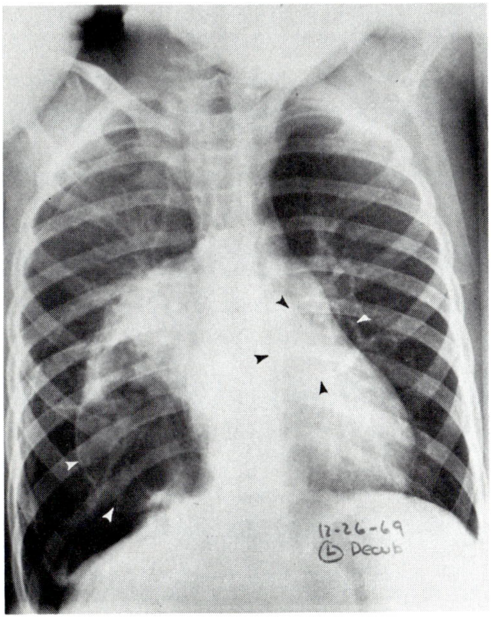

B

FIG. 19-83. Cyst formation in pulmonary metastases from Wilms' tumor.

A, Round metastatic masses are present posterior to both hilar structures.

B, Within 6 months, they have enlarged and become thin-walled cysts. A pneumothorax has been produced on the right.

predilection for forming fungus balls within the cyst.[23] These lesions should be differentiated from similar cystic lesions produced by septic emboli. In Figure 19-84, the child, who has leukemia in remission, had positive blood cultures of *E. coli.* The roentgenogram shows lesions that have a bull's-eye appearance and resemble fungus balls. However, the child was lying in the left side down decubitus position, in which fungus balls would move to a dependent position against the cyst wall. These lesions remain centrally located within the cyst.

Infiltrative Diseases

PNEUMONIA

The roentgenologic protocol for investigation of repeated pneumonias in an infant or child depends on the diagnosis entertained clinically. For instance, respiratory difficulties encountered during feeding of an infant may be caused by aspiration or may be due to the breathlessness of heart failure. On the other hand, a poorly coordinated swallowing mechanism may be at fault. Consideration of the possibility of an *H-type tracheoesophageal fistula* is always on the list of diagnoses. An esophagogram usually shows the lesion. The study should be done with a feeding tube

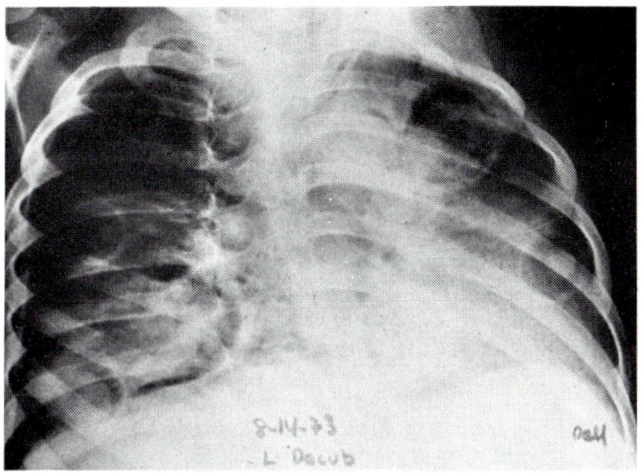

FIG. 19-84. Septic emboli with cyst formation. The child had leukemia in remission and positive blood cultures for *E. coli.* The typical "bulls-eye" lesions are clearly demonstrated. The roentgenogram was made in the left decubitus position and, unlike fungus balls, which fall to the side of the cyst that is dependent, the central mass remains fixed in position.

placed down to about the level of the second thoracic vertebra because this type of fistula is almost always at or near the level of the thoracic inlet. A thin suspension of barium with the consistency of milk is injected under fluoroscopic control, with the patient positioned so that the trachea can be seen clearly separated from the esophagus. The patency of the fistula is probably determined by the pressure gradient across its wall, which in turn is determined by the pressure in the mediastinum and the patency of the glottis. Therefore careful, continuous injections are made under fluoroscopic control while the patient's breathing pattern is permitted to vary from quiet to deep breathing (crying included). This process should be repeated several times, with some method of continuous or rapid-interval recording when necessary.

Feeding the barium by bottle allows for uncontrolled aspiration, and if the fistula happens to be large, barium may flood the lungs (Fig. 19-85). Full-strength water-soluble contrast agents should never be used for this purpose because of the high osmolality (1600 to 1900 mOsm/l) of the media; pulmonary edema is induced when these media are placed in the lung. In addition, the presence of Tween-80 in one of these agents (Gastrografin) precludes its use even in the diluted form.

The classic lobar consolidation is not seen ordinarily in children today, probably because development of the relevant pulmonary lesions is aborted by the early institution of appropriate antibiotics. When lobar pneumonias do appear, unusual circumstances or unusual organisms must be considered as possibly contributory. Among the latter are those that cause a dense roentgen opacity related to the production of large quantities of mucopurulent material, as in Klebsiella[23] or staphylococcal pneumonia. Some pneumonias produce initial symptoms that are not so debilitating, and so allow time for the roentgenographic consolidation to take place. Included in this group are some viruses, mycoplasma, and tuberculosis. Unusual circumstance, such as the coincidence of another disease that produces pulmonary symptoms, is a predisposing factor. For instance, the patient with sickle cell disease may initially have mild pulmonary symptoms and display a segmental or lobar type of opacity. The presence of this type of pneumonic density should always raise the question of sickle cell anemia in a susceptible black patient. The differentiation between infarction and pneumonia cannot be decided accurately on the basis of the roentgenogram's appearance. The patient in Figure 19-86 shows several large round densities, which could possibly be mistaken for metastic lesions except that the borders are not sharp. These densities are multiple foci of *pneumonia due to pneumococcus.* Response to penicillin and the subsequent course was typical. This unusual circumstance developed because the child had measles and the pulmonary symptoms initially were ascribed to measles.

The roentgenographic presentation of lobar pneumonia should always suggest obstruction of the bronchus. Infections of certain kinds may be productive of enough mucopurulent material to prevent volume loss. In small children, foreign body and *tuberculosis* (Fig. 19-87) should be considered. The appropriate radiologic work-up of obstruction and its integration with other studies have been discussed previously (p. 601ff). The more diffuse pattern of bronchopneumonia is demonstrated by a severe case of *mycoplasma* infection (Fig. 19-88). The confidence level of correct diagnosis made from any single pattern of radiographic findings is felt to be fair to poor if the object is to determine the etiologic agent. It improves when the observer is experienced and when other pertinent information is considered.

Figure 19-89 is typical of the changes produced by infection with *Pneumocystis carinii.*[9,17] The patient is a 4-month-old Vietnamese infant who was born prematurely

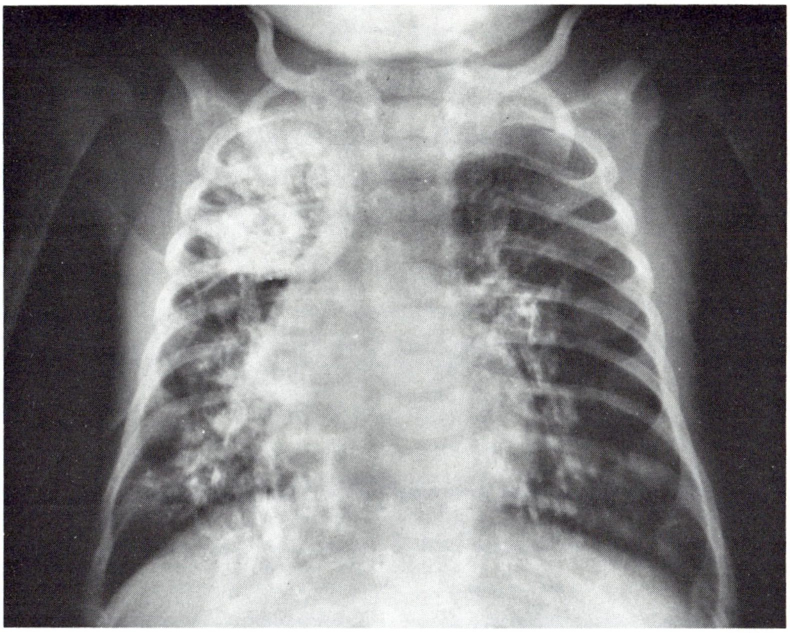

A

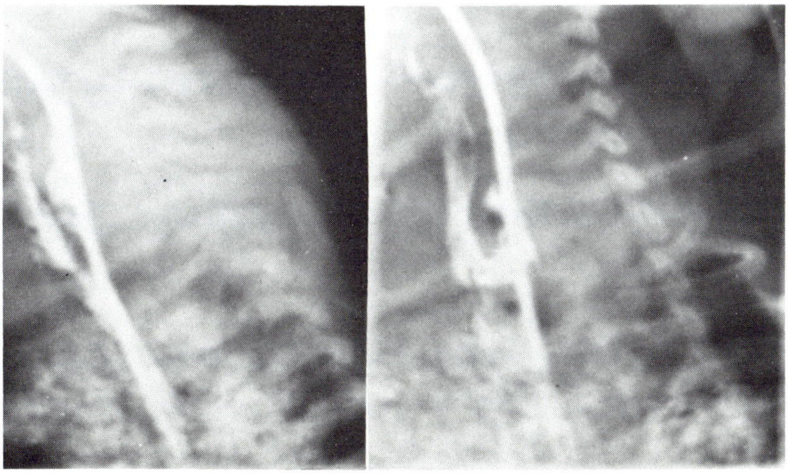

B

FIG. 19-85. H-type tracheoesophageal fistula.

A, Roentgenogram of a child with a large fistula. He had been studied for an H-type fistula by means of a bottle. Large amounts of barium entered the lung through the fistula. After 5 years, no barium is seen on his roentgenogram.

B, Fistula opacified under fluoroscopic control with a feeding tube in place. Notice that the fistula changes size considerably in varying phases of ventilation.

and later adopted and brought to this country. However, the roentgenographic changes are not specific and cannot readily be distinguished from abnormal patterns produced on the roentgenograms of children the same age with pneumonias of other cause. Indeed,

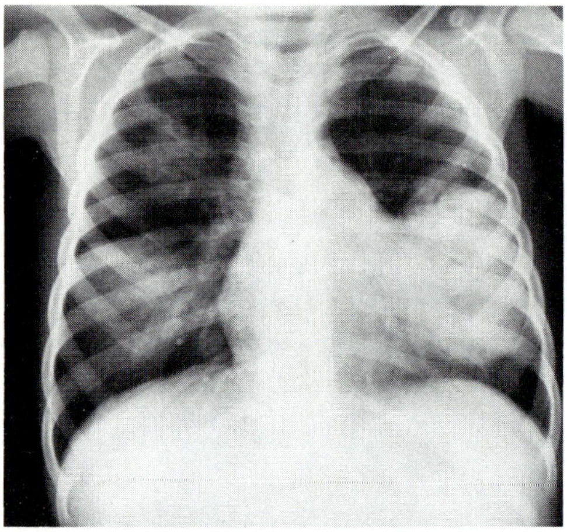

FIG. 19-86. Pneumococcal pneumonia in a patient whose diagnosis was delayed because he had measles.

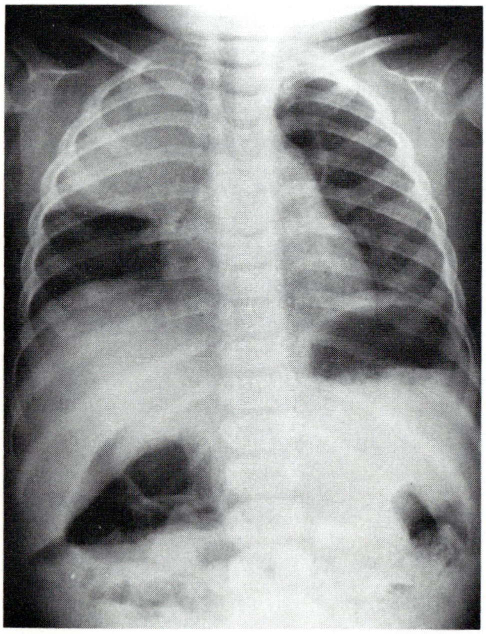

FIG. 19-87. Tuberculosis. Right upper lobe density without volume loss or an air bronchogram suggests that pneumonia has occurred secondarily in the presence of the obstructed bronchus. Endobronchial tuberculosis is the cause of the obstruction in this child.

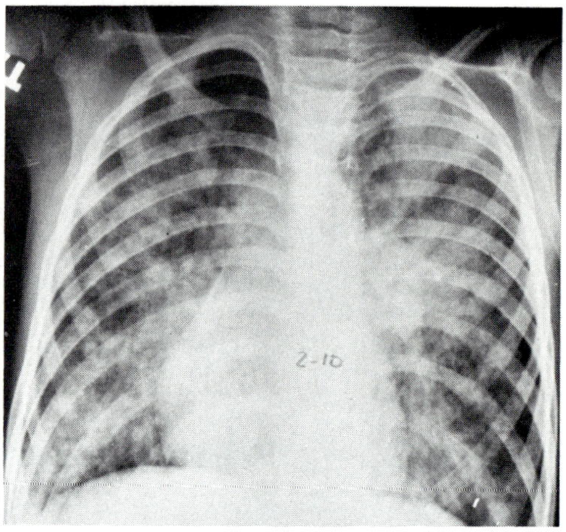

FIG. 19-88. Mycoplasma pneumoniae. Diffuse involvement of both lungs is present; however, mycoplasma infection may give either an interstitial pattern or occasionally a lobar consolidation.

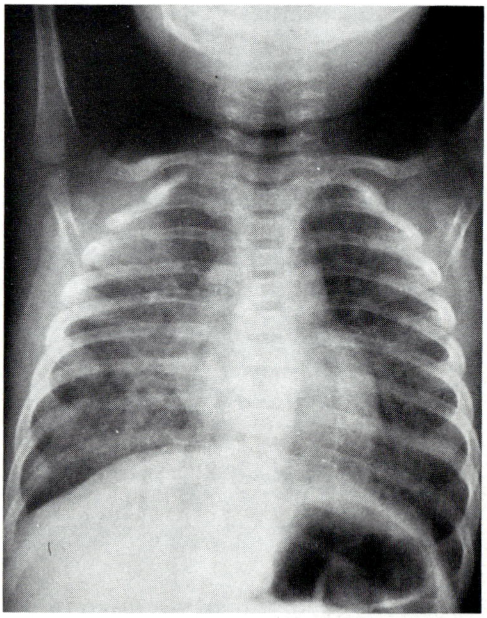

FIG. 19-89. Pneumocystis carinii pneumonia. The patient was a premature infant born in Vietnam; the disease developed when the infant was 4 months of age.

since *P. carinii* infections often occur in a setting of chronic debility and serious systemic disease with lung involvement by leukemic infiltration, nephritic edema, or rheumatic changes (see also Chapter 18), the presenting roentgenographic pattern of

P. carinii may be quite altered by these other factors.

The pattern of bilateral densities seen in the film in Figure 19-90, which developed over a period of several weeks, followed two separate episodes of transient pleural effusion, which were the result of *multiple pulmonary emboli* (diagnosis by lung biopsy). However, though entirely consistent and even typical of that diagnosis, infection had been the favored radiographic diagnosis. Since the child had lupus nephritis and had been treated with steroids, an opportunistic infection, namely, *P. carinii*, was the erroneous clinical diagnosis. These two cases should serve to remind one of the limitations of the method.

On the other hand, these diffuse roentgenographic patterns do offer information of value. The device of separating diseases into those that display a *reticulonodular pattern* and therefore are interstitial in nature and those that are more confluent and therefore involve the airspace is popular and useful. The limitations of this classification are becoming more evident. However, certain empirically established patterns are useful in quickly reducing the number of diagnostic choices.

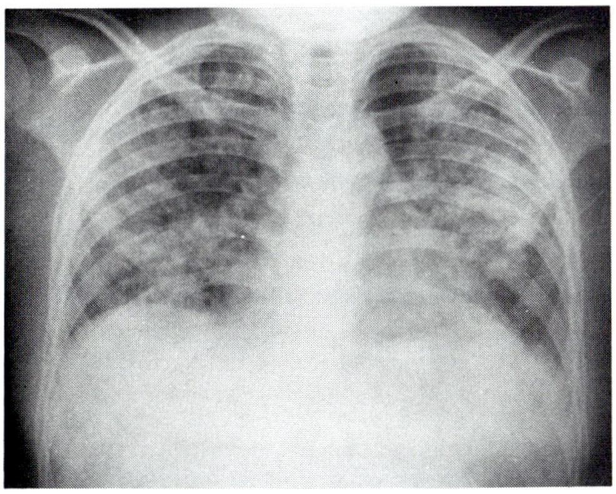

FIG. 19-90. Multiple pulmonary emboli. Bilateral pulmonary densities associated with small lung volumes are findings compatible with the diagnosis, but the diagnosis of pulmonary emboli ordinarily must be made in conjunction with clinical findings.

Figure 19-91 exhibits the nodular pattern of *miliary tuberculosis*. The adenopathy on the right is somewhat obscured.

The reticulonodular pattern can suggest a storage disease, such as *Niemann-Pick disease* in Fig. 19-92[43] or *glycogen storage disease* in Figure 19-93 (see also Chapter 18). The wide distribution of small punctate calcifications in Figure 19-94 ordinarily suggests healed granulomatous disease such as tuberculosis or

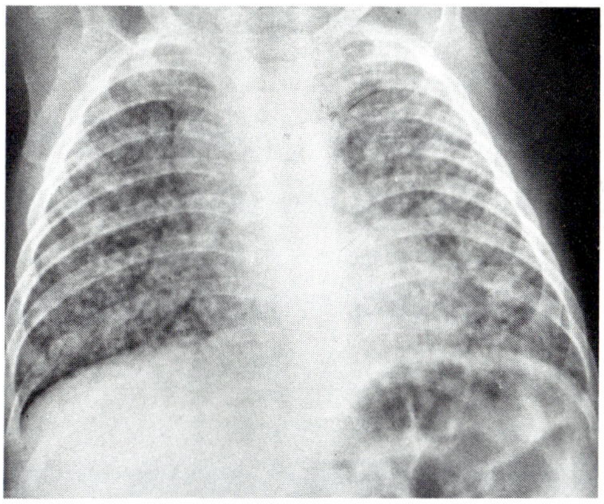

FIG. 19-91. Miliary tuberculosis.

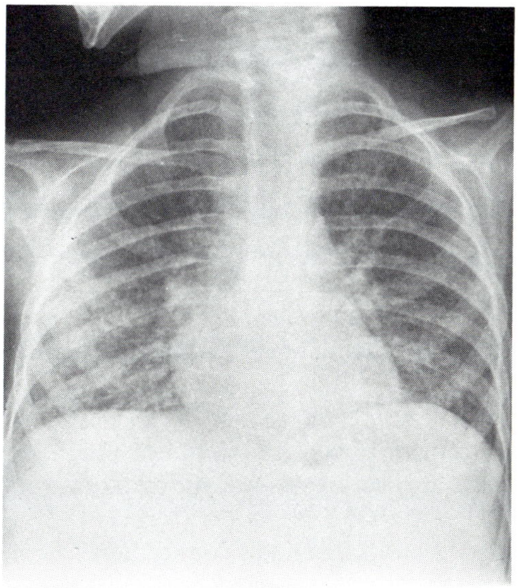

FIG. 19-92. Niemann-Pick disease. A fine reticulonodular pattern appears throughout the lungs.

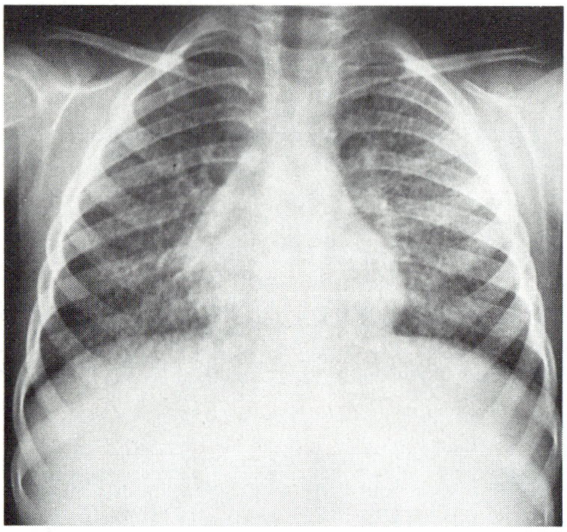

FIG. 19-93. Glycogen storage disease. The lung is involved diffusely as shown by a fine reticulonodular pattern.

histoplasmosis, but has been described in post-viral pneumonias such as chickenpox. In the case in Figure 19-94, a chest film was reported to have shown these calcifications in the newborn period. This film was made at 1 year of age; the child had markedly elevated titers for cytomegalic inclusion disease.[18]

PULMONARY EDEMA

The central location of the radiodensity seen in pulmonary edema, involving the hilar, perihilar, and midzones of the lung but sparing the outer or peripheral zone, is the hallmark that leads to its diagnosis.[34] The density is mostly confluent, imparting a somewhat hazy quality to the area. The hilar and midzone vessels can be seen but lose their sharp definition. Linear channels emanating from the hilum have increased in number and probably represent dilated lymphatics. Air bronchograms may be seen but are not a prominent feature; if bronchi are seen, they usually show evidence of "peribronchial cuffing" or "thickening" due to the accumulation of fluid in the interstices.

Figure 19-95 shows the aforementioned changes in a child in heart failure due to hypertension and glomerulonephritis. Note particularly the lack of change in distribution of the pulmonary fluid when the position is changed from the erect to left decubitus posi-

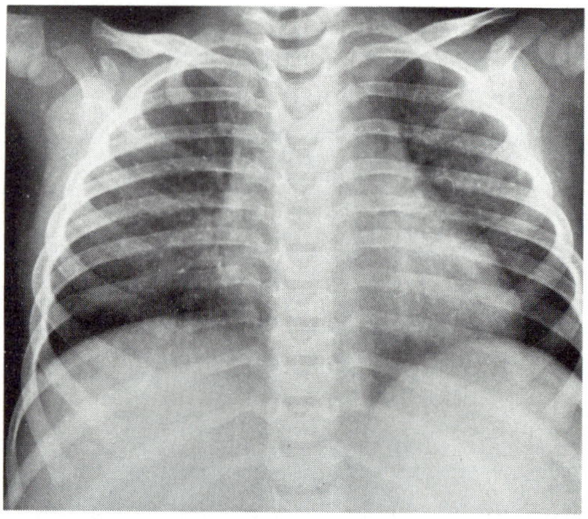

A

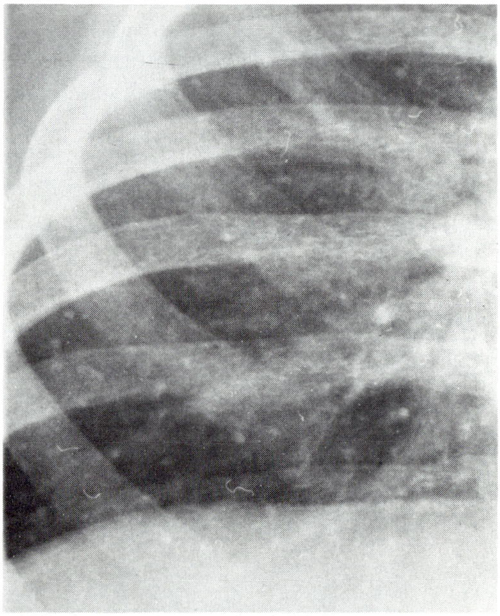

B

FIG. 19-94. Cytomegalic inclusion disease. Punctate calcifications are seen in this 12-month-old child who had elevated titers for cytomegalic inclusion disease. Skull roentgenograms were normal. He was reported to have had these calcifications on his chest roentgenogram in the neonatal period.

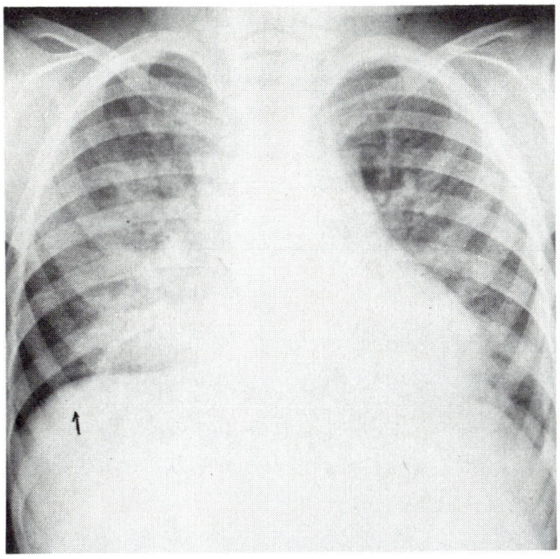

A

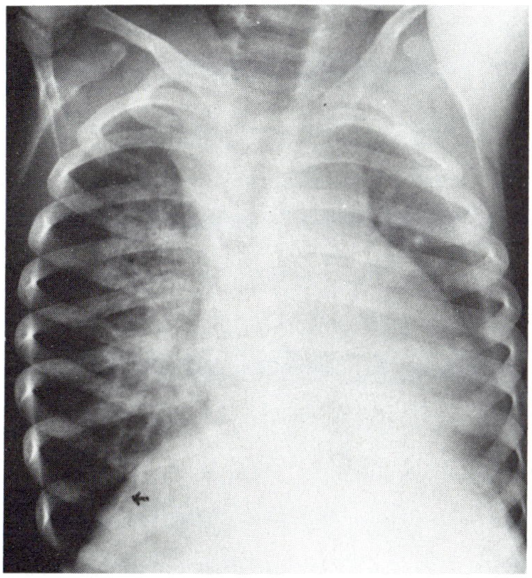

B

FIG. 19-95. *A*, Pulmonary edema due to hypertension in a child with glomerulonephritis. The central location of the density is typical.

B, In the left decubitus position, the "medullary" distribution of the fluid in the interstices of the right lung is clearly shown.

tion. The historically interesting concept of "medulla-cortex" of the lung is beautifully demonstrated in this decubitus film.

In the erect position, the edema fluid accumulates in the lower lung preferentially because of the hydrostatic pressure gradient down the chest. In Figure 19-96, the haziness (fluid) is confined to the lower lobes, and as a consequence, the upper lobe vessels and the hilar structures have sharp borders while the lower lobe vessels are poorly defined. In addition, the lower lobe vessels are small while the upper lobe vessels are larger. This reversal of the normal relationship signals the presence of a diversion of blood flow to the upper lungs because of the edema. An increase in flow will cause the vein to dilate (see arrow) when left atrial pressure increases. The cause for heart failure in this child in Figure 19-96 was acute rheumatic fever.

Although not well understood, pulmonary edema due to heart failure may also present as a localized density simulating pneumonia (Fig. 19-97). The problem of identification of an area of pneumonia in a child with intermittent or chronic congestive heart failure is virtually impossible. The dilemma is most often encountered when heart failure is a consequence of a large left-to-right shunt.

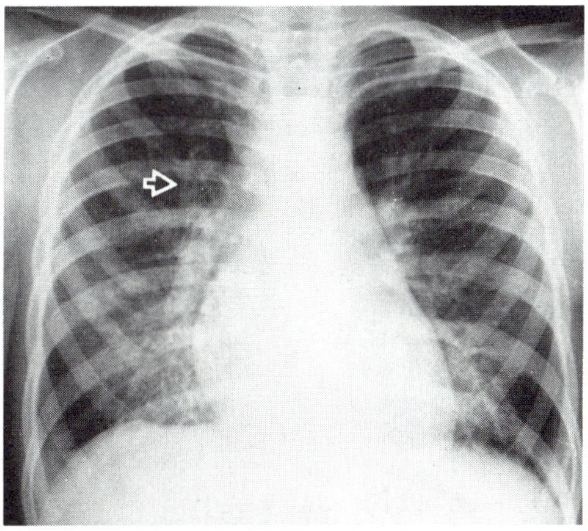

FIG. 19-96. Pulmonary edema. In the erect position, the edema accumulates in the lower lung because of the increase in hydrostatic pressure; blood flow to the area is decreased, with the result that the vessels are smaller and poorly seen. Blood flow is diverted to the upper lung and the vessels are larger (arrows) than the lower lobe vessels. The patient was in heart failure because of acute rheumatic fever.

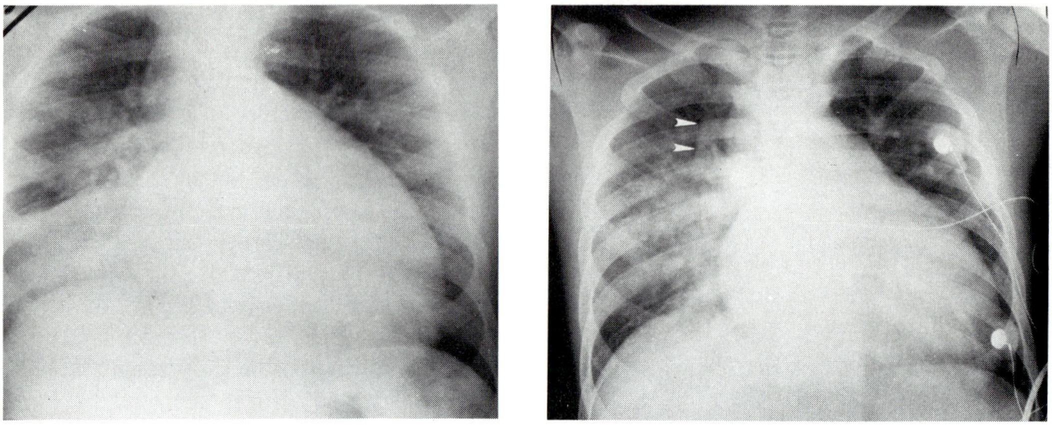

A B

FIG. 19-97. *A*, Lobar pulmonary edema. Initially this patient with marked cardiomegaly developed a lobar density on the right, simulating pneumonia. Treatment for heart failure was begun, with improvement.

B, In less than 24 hours, the density cleared and a typical pulmonary edema pattern is seen. Arrows indicate a large upper lobe vein.

Transient localized areas of pulmonary edema, which may result in segmental or subsegmental atelectasis (Fig. 19-98), cannot be distinguished from pneumonia. Usually, the decision to treat pneumonia or heart failure (or both) must be based on clinical determinants. Another cause for confusion is the remarkable similarity in appearance of the 2-week-old premature infant with a patent ductus arteriosus in heart failure and another 2-week-old premature infant whose diagnosis is the Wilson-Mikity syndrome[72] (Fig. 19-99).

Histiocytosis, sarcoidosis, and, occasionally,

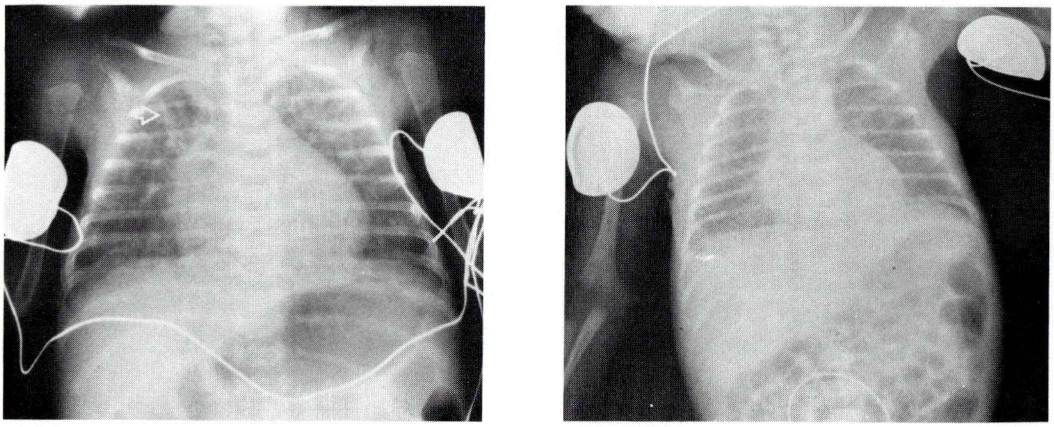

A B

FIG. 19-98. *A*, Infant, 3 weeks old, with a large left-to-right shunt because of a ventricular septal defect. Heart failure ensued. A typical segmental atelectasis in the right upper lobe (arrow) may or may not be related to infection.

B, Normal roentgenogram at 3 days of age.

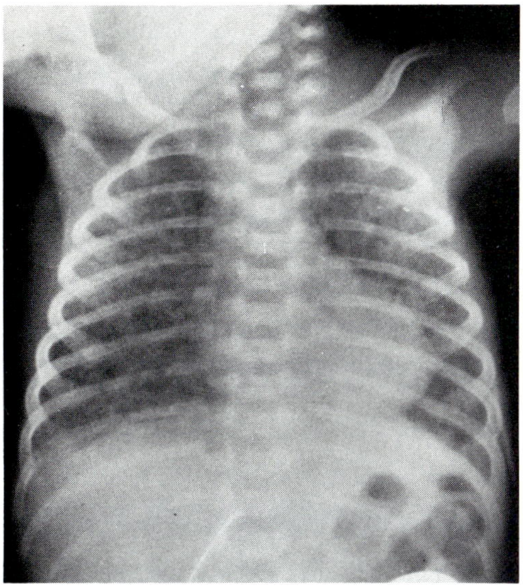

A

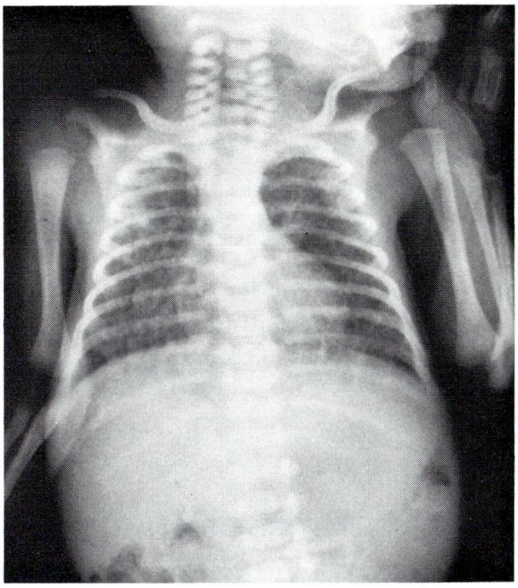

B

FIG. 19-99. *A*, Two-week-old premature infant with a patent ductus arteriosus. The lungs are large and the markings increased. The heart size is at the upper limits of normal.

B, Two-week-old premature infant with Wilson-Mikity syndrome. The roentgenograms are virtually indistinguishable.

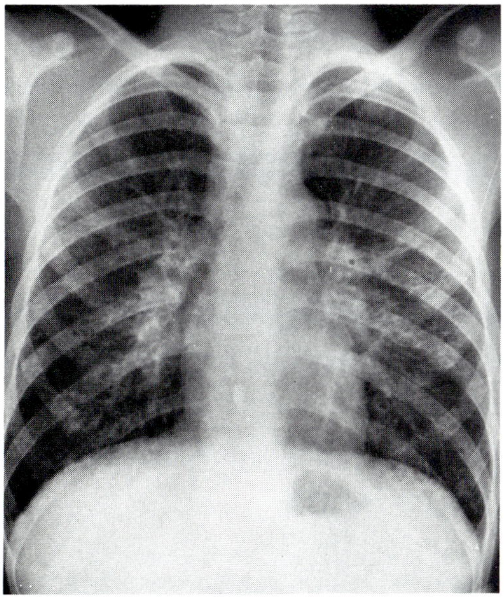

A

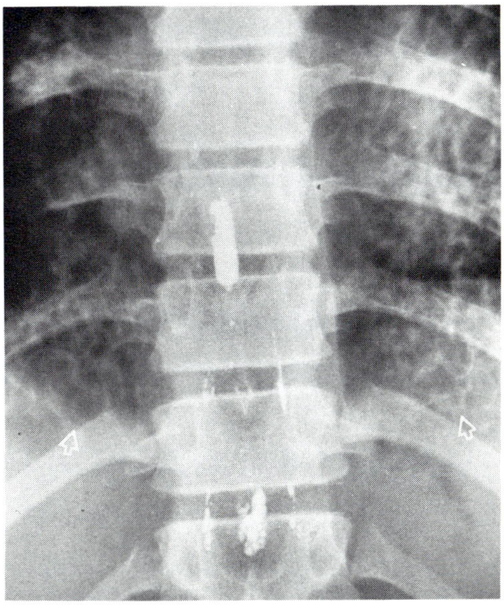

B

FIG. 19-100. *A*, Histiocytosis. A 14-year-old male had solitary vertebral involvement 1 year previously. The chest roentgenogram shows hilar adenopathy, peribronchial cuffing, and a diffuse interstitial pattern. He has since had involvement of several other areas of osseous involvement. Lesions have all resolved with treatment.

B, Coned-down view to show reticular pattern with distortion by scarring to produce a honeycombed pattern. Residual myelographic material appears in the spinal canal.

Hodgkin's disease may produce a roentgenographic pattern consistent with interstitial disease. The presence of hilar lymph node enlargement suggests the possibility that the interstitial roentgen changes reflect lymphatic dilatation in part due to obstruction to flow through the abnormal nodes. This pattern may also be seen in heart failure where the obstruction to lymph flow is due to elevated pressures in the superior vena cava. In Figure 19-100, the changes result from histiocytosis involving the skeletal system and the lungs in a 14-year-old boy. The very large hilar nodes present are accompanied by peribronchial thickening and a diffuse reticular pattern. The film of a 12-year-old girl with Hodgkin's disease displays a mild reticular pattern throughout the lungs and septal lines (Kerley B lines) (Fig. 19-101).

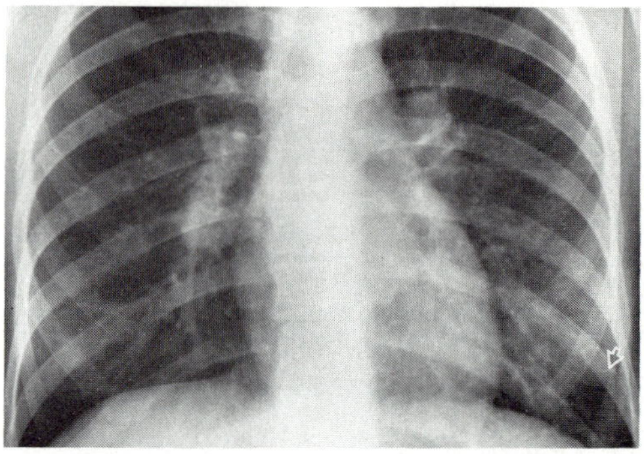

FIG. 19-101. Hodgkin's disease. Hilar adenopathy is seen in combination with a diffuse interstitial pattern, including septal lines (arrow).

Septal lines are short, straight thin lines that lie approximately at right angles to their intercept on the pleural surface. They reflect accumulation of fluid in the interlobular septa of the lung; in chronic states, the septal lines become permanent. The lines are seen classically in mitral stenosis and often in acute congestive failure of any cause. Their presence in these situations correlates well with an increase in pulmonary venous pressure. Septal lines may be seen (as in Fig. 19-102) in any situation of local or generalized dilatation of lymphatics, whether due to obstruction, overproduction of lymph, or stasis due to failure of the transport system.

An acute shift of fluid into the lung parenchyma may be caused by many different factors and agents other than hydrostatic pressure. The "integrity" of the endothelium of the microcirculation is affected so that, in any given instance, one or more of the elements of the circulation may traverse the wall along

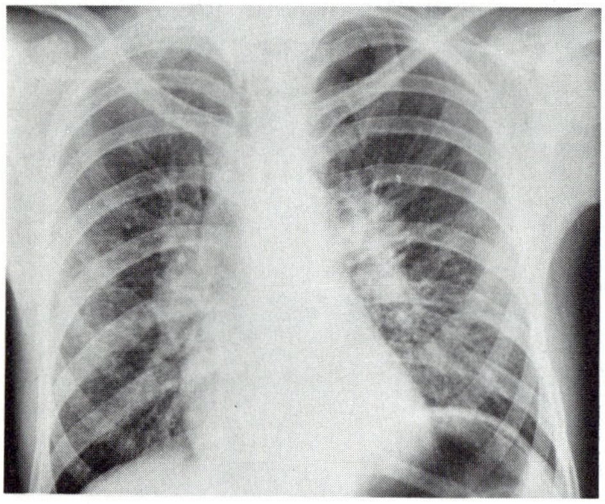

A

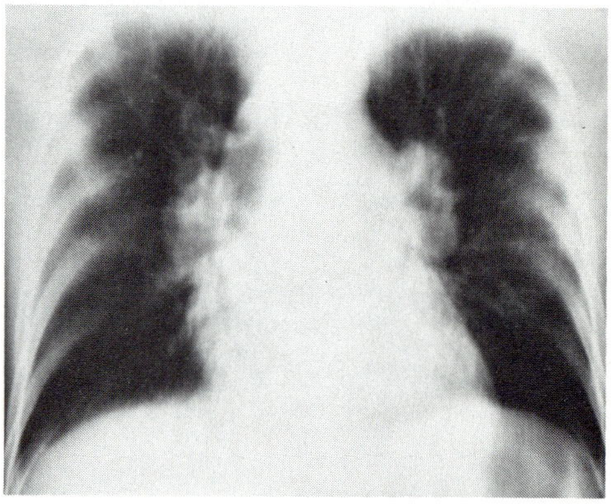

B

FIG. 19-102. *A*, Sarcoidosis. Hilar adenopathy and a diffuse interstitial pattern in this 14-year-old boy makes this condition virtually indistinguishable from histiocytosis and even, at times, Hodgkin's disease.
B, Tomography shows the hilar adenopathy to good advantage.

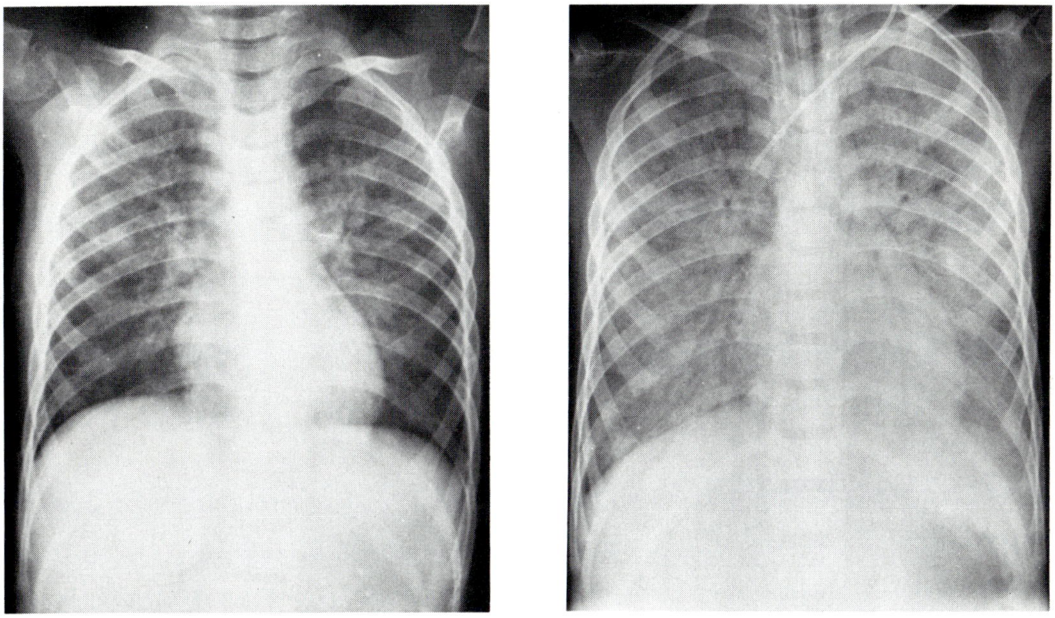

A B

FIG. 19-103, Chicken pox pneumonia (A) leading to acute respiratory failure (B). The second roentgenogram followed the first by 24 hours.

with the fluid. The particulate elements and the fluid, in combination, tend generally to render the lung quite opaque, with relative sparing of the inner or central zones of the lung.

Frequently an infection is present, as was the case in the child with *chickenpox* whose films are shown in Figure 19-103. The first film, showing minimal nonspecific changes consistent with a viral *bronchopneumonia,* precedes the second film by 24 hours. The child was in *acute respiratory failure.*[51] On the other hand, another child, who had *leukemia* (Fig. 19-104), virtually cleared her lungs within 12 hours after steroids were given. She had also been given antibiotics.

The *pulmonary pathology of sickle cell disease* may sometimes result from an acute shift of fluid and cells due to "injury" to the capillary endothelium (Fig. 19-105). Both thrombus and infection could account for the changes. This 10-year-old girl had only a few

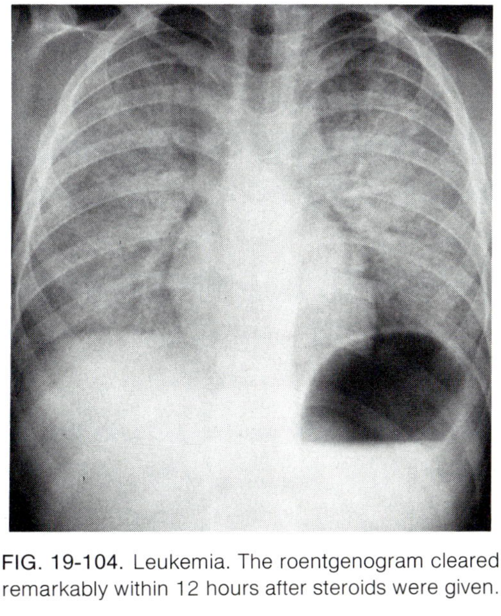

FIG. 19-104. Leukemia. The roentgenogram cleared remarkably within 12 hours after steroids were given.

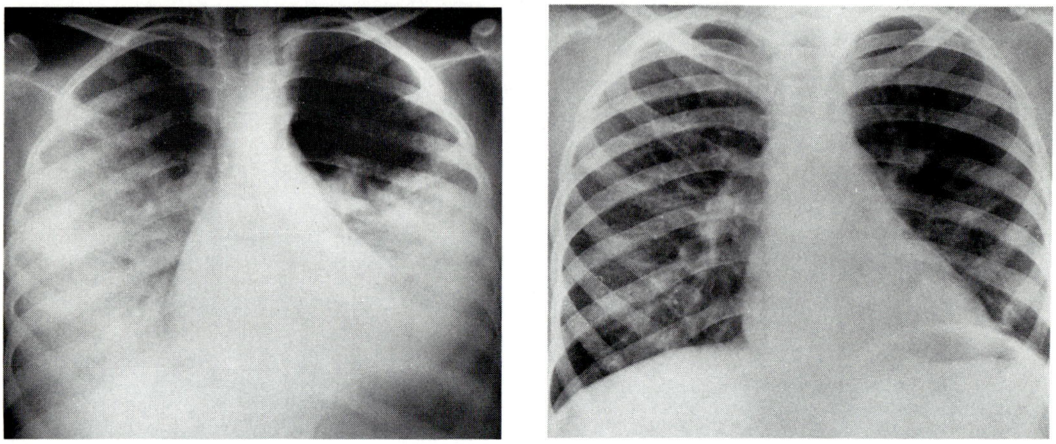

A B

FIG. 19-105. Sickle cell "pulmonopathy": *A*, Roentgenogram showed progressive opacification over a 12-hour period to the point reached in this film.
B, Six days later. Actually considerable improvement occurred within 2 days.

minor areas of density 12 hours before. She survived and most of the fluid in the lung cleared within 48 hours. The second film was made 6 days later.

Hemorrhage may result in an interesting pattern in which the midzones of the lung are involved, with the inner (hilar) zone and the outer (cortical) zones apparently spared. Classically Goodpasture's syndrome appears this way.[60] Two cases illustrate this midzonal pattern:

Figure 19-106 with *Henoch-Schönlein syndrome* and Figure 19-107 with *hemosiderosis.* These conditions cleared quickly. With repeated episodes of bleeding, minute fibrotic nodules may be formed, giving an appearance of nodular interstitial disease.

Trauma to the thorax leading to hemor-

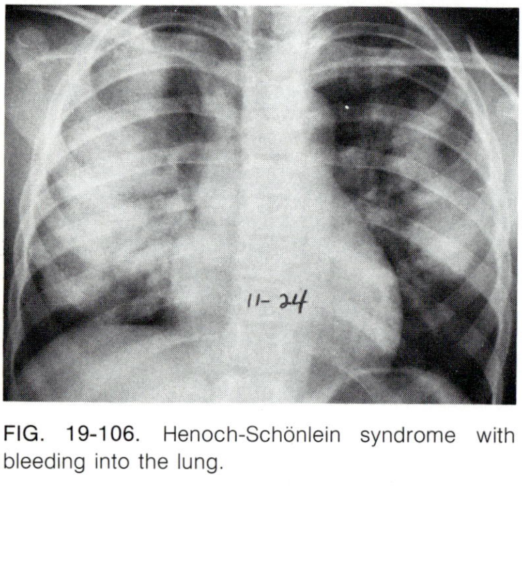

FIG. 19-106. Henoch-Schönlein syndrome with bleeding into the lung.

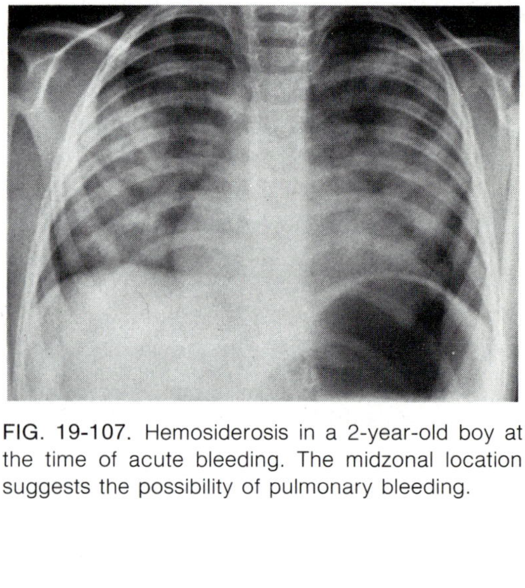

FIG. 19-107. Hemosiderosis in a 2-year-old boy at the time of acute bleeding. The midzonal location suggests the possibility of pulmonary bleeding.

rhage may give a similar appearance (Fig. 19-108). Clearance takes place within a few days, though complications such as pneumatoceles may arise. However, these complications usually resolve without incident.

Finally, persistence of the fetal lung fluid after birth as a kind of "edema" state is a

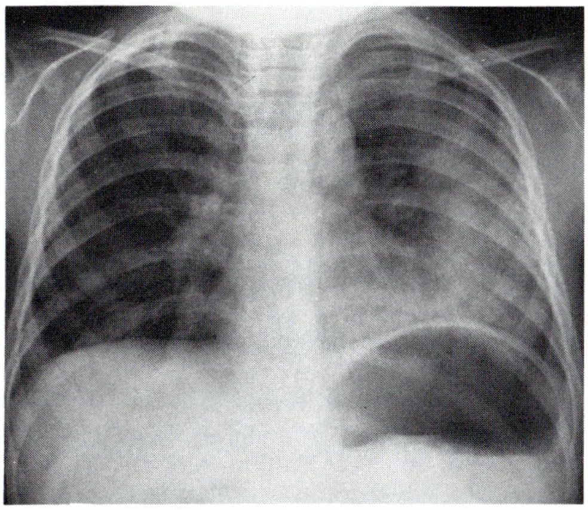

FIG. 19-108. Contusion with pulmonary bleeding.

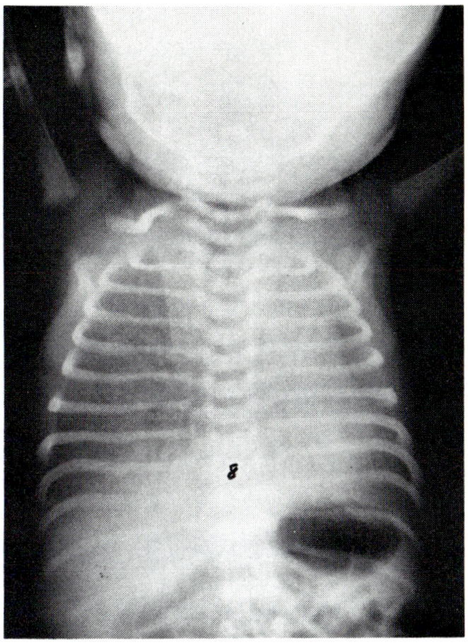

FIG. 19-109. Severe fetal pulmonary fluid retention in a child delivered by cesarean section.

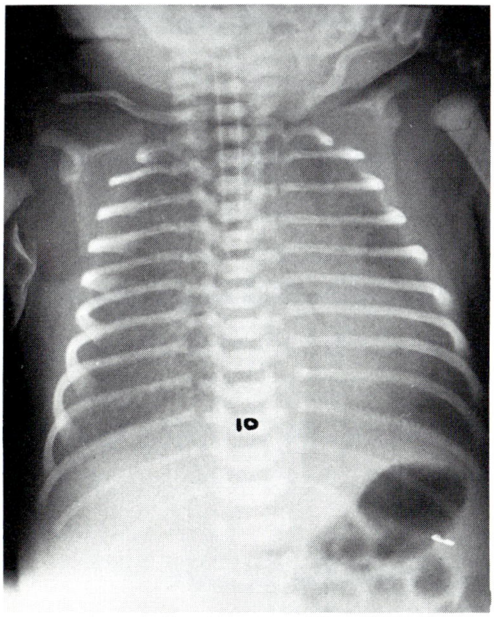

A

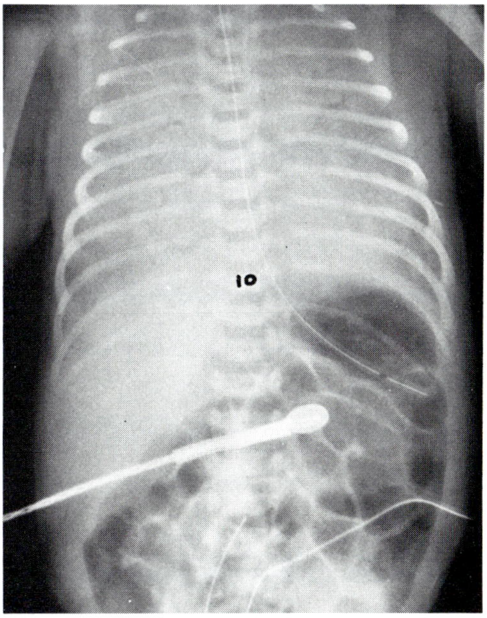

B

FIG. 19-110. Severe respiratory distress syndrome in a newborn child who had no measurable thyroid function.
A, Roentgenogram on day 1.
B, Day 2.

major reason for the opacities encountered in the newborn. This problem is seen chiefly in the syndrome, transient tachypnea of the newborn[2] (see Fig. 19-43). However, with more serious diseases, the lungs may be virtually opaque, as in Figure 19-109, a child who was born by cesarean section and had a very low Apgar score. Notice that the level of the diaphragm is normal so that atelectasis can be discounted as a major reason for the opacity. The full-term newborn infant proved to have no measurable thyroid function (Fig. 19-110). The films were made on the first and second day of life and show the diaphragm to be low (between the ninth and tenth ribs). The first film shows changes of residual fluid. The relationship of thyroid deficiency and respiratory distress syndrome has been suggested, although a clear understanding of this relationship is not yet available.

BIBLIOGRAPHY

1. Anderson, R. C., F. Char and P. Adams, Jr.: Proximal interruption of a pulmonary arch (absence of one pulmonary artery): case report and a new embryologic interpretation. *Dis. Chest 34*:73, 1958.
2. Avery, M. E., O. D. Gatewood and G. Brumley: Transient tachypnea of the newborn: possible delayed resorption of fluid at birth. *Am. J. Dis. Child. 111*:380, 1966.
3. Avnet, N. L.: Roentgenologic features of congenital bilateral anterior diaphragmatic eventration. *Am. J. Roentgenol. 88*:743, 1962.
4. Barnhard, H. J., J. A. Pierce, J. W. Joyce and J. H. Bates: Roentgenographic determination of total lung capacity. A new method evaluated in health, emphysema, and congestive heart failure. *Am. J. Med. 42*:547, 1967.
5. Baxter, J. D. and J. S. Dunbar: Tracheomalacia. *Ann. Otol. Rhinol. Laryngol. 72*:1013, 1963.
6. Berdon, W. E. and D. H. Baker: Vascular anomalies and the infant lung: rings, slings, and other things. *Seminars in Roentgenology,* Vol. 7, No. 1 (Jan.), 1972.
7. Brunner, S.: Tracheography and bronchography: techniques and indications during infancy and childhood. In *Progress in Pediatric Radiology,* Vol. 1. Karger, Basel, p. 45, 1967.
8. Caffey, J.: On the natural regression of pulmonary cysts during early infancy. *Pediatrics 11*:48, 1953.
9. Capitanio, M. A. and J. A. Kirkpatrick, Jr.: Pneumocytosis carinii pneumonia. *Am. J. Roentgenol., 97*:174, 1966.
10. Capitanio, M. A. and J. A. Kirkpatrick: Lateral decubitus film: an aid in determining air-trapping in children. *Radiology 103*:460, 1972.
11. Christiaens L., G. Decroix, B. Gaudier, G. Fontaine, R. Walbum and J. P. Farriaux: Hemangiomas of the larynx and of the trachea in infants: six cases. *Arch. Fr. Pediatr. 22*:513, 1965.
12. Coussemart, A. M. and C. A. Gooding: Cavitating pulmonary metastatic disease in children. *Am. J. Roentgenol. 117*:833, 1973.
13. Craig, J. M., J. Kirkpatrick and E. B. D. Neuhauser: Congenital cystic adenomatoid malformation of lungs in infants. *Am. J. Roentgenol. 76*:516, 1956.
14. Davis, W. S. and R. P. Allen: Accessory diaphragm: duplication of the diaphragm. *Radiol. Clin. North Am. 6*:258, 1968.
15. Dunbar, J. S.: Upper respiratory tract obstruction in infants and children. Caldwell lecturer, 1969: *Am. J. Roentgenol. 109*:225, 1970.
16. Dunbar, J. S.: Epiglottitis and croup. *J. Can. Assoc. Radiol. 12*:86, 1961.
17. Ebel, Kl-D., and H. Fendel: The roentgen changes of pneumocystis pneumonia and their anatomic basis. In *Progress in Pediatric Radiology,* Vol. 1. Karger, Basel, p. 177, 1967.
18. Emanuel, I. and G. W. Kenny: Cytomegalic inclusion disease of infancy. *Pediatrics 38*:957, 1966.
19. Fagan, C. J.: Traumatic lung cyst. *Am. J. Roentgenol. 97*:186, 1966.
20. Felson, B.: Accessory diaphragm. In *Chest Roentgenology.* W. B. Saunders Co., Philadelphia, p. 89, 1973.
21. Felson, B.: The mediastinal lines. In *Chest Roentgenology.* W. B. Saunders Co., Philadelphia, p. 409, 1973.
22. Felson, B.: Pulmonary agenesis and related anomalies. In *Seminars in Roentgenology,* Vol. VII, No. 1, p. 17, Jan. 1972.
23. Felson, B., L. S. Rosenberg and M. Hamburger, Jr.: Roentgen findings in acute Friedlander's pneumonia. *Radiology 53*:559, 1949.
24. Fraser, R. G. and J. A. P. Paré: *Diagnosis of Diseases of the Chest.* W. B. Saunders Co., Philadelphia, p. 581, 1970.
25. Fraser, R. G. and J. A. P. Paré: *Diagnosis of Diseases of the Chest.* W. B. Saunders Co., Philadelphia, p. 1240, 1970.
26. Fraser, R. G. and J. A. P. Paré: Unilateral or lobar emphysema (Swyer-James or MacLeod's syndrome). In *Diagnosis of Diseases of the Chest.* W. B. Saunders Co., Philadelphia, p. 1033, 1970.
27. Friedman, P. S., L. Solis-Cohen and S. Levine:

Accessory lobe of the liver and its significance in roentgen diagnosis. *Am. J. Roentgenol. 57*:601, 1947.
28. Gerle, R. D., A. Jeretski, III, C. A. Ashley and A. S. Berne: Congenital broncho-pulmonary foregut malformation; pulmonary sequestration communicating with the gastrointestinal tract. *N. Engl. J. Med. 278*:1413, 1968.
29. Gold, W. M. and K. R. McKormack: Pulmonary function response to radioisotope scanning of the lung. *J.A.M.A. 197*:146, 1966.
30. Goldman, H. S. and M. Zelefsky: Utility of the decubitus position in children. *Presentation Radiologic Society North America,* Chicago, Nov., 1968.
31. Goris, M. L., S. G. Daspito, J. P. Walter, J. McRae and J. Lamb: Applications of ventilation lung imaging with ^{81m}-Krypton. *Radiology 122*:399, 1977.
32. Griscom, N. T., G. P. C. Harris, M. E. B. Wohl, G. F. Vawter and A. J. Eraklin: Fluid-filled lung due to airway obstruction in the newborn. *Pediatrics 43*:388, 1969.
33. Heikel, P. E. and M. Pasila: Intralobar sequestration of the lung. In *Progress in Pediatric Radiology.,* Vol. 1. Year Book Medical Publishers, Chicago, p. 256, 1967.
34. Heitzman, E. R.: Pulmonary edema and hemorrhage. In *The Lung. Radiologic-Pathologic Correlations.* C. V. Mosby Co., St. Louis, 1973.
35. Hendren, W. H., III, and R. V. Haggerty: Staphylococcic pneumonia in infancy and childhood: analysis of seventy-five cases. *J.A.M.A. 168*:6, 1968.
36. Hoffman, J. I. E.: The normal pulmonary circulation. In *Pulmonary Physiology of the Fetus, Newborn and Child,* E. M. Scarpelli (Ed.). Lea & Febiger, Philadelphia, p. 271, 1975.
37. Holman, C. B. and W. E. Miller: Juvenile nasopharyngeal fibroma. *Am. J. Roentgenol. Radium Ther. 94*:292, 1965.
38. Hudson, H. L. and W. H. McAlister: Obstructing tracheal hemangioma in infancy. *Am. J. Roentgenol. 93*:428, 1965.
39. Joseph, P. M., W. E. Berdon, D. H. Baker, T. L. Slovis and J. O. Haller: Upper airway obstruction in infants and small children. *Radiology 121*:143, 1976.
40. Kartagener, M. and P. Stucki: Bronchiectasis with situs inversus. *Arch. Pediatr. 79*:193, 1962.
41. Kassner, E. G., H. S. Goldman and A. Elguezabel: Cavitating lung nodules and pneumothorax in children with metastatic Wilms' tumor. *Am. J. Roentgenol. 126*:728, 1976.
42. Keats, T. E. and J. S. Crane: Cystic changes of the lungs in histiocystosis. *Am. J. Dis. Child. 88*:764, 1954.
43. Kittredge, R. D., A. Geller and N. Finby: The reticuloendothelioses in the lung. *Am. J. Roentgenol. 100*:588, 1967.
44. Krause, G. R. and M. Lubert: Patterns of lobar collapse as observed radiographically. *Radiology 56*:165, 1951.
45. Loyd, H. M., S. T. String and A. B. Du Bois: Radiographic and plethysmographic determination of total lung capacity. *Radiology 86*:7, 1966.
46. Lubert, M. and G. R. Krause: Further observations on lobar collapse. *Radiol. Clin. North Am. 1*:331, 1963.
47. MacEwan, D. W., J. S. Dunbar, R. D. Smith and B. St.-J. Brown: Pneumothorax in the neonate (its recognition and evaluation). *Am. Radiol. 7*:459, 1964.
48. MacKellar, A. and J. C. Kennedy: Congenital diverticulum of the pharynx simulating esophageal atresia. *J. Pediatr. Surg. 7*:408, 1972.
49. MacLeod, W. M.: Abnormal transradiancy of one lung. *Thorax 9*:147, 1954.
50. Macguire, G. H.: The larynx: simplified radiological examination using heavy filtration and high voltage. *Radiology 87*:102, 1966.
51. Meschan, I., C. R. De Armas and M. Scharyj: Adult bronchopulmonary dysplasia: the simularity in roentgen and histopathologic appearance between some cases of oxygen toxicity, radiation pneumonitis, and postcytotoxic nonspecific bronchopneumonia. *Radiology 92*:612, 1969.
52. Moskowitz, P. S. and N. T. Griscom: The medial pneumothorax. *Radiology 120*:143, 1976.
53. Moyer, J. H., G. Glantz and A. N. Brest: Pulmonary arteriovenous fistulas. Physiologic and clinical considerations. *Am. J. Med. 32*:417, 1962.
54. Nadel, J. A., W. G. Wolff and P. D. Graf: Powdered tantalum as a medium for bronchography in canine and human lungs. *Invest. Radiol., 3*:229, 1968.
55. Osterman, F. A., Jr., B. W. Gayler, G. H. Zeman, B. G. Kirk and H. Kashima: The larynx and pharynx: xeroradiographic technique. *Appl. Radiol. 5*:53, 1976.
56. Patriquin, H. B.: The roentgen evaluation of childhood speech disorders: basic principles and techniques, with special reference to movements of the lateral pharyngeal walls. *Am. Radiol. 16*:273, 1973.
57. Roehm, J. O. F., Jr., K. L. Jue and K. Amplatz: Radiographic features of the scimitar syndrome. *Radiology 86*:856, 1966.
58. Rogers, L. F. and J. C. Osmer: Bronchogenic cysts—a review of 46 cases. *Am. J. Roentgenol. 91*:273, 1964.
59. Sane, S. M. and B. R. Girdany: Cysts and neoplasms in the infant lung. In *Seminars in Roentgenology,* Vol. 7, No. 2, p. 122, April 1972.
60. Schwartz, E. E., J. G. Teplick, O. Gaddo and A. B. Schwartz: Pulmonary hemorrhage in renal disease: Goodpasture's syndrome and other causes. *Radiology 122*:39, 1977.
61. Simon, G. and L. Reid: Atresia of apical bronchus

of the left upper lobe—report of three cases. *Br. J. Dis. Chest 57*:126, 1963.

62. Singleton, E. B. and M. L. Wagner: Fluid in congenital lobar emphysema. In *Radiologic Atlas of Pulmonary Abnormalities in Children.* W. B. Saunders Co., Philadelphia, p. 73, 1971.
63. Singleton, E. B. and M. L. Wagner: *Radiologic Atlas of Pulmonary Abnormalities in Children:* W. B. Saunders Co., Philadelphia, p. 4, 1971.
64. Smith, P. L. and B. Gerald: Empyema in childhood followed roentgenographically: decortication seldom needed. *Am. J. Roentgenol. 106*:114, 1969.
65. Swischuk, L. E.: Bubbles in hyaline membrane disease. *Radiology 122*:417, 1977.
66. Swyer, P. R. and G. C. W. James: A case of unilateral pulmonary emphysema. *Thorax 8*:133, 1953.
67. Taplin, G. V., D. E. Johnson, J. C. Kennedy, E. K. Dore, N. D. Poe, L. A. Swanson and A. Greenberg: Aggregated albumin labeled with various isotopes. In *Radioactive Pharmaceuticals,* G. A. Andrews, R. M. Kniseley, and H. N. Wagner, Jr. (Eds.). AEC Sympos. SCR. 6, USAEC Div. of Tech. Inf. p. 525, 1966.
68. Turk, L. N., III and G. E. Lindskog: The importance of angiographic diagnosis in intralobar pulmonary sequestration. *J. Thorac. Cardiovasc. Surg. 41*:299, 1961.
69. Weber, A. L., K. T. Bird and M. L. Janower: Primary tuberculosis in childhood with particular emphasis on changes affecting the tracheobronchial tree. *Am. J. Roentgenol. 103*:123, 1968.
70. West, J. B.: Measurement of pulmonary blood flow and ventilation with radioactive gases. In *Nuclear Medicine,* W. H. Blahd (Ed.). McGraw Hill, New York, p. 313, 1965.
71. White, H. and W. F. Rowley: Cystic fibrosis of the pancreas: clinical and roentgenographic manifestations. *Radiol. Clin. North Am. 1*:539, 1963.
72. Wilson, M. G. and V. G. Mikity: New form of respiratory disease in premature infants. *Am. J. Dis. Child. 99*:488, 1960.
73. Woesnor, M., E. Brown and I. Sanders: Xeroradiographic zonography of the larynx and hypopharynx. *Am. Otol. 83*:42, 1974.

Index